DISEASES AND DISORDERS

A NURSING THERAPEUTICS MANUAL

Second Edition

DISEASES AND DISORDERS

A NURSING THERAPEUTICS MANUAL

Second Edition

Marilyn Sawyer Sommers, RN, PhD, FAAN
Professor
University of Cincinnati
Cincinnati, Ohio

Susan A. Johnson, RN, PhD
Assistant Professor
College of Mount St. Joseph
Cincinnati, Ohio

 F. A. Davis Company • Philadelphia

Acquisitions Editor: Joanne P. DaCunha, RN, MSN
Developmental Editor: Ron Watson
Cover Designer: Lewis J. Forgione

As new scientific information becomes available through basic and clinical research, recommended treatments and drug therapies undergo changes. The author(s) and publisher have done everything possible to make this book accurate, up to date, and in accord with accepted standards at the time of publication. The author(s), editors, and publisher are not responsible for errors or omissions or for consequences from application of the book, and make no warranty, expressed or implied, in regard to the contents of the book. Any practice described in this book should be applied by the reader in accordance with professional standards of care used in regard to the unique circumstances that may apply in each situation. The reader is advised always to check product information (package inserts) for changes and new information regarding dose and contraindications before administering any drug. Caution is especially urged when using new or infrequently ordered drugs.

ISBN 0–8036-0811-X

DEDICATION

To the home team, with love.

MSS

To my two wonderful sisters: Debbie, the finest nurse I know, and Lisa, who always makes me feel special. And in memory of our mother, Bernadine Nelson, who taught us everything we really need to know in life.

SAJ

PREFACE

The first edition of this book, *Davis's Manual of Nursing Therapeutics for Diseases and Disorders,* was conceived as a text to provide distilled, up-to-date information to nursing students and staff nurses about many conditions and diagnoses encountered in nursing practice. With the second edition, along with its new title, *Diseases and Disorders: A Nursing Therapeutics Manual,* we have responded to the ever-changing health care environment as well as to the recommendations of our readers and editors. We have held true to our initial purpose in this second edition: to provide a ready source of information for nurses in a time of short staffing, brief lengths of stay, and increasing patient acuity both in the hospital and in the home.

As in the first edition, we have a commitment to concise explanations of pathophysiology and therapeutic interventions that have a sound scientific basis. In addition, we have increased our gender-specific content in the section, **Gender and Life Span Considerations,** because we believe that the role of gender has been underexplored in the nursing literature. Importantly, we have maintained our view that information should be organized by the nursing process; we have emphasized nursing diagnoses, outcomes, and independent interventions that are the essence of professional nursing practice.

Each entry begins with the Diagnosis Related Group (DRG) category. DRGs were initiated by the Health Care Financing Administration to serve as an organizing framework to group-related conditions and to stabilize reimbursements. Because they provide a convenient standard to evaluate hospital care, DRGs are used by institutions and disciplines to measure utilization and to allocate resources. We have included DRGs to indicate the expected norms in average length of stay for each entry. Each entry follows the nursing process, with assessment information incorporated in the **History** and **Physical Assessment** sections, the **Psychosocial Assessment,** and **Diagnostic Highlights**. Based on requests from our readers and reviewers, we have supplemented information on diagnostic testing from the first edition to provide normal and abnormal values for the most important diagnostic tests. We have also added a section to explain the rationale for the test. These detailed, specific sections provide the foundation needed to perform a comprehensive assessment of the patient's condition so that a **Primary Nursing Diagnosis** can be formulated appropriate to the patient's specific needs. In the second edition, we have used the Nursing Outcomes Classification (Iowa Outcomes Project; Johnson, Maas, & Moorhead, 1999) and the Nursing Interventions Classification (Iowa Intervention Project; McCloskey & Bulechek, 1999) to expand the Nursing Diagnosis section. The Nursing Outcomes Classification uses specific labels to provide standardization of expected patient outcomes. The Nursing Interventions Classification standardizes, defines, and facilitates the appropriate selection of nursing interventions for nurses.

The **Planning and Implementation** section is divided into **Collaborative** and **Independent** interventions. The intent of the Collaborative section is to detail the goals of a multidisciplinary plan of care to manage the condition or disease. The second edition contains an expanded section on **Pharmacologic Highlights** that explores commonly used drugs, their doses, mechanisms of action, and rationales for use. The Independent section focuses on independent nursing interventions that demonstrate the core of the art and science of nursing. Each entry then finishes with **Documentation Guidelines** and **Discharge and Home Healthcare Guidelines** to help nurses evaluate the outcomes of care and to prepare hospitalized patients for discharge.

As with the first edition, the idea for the book originated with Joanne Patzek DaCunha, Acquisitions Editor at F.A. Davis. The authors salute her creativity, perseverance, enthusiasm, and vision for the first and second editions. More importantly, her gracious friendship and support enabled us to accomplish this revision with a minimum of difficulty. We also owe a debt of gratitude to Jeff Sommers for his assistance with manuscript development, editing, proofreading, and supportive cheerleading.

The entire reason to revise this book is to provide practicing nurses a concise and yet scientifically sound text to guide the professional practice of nursing. The provision of nursing care in the 21st century presents us with overwhelming challenges, and yet nursing is the discipline of choice for millions of practitioners. We hope this book honors the science of nursing and makes it easier to practice the art of nursing.

MSS

SAJ

CONSULTANTS

Dianne V. Benton, RN, MS
Instructor, Senior Level Medical-Surgical Nursing
Louise Obici School of Nursing
Suffolk, Virginia

Barbara Dunn, RN, MSN
Professor, Nursing
New Hampshire Technical Institute
Concord, New Hampshire

Mary Taylor Martof, RN, EdD
Associate Professor
Louisiana State Health Sciences Center
New Orleans, Louisiana

Christine C. Mihal, RN, MSN
Lecturer of Nursing
Associate Director of Baccalaureate Nursing
Farleigh Dickinson University
Teaneck, New Jersey

Anne Pithan, RN, MSN
Nursing Faculty
St. Luke's College of Nursing
Sioux City, Iowa

Sylvia J. Sheffler, RN, DNSc
Associate Professor
Delaware State University
Dover, Delaware

Susan Wilkinson, RN, MSN, PhD(c)
Professional Specialist, Department of Nursing
Angelo State University
San Angelo, Texas

CONTRIBUTORS

At the time of publication, the contributors to the first edition held the following positions.

Carol D. Abeyta, RN, MSN
Assistant Professor
College of Mount St. Joseph
Cincinnati, Ohio

Margaret M. Anderson, EdD, RN,C, CNAA
Assistant Professor, Nursing
BSN/MSN Program
Northern Kentucky University
Highland Heights, Kentucky

Phyllis B. Augspurger, RN, PhD
Assistant Professor
Xavier University
Cincinnati, Ohio

Shirley D. Bartley, MEd, BN, RN
Instructor
Red River Community College
Winnipeg, Manitoba, Canada

Terry Beery, RN, MS, CCRN
Doctoral Candidate
University of Cincinnati
Cincinnati, Ohio

Marianne Benjamin, RN, BSN
Master's Candidate
Unit Director
Indiana University Medical Center
Indianapolis, Indiana

Kathleen M. Blade, RN, MS
Junior Level Faculty
St. Joseph Hospital School of Nursing
North Providence, Rhode Island

Wendy P. Blakely, RN, MN, CCRN
Assistant Professor, Medical-Surgical
Nursing
Montana State University College of
Nursing
Billings, Montana

Kathleen Boyle, RN, EdD
Assistant Professor
University of Cincinnati
Cincinnati, Ohio

Susan V. Brammer, RN,C, MA
Instructor, Department of Nursing
Thomas More College
Crestview Hills, Kentucky

Robert Brautigan, RN, MSN
Assistant Professor of Nursing
Northern Kentucky University
Highland Heights, Kentucky

LCDR Bonnie Ann Bulach, NC, RN, MSN
United States Navy

Stephanie Lennon-Catron, RN, MSN
Assistant Professor of Nursing
Montana State University—Northern
Great Falls, Montana

Elizabeth Chapman, RN, MS, CCRN
ICU/CCU Charge Nurse
Garden Park Community Hospital
Nursing Faculty
Mississippi Gulf Coast Community
College
Jefferson Davis Campus
Gulfport, Mississippi

Joy Churchill, RN, MSN
Assistant Professor of Nursing
Northern Kentucky University
Highland Heights, Kentucky

Maureen A Courtade, RN, MSN
Doctoral Student
University of Cincinnati
Cincinnati, Ohio

Lona W. Crane, RN,C, MSN
Nursing Instructor
Xavier University
Cincinnati, Ohio

Grace Cumberbatch, RN, MA Nursing
Associate Professor
La Guardia Community College—
CUNY
Long Island City, New York

Carolyn W. DeVore, RNCS, PhD
Assistant Professor
University of Cincinnati
Cincinnati, Ohio

M. Joyce Dienger, RN, MSN, OCN
Assistant Professor
Department of Nursing
College of Mount Saint Joseph
Cincinnati, Ohio

Colleen Doherty, RN, MSN, CCRN
Clinical Nurse Specialist, Critical Care
St. Elizabeth Medical Center
Edgewood, Kentucky

Mary Louise Drake, RN, EdD
Professor
University of Windsor
Windsor, Ontario, Canada

Janice M. Dyehouse, RN, PhD
Associate Professor
University of Cincinnati
Cincinnati, Ohio

Dawn Marie Ferguson, RN
Staff Nurse, Bone Marrow Transplant
Unit
Indiana University Medical Center
Indianapolis, Indiana

Sara Fickle, RN, MSN
Unit Director
Indiana University Medical Center
Indianapolis, Indiana

Donna K. Garrett, RN, MSN, CCRN
Clinical Nurse Specialist, Critical
Care
Grand Rapids, Michigan

Alice C. Geissler, RN, BSN, CCRN
Contract Practitioner
Colorado Springs, Colorado

Sharon Ivy Gordon, RN, MSN, CNOR
Instructor of Nursing
Mississippi Gulf Coast Community
College
Gulfport, Mississippi

Doreen J. Gudlin, RN, MSN, CCRN
Nursing Education Specialist
St. Mary's Hospital
Rochester, Minnesota

Sharon A. Haines, RN, MSN, FNP
Section Head, Clinical Operations,
Clinical and Medical Affairs
Procter & Gamble Pharmaceuticals
Cincinnati, Ohio

Marcia J. Hern, RN, EdD
Associate Professor of Nursing
University of Cincinnati
Cincinnati, Ohio

**Cheryl Schneider Hickey, RN, MSN,
CCRN**
Critical Care Clinical Nurse Specialist
Bethesda North Hospital
Montgomery, Ohio

Katherine Voorhees Hieber, RNCS, MS
Assistant Professor of Nursing
Miami University—Middletown
Middletown, Ohio

Kathleen Holmes, RN, MSN
Unit Director
Indiana University Medical Center
Indianapolis, Indiana

Sandi Hurley, RN, CCRN
Primary RN, ICU
Miami Valley Hospital
Dayton, Ohio

Susan A. Johnson, RN, PhD
Assistant Professor
College of Mount St. Joseph
Cincinnati, Ohio

Mary C. Kishman, RN, MSN
Assistant Professor
College of Mount St. Joseph
Cincinnati, Ohio

Adrianne J. Lane, RN,C, EdD
Assistant Professor of Nursing
University of Cincinnati
Cincinnati, Ohio

Denise R. Lucas, RN,C, MSN
Perinatal Clinical Nurse Specialist
Bethesda Hospital
Cincinnati, Ohio

Von Matheny, RN
Colorado Springs, Colorado

Lenora M. Maze, RN, BSN, CCRN
Clinical Service Facilitator, Neuro-
science ICU
Indiana University
Indianapolis, Indiana

Cheryl McKenzie, RN,C, MN, FNP
Assistant Professor, Nursing
Northern Kentucky University
Highland Heights, Kentucky

Diane McPhillips, RN, MSN, CCRN
Nurse Clinician
University of Cincinnati
Cincinnati, Ohio

I. Donna Meder, RN, BN, MN
Coordinator, Nursing—Prior
Learning Assessment
Red River Community College
Winnipeg, Manitoba, Canada

Linda Weaver Moore, RN, MSN
Assistant Professor
Xavier University
Cincinnati, Ohio

Pamela Mullen, RN, MSN
Instructor
Miami University—Hamilton
Hamilton, Ohio

Mary Myers, RN, BSN
Unit Director, Surgical Intensive Care
Unit
Indiana University Medical Center
Indianapolis, Indiana

Arianna Newman, RN, MSN
University of Cincinnati
Cincinnati, Ohio

Jane L. Niday, RN, CCRN
Primary Nurse I
Miami Valley Hospital
Dayton, Ohio

Mary A. O'Shea, RN, MN
Nursing Informatics Coordinator
Department of Veterans Affairs
Medical Center
Kansas City, Missouri

JoAnn Randolph, RN, BSN, MS, PhD(c)
Office Manager/Office Nurse
Mid-west Occupational Health Center
Cincinnati, Ohio

Linda S. Reig, RN, MSN, MBA
Associate Professor
Xavier University
Cincinnati, Ohio

Denise L. Robinson, RN, PhD, CCRN
Associate Professor, Director RN-
BSN Program
Northern Kentucky University
Highland Heights, Kentucky

Anne C. Russell, RN, MSN, CCRN
Trauma Clinical Associate
Miami Valley Hospital
Dayton, Ohio

Denise A. Sadowski, RN, MSN
Independent Consultant and Educator
Cincinnati, Ohio

Linda A. Schmid, RN, MSN
Assistant Professor
Xavier University
Cincinnati, Ohio

Deborah Jane Schwytzer, RN, MSN, CEN
Instructor
University of Cincinnati
Cincinnati, Ohio

Jeannine A. Shaner, RN, MSN
Nursing Faculty
Mississippi Gulf Coast Community
College
Gulfport, Mississippi

Susan Skelton-Smith, RN, MSN, CCRN
Critical Care Clinical Nurse Specialist
Department of Veterans Affairs
Medical Center
Kansas City, Missouri

Patricia A. Slater, RN, MSN
Assistant Professor
College of Mount St. Joseph
Cincinnati, Ohio

Marilyn Sawyer Sommers, RN, PhD
Associate Professor
University of Cincinnati
Cincinnati, Ohio

Anne Spanier, RN, MSN, EdD
Clinical Nurse Specialist Long Term
Care/Chronic Illness
Assistant Professor, RN-MSN
Coordinator
College of Mount St. Joseph
Cincinnati, Ohio

Lynette Leeseberg Stamler, RN, PhD
Assistant Professor
University of Windsor
Windsor, Ontario, Canada

Jill Hoblitzell Strub, RN, CSN, MSN
Instructor
University of Cincinnati
Cincinnati, Ohio

Dena J. Sutermaster, RN, MSN
Assistant Professor
Montana State University
Billings, Montana

Lois N. Tessler, RN, BN
Instructor of Nursing
Red River Community College
Winnipeg, Manitoba, Canada

Janet Trigg, RN, EdD
Associate Professor
University of Cincinnati
Cincinnati, Ohio

Diane Twedell, RN, BSN, CCRN, CEN
Nurse Manager, Emergency Services
Mayo Medical Center
Rochester, Minnesota

Sandra R. Urquhart, RN,C, MSN
Assistant Professor
College of Mount St. Joseph
Cincinnati, Ohio

Darla Vale, RN, MSN, CCRN
Assistant Professor
College of Mount St. Joseph
Cincinnati, Ohio

Tina M. Volz, RN, MSN
Doctoral Student
University of Cincinnati
Cincinnati, Ohio

Jennifer Vonnahme, RN, MA, OCN
Assistant Professor of Nursing
Miami University
Oxford, Ohio

Sandy Warner, RN,C, MSN
Adjunct Clinical Instructor
College of Mount St. Joseph
Staff Nurse
Good Samaritan Hospital
Cincinnati, Ohio

Tina Leigh Weitkamp, RN,C, MSN
Associate Professor of Clinical
Nursing
University of Cincinnati
Staff Nurse
Mercy Hospital Anderson
Cincinnati, Ohio

Kathryn F. Wekselman, RN,C, BSN, MLn, PhD(c)
Doctoral Candidate
University of Cincinnati
Cincinnati, Ohio

Deborah Wendt, RN, MSN, CS
Assistant Professor
College of Mount St. Joseph
Cincinnati, Ohio

Janalyce Willis, RN, MSN
Surgical and Critical Care Staff
  Development Coordinator
University Hospital
Indiana University Medical Center
Indianapolis, Indiana

Cheryl Lynn Wolverton, RN, MSN, CCRN
Clinical Nurse Specialist,
  Cardiovascular/Cardiology
University Hospital
Indiana University Medical Center
Indianapolis, Indiana

Donna Polk Workman, RN, MSN
Assistant Professor
College of Mount St. Joseph
Cincinnati, Ohio

CONTENTS

Abdominal Aortic Aneurysm

DRG Category: 130
Mean LOS: 5.8 days
Description: MEDICAL: Peripheral Vascular Disorder with CC
DRG Category: 110
Mean LOS: 9.1 days
Description: SURGICAL: Major Cardiovascular Procedures with CC

An abdominal aortic aneurysm is a localized outpouching or dilatation of the arterial wall in the latter portion of the descending segment, the abdominal aorta. Aneurysms of the abdominal aorta occur more frequently than those of the thoracic aorta. Abdominal aortic aneurysms may be fusiform (shaped like a spindle) or saccular (looks like a pouch) in shape. A fusiform aneurysm in which the dilated area encircles the entire aorta is most common. A saccular aneurysm has a dilated area on only one side of the vessel.

The outpouching of the wall of the aorta occurs when the musculoelastic middle layer or media of the artery becomes weak (often caused by plaque and cholesterol deposits) and degenerative changes occur. There is also a stretching of the inner and outer layers of the arterial wall. As the pulsatile force of the blood continues to rush through the aorta, the vessel wall becomes increasingly weak, and the aneurysm enlarges. Abdominal aneurysms can be fatal. More than half of people with untreated aneurysms die of aneurysm rupture within 2 years.

CAUSES

Most authorities believe that the most common cause of abdominal aneurysms is atherosclerosis. The atherosclerotic process causes the buildup of plaque, which alters the integrity of the aortic wall. Other causes include high blood pressure, heredity, connective tissue disorders, trauma, and infections (syphilis, tuberculosis, and endocarditis). Smoking is also a contributing cause.

GENDER AND LIFE SPAN CONSIDERATIONS

Abdominal aneurysms are far more common in hypertensive men than women; from three to eight times as many men as women develop abdominal aortic aneurysms. The incidence of abdominal aortic aneurysm increases with age. The occurrence is rare before the age of 50 and common between the ages of 60 and 80, when the atherosclerotic process tends to become more pronounced.

◻ ASSESSMENT

HISTORY. When the aorta enlarges and compresses the surrounding structures, patient complaints may include flank and back pain, epigastric discomfort, or altered bowel elimination. The pain may be deep and steady with no change if the patient shifts position. If the patient reports severe back and abdominal pain, rupture of the abdominal aortic aneurysm may be imminent.

1

PHYSICAL EXAMINATION. Inspect the patient's abdomen for a pulsating abdominal mass in the periumbilical area, slightly to the left of midline. Auscultate over the pulsating area for an audible bruit. Gently palpate the area to determine the size of the mass and whether tenderness is present.

Watch for signs that may indicate impending aneurysm rupture. Note subtle changes such as a change in the characteristics and quality of peripheral pulses, changes in neurologic status, and changes in vital signs such as a drop in blood pressure, increased pulse, and increased respirations.

Because emergency surgery is indicated for both a rupture and a threatened rupture, careful assessment is very important. When the aneurysm ruptures into the retroperitoneal space, hemorrhage is confined by surrounding structures, preventing immediate death by loss of blood. Examine the patient for signs of shock, including decreased capillary refill, increased pulse and respirations, a drop in urine output, weak peripheral pulses, and cool and clammy skin. When the rupture occurs anteriorly into the peritoneal cavity, rapid hemorrhage generally occurs. The patient's vital signs and vital functions diminish rapidly. Death is usually imminent because of the rapidity of events.

PSYCHOSOCIAL. In most cases the patient with an abdominal aortic aneurysm faces hospitalization, a serious surgical procedure, a stay in an intensive care unit, and a substantial recovery period. Therefore, assess the patient's coping mechanisms and existing support system. Assess the patient's anxiety level regarding surgery and the recovery process.

DIAGNOSTIC HIGHLIGHTS

General Comments: Because this condition causes no symptoms, it is often diagnosed through routine physical exams or abdominal x rays.

Test	Normal Result	Abnormality with Condition	Explanation
Standard test: Computed tomography (CT) scan	Negative study	Locates outpouching within the aortic wall	Assesses size and location of aneurysm
Abdominal x ray	Negative study	May show location of aneurysm with an "eggshell" appearance	Assesses size and location of aneurysm

Other Tests: Ultrasound of the abdomen; magnetic resonance imaging (MRI); aortography

PRIMARY NURSING DIAGNOSIS

Risk for fluid volume deficit related to hemorrhage

OUTCOMES. Fluid balance; Circulation status; Cardiac pump effectiveness; Hydration

INTERVENTIONS. Bleeding reduction; Fluid resuscitation; Blood product administration; Intravenous therapy; Circulatory care; Shock management

□ PLANNING AND IMPLEMENTATION

Collaborative

PREOPERATIVE. The treatment of choice for aneurysms 6 cm or greater in size is surgical repair. When aneurysms are smaller, some controversy exists regarding treatment. Some authorities suggest the smaller aneurysm should just be evaluated frequently by ultrasound examination, with surgical intervention only if the aneurysm expands. Others suggest elective surgical repair regardless of aneurysm size. If the aneurysm is leaking or about to rupture, immediate surgical intervention is required to improve survival rates.

SURGICAL. The type and extent of surgery depend on the location of the aneurysm. Typically, an abdominal incision is made, the aneurysm is opened, clots and debris are removed, and a synthetic graft is inserted within the natural arterial wall and then sutured. During this procedure, the aorta is cross-clamped proximally and distally to the aneurysm to allow the graft to take hold. The patient is treated with heparin during the procedure to decrease the clotting of pooled blood in the lower extremities.

POSTOPERATIVE. The patient will typically spend 2 to 3 days in the intensive care setting until her or his condition stabilizes. Monitor patient cardiac and circulatory status closely, and pay particular attention to make sure the peripheral pulses are present and the patient's feet are warm and pink. Immediately report to the physician any absent or diminished pulse or cool, pale, mottled, or painful extremity. These signs could indicate an obstructed graft. Ventricular dysrhythmias are common in the postoperative period because of hypoxemia (deficient oxygen in the blood), hypothermia (temperature drop), and electrolyte imbalances. An endotracheal tube may be inserted to support ventilation. An arterial line, central venous pressure line, and peripheral intravenous lines are all typically ordered to maintain and monitor fluid balance. Adequate blood volume is supported to ensure patency of the graft and to prevent clotting of the graft as a result of low blood flow. Foley catheters are also used to assist with urinary drainage, as well as with accurate intake and output measurements. Monitor for signs of infection; watch for temperature and white blood cell count elevations. Observe the abdominal wound closely, noting poor wound approximation, redness, swelling, drainage, or odor. Also report pain, tenderness, and redness in the calf of the patient's leg. These symptoms may indicate thrombophlebitis from clot formation. If the patient develops severe postoperative back pain, notify the surgeon immediately; pain may indicate that a graft is tearing.

EXPERIMENTAL THERAPY. Several medical centers are using an experimental graft that is inserted through a groin artery into the area of the aneurysm. This device, a stainless steel stent that is covered with woven Dacron, is expandable and carries blood past the weakened portion of the aneurysm. The procedure can be performed without extensive surgery but at this time will need several years of evaluation before it can be used generally.

PHARMACOLOGIC HIGHLIGHTS

Medication or Drug Class	Dosage	Description	Rationale
Morphine	1–10 mg IV	Opioid analgesic	Relieves surgical pain
Fentanyl	50–100 mcg IV	Opioid analgesic	Relieves surgical pain
Antihypertensives and/or diuretics	Varies by drug		Rising BP may stress graft suture lines

Independent

PREOPERATIVE. Teach the patient about the disease process, breathing and leg exercises, the surgical procedure, and postoperative routines. Support the patient by encouraging him or her to share fears, questions, and concerns. When appropriate, include support persons in the discussions. Note that the surgical procedure may be performed on an emergency basis, which limits the time available for preoperative instruction. If the patient is admitted in shock, support airway, breathing, and circulation, and expedite the surgical procedure.

POSTOPERATIVE. Keep the incision clean and dry. Inspect the dressing every hour to check for bleeding. Use sterile techniques for all dressing changes. To ensure adequate respiratory function and to prevent complications, assist the patient with coughing and deep breathing after extubation. Splint the incision with pillows, provide adequate pain relief prior to coughing sessions, and position the patient with the head of the bed elevated to facilitate coughing. Turn the patient side to side every 2 hours to promote good ventilation and to limit skin breakdown.

Remember that emergency surgery is a time of extreme anxiety for both the patient and significant others. Answer all questions, provide emotional support, and explain all procedures carefully. If the patient or family is not able to cope effectively, you may need to refer them for counseling.

DOCUMENTATION GUIDELINES

- Location, intensity, and frequency of pain, and the factors that relieve pain
- Appearance of abdominal wound (color, temperature, intactness, drainage)
- Evidence of stability of vital signs, hydration status, bowel sounds, electrolytes
- Presence of complications: Hypotension, hypertension, cardiac dysrhythmias, low urine output, thrombophlebitis, infection, graft occlusion, changes in consciousness, aneurysm rupture, excessive anxiety, poor wound healing

DISCHARGE AND HOME HEALTHCARE GUIDELINES

WOUND CARE. Explain the need to keep the surgical wound clean and dry. Teach the patient to observe the wound and report to the physician any increased swelling, redness, drainage, odor, or separation of the wound edges. Also instruct the patient to notify the physician if a fever develops.

ACTIVITY RESTRICTIONS. Instruct the patient to lift nothing heavier than 5 pounds for about 6 to 12 weeks and to avoid driving until his or her physician permits. Braking while driving may increase intra-abdominal pressure and disrupt the suture line. Most surgeons temporarily discourage activities that require pulling, pushing, or stretching—activities such as vacuuming, changing sheets, playing tennis and golf, mowing grass, and chopping wood.

COMPLICATIONS FOLLOWING SURGERY. Discuss with the patient the possibility of clot formation or graft blockage. Symptoms of a clot may include pain or tenderness in the calf, and these symptoms may be accompanied by redness and warmth in the calf. Signs of graft blockage include a diminished or absent pulse and a cool, pale extremity. Tell patients to report such signs to the physician immediately.

COMPLICATIONS FOR PATIENTS NOT REQUIRING SURGERY. Compliance with the regime of monitoring the size of the aneurysm by computed tomography over time is essential. The patient needs to understand the prescribed medication to control hypertension and, when necessary and possible, needs to attend smoking cessation classes. Advise the patient to report abdominal fullness or back pain, which may indicate a pending rupture.

Abdominal Trauma

DRG Category: 188
Mean LOS: 4.9 days
Description: MEDICAL: Other Digestive System Diagnoses, Age > 17 with CC
DRG Category: 154
Mean LOS: 13.3 days
Description: SURGICAL: Stomach, Esophageal, and Duodenal Procedures, Age > 17 with CC

Abdominal trauma accounts for approximately 15% of all trauma-related deaths. Intra-abdominal trauma is usually not a single organ system injury; as more organs are injured, the risks of organ dysfunction and death climb. The abdominal cavity contains solid, gas-filled, fluid-filled, and encapsulated organs. These organs are at greater risk for injury than are other organs of the body because they have few bony structures to protect them. Although the last five ribs serve as some protection, if they are fractured, the sharp-edged bony fragments can cause further organ damage from lacerations or organ penetration (Table 1).

Abdominal trauma can be blunt or penetrating. *Blunt injuries* occur when there is no break in the skin; they often occur as multiple injuries. In blunt injuries, the spleen and liver are the most commonly injured organs. Injury occurs because of the crushing, shearing, and bursting forces that are related to the impact velocity and abdominal compression. *Penetrating injuries* are those associated with foreign bodies set into motion. The foreign object penetrates the organ and dissipates energy into the organ and surrounding areas. The most commonly involved abdominal organs with penetrating trauma include the intestines, liver, and spleen. Complications following abdominal trauma include profuse bleeding from aortic dissection or other vascular structures, hemorrhagic shock, peritonitis, abscess formation, septic shock, paralytic ileus, ischemic bowel syndrome, acute renal failure, liver failure, adult respiratory distress syndrome, disseminated intravascular coagulation, and death.

CAUSES

At least half of the cases of blunt abdominal trauma are caused by motor vehicle crashes (MVCs). These injuries are often associated with head and chest injuries as well. Other causes of blunt injury include falls, aggravated assaults, and contact sports. Penetrating injuries can occur from gunshot wounds, stab wounds, or impalements.

GENDER AND LIFE SPAN CONSIDERATIONS

Traumatic injuries, which are usually preventable, are the leading cause of death in the first four decades of life. Most blunt abdominal trauma is associated with MVCs, which in the 15- to 24-year-old age group are three times more common in males than females. In the 15- to 34-year-old age group, European-Americans have a death rate from MVCs that is 40% higher than that of African-Americans. Penetrating injuries from gunshot wounds and stab wounds, which are on the increase

TABLE 1 | **Injuries to the Abdomen**

ORGAN OR TISSUE	COMMON INJURIES	SYMPTOMS
Diaphragm	Partially protected by bony structures, diaphragm is most commonly injured by penetrating trauma (particularly gunshot wounds to the lower chest) Automobile deceleration may lead to rapid rise in intra-abdominal pressure and a burst injury Diaphragmatic tear usually indicates multiorgan involvement	· Decreased breath sounds · Abdominal peristalsis heard in thorax · Acute chest pain and shortness of breath may indicate diaphragmatic tear · May be hard to diagnose because of multisystem trauma, or the liver may "plug" the defect and mask it
Esophagus	Penetrating injury is more common than blunt injury May be caused by knives, bullets, foreign body obstruction May be caused by iatrogenic perforation May be associated with cervical spine injury	· Pain at site of perforation · Fever · Difficulty swallowing · Cervical tenderness · Peritoneal irritation
Stomach	Penetrating injury is more common than blunt injury; in one-third of patients, both the anterior and posterior walls are penetrated May occur as a complication from cardiopulmonary resuscitation or from gastric dilation	· Epigastric pain · Epigastric tenderness · Signs of peritonitis · Bloody gastric drainage
Liver	Most commonly injured organ (both blunt and penetrating injuries); blunt injuries (70% of total) usually occur from motor vehicle crashes and steering wheel trauma Highest mortality from blunt injury (more common in suburban areas); gunshot wounds (more common in urban areas) Hemorrhage is most common cause of death from liver injury; overall mortality 10%–15%	· Persistent hypotension despite adequate fluid resuscitation · Guarding over right lower quadrant 6 ribs or right upper quadrant · Dullness to percussion · Abdominal distention and peritoneal irritation · Persistent thoracic bleeding
Spleen	Most commonly injured organ with blunt abdominal trauma Injured in penetrating trauma of the left upper quadrant	· Hypotension, tachycardia, shortness of breath · Peritoneal irritation · Abdominal wall tenderness · Left upper quadrant pain · Fixed dullness to percussion in left flank; dullness to percussion in right flank that disappears with change of position

continued on the following page

TABLE 1 | **Injuries to the Abdomen (*Continued*)**

ORGAN OR TISSUE	COMMON INJURIES	SYMPTOMS
Pancreas	Most often penetrating injury (gunshot wounds at close range) Blunt injury from deceleration; injury from steering wheel Often associated (40%) with other organ damage (liver, spleen, vessels)	· Pain over pancreas · Paralytic ileus · Symptoms may occur late (after 24 hours); epigastric pain radiating to back; nausea, vomiting · Tenderness to deep palpation
Small intestines	Duodenum, ileum, and jejunum; hollow viscous structure most often injured by penetrating trauma Gunshot wounds account for 70% of cases Incidence of injury is third only to liver and spleen injury When small bowel ruptures from blunt injury, rupture occurs most often at proximal jejunum and terminal ileum.	· Testicular pain · Referred pain to shoulders, chest, back · Mild abdominal pain · Peritoneal irritation · Fever, jaundice, intestinal obstruction
Large intestines	One of the more lethal injuries because of fecal contamination; occurs in 5% of abdominal injuries More than 90% of incidences are penetrating injuries Blunt injuries are often from safety restraints in motor vehicle crashes	· Pain, muscle rigidity · Guarding, rebound tenderness · Blood on rectal exam · Tenderness, fever

in U.S. preteens and young adults, are more common in African-Americans than European-Americans.

□ ASSESSMENT

HISTORY. For patients who have experienced abdominal trauma, establish a history of the mechanism of injury by including a detailed report from the pre-hospital professionals, witnesses, or significant others. Information regarding the type of trauma (blunt or penetrating) is helpful. If the patient was in an MVC, determine the speed and type of the vehicle, whether the patient was restrained, the patient's position in the vehicle, and whether the patient was thrown from the vehicle on impact. If the patient was injured in a motorcycle crash, determine whether the patient was wearing a helmet. In cases of traumatic injuries from falls, determine the point of impact, the distance of the fall, and the type of landing surface. If the patient has been shot, ask the paramedics or police for ballistics information, including the caliber of the weapon and the range at which the person was shot.

PHYSICAL EXAMINATION. The patient's appearance may range from anxious but healthy to critically injured with a full cardiopulmonary arrest. If the patient is hemorrhaging from a critical abdominal injury, he or she may be profoundly hypotensive with the symptoms of hypovolemic shock (see **Hypovolemic/ Hemorrhagic Shock**, p. 529). The initial evaluation or primary survey of the trauma patient is centered on assessing the airway, breathing, circulation, disability (neurological status), and exposure (by completely undressing the patient). Life-saving interventions may accompany assessments made during the primary survey in the presence of life- and limb-threatening injuries. The primary survey is followed by a secondary survey, a thorough head-to-toe assessment of all organ systems. The assessment of the injured patient should be systematic, constant, and with re-evaluation.

When you inspect the patient's abdomen, note any disruption from the normal appearance such as distension, lacerations, ecchymoses, and penetrating wounds. Inspect for any signs of obvious bleeding such as ecchymoses around the umbilicus (Culles sign) or over the left upper quadrant, which may occur with a ruptured spleen. Grey-Turner's sign, bruising of the flank area, may indicate retroperitoneal bleeding. Inspect the perineum for accompanying urinary tract injuries that may lead to bleeding from the urinary meatus, vagina, and rectum. If the patient is obviously pregnant, determine the fetal age and monitor the patient for premature labor.

Auscultate all four abdominal quadrants for 2 minutes per quadrant to determine the presence of bowel sounds. Although the absence of bowel sounds can indicate underlying bleeding, their absence does not always indicate injury. Bowel sounds heard in the chest cavity may indicate a tear in the diaphragm. Trauma to the large abdominal blood vessels may lead to a friction rub or bruit. Percussion of the abdomen identifies air, fluid, or tissue intra-abdominally. Air-filled spaces produce tympanic sounds as heard over the stomach. Abnormal hyper-resonance can indicate free air; abnormal dullness may indicate bleeding. When you palpate the abdomen and flanks, note any increase in tenderness that can be indicative of an underlying injury. Note any masses, rigidity, pain, and guarding. Kehr's sign—radiating pain to the left shoulder when you palpate the left upper quadrant—is associated with injury to the spleen. Palpate the pelvis for injury.

PSYCHOSOCIAL. Changes in lifestyle may be required, depending on the type of injury. Large incisions and scars may be present. If injury to the colon has occurred, a colostomy, whether temporary or permanent, alters the patient's body image and lifestyle. The sudden alteration in comfort, potential body image changes, and possible impaired functioning of vital organ systems can often be overwhelming and lead to maladaptive coping.

DIAGNOSTIC HIGHLIGHTS

Test	Normal Result	Abnormality with Condition	Explanation
Computed tomography (CT) scan	Normal and intact abdominal structures	Injured or ruptured organs, accumulation of blood or air in the peritoneum, in the retroperitoneum, or above the diaphragm	Provides detailed pictures of the intra-abdominal and retroperitoneal structures, the presence of bleeding, hematoma formation, and the grade of injury

| Diagnostic peritoneal lavage (DPL) | Negative lavage without presence of excessive bleeding or bilious or fecal material | Direct aspiration of 5–10 mL of blood, bile, or fecal material from a peritoneal catheter. Following lavage with 1 L of normal saline, the presence of 100,000 red cells or 500 white cells per μL is a positive lavage. This is 90% sensitive for detecting intra-abdominal hemorrhage | Determines presence of intra-abdominal hemorrhage or rupture of hollow organs; contraindicated when there are existing indications for laparotomy |

Other Tests: Serum complete blood counts; serum chemistries; serum amylase; abdominal, chest, and cervical spine radiographs; excretory urograms; and arteriography

PRIMARY NURSING DIAGNOSIS

Ineffective breathing pattern related to pain and abdominal distension

OUTCOMES. Respiratory status: Gas exchange; Respiratory status: Ventilation; Symptom control behavior; Treatment behavior: Illness or injury; Comfort level

INTERVENTIONS. Airway management; Anxiety reduction; Oxygen therapy; Airway suctioning; Airway insertion and stabilization; Cough enhancement; Mechanical ventilation; Positioning; Respiratory monitoring

☐ PLANNING AND IMPLEMENTATION

Collaborative

The initial care of the patient with abdominal trauma follows the ABCs of resuscitation. Measures to ensure adequate oxygenation and tissue perfusion include the establishment of an effective airway and a supplemental oxygen source, support of breathing, control of the source of blood loss, and replacement of intravascular volume. As with any traumatic injury, treatment and stabilization of any life-threatening injuries are completed immediately.

SURGICAL. Surgical intervention is needed for specific injuries to organs. Diaphragmatic tears are repaired surgically to prevent visceral herniation in later years. Esophageal injury is often managed with gastric decompression with a nasogastric tube, antibiotic therapy, and surgical repair of the esophageal tear. Gastric injury is managed similarly to esophageal injury, although a partial gastrectomy may be needed if extensive injury has occurred. Liver injury may be managed nonoperatively or operatively, depending on the degree of injury and the amount of bleeding. Patients with liver injury are apt to experience problems with albumin formation, serum glucose levels (hypoglycemia in particular), blood coagulation, resistance to infection, and nutritional balance. Management of injuries to the spleen depends on the patient's age, stability, associated injuries, and type of splenic injury. Because removal of the spleen places the patient at risk for immune compromise, splenectomy is the treatment of choice only when the spleen is totally separated from the blood supply, when the patient is markedly hemodynamically unstable, or when the spleen is totally macerated. Treatment of pancreatic injury depends on the degree of pancreatic damage, but drainage of the area is usually necessary to prevent pancreatic fistula formation and surrounding tissue damage from pancreatic enzymes. Small- and large-bowel perforation or lacerations are managed by surgical exploration and repair. Preoperative and postoperative antibiotics are administered to prevent sepsis.

NUTRITIONAL. Nutritional requirements may be met with the use of a small-bore feeding tube placed in the duodenum during the initial surgical procedure or at the bedside under fluoroscopy. It may be necessary to eliminate gastrointestinal feedings for extended periods of time, depending on the injury and the surgical intervention required. Total parenteral nutrition may be used to provide nutritional requirements.

PHARMACOLOGIC HIGHLIGHTS

Medication or Drug Class	Dosage	Description	Rationale
Histamine-2 blockers	Varies with drug	Ranitidine (Zantac); cimetidine (Tagamet); famotidine (Pepcid); nizatidine (Axid)	Block gastric secretion and maintain pH of gastric contents above 4.0, thereby decreasing inflammation

Other Therapies: Narcotic analgesia to manage pain and limit atelectasis and pneumonia, and antibiotic therapy as indicated

Independent

The most important priority is the maintenance of an adequate airway, oxygen supply, breathing patterns, and circulatory status. Be prepared to assist with endotracheal intubation and mechanical ventilation by maintaining an intubation tray within immediate reach at all times. Maintain a working endotracheal suction at the bedside as well. If the patient is hemodynamically stable, position the patient for full lung expansion, usually in the semi-Fowler position with the arms elevated on pillows. If the cervical spine is at risk after an injury, maintain the body alignment and prevent flexion and extension by using a cervical collar or other strategy as dictated by trauma service protocol.

The nurse is the key to providing adequate pain control. Encourage the patient to describe and rate the pain on a scale of 1 through 10 to help you evaluate whether the pain is being controlled successfully. Consider using nonpharmacologic strategies, such as diversionary activities or massage, to manage pain as an adjunct to analgesia.

Emotional support of the patient and family is also a key nursing intervention. Patients and their families are often frightened and anxious. If the patient is awake as you implement strategies to manage the ABCs, provide a running explanation of the procedures to reassure the patient. Remember to hold the patient's hand to offer reassurance when possible. Explain to the family the treatment alternatives and keep them updated as to the patient's response to therapy. Notify the physician if the family needs to speak to him or her about the patient's progress. If blood component therapy is essential to manage bleeding, answer the patient's and family's questions about the risks of hepatitis and human immunodeficiency virus (HIV) transmission.

DOCUMENTATION GUIDELINES

- Abdominal assessment: Description of wounds or surgical incisions, wound healing, presence of bowel sounds, location of bowel sounds, number and quality of bowel movements, patency of drainage tubes, color of urine, presence of bloody urine or clots, amount of urine, appearance of catheter insertion site, fluid balance (intake and output, patency of intravenous catheters, speed of fluid resuscitation)
- Comfort: Location, duration, precipitating factors of pain; response to medications; degree of pain control
- Presence of complications: Pulmonary infection, hemorrhage, wound infection, alcohol withdrawal
- Assessment of level of anxiety, degree of understanding, adjustment, family or partner's response, and coping skills
- Understanding of and interest in patient teaching

DISCHARGE AND HOME HEALTHCARE GUIDELINES

Provide a complete explanation of all emergency treatments and answer the patient's and family's questions. Explain the possibility of complications to recovery, such as poor wound healing, infection, and bleeding. Explain the risks of blood transfusions, and answer any questions about exposure to blood-borne infections. If needed, provide information about any follow-up laboratory procedures that might be required after discharge. Provide the dates and times that the patient is to receive follow-up care with the primary healthcare provider or the trauma clinic. Give the patient a phone number to call with questions or concerns. Provide information on how to manage any drainage systems, colostomy, intravenous therapies, or surgical wounds.

Abortion, Spontaneous

DRG Category: 380
Mean LOS: 4.16 days
Description: MEDICAL: Abortion without Dilation and Curettage
DRG Category: 381
Mean LOS: 1.7 days
Description: SURGICAL: Abortion with Dilation and Curettage, Aspiration Curettage, or Hysterotomy

Spontaneous abortion (SAB) is defined as the termination of pregnancy from natural causes before the fetus is viable. Viability is defined as 20 to 24 weeks' gestation or a fetal weight of more than 500 g. SABs are a common occurrence in human reproduction, occurring in approximately 15% to 22% of all pregnancies. There are five types of SABs, classified according to symptoms (Table 2): threatened, inevitable, incomplete, complete, and missed. A threatened abortion occurs when there is slight bleeding and cramping very early in the pregnancy;

about 50% of women in this category abort. An inevitable abortion occurs when the membranes rupture, the cervix dilates, and bleeding increases. An incomplete abortion occurs when the uterus retains parts of the products of conception and the placenta. Sometimes, the fetus and placenta are expelled, but part of the placenta may adhere to the wall of the uterus and lead to continued bleeding. A complete abortion occurs when all the products of conception are passed through the cervix. A missed abortion occurs when the products of conception are retained for 2 months or more after the death of the fetus. Signs and symptoms of these five types of abortion involve varying degrees of vaginal bleeding, cervical dilatation, and uterine cramping.

TABLE 2 | **Types of SABs**

TYPE OF ABORTION	BLEEDING	PAIN	CERVICAL DILATION	TISSUE PASSAGE
Threatened	Slight	Mild cramping	No	No
Inevitable	Moderate	Moderate cramping	Yes	No
Incomplete	Heavy	Severe cramping	Yes	Yes
Complete	Decreased; slight	Mild cramping	No	Yes
Missed	None; slight	None	No	No

CAUSES

The majority of SABs are caused by chromosomal abnormalities that are incompatible with life; the majority also have autosomal trisomies. Maternal infections, such as listeriosis, toxoplasmosis, and rubella, increase the risk for an SAB. Inherited disorders or abnormal embryonic development resulting from environmental factors (teratogens) may also play a role. Patients who are classified as habitual aborters (three or more consecutive SABs) usually have an incompetent cervix—that is, a situation in which the cervix is weak and does not stay closed to maintain the pregnancy. Occupation may also be a consideration if the woman is exposed to teratogens.

GENDER AND LIFE SPAN CONSIDERATIONS

SABs usually occur prior to 8 weeks' gestation and are more common in teens, elderly primigravidas, and those women who engage in high-risk behaviors, such as drug and alcohol use or multiple sex partners.

□ ASSESSMENT

HISTORY. Obtain a complete obstetric history. Determine the date of the last menstrual period to calculate the fetus's gestational age. Vaginal bleeding is usually the first symptom that signals the onset of a spontaneous abortion; question the patient as to the onset and amount of bleeding. Inquire further about a small gush of fluid, which indicates a rupture of membranes, although at this early point in gestation, there is only a small amount of amniotic fluid expelled. Ask the patient to describe the duration, location, and intensity of her pain. Pain varies from a mild cramping to severe abdominal pain, depending on the type of abortion; pain can also occur as a backache or pelvic pressure. Although it is a sensitive topic, ask the patient about the passage of fetal tissue. If possible, the patient should bring the tissue passed at home into the hospital because sometimes laboratory pathologic analysis can reveal the cause of the abortion. With a missed abortion, early signs of pregnancy cease; thus, inquire about nausea, vomiting, breast tenderness, urinary frequency, and leukorrhea (white or yellow mucous discharge from the vagina).

PHYSICAL EXAMINATION. Temperature is elevated above 100.4°F if a maternal infection is present. Additionally, pallor, cool and clammy skin, and changes in the level of consciousness are symptoms of shock. Examine the patient's peripad for blood loss, and determine if any tissue has been expelled. Sometimes tissue can be observed at the introitus, but do not perform a vaginal examination if that situation occurs.

PSYCHOSOCIAL. Assess the patient's emotional status, as well as that of the baby's father and other family members. Often this hospital admission is the first one for the patient, and it may cause anxiety and fear. The father may withhold expressing his grief, feeling he needs to "be strong" for the mother.

DIAGNOSTIC HIGHLIGHTS

General Comments: Most of the time, diagnosis of SAB is made based on patient symptoms and the documentation of a positive pregnancy test.

Test	Normal Result	Abnormality with Condition	Explanation
Human chorionic gonadotropin (hCG)	Negative <5 m IU/mL	>5 m IU/mL, increases as the gestation progresses	HCG normally is not present in non-pregnant women
Ultrasound (transvaginal, transabdominal)	Positive fetal heart beat; growth within normal limits	Heart beat absent; gestational sac appears shriveled, or shrinking	Used to diagnose a missed abortion
Red blood cells; HGB; HCT	4.2–5.4 mL/mm³; 12–16 g/dL; 37%–47%	These three values will decrease several hours after significant blood loss has occurred	With active bleeding, red blood cells are lost

HCT = hematocrit; HGB = hemoglobin; IU = international units.

Other Tests: Blood type and crossmatch, white blood cells; habitual aborters should also undergo additional testing to rule out causes other than an incompetent cervix (thyroid stimulating hormone, mid-luteal phase serum progesterone measurement, hysterosalpingogram, and screening for lupus anticoagulant).

PRIMARY NURSING DIAGNOSIS

Anticipatory grieving related to an unexpected pregnancy outcome

OUTCOMES. Grief resolution

INTERVENTIONS. Grief work facilitation; Active listening; Presence; Truth telling; Support group

☐ PLANNING AND IMPLEMENTATION

Collaborative

MEDICAL. Threatened abortions are treated conservatively with bed rest at home. Patients are instructed to abstain from intercourse for at least 2 weeks following the cessation of bleeding. Approximately 50% of patients who are diagnosed with a threatened abortion carry their pregnancies to term. Inevitable and incomplete abortions are considered obstetric emergencies. Intravenous (IV) fluids are started immediately for fluid replacement, and narcotic analgesics are administered to decrease the pain. Oxytocics, when given IV, help decrease the bleeding. With any type of abortion, it is critical to determine the patient's blood Rh status. Any patient who is Rh-negative is given an injection of an $Rh_o(D)$ immune globulin (rhoGAM) to prevent Rh isoimmunization in future pregnancies. To determine the patient's response to treatment, monitor the patient's vital signs, color, level of consciousness, and response to fluid replacement.

SURGICAL. A dilation and curettage (D&C) is usually indicated. This procedure involves dilating the cervix and scraping the products of conception out of the uterus with a curette. The nurse's role in this procedure is to explain the procedure to the patient and family, assist the patient to the lithotomy position in the operating room, perform the surgical prep, and support the patient during the procedure.

A D&C is not indicated in the case of a complete abortion, since the patient has passed all tissue. Bleeding and cramping are minimal. Monitor the patient for complications, such as excessive bleeding and infection. With a missed abortion, the physician can wait for up to 1 month for the products of conception to pass independently; however, disseminated intravascular coagulation (DIC) or sepsis may occur during the wait. Clotting factors and white blood cell (WBC) counts should be monitored during this waiting time. The physician can remove the products of conception if an SAB does not occur.

PHARMACOLOGIC HIGHLIGHTS

Medication or Drug Class	Dosage	Description	Rationale
Oxytocin (Pitocin)	10–20 U IV after passage of tissue	Oxytocic	Stimulates uterine contractions to decrease postpartum bleeding
RhD immunoglobulin (RhoGAM)	120 μg (prepared by blood bank)	Immune serum	Prevents Rh isoimmunizations in future pregnancies; given if mother is Rh negative and infant is Rh positive

Independent

PREOPERATIVE. Monitor for shock in patients who are bleeding. Nursing interventions are complex because of the profound physiologic and psychological changes that a woman experiences with a spontaneous abortion. Monitor emotional status. Emotional support of this patient is very important. In cases of a threatened abortion, avoid offering false reassurance because the patient may lose the pregnancy despite taking precautions. Phrases such as "I'm sorry" and "Is there anything I can do?" are helpful. It is not helpful to say, "If the baby had lived, he or she would probably be mentally retarded," or "You are young; you can get pregnant again." Inform the patient of perinatal grief support groups.

POSTOPERATIVE. Expect the patient to experience very mild uterine cramping and minimal vaginal bleeding. Patients are very drowsy from the anesthesia; assure that a call light is within easy reach and side rails are up for safety. Assist the patient to the bathroom; syncope is possible because of anesthesia and blood loss.

DOCUMENTATION GUIDELINES

- Amount and characteristics of blood loss, passage of fetal tissue, severity and location of pain, vital signs
- Signs of hypovolemic shock (pallor; cold, clammy skin; change in level of consciousness)
- Patient's (and father's) emotional response to losing the pregnancy

DISCHARGE AND HOME HEALTHCARE GUIDELINES

PREVENTION. Use extreme caution not to make the patient feel guilty about the cause of the SAB; however, it is important that she be made aware of factors that might contribute to the occurrence of an SAB (such as cigarette smoking; alcohol and drug usage; exposure to x rays or environmental teratogens). Preconceptual care should be encouraged, should the patient decide to become pregnant again.

COMPLICATIONS. Teach the patient to notify the physician of an increase in bleeding, return of painful uterine cramping, malodorous vaginal discharge, temperature greater than 100.4°F, or persistent feelings of depression.

HOME CARE. Teach the patient to avoid strenuous activities for a few days. Encourage the patient to use peripads instead of tampons for light vaginal discharge to decrease the likelihood of an infection. Explain that the patient should avoid intercourse for at least 1 week and then use some method of birth control until a future pregnancy can be discussed with the physician.

Abruptio Placentae

DRG Category: 372
Mean LOS: 2.7 days
Description: MEDICAL: Vaginal Delivery with Complicating Diagnosis

Abruptio placentae is the premature separation of a normally implanted placenta before the delivery of the baby. It is characterized by a triad of symptoms: vaginal bleeding, uterine hypertonus, and fetal distress. It can occur during the prenatal or intrapartum period. In a marginal abruption, separation begins at the periphery and bleeding accumulates between the membranes and the uterus and eventually passes through the cervix, becoming an external hemorrhage. In a central abruption, the separation occurs in the middle, and bleeding is trapped between the detached placenta and the uterus, concealing the hemorrhage. Frank vaginal bleeding also does not occur if the fetal head is tightly engaged. Since bleeding can be concealed, note that the apparent bleeding does not always indicate actual blood loss. If the placenta completely detaches, massive vaginal bleeding is seen. Abruptions are graded according to the percentage of the placental surface that detaches (Table 3). Destruction and loss of function of the placenta result in fetal distress.

CAUSES

The cause of abruptio placentae is unknown; however, any condition that causes vascular changes at the placental level may contribute to premature separation of the placenta. Chronic hypertension and pregnancy-induced hypertension are the most common associated factors. Also implicated are malnutrition, cigarette smoking, alcohol ingestion, and cocaine and crack use, as

TABLE 3 | **Grading System for Abruptions**

Grade 0	Less than 10% of the total placental surface has detached; the patient has no symptoms; however, a small retroplacental clot is noted at birth.
Grade I	Approximately 10%–20% of the total placental surface has detached; vaginal bleeding and mild uterine tenderness are noted; however, the mother and fetus are in no distress.
Grade II	Approximately 20%–50% of the total placental surface has detached; the patient has uterine tenderness and tetany; bleeding can be concealed or is obvious; signs of fetal distress are noted; the mother is not in hypovolemic shock.
Grade III	More than 50% of the placental surface has detached; uterine tetany is severe; bleeding can be concealed or is obvious; the mother is in shock and often experiencing coagulopathy; fetal death occurs.

well as such conditions as fibroids (especially those located behind the placental implantation site), severe diabetes or renal disease, and vena caval compression.

GENDER AND LIFE SPAN CONSIDERATIONS

Increased incidence of abruption is noted in those with grand multiparity and advanced maternal age. Additionally, the risk of recurrence in a subsequent pregnancy is increased. Abruptions occur in one of 120 deliveries and are responsible for 15% of third-trimester stillbirths. Severe abruptions are associated with a 25% to 35% perinatal mortality rate.

☐ ASSESSMENT

HISTORY. Obtain an obstetric history. Determine the date of the last menstrual period to calculate the estimated day of delivery and gestational age of the infant. Inquire about alcohol, tobacco, and drug usage during pregnancy. Ask the patient to describe the onset of bleeding (the circumstances, amount, and presence of pain). When obtaining a history from a patient with an abruption, recognize that it is possible for her to be disoriented from blood loss and/or cocaine or other drug usage. Generally, patients have one of the risk factors, but sometimes no clear precursor is identifiable.

PHYSICAL EXAMINATION. Assess the amount and character of vaginal bleeding; blood is often dark red in color, and the amount may vary, depending on the location of abruption. Palpate the uterus; patients complain of uterine tenderness and pain. The fundus is woodlike, and you can note poor resting tone. With a mild placental separation, contractions are usually of normal frequency, intensity, and duration. If the abruption is more severe, strong, erratic contractions occur. Assess for signs of concealed hemorrhage: slight or absent vaginal bleeding; an increase in fundal height; a rigid, boardlike abdomen; poor resting tone; constant abdominal pain; and late decelerations or decreased variability of the fetal heart rate. A vaginal exam should not be done until an ultrasound is performed to rule out placenta previa.

Using electronic fetal monitoring, determine the baseline fetal heart rate and presence or absence of accelerations, decelerations, and variability. Ask the patient if she feels the fetal movement. Fetal position and presentation can be assessed by Leopold's maneuvers. Assess the contraction status, and view the fetal monitor strip to note the frequency and duration of contractions. Throughout labor, monitor the patient's bleeding, vital signs, color, urine output, level of consciousness, uterine resting tone and contractions, and cervical dilation. If placenta previa has been ruled out, perform sterile vaginal exams to determine the progress of labor. Assess the patient's abdominal girth hourly by placing a tape measure at the level of the umbilicus. Maintain continuous fetal monitoring.

PSYCHOSOCIAL. Assess the patient's understanding of the situation and also the significant other's degree of anxiety, coping ability, and willingness to support the patient.

DIAGNOSTIC HIGHLIGHTS

General Comments: Abruptio placentae is diagnosed based on the clinical symptoms, and the diagnosis is confirmed after delivery by examining the placenta.

Test	Normal Result	Abnormality with Condition	Explanation
Pelvic ultrasound	Placenta is visualized in the fundus of the uterus	None; ultrasound is used to rule out a previa	If the placenta is in the lower uterine segment, a previa (not an abruption) exists

Other Tests: Complete blood count (CBC); coagulation studies; type and cross-match

PRIMARY NURSING DIAGNOSIS

Fluid volume deficit related to blood loss

OUTCOMES. Fluid balance; Hydration; Circulation status

INTERVENTIONS. Bleeding reduction; Blood product administration; Intravenous therapy; Shock management

☐ PLANNING AND IMPLEMENTATION

Collaborative

If the fetus is immature (less than 37 weeks) and the abruption is mild, conservative treatment may be indicated. However, conservative treatment is rare because the benefits of aggressive treatment far outweigh the risk of the rapid deterioration that can result from an abruption. Conservative treatment includes bed rest, tocolytic (inhibition of uterine contractions) therapy, and constant maternal and fetal surveillance. If a vaginal delivery is indicated and no regular contractions are occurring, the physician may choose to cautiously infuse oxytocin to induce the labor.

If the patient's condition is more severe, aggressive, expedient, and frequent assessments of blood loss, vital signs, and fetal heart rate pattern and variability are performed. Give lactated Ringer's solution intravenously (IV) via a large-gauge peripheral catheter. At times, two intravenous catheters are needed, especially if a blood transfusion is anticipated and the fluid loss has been great. If there has been an excessive blood loss, blood transfusions and central venous pressure (CVP) monitoring may be ordered. A normal CVP of 10 cm H_2O is the goal. CVP readings may indicate fluid volume deficit (low readings) or fluid overload and possible pulmonary edema following treatment (high readings).

If the mother or fetus is in distress, an emergency cesarean section is indicated. If any signs of fetal distress are noted (flat variability, late decelerations, bradycardia, tachycardia), turn the patient to her left side, increase the rate of her IV infusion, administer oxygen via face mask, and notify the physician. If a cesarean section is planned, see that informed consent is obtained in accordance with unit policy, prepare the patient's abdomen for surgery, insert a Foley catheter, administer preoperative medications as ordered, and notify the necessary personnel to attend the operation.

After delivery, monitor the degree of bleeding and perform fundal checks frequently. The fundus should be firm, midline, and at or below the level of the umbilicus. Determine the Rh status of the mother; if the patient is Rh-negative and the fetus is Rh-positive with a negative Coombs' test, administer $Rh_o(D)$ immune globulin (rhoGAM).

PHARMACOLOGIC HIGHLIGHTS

Medication or Drug Class	Dosage	Description	Rationale
Magnesium sulfate	4–6 g IV loading dose, 1–4 g/hr IV maintenance	Anticonvulsant	Effective tocolytic; relaxes the uterus, slowing the abruption
Oxytocin (Pitocin)	10–20 U in 500–1000 mL of IV fluid	Oxytocic	Assists the uterus to contract after delivery to prevent hemorrhage

Independent

During prenatal visits, explain the risk factors and the relationship between alcohol and substance abuse to the condition. Teach the patient to report any signs of abruption, such as cramping and bleeding. If the patient develops abruptio placentae and a vaginal delivery is chosen as the treatment option, the mother may not receive analgesics because of the fetus's prematurity; regional anesthesia may be considered. The labor, therefore, may be more painful than most mothers experience; provide support during labor. Keep the patient and the significant others informed of the progress of labor, as well as the condition of the mother and fetus.

Offer as many choices as possible to increase the patient's sense of control. Reassure the significant others that both the fetus and mother are being monitored for complications and that surgical intervention may be indicated. Provide the patient and family with an honest commentary about the risks. Discuss the possibility of an emergency cesarean section or the delivery of a premature infant. Answer the patient's questions honestly about the risk of a neonatal death. If the fetus does not survive, support the patient and listen to her feelings about the loss.

DOCUMENTATION GUIDELINES

- Amount and character of bleeding: Uterine resting tone; intensity, frequency, and duration of contractions and uterine irritability
- Response to treatment: Intravenous fluids, blood transfusion, medications, surgical interventions
- Fetal heart rate baseline, variability, absence or presence of accelerations or decelerations, bradycardia, tachycardia

DISCHARGE AND HOME HEALTHCARE GUIDELINES

Discharge before delivery (if the fetus is very immature and the mother and infant are stable).

MEDICATIONS. Instruct the patient not to miss a dose of the tocolytic medication; usually the medication is prescribed for every 4 hours and is to be taken throughout the day and night. Tell her to expect side effects of palpitations, fast heart rate, and restlessness. Teach the patient to notify the doctor and come to the hospital immediately if she experiences any bleeding or contractions. Note that being on tocolytic therapy may mask contractions. Therefore, if she feels any uterine contractions, she may be developing abruptio placentae.

POSTPARTUM. Give the usual postpartum instructions for avoiding complications. Inform the patient that she is at much higher risk of developing abruptio placentae in subsequent pregnancies. Instruct the patient on how to provide safe care of the infant. If the fetus has not survived, provide a list of referrals to the patient and significant others to help them manage their loss.

Acid-Base Imbalances: Metabolic Acidosis and Alkalosis

DRG Category: 296
Mean LOS: 5.4 days
Description: MEDICAL: Nutritional and Miscellaneous Metabolic Disorders, Age > 17 with CC
DRG Category: 244
Mean LOS: 4.9 days
Description: MEDICAL: Nutritional and Miscellaneous Metabolic Disorders, Age > 17 with CC

The hydrogen ion concentration ($[H+]$) of the body, described as the pH or negative log of the $[H+]$), is maintained in a narrow range to promote health and homeostasis. The body has many regulatory mechanisms that counteract even a slight deviation from normal pH. Acid-base imbalance can alter many physiologic processes and lead to serious problems or, if left untreated, to coma and death. A pH below 7.35 is considered acidosis and above 7.45 is alkalosis. Alterations in hydrogen ion concentration can be metabolic or respiratory in origin, or they may have a mixed origin.

Metabolic acidosis, a pH below 7.35, results from any nonpulmonary condition that leads to an excess of acids over bases. Renal patients with chronic acidemia may show signs of skeletal problems as calcium and phosphate are released from bone to help with the buffering of acids. Children with chronic acidosis may show signs of impaired growth. Metabolic alkalosis, a pH above 7.45, results from any nonpulmonary condition that leads to an excess of bases over acids. Metabolic alkalosis results from one of two mechanisms: an excess of bases or a loss of acids. Patients with a history of congestive heart failure and hypertension, who are on sodium-restricted diets and diuretics, are at greatest risk for metabolic alkalosis.

Respiratory acidosis is a pH imbalance that results from alveolar hypoventilation and an accumulation of carbon dioxide. It can be classified as either acute or chronic. Acute respiratory acidosis is associated with a sudden failure in ventilation. Chronic respiratory acidosis is seen in patients with chronic pulmonary disease, in whom long-term hypoventilation results in a chronic elevation (> 45 mm Hg) of $PaCO_2$ levels (hypercapnia), which renders the primary mechanism of inspiration, an elevated $PaCO_2$, unreliable. The major drive for respiration in chronic pulmonary disease patients becomes a low oxygen level (hypoxemia). Respiratory alkalosis is a pH imbalance that results from the excessive loss of carbon dioxide through hyperventilation ($PaCO_2 < 35$ mm Hg). Respiratory alkalosis is the most frequently occurring acid-base imbalance of hospitalized patients. Patients with respiratory alkalosis are at risk for hypokalemia, hypocalcemia, and hypophosphatemia.

CAUSES

See Table 4.

GENDER AND LIFE SPAN CONSIDERATIONS

Metabolic acidosis occurs primarily in patients with insulin-dependent diabetes mellitus (IDDM) and chronic renal failure, regardless of age. Metabolic acidosis from severe diarrhea can occur at any age, but children and the elderly are at greater risk because of associated fluid imbalances. Young women are at an increased risk of metabolic acidosis because of the popular fad diets of starvation.

Metabolic alkalosis is a common disorder of adult hospitalized patients. Elderly patients are at risk for metabolic alkalosis because of their delicate fluid and electrolyte status. Young women who practice self-induced vomiting to lose weight are also at risk for developing metabolic alkalosis. Finally, middle-aged men and women with chronic hypercapnia respiratory failure are at risk for metabolic alkalosis if their $PaCO_2$ levels are rapidly decreased with mechanical ventilation, corticosteroids, or antacids.

Patients of all ages are at risk for acute respiratory acidosis when an injury or illness results in alveolar hypoventilation. The elderly are at high risk for electrolyte and fluid imbalances, which can lead to respiratory depression. Patients with chronic obstructive pulmonary disease (COPD) are at highest risk for chronic respiratory acidosis. The typical COPD patient is a middle-aged man with a history of smoking. Older children and adults are at risk for respiratory alkalosis with large-dose salicylate ingestion. The elderly are at an increased risk for respiratory alkalosis because of the high incidence of pulmonary disorders, specifically pneumonia, in the elderly population. Identification of a respiratory alkalosis may be more difficult in the older patient because the early symptoms of increased respirations and altered neurological status may be attributed to other disease processes.

TABLE 4	**Common Causes of Acid-Base Disorders**
ACID-BASE DISORDER	**COMMON CAUSES**
Metabolic acidosis	Decreased acid excretion: chronic renal disease results in decreased acid excretion and is the most common cause of chronic metabolic acidosis Excessive acid production: oxygen tissue deprivation with shock and cardiopulmonary arrest, vigorous exercise (transient), prolonged periods of fever, ketoacidosis in insulin-dependent diabetics, alcoholic ketoacidosis, and ingestion of drugs and chemicals (methanol, ethylene glycol, aspirin) Underproduction of bicarbonate: pancreatitis Excessive loss of bicarbonate: severe diarrhea; intestinal obstruction; small bowel, pancreatic, ileostomy, or biliary fistula drainage Hyperchloremic acidosis, an increase in the extracellular concentration of chloride, also promotes bicarbonate loss
Metabolic alkalosis	Most common: vomiting and nasogastric suctioning. Other: ingestion of bicarbonates, carbonates, acetates, citrates, and lactates found in total parenteral nutrition solutions, Ringer's lactate, and sodium bicarbonate administration; rapid administration of stored blood and volume expanders with high citrate and acetate levels; excessive intake of antacids, which are composed of sodium bicarbonate or calcium carbonate; loss of acids (gastric fluid loss, diuretic therapy, excessive mineralocorticoid release); hypercalcemia; diuretic therapy; aldosterone excess.
Respiratory acidosis	Depression of respiratory center in the medulla: head injury, drug ingestion (anesthetics, opiates, barbiturates, ethanol) Decreased amount of functioning lung tissue: bronchial asthma, chronic bronchitis, emphysema, pneumonia, hemothorax, pneumothorax, pulmonary edema Airway obstruction: foreign body aspiration, sleep apnea, bronchospasm, laryngospasm Disorders of chest wall: flail chest, impaired diaphragm movement (pain, splinting, chest burns, tight chest or abdominal dressings) Abdominal distension: obesity, ascites, bowel obstruction Disorders of respiratory muscles: severe hypokalemia, amyotrophic lateral sclerosis, Guillain-Barré syndrome, poliomyelitis, myasthenia gravis, drugs (curare, succinylcholine)
Respiratory alkalosis	Hyperventilation due to hypoxemia (a decrease in the oxygen content of blood): anemia; hypotension; high altitudes; and pulmonary disease, such as pneumonia, interstitial lung disease, pulmonary vascular disease, and acute asthma Direct stimulation of the central respiratory center: anxiety, pain, fever, sepsis, salicylate ingestion, head trauma, central nervous system (CNS) disease (inflammation, lesions)
Examples of mixed disorders	Respiratory acidosis and metabolic alkalosis: chronic obstructive pulmonary disease (COPD) produces chronically elevated $PaCO_2$ levels and high HCO_3 levels as a compensatory mechanism. If the chronically elevated $PaCO_2$ is rapidly decreased, as it would be with aggressive mechanical ventilation, HCO_3 levels remain elevated, causing metabolic alkalosis

continued on the following page

TABLE 4 | **Common Causes of Acid-Base Disorders (*Continued*)**

ACID-BASE DISORDER	COMMON CAUSES
	Respiratory alkalosis and metabolic acidosis: salicylate ingestion directly stimulates the respiratory center, resulting in an increased rate and depth of breathing; ingestion of large amounts of salicylates can also produce metabolic acidosis; respiratory alkalosis results from the "blowing off" of CO_2

□ ASSESSMENT

HISTORY.

Metabolic Acidosis: Establish a history of renal disease, IDDM, or hepatic or pancreatic disease. Determine if the patient has experienced seizure activity, starvation, shock, acid ingestion, diarrhea, nausea, vomiting, anorexia, or abdominal pain or dehydration. Ask if the patient has experienced dyspnea with activity or at rest, as well as weakness, fatigue, headache, or confusion.

Metabolic Alkalosis: Establish a history of prolonged vomiting, nasogastric (NG) suctioning, hypercalcemia, hypokalemia, or hyperaldosteronism. Determine if the patient has been taking thiazide diuretics, has been receiving potassium-free intravenous (IV) infusions, eats large quantities of licorice, or regularly uses nasal sprays. Elicit a history of lightheadedness; agitation; muscle weakness, cramping, and twitching or tingling; or circumoral paresthesia. Ask the patient if he or she has experienced anorexia, nausea, or vomiting.

Respiratory Acidosis: Establish a history of impaired ventilation or breathlessness. The initial manifestations of respiratory acidosis involve changes in a patient's behavior. Investigate early signs of confusion, impaired judgment, motor incoordination, and restlessness. Determine if the patient has experienced headache, lethargy, blurred vision, confusion, or nausea.

Respiratory Alkalosis: Establish a history of hyperventilation from anxiety or mechanical overventilation. Early manifestations involve changes in neurological and neuromuscular status due to decreased $PaCO_2$ levels (hypocapnia), which may lead to decreased cerebral perfusion. Determine if the patient has experienced lightheadedness, anxiety, the inability to concentrate, or confusion. Elicit a patient history of muscle cramps, spasms, tingling (paresthesia) of the extremities, and circumoral (around the mouth) numbness. Other possible symptoms are nausea and vomiting, caused by a low potassium level.

PHYSICAL EXAMINATION.

Metabolic Acidosis: Inspect the patient's skin, noting if it feels warm. Note a flushed appearance. Assess the patient's breathing pattern for Kussmaul's respirations, a compensatory mechanism that the body uses to attempt to balance the pH by blowing off carbon dioxide. Check for an increased heart rate caused by stimulation of the sympathetic nervous system. To detect changes in cardiac performance, use a cardiac monitor for patients with a pH less than 7 and a potassium level greater than 5 mEq/L. Assess for changes in heart rate, ventricular ectopics, T-wave configuration, QRS, and P-R intervals. Include neurological status checks at least every 4 hours, or more frequently if the patient is confused or lethargic.

Metabolic Alkalosis: The patient with metabolic alkalosis demonstrates signs associated with the accompanying electrolyte imbalances. If hypocalcemia is present, the patient may demonstrate positive Chvostek's and Trousseau's signs (see **Hypocalcemia,** p. 495). Hypocalcemia and hypokalemia affect muscle strength and irritability. Assess the strength of the patient's hand grasps. Observe the patient's gait for unsteadiness, and note the presence of any hyperactive reflexes such as spasms and seizures. Observe the patient's breathing patterns for a compensatory decrease in the rate and depth of breathing. Use continuous cardiac monitoring, and check for an increased heart rate or ventricular dysrhythmias. Assess the patient for atrial tachycardias, ventricular dysrhythmias, and a prolonged Q-T interval.

Respiratory Acidosis: Assess the patient for an increased heart rate. As PaO_2 decreases and $PaCO_2$ increases, the sympathetic nervous system is stimulated, resulting in a release of catecholamines, epinephrine, and norepinephrine, which causes an increase in heart rate and cardiac output. Note cardiovascular abnormalities, such as tachycardia, hypertension, and atrial and ventricular dysrhythmias. During periods of acute respiratory acidosis, monitor the cardiac rhythm continuously. Take the patient's pulse, noting a bounding quality characteristic of hypercapnia. If the cause of the respiratory acidosis is respiratory center depression or respiratory muscle paralysis, respirations are slow and shallow. As respiratory acidosis worsens and respiratory muscles fail, the rate of respirations decreases.

Respiratory Alkalosis: The hallmark sign of respiratory alkalosis is hyperventilation; the patient may be taking 40 or more respirations per minute and may manifest a breathing pattern that is reminiscent of Kussmaul's breathing caused by diabetic acidosis. Check the patient for an increased heart rate, caused by hypoxemia. Test the patient's hand grasps for signs of weakness. Observe the patient's gait for unsteadiness, and note any indications of hyperactive reflexes such as spasms, tetany, and seizures. The presence of a positive Chvostek's or Trousseau's sign may indicate hypocalcemia (see **Hypocalcemia,** p. 495), which may occur from lower amounts of ionized calcium during periods of alkalosis.

PSYCHOSOCIAL. Acid-base imbalances frequently affect patients with both acute and chronic illnesses. Their response to yet another problem is at best unpredictable. Neurological changes such as confusion, agitation, or psychosis are upsetting if they occur, as are electrolyte disturbances. Anticipate the patient's feeling powerless, and plan care to support all psychological needs.

DIAGNOSTIC HIGHLIGHTS

Test	Normal Result	Abnormality with Condition	Explanation
Arterial blood gases	pH 7.35–7.45; PaO_2 80–100 mm Hg; $PaCO_2$ 35–45 mm Hg; SaO_2 > 95%; HCO_3 22–26 mEq/L	*Metabolic acidosis:* pH < 7.35; HCO_3 < 22 mEq/L; *Metabolic alkalosis:* pH > 7.45; HCO_3 > 26 mEq/L; *Respiratory acidosis:* pH < 7.35; $PaCO_2$ > 45 mm Hg; *Respiratory alkalosis:* pH > 7.45; $PaCO_2$ < 35 mm Hg	All values are prior to compensation

Anion gap	12–16 mEq/L	*Metabolic acidosis:* increased; *Metabolic alkalosis:* decreased	Calculation of difference between major cations and anions in blood

Other Tests: Electrocardiogram; serum electrolyte levels (sodium, chloride, calcium, potassium, magnesium); glucose; lactate; total protein; blood urea nitrogen; creatinine; urine pH

PRIMARY NURSING DIAGNOSIS

Altered health maintenance related to acid-base imbalances

OUTCOMES. Knowledge: Diet; Disease process; Health behaviors; Medication: Treatment regime; Nutritional status; Electrolyte and acid-base balance

INTERVENTIONS. Acid-base management; Acid-base monitoring; Heath education; Risk identification; Teaching: Disease process; Referral; Medication management; Nutritional management

▢ PLANNING AND IMPLEMENTATION

Collaborative

GENERAL. The highest priority for all patients with acid-base imbalances is to maintain the adequacy of airway, breathing, and circulation. An important focus for collaborative treatment is to deliver oxygen, remove carbon dioxide, and monitor gas exchange. Treatment is focused on correcting the cause and restoring fluids and electrolytes to a normal range. Provide constant cardiac monitoring for patients with hypokalemia, hypocalcemia, and hypomagnesemia. Consult with a dietitian to provide foods that can help restore electrolyte balance and increase oral intake. If a patient demonstrates impaired physical mobility, consult a physical therapist to evaluate the patient's abilities and to recommend needed strengthening exercises and assist devices.

Metabolic Acidosis: Sodium bicarbonate may be administered to treat normal anion gap metabolic acidosis but is controversial in treating increased anion gap metabolic acidosis. Research has shown that administering sodium bicarbonate may inhibit hemoglobin release of oxygen to the tissues, thus increasing the acidosis. Sodium bicarbonate is recommended if the pH is greatly reduced (<7.2). Sodium bicarbonate may be administered by intravenous drip or by intravenous push. Overmedication of sodium bicarbonate may cause metabolic alkalosis, fluid volume overload, hypokalemia, and worsened acidosis. Potassium-sparing diuretics, amphotericin B, and large quantities of isotonic saline solutions should not be administered to patients with suspected renal failure. These drugs may contribute to the development of metabolic acidosis.

Metabolic Alkalosis: Pharmacologic therapy may include IV saline solutions, potassium supplements, histamine antagonists, and carbonic anhydrase inhibitors. IV saline solutions (0.9% or 0.45%) may be used to replace lost volume and chloride ions. Causes of metabolic alkalosis that respond favorably to saline therapy include vomiting, NG suctioning, post chronic hypercapnia, and diuretic therapy. The causes of metabolic alkalosis that do not respond favorably to the administration of saline include hypokalemia and mineralocorticoid excess. Potassium chloride is used to treat hypokalemia in a patient with metabolic alkalosis. Dietary supplements of potassium are not effective unless chloride levels are stabilized.

Histamine H_2 receptor antagonists, particularly cimetidine and ranitidine, reduce the production of hydrochloric acid in the stomach and may prevent the occurrence of metabolic alkalosis in patients with NG suctioning and vomiting.

The carbonic anhydrase inhibitor acetazolamide (Diamox) is useful for correcting metabolic alkalosis in patients with congestive heart failure who cannot tolerate fluid volume administration. Acetazolamide promotes the renal excretion of bicarbonate. Severe metabolic alkalosis may require the administration of weak acid solutions. Because acetazolamide promotes the excretion of potassium, it is not given until serum potassium levels are evaluated as safe.

Potassium-sparing diuretics, such as spironolactone, may be used if diuretics are needed. Anticonvulsants are usually not needed because the risk for seizures decreases as fluid and electrolyte imbalances are corrected.

Respiratory Acidosis: Although oxygen therapy is required to treat the hypoxemia that accompanies respiratory acidosis, a fraction of inspired air (FiO_2) of less than 0.40 is desirable. Oxygen concentrations greater than 0.80 are toxic to the lung in 5 to 6 days. Caution: The use of oxygen for patients with COPD and hypercapnia may remove the stimulus for respiration and result in respiratory depression. If the $PaCO_2$ is greater than 60 mm Hg or the PaO_2 is less than 50 mm Hg with high levels of supplemental oxygen, intubation and mechanical ventilation are required. Pharmacologic therapy for respiratory acidosis depends on the cause and severity of acidosis. The administration of sodium bicarbonate is controversial for a pH greater than 7.0. If the pH is below 7.0, sodium bicarbonate administration is recommended. Bronchodilators may be used to decrease bronchospasms. Antibiotics are prescribed for respiratory infections, but sedatives that depress respirations are limited.

Respiratory Alkalosis: Because the most common cause of respiratory alkalosis is anxiety, reassurance and sedation may be all that is needed. Pharmacologic therapy most likely includes the administration of antianxiety medications and potassium supplements. Benzodiazepines, commonly used to control acute anxiety attacks, are administered intramuscularly or intravenously. If the anxiety is more severe and the respiratory alkalosis is pronounced, rebreathing small amounts of exhaled air with a paper bag or a rebreather mask helps increase arterial $PaCO_2$ levels and decrease arterial pH. If the cause of the hyperventilation is hypoxemia, oxygen therapy is needed. Overventilation by mechanical ventilation can be easily remedied by decreasing the respiratory rate or tidal volume. If ventilator changes do not decrease the pH, dead space can be added to the ventilator tubing. Dead space provides a smaller volume of air so that less CO_2 can be expired.

Independent

For patients who are acutely ill, the priority is to maintain a patent airway, which can be managed through positioning or the use of an oral airway or endotracheal tube. Position patient in a semi-Fowler position to allow for optimal chest wall expansion, patient comfort, and adequate gas exchange. Aggressive pulmonary hygiene techniques are used to mobilize secretions and increase alveolar ventilation. These measures should include turning, coughing, and deep breathing every 2 hours; postural drainage and percussion every 4 hours; and sitting up in a chair twice per day.

Orient a confused patient to person, time, and place. Use clocks, calendars, family photos, and scheduled rest periods to help maintain orientation. Assist the patient in using hearing aids and glasses to ensure an accurate interpretation of surroundings. Consider using restraints if the risk for injury is high. Remove the restraints every 2 hours to allow for range-of-motion exercises. Incorporate the patient's normal sleep routines into the care plan. Schedule collaborative activities to allow at least two 1-hour rest periods during the day and one 4-hour rest period at night.

Provide assistance as needed in feeding, bathing, toileting, and dressing. Provide frequent mouth care (every 2 hours) to ensure patient comfort. If the patient is able to swallow, offer sips of water or ice chips every hour. Avoid lemon glycerine swabs, which may cause dryness. The patient is not discharged until the cause of the acid-base alteration has been resolved; in many patients, however, underlying organ diseases may not be resolved.

DOCUMENTATION GUIDELINES

- Physical findings: Flushed, dry, warm skin; mental status (presence of disorientation or confusion); respiratory rate and pattern, breath sounds; cardiac rhythm and rate, blood pressure, quality of pulses, urine output; level of consciousness, orientation, ability to concentrate, motor strength, and seizure activity (if seizures are present, the following information should be charted: time the seizure began, parts of the body involved in the seizure, progression of the seizure, type of body movements, pupil size and reaction, eye movements, vital signs during seizure and postictal state)
- Response to therapy: Medications, activity, interventions
- Laboratory values: Arterial blood gases (ABGs) and serum potassium, calcium, sodium, chloride, and magnesium

DISCHARGE AND HOME HEALTHCARE GUIDELINES

The patients at highest risk for a recurrence of acid-base imbalances are those who consume large quantities of thiazide diuretics, antacids, and licorice, as well as those who have chronic renal, pulmonary, cardiac, and neurological disorders and IDDM. Make sure these patients understand the importance of maintaining the prescribed treatment regimen. Teach patients on diuretic therapy the signs and symptoms of the associated fluid and electrolyte disturbances of hypovolemia and hypokalemia. Teach patients the action, dose, and side effects of all medications. Teach the patient with mild-to-moderate anxiety progressive muscle relaxation, therapeutic breathing, and visualization techniques to control anxiety.

Acquired Immunodeficiency Syndrome

DRG Category: 490
Mean LOS: 5.1 days
Description: MEDICAL: HIV with or without Related Conditions
DRG Category: 489
Mean LOS: 8.3 days
Description: MEDICAL: HIV with Major Related Conditions

Acquired immunodeficiency syndrome (AIDS) is the final result of an infection with a retrovirus, the human immunodeficiency virus (HIV). The Centers for Disease Control and Prevention (CDC) first described AIDS in 1981, and since then the disease has become one of the most widely publicized and feared diseases of our time. Experts suggest that more than 1 million Americans and 40 million people worldwide are infected with HIV. More than 90% of those people infected are in developing nations.

The CDC proposed a four-stage classification for the phases of HIV infection. (See Table 5.)

TABLE 5 | **Proposed CDC Four-Stage Classification for the Phases of HIV Infection**

CLASSIFICATION	DESCRIPTION	COMMENTS
Group I	Acute infection	Early, acute phase in an immunocompetent person to an HIV infection. Widespread level of viral production occurs with widespread seeding of lymph tissues. Symptoms are generally nonspecific, such as sore throat, myalgia, fever, weight loss, and fatigue. Symptoms occur 3–6 weeks after infection and resolve 2–4 weeks later
Group II	Asymptomatic infection	In the middle phases of disease, patients may remain asymptomatic (Group II) or may develop a persistent generalized lymphadenopathy. In either case, HIV replication occurs primarily in the lymphoid tissues.
Group III	Persistent generalized lymphadenopathy	Patients may remain in Group II or Group III, which are middle, chronic phases. Patients may also experience opportunistic infections such as herpes zoster and candida. Most but not all people progress to AIDS in 7 to 10 years.

continued on the following page

TABLE 5	**Proposed CDC Four-Stage Classification for the Phases of HIV Infection**

CLASSIFICATION	DESCRIPTION	COMMENTS
Group IV	Final crisis phase with constitutional disease, neurological disease, secondary infection or neoplasm, or other conditions	Final crisis phase characterized by a breakdown of immune defenses, increased viral counts, and multiple clinical signs such as persistent fever, fatigue, weight loss, diarrhea, and serious opportunistic infections (protozoal, helminthic, fungal, bacterial, viral) and neoplasms such as Kaposi's sarcoma and primary lymphoma of the brain.

HIV infection of lymphocytes and other cells that bear specific protein markers leads to lymphopenia and impaired T and B cell function.

CAUSES

HIV causes AIDS. Two HIV strains have been identified: HIV-1 and HIV-2. HIV-1 is the prototype virus and is responsible for most cases of AIDS in the United States. HIV-2 is found chiefly in West Africa, appears to be less easily transmitted, and has a longer incubation period. Susceptibility to infection is unclear. The presence of sexually transmitted diseases (STDs) with open lesions, such as herpes and syphilis, may increase the patient's susceptibility to viral entry. People with cytomegalovirus and Epstein-Barr virus infections may also be more susceptible because of an increased number of target cells. Routes of transmission are through sexual contact (male to male, male to female, female to male, and female to female); by blood to blood or transfusion contact (generally blood products given between 1977 and 1985); through the use of needles contaminated by an HIV-infected person; by blood or other HIV-infected fluids coming in contact with open lesions or mucous membranes; and by mother to child during the in utero period, during delivery, or by breastfeeding.

GENDER AND LIFE SPAN CONSIDERATIONS

HIV is the leading cause of death in the United States for men ages 25 to 44 years and is the third leading cause of death in women of the same age range. Individuals can contract HIV at any time during their life span, including infancy. The average time between exposure and diagnosis in adults is from 8 to 10 years, although the incubation period varies among people. In children, the incubation period is approximately 18 months. Children are likely to have a history of repeated bacterial infections such as middle ear infections and pneumonia. Approximately 2% of all AIDS cases occur in children under the age of 13 years. Most of the AIDS cases in children are the result of maternal-child transmission or from exposure to blood or blood products.

◻ ASSESSMENT

HISTORY. Common symptoms include night sweats, lymphadenopathy, fever, weight loss, fatigue, and rash. Gastrointestinal (GI) disturbances such as nausea, vomiting, diarrhea, and anorexia are common. The patient may describe neurologic manifestations, including headache, lightheadedness, memory loss, word-finding difficulty, inability to concentrate, and mood swings. Patients may notice gait disturbance, a "stiff" neck and pain, burning, numbness, and tingling in the extremities. A history of infections such as tuberculosis, herpes, hepatitis B, fungal infections, or STDs is common in the HIV and AIDS population.

PHYSICAL EXAMINATION. Patients with HIV and AIDS are at risk for opportunistic infections that affect all systems and diseases common to their age group. (See Box 1.) Wasting syndrome is common to AIDS patients. Fever may or may not be present. The patient's skin may have a generalized rash or lesions from herpes or Kaposi's sarcoma (a metastasizing skin cancer). Ask the patient to walk during the examination to examine the patient's gait. Note ataxia, motor weakness, gait disturbance, and hemiparesis. Palpate the patient's lymph nodes to determine if lymphadenopathy is present, particularly in two or more extrainguinal sites.

BOX 1 SYMPTOMS IN AIDS PATIENTS REQUIRING MEDICAL ATTENTION
New cough
Shortness of breath or dyspnea on exertion
Increased fatigue or malaise
Fever
Night sweats
Headache or stiff neck
Visual changes: Floaters, blurring, photophobia, changes in visual fields
Mental status alteration: Change in level of consciousness, loss of memory, forgetfulness, loss of concentration, depression, mood swings
New onset of diarrhea
Sudden weight loss
Increased size of or pain in lymph nodes
Skin lesions
Pain

PSYCHOSOCIAL. Diagnosis of HIV is a crisis, and the crisis may exacerbate any underlying psychiatric disorders. A person may be in a state of denial or have anxiety, psychologic numbness, depression, or suicidal ideation. Remember that in this state people cannot focus and do not hear what healthcare professionals tell them. The patient undergoes a fear of the loss of sex life, contaminating others, rejection, and stigma. Fears about loss of employment, financial independence, and insurance are realities. As the disease progresses, grief over losses, hopelessness, suicidal ideation, and emotional exhaustion may occur. The patient deals with stress over the demands of treatment, embarrassment because of physical symptoms, and loneliness.

DIAGNOSTIC HIGHLIGHTS

Test	Normal Result	Abnormality with Condition	Explanation
Enzyme-linked immunosorbent assay (ELISA)	Negative for HIV antibodies	Positive for HIV antibodies	Positive test is confirmed by a Western blot
T lymphocyte and B lymphocyte subsets	B cells: 65–4785/ml; CD4 T cells: 450–1400/ml; CD4 to CD8 T cell ratio: 1–3.5	B and T cell values decreased. CD4 counts less than 500/mL are generally associated with symptoms; CD4 counts less than 200mL are associated with severe immune suppression. Any HIV-infected person with a CD4 level less than 200/mL is considered to have AIDS	HIV infects cells with the CD4 protein marker
Viral load: polymerase chain reaction (PCR)	Negative	Detects number of copies/ml; test has a lower limit of 400 copies/mL but can reach levels at 30,000 copies/mL and higher	Quantitative assay that measures amount of HIV-1 RNA in plasma

Other Tests: Complete blood count; HIV p24 antigen or viral culture

PRIMARY NURSING DIAGNOSIS

Risk for infection related to immune deficiency

OUTCOMES. Immune status; Respiratory status: Gas exchange; Respiratory status: Ventilation; Thermoregulation

INTERVENTIONS. Infection control; Infection protection; Respiratory monitoring; Temperature regulation

☐ PLANNING AND IMPLEMENTATION

Collaborative

Much of the collaborative management is based on pharmacologic therapy (see below). Supportive management consists of treatment of malignancies with chemotherapy and irradiation, treatment of infections as they develop, and the management of discomfort with analgesia. Surgical management may be needed to excise lesions from Kaposi's sarcoma or to drain abscesses. If the patient becomes short of breath, oxygen is often prescribed to improve gas exchange. Dietary support is important in the treatment of HIV infection and AIDS throughout the progression of the illness.

PHARMACOLOGIC HIGHLIGHTS

Antiretroviral therapies are grouped into three categories and should always be used in combination. Drugs have important interactions with other medication. Interactions need to be reviewed carefully.

Medication or Drug Class	Dosage	Description	Rationale
Antiretroviral therapy: nucleoside analogs such as zidovudine, dideoxynosine, dideoxycytidine	Zidovudine 300 mg po bid	Nucleoside analog	Decreases HIV replication by incorporation into the strand of DNA, causing chain termination
Antiretroviral therapy: protease inhibitors such as ritonavir	Saquinavir 600 mg po tid for original formulation; 1200 po saquinavir, indinavir, tid for soft-gel	Protease inhibitor	Blocks the action of the viral protease required for protein processing late in the viral cycle
Antiretroviral therapy: non-nucleoside reverse transcriptase inhibitors such as nevirapine, delavirdine	Nevirapine 400 mg po QD	Non-nucleoside reverse transcriptase inhibitors	Inhibits HIV by binding non-competitively to the reverse transcriptase

Independent

Nursing interventions are complex because of the many physical, psychologic, and social effects that occur from HIV infection and AIDS. During the more acute stages of the illness, focus on maximizing the patient's health and promoting comfort. Educate the patient and significant others regarding self-care by keeping any lesions and the skin clean and dry. Diarrhea can limit activities and also cause pain, both abdominal and perianally, if any lesions are present. Keep the perianal area clean, and assist the patient to clean himself or herself immediately. Instruct the patient about the food substances that are GI irritants. Explain that diarrhea can cause dehydration, electrolyte disturbances, and malabsorption; provide the patient with ways to maintain fluid and electrolyte balance. All patients need to be instructed to perform frequent and thorough oral care. Teach patients to avoid toothbrushes. Tell them to clean the teeth, gums, and membranes with a soft gauze pad; to use mouthwashes without alcohol; to lubricate the lips; and to avoid foods that are spicy, acidic, thermally hot, and hard to chew. Also explain the need to seek treatment for candida and herpes and to use xylocaine for discomfort.

Explain the mechanisms for HIV transmission and teach the patient and significant others the precautions regarding transmission both by casual and sexual routes. Explain that if the patient has spills of blood or secretion, they should be cleaned up with a 1:10 solution of bleach and water to limit the risk of infection to others. Use universal precautions whenever you are exposed to blood, body fluids, or secretions, and teach the patient's significant others to do the same.

Note that the best outcomes result from early intervention. Many times the patient's family members are unaware of his or her bisexual or homosexual orientation. The diagnosis of AIDS may increase the distance between friends and family members. Social isolation often occurs because others avoid the patient out of the fear of being infected. Allow the patient to talk about the diagnosis and isolation. Use touch and encourage others to touch, hug, hold hands, and give back rubs to the patient to help fulfill the patient's need for touch. Encourage the patient's participation in support groups and use of volunteer "friends." The patient may experience anger, denial, anxiety, hopelessness, and depression. Ensure that the needed support services are available for home health care; make sure the patient has support for meals, financial assistance, and hygienic care.

DOCUMENTATION GUIDELINES

- Physical changes: Weight, mental status, vital signs, skin integrity, bowel habits
- Tolerance to activity, fatigue, ability to sleep, ability to manage self-care
- Emotional response, coping, signs of ineffective coping, support from family and friends
- Presence of opportunistic infections, complications of infections, medications, resistance, recurrence
- Requests for management of the critical phases of disease, and pertinent information about the patient's wishes regarding the final stages of life

DISCHARGE AND HOME HEALTHCARE GUIDELINES

PREVENTION. Teach the patient or caregiver universal precautions at home; adequate nutritional strategies; the names and telephone numbers for support organizations; self-assessments daily for temperature elevations; signs of thrush (candida), herpes, and other opportunistic infections; symptoms of complications such as cough, lesions, and fever; strategies to limit situations with high infection potential (crowds, people with colds or flu).

TRANSMISSION. Teach the patient strategies to practice safe sex. Inform the patient that the disease can be transmitted during high-risk sexual practices that expose partners to body fluids. These practices include vaginal and anal intercourse without a condom, or oral sex without protection. Encourage the patient to use safe sex practices such as hugging, petting, mutual masturbation, and protected anal and vaginal sex.

Encourage the patient to notify any sexual partners and healthcare providers that he or she has an HIV infection. Explain that the patient should not donate blood, blood products, or organs, tissues, or sperm. If the patient continues to abuse intravenous drugs, make sure the patient knows never to share needles.

Explain to women of childbearing age that any pregnancy may result in an infant with an HIV infection. Explain that HIV may also infect an infant during delivery or during breastfeeding. Encourage the woman to notify her physician as soon as pregnancy occurs to allow preventative treatment to limit the risk to the fetus.

SUPPORT SYSTEMS. Inform the patient about the possible physiologic, emotional, and mental effects of the disease, along with the treatments and resources that are available to them. Encourage the patient to explore hospice care early in the treatment cycle to establish a possible long-term relationship as the disease progresses.

Acromegaly

DRG Category: 300
Mean LOS: 6.3 days
Description: MEDICAL: Endocrine Disorders with CC

Acromegaly is a rare, chronic, and disabling disorder of body growth and endocrine dysfunction in adults (after closure of the epiphyses) that is caused by excessive levels of growth hormone (GH). In adults, it is almost always due to a growth hormone–secreting pituitary adenoma. The excess production of GH causes enlargement of tissues and an altered production of glucocorticoids, mineralocorticoids, and gonadotropins. Left untreated, acromegaly causes gross physical deformities, crippling neuromuscular alterations, major organ dysfunctions, and decreased visual acuity. Acromegaly increases an individual's risk for heart disease, diabetes mellitus, and gallstones. The resultant cardiac disease reduces life expectancy.

CAUSES

The overproduction of GH is a result of hyperpituitarism. More than 90% of patients have a pituitary adenoma. The etiology of adenomas is unknown. Hyperpituitarism can also occur with lung, gastric, breast, and ovarian cancers and may have a genetic cause.

GENDER AND LIFE SPAN CONSIDERATIONS

Diagnosis of acromegaly usually occurs after the age of 40 in men and 45 in women.

☐ ASSESSMENT

HISTORY. The course of acromegaly is slow, with very gradual changes over 7 to 10 years. Reviewing a patient's old photographs may reveal the progressive changes in facial features. Determine if the patient has had a change in hat, glove, ring, or shoe size because of an overgrowth of the hands and feet. Ask the patient if he or she has had headaches or visual disturbances, which in acromegaly are caused by the growth of the adenoma, which exerts pressure on brain tissue and cranial nerves III, IV, and VI. Establish a history of altered sexual function, which may be an indicator of decreased gonadotropin production. Ask about the presence of pain in the hands, feet, and spine, which is probably caused by bone growths; also ask about problems with chewing, swallowing, or talking, which may be caused by tongue, jaw, and teeth enlargement. Note the presence of a deepening of the voice, recurrent bronchitis, excessive sweating, heat intolerance, fatigue, and muscle weakness. Check for a family history of pituitary tumors.

PHYSICAL EXAMINATION. The initial physical changes that occur with acromegaly result from an enlargement of the bones in the head, hands, and feet. The parts of the head that may be enlarged by acromegaly include the jaw, forehead, nose, tongue, and teeth. Observe the patient's facial appearance, noting an enlarged supraorbital ridge, thickened ears and nose, or jutting of the jaw (prognathism). If the patient has an enlarged tongue, note any respiratory alterations.

Examine the patient's fingers for signs of thickening. Inspect the patient's torso, noting a barrel chest or kyphosis. Note any signs of bowed legs. Assess the patient's skin for signs of oiliness or excessive sweating (diaphoresis). Assess the patient's hand strength. Test the patient's vision for bitemporal hemianopia and loss of visual acuity. Note a deep, hollow-sounding voice.

PSYCHOSOCIAL. Patients with acromegaly undergo some dramatic physical changes that can lead to permanent dysfunctions. These changes affect the patient's self-concept and ability to perform expected roles. Note any irritability or hostility.

DIAGNOSTIC HIGHLIGHTS

Test	Normal Result	Abnormality with Condition	Explanation
Plasma somato-medin C (insulin-like growth factor)	Adult females: 24–253 ng/mL; Males: 43–178 ng/mg	Increased; if levels are only moderately elevated, diagnosis is confirmed by giving 75 mg of glucose orally and measuring serum growth hormone q 30 minutes for 2 hours. Failure to suppress growth hormone confirms diagnosis of acromegaly	Small polypeptide produced in the liver; directly stimulates growth and proliferation of normal cells and predicts over-production of growth hormone

Other Tests: Pituitary imaging; x rays of skull, hands, feet

PRIMARY NURSING DIAGNOSIS

Body image disturbance related to anxiety over thickened skin and enlargement of face, hands, and feet

OUTCOMES. Self-esteem; Body image; Anxiety control

INTERVENTIONS. Body image enhancement; Coping enhancement; Emotional support; Self-esteem enhancement; Support group; Anxiety reduction

☐ PLANNING AND IMPLEMENTATION

Collaborative

SURGICAL. The goal of treatment is to normalize pituitary function. Pituitary adenomas are frequently removed by a transsphenoidal hypophysectomy through an incision in the upper lip. After the gland is removed, a muscle graft is used to pack the dura and prevent leakage of cerebral spinal fluid. When the incision is closed, nasal packing and a mustache dressing are used to tamponade the area. A transfrontal craniotomy may be used if the tumor is large or if a transsphenoidal approach is contraindicated. Because many patients have macroadenomas, complete tumor resection with cure of acromegaly may be impossible and radiotherapy may be used to prevent regrowth and control symptoms.

POSTOPERATIVE. After surgery, assess the patient's neurologic status and report significant changes. Also check for the presence of pain. Antibiotics, antipyretics, and analgesics may be used to control infection and pain. Check nasal drainage for the presence of glucose, which indicates cerebrospinal fluid drainage. Monitor blood glucose. Growth hormone levels generally fall rapidly after surgery, thus removing an insulin-antagonist effect and possibly causing hypoglycemia. Pituitary dysfunction occurs in about one-fifth of patients after surgery and requires glucocorticoids, gonadotropins, and thyroid replacement hormone therapy.

PHARMACOLOGIC HIGHLIGHTS

Medication or Drug Class	Dosage	Description	Rationale
Octreotide	100 μg sc tid	Somatostatin analog	Suppresses growth hormone secretion while the effect of radiation is being awaited after surgery

Independent

PREOPERATIVE. At the time of diagnosis, the patient requires education and emotional support. Focus education on the cause of the disease, the prescribed medical regimen, and preparation for surgery. Encourage the patient to interact with family and significant others. Reassure the patient that treatment reverses some of the physical deformities. If you note disabling behavior, refer the patient to psychiatric resources.

Prepare the patient and family for surgery. Explain the preoperative diagnostic tests and examinations. For a patient who is undergoing a transsphenoidal hypophysectomy or a transfrontal craniotomy, explain the postoperative need for nasal packing and a mustache dressing.

POSTOPERATIVE. Elevate the patient's head to facilitate breathing and fluid drainage. Do not encourage the patient to cough, as this interferes with the healing of the operative site. Provide frequent mouth care, and keep the skin dry. To promote maximum joint mobility, perform or assist with range-of-motion exercises. Encourage the patient to ambulate within 1 to 2 days of the surgery. To assure healing of the incision site, explain the need to avoid activities that increase intracranial pressure, such as toothbrushing, coughing, sneezing, nose blowing, and bending.

DOCUMENTATION GUIDELINES

- Physical findings: Respiratory rate and pattern; nasal drainage: color, amount, and presence of glucose
- Neurologic status: Level of consciousness, motor strength, sensation, and vision
- Presence of postoperative complications: Diabetes insipidus, hypopituitarism, meningitis
- Psychosocial assessment: Self-esteem, coping, interpersonal relationships, and sexual dysfunction

DISCHARGE AND HOME HEALTHCARE GUIDELINES

REFERRALS. Refer patients with advanced acromegaly who experience arthritic changes and require assist devices for ambulation and activities of daily living to a physical therapist.

ACTIVITY RESTRICTIONS. Instruct the patient to avoid activities that increase intracranial pressure for up to 2 months after surgery. Toothbrushing can be resumed in 2 weeks. Instruct the patient to report increased nasal drainage. Incisional numbness and altered olfaction may occur for 4 months after surgery.

MEDICATIONS. If octreotide is prescribed, the patient will need to be able to demonstrate how to administer a subcutaneous injection.

FOLLOW-UP. Patients need to be monitored for development of cardiac disease, diabetes mellitus, and gallstones and a recurrence of symptoms. Advise the patient to wear a medical identification bracelet.

Acute Adrenal Crisis

DRG category: 300
Mean LOS: 6.3 days
Description: MEDICAL: Endocrine Disorders with CC

Acute adrenal crisis is a life-threatening endocrine emergency caused by a deficit of glucocorticoids (primarily cortisol) or mineralocorticoids (primarily aldosterone). The anterior pituitary gland produces adrenocorticotropic hormone (ACTH), which causes the adrenal cortex to produce corticosteroid and aldosterone hormones.

A deficiency of cortisol produces many metabolic abnormalities, such as decreases in glucose production, protein and fat metabolism, appetite, and digestion. Serious systemic effects include a decrease in vascular tone and a diminished effect of catecholamines such as epinephrine and norepinephrine. Normally a body under stress releases corticosteroids. The decrease in both the vascular tone of the blood vessels and the decreased effect of catecholamines in an individual in an adrenal crisis can cause shock. The deficiency of aldosterone results in profound fluid and electrolyte imbalances: a decrease in sodium and water retention, a decrease in circulating blood volume, and an increase in both potassium and hydrogen ion reabsorption.

CAUSES

Acute adrenal insufficiency is most commonly caused by acute withdrawal of chronic corticosteroid therapy. It can also occur from immune destruction of the adrenal cortex or adrenal hemorrhage, or from infiltration by metastatic carcinoma. Before signs and symptoms appear, at least 90% or more of the adrenal cortex is damaged. The disorders result in deficiencies of both glucocorticoid and mineralocorticoid hormones.

GENDER AND LIFE SPAN CONSIDERATIONS

Acute adrenal crisis may occur at any age, without regard to gender, and may be associated with developmental or genetic abnormalities. In children, the most common cause of acute adrenal crisis is an overwhelming infection with Pseudomonas or meningococcal meningitis (also known as Waterhouse-Friderichsen syndrome). In adults, acute adrenal crisis is more commonly associated with hemorrhagic destruction because of anticoagulant therapy or aggravation of adrenal hypofunction during periods of major stress.

☐ ASSESSMENT

HISTORY. Elicit a medication history, with particular attention to such medications as corticosteroids, phenytoin, barbiturates, anticoagulants, and rifampin. Note a history of cancer, autoimmune diseases requiring treatment with corticosteroids, or radiation to the head or abdomen. A family history of either Addison's disease or an autoimmune disease may be important.

Inquire about a recent decrease in appetite, abdominal pain, weight loss, or salt craving. Often in crisis, the patient or family may describe fever, nausea, and vomiting. Determine if the patient has experienced signs and symptoms such as generalized fatigue, apathy, dizziness, weakness, headache, or changes in skin pigmentation. Some patients describe central nervous system effects such as confusion, irritability, psychoses, emotional lability, or even seizures. Women may describe a decreased libido and amenorrhea.

PHYSICAL EXAMINATION. The patient appears to be critically ill. Because of decreased fluid volume caused by a decrease in water reabsorption, the patient may arrive at the hospital in shock with severe hypotension; tachycardia; decreased cardiac output; weak and rapid pulses; and cool, pale skin. Peripheral pulses may be weak and irregular. Urine output is usually quite low. The blood pressure may be very hard to maintain because a decrease in the catecholamines can result in decreased vascular tone.

An increase in skin pigmentation (bronze color) is noticeable in European-Americans. Areas most often affected include the mucous membranes and areas over joints and scars. A loss of pubic hair may also occur from a decreased level of adrenal androgens.

PSYCHOSOCIAL. Assess the patient's and significant others' ability to cope with a critical illness and the presence of a social network to support them.

DIAGNOSTIC HIGHLIGHTS

Test	Normal Result	Abnormality with Condition	Explanation
Serum cortisol level	6 to 8 AM, 5–23 μg/dL	Decreased	Determines the ability of the adrenal gland to produce gluco-corticoids
Serum electrolytes and chemistries	Sodium 136–145 mEq/L; potassium 3.5–5.1 mEq/L; blood urea nitrogen 5–20 mg/dL; glucose 70–105 mg/dL	Hyponatremia; hyperkalemia; azotemia; hypoglycemia	Values reflect sodium loss from a deficit in mineralo-cortocoids with loss of fluids, and poor glucose control because of decreased gluconeogenesis

Other Tests: ACTH, ACTH stimulation test; complete blood count; skull x rays; pituitary and adrenal imaging

PRIMARY NURSING DIAGNOSIS

Fluid volume deficit related to water loss and insufficient ability to reabsorb water

OUTCOMES. Fluid balance; Circulation status; Cardiac pump effectiveness; Hydration; Nutritional status

INTERVENTIONS. Fluid/electrolyte management; Hypoglycemia management; Intravenous therapy; Fluid monitoring; Medication administration

◻ PLANNING AND IMPLEMENTATION

Collaborative

Pharmacologic treatment centers on fluid and electrolyte replacement and hormonal supplements (see Pharmacologic Highlights box). Fluid replacement with dextrose- and sodium-containing solutions allows for correction of hypovolemia and hypoglycemia. As much as 5 L or more of fluid may be needed to maintain an adequate blood pressure, circulation, and urine output and to replace the fluid deficit.

PHARMACOLOGIC HIGHLIGHTS

Medication or Drug Class	Dosage	Description	Rationale
Dexamethasone	4 mg IV	Corticosteroid	Substitution therapy in deficiency state
Hydrocortisone sodium succinate	100 mg IV q 6–8 hours	Corticosteroid	Substitution therapy in deficiency state

Other Therapies: Cortisone acetate (Cortone); fludrocortisone acetate (Florinef)

Independent

During the initial hours of managing a patient with acute adrenal crisis, the first priority is to maintain airway, breathing, and circulation. Patients who receive large amounts of room-temperature fluids are at risk for hypothermia. Keep the temperature of the room warm and the bed linens dry. If possible, keep the patient fully covered. During massive fluid replacement, administer warmed (body-temperature) fluids if possible.

Teach the patient on corticosteroids about the medication and the need to continue to take it until the physician tapers the dose and then finally discontinues it. Explain the symptoms of adrenal crisis to any patient who is undergoing anticoagulant therapy. Explain the effects of stress on the disease and the need for adjustment of medications during times of stress.

Patients with altered tissue perfusion require frequent skin care. If the patient is immobile, perform active and passive range-of-motion exercises at least every 8 hours. Encourage coughing and deep breathing to limit the complications from immobility. Provide small, frequent meals and make referrals to the dietitian early in the hospitalization.

DOCUMENTATION GUIDELINES

- Physical findings: Vital signs; pulmonary artery catheter pressure readings; monitoring of airway, breathing, circulation; urine output; mental status
- Important changes in laboratory values: Plasma cortisol, serum glucose, serum sodium and potassium, pH, oxygen saturation

- Presence of complications: Infection, cardiac dysrhythmias, fluid and electrolyte imbalance, weight loss
- Response to therapy: Daily weights, appetite, level of hydration

DISCHARGE AND HOME HEALTHCARE GUIDELINES

PATIENT TEACHING. Teach the patient and significant others about the disease and the factors that aggravate it. Provide suggestions about rest and activity and stress reduction. Explain the signs and symptoms that may lead to crisis.

PREVENTION. Identify the stressors and the need to increase medication during times of stress. Teach the patient and family when the physician needs to be notified.

MEDICATIONS. Teach the patient the name, dosage, action, and side effects of drugs and the need to continue using them for life. Provide written instruction about medications and follow up physician's appointments.

Acute Alcohol Intoxication

DRG Category: 434
Mean LOS: 4.9 days
Description: MEDICAL: Alcohol/Drug Abuse or Dependence, Detoxification, or Other Symptoms Treated with CC

Acute alcohol intoxication occurs when a person consumes large quantities of alcohol. In many states, legal intoxication is 100 mg/dL, or 0.1 g/dL. Acute alcohol intoxication leads to complex physiologic interactions. Alcohol is a primary and continuous depressant of the central nervous system (CNS). The patient may seem stimulated initially because alcohol depresses inhibitory control mechanisms. Effects on the CNS include loss of memory, concentration, insight, and motor control. Advanced intoxication can produce general anesthesia, while chronic intoxication may lead to brain damage, memory loss, sleep disturbances, and psychoses. Respiratory effects also include apnea, decreased diaphragmatic excursion, diminished respiratory drive, impaired glottal reflexes, and vascular shunts in lung tissue. The risk of aspiration and pulmonary infection increases while respiratory depression and apnea occur.

The cardiovascular system becomes depressed, leading to depression of the vasomotor center in the brain and to hypotension. Conversely, in some individuals intoxication causes the release of catecholamines from adrenal glands, which leads to hypertension. Intoxication depresses leukocyte movement into areas of inflammation, depresses platelet function, and leads to fibrinogen and clotting factor deficiency, thrombocytopenia, and decreased platelet function.

The effects on the gastrointestinal (GI) system include stimulation of gastric secretions, mucosal irritation, cessation of motor function of the gut, and delayed absorption. Pylorospasm and vomiting may occur.

CAUSES

Alcohol intoxication occurs when a person ingests alcohol at a rate faster than his or her body can metabolize it. Alcohol is metabolized at a rate of approximately

15 g/hour. One standard drink (12 ounces of beer or 1 ounce of whiskey) provides about 14 g of alcohol. When a person drinks faster than the body metabolizes alcohol, he or she becomes intoxicated when blood alcohol levels reach 100 mg/dL, although the physiologic effects occur at levels as low as 40 mg/dL.

GENDER AND LIFE SPAN CONSIDERATIONS

Acute alcohol intoxication can affect people of any age, gender, race, or socioeconomic background. Alcohol use should be considered when a patient is seen for trauma, acute abdominal pain, cardiac dysrhythmias, cardiomyopathy, encephalopathy, coma, seizures, pancreatitis, sepsis, anxiety, delirium, depression, or suicide attempt.

TEENAGERS AND YOUNG ADULTS. The use of alcohol is seen as a part of growing up for many individuals. Binge drinking is common and dangerous. The combination of alcohol and potentially risky activities, such as driving or sex, is a source of high morbidity and mortality for teens.

PREGNANT WOMEN. Alcohol is a potent teratogen. Binge drinking and moderate to heavy drinking have been associated with many fetal abnormalities. There is no currently known safe drinking level during pregnancy.

ELDERLY. Loss of friends and family, loss of income, decreased mobility, and chronic illness or pain may increase isolation and loneliness and lead to an increased use of alcohol by the elderly.

☐ ASSESSMENT

HISTORY. Ask the patient how much alcohol he or she consumed and over what period of time. Elicit a history of past patterns of alcohol consumption. You may need to consult other sources, such as family or friends, to obtain accurate information when the patient is acutely intoxicated on admission.

PHYSICAL EXAMINATION. The intoxicated individual needs to have a careful neurologic, respiratory, and cardiovascular evaluation. In life-threatening situations, conduct a brief survey to identify serious problems and begin stabilization. Begin with assessment of the airway, breathing, and circulation (the ABCs).

RESPIRATORY. Assess the patency of the patient's airway. Check the patient's respiratory rate and rhythm, and listen to the breath sounds. Monitor the patient carefully for apnea throughout the period of intoxication. Determine the adequacy of the patient's breathing.

CARDIOVASCULAR. Check the strength and regularity of the patient's peripheral pulses. Take the patient's blood pressure to ascertain if there are any orthostatic changes. Check the patient's heart rate, rhythm, and heart sounds. Inspect for jugular distension, and assess the patient's skin color, temperature, and capillary refill.

NEUROLOGIC. Assess the patient's level of consciousness. The brief mental status examination includes general appearance and behavior, levels of consciousness and orientation, emotional status, attention level, language and speech, and memory. Conduct an examination of the cranial nerves. Assess the patient's deep tendon and stretch reflexes. Perform a sensory examination by assessing the patient's response to painful stimuli, and check for autonomic evidence of sympathetic stimulation. Check the adequacy of the gag reflex.

PSYCHOSOCIAL. Individuals admitted to the hospital during episodes of acute alcohol intoxication need both a thorough investigation of the physiologic responses and a careful assessment of their lifestyle, attitudes, and stressors. Binge drinkers and dependent drinkers have complex psychosocial needs. Identify the patient's support systems (family and friends), and assess the effect of those systems on the patient's health maintenance.

DIAGNOSTIC HIGHLIGHTS

Test	Normal Result	Abnormality with Condition	Explanation
Blood alcohol concentration	Negative (< 10 mg/ dL or 0.01 g/dL)	Positive (> 10 mg/ dL or 0.01 g/dL)	Legal intoxication is most states is 80–100 mg/dL
Liver function gamma-glutamyl transpeptidase (GGT)	4–25 units (females); 7–40 units (males)	Elevated above normal	Evidence of liver disease or alcoholism
Aspartate aminotransferase (AST)	8–20 units/L	Elevated above normal	Evidence of liver disease or alcoholism
Alanine aminotransferase (ALT)	8–10 units/L	Elevated above normal	Evidence of liver disease or alcoholism

Other Tests: Blood glucose levels: Elevated or low blood glucose levels without a family history of diabetes mellitus indicate chronic alcohol use.

PRIMARY NURSING DIAGNOSIS

Altered thought processes related to CNS depression

OUTCOMES. Cognitive orientation; Cognitive ability; Electrolyte and acid-base balance; Fluid balance; Neurologic status; Safety behavior

INTERVENTIONS. Airway management; Aspiration precautions; Behavior management; Delusion management; Environmental management; Surveillance

☐ PLANNING AND IMPLEMENTATION

Collaborative

MEDICAL. Electrolyte replacement, especially magnesium and potassium, may be necessary. Dehydration is a common problem, and adequate fluid replacement is important. Intravenous fluids may be necessary. During periods of acute intoxication, use care in administering medications that potentiate the effects of alcohol, such as sedatives and analgesics. Calculate when the alcohol will be fully metabolized and out of the patient's system by dividing the blood alcohol level on admission by 20 mg/dL. The result is the number of hours the patient needs to metabolize the alcohol fully.

Anticipate withdrawal syndrome with any intoxicated patient. Formal withdrawal assessment instruments are available to help guide the use of benzodiazepines. If the patient is a dependent drinker, an alcohol referral to social service, psychiatric consultation service, or a clinical nurse specialist is important.

PHARMACOLOGIC HIGHLIGHTS

Medication or Drug Class	Dosage	Description	Rationale
Thiamine	100 mg IV	Vitamin supplement	Counters effects of nutritional deficiencies
Benzodiazepines	Varies by drug	Antianxiety	Manage alcohol withdrawal

Independent

Create a safe environment to reduce the risk of injury. Reorient the patient frequently to people and the environment as the level of intoxication changes. Create a calm, nonjudgmental atmosphere to reduce anxiety and agitation.

Alcoholic withdrawal can occur as early as 48 hours after the blood alcohol level has returned to normal or, more unusually, as long as 2 weeks later. Monitor for early signs such as agitation, restlessness, and confusion. Keep the room dark and decrease environmental stimulation. Avoid using the intercom. Remain with the patient as much as possible. Encourage the patient to take fluids to diminish the effects of dehydration. Avoid using restraints unless the patient is at risk for injuring himself or herself or others.

As the patient recovers, perform a complete nutritional assessment with a dietary consultation if appropriate.

DOCUMENTATION GUIDELINES

- Physical findings: Initial neurologic, respiratory, and cardiovascular function, and ongoing monitoring of these systems
- Alcohol history, assessment, and interventions (Note that history may need to be kept confidential)
- Response to referral to substance abuse screening and diagnosis if appropriate
- Symptoms of withdrawal and response to treatment
- Response to nutrition counseling

DISCHARGE AND HOME HEALTHCARE GUIDELINES

PREVENTION. Focus teaching on the problems associated with intoxication and strategies to avoid further intoxication. Encourage the patient to adapt proper nutrition.

REFERRALS. Refer the patient to appropriate substance abuse support groups such as Alcoholics Anonymous (AA).

Acute Respiratory Distress Syndrome

DRG Category: 087
Mean LOS: 5.5 days
Description: MEDICAL: Pulmonary Edema and Respiratory Failure
DRG Category: 475
Mean LOS: 9.5 days
Description: MEDICAL: Respiratory System Diagnosis with Ventilator Support
DRG Category: 483
Mean LOS: 41.9 days
Description: SURGICAL: Tracheostomy Except for Face, Mouth, and Neck Diagnoses

The term adult respiratory distress syndrome (ARDS) was first coined by Ashbaugh and Petty in 1971. Previously, terms such as stiff lung, wet lung, shock lung, adult hyaline-membrane disease, and other terms were used to describe this syndrome. In 1992 the American-European Consensus Conference on ARDS recommended changing the name back to what Ashbaugh and Petty originally named it in 1967, acute respiratory distress syndrome, because this condition affects children, teenagers, and adults.

ARDS is defined as noncardiogenic pulmonary edema that occurs despite low to normal pressures in the pulmonary capillaries. Many theories and hypotheses are currently under investigation. Patients with ARDS are characterized as having high-permeability pulmonary edema (HPPE) in contrast to cardiogenic pulmonary edema. In ARDS, the alveolar-capillary membrane is damaged, and both fluid and protein leak into the interstitial space and alveoli. Recent research has focused on possible mediators of the membrane damage, such as neutrophils, tumor necrosis factor (TNF), bacterial toxins, and oxygen free radicals, among others.

As ARDS progresses, patients exhibit decreased lung volumes and markedly decreased lung compliance. Type II pneumocytes, the cells responsible for surfactant production, are damaged. This deficiency is thought to be partly responsible for the alveolar collapse and the decrease in lung volumes that occur. Refractory hypoxemia occurs as the lungs are perfused but not ventilated (a condition called capillary shunting) due to the damage to the alveoli. As ARDS progresses, respiratory failure and cardiopulmonary arrest can develop.

CAUSES

Various conditions can predispose a patient to ARDS, but they usually represent a sudden, catastrophic situation. These conditions can be classified into two categories: direct lung injury and indirect lung injury. Direct injury occurs from gastric aspiration, near drowning, chemical inhalation, and oxygen toxicity. Indirect injury occurs from mediators released during sepsis, multiple trauma, thermal injury, hypoperfusion or hemorrhagic shock, disseminated intravascular coagulation, drug overdose, and massive blood transfusions. The most common risk factor for ARDS is sepsis from an abdominal source. Approximately 150,000 new cases of ARDS occur each year. Mortality rates vary and have been estimated to be between 50% and 70%.

GENDER AND LIFE SPAN CONSIDERATIONS

ARDS can occur equally across genders and at any age, including during child-hood, to those who have been subjected to severe physiologic stresses such as sepsis, burns, or trauma.

◻ ASSESSMENT

HISTORY AND PHYSICAL EXAMINATION. The patient with ARDS appears in acute res-piratory distress with a marked increase in the work of breathing that may lead to nasal flaring, the use of accessory muscles to breathe, and profound di-aphoresis. The respiratory rate may be more than 30 to 40 breaths per minute. If ARDS has progressed, the patient may have a dusky appearance with cyanosis around the lips and nail beds, or the patient may be very pale. Hy-poxemia usually leads to restlessness, confusion, agitation, and even combat-ive behavior.

Palpation of the peripheral pulses reveals rapid, sometimes thready, pulses. Blood pressure may be normal or elevated initially, then decreased in the later stages. Auscultation of the lungs differs, depending on the stage of ARDS. In the early stage, the lungs have decreased breath sounds. In the mid-dle stages of ARDS, the patient may have basilar crackles or even coarse crack-les. In the late stage of ARDS, if the disease has been left untreated, the patient may have bronchial breath sounds or little gas exchange with no breath sounds. If airway and breathing are not maintained, the patient becomes fa-tigued and apneic. When the patient is intubated and mechanically ventilated, the lungs may sound extremely congested, with wheezes and coarse crackles throughout.

Diagnosis involves excluding other causes of acute respiratory failure. A con-sensus conference has defined ARDS as having the following features: acute bi-lateral lung infiltrates; a ratio of PaO_2 to inspired oxygen concentration (FiO_2) of less than 200; no evidence of heart failure or volume overload.

PSYCHOSOCIAL. Patients may exhibit anxiety and fear because of hypoxemia and the real threat of death. Feelings of social isolation and powerlessness can occur as the patient is placed on mechanical ventilation and is unable to verbalize.

DIAGNOSTIC HIGHLIGHTS

General Comments: The diagnosis of ARDS can be controversial and is one of exclusion. There are no specific markers that identify alveolar-capillary mem-brane damage. Early in ARDS, the pH is elevated and the $PaCO_2$ is decreased be-cause of hyperventilation. In the later stages, the $PaCO_2$ is elevated and the pH is decreased. Other supporting tests include pulmonary function tests, pulse oximetry, and pulmonary capillary wedge pressure.

Test	Normal Result	Abnormality with Condition	Explanation
Chest x ray	Clear lung fields	Diffuse infiltrates without cardiomeg-aly or pulmonary vascular redistribu-tion	Findings reflect non-cardiogenic pulmonary edema

Arterial blood gases	Pao$_2$ 80–100 mm Hg; Paco$_2$ 35–45 mm Hg; Sao$_2$ > 95%	Pao$_2$ < 80 mm Hg; Paco$_2$ varies; Sao$_2$ < 95%	Poor gas exchange leads to hypoxemia and, as respiratory failure progresses, to hypercapnea

PRIMARY NURSING DIAGNOSIS

Impaired gas exchange related to increased alveolar-capillary permeability, interstitial edema, and decreased lung compliance

OUTCOMES. Respiratory status: Gas exchange; Respiratory status: Ventilation; Comfort level; Anxiety control

INTERVENTIONS. Airway insertion and stabilization; Airway management; Respiratory monitoring; Oxygen therapy; Mechanical ventilation; Anxiety reduction

☐ PLANNING AND IMPLEMENTATION

Collaborative

MECHANICAL VENTILATION. The treatment for ARDS is directed toward the underlying cause and maintaining oxygenation. To this end almost all patients with ARDS require endotracheal intubation and mechanical ventilation with a variety of positive-pressure modes. Common methods for mechanical ventilation include pressure-controlled ventilation with an inverse inspiratory-expiratory ratio. This mode prolongs aspiration and controls the amount of pressure in each breath to stabilize the alveoli and to re-establish the functional residual capacity (FRC) to normal levels. If possible, the physician attempts to limit the fraction of inspired oxygen (Fio) to less than 0.50 (50%) to limit complications from oxygen. Positive end–expiratory pressure (PEEP) is often added to the ventilator settings to increase the FRC and to augment gas exchange.

PHARMACOLOGIC HIGHLIGHTS

General Comments: Use of genetically engineered surfactant has been studied in ARDS but has not demonstrated the success that has occurred in premature infants with surfactant deficiency. Corticosteroids have been widely used in ARDS, yet studies have not demonstrated any improvement in patient outcomes and remain controversial. If the patient is difficult to ventilate, he or she may receive skeletal muscle relaxants such as vecuronium (Norcuron), which are neuromuscular blocking agents that paralyze the patient's skeletal muscles. These medications are used only when the patient's gas exchange is so poor as to threaten his or her life. Neuromuscular blocking agents paralyze the patient without affecting mental status, so the patient requires sedation to counteract the accompanying fear and anxiety that occur when the patient is unable to move.

Medication or Drug Class	Dosage	Description	Rationale
Nitric oxide	Inhalation route; dosage varied	Pulmonary vascular vasodilator	Decreases pulmonary vascular resistance with increased perfusion to ventilated areas

Independent

To augment gas exchange, the patient needs endotracheal suctioning periodically. Prior to suctioning, hyperventilate and hyperoxygenate the patient to prevent the ill effects of suctioning, such as cardiac dysrhythmias or hypotension. Turn the patient as often as possible, even every hour, to increase ventilation and perfusion to all areas of the lung. If the patient has particularly poor gas exchange, consider a rocking bed that constantly changes the patient's position. If the patient's condition allows, even if the patient is intubated and on a ventilator, get the patient out of bed for brief periods. Evaluate the patient's condition to determine if soft restraints are appropriate. Although restraints are frustrating for the patient, they may be necessary to reduce the risk of self-extubation.

If the patient requires medications for skeletal muscle paralysis, provide complete care. Use artificial tears to moisten the patient's eyes because the patient loses the blink reflex. Provide passive range-of-motion exercises every 8 hours to prevent contractures. Reposition the patient at least every 2 hours for comfort and adequate gas exchange, and to prevent skin breakdown. Provide complete hygiene, including mouth care as needed. Assist the patient to conserve oxygen and limit oxygen consumption by spacing all activities, limiting interruptions to enhance rest, and providing a quiet environment.

The patient and family may be fearful and anxious. Acknowledge their fear without providing false reassurance. Explain the critical care environment and technology but emphasize the importance of the patient's humanness over and above the technology. Maintain open communication among all involved. Answer all questions and provide methods for the patient and family to communicate, such as a magic slate or point board.

DOCUMENTATION GUIDELINES

- Respiratory status of the patient: respiratory rate, breath sounds, and the use of accessory muscles; arterial blood gas (ABG) levels; pulse oximeter and chest x ray results
- Response to treatment, mechanical ventilation, immobility, and bed rest
- Presence of any complications (depends on the precipitating condition leading to ARDS)

DISCHARGE AND HOME HEALTHCARE GUIDELINES

PREVENTION. Prompt attention for any infections may decrease the incidence of sepsis, which can lead to ARDS.

COMPLICATIONS. If patients survive ARDS, few residual effects are seen. Complications are directed to any other conditions the patient may have.

Adrenal Insufficiency (Addison's Disease)

DRG Category: 300
Mean LOS: 6.3 days
Description: MEDICAL: Endocrine Disorders with CC

Addison's disease, primary adrenal insufficiency, occurs rarely. The adrenal glands consist of the medulla and the cortex. The medulla is responsible for the secretion of the catecholamines epinephrine and norepinephrine; the cortex is responsible for the secretion of glucocorticoids, mineralocorticoids, and androgen. The principal glucocorticoid, cortisol, helps regulate blood pressure, metabolism, anti-inflammatory response, and emotional behavior. The principal mineralocorticoid, aldosterone, is important for regulating sodium levels. Adrenal insufficiency is characterized by the decreased production of cortisol, aldosterone, and androgen. Cortisol deficiency causes altered metabolism, decreased stress tolerance, and emotional lability. Aldosterone deficiency causes urinary loss of sodium, chloride, and water, resulting in dehydration and electrolyte imbalances. Androgen deficiency leads to the loss of secondary sex characteristics.

CAUSES

Idiopathic adrenal atrophy is the most common cause of adrenal insufficiency. It is not known exactly why this occurs, but it is believed to be related to an autoimmune response that results in the slow destruction of adrenal tissue. Tuberculosis, histoplasmosis, acquired immunodeficiency syndrome (AIDS), and hemorrhage into the adrenal glands have all been associated with destruction of the adrenal glands. All patients with adrenal insufficiency or steroid-dependent disorders are at risk for an acute adrenal crisis. Secondary adrenal failure can also occur with adrenocorticotropic hormone (ACTH) deficiency caused by disorders of the pituitary or hypothalamus or suppression because of glucocorticoid therapy.

GENDER AND LIFE SPAN CONSIDERATIONS

Addison's disease affects males and females of all ages equally and can occur at any age.

◻ ASSESSMENT

HISTORY. Determine if the patient has a history of recent infection, steroid use, or adrenal or pituitary surgery. Establish a history of poor tolerance for stress, weakness, fatigue, and activity intolerance. Ask if the patient has experienced anorexia, nausea, vomiting, or diarrhea as a result of altered metabolism. Elicit a history of craving for salt or an intolerance to cold. Determine presence of altered menses in females and impotence in males.

PHYSICAL EXAMINATION. Assess the patient for signs of dehydration such as tachycardia, altered level of consciousness, dry skin with poor turgor, dry mucous membranes, weight loss, and weak peripheral pulses. Check for postural hypotension—that is, a drop in systolic blood pressure greater than 15 mm Hg when the patient is moved from a lying to a sitting or standing position.

Inspect the skin for pigmentation changes caused by an altered regulation of melanin, noting if surgical scars, skin folds, and genitalia show a characteristic bronze color. Inspect the patient's gums and oral mucous membranes to see if they are bluish-black. Take the patient's temperature to see if it is subnormal. Note any loss of axillary and pubic hair that could be caused by decreased androgen levels.

PSYCHOSOCIAL. Because an acute adrenal crisis may be precipitated by emotional stress, periodic psychosocial assessments are necessary for patients with adrenal insufficiency. Patients with an adrenal insufficiency frequently complain of weakness and fatigue, which are also characteristic of an emotional problem. However, weakness and fatigue of an emotional origin seem to have a pattern of being worse in the morning and lessening throughout the day, while the weakness and fatigue of adrenal insufficiency seem to be precipitated by activity and lessen with rest. Patients with adrenal insufficiency may show signs of depression and irritability from decreased cortisol levels.

DIAGNOSTIC HIGHLIGHTS

General Comments: To determine if a cortisol deficit exists, a plasma cortisol level is drawn in the morning; less than 10 µg/dL suggests adrenal insufficiency.

Test	Normal Result	Abnormality with Condition	Explanation
Serum cortisol level	6–8 AM, 5–23 µg/dL	Decreased	Determines the ability of the adrenal gland to produce glucocorticoids
Serum electrolytes and chemistries	Sodium 136–145 mEq/L; potassium 3.5–5.1 mEq/L; blood urea nitrogen 5–20 mg/dL; glucose 70–105 mg/dL	Hyponatremia; hyperkalemia; azotemia; hypoglycemia	Values reflect sodium loss from a deficit in mineralocortocoids with loss of fluids, and poor glucose control because of decreased gluconeogenesis

Other Tests: Adrenocorticotropin hormone (ACTH) stimulation test; metyrapone suppression test; urine 17-hydroxycorticosteroids (17-OHCS) and 17-ketosteroids (17-KS); electrocardiogram (ECG); and computed tomography

PRIMARY NURSING DIAGNOSIS

Altered nutrition: Less than body requirements related to anorexia, vomiting, and nausea

OUTCOMES. Fluid balance; Hydration; Nutritional status: Food and fluid intake; Nutritional status: Energy

INTERVENTIONS. Fluid/electrolyte management; Hypoglycemia management; Nutritional management; Nutritional counseling

☐ PLANNING AND IMPLEMENTATION

Collaborative

Collaborative treatment of adrenal insufficiency focuses on restoring fluid, electrolyte, and hormone balance. The fluid used for adrenal insufficiency will most likely be 5% dextrose in 0.9% sodium chloride to replace fluid volume and serum sodium. Patients with adrenal insufficiency will require lifelong replacement steroid therapy. Patients with diabetes mellitus will require insulin adjustments for elevated serum glucose levels.

PHARMACOLOGIC HIGHLIGHTS

General Comments: Fludrocortisone promotes kidney reabsorption of sodium and the excretion of potassium. Overtreatment can result in fluid retention and possibly congestive heart failure; therefore, monitor serum potassium and sodium levels frequently during fludrocortisone administration.

Medication or Drug Class	Dosage	Description	Rationale
Glucocorticoids such as dexamethasone and prednisone	Varies by drug	Corticosteroid	Replacement therapy in deficiency state
Fludrocortisone	0.1 mg po qid	Mineralocorticoid	Replacement therapy in deficiency state

Independent

Because of the negative effect of physical and emotional stress on the patient with adrenal insufficiency, promote strategies that reduce stress. Teach the patient to rest between activities to conserve energy and to wear warm clothing to increase comfort and limit heat loss. To limit the risk of infection, encourage the patient to use good hand-washing techniques and to limit exposure to people with infections. To prevent complications, teach the patient to avoid using lotions that contain alcohol to prevent skin dryness and breakdown and to eat a nutritious diet that has adequate proteins, fats, and carbohydrates to maintain sodium and potassium balance.

Finally, the prospect of a chronic disease and the need to avoid stress may lead patients to impaired social interaction and ineffective coping. Discuss with the patient the presence of support systems and coping patterns. Provide emotional support by encouraging the patient to verbalize feelings about an altered body image and anxieties about the disease process. Incorporate the patient's unique positive characteristics and strengths into the care plan. Encourage the patient to interact with family and significant others. Before discharge, refer patients who exhibit disabling behaviors to therapists, self-help groups, or crisis intervention centers.

DOCUMENTATION GUIDELINES

- Physical findings: Cardiovascular status, including blood pressure and heart rate; tissue perfusion status, including level of consciousness, skin tempera-

ture, peripheral pulses, and urine output; fluid volume status, including neck vein assessment, daily weights, and fluid input and output
- Laboratory findings: Blood levels of potassium, sodium, hematocrit, and blood urea nitrogen (BUN)

DISCHARGE AND HOME HEALTHCARE GUIDELINES

PREVENTION. To prevent acute adrenal crisis, teach patients how to avoid stress. Emphasize the need to take medications as prescribed and to contact the physician if the patient becomes stressed or unable to take medications.

MEDICATIONS. Be sure the patient understands the reason for steroids prescribed. (See Box 2 for full explanation.)

RESOURCES. Referrals may be necessary to identify potential physical and emotional problems. Notify the hospital's social service department before patient discharge if you have identified obvious environmental stressors. Initiate home health nursing to assure compliance with medical therapy and early detection of complications. If you identify emotional problems, refer the patient to therapists or self-help groups.

BOX 2   PATIENT TEACHING FOR CORTICOSTEROIDS

- Emphasize the lifetime nature of taking corticosteroids.
- Provide name, dosage, and action of the prescribed medication.
- Explain the common side effects of weight gain, swelling around the face and eyes, insomnia, bruising, gastric distress, gastric bleeding, and petechiae.
- Advise the patient to take the medication with meals to avoid gastric irritation and to take the medication at the time of day prescribed, usually in the morning.
- Suggest the patient weigh self daily, at the same time each day, and call the healthcare provider if weight changes by ±5 pounds.
- Emphasize that the patient should always take the medication. Not taking it can cause life-threatening complications. Tell patient to call the healthcare provider if he or she is unable to take medication for more than 24 hours.
- Explain that periods of stress require more medication. Tell the patient to call the healthcare provider for changes in dose if he or she experiences extra physical or emotional stress. Illness and temperature extremes are considered stressors.
- Explain preventative measures. Tell the patient that, to prevent getting ill, he or she should avoid being in groups with people who are ill and environments where temperatures change from very hot to very cold.
- Teach the patient to recognize signs of undermedication: weakness, fatigue, and dizziness. Emphasize the need to report underdosing to the healthcare provider.
- Teach the patient to avoid dizziness by moving from a sitting to a standing position slowly. Urge the patient to always wear a medical alert necklace or bracelet to inform healthcare professionals of the diagnosis.

Air Embolism

DRG Category: 078
Mean LOS: 7.8 days
Description: MEDICAL: Pulmonary Embolism

An air embolism is an obstruction in a vein or artery caused by a bubble of gas. Air enters the circulatory system when the pressure gradient favors movement of air or gas from the environment into the blood. A venous air embolism is the most common form of air embolism. It occurs when air enters the venous circulation, passes through the right side of the heart, and then proceeds to the lungs. In relatively small amounts, the lungs can filter the air; it is absorbed without complications. When large amounts of air (80 to 100 mL) are introduced into the body, however, the lungs no longer have the capacity to filter the air, and the patient has serious or even lethal complications. One of the most serious complications is when the large air bubble blocks the outflow of blood from the right ventricle into the lungs, preventing the blood from moving forward. The patient develops cardiogenic shock because of insufficient cardiac output. Experts have found that the risk from air embolism increases as both the volume and the speed of air injection increase.

An arterial embolism occurs when air gains entry into the pulmonary venous circulation and then passes through the heart and into the systemic arterial circulation. An arterial embolism can also form in the patient who has a venous embolism and a right-to-left shunt (often caused by a septal defect in the heart) so that the air bubble moves into the left ventricle without passing through the lungs. Pulmonary capillary shunts can produce the same effect. The arterial embolism may cause serious or even lethal complications in the brain and heart. Scientists have found that as little as 0.05 mL of air in the coronary arteries can cause death.

CAUSES

The two major causes of air embolism are iatrogenic and environmental. Iatrogenic complications are those that occur as a result of a diagnostic or therapeutic procedure. Situations where iatrogenic injury is a possibility include insertion, maintenance, or removal of the central line. The risk is highest during catheter insertion because the large-bore needle, which is in the vein, is at the hub while the catheter is threaded into the vein. Air can be pulled into the circulation whenever the catheter is disconnected for a tubing change or the catheter-tubing system is accidentally disconnected or broken. When the catheter is removed, air can also enter the fibrin tract that was caused by the catheter during the brief period between removal and sealing of the tract. Other procedures that can lead to air embolism are cardiac catheterization, coronary arteriography, transcutaneous angioplasty, embolectomy, and hemodialysis. Some surgical procedures also place the patient at particular risk, including orthopedic, urologic, gynecologic, open heart, and brain surgery, particularly when the procedure is performed with the patient in an upright position. Conditions such as multiple trauma, placenta previa, and pneumoperitoneum have also been associated with air embolism.

Environmental causes occur when a person is exposed to atmospheric pressures that are markedly different from atmospheric pressure at sea level. Two such examples are deep-sea diving (scuba diving) and high-altitude flying.

Excessive pressures force nitrogen, which is not absorbable, into body tissues and the circulation. Nitrogen accumulates in the extracellular spaces, forms bubbles, and enters into the bloodstream as emboli.

GENDER AND LIFE SPAN CONSIDERATIONS

An air embolism can occur with either gender and at any age if the individual is placed at risk for either an iatrogenic or an environmental cause.

□ ASSESSMENT

HISTORY. The patient may have been scuba diving or flying at the onset of symptoms. Usually patients who develop an iatrogenic air embolism are under the care of the healthcare team, who assesses the signs and symptoms of air embolism as a complication of treatment. Some patients have a gasp or cough when the initial infusion of air moves into the pulmonary circulation. Suspect an air embolism immediately when a patient becomes symptomatic following insertion, maintenance, or removal of a central access catheter. Patients suddenly become dyspneic, dizzy, nauseated, confused, and anxious, and they may complain of substernal chest pain. Some patients describe the feeling of "impending doom."

PHYSICAL EXAMINATION. On inspection, the patient may appear in acute distress with cyanosis, jugular neck vein distension, or even seizures and unresponsiveness. Some reports explain that more than 40% of patients with an air embolism have central nervous system effects such as altered mental status or coma. When auscultating the patient's heart, listen for a "mill-wheel murmur" produced by air bubbles in the right ventricle and heard throughout the cardiac cycle. The murmur may be loud enough to be heard without a stethoscope but is only temporarily audible and is usually a late sign. More common than the mill-wheel murmur is a harsh systolic murmur or normal heart sounds. Most patients have a rapid apical pulse and low blood pressure. You may also hear wheezing from acute bronchospasm. The patient may have increased central venous pressure, pulmonary artery pressures, increased systemic vascular resistance, and decreased cardiac output.

PSYCHOSOCIAL. Most patients respond with fear, confusion, and anxiety. The family or significant others are understandably upset as well. Evaluate the patient's and family's ability to cope with the crisis and provide the appropriate support.

DIAGNOSTIC HIGHLIGHTS

Test	Normal Result	Abnormality with Condition	Explanation
Arterial blood gases	PaO_2 80–100 mm Hg; $PaCO_2$ 35–45 mm Hg; $SaO_2 > 95\%$	$PaO_2 < 80$ mm Hg; $PaCO_2$ varies; $SaO_2 < 95\%$	Poor gas exchange leads to hypoxemia and hypercapnea from dead-space ventilations

Other Tests: Supporting tests include electrocardiogram (ECG) and chest x ray.

PRIMARY NURSING DIAGNOSIS

Decreased cardiac output related to blocked left ventricular filling

OUTCOMES. Cardiac pump effectiveness; Circulation status; Tissue perfusion: Cerebral, Peripheral, Cardiac

INTERVENTIONS. Cardiac care; Circulatory care; Shock management; Hemodynamic regulation

□ PLANNING AND IMPLEMENTATION

Collaborative

PREVENTION. Several strategies can help prevent development of air embolism. First, maintain the patient's level of hydration because dehydration predisposes the patient to decreased venous pressures. Second, some clinicians recommend that you position the patient in Trendelenburg's position during central line insertion because the position increases central venous pressure. Third, instruct the patient to perform Valsalva's maneuver on exhalation during central line insertion or removal to increase intrathoracic pressure and thereby to increase central venous pressure.

Prime all tubings with intravenous fluid prior to connecting the system to the catheter. Immediately apply an occlusive pressure dressing after catheter removal, and maintain the site with a occlusive dressing for at least 24 hours. To prevent air embolism during surgical procedures, the surgeon floods the surgical field with liquid in some situations so that liquid rather than air enters the circulation.

TREATMENT. If an air embolus occurs, the first efforts are focused on preventing more air from entering the circulation. Place the patient on 100% oxygen immediately to facilitate the washout of nitrogen from the bubble of atmospheric gas. Place the patient in the left lateral decubitus position. This position allows the obstructing air bubble in the pulmonary outflow tract to float toward the apex of the right ventricle, which relieves the obstruction. Use Trendelenburg's position to relieve the obstruction caused by air bubbles. Other suggested strategies are to aspirate the air from the right atrium, to use closed-chest cardiac compressions, and to administer fluids to maintain vascular volume. Hyperbaric oxygen therapy may improve the patient's condition as well: This therapy increases nitrogen washout in the air bubble, thereby reducing the bubble's size and the absorption of air. Note that if the patient has to be transferred to a hyperbaric facility, the decrease in atmospheric pressure that occurs at high altitudes during fixed-wing or helicopter transport may worsen the patient's condition because of bubble enlargement or "bubble explosion." Ground transport or transport in a low-flying helicopter is recommended, along with administering 100% oxygen and adequate hydration during transport.

Independent

If the patient suddenly develops the symptoms of an air embolism, place the patient on the left side with the head of the bed down to allow the air to float out of the outflow track. Notify the physician immediately, and position the resuscitation cart in close proximity. Initiate 100% oxygen via a nonrebreather mask immediately before the physician arrives, according to unit policy. Be prepared for a sudden deterioration in cardiopulmonary status and potential for cardiac arrest.

The patient and family need a great deal of support. Remain in the patient's room at all times, and if the patient finds touch reassuring, hold the patient's hand. Provide an ongoing summary of the patient's condition to the family. Expect the patient to be extremely frightened and the family to be anxious or even angry. Ask the chaplain, clinical nurse specialist, nursing supervisor, or social worker to remain with the family during the period of crisis.

DOCUMENTATION GUIDELINES

- Physical findings: Changes in vital signs, cardiopulmonary assessment, skin color, capillary blanch, level of activity, changes in level of consciousness
- Pain: Location, duration, precipitating factors, response to interventions
- Responses to interventions: Positioning, oxygen, hyperbaric oxygen, evacuation of air, cardiopulmonary resuscitation
- Development of complications: Seizures, cardiac arrest, severe anxiety, ineffective patient or family coping

DISCHARGE AND HOME HEALTHCARE GUIDELINES

PREVENTION. Instruct the patient to report any signs of complications. Make sure that the patient and family are aware of the next follow-up visit with the healthcare provider. If the patient is being discharged with central intravenous access, make sure that the caregiver understands the risk of air embolism and can describe all preventive strategies to limit the risk of air embolism.

Alcohol Withdrawal

DRG Category: 434
Mean LOS: 4.9 days
Description: MEDICAL: Alcohol or Drug Abuse or Dependence, Detoxification, or Other Symptoms Treated with CC

Withdrawal is a pattern of physiologic responses to the discontinuation of a drug. Although most central nervous system (CNS) depressants produce similar responses, alcohol is the only one in which withdrawal is life threatening, with a mortality rate of about 25%. Withdrawal symptoms should be anticipated with any patients who have been drinking the alcohol equivalent of a six-pack of beer on a daily basis for a period of 6 months; smaller patients who have drunk less may exhibit the same symptoms. Alcohol withdrawal involves CNS excitation, respiratory alkalosis, and low serum magnesium levels, leading to an increase in neurologic excitement. (See Table 6.)

Approximately 30% of the patients on a general hospital unit are alcoholic; however, only 2% of them have a diagnosis of alcoholism. The other 28% have been admitted for a variety of reasons. Illnesses such as esophagitis, gastritis, ulcers, hypoglycemia, pancreatitis, and some anemias can be attributed directly to alcohol usage. Chronic alcoholism is the most common cause of cardiomyopathy. There is also an increased incidence of injuries, falls, and hip fractures related to high blood alcohol levels.

Alcohol withdrawal is a life-threatening condition. It can begin within 12 to 24 hours of admission or as late as 5 days after admission. Early-stage withdrawal usually occurs within 48 hours of the patient's last drink, with generally mild symptoms. Late-stage alcohol withdrawal, or alcohol withdrawal delirium, begins 72 to 96 hours after the patient's last drink. It occurs in approximately 5% of all hospitalized alcoholics and is the most acute phase of alcohol withdrawal.

TABLE 6 | **Pathophysiology of Alcohol Withdrawal**

MECHANISM	EXPLANATION
Respiratory alkalosis	Alcohol produces a depressant effect on the respiratory center, depressing a person's respirations and increasing the level of CO_2. Once the person ceases intake of alcohol, the respiratory center depressions cease, leaving an increased sensitivity to CO_2. This increase in sensitivity produces an increase in the rate and depth of the person's respirations (hyperventilation) and lowered levels of CO_2 (respiratory alkalosis).
Low magnesium levels	Many chronic alcoholics have low magnesium intake because of inadequate nutrition. Compounding the problem is the loss of magnesium from the gastrointestinal tract that is caused by alcohol-related diarrhea and the loss of magnesium in the urine that is caused by alcohol-related diuresis. Maintaining magnesium levels in the normal range of 1.8 to 2.5 mEq/L decreases neuromuscular irritability during withdrawal.
CNS excitation	Chronic alcohol use alters cell membrane proteins that normally open and close ion channels to allow electrolytes to enter and exit the cell. With the cessation of alcohol intake, the altered proteins produce an increase in neurologic excitement.

CAUSES

When a heavy drinker takes a drink, there is a calming effect, a sense of tranquility. As alcohol consumption continues, the CNS is increasingly depressed, leading to a sleep state. The brain (reticular activating system) attempts to counteract sleepiness and the depression with a "wake-up" mechanism. The reticular activating system works through chemical stimulation to keep the body and mind alert. The individual who drinks on a daily basis builds a tolerance to the alcohol, requiring increasing amounts to maintain the calming effect. If no alcohol is consumed for 24 hours, the reticular activating system nonetheless continues to produce the stimulants to maintain alertness, which leads the individual to experience an overstimulated state and the development of alcohol withdrawal symptoms after 48 hours.

GENDER AND LIFE SPAN CONSIDERATION

Overuse and abuse of alcohol are seen in all age groups and in females and males. More and more teens are identified as alcoholic and should have their drug or alcohol usage assessed on admission to the hospital or clinic. Binge drinking (more than five drinks at one time) is a growing problem among college students. Although 70% of alcoholics are thought to be male, women are more likely to hide their problem. Of growing concern is the number of elderly who are abusing alcohol as a way to deal with their grief, loneliness, and depression.

☐ ASSESSMENT

HISTORY. Determine when the patient had his or her last drink to assess the risk of alcohol withdrawal. Do not ask "Do you drink?" but, rather, "When did you have your last drink?" Asking the patient's significant others about his or her alcohol use may be another way to establish a history of alcohol abuse; however, the significant others may also be unwilling to answer potentially embarrassing questions honestly.

PHYSICAL EXAMINATION. Use the CAGE questionnaire, an alcoholism screening instrument, CAGE being an acronym for key words in the questions. Affirmative answers to two or more of the CAGE screening questions identify individuals who require more intensive evaluation. Ask the following questions:
- Have you ever felt the need to CUT down on drinking?
- Have you ever felt ANNOYED by criticisms of your drinking?
- Have you ever had GUILTY feelings about drinking?
- Have you ever taken a morning EYE opener?

Determine if the patient has a history of poor nutrition or an illness or infection that has responded poorly to treatment; these are possible signs of alcoholism. Ask the patient if he or she has experienced any agitation, restlessness, anxiety, disorientation, or tremors in the past few hours, which are signs of the onset of early-stage alcohol withdrawal. Determine if the patient has been sweating excessively; feeling weak in the muscles; or experiencing rapid breathing, vomiting, or diarrhea.

Use caution in the amount of information you document regarding an alcohol history. The information is more appropriately placed in a confidential file that is not a part of the formal patient record to protect the patient's confidentiality. Patients have lost medical coverage when insurance agents or attorneys have obtained access to written confidential information on the patient record. Recommend strategies for care in writing, but do not detail a confidential patient drinking history in the legal patient record.

Although many alcoholics appear normal, look for clues of alcohol use, particularly if the patient has not been forthcoming during the history taking. Note the odor of alcohol on the breath or clothing. Inspect arms and legs for bruising or burns that may have been caused by injury. Inspect for edema around the eyes or tibia and a flushed face from small-vessel vasodilatation. Observe general appearance, noting if the patient appears haggard or older than the stated age.

The first symptoms of alcohol withdrawal can appear as soon as 4 hours after the last drink. Note any comments made by the patient about drinking, even in jest. Observe any defensiveness or guarded responses to questions about drinking patterns. Note if the patient requests sedation. If you suspect that a patient may have been abusing alcohol, assess the vital signs every 2 hours for the first 12 hours. If the patient remains stable, vital signs can be assessed less frequently; however, monitor the patient carefully for signs of mild anxiety or nervousness that could indicate alcohol withdrawal. Temperature, blood pressure, and heart rate begin to elevate. Hyperalertness and irritability increase. The patient may remark that he or she feels "trembly" or nervous on the "inside" (internal tremors). Temperature, blood pressure, and heart rate continue to elevate. Mild disorientation and diaphoresis are present. External tremors are visible. Delirium tremens (DTs) is the name associated with the symptoms of confusion and tremors. If the brain is still not sedated, the patient can have seizures, cardiac failure, and death unless medication protocols are instituted.

PSYCHOSOCIAL. Patients who have previously experienced active withdrawal may have little trust or confidence that the nurse will treat them any differently. Individuals who are alcohol-dependent may be in denial or very embarrassed at having their drinking exposed. Maintain a nonjudgmental, supportive approach. The patient needs to feel secure that you will be there to keep him or her safe. Assess the patient's coping mechanisms and support system.

DIAGNOSTIC HIGHLIGHTS

Test	Normal Result	Abnormality with Condition	Explanation
Blood alcohol concentration	Negative (< 10 mg/ dL or 0.01 g/dL)	Positive (> 10 mg/ dL or 0.01 g/dL)	Legal intoxication is most states is 80– 100 mg/dL
Liver function gamma-glutamyl transpeptidase (GGT)	4–25 units (females); 7–40 units (males)	Elevated above normal	Evidence of liver disease or alcoholism
Aspartate aminotransferase (AST)	8–20 units/L	Elevated above normal	Evidence of liver disease or alcoholism
Alanine aminotransferase (ALT)	8–10 units/L	Elevated above normal	Evidence of liver disease or alcoholism

Other Tests: Blood glucose levels: Elevated or low blood glucose levels without a family history of diabetes mellitus indicate chronic alcohol use

PRIMARY NURSING DIAGNOSIS

Fluid volume deficit related to water loss

OUTCOMES. Fluid balance; Circulation status; Cardiac pump effectiveness; Hydration; Nutrition management; Nutrition therapy

INTERVENTIONS. Fluid/electrolyte management; Fluid monitoring; Shock management: Volume; Medication administration; Circulatory care

☐ PLANNING AND IMPLEMENTATION

Collaborative

Upon assessment of a pattern of heavy drinking, the patient is often placed on prophylactic benzodiazepines. These medications are particularly important if the patient develops early signs of withdrawal, such as irritability, anxiety, tremors, restlessness, confusion, mild hypertension (blood pressure greater than 140/90), tachycardia (heart rate greater than 100), and a low-grade fever (temperature greater than 100 °F). Keeping the patient safe during the withdrawal process depends on managing the physiologic changes, the signs and symptoms, and the appropriate drug protocols. The goal is to keep the patient mildly sedated or in a calm and tranquil state but still allow for easy arousal.

Once the patient's nausea and vomiting have been controlled, encourage a well-balanced diet. Monitor the patient continually for signs of dehydration, such as poor skin turgor, dry mucous membranes, weight loss, concentrated urine, and hypotension. Record intake and output. If the patient's blood pressure drops below 90 mm Hg, a significant fluid volume loss has occurred; notify the physician immediately.

PHARMACOLOGIC HIGHLIGHTS

Medication or Drug Class	Dosage	Description	Rationale
Thiamine; multivitamin supplements	100 mg IV; 1 amp multivitamin	Vitamin supplement	Counters effects of nutritional deficiencies
Benzodiazepines	Varies by drug	Antianxiety	Manages alcohol withdrawal; prescribed for their sedating effect and to control the tremors or seizures, which can be life-threatening.

Independent

Managing fluid volume deficit is a top priority in nursing care. Encourage the patient to drink fluids, particularly citrus juices, to help replace needed electrolytes. Caution the patient to avoid caffeine, which stimulates the CNS. Maintain a quiet environment to assist in limiting sensory or perceptual alterations and sleep pattern disturbance.

An appropriately sedated patient should not undergo acute withdrawal. If symptoms occur, however, stay at the bedside during episodes of extreme agitation to reassure the patient. Avoid using restraints. However, if they become necessary, position the patient to prevent aspiration. Use soft rather than leather restraints to reduce the risk for skin abrasions and circulatory insufficiency. During restraint, check the patient's circulation every 2 hours or more often.

When the patient is awake, alert, and appropriately oriented, discuss his or her drinking and the effect of drinking on the patient's illness. Encourage the patient to seek help from Alcoholics Anonymous (AA) or to see a counselor or attend a support group. Refer the patient to a clinical nurse specialist if appropriate.

DOCUMENTATION GUIDELINES

- Physical findings: Vital signs, fluid intake and output, skin turgor, presence of tremors or seizures
- Mental status: Anxiety level, auditory-visual hallucinations, confusion, violent behavior
- Reactions to the alcohol withdrawal experience

DISCHARGE AND HOME HEALTHCARE GUIDELINES

TEACHING. Teach the patient to eat a well-balanced diet with sufficient fluids. Emphasize the value of exercise and adequate rest. Encourage the patient to develop adequate coping strategies.

FOLLOW-UP. Following an alcohol withdrawal experience, the patient may be able to accept that he or she has a problem with alcohol abuse. Discharge plans may include behavior modification programs, sometimes in conjunction with disulfiram (Antabuse) or participation in AA. Families must also be involved in the treatment planning to gain an understanding of the part that family dynamics play in the alcoholic's problems.

Allergic Purpura

DRG Category: 397
Mean LOS: 5.0 days
Description: MEDICAL: Coagulation Disorders

Allergic purpura is an allergic reaction that leads to acute or chronic inflammation of the vessels of the skin, joints, gastrointestinal (GI) tract, and genitourinary (GU) tract. It occurs as an acquired, abnormal immune response to a variety of agents that normally do not cause allergy, and it is manifested by bleeding into the tissues, organs, and joints, which leads to organ dysfunction, discomfort, and immobility. An acute attack of allergic purpura can last for several weeks, but usually episodes of the disease subside without treatment within 1 to 6 weeks. Patients with chronic allergic purpura can have a persistent and debilitating disease. The most severe complications are acute glomerulonephritis and renal failure. Hypertension often complicates the course, and, if bleeding is excessive, the patient can develop a fluid volume deficit. On rare occasions patients may be at risk for airway compromise from laryngeal edema.

CAUSES

Allergic purpura occurs in response to agents such as bacteria, drugs, food, or bee stings. The allergic reaction, probably an autoimmune response directed against the vessel walls, may be triggered by a bacterial infection. Most patients have experienced an upper respiratory infection, particularly a streptococcal infection, 1 to 3 weeks prior to the development of allergic purpura. Experts suggest that other causes, such as allergic reactions to drugs and vaccines, insect bites, and foods (wheat, eggs, chocolate, milk) may lead to the condition.

GENDER AND LIFE SPAN CONSIDERATIONS

Allergic purpura can occur at any age, but it is most common in children between the ages of 3 and 7; the condition is more common in males than females. In children the condition is called Henoch-Schonlein purpura. Children have a better prognosis for complete recovery than do adults.

◻ ASSESSMENT

HISTORY. Approximately one to two out of four patients with allergic purpura have GU symptoms such as dysuria and hematuria. Other symptoms include headaches; fever; peripheral edema; and skin lesions accompanied by pruritus, paresthesia, and angioedema (swelling of the skin, mucous membranes, or organs). Other patients describe severe GI symptoms (spasm, colic, constipation, bloody vomitus, bloody stools) and joint pain.

PHYSICAL EXAMINATION. Inspect the patient's skin for the typical skin lesions—patches of purple macular lesions of various sizes that result from vascular leakage into the skin and mucous membranes. These lesions most commonly occur on the hands and arms. Note that in children, the lesions more commonly start as urticarial areas that then expand into hemorrhagic lesions. Determine if the patient has any peripheral swelling, particularly in the hands and face. Perform gentle range of motion of the extremities to determine the presence and location of joint pain. Assess the color of the patient's urine and stool, and note any bleeding.

PSYCHOSOCIAL. The patient may experience a disturbance in body image because of the disfigurement caused by the rash and swelling. Determine the patient's response to his or her appearance, and identify whether the changes interfere with implementing various roles such as parenting or work.

DIAGNOSTIC HIGHLIGHTS

No single laboratory test identifies allergic purpura. Supporting tests include complete blood count (CBC), erythrocyte sedimentation rate (ESR), urinalysis, blood urea nitrogen (BUN), creatinine, and coagulation profile.

PRIMARY NURSING DIAGNOSIS

Impaired skin integrity related to damage and inflammation of vessels

OUTCOMES. Tissue integrity: Skin and mucous membranes; Wound healing; Body image

INTERVENTIONS. Skin surveillance; Wound care; Body image enhancement

□ PLANNING AND IMPLEMENTATION

Collaborative

The treatment prescribed is based on the acuity and severity of the symptoms. Some patients are treated pharmacologically with corticosteroids to relieve edema and analgesics to manage joint and GI discomfort. Allergy testing to identify the provocative allergen is usually performed. If the allergen is a food or medication, the patient needs to avoid ingesting the allergen for the rest of his or her life. Patients who are placed on corticosteroids or immunosuppressive therapy need an environment that protects them as much as possible from secondary infection. If the patient is on corticosteroids, monitor him or her for signs of Cushing's syndrome and the complications of corticosteroids, such as labile emotions, fluid retention, hyperglycemia, and osteoporosis.

PHARMACOLOGIC HIGHLIGHTS

Medication or Drug Class	Dosage	Description	Rationale
Glucocorticoids	Varies by drug	Corticosteroid	Relieves edema and analgesics to manage joint and GI discomfort.
Azathioprine	Varies by age and whether it is initial or maintenance dose	Immunosupressant	Suppresses cell-mediated hypersensitivity

Independent

Protect open or irritated skin lesions from further tissue trauma and infection. Apply unguents and soothing creams, if appropriate, to manage discomfort. Assist the patient with colloidal baths and activities of daily living if joint pain and the lesions give the patient limited activity tolerance. Reassure the patient that the lesions are of short duration prior to healing. Explore possible sources of the allergy. Allow the patient time to discuss concerns about the disease. If the patient or significant other appears to be coping ineffectively, provide a referral to a clinical nurse specialist or counselor.

DOCUMENTATION GUIDELINES

- Extent, location, and description of erythema; degree of discomfort; signs of wound infection; presence and description of edema
- Response to allergy testing and withdrawal of the provocative agent if identified
- Response to treatments: Medications, creams, and colloidal baths
- Emotional response to the condition; problems coping; body image disturbance

DISCHARGE AND HOME HEALTHCARE GUIDELINES

PREVENTION. Teach the patient about the disease and its cause. If the allergen is identified, assist the patient in eliminating the allergen if possible. Teach the patient to protect lesions from additional trauma by wearing long-sleeved blouses or shirts. Teach the patient to pay particular attention to edematous areas where skin breaks down easily if injured. Encourage the patient to prevent secondary infections by avoiding contact with others and by using good hand washing techniques. Encourage the patient to report recurrent signs and symptoms, which are most likely to occur 6 weeks after the initial onset of symptoms.

MEDICATIONS. Provide the patient with information about the medications, including dosage, route, action, and side effects. Provide the patient with written information so that the patient can refer to it for questions at home.

Alzheimer's Disease

DRG Category: 012
Mean LOS: 6.3 days
Description: MEDICAL: Degenerative Nervous System Disorders

Alzheimer's disease is a degenerative disorder of the brain that is manifested by dementia and progressive physiologic impairment. It is the most common cause of dementia in the elderly. Dementia involves progressive decline in two or more of the following areas of cognition: memory, language, calculation, visual-spatial perception, judgment, abstraction, and behavior. Dementia of the Alzheimer's type (DAT) accounts for approximately half of all dementias. The average time from onset of symptoms to death is 8 to 10 years. The pathophysiologic changes that occur in DAT include the following:

1. Presence of neurofibrillary tangles, neuritic plaques, and amyloid angiopathy
2. Accumulation of lipofuscin granules and granulovacuolar organelles in the cytoplasm of the neurons
3. Structural changes in the dendrites of the neurons and in the cell bodies
4. Predominant neuronal degeneration in the cortical association areas of the basal ganglia
5. Gross cortical atrophy and widening of the sulci
6. Enlargement of the ventricles
7. Decrease in neurotransmitters (acetylcholine, dopamine, norepinephrine, serotonin), somatostatin, and neuropeptide substance P

CAUSES

The cause of Alzheimer's disease is unknown. A hereditary link has not been proven; however, there is evidence of a hereditary autosomal dominance in 10% of reported cases. A relationship between Alzheimer's disease and a defect in chromosome 21 has been found in the majority of patients studied with familiar DAT. Patients with Down syndrome eventually develop DAT if they live long enough. There is a higher-than-normal concentration of aluminum in the brain of a person with DAT, but the effect is unknown.

A distinct protein, AZ-50, has been identified at autopsy in the brains of DAT patients. This protein has been isolated from neurons that were not yet damaged, suggesting that its presence early in the degenerative process might cause the neuronal damage. The life expectancy of a DAT patient is reduced 30% to 60%.

GENDER AND LIFE SPAN CONSIDERATIONS

The onset of DAT may occur at any age but is rare before age 50; the average onset occurs after age 65. Currently, dementia is the fourth leading cause of death in individuals older than 65, and its prevalence is increasing with the aging of the population: 2% to 4% of the population over age 65 has DAT; after age 85, 20% of the population is affected; more females than males have the disease.

☐ ASSESSMENT

HISTORY. DAT is a slowly progressing disease, and secondary sources are used for diagnosis because the patient is often unaware of a thought-processing problem. Past medical history should be evaluated for previous head injury, surgery, recent falls, headache, and family history of DAT.

PHYSICAL EXAMINATION. The history will help determine which stage the disease process has reached at the time of patient assessment. The following four-stage scale reflects the progressive symptoms of DAT:

Stage 1 is characterized by recent memory loss, increased irritability, impaired judgment, loss of interest in life, decline of problem-solving ability, and reduction in abstract thinking. Remote memory and neurologic exam remain unchanged from baseline.

Stage 2 lasts 2 to 4 years and reveals a decline in the patient's ability to manage personal and business affairs, an inability to remember shapes of objects, continued repetition of a meaningless word or phrase (perseveration), wandering or circular speech patterns (circumlocution dysphasia), wandering at night, restlessness, depression, anxiety, and intensification of cognitive and emotional changes of stage 1.

Stage 3 is characterized by impaired ability to speak (aphasia), inability to recognize familiar objects (agnosia), inability to use objects properly (apraxia), inattention, distractibility, involuntary emotional outbursts, urinary or fecal incontinence, lint-picking motion, and chewing movements. Progression through stages 2 and 3 varies from 2 to 12 years.

Stage 4, which lasts approximately 1 year, reveals a patient with a masklike facial expression, no communication, apathy, withdrawal, eventual immobility, assumed fetal position, no appetite, and emaciation.

The neurologic examination remains almost normal except for increased deep tendon reflexes and the presence of snout, root, and grasp reflexes that appear in stage 3. In stage 4, there may be generalized seizures and immobility, which precipitate flexion contractures.

Appearance may range from manifesting normal patient hygiene in the early stage to a total lack of interest in hygiene in the later stages. Some patients also demonstrate abusive language, inappropriate sexual behaviors, and paranoia. The Folstein-mini mental exam is a quick evaluation tool that can assist in diagnosis and monitoring of the disease's progression.

PSYCHOSOCIAL. The nurse needs to assess the family for its ability to cope with this progressive disease, to provide physical and emotional care for the patient, and to meet financial responsibilities. A multidisciplinary team assessment approach is recommended for the patient and family.

DIAGNOSTIC HIGHLIGHTS

Test	Normal Result	Abnormality with Condition	Explanation
Brain biopsy upon autopsy	Negative	Positive for cellular changes that are associated with the disease	The U.S. Department of Health and Human Services cites the clinical criteria for diagnosis of DAT as follows: (1) presence of at least two cognitive deficits, (2) onset occurring between ages 40 and 90, (3) progressive deterioration, and (4) all other causes ruled out.

Other Tests: Supporting tests include computed tomography (CT) scan; magnetic resonance imaging (MRI); positron emission tomography (PET).

PRIMARY NURSING DIAGNOSIS

Self-care deficit related to impaired cognitive and motor function

OUTCOMES. Self-care: Activities of daily living—Bathing, Hygiene, Eating, Toileting; Cognitive ability; Comfort level; Role performance; Social interaction skills; Hope

INTERVENTIONS. Self-care assistance: Bathing and Hygiene; Oral health management; Behavior management; Body image enhancement; Emotional support; Mutual goal setting; Exercise therapy; Discharge planning

□ PLANNING AND IMPLEMENTATION

Collaborative

The initial management of the patient begins with education of the family and caregivers regarding the disease, the prognosis, and changes in lifestyle that are necessary as the disease progresses. Basic collaborative principles include:
• Keep requests for the patient simple
• Avoid confrontation and requests that might lead to frustration
• Remain calm and supportive if the patient becomes upset
• Maintain a consistent environment
• Provide frequent cues and reminders to reorient the patient
• Adjust expectations for the patient as he or she declines in capacity

PHARMACOLOGIC HIGHLIGHTS

Generally, therapy is focused on symptoms with an attempt to maintain cognition.

Medication or Drug Class	Dosage	Description	Rationale
Donepezil	5–10 mg po qd	Cholinesterase inhibitor	Improves cognitive symptoms; improves cognitive function in the early stages of the disease only; drug effects diminish as the disease progresses
Vitamin E	1000 IU po bid	Vitamin supplement	Antioxidant to decrease effects of oxygen-free radicals

Other Therapies: Secondary treatments are aimed at treating depression, psychosis, and agitation. To control night wandering and behavioral outbursts, physicians prescribe mild sedatives such as diphenhydramine. Barbiturates are avoided because they can precipitate confusion. Depression is treated with antidepressants (trazodone), and agitation is controlled by anxiolytics (oxazepam or diazepam). Psychotic behaviors are treated with antipsychotics (chlorpromazine or haloperidol).

Independent

Promote patient activities of daily living to the fullest, considering the patient's functional ability. Give the patient variable assistance or simple directions to perform those activities. Anticipate and assess the patient's needs mainly through nonverbal communication because of the patient's inability to communicate meaningfully through speech. Many times emotional outbursts or changes in behavior are a signal of the patient's toileting needs, discomfort, hunger, or infection.

To maximize orientation and memory, provide a calendar and clock for the patient. Encourage the patient to reminisce, since loss of short-term memory triggers anxiety in the patient. Emotional outbursts usually occur when the patient is fatigued, so it is best to plan for frequent rest periods throughout the day.

Maintain physical safety of the patient by securing loose rugs, supervising electrical devices, and locking doors and windows. Lock up toxic substances and medications. Supervise cooking, bathing, and outdoor recreation. Be sure that the patient wears appropriate identification in case he or she gets lost. Terminate driving by removing the car keys or the car. Provide a safe area for wandering. Encourage and anticipate toileting at 2- to 3-hour intervals. Change incontinence pads as needed, but use them only as a last resort. Bowel and bladder programs can be beneficial in the early stage of the disease.

Provide structured activity during the day to prevent night wandering. If confusion and agitated wandering occur at night, provide toileting, fluids, orientation, night lights, and familiar objects within a patient's view. Some patients respond calmly when given the security of a stuffed animal or a familiar blanket.

Encourage family members to verbalize their emotional concerns, coping strategies, and other aspects of caregiver role strain. Discuss appropriate referrals to local support groups, clergy, social workers, respite care, day care, and attorneys. Provide information about advanced directives (living wills and durable power of attorney for healthcare).

DOCUMENTATION GUIDELINES

- Any changes in cognitive function: Confused orientation (time, place, person), emotional outbursts, forgetfulness, paranoia, decreased short-term memory, impaired judgment, loss of speech, disturbed affect, decline of problem-solving ability, and reduction in abstract thinking
- Response to medications (anxiolytics, antipsychotics, cholinesterase inhibitors, antidepressants, sedatives)
- Verbal and nonverbal methods that effectively meet or communicate the patient's needs
- Caregiver response to patient behaviors and information about DAT
- Ability to perform the activities of daily living

DISCHARGE AND HOME HEALTHCARE GUIDELINES

MEDICATIONS. Be sure the caregiver understands all medications, including the dosage, route, action, and adverse effects.

SAFETY. Explain the need to supervise outdoor activity, cooking, and bathing. Lock doors and windows, and lock up medications and toxic chemicals. Make sure the patient wears identification to provide a safe return if he or she becomes lost. Commercially made products are available that trigger an alarm if the patient wanders out of safe territory.

Amputation

DRG Category: 113
Mean LOS: 12.7 days
Description: SURGICAL: Amputation for Circulation System Disorders, Except Upper Limb and Toe
DRG Category: 442
Mean LOS: 5.8 days
Description: SURGICAL: Other Operating Room Procedures for Injuries with CC

Amputation is the surgical severing of any body part. Amputations can be surgical (therapeutic) or traumatic (emergencies resulting from injury). Some of the most poignant stories of the American Civil War are of healthy young soldiers whose legs were so injured they required removal. The type of amputation performed in that era by a surgeon called a "sawbones" was straight across the leg, with all bone and soft tissue severed at the same level. That procedure, known as a guillotine (or open) amputation, is still seen today.

A traumatic amputation is usually the result of an industrial accident, in which blades of heavy machinery sever part of a limb. A healthy young person who suffers a traumatic amputation without other injuries is often a good candidate for limb salvage. Reattachment of a limb will take place as soon as possible following the injury. The chief problems are hemorrhage and nerve damage. A closed amputation is the most common surgical procedure today. The bone is severed somewhat higher than the surrounding tissue, with a skin flap pulled over the bone end, usually from the posterior surface. This procedure provides more even pressure for a weight-bearing surface, promoting healing and more successful use of a prosthesis. (See Table 7 for levels of amputations.)

CAUSES

Peripheral vascular disease is much more frequently the cause of amputation than are accidents. Poor foot care, impaired circulation, and peripheral neuropathy combine to engender serious ulcerations, which may be undetected until it is too late to salvage the foot or even the entire limb. Congenital deformity, severe burns, and crushing injuries that render a limb permanently unsightly, painful, or nonfunctional may be treated with surgical amputation. Tumors (usually malignant) and chronic osteomyelitis that does not respond to other treatment may also necessitate amputation.

GENDER AND LIFE SPAN CONSIDERATIONS

Amputations are seen in people of all ages. Youngsters who have an amputation very early in life, and are fitted with new and appropriate prostheses as they outgrow the old ones, have the best physical and psychological adjustment to amputation. In young adulthood, more men than women suffer traumatic amputations brought about by hazardous conditions in both the workplace and recreation. The greatest number of amputations is performed in older adults, especially men over 60.

TABLE 7 | **Levels of Amputation**

TYPE	DESCRIPTION
Below the knee	Most common surgical site, performed rather than above-the-knee amputation whenever possible because the higher the amputation performed, the greater the energy required for mobility
Syme procedure	Partial amputation with salvage of the ankle; has advantages over loss of the limb higher up because it does not require a prosthesis and produces less weight-bearing pain
Transmetatarsal/ toe amputation	Involves removal of limited amount of limb; requires little rehabilitation; often followed by additional surgery at a higher level because of inadequate healing when used for patients with peripheral vascular disease
Hip disarticulation/ extensive hemipelvectomy	Usually performed for malignancies; because of the surgery involved and the extremely bulky prosthesis required for ambulation, these procedures are used either as life-saving measures in young patients or as a surgery of last resort for pain control
Upper extremity	Performed with salvage of as much normal tissue as possible. Function of the upper extremity is vital to normal activities of daily living. Much research is being conducted at the current time to manufacture and refine protheses that can substitute for the patient's arm and hand, providing both gross and fine movement. Cosmetic considerations are extremely important in the loss of the upper extremity for many patients.

◻ ASSESSMENT

HISTORY. Seek information in such areas as control of diabetes and hypertension, diet, smoking, and any other activities that may affect the condition and rehabilitation of the patient.

PHYSICAL EXAMINATION. Inspection of the limb prior to surgery should focus on the area close to the expected site of amputation. Because of limited circulation, the limb often feels cool to the touch. Any lacerations, abrasions, or contusions may indicate additional problems with healing and should be made known to the surgeon.

PSYCHOSOCIAL. The young patient with a traumatic amputation may be in the denial phase of grief. The older patient with a long history of peripheral vascular problems, culminating in loss of a limb, may fear the loss of independence. Patients may show hostility or make demands of the nurse that seem unreasonable. Incomplete grieving, along with depression and false cheerfulness, can indicate psychological problems that predispose to phantom limb pain and prolong rehabilitation.

Those patients who are reluctant to have visitors while they are hospitalized following an amputation are most apt to have problems with depression later.

DIAGNOSTIC HIGHLIGHTS

Test	Normal Result	Abnormality with Condition	Explanation
Ankle arm index (AAI)	AAI >1.0	AAI < 0.6	Ratio of the blood pressure in the leg to that in the arm; identifies people with severe aortoiliac occlusive disease

Other Tests: Limb blood pressure; Doppler ultrasonography; ultrasonic duplex scanning; plethysmography; computed tomography

PRIMARY NURSING DIAGNOSIS

Impaired mobility related to loss of lower extremity

OUTCOMES. Balance; Body positioning; Ambulation; Bone healing; Comfort level; Joint movement;, Mobility level; Muscle function; Pain level; Wound healing; Safety behavior: Fall prevention

INTERVENTIONS. Positioning; Body image enhancement; Fall prevention; Exercise promotion; Exercise therapy: Ambulation and balance; Pain management; Positioning; Prosthesis care; Skin surveillance; Wound care

◻ PLANNING AND IMPLEMENTATION

Collaborative

MANAGEMENT OF TRAUMATIC AMPUTATION. If complete amputation of a body part occurs, flush the wound with sterile normal saline, apply a sterile pressure dressing, and elevate the limb. Do not apply a tourniquet to the extremity. Wrap the amputated body part in a wet sterile dressing that has been soaked with sterile normal saline solution. Place the body part in a clean, dry plastic bag, label the bag, and seal it. Place the bag in ice, and transport it with the trauma patient. Do not store the amputated part on dry ice or in normal saline. Following reimplantation surgery, assess the color, temperature, peripheral pulses, and capillary refill of the reimplanted body part every 15 minutes. If the skin temperature declines below the recommended temperature or if perfusion decreases, notify the surgeon immediately.

POSTOPERATIVE MANAGEMENT. Many interventions can help improve the patient's mobility—for example, care of the surgical wound, control of pain, and prevention of further injury. If any excessive bleeding occurs, notify the surgeon immediately and place direct pressure on the area of hemorrhage. Occasionally, a patient returns from surgery with either a Jobst air splint or an immediate postsurgical fitted prosthesis already in place. Explain that the device is intended to aid ambulation and prevent the complications of immobility.

A particular danger to mobility for the patient with a lower limb amputation is contracture of the nearest joint. Elevate the stump on a pillow for the first 24 hours following surgery to control edema. However, after 24 hours do not elevate the stump any longer, or the patient may develop contractures. To prevent contractures, turn the patient prone for 15 to 30 minutes twice a day with the limb extended if the patient can tolerate it. If not, keep the joints extended rather than flexed.

PHARMACOLOGIC HIGHLIGHTS

Medication or Drug Class	Dosage	Description	Rationale
Analgesia	Varies by drug	The amputation procedure is painful and generally requires narcotic analgesia	Relieve pains and tallows for increasing mobility to limit surgical complications

Other Therapies: Intense burning, crushing, or knifelike pain responds to anticonvulsants such as phenytoin (Dilantin) and carbamazepine (Tegretol). The severe muscle cramps or spasmodic sensations that other patients experience respond better to a central-acting skeletal muscle relaxant such as baclofen (Lioresal). Besides the usual narcotics, a beta blocker such as propranolol may be used for the constant, dull, burning ache.

Independent

Postoperative pain located specifically in the stump can be severe and is not usually aided by positioning, distraction, or other nonpharmacologic measures. True stump pain should be short term and should decrease as healing begins. Stump pain that continues to be severe after healing progresses may indicate infection and should be investigated. Phantom limb pain, very real physical discomfort, usually begins about 2 weeks after surgery. It may be triggered by multiple factors, including neuroma formation, ischemia, scar tissue, urination, defecation, and even a cold temperature of the limb. The sensations of phantom limb pain may be described in two basic patterns and are treated with different types of medication. Some nonpharmacologic treatments have also shown success, especially transcutaneous electrical nerve stimulation, hypnosis, whirlpool, and massage therapy.

Grieving over loss of a body part is a normal experience and a necessary condition for successful rehabilitation. It becomes excessive when it dominates the person's life and interferes seriously with other functions. Explore concerns, and help the patient and family determine which are real and which are feared.

Looking at the stump when the dressing is first changed is usually difficult for the patient. It triggers a body image disturbance that may take weeks or months to overcome. The nurse's calm manner in observing and caring for the stump encourages the patient to move toward accepting the changes in her or his body.

Regardless of the type of dressing, stump sock, or temporary prosthesis, inspect the surgical area of an amputation every 8 hours for healing. The goal of bandaging is to reduce edema and shrink the stump into shape for a future prosthesis. Keep the wound clean and free of infection.

Many problems of safety or potential for injury exist for the patient who reestablishes his or her center of balance and relearns ambulation. Urge caution, especially with the young patient who denies having any disability. Safety concerns play a prominent role in planning for discharge. The nurse or physical therapist assesses the home situation.

DOCUMENTATION GUIDELINES

- Condition of the surgical site, including signs of irritation, infection, edema, and shrinkage of tissue
- Control of initial postoperative pain by pain medication

- Measures, both effective and ineffective, in control of phantom limb pain
- Ability to look at the stump and take part in its care
- Participation in physical therapy, including reluctance to try new skills
- Presence of any complication: Bleeding, thrombophlebitis, contractures, infection, return of pain after initial postoperative period

DISCHARGE AND HOME HEALTHCARE GUIDELINES

PREVENTION OF COMPLICATIONS. Teach the patient to wash the stump daily with plain soap and water, inspecting for signs of irritation, infection, edema, or pressure. Remind him or her not to elevate the stump on pillows, as a contracture may still occur in the nearest joint.

PHANTOM LIMB PAIN. Teach the patient to apply gentle pressure to the stump with the hands to control occasional phantom limb pain and to report frequent phantom limb pain to the physician.

PHYSICAL THERAPY. Give the patient the physical therapy or exercise schedule he or she is to follow and make sure she or he understands it. If the patient needs to return to the hospital for physical therapy, check on the availability of transportation.

SUPPLIES AND EQUIPMENT. Make sure that the patient is provided with needed supplies and equipment, for example, stump socks and a well-fitting prosthesis.

ENVIRONMENT. Instruct the patient to avoid environmental hazards, for example, throw rugs and steps without banisters.

SUPPORT SERVICES. Many communities have support services for amputees and for patients who have suffered a loss (including a body part). Help the patient locate the appropriate service, or refer him or her to the social service department for future support.

Amyloidosis

DRG Category: 240
Mean LOS: 6.4 days
Description: MEDICAL: Connective Tissue Disorders with CC

Amyloidosis is a rare, chronic metabolic disorder that is characterized by the extracellular deposition of the fibrous protein amyloid in one or more sites of the body. Accumulation of amyloid eventually compromises vital functions of the affected organs and tissues. Accumulation and infiltration of amyloid into tissues puts pressure on surrounding tissues, causing atrophy of cells. Some forms of amyloidosis cause reticuloendothelial cell dysfunction and abnormal immunoglobulin synthesis.

The associated disease states may be inflammatory, hereditary, or neoplastic; deposition can be localized or systemic. Although primary amyloidosis is not associated with a chronic disease, secondary amyloidosis is associated with such chronic diseases as tuberculosis, syphilis, Hodgkin's disease, and rheumatoid arthritis, and with extensive tissue destruction. The spleen, liver, kidneys, and adrenal cortex are most frequently involved. For a patient with generalized amyloidosis, the average survival rate is 1 to 4 years. Some patients have lived longer, but amyloidosis can result in permanent or life-threatening organ damage. The major cause of death is renal failure.

CAUSES

The precise causes of amyloidosis are unknown, although some experts suspect an immunobiologic basis for the disease. The disease has complex causes, with both immune and genetic factors involved. It may be due to an enzyme defect or an altered immune response. Some forms of amyloidosis appear to have a genetic cause. Another form of amyloidosis appears to be related to Alzheimer's disease.

GENDER AND LIFE SPAN CONSIDERATIONS

Amyloidosis is seen more in adult populations. Elderly individuals, especially those with Alzheimer's disease, are also at risk. Little is known about gender considerations. Patients whose origins are Portuguese, Japanese, Swedish, Greek, and Italian seem to be more susceptible. Some studies show that African Americans have a higher risk for cardiac-related amyloidosis leading to cardiomyopathy than do other populations.

◘ ASSESSMENT

HISTORY. Establish a history of weakness, weight loss, lightheadedness, or fainting (syncope). Ask the patient if he or she has experienced difficulty breathing. Determine if the patient has experienced difficulty in swallowing, diarrhea, or constipation, which are signs of gastrointestinal (GI) involvement. Determine if the patient has experienced joint pain, which is a sign of amyloid arthritis. Elicit a history of potential risk factors.

PHYSICAL EXAMINATION. Assess for kidney involvement by inspecting the patient's feet for signs of pedal edema and the patient's face for signs of periorbital edema. Take the patient's pulse, noting changes in rhythm and regularity. Note any changes in the patient's blood pressure. Auscultate the patient's heart sounds for the presence of dysrhythmias, murmurs, or adventitious sounds. Auscultate the breath sounds and observe for dyspnea.

Observe the patient's tongue for swelling and stiffness, and assess the patient's ability to speak and swallow. Auscultate bowel sounds, noting hypoactivity. Palpate the patient's abdomen, noting any enlargement of the liver. Observe the patient for signs of abdominal pain, and check the patient's stool for blood.

Assess the patient's skin turgor and color, noting any evidence of jaundice. Malabsorption occurs with GI involvement, leading to malnourishment. Observe the patient's skin for the presence of lesions that may indicate nutrient or vitamin deficiencies. Palpate the axillary, inguinal, and anal regions for the presence of plaques or elevated papules. Inspect the patient's neck and mucosal areas, such as the ear or tongue, for lesions. Observe the patient's eyes, noting any periorbital ecchymoses ("black-eye syndrome"). Neurologic testing may reveal decreased pain sensation and muscle strength in the extremities.

PSYCHOSOCIAL. Because the patient with amyloidosis may be asymptomatic, the suddenness of the revelation of the disease can be traumatic. Patients with facial lesions may be upset at the change in their appearance.

DIAGNOSTIC HIGHLIGHTS

Test	Normal Result	Abnormality with Condition	Explanation
Biopsy: usually taken from the rectal mucosa, abdominal fat pads, skin, and gums	Negative	Positive for amyloid usually with Congo red staining techniques	Identifies the presence of amyloid with appropriate stains

Other Tests: Electrocardiogram; serum alkaline phosphatase; urinalysis

PRIMARY NURSING DIAGNOSIS

Ineffective airway clearance related to tongue obstruction (macroglossia)

OUTCOMES. Respiratory status: gas exchange and ventilation; Oral health

INTERVENTIONS. Airway insertion; Airway management; Airway suctioning; Oral health promotion; Respiratory monitoring; Ventilation assistance

☐ PLANNING AND IMPLEMENTATION

Collaborative

Therapy is targeted to amelioration of the underlying organ dysfunction through pharmacological therapy, but there is no known cure. Surgical procedures may be used to treat severe symptoms. The patient may develop a complication of the tongue called macroglossia. If this occurs, a tracheotomy may be necessary to maintain oxygenation. Patients with severe renal amyloidosis and azotemia may undergo bilateral nephrectomy and renal transplantation followed by immune therapy, although the donor kidney may be susceptible to amyloidosis as well.

OTHER MANAGEMENT. A dietary consultation can provide the patient with a plan to supplement needed nutrients and bulk-forming foods based on the patient's symptoms. Unless the patient requires fluid restriction, he or she needs to drink at least 2 L of fluid per day. A referral to a speech therapist may be necessary if the patient's tongue prevents clear communication.

PHARMACOLOGIC HIGHLIGHTS

Medication or Drug Class	Dosage	Description	Rationale
Colchicine; melphalan; prednisone	Varies with drug	Varies with drug	Decreases amyloid deposits; no known effective therapy to reverse amyloidosis

Other Therapies: Dimethylsulfoxide (DMSO) has been used at times to decrease amyloid deposits. To prevent serious cardiac complications in patients with cardiac amyloidosis, antidysrhythmic agents are prescribed. Digitalis is avoided because patients are susceptible to toxicity. Vitamin K is used to treat coagulation problems, and analgesics are prescribed for pain. As the disease progresses and malabsorption develops secondary to GI involvement, parenteral nutrition is used to meet nutritional needs.

Independent

Maintain a patent airway when the patient's tongue is involved. Prevent respiratory tract complications by gentle and adequate suctioning when necessary. Keep a tracheotomy tray at the patient's bedside in case of airway obstruction. When the patient is placed on bed rest, institute measures to prevent atrophy of the muscles, development of contractures, and formation of decubitus ulcers.

Provide a pleasant environment to stimulate the patient's appetite. Give oral hygiene before and after meals and assist the patient as needed with feeding. Note that the disease puts tremendous stressors on the family and patient as they cope with a chronic disease without hope of recovery. Encourage the patient to verbalize his or her feelings. Involve loved ones in the care of the patient, and involve the patient in all discussions surrounding his or her care. Present a realistic picture of the prognosis of the illness, but do not remove all the patient's hope. Refer the patient and family to the chaplain or a clinical nurse specialist for counseling if appropriate.

DOCUMENTATION GUIDELINES

- Physical findings: Adequacy of airway, degree of hydration or dehydration, presence of lesions, macroglossia, edema
- Ability to use extremities: Range of motion, weakness, gait, activity tolerance
- Nutritional status
- Changes in heart and lung sounds, presence of dysrhythmias
- Response to medications, speech therapy, counseling, surgery
- Emotional responses to disease: Degree of hope, resiliency, family support, ability to cope
- Understanding of and interest in patient teaching

DISCHARGE AND HOME HEALTHCARE GUIDELINES

MEDICATIONS. Teach the patient the purpose, dosage, schedule, precautions and potential side effects, interactions, and adverse reactions of all prescribed medications.

COMPLICATIONS. Teach the patient to examine his or her legs daily for signs of swelling. Instruct the patient to monitor urinary output for a decrease in quantity. Teach the patient to test the stool for bleeding. Advise the patient to report breathing difficulties or irregular heart beats.

FOLLOW-UP. Explain to the patient and significant others that a variety of counseling and social supports are available to help as the disease progresses. Give the patient a phone number to call if some health assistance is needed.

Amyotrophic Lateral Sclerosis

DRG Category: 012
Mean LOS: 6.3 days
Description: MEDICAL: Degenerative Nervous System Disorders

Amyotrophic lateral sclerosis (ALS) is the most common progressive motor neuron disease of muscular atrophy. Approximately 30,000 Americans have the disease, which is often referred to as Lou Gehrig's disease after the baseball player who died from it. ALS is characterized by a progressive loss of motor neurons (in both the cerebral cortex and the spinal cord). The muscular atrophy is designated by the term "amyotrophy." As motor neurons are destroyed in the cerebral cortex, the long axons and the myelin sheaths that make up the corticospinal nerve tracts disappear. The loss of fibers in the nerve tracts and development of a firmness in the tissues leads to the designation of "lateral sclerosis." One important feature of the disease is the selective nature of neuronal cell death. The sensory networks and the portions of the brain needed for control and regulation of movement, intellect, and thinking are not affected. The most common complications of ALS are respiratory. Death often occurs 3 to 5 years after the onset of the disease because of pneumonia, respiratory failure, or aspiration, although some patients live as long as 10 or 15 years.

CAUSES

The precise cause is unknown. Approximately 10% of ALS patients have an inherited form of the disease. Theories of disease development include a viral infection that creates a metabolic disturbance in motor neurons, or an autoimmune response directed against motor neurons. Precipitating factors include physical exhaustion, severe stress, viral infections, and conditions such as myocardial infarction, malnutrition, and traumatic injury.

GENDER AND LIFE SPAN CONSIDERATIONS

There is a higher incidence of ALS in men than in women. The onset of the disease usually occurs in middle age, predominantly in the fifth or sixth decade. If the symptoms develop during the teenage years, the patient probably has an inherited form of the disease.

◻ ASSESSMENT

HISTORY. Because the first evidence of the disease is often gradually developing asymmetric weakness in one limb, establish a recent history of muscle weakness or involuntary contractions (fasciculations) of the muscles, especially in the feet and hands. Ask whether the patient has lost weight, experienced difficulty in chewing or swallowing, or if he or she has been drooling. Elicit a history of breathing difficulties or choking. Ask if the patient has experienced any crying spells or periods of inappropriate laughter, which can be caused by progressive bulbar palsy (degeneration of upper motor neurons in the medulla oblongata).

PHYSICAL EXAMINATION. Determine how the disease is affecting the patient's functioning and ability to carry out the activities of daily living. Assess for the characteristic atrophic changes such as weakness or fasciculation in the muscles of the forearms, hands, and legs. One side of the body may have more muscle involvement than the other. Assess the patient's respiratory status, noting rate and pattern and the patient's breath sounds.

As the disease progresses, muscle weakness that began asymmetrically becomes symmetrical. Muscles of chewing, swallowing, and tongue movement are affected. Note facial symmetry, the presence or absence of a gag reflex, slurred speech, and the ability to swallow. Note any tendency to drool or any tongue tremors.

PSYCHOSOCIAL. The patient with ALS is confronted with a progressive fatal illness. Because mental capacity is not affected by this disease, the patient remains alert even in the late stages of the disease. Patients with ALS usually experience depression and need a great deal of emotional support.

DIAGNOSTIC HIGHLIGHTS

General Comments: Because ALS is currently untreatable, it is essential that other potential causes of motor neuron dysfunction be excluded by diagnostic testing.

Test	Normal Result	Abnormality with Condition	Explanation
Electromyography	Normal conduction velocity 40–80 meters per second after a nerve is stimulated	Decrease in conduction velocity of motor units of affected muscles	Rules out other muscle diseases; often reflects a decrease in motor units of the affected muscles

Other Tests: Muscle biopsy; cerebrospinal fluid analysis; pulmonary function tests; computed tomography (CT) scan, magnetic resonance imaging (MRI), and other conduction studies

PRIMARY NURSING DIAGNOSIS

Ineffective airway clearance because of weakened cough effort

OUTCOMES. Respiratory status: Gas exchange and ventilation; Oral health

INTERVENTIONS. Airway insertion; Airway management; Airway suctioning; Oral health promotion; Respiratory monitoring; Ventilation assistance

◻ PLANNING AND IMPLEMENTATION

Collaborative

Management of ALS is focused on the treatment of symptoms and rehabilitation measures. No specific treatment for the disease exists that will influence the underlying pathophysiology.

REHABILITATION. Rehabilitation aids are available to overcome the effects of muscular disability and to support weakened muscles. A planned program of exercise helps patients function for a longer period of time.

AIRWAY MANAGEMENT. Supporting the patient's airway and breathing becomes essential as the disease progresses. The patient's deteriorating respiratory status may eventually require mechanical ventilation. If a ventilator is being used at home, patient and significant others will need instructions on ventilatory management.

NUTRITION. When the patient can no longer maintain nutrition, enteral or parenteral feedings may be initiated. Long-term nutritional management may require a gastrostomy or cervical esophagostomy.

PHARMACOLOGIC HIGHLIGHTS

Medication or Drug Class	Dosage	Description	Rationale
Diazepam	5 mg po prn	Benzodiazepine	Manages muscle spasticity
Baclofen	5 mg po tid	Skeletal muscle relaxant	Manages muscle spasticity

Other Therapies: Quinine can also be used for relief of painful muscle cramps and spasms.

Independent

MANAGING THE DISEASE. Teach the patient breathing exercises, methods to change positions, chest physical therapy techniques, and incentive spirometry. Explore measures to reduce the risk of aspiration. Encourage rest periods prior to meals to decrease muscle fatigue. Have the patient sit in an upright position with his or her neck slightly flexed during meals, use a neck support such as a cervical collar, and serve foods with a soft consistency. Encourage the patient to remain in an upright position for at least 30 minutes after a meal. If the patient is having problems handling oral secretions, teach him or her how to use oral suction.

As the disease worsens, the patient may lose the ability to speak. Work with the patient and family to develop alternate methods of communication, such as eye blinks, a picture or word chart, or computers with artificial speech or synthesizers. When the patient's immobility increases, teach the family to provide skin care to all pressure points. The patient needs to be turned and positioned frequently. The use of a pressure-reducing mattress will also help maintain skin integrity.

ACTIVITIES OF DAILY LIVING. To achieve maximum mobility and independence, institute an exercise regimen with active or passive range-of-motion (ROM) exercises. Use supportive devices for mobility and transfer, and instruct the patient on the use of splints. Establish regular bowel and bladder routines. Work with the patient and significant others to develop a pattern for activities of daily living that allows the patient to participate but not to become overly fatigued. As mobility decreases, help the patient obtain equipment such as a walker, a wheelchair, or a lift. Ask the patient or family to describe the living environment (or perform a home assessment) to identify areas that may cause potential injury or to recommend modifications to the environment.

EMOTIONAL SUPPORT. Early in the disease process, expect the patient and family to be angry, deny the probable disease outcome (death), or show extreme anxiety. The patient and family will most likely experience periods of depression and may need a referral to a counselor or support group. Most communities have local chapters of the Amyotrophic Lateral Sclerosis Association.

DOCUMENTATION GUIDELINES

- Physical findings related to the patient's respiratory status, including respiratory rate, depth, rhythm, breathing pattern, respiratory excursion, breath sounds, and cough effort
- Responses to the nursing interventions taken to support the patient's respiratory function, such as coughing, deep breathing, frequent position changes, and incentive spirometry
- Nutritional status: Patient's weight, measure to maintain nutrition (feeding patient, soft or pureed food, tube feeding)
- Patient's ability to perform activities of daily living
- Responses to all ROM exercises or active exercises
- Responses to equipment or assistive devices such as splints necessary in patient care

DISCHARGE AND HOME HEALTHCARE GUIDELINES

PREVENTION OF ASPIRATION. Teach the family or caregivers how to protect the patient's airway and dislodge food if the patient aspirates. Teach the patient or family how to suction the patient.

TREATMENT. Provide information regarding home healthcare products that are available and explain how to get them. Explain to the patient and family treatment options such as mechanical ventilation and tracheostomy.

EMOTIONAL. Explore coping strategies. Support groups for ALS patients are available in many cities. Refer the patient or family to Respite Care or the ALS Association.

Anaphylaxis

DRG Category: 447
Mean LOS: 2.3 days
Description: MEDICAL: Allergic Reactions, Age > 17

Anaphylactic shock, or anaphylaxis, is an immediate, life-threatening allergic reaction that is caused by a systemic antigen-antibody immune response to a foreign substance (antigen) introduced into the body. It is caused by a type I, immunoglobulin E–mediated reaction. The antigen combines with immunoglobulin E (IgE) on the surface of the mast cells, and this precipitates a release of histamine and other chemical mediators such as serotonin and slow-reacting substance of anaphylaxis (SRS-A). The resulting increased capillary permeability, smooth muscle contraction, and vasodilation account for the cardiovascular collapse.

Bronchoconstriction, bronchospasm, and relative hypovolemia result in impaired airway, breathing, and circulation; death may follow if anaphylaxis is not promptly reversed. Although a delayed reaction may occur 24 hours after the exposure to an antigen, most reactions occur within minutes after exposure, and a recurrence of symptoms may occur after 4 to 8 hours. The most common causes of death from anaphylaxis are airway obstruction and hypotension.

CAUSES

Although anaphylaxis can result from a variety of causes, the most common is penicillin, which induces a reaction in 1 to 4 of every 10,000 people who receive it. Other common sources are other antibiotics, bee stings, iodine-based contrast materials, and medications that have been derived from biologic protein sources. These medications can include those derived from horse sera, vaccines, enzymes, and hormones. Foods such as fish, eggs, peanuts, milk products, and chocolate can cause allergic reactions and anaphylaxis.

GENDER AND LIFE SPAN CONSIDERATIONS

Anaphylactic shock can occur at any age and in both men and women. To prevent infants and children from experiencing severe allergic reactions, pediatricians carefully plan vaccines and diet to limit the risk of allergic reaction until a child's immune system is more mature.

◻ ASSESSMENT

HISTORY. Obtain information about any recent food intake, medication ingestion, or known allergies. The earlier the signs and symptoms begin, the more severe the reaction. Often the symptoms include weakness, a sense of impending doom, sweating, sneezing, nasal itchiness, shortness of breath, and rash. If the patient describes a "lump in the throat," it may indicate laryngeal edema, which necessitates initiating emergency airway management immediately. Some patients describe lightheadedness, tachycardia, syncope, and gastrointestinal symptoms (nausea, vomiting, and pain). Ask the members about a family history of drug allergies or a history of previous reactions.

PHYSICAL EXAMINATION. Note any hives, which appear as well-defined areas of redness with raised borders and blanched centers. Generalized symptoms include flushing, tingling, and angioedema around the mouth, tongue, eyes, and hands. Wheezing, stridor, and difficulty breathing indicate laryngeal edema and bronchospasm and may indicate the need for emergency intubation. Auscultate the patient's blood pressure with a high suspicion for hypotension. Auscultate the patient's heart to identify cardiac dysrhythmias, which may precipitate vascular collapse. Palpate the patient's extremities for signs of cardiovascular compromise, such as weak peripheral pulses and delayed capillary refill.

PSYCHOSOCIAL. The patient who is experiencing an anaphylactic reaction is often panicky and fearful. Although alert, the patient may express a feeling of helplessness, loss of control, and impending doom. In addition, the family, parents, or significant others are apt to be fearful and severely anxious.

DIAGNOSTIC HIGHLIGHTS

No specific laboratory tests are required to make the diagnosis of anaphylactic shock, although diagnostic tests may be performed to rule out other causes of the symptoms, such as congestive heart failure, myocardial infarction, or status asthmaticus.

PRIMARY NURSING DIAGNOSIS

Ineffective airway clearance related to laryngeal edema and bronchospasm

OUTCOMES. Respiratory status: Gas exchange and ventilation; Safety status: Physical injury

INTERVENTIONS. Airway insertion; Airway management; Airway suctioning; Oral health promotion; Respiratory monitoring; Ventilation assistance

☐ PLANNING AND IMPLEMENTATION

Collaborative

The plan of care depends on the severity of the reaction. Discontinue the administration of any possible allergen immediately. Complete an assessment of the patient's airway to ensure patency and adequate breathing. If the patient has airway compromise, endotracheal intubation and mechanical ventilation with oxygenation may be necessary. More severe or prolonged cases of anaphylactic shock are aggressively treated with the establishment of IV access and a normal saline infusion and supplemental oxygen therapy. The patient may require urinary catheterization to monitor urinary output during periods of instability.

PHARMACOLOGIC HIGHLIGHTS

Medication or Drug Class	Dosage	Description	Rationale
Epinephrine	Aqueous solution of 1 mg/mL (1:1000) at a dose of 0.01 mL/kg subcutaneously and repeated at 10–20 minute intervals. If airway is not patent, a dose of 3–5 mL of a 1:10,000 solution is diluted with 10 mL normal saline and given by intravenous (IV) push in femeral or jugular vein. May also be given down the endotracheal tube. For protracted cases, an epinephrine drip may be used intravenously	Catecholamine	Decreases inflammation and allergic response
Diphenhydramine (Benadryl) may be given to inhibit further histamine release.	25–50 mg IV	Antihistamine	Inhibits histamine release and relieves skin symptoms

Other Medications: Corticosteroids (hydrocortisone) and aminophylline for swelling and bronchospasm; severe hypotension can be treated with vasopressor agents such as norepinephrine (Levophed).

Independent

The most important priority for nurses is to ensure adequacy of the airway, breathing, and circulation. Keep intubation equipment available for immediate use. Insert an oral or nasal airway if the patient is at risk for airway occlusion but has adequate breathing. Use an oral airway for unresponsive patients and a nasal airway for patients who are responsive. If endotracheal intubation is necessary, secure the tube firmly and suction the patient as needed to maintain the airway. If the patient has a compromised circulation that does not respond to pharmacologic intervention, begin cardiopulmonary resuscitation with chest compressions.

Teach the patient and family how to prevent future allergic reactions. Explain the nature of the allergy, the signs and symptoms to expect, and measures to perform if the patient is exposed to the allergen. Teach the patient that if shortness of breath, difficulty swallowing, or the formation of the "lump in the throat" occurs, he or she should go to an emergency department immediately. If the allergen is a medication, make sure the patient and family understand that they must avoid the various sources of the medication in both prescription drugs and available over-the-counter preparations. Encourage the patient to notify all healthcare providers of the allergy prior to treatment.

DOCUMENTATION GUIDELINES

- Adequacy of airway: Patency of airway, ease of respirations, chest expansion, respiratory rate, presence of stridor or wheezes
- Cardiovascular assessment: Changes in vital signs (particularly blood pressure and heart rate), skin color, cardiac rhythm.
- Assessment of level of anxiety, degree of understanding, adjustment, and coping skills.

DISCHARGE AND HOME HEALTHCARE GUIDELINES

FOLLOW-UP. Provide a complete explanation of all allergic responses and how to avoid future reactions. If the patient has a reaction to a food or medication, instruct the patient and family about the substance itself and all potential sources. If the patient has a food allergy, you may need to include a dietician in the patient teaching. Encourage the patient to carry an anaphylaxis kit with epinephrine. Teach the patient to administer subcutaneous epinephrine in case of emergencies. Encourage the patient to wear an identification bracelet at all times that specifies the allergy.

Angina Pectoris

DRG Category: 140
Mean LOS: 3.2 days
Description: MEDICAL: Angina pectoris
DRG Category: 124
Mean LOS: 4.2 days
Description: MEDICAL: Circulatory Disorders, Except AMI, W Card Cath, and Complex

Angina pectoris is a symptom of ischemic heart disease that is characterized by paroxysmal and usually recurring substernal or precordial chest pain or discomfort. Angina pectoris is caused by varying combinations of increased myocardial demand and decreased myocardial perfusion. The imbalance between supply and demand is caused either by a primary decrease in coronary blood flow or by a disproportionate increase in myocardial oxygen requirements. Blood flow through the coronary arteries is partially or completely obstructed because of coronary artery spasm, fixed stenosing plaques, disrupted plaques, thrombosis, platelet aggregation, and embolization.

Angina can be classified as chronic exertional (stable, typical) angina, variant angina (Prinzmetal's), or unstable or crescendo an gina. (See Table 8.) Chronic exertional angina is usually caused by obstructive coronary artery disease that causes the heart to be vulnerable to further ischemia whenever there is increased demand or workload. Variant angina may occur in people with normal coronary arteries who have cyclically recurring angina at rest, unrelated to effort. Unstable angina is diagnosed in patients who report a changing character, duration, and intensity of their pain. Experts are also recognizing that not all ischemic events are perceived by patients, even though such events, called silent ischemia, may have adverse implications for the patient.

TABLE 8 | **Classification of Angina Pectoris**

TYPE	CAUSE	DESCRIPTION	DURATION	CESSATION
Stable (typical)	Reduction of coronary perfusion by chronic stenosing coronary atherosclerosis; related to activities that increase myocardial demand	Chest discomfort is produced by exertion and relieved by rest; pain may occur after meals or be brought on by emotional tension.	3–15 minutes	Relieved by rest and/or nitroglycerin
Prinzmetal variant angina	Coronary artery spasm without increased myocardial oxygen demand	Occurs at rest, often during sleep in early morning hours; associated with elevation of the ST segment of	Tends to last longer than other forms of angina	May subside with exercise

continued on the following page

TABLE 8	Classification of Angina Pectoris (*Continued*)			
TYPE	CAUSE	DESCRIPTION	DURATION	CESSATION
		the ECG, which indicates transmural ischemia		
Unstable angina	Disruption of an atherosclerotic plaque or vasospasm or both	Pattern of pain with progressively increasing frequency and precipitated with progressively less effort	Prolonged duration longer than that of stable angina	May not be relieved by nitroglycerin (NTG) or rest; 10%–20% of untreated patients may progress to MI

CAUSES

Most recurrent angina pectoris is caused by atherosclerosis, which is the most common cause of coronary artery disease (CAD) and continues to be the leading cause of death for both women and men in the United States. However, it may occur in patients with normal coronary arteries as well. Approximately 90% of patients with recurrent angina pectoris have hemodynamically significant stenosis or occlusion of a major coronary artery.

GENDER AND LIFE SPAN CONSIDERATIONS

The risk of ischemic heart disease increases with age and when predispositions to atherosclerosis (smoking, hypertension, diabetes mellitus, hyperlipoproteinemia) are present. Nearly 10% of myocardial infarctions (MI) occur in people under age 40, however, and 45% occur in people under age 65. Men are at greater risk for MI than women are, but the differential progressively declines with advancing age.

☐ ASSESSMENT

HISTORY. Ask the patient to describe past chest discomfort in terms of quality (aching, sharp, tingling, knifelike, choking, squeezing), location and radiation, precipitating factors (activity), duration, alleviating factors (relieved by rest), and associated signs and symptoms during the attack (dyspnea, anxiety, diaphoresis, nausea). Obtain information regarding the medications, family history, and modifiable risk factors such as eating habits, lifestyle, and physical activity. If chest discomfort is present at the time of the interview, delay collection of historical data until you implement appropriate interventions for ischemic chest pain and the patient is pain-free.

PHYSICAL EXAMINATION. During anginal attacks, chest discomfort is often described as an ache, rather than an actual pain, and may be characterized as a heaviness, pressure, tightness, squeezing sensation, or indigestion. The discomfort is typically located in the substernal region or across the anterior upper chest. Often, the area of pain is the size of a clenched fist and the patient may place his or her fist over the area of discomfort (Levine's sign). The sensation may radiate to the neck, jaw, or tongue; to either arm, elbow, wrist, or hand; or to the upper abdomen. Anginal discomfort is typically of short duration, usually 3 to 5 minutes, but can last up to 30 minutes or longer. The discomfort may have been brought on by physical or emotional stress, exposure to extreme temperatures, or eating a heavy meal. Termination of the precipitating factor may bring about alleviation of the discomfort. Frequently, the patient is anxious, pale, diaphoretic, lightheaded, dyspneic, tachycardiac, and nauseated. Upon auscultation, the patient may have atrial or ventricular gallops (S_3, S_4).

PSYCHOSOCIAL. Patients often rationalize that their symptoms are the result of indigestion or overexertion. Denial can interfere with identification of a symptom and be harmful to the patient. Chest pain and all the surrounding implications can be extremely stressful and anxiety-producing to the patient and family.

DIAGNOSTIC HIGHLIGHTS

Diagnostic data are not collected to diagnose and confirm angina pectoris (a symptom) but, rather, to diagnose the underlying cause of angina pectoris. The majority of testing is done to determine any damage that may have occurred during an acute anginal episode, such as a myocardial infarction (MI).

Test	Normal Result	Abnormality with Condition	Explanation
Electrocardiogram	Normal PQRST pattern	ST segment depression, T wave inversion. May have transient ST elevation (less frequent); ECG may be normal	Assesses the electrical conduction system, which is adversely affected by myocardial ischemia
Creatine kinase isoenzyme (MB-CK)	0%–6% to total CK	Elevated in some patients with unstable angina	One-third of patients with unstable angina may have elevations due to tissue damage
Troponin I Troponin T	< 3.1 µg/L <0.2 µg/L	Elevated in MI	Differentiates between angina and MI

Other Tests: Cholesterol (total, low-density lipoprotein, high-density lipoprotein); exercise stress testing; cardiac catheterization

PRIMARY NURSING DIAGNOSIS

Altered tissue perfusion (myocardial) related to narrowing of the coronary artery(ies) and associated with atherosclerosis, spasm, or thrombosis

OUTCOMES. Cardiac pump effectiveness; Circulation status; Comfort level; Pain control behavior; Pain level; Tissue perfusion: Cardiac

INTERVENTIONS. Cardiac care; Cardiac precautions; Oxygen therapy; Pain management; Medication administration; Circulatory care; Positioning

☐ PLANNING AND IMPLEMENTATION

Collaborative

For any patient who is experiencing an acute anginal episode, pain management is the priority, not only for patient comfort but also to decrease myocardial oxygen consumption. The physician orders selected therapies that either decrease myocardial oxygen demand or increase coronary blood and oxygen supply. These therapies may include short-term bed rest; oxygen therapy; cardiac monitoring to prevent potential complications; and small, frequent, easily digested meals.

DIET. A collaborative effort among the patient, dietician, physician, and nurse plans for a diet low in cholesterol, fat, calories, and sodium. Drinks in the coronary care unit or step-down unit are usually decaffeinated and not too hot or cold.

VITAL SIGNS. During unstable periods, the nurse and physician closely monitor the patient's vital signs and his or her response to pain-relieving therapies (narcotics, nitrates). Often the patient is placed on a cardiac monitor to determine if life-threatening dysrhythmias occur during an anginal episode, particularly if the angina may be a symptom that the patient is having an MI.

PHARMACOLOGIC HIGHLIGHTS

Medication or Drug Class	Dosage	Description	Rationale
Nitroglycerin (NTG)	0.3–0.6 mg prn SL for stable angina; IV for unstable angina—IV dose varies	Nitrate	Relieves ischemic symptoms by vasodilation of coronary arteries; reduces left ventricular preload and afterload
Aspirin	160–325 mg po qd	Nonsteroidal anti-inflammatory	Inhibits platelet aggregation to reduce risk of coronary artery blockage
Beta-adrenergic antagonists (atenolol, propranolol, metoprolol, etc)	Varies by drug	Beta-adrenergic antagonists	Reduces myocardial oxygen demands by decreasing heart rate, BP, and contractility

Other Therapy: There are numerous drugs to decrease myocardial oxygen consumption: intravenous nitroglycerin (NTG) by infusion, long-acting nitrates, narcotics for pain control, beta-adrenergic blocking agents, calcium-channel blocking agents, vasodilators, diuretics, antihypertensive agents, and anticoagulants.

Independent

To decrease oxygen demand, encourage the patient to maintain bed rest until the pain subsides; even though bed rest is usually short term, a sheepskin, air mattress, foam pad, foot cradle, or heel pads can reduce the risk of skin breakdown and increase patient comfort. Encourage rest throughout the entire hospitalization.

Because anxiety and fear are common among both patients and families, attempt to have them discuss concerns and express their feelings. With the patient and family, discuss the diagnosis, the activity and diet restrictions, and the medical treatment. Refer the patient to a smoking cessation program if appropriate. Numerous lifestyle changes may be needed. Cardiac rehabilitation is helpful in limiting risk factors and providing additional guidance, social support, and encouragement. Adequate education and support are essential if the patient is to adhere to the prescribed therapy and treatment plan.

DOCUMENTATION GUIDELINES

- Description of pain: Onset (sudden, gradual), character (aching, sharp, burning, pressure), precipitating factors, associated symptoms (anxiety, dyspnea, diaphoresis, dizziness, nausea, cyanosis, pallor), duration, and alleviating factors of the anginal episode
- Response to prescribed medications
- Reaction to bed rest or limitation in activity

DISCHARGE AND HOME HEALTHCARE GUIDELINES

PREVENTION. Teach the patient factors that may precipitate anginal episodes and the appropriate measures to control episodes. Teach the patient the modifiable cardiovascular risk factors and ways to reduce them.

MEDICATIONS. Be sure the patient understands all medications, including the dose, route, action, and adverse effects. If the patient's physician prescribes sublingual NTG, instruct the patient to lie in semi-Fowler position and take up to three tablets 5 minutes apart to relieve chest discomfort. Instruct the patient that if relief is not obtained after ingestion of the three tablets, he or she should seek medical attention immediately. Remind the patient to check the expiration date on the NTG tablets and to replace the bottle, once it is opened, every 3 to 5 months.

COMPLICATIONS. Teach the patient the importance of not denying or ignoring anginal episodes and of reporting them to the healthcare provider immediately.

Anorectal Abscess and Fistula

DRG Category: 188
Mean LOS: 4.9 days
Description: MEDICAL: Other Digestive System Diagnoses, Age > 17 with CC
DRG Category: 157
Mean LOS: 4.4 days
Description: SURGICAL: Anal and Stomal Procedures with CC

An anorectal abscess, sometimes called a perirectal abscess, is the formation of pus in the soft tissue that surrounds the anal canal or lower rectum. Perianal abscess is the most common form, affecting four out of five patients; ischiorectal (abscess in the ischiorectal fossa in the fatty tissue on either side of the rectum) and submucosal or high intermuscular abscesses account for most of the remaining cases of anorectal abscess. A rare form of anorectal abscess is called pelvirectal abscess, which extends deeply into pelvic regions from the rectum.

Anorectal abscesses can lead to anal fistulas, also known as fistula in ano. An anal fistula is the development of an abnormal tract or opening between the anal canal and the skin outside the anus. It should not to be confused with an anal fissure, which is an elongated ulcer located just inside the anal orifice, caused by the traumatic passage of large, hard stools.

CAUSES

Perirectal abscesses are usually caused by an infection in an anal gland or the surrounding lymphoid tissue. Lesions that can lead to anorectal abscesses and fistulas can be caused by infections of the anal fissure; infections through the anal gland; ruptured anal hematoma; prolapsed thrombosed internal hemorrhoids; and septic lesions in the pelvis, such as acute salpingitis, acute appendicitis, and diverticulitis. Ulcerative colitis and Crohn's disease are systemic illnesses that can cause abscesses, and people who are immunosupprsssed are more susceptible to abscesses.

GENDER AND LIFE SPAN CONSIDERATIONS

The elderly are more prone to the condition because of their increased incidence of constipation, hemorrhoids, and diabetes mellitus. Women are more commonly affected by constipation than are men. An anorectal fistula is a rare diagnosis in children.

☐ ASSESSMENT

HISTORY. Ask the patient to describe the kind of pain and the precise location. Determine if the pain is exacerbated by sitting or coughing. Ask if the patient has experienced rectal itching. Elicit a history of signs of infection such as fever, chills, nausea, vomiting, malaise, or myalgia. Ask the patient if he or she has experienced constipation, which is a common symptom because of the patient's attempts to avoid pain by preventing defecation.

PHYSICAL EXAMINATION. Inspect the patient's anal region. Note any red or oval swelling close to the anus. Digital examination may reveal a tender induration that bulges into the anal canal in the case of ischiorectal abscess, or a smooth swelling of the upper part of the anal canal or lower rectum in the case of submucous or high intermuscular abscess. Digital examination may reveal a tender mass high in the pelvis, even extending into one of the ischiorectal fossae if the patient has a pelvirectal abscess. Examination of a perianal abscess generally reveals no abnormalities. Examination may not be possible without anesthesia. Note any pruritic drainage or perianal irritation, which are signs of a fistula.

On inspection, the external opening of the fistula is usually visible as a red elevation of granulation tissue with purulent or serosanguinous drainage on compression. Palpate the tract, noting that there is a hardened cordlike structure.

PSYCHOSOCIAL. Patients with perirectal abscesses and fistulas may delay seeking treatment because of embarrassment relating to the location, the odor, or the sight of the lesion. Provide privacy and foster dignity when interacting with these patients. Inform the patient of every step of the procedure. Provide comfort during the examination.

DIAGNOSTIC HIGHLIGHTS

Test	Normal Result	Abnormality with Condition	Explanation
White blood cell (WBC) count	Adult males and females 4,500–11,000/μL	Elevated	Infection and inflammation may elevate the WBC count

Other Tests: Barium studies; sigmoidoscopy; colonoscopy

PRIMARY NURSING DIAGNOSIS

Pain (acute) related to inflammation of the perirectal area

OUTCOMES. Comfort level; Pain control behavior; Pain level; Wound healing

INTERVENTIONS. Pain management; Medication administration; Positioning; Teaching: Prescribed medication

☐ PLANNING AND IMPLEMENTATION

Collaborative

SURGICAL. The abscess is incised and drained surgically. For patients with fistulas, fistulotomies are performed to destroy the internal opening (infective source) and establish adequate drainage. The wound is then allowed to heal by secondary intention. Frequently, this procedure requires incision of sphincter fibers. Fistulectomy may be necessary, which involves the excision of the entire fistulous tract.

POSTOPERATIVE. Encourage the patient to urinate, but avoid catheterization and the use of suppositories. Postoperatively, a bulk laxative or stool softener is often prescribed on the day of the surgery. Intramuscular injections of analgesics are given to control pain. Assess the perirectal area hourly for bleeding for the first 12 to 24 hours postoperatively. When open fistula wounds are left, as in a fistulotomy, the anal canal may be packed lightly with oxidized cellulose.

Encourage the patient to drink clear liquids after any nausea has passed. Once clear liquids have been taken without nausea or vomiting, remove the intravenous fluids, and encourage the patient to begin to drink a full liquid diet the day after surgery. From there the patient can progress to a regular diet by the third day after surgery. The most common complications are incontinence (if sphincter fibers were incised during surgery) and hemorrhage.

PHARMACOLOGIC HIGHLIGHTS

Medication or Drug Class	Dosage	Description	Rationale
Antibiotics	Varies by drug	Antibiotics to cover GI infections: ampicillin plus aminoglycosides plus	Provide antimicrobials directed against bowel flora, particularly in

| either clindamycin or metronidazole; cefoxitin or cefotetan alone; aminoglycoside and cefoxitin | people who are immunosuppressed |

Independent

POSTOPERATIVE. Immediately following the procedure and before the patient enters the post-anesthesia care unit, place a dry, sterile dressing on the surgical site. Provide sitz baths twice a day for comfort and cleanliness, and place a plastic inflatable doughnut on a chair or bed to ease the pain of sitting. As soon as the patient tolerates activity, encourage ambulation to limit postoperative complications.

PATIENT TEACHING. Teach the patient how to keep the perianal area clean; teach the female patient to wipe the perineal area from front-to-back after a bowel movement in order to prevent genitourinary infection. Teach the patient about the need for a high-fiber diet that helps prevent hard stools and constipation. Explain how constipation can lead to straining that increases pressure at the incision site. Unless the patient is on fluid restriction, encourage him or her to drink at least 3 L of fluid a day.

DOCUMENTATION GUIDELINES

- Physical findings of perirectal area: Drainage, edema, redness, tenderness
- Response to comfort measures: Sitz baths, inflatable doughnuts, analgesia
- Reaction to ambulation postoperatively
- Presence of surgical complications: Poor wound healing, bleeding, foul wound drainage, fever, unrelieved pain
- Output (stool): Appearance, consistency, odor, amount, color, frequency

DISCHARGE AND HOME HEALTHCARE GUIDELINES

PATIENT TEACHING. Teach female patients to wipe from front to back to avoid the contamination of the vagina or urethra with drainage from the perirectal area. Teach the patient to avoid using bar soap directly on the anus because it can cause irritation to the anal tissue. Teach patients to dilute the soap with water on a washcloth to cleanse the area.

DIET. Explain the need to remain on a diet that will not cause physical trauma or irritation to the perirectal area. A diet high in fiber and fluids will help soften the stools, and bulk laxatives can help prevent straining. Emphasize to the patient the need to avoid spicy foods and hot peppers to decrease irritation to the perirectal area upon defecation.

MEDICATION. Teach the patient the purpose, dosage, schedule, precautions and potential side effects, interactions, and adverse reactions of all prescribed medications. Encourage the patient to complete the entire prescription of antibiotics that are prescribed.

Anorexia Nervosa

DRG Category: 428
Mean LOS: 5.7 days
Description: MEDICAL: Disorders of Personality and Impulse Control

Anorexia nervosa is an eating disorder of complex and life-threatening proportions. It is an illness of starvation that is brought on by a severe disturbance of body image and a morbid fear of obesity. One in 250 adolescents is affected, and, tragically, about 5% of those affected die. Anorexia nervosa is characterized by a person's refusal to maintain a minimally normal body weight for his or her height and age. This is done through inadequate food intake with no medical reason to account for weight loss. A distorted body image, dominated by an intense fear of obesity, leads to a relentless pursuit of an unreasonable and unhealthy thinness.

Weight is lost three ways in this condition: by restricting food intake, by excessive exercise, or by purging either with laxatives or by vomiting. Initially patients receive attention and praise for their extreme self-control over food intake, but as the illness progresses this attention is replaced by worry and efforts to monitor the patient's food intake. The increased negative attention and attempts at control of the patient serve to reinforce the patient's need for control and contribute to the progression of the illness. Adverse consequences of anorexia nervosa include possible atrophy of the cardiac muscle and cardiac dysrhythmias, alteration in thyroid metabolism, and estrogen deficiencies (those with long-standing estrogen deficiencies may develop osteoporosis). Refeeding may lead to slowed peristalsis, constipation, bloating, and fluid retention.

CAUSES

The causes of anorexia nervosa are not well understood, but are probably a combination of biological, psychological, and social factors. Abnormalities in central neurotransmitter activity are suggested by an alteration in serotonin metabolism. Psychological factors are the most frequently offered explanations. Onset usually occurs during early adolescence, a time when emerging sexuality, individuality, and separation from the family become central issues for the individual, especially the female. Anorexia nervosa is generally associated with an enmeshed family system where there are high performance expectations, rigid rules, and disturbed communication patterns. Another theory posits that anorexia nervosa occurs at the time of puberty as a person's way of avoiding adult responsibility and body image. The incidence of anorexia nervosa has increased in recent years, leading to the concern that it is a way for young women to rebel against the conflicted messages of the socialization roles of women.

GENDER AND LIFE SPAN CONSIDERATIONS

Anorexia nervosa generally occurs in adolescent females between the ages of 12 and 18, usually before the onset of puberty.

☐ ASSESSMENT

HISTORY. The patient typically claims to feel well and appears unconcerned about his or her weight loss. Obtain a diet and weight history. Assess the patient for both gradual and abrupt weight loss, and compare the values to normals for his or her age and height. Assess the current food intake; develop a diet history; elicit a description of exercise patterns; and assess for the amount and frequency of binging, purging, and laxative and diuretic use.

Assess the patient's perception of his or her body image. Although patients appear emaciated, they view themselves as fat. Hunger is not a complaint. Complaints include difficulty sleeping, abdominal discomfort and bloating after eating, constipation, cold intolerance, and polyuria; therefore, assess all of these dimensions. Unlike other starving individuals, anorexic people are not fatigued until malnutrition is severe. Most are restless and active, and some exercise excessively. Assess how the patient views food to determine the intensity of the fear of weight gain and his or her preoccupation with restricting food. Obtain a history of menses in females because usually the patient has a history of amenorrhea or a delayed onset of menses.

PHYSICAL EXAMINATION. On examination, the person appears extremely thin—if not emaciated—but animated. Obtain the patient's weight, which for diagnosis should be 15% below normal body weight for her or his age and height. You may note bradycardia, postural hypotension, and hypothermia. The patient's skin may appear dry, pale, and yellow-tinged, and the face and arms may be covered by a fine, downy hair (lanugo). The nails are generally brittle, and there is a loss of or thinning of hair. There is usually delayed sexual maturation. Breasts may be atrophied or poorly developed. Amenorrhea may precede or accompany the weight loss. Bowel sounds may be hypoactive.

PSYCHOSOCIAL. Psychosocial assessment should include assessment of self-esteem, peer relationships, changes in school performance, involvement in sports, perception of self as a sexual being, fear of sexual maturity, and perception of body image. Because anorexic patients are preoccupied with food, they often isolate themselves from peers and friends. When assessing body image, it is helpful to have the female patient take a female body outline and color in those areas that are pleasing and those that are displeasing.

Assess family communication patterns to determine who talks for whom, how decision-making and conflict are handled, and how parents view the current problem. Assess recent family crises and recent counseling experiences.

DIAGNOSTIC HIGHLIGHTS

General Comments: No laboratory test is able to diagnose anorexia nervosa, but supporting tests are used to follow the response to treatment and the progression of the illness.

Test	Normal Result	Abnormality with Condition	Explanation
Complete blood count	Red blood cells (RBC) 4.0–5.5 million/μL; white blood cells (WBC) 4,500–11,000/μL; hemoglobin (Hg) 12–18 g/dL; hematocrit (Hct) 37%–54%; reticulocyte count	Anemia; RBC < 4.0; hematocrit < 35%; hemoglobin < 12 g/dL	Caused by protracted under-nutrition

	0.5%–2.5% of total RBCs; platelets 150,000–400,000/µL		
Albumin	3.5–5.0 g/dL	Hypoalbuminemia; albumin < 3.5 g/dL	Caused by protracted undernutrition

Other Tests: Serum electrolytes may show hypokalemia, hypochloremia, hypomagnesemia, hypocalcemia, or hypoglycemia. Other laboratory tests include cholesterol (elevated), serum amylase (elevated), luteinizing hormone (decreased), testosterone (decreased), thyroxine (mildly decreased), electrocardiogram, blood urea nitrogen.

PRIMARY NURSING DIAGNOSIS

Altered nutrition: Less than body requirements related to an intense fear of becoming fat; denial of being (too) thin; excessive exercise

OUTCOMES. Nutritional status: Food and fluid intake; Nutrient intake; Body mass; Energy

INTERVENTIONS. Eating disorders management; Nutrition management; Nutritional counseling; Nutritional monitoring; Weight management

☐ PLANNING AND IMPLEMENTATION

Collaborative

If malnutrition is critical, the patient may need hospitalization. In the early stages of hospitalization, the patient may need tube feedings or hyperalimentation when intake is not sufficient to sustain metabolic needs and to prevent malnutrition or death. Usually the physician prescribes an initial diet of 1200 to 1600 kcal/day. Usually a target weight is chosen by the treatment team. Calories are increased slowly to ensure a steady weight gain of 2 to 4 pounds per week. Intravenous fluids may be used for severe dehydration to replace vascular volume and total body water.

The nurse collaborates with the dietitian to determine appropriate weight gain expectations. As refeeding takes place, the patient is involved in group therapy to talk about his or her feelings, learn new coping behaviors, decrease social isolation, develop a realistic perception of body image, and learn age-appropriate behaviors. Concurrently, both the individual patient and the family are involved in sessions to educate them on the nature and processes of the disease and the prognosis and treatment plan. Family therapy facilitates learning new ways of handling conflict, solving problems, and supporting the patient's move toward independence.

PHARMACOLOGIC HIGHLIGHTS

Medication or Drug Class	Dosage	Description	Rationale
Multivitamins	1 capsule per day po	Combination of water and fat-soluble organic	Provide for growth, reproduction, and health

> substances needed for good
> nutrition

Other Therapy: Symptoms may be managed with antacids, acetaminophen, bulk laxatives, stool softeners, anxiolytics agents (Ativan, Novolorazem)

Independent

The primary goal for the nurse is to establish a therapeutic, nonjudgmental, trusting relationship with the patient. The most important nursing intervention is to facilitate refeeding, thus helping the patient meet his or her weight goal and daily nutritional requirements. If tube feedings are needed, use a consistent and matter-of-fact approach. Be alert to possible disconnecting of the tube or signs of suicidal ideation or behavior.

Once tube feedings and total parenteral nutrition are no longer necessary, create a pleasant environment during meals. Smaller meals and supplemental snacks can be an effective strategy. Having a menu available for choice increases a sense of control for the patient. Maintain a regular weighing schedule. To avoid fear of weight gain, weigh patients with their back to the scale. Monitor the exercise program and set limits on physical activities. Work with the patient to develop strategies to stop vomiting and laxative and diuretic abuse as necessary.

Work with the family individually or in a group to educate about the disease prognosis and treatment process. Parents are educated in ways to encourage their adolescent without limiting his or her growth and independence. Identify family interaction patterns, and encourage each family member to speak for himself or herself. Communicate a message that it is acceptable for family members to be different from each other and that individuation is an important growth step. Assist parents in learning new ways to handle family and marital conflict. Teaching family negotiation skills is important.

DOCUMENTATION GUIDELINES

- Nutrition: Food and fluid intake for each meal; daily weights.
- Response to care and teaching: Understanding of the disease process and need for treatment (patient and family); understanding of ways to identify and cope with anxiety and anger; assessment of own body image
- Family meetings: Family interaction patterns
- Verbalizations of increased self-esteem as indicated by positive self-statements concerning appearance, accomplishments, or interactions with peers and family

DISCHARGE AND HOME HEALTHCARE GUIDELINES

Teach the patient how to maintain adequate nutrition and hydration. Explore non-food-related coping mechanisms and ways to have decreased association between food and emotions. Explore ways to recognize maladaptive coping behaviors and stressors that precipitate anxiety. Teach the patient strategies to increase self-esteem and to maintain a realistic perception of body image. Explore ways to maintain increased independence and age-appropriate behaviors.

Aortic Insufficiency

DRG Category: 135
Mean LOS: 4.3 days
Description: MEDICAL: Cardiac Congenital and Vascular Disorders, Age > 17 with CC

Aortic insufficiency (AI) is the incomplete closure of the aortic valve leaflets, which allows blood to regurgitate backward from the aorta into the left ventricle. The retrograde blood flow occurs during ventricular diastole when ventricular pressure is low and aortic pressure is high. The backflow of blood into the ventricle decreases forward flow in the aorta and increases left ventricular volume and pressure. In compensation, the left ventricle dilates and hypertrophies to accommodate the increased blood volume. Eventually, the increase in left ventricular pressure is reflected backward into the left atrium and pulmonary circulation.

Most patients with AI experience left ventricular failure. If heart failure is serious, the patient may develop pulmonary edema. If the patient is overtaxed by an infection, fever, or cardiac dysrhythmia, myocardial ischemia may also occur.

CAUSES

AI may result either from an abnormality of the aortic valve or from dilation and distortion of the aortic root. Common causes of valvular AI are rheumatic heart disease, endocarditis, trauma, and congenital anatomic abnormalities. Dilation or distortion of the aortic root may be due to systemic hypertension, aortic dissection, syphilis, Marfan's syndrome, and ankylosing spondylitis. Rheumatic heart disease and endocarditis cause the valve cusps to become thickened and retracted, whereas an aortic aneurysm causes dilation of the annulus (the valve ring that attaches to the leaflets). Chronic high blood pressure causes an increased pressure on the aortic valve, which may weaken the cusps. All of these conditions inhibit the valve leaflets from closing tightly, thus allowing backflow of blood from the high-pressure aorta.

GENDER AND LIFE SPAN CONSIDERATIONS

Symptoms do not usually occur until age 40 to 50 years. AI is more common in males unless it is associated with mitral valve disease, when it is then more common in women. Mild aortic regurgitation is probably quite common in the elderly but is usually overlooked.

☐ ASSESSMENT

HISTORY. A history of rheumatic fever suggests possible cardiac valvular malfunction; however, many patients who have had rheumatic fever do not remember having the condition. The most common symptom of AI is labored breathing on exertion, which may be present for many years before progressive symptoms develop. Angina with exertion, orthopnea, and paroxysmal nocturnal dyspnea are also principal complaints. Patients with severe AI often complain of an uncomfortable awareness of their heartbeat (palpitations), especially when lying down.

PHYSICAL EXAMINATION. Inspection of the thoracic wall may reveal a thrusting apical pulsation. Palpation of the precordium reveals the apical pulse to be bounding and displaced to the left. Auscultation of heart sounds reveals the classic decrescendo diastolic murmur. The duration of the murmur correlates with the severity of the regurgitation. Auscultation of breath sounds may reveal fine crackles (rales) if pulmonary congestion is present from left-sided heart failure. The pulmonary congestion will vary with the amount of exertion, the degree of recumbency, and the severity of regurgitation. Assessment of vital signs reveals a widened pulse pressure caused by the low diastolic blood pressure (often close to 40 mm Hg). The heart rate may be elevated, in an attempt to increase the cardiac output and decrease the diastolic period of backflow.

PSYCHOSOCIAL. The symptoms of AI usually develop gradually. Most people have already made adjustments in their lifestyle to adapt, not seeking treatment until the symptoms become debilitating. Assess what the patient has already done to cope with this condition.

DIAGNOSTIC HIGHLIGHTS

Test	Normal Result	Abnormality with Condition	Explanation
Cardiac catheterization	Normal aortic valve	Diastolic regurgitant flow from the aorta into the left ventricle; increased left ventricular end-diastolic volume/pressure	Aortic valve is incompetent and during diastolic phase, blood flows backward into the left ventricle
Doppler echocardiography	Normal aortic valve	Incompetent aortic valve	Aortic valve is incompetent and during diastolic phase, blood flows backward into the left ventricle

Other Tests: Echocardiography to assess aortic valve's structure and mobility electrocardiogram (ECG); chest radiography

PRIMARY NURSING DIAGNOSIS

Activity intolerance related to imbalance between oxygen supply and demand

OUTCOMES. Endurance; Energy conservation; Self-care; Ambulation: Walking; Circulation status; Cardiac pump effectiveness; Rest; Respiratory status; Symptom severity; Nutritional status: Energy

INTERVENTIONS. Activity therapy; Energy management; Circulatory care; Exercise therapy: ambulation; Oxygen therapy; Self-care assistance; Nutrition management

◻ PLANNING AND IMPLEMENTATION

Collaborative

MEDICAL. Medical management focuses initially on treating the underlying cause, such as endocarditis or syphilis. Patients are encouraged to limit strenuous physical activity. Fluid restrictions and diuretics may be ordered to reduce pulmonary congestion. Supplemental oxygenation will enhance oxygen levels in the blood to decrease labored breathing and chest pain.

SURGICAL. Most patients can be stabilized with medical treatment, but early elective valve surgery should be considered because the outlook for medically treated symptomatic disease is poor. Surgical repair or replacement is the most common treatment of AI.

The incompetent valve can be replaced with a synthetic or biologic valve, such as a pig valve. The choice of valve type is based on the patient's age and potential for clotting problems. The biologic valve usually shows structural deterioration after 6 to 10 years and needs to be replaced. The synthetic valve is more durable but also more prone to thrombi formations.

PHARMACOLOGIC HIGHLIGHTS

Medication or Drug Class	Dosage	Description	Rationale
Digoxin	0.25 mg po qd	Cardiotonic	Increases force of contraction in people with left ventricular dysfunction
Nifedipine	10–30 mg TID po or SL	Calcium channel blocker; systemic vasodilators	Decreases afterload (pressure that the left ventricle has to pump against) and decreases regurgitant blood flow.
Diuretics	Varies with drug	Thiazides; loop diuretics	Enhance pumping ability of the heart

Other Medications: If the incompetent valve is replaced surgically with a synthetic valve, patients are prescribed long-term anticoagulation therapy such as warfarin (Coumadin) to prevent thrombi from forming on the synthetic valve. Initially, heparin is given along with the warfarin, and the prothrombin time (PT) is monitored. As the PT value becomes therapeutic, the heparin is discontinued.

Independent

Physical and psychological rest decreases cardiac workload, which reduces the metabolic demands on the myocardium. Physical rest is enhanced by providing assistance with activities of daily living and encouraging activity restrictions. Most patients with advanced AI are placed on activity restrictions to decrease cardiac workload. If the patient is on bed rest, advise him or her to use the bedside commode, because research has shown it creates less workload for the heart than using the bedpan. If the patient can tolerate some activities, those that increase isometric work, such as lifting heavy objects, are more detrimental than activities such as walking or swimming.

Encourage the patient to avoid sudden changes in position to minimize increased cardiac demand. If the patient is hospitalized, instruct the patient to sit on the edge of the bed before standing. If pulmonary congestion is present, elevate the head of the bed slightly to enhance respiration.

Reducing psychological stress is a challenge. Approach the patient and family in a calm, relaxed manner. Decrease the fear of the unknown by providing explanations and current information and encouraging questions. To help the patient maintain or re-establish a sense of control, permit the patient to participate in decisions about aspects of care within his or her knowledge. If the patient decides to have valve surgery, offer to let him or her speak with someone who has already had the surgery. Seeing and talking with someone who has undergone surgery and lives with a replacement valve is usually very therapeutic.

DOCUMENTATION GUIDELINES

- Physical findings: Diastolic murmur, bounding apical pulse, rales in the lungs, presence or absence of pain, quality of pulses
- Response to diuretics, cardiotonics, vasodilators, and inotropic agents
- Reaction to activity restrictions, fluid restrictions, and cardiac diagnosis
- Presence of complications: Chest pain, bleeding, fainting

DISCHARGE AND HOME HEALTHCARE GUIDELINES

MEDICATIONS. Be sure the patient understands all medications, including the dose, route, action, adverse effects, and need for routine laboratory monitoring for anticoagulants.

COMPLICATIONS OF ANTICOAGULANTS. Explain the need to avoid activities that may predispose the patient to excessive bleeding. Teach the patient to hold pressure on bleeding sites to assist in clotting. Remind the patient to notify healthcare providers of anticoagulant use before procedures. Identify foods high in vitamin K (fats, fish meal, grains), which should be limited so that the effect of anticoagulants is not reversed.

TEACHING. Instruct the patient to report the recurrence or escalation of signs and symptoms of AI, which could indicate that the medical therapy needs readjusting or the replaced valve is malfunctioning. Patients with synthetic valves may hear an audible click like a ticking watch from the valve closure.

PREVENTION OF BACTERIAL ENDOCARDITIS. Patients who have had surgery are susceptible to bacterial endocarditis, which will cause scarring or destruction of the heart valves. Bacterial endocarditis may result from dental work, surgeries, and invasive procedures, so people who have repaired or replaced heart valves should be given antibiotics before and after these treatments.

Aortic Stenosis

DRG Category: 135
Mean LOS: 4.3 days
Description: MEDICAL: Cardiac Congenital and Vascular Disorders, Age > 17 with CC

Aortic stenosis is a narrowing of the aortic valve orifice, which obstructs outflow from the left ventricle during systole. The left ventricle must overcome the increased resistance to ejection by generating a higher-than-normal pressure during systole, which is achieved by stretching and generating a more forceful contraction. The blood is propelled through the narrowed aortic valve at an increased velocity.

As the stenosis in the aortic valve progresses, two sequelae occur. One is that cardiac output becomes fixed, making increases even with exertion impossible. The other is left-sided heart failure. Pressure overload of the heart occurs with concentric hypertrophy of the left ventricle. Left ventricular end diastolic pressure rises, myocardial oxygen demand increases, and left ventricular mass and wall stress are increased. The increase in left ventricular pressure is reflected backward into the left atrium. Because the left atrium is unable to empty adequately, the pulmonary circulation becomes congested. Eventually, right-sided heart failure can develop as well.

CAUSES

The predominant causative factor in aortic stenosis is congenital malformation of the aortic valve. Congenital causes can lead to unicuspid and bicuspid or malformed valves. When they become calcified, symptoms may occur. Stenosis can also occur with narrowing of the subvalvular outflow tract by fibroelastic membranes or muscle tissue. Rheumatic heart disease and degenerative calcification are other causes of aortic stenosis. The patient's age when the condition manifests itself usually suggests the cause.

GENDER AND LIFE SPAN CONSIDERATIONS

Aortic stenosis can occur at any age, depending on the cause. Congenital stenosis is usually seen in patients younger than 30 years old. In patients between the ages of 30 and 70 years, the cause is equally attributed to congenital malformation and rheumatic heart disease. Atherosclerosis and degenerative calcification of the aortic valve are the predominant causes for stenosis in people older than 70 years. Approximately 80% of people with aortic stenosis are male.

◻ ASSESSMENT

HISTORY. A history of rheumatic fever suggests possible cardiac valvular malfunction; however, many patients who have had rheumatic fever do not remember having had the condition; the diagnosis therefore is usually based on symptoms. Given the potential genetic causes, a family history of aortic stenosis can be significant.

PHYSICAL EXAMINATION. The classic symptoms of aortic stenosis are chest pain, fainting on exertion (syncope), and labored breathing on exertion due to heart failure. Inspection of the thoracic wall may reveal a thrusting apical pulsation. A systolic thrill (vibrations felt from turbulent blood flow) may be palpated over the second intercostal space to the right of the sternum. A lift or heave may be palpated over the apex of the heart.

Auscultation of heart sounds reveals a harsh systolic crescendo-decrescendo murmur. The murmur, referred to as diamond-shaped, is considered the hallmark of aortic stenosis. Auscultation of breath sounds may reveal fine crackles (rales) if pulmonary congestion is present in left-sided heart failure. The pulmonary congestion will vary with the amount of exertion and severity of stenosis.

PSYCHOSOCIAL. Because the symptoms of aortic stenosis are usually gradual, most people have already made adjustments in their lifestyle to adapt and do not seek treatment until the symptoms become debilitating. Assess what the patient has already done to cope with this condition. In addition, assess the patient's degree of anxiety about a diagnosed heart condition and potential treatment.

DIAGNOSTIC HIGHLIGHTS

Test	Normal Result	Abnormality with Condition	Explanation
Cardiac catheterization	Normal aortic valve	Opening in the aortic valve is obstructed and narrowed	Aortic valve is narrowed with the pressure gradient across the valve directly related to the degree of obstruction
Doppler echocardiography	Normal aortic valve	Stenosed aortic valve	Reveals abnormal blood flow patterns

Other Tests: Echocardiography to assess the aortic valve's structure and mobility; electrocardiogram (ECG); chest radiography

PRIMARY NURSING DIAGNOSIS

Activity intolerance related to imbalance between oxygen supply and demand

OUTCOMES. Endurance; Energy conservation; Self-care; Ambulation: Walking; Circulation status; Cardiac pump effectiveness; Rest; Respiratory status; Symptom severity; Nutritional status: Energy

INTERVENTIONS. Activity therapy; Energy management; Circulatory care; Exercise therapy: Ambulation; Oxygen therapy; Self-care assistance; Nutrition management

◻ PLANNING AND IMPLEMENTATION

Collaborative

MEDICAL. Most patients with aortic stenosis are placed on activity restrictions to decrease cardiac workload. Patients on bed rest should use the bedside commode because research has shown it creates less workload for the heart than using the bedpan. Fluid restrictions and diuretics may be ordered to reduce pulmonary congestion. Supplemental oxygenation will enhance oxygen levels in the blood to decrease labored breathing and chest pain.

SURGICAL. Surgical repair or replacement is the most common treatment of aortic stenosis. The average survival rate after the appearance of symptoms is less than 5 years for patients with aortic stenosis who are treated medically. Surgical treatment increases the survival rate dramatically. The stenotic valve can be replaced with a synthetic valve or a biologic valve, such as a pig valve. The choice of valve type is based on the patient's age and the potential for clotting problems. The biologic valve usually shows structural deterioration after 6 to 10 years and needs to be replaced. The synthetic valve is more durable but also more prone to thrombi formation.

PHARMACOLOGIC HIGHLIGHTS

Medication or Drug Class	Dosage	Description	Rationale
Digoxin	0.25 mg po qd	Cardiotonic	May be useful in the presence of heart failure and left ventricular dilation and impaired systolic function

Other Therapy: Diuretics. Nitrates and other vasodilators are to be avoided if possible because they reduce filling pressures and may lower systolic blood pressure. If the stenotic valve is replaced surgically with a synthetic valve, patients are prescribed long-term anticoagulation therapy such as warfarin (Coumadin) to prevent thrombi from forming on the synthetic valve. Initially, heparin is given along with the warfarin, and the prothrombin time (PT) is monitored. As the PT value becomes therapeutic, the heparin is discontinued.

Independent

Physical and psychological rest decreases cardiac workload, which reduces the metabolic demands of the myocardium. Physical rest is enhanced by providing assistance with activities of daily living and encouraging activity restrictions. Reducing psychological stress can also be difficult. Decrease the fear of the unknown by providing explanations and current information, and encouraging questions. To help the patient maintain or re-establish a sense of control, permit the patient to participate in decisions about aspects of care within his or her knowledge. If the patient decides on surgery, offer to let him or her speak with someone who has already had the surgery.

Discourage sudden changes in position to minimize increased cardiac demand. Instruct the patient to sit on the edge of the bed before standing. Elevate the head of the bed slightly if pulmonary congestion is present, to enhance respiration.

Monitoring physical status is a priority for nursing care. Assess for episodes of dizziness or fainting. The episodes may occur because of decreased cardiac output or cardiac dysrhythmias, so patients should be told to report occurrence of these symptoms promptly. Dizziness and fainting are correlated with sudden death, which, according to recent research, occurs in 10% to 20% of all patients with advanced aortic stenosis. Maintain a safe physical environment for the patient by removing obstructions in the patient's room.

DOCUMENTATION GUIDELINES

- Physical findings of systolic murmur, systolic thrill, and rales in the lungs
- Response to diuretics, nitrates, and rest
- Reaction to activity restrictions, fluid restrictions, and cardiac diagnosis
- Presence of complications: Chest pain, bleeding tendencies, labored breathing, fainting

DISCHARGE AND HOME HEALTHCARE GUIDELINES

MEDICATIONS. Be sure the patient understands all medications, including the dose, route, action, adverse effects, and need for routine laboratory monitoring for anticoagulants.

COMPLICATIONS OF ANTICOAGULANTS. Explain the need to avoid activities that may predispose the patient to excessive bleeding. Teach the patient to hold pressure on bleeding sites to assist in clotting. Remind the patient to notify healthcare providers of anticoagulant use before medical, surgical, or dental procedures. Identify foods high in vitamin K (green, leafy vegetables; oats; wheat; rye), which need to be eaten in a consistent amount, no binging, so the effect of anticoagulants is not reversed.

TEACHING. Instruct the patient to report the recurrence or escalation of signs and symptoms of aortic stenosis, which could indicate that the medical therapy needs readjusting or the replaced valve is malfunctioning. Patients with synthetic valves may hear an audible click like a ticking watch from the valve closure.

PREVENTION OF BACTERIAL ENDOCARDITIS. Patients who have had surgery are susceptible to bacterial endocarditis, which will cause scarring or destruction of the heart valves. Because bacterial endocarditis may result from dental work, surgeries, and invasive procedures, people who have repaired or replaced heart valves should be given antibiotics before and after these treatments.

Aplastic Anemia

DRG Category: 395
Mean LOS: 4.3 days
Description: MEDICAL: Red Blood Cell Disorders, Age > 17

Aplastic or hypoplastic anemia is a clinical syndrome that is characterized by a decrease in all formed elements of peripheral blood and its bone marrow. If all elements are suppressed—resulting in loss of production of healthy erythrocytes, platelets, and granulocytes—the condition is known as pancytopenia. Onset is often insidious and may become chronic; however, onset may be rapid and overwhelming when the cause is a myelotoxin (a poison that damages the bone marrow).

With complete bone marrow suppression, leukocytic failure may result in fulminating infections, greatly reducing the chances for complete recovery. Less severe cases may have an acute transient course or a chronic course with ultimate recovery, although the platelet count may remain subnormal, thus requiring a lifetime of precautions against bleeding. Aplastic anemia may produce fatal bleeding or infection, however, especially if it is idiopathic or stems from chloramphenicol or infectious hepatitis. Between 80% and 90% of patients with severe pancytopenia die.

CAUSES

Aplastic anemia often develops from an injury or damage to the stem cells that inhibit red blood cell (RBC) production. A less common development occurs when damaged bone marrow microvasculature creates an unfavorable environment for cell growth and maturation, resulting in aplastic anemia. Approximately 50% of aplastic anemias are caused by drugs such as antibiotics and anticonvulsants, toxic agents such as benzene and chloramphenicol, or radiation. Other causes include severe disease such as hepatitis and preleukemic and neoplastic infiltration of the bone marrow. Some forms of aplastic anemia are congenital, such as congenital hypoplastic anemia, Fanconi's anemia, and anemia of Blackfan and Diamond.

GENDER AND LIFE SPAN CONSIDERATIONS

Incidence of the condition is fairly low, without apparent sex or age preference. Congenital hypoplastic anemia occurs in infants in the third month of life, and Fanconi's anemia occurs in children under the age of 10.

□ ASSESSMENT

HISTORY. Determine if the patient has recently been exposed to known risk factors, such as recent treatment with chemotherapeutic drugs or antibiotics known to cause bone marrow suppression, radiation therapy, or accidental exposure to organic solvents. Establish a history of dyspnea, headache, intolerance for activity, progressive fatigue, malaise, chills and possibly fever, easy bruising, or frank bleeding.

PHYSICAL EXAMINATION. Examine the patient's skin for pallor or a jaundiced appearance. Inspect the patient's mucous membranes for bleeding. Inspect the patient's mouth and throat for lesions. Palpate the patient's lymph nodes to see if they are enlarged. Palpate the patient's liver and spleen, and note any enlargement. Auscultate the patient's chest for tachycardia and adventitious lung sounds.

PSYCHOSOCIAL. Assess the patient's mental status as an indicator of cerebral perfusion; assess the sensorimotor status to evaluate nervous system oxygenation. Patients may be anxious or fearful because of their low level of energy. Discomfort caused by mouth pain may cause the patient to feel irritable. The parents of an infant with a congenital form of aplastic anemia may be quite agitated over the child's illness.

DIAGNOSTIC HIGHLIGHTS

Test	Normal Result	Abnormality with Condition	Explanation
Complete blood count	Red blood cells (RBCs) 4.0–5.5 million/μL	Decreased to less than 1.0 million/μL; usually normochromic and normocytic, but may be macro-	Injury to the stem cells decreases production of blood cells

	cytic (enlarged) and anisocytotic (excessive variation in erythrocyte size)
White blood cells 4,500–11,000/μL	Decreased
Reticulocyte count 0.5–2.5% of total RBCs	Decreased
Platelets 150,000–400,000/μL	

Other Tests: Serum iron; coagulation tests; bone marrow biopsy.

PRIMARY NURSING DIAGNOSIS

Risk for infection related to inadequate secondary defenses (decreased hemoglobin and leukopenia), immunosuppression, pharmaceutic agents, chronic disease, malnutrition, or invasive procedures

OUTCOMES. Immune status; Knowledge: Infection control; Risk control; Risk detection; Nutritional status; Tissue integrity: Skin and mucous membranes

INTERVENTIONS. Environmental management; Infection control; Infection prevention; Medication prescribing; Nutritional management; Surveillance; Medication management

◻ PLANNING AND IMPLEMENTATION

Collaborative

MEDICAL. If anemia is caused by a particular agent or drug, withdrawing it is usually the first step in treatment. Clinical research studies have indicated some promising results with colony-stimulating factors (CSFs) such as interleukin-3 to encourage growth of specific blood elements. Oxygen is administered to ensure cellular oxygenation. Transfusion of packed RBCs and platelets may be required as supportive measures and to prevent bleeding. Platelets are sometimes given prophylactically when the anemia is chronic.

SURGICAL. Bone marrow transplantation is the treatment of choice for severe aplastic anemia. Protocols may vary slightly but generally indicate that the recipient must have a human leukocyte antigen (HLA) identical to that of the bone marrow donor (such as a sibling or twin) and receive a preparatory regimen of immunosuppression and radiation therapies.

POSTOPERATIVE. Postoperatively, relieve pain with analgesics and ice packs as needed. Monitor the patient for fever or chills, sore throat, or red or draining wounds, and administer prophylactic antibiotics as prescribed. Treat the patient's reactions to postoperative chemotherapy or radiation therapy as prescribed, by administering antiemetics to control nausea and vomiting. Administer allopurinol as prescribed, to prevent hyperuricemia that results from tumor breakdown products, and maintain the patient on the prescribed immunosuppressive regime. The physician may also prescribe vitamins, steroids, iron supplements, and folic acid supplements. Monitor postoperative patients for signs of graft-versus-host (GVH) reaction, including maculopapular rash, pancytopenia, jaundice, joint pain, and anasarca.

PHARMACOLOGIC HIGHLIGHTS

Medication or Drug Class	Dosage	Description	Rationale
Corticosteroids	Varies by drug	Glucocorticoids such as prednisone	Stimulates erythroid production

Other Therapy: Immunosuppression therapy with such agents as antithymo-cyte and antilymphocyte globulin or cyclosporine may be tried in patients who are not candidates for bone marrow transplant. Antibiotics may be given if infection or sepsis is present. Androgens, a controversial treatment, may be prescribed to stimulate bone marrow function.

Independent

Perform meticulous hand washing before patient contact. If protective or reverse isolation is required, use gloves, gown, and mask, and make sure that visitors do the same. Report any signs of systemic infection, and obtain the prescribed cultures. Provide frequent skin care, oral care, and perianal care to prevent both infection and bleeding. Avoid invasive procedures, if possible. When invasive procedures are necessary, maintain strict aseptic techniques and monitor the sites for signs of inflammation or drainage. Teach the patient and significant others symptoms of infection and to report them immediately to healthcare providers.

To help combat fatigue and conserve patient energy, plan frequent rest periods between activities. Instruct the patient in energy-saving techniques. Encourage the patient to increase activities gradually to the level of maximum tolerance.

Some patients with aplastic anemia undergo bone marrow transplants. Preoperatively, teach the patient about the procedure. Explain that chemotherapy and possible radiation treatments are necessary to remove cells that may cause the body to reject the transplant. Offer support and reassurance.

DOCUMENTATION GUIDELINES

- Laboratory findings: Complete blood count, platelet count, coagulation studies
- Physical findings: Skin color, presence of jaundice or ecchymoses, appearance of mouth and throat lesions, vital signs, presence of adventitious breath sounds
- Responses to interventions: Medications, bone marrow transplantation
- Progress toward desired outcomes: Activity tolerance, ability to maintain self-care

DISCHARGE AND HOME HEALTHCARE GUIDELINES

PREVENTION. Teach the patient the importance of avoiding exposure to individuals who are known to have acute infections. Emphasize the need for preventing trauma, abrasions, and breakdown of the skin. Be sure the patient understands the need to maintain a good nutritional intake to enhance the immune system and resistance to infections. Teach the patient the potential for bleeding and hemorrhage, and offer instruction in measures to prevent bleeding, including the use of a soft toothbrush and an electric razor. Discuss the need for regular dental examinations. Explain the importance of maintaining regular bowel movements to prevent straining and rectal bleeding. Instruct the patient to avoid enemas and rectal thermometers because of the risk of rectal perforation.

MEDICATIONS. Teach the patient the purpose, dosage, schedule, precautions and potential side effects, interactions, and adverse reactions of all prescribed medications.

COMPLICATIONS. Teach the patient to recognize the indicators of a systemic infection. Stress the fact that fever and usual wound infection signs may or may not be present since the immune system may be depressed. Instruct the patient about the symptoms that require immediate medical intervention, and make sure the patient knows who to notify. Stress the importance of reporting increased symptoms of anemia, including progressive fatigue, weakness, paresthesias, blurred vision, palpitations, and dizziness.

Appendicitis

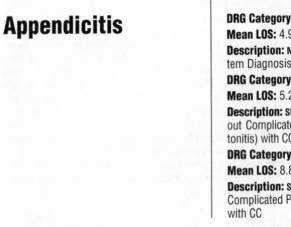

DRG Category: 188
Mean LOS: 4.9 days
Description: MEDICAL: Other Digestive System Diagnosis, Age > 17 with CC
DRG Category: 166
Mean LOS: 5.2 days
Description: SURGICAL: Appendectomy without Complicated Principal Diagnosis (Peritonitis) with CC
DRG Category: 164
Mean LOS: 8.8 days
Description: SURGICAL: Appendectomy with Complicated Principal Diagnosis (Abscess) with CC

Appendicitis is an acute inflammation of the veriform appendix, a narrow, blind tube that extends from the inferior part of the cecum. The appendix has no known function but does fill and empty as food moves through the gastrointestinal tract. Appendicitis begins when the appendix becomes obstructed or inflamed. Irritation and inflammation lead to engorged veins, stasis, and arterial occlusion. Eventually bacteria accumulate, and the appendix can develop gangrene. Appendicitis is the most common cause of acute inflammation in the right lower quadrant of the abdominal cavity and is the most common surgical emergency. If left undiagnosed, appendicitis can progress to appendiceal perforation and then to peritonitis, a life-threatening process.

CAUSES

Appendicitis is generally caused by obstruction. Since the appendix is a small, fingerlike appendage of the cecum, it is prone to obstruction as it regularly fills and empties with intestinal contents. The obstruction may be caused by a fecalith (a hard mass of feces), a foreign body in the lumen of the appendix, fibrous disease of the bowel wall, infestation of parasites, or twisting of the appendix by adhesions. Of all cases, approximately 60% are associated with hyperplasia of the submucosal lymphoid follicles and 35% to fecal stasis or fecalith.

GENDER AND LIFE SPAN CONSIDERATIONS

Twice as many men as women develop appendicitis, which occurs in approximately 10% of the population in Western countries. Appendicitis is rare before the age of 2 years, with the peak incidence of appendicitis occurring between 20 and 30 years of age. However, appendicitis in the elderly population is being reported with increasing frequency as life expectation increases. Unfortunately, appendicitis in the elderly tends to progress to perforation more rapidly, with fewer symptoms than expected. Older patients usually experience decreased pain sensations, very minor leukocyte elevations, and temperature elevations that are minimal when compared with younger patients.

◻ ASSESSMENT

HISTORY. Most patients with appendicitis report a history of midabdominal pain that initially comes in waves. In addition, early in the disease process, many patients report a discomfort that creates an urge to defecate to obtain relief. As the disease process progresses, patients usually complain of a constant epigastric or periumbilical pain that eventually localizes in the right lower quadrant of the abdomen. Some patients may report a more diffuse lower abdominal pain or referred pain. Should perforation of the appendix occur, pain may subside to generalized abdominal discomfort. In addition to pain, patients often complain of anorexia, nausea, vomiting, abdominal distension, and temporary constipation. Temperature elevations may also be reported (usually 100°F to 101°F).

PHYSICAL EXAMINATION. Observe the patient for typical signs of pain, including facial grimacing, clenched fists, diaphoresis, tachycardia, and shallow but rapid respirations. In addition, patients with appendicitis commonly guard the abdominal area by lying still with the right leg flexed at the knee. This posture diminishes tension on the abdominal muscles and increases comfort. Slight abdominal distension may also be observed.

Early palpation of the abdomen reveals slight muscular rigidity and diffuse tenderness around the umbilicus and midepigastrium. Later, as the pain shifts to the right lower quadrant, palpation generally elicits tenderness at McBurney's point (a point midway between the umbilicus and the right anterior iliac crest). Right lower quadrant rebound tenderness (production of pain when palpation pressure is relieved) is typical. Also, a positive Rovsing's sign may be elicited by palpating the left lower quadrant, which results in pain in the right lower quadrant.

PSYCHOSOCIAL. The patient with appendicitis faces an unexpected hospitalization and surgical procedure. Assess the patient's coping ability, typical coping mechanisms, stress level, and support system. Also, assess the patient's anxiety level regarding impending surgery and the recovery process.

DIAGNOSTIC HIGHLIGHTS

General Comments: Note that the diagnosis of appendicitis is made by clinical evaluation with the diagnostic tests of secondary importance.

Test	Normal Result	Abnormality with Condition	Explanation
Complete blood count	Adult males and females 4,500–11,000/μL	Infection and inflammation may elevate the WBC count	Leukocytosis may range from 10,000 to 16,000/μL. Neutrophil count is frequently elevated above 75%. In 10% of cases, leukocyte and differential cell counts are normal.

Other Tests: Flat-plate abdominal x ray to confirm the diagnosis; urinalysis in 25%–40% of people with appendicitis indicates pyria, albumininuria, and hematuria; serum electrolytes, blood urea nitrogen, and serum creatinine identify dehydration; abdominal ultrasound (particularly useful in women to rule out gynecological causes); abdominal computed tomography (CT) scan; barium enema; diagnostic laparoscopy.

PRIMARY PREOPERATIVE NURSING DIAGNOSIS

Pain (acute) related to inflammation

OUTCOMES. Comfort level; Pain control behavior; Pain level; Symptom severity

INTERVENTIONS. Analgesic administration; Anxiety reduction; Environmental management: Comfort; Pain management; Medication management; Patient-controlled analgesia assistance

PRIMARY POSTOPERATIVE NURSING DIAGNOSIS

Risk for infection related to the surgical incision

OUTCOMES. Immune status; Knowledge: Infection control; Risk control; Risk detection; Tissue integrity: Skin; Nutritional status

INTERVENTIONS. Infection control; Infection protection; Medication prescribing; Surveillance; Wound care; Nutritional management; Fluid/electrolyte management

☐ PLANNING AND IMPLEMENTATION

Collaborative

SURGICAL. An appendectomy (surgical removal of the appendix) is the preferred method of management for acute appendicitis if the inflammation is localized. If the appendix has ruptured and there is evidence of peritonitis or an abscess, conservative treatment consisting of antibiotics and intravenous (IV) fluids is given 6 to 8 hours prior to an appendectomy. Generally, an appendectomy is performed within 24 to 48 hours after the onset of symptoms under either general or spinal anesthesia. Preoperative management includes IV hydration, antipyretics, antibiotics, and, after definitive diagnosis, analgesics.

POSTOPERATIVE. Postoperatively, patient recovery from an appendectomy is usually uncomplicated, with hospital discharge in 24 to 72 hours (sometimes sooner if the laser technique is used). The development of peritonitis complicates recovery, and hospitalization may extend 5 to 7 days. The physician generally orders oral fluids and diet as tolerated within 24 to 48 hours after surgery.

Prescribed pain medications are given by the intravenous or intramuscular routes until the patient can take them orally. Antibiotics may continue postoperatively as a prophylactic measure. Ambulation is started the day of surgery or the first postoperative day.

PHARMACOLOGIC HIGHLIGHTS

Medication or Drug Class	Dosage	Description	Rationale
Crystalloid intravenous fluids	100–500 mL/hr of IV, depending on volume state of the patient	Isotonic solutions such as normal saline solution or lactated Ringers solution	Replaces fluids and electrolytes lost through fever and vomiting; replacement continues until urine output is 1 cc/kg of body weight and electrolytes are replaced
Antibiotics	Varies with drug	Broad-spectrum antibiotic coverage	Controls local and systemic infection and reduces the incidence of postoperative wound infection

Independent

PREOPERATIVE. Preoperatively, several nursing interventions focus on promoting patient comfort. Avoid applying heat to the abdominal area, which may cause appendiceal rupture. Permit the patient to assume the position of comfort while maintaining bed rest. Reduce the patient's anxiety and fear by carefully explaining each test, what to expect, and the reasons for the tests. Answer the patient's questions concerning the impending surgery, and provide the patient with instructions regarding splinting the incision with pillows during coughing, deep breathing, and moving.

POSTOPERATIVE. Postoperatively, assess the surgical incision for adequate wound healing. Note the color and odor of the drainage, any edema, the approximation of the wound edges, and the color of the incision. Encourage the patient to splint the incision during deep-breathing exercises. Assist the patient to maintain a healthy respiratory status by encouraging deep breathing and coughing 10 times every 1 to 2 hours for 72 hours. Turn the patient every 2 hours, and continue to monitor the breath sounds. Encourage the patient to assume a semi-Fowler position while in bed to promote lung expansion.

DOCUMENTATION GUIDELINES

- Location, intensity, frequency, and duration of pain
- Response to pain medication, ice applications, and position changes
- Patient's ability to ambulate and tolerate food
- Appearance of abdominal incision (color, temperature, intactness, drainage)

DISCHARGE AND HOME HEALTHCARE GUIDELINES

MEDICATIONS. Be sure the patient understands any pain medication prescribed, including doses, route, action, and side effects. Make certain the patient understands that he or she should avoid operating a motor vehicle or heavy machinery while taking such medication.

INCISION. Sutures are generally removed in the physician's office in 5 to 7 days. Explain the need to keep the surgical wound clean and dry. Teach the patient to observe the wound and report to the physician any increased swelling, redness, drainage, odor, or separation of the wound edges. Also instruct the patient to notify the doctor if a fever develops. The patient needs to know these may be symptoms of wound infection. Explain that the patient should avoid heavy lifting and should question the physician about when lifting can be resumed.

COMPLICATIONS. Instruct the patient that a possible complication of appendicitis is peritonitis. Discuss with the patient symptoms that indicate peritonitis, including sharp abdominal pains, fever, nausea and vomiting, and increased pulse and respiration. The patient must know to seek medical attention immediately should these symptoms occur.

NUTRITION. Instruct the patient that diet can be advanced to his or her normal food pattern as long as no gastrointestinal distress is experienced.

Arterial Occlusive Disease

DRG Category: 130
Mean LOS: 5.8 days
Description: MEDICAL: Peripheral Vascular Disorders with CC
DRG Category: 478
Mean LOS: 6.3 days
Description: SURGICAL: Other Vascular Procedures with CC

Arterial occlusive disease is characterized by reduced blood flow through the major blood vessels of the body because of an obstruction or narrowing of the lumen of the aorta and its major branches. Changes in the arterial wall include the accumulation of lipids, calcium, blood components, carbohydrates, and fibrous tissue in the endothelial lining. Arterial occlusive disease, which may be chronic or acute, may affect the celiac, mesenteric, innominate, subclavian, carotid, and vertebral arteries. Arterial disorders that may lead to arterial obstruction include arteriosclerosis obliterans, thromboangiitis obliterans, arterial embolism, and an aneurysm of the lower extremity. A sudden occlusion usually causes tissue ischemia and death, whereas a gradual blockage allows for the development of collateral vessels. Usually arterial occlusive diseases are only part of a complex disease syndrome that affects the entire body. Complications include severe ischemia, skin ulceration, gangrene, leg amputation, and sepsis.

CAUSES

Arteries can become occluded by atherosclerotic plaque, thrombi, or emboli. The most common cause of acute arterial insufficiency is embolization, with cardiac sources accounting for more than 70% of emboli. Subsequent obstruction and damage to the vessels can follow chemical or mechanical trauma and infections or inflammatory processes. Arteriosclerosis obliterans is marked by plaque formation on the intimal wall of medium-sized arteries, causing partial occlusion. In addition, there is calcification of the media and a loss of elasticity that predisposes the patient to dilation or thrombus formation. Thromboangiitis obliterans (Buerger's disease), which is characterized by an inflammatory infiltration of vessel walls, develops in the small arteries and veins (hands and feet) and tends to be episodic. Risk factors include hyperlipidemia, hypertension, and smoking.

GENDER AND LIFE SPAN CONSIDERATIONS

Thromboangiitis obliterans, a causative factor for arterial occlusive disease, typically occurs in male smokers between the ages of 20 and 40. Arterial insufficiency usually occurs in individuals over 50 years of age.

☐ ASSESSMENT

HISTORY. Elicit a history of previous illnesses or surgeries that were vascular in nature; ask if the patient has been diagnosed with arterial occlusive disease in the past. Determine if a positive family history exists for hypertension or vascular disorders in first-order relatives. Ask if the patient smokes cigarettes; eats a diet high in fats; leads a sedentary lifestyle; or is subject to emotional stress, anxiety, or ulcers. Determine if the patient has experienced any pain, swelling, redness, or pallor. Establish a history of signs and symptoms that may point to the site of occlusion. Determine if the patient has experienced any transient ischemic attacks (TIAs) because of reduced cerebral circulation. Elicit a history of such signs and symptoms as unilateral sensory or motor dysfunction, difficulty in speaking (aphasia), confusion, difficulty with concentration, or headaches, all of which are signs of possible carotid artery involvement. Ask if the patient has experienced signs of vertebrobasilar artery involvement, such as binocular visual disturbances, vertigo, dysarthria, or episodes of falling down. Determine if the patient has experienced lameness in the right arm (claudication), which is a sign of possible innominate artery involvement. The specific finding in peripheral arterial insufficiency is intermittent claudication. The pain is insidious in onset, occurring with exercise and relieved by rest.

Determine if the patient's mesenteric artery is involved by asking if he or she has experienced acute abdominal pain, nausea, vomiting, or diarrhea. Ask the patient if he or she has experienced numbness, tingling (paresthesia), paralysis, muscle weakness, or sudden pain in both legs, which are all signs of aortic bifurcation occlusion. Determine if the patient has experienced sporadic claudication of the lower back, buttocks, and thighs or impotence in male patients, all of which are indicators of iliac artery occlusion. Elicit a history of sporadic claudication of the patient's calves after exertion; ask if the patient has experienced pain in the feet—these are signs of femoral and popliteal artery involvement.

PHYSICAL EXAMINATION. Observe both legs, noting alterations in color or temperature of the affected limb. Cold, pale legs may suggest aortic bifurcation occlusion. Inspect the patient's legs for signs of cyanosis, ulcers, or gangrene. Limb perfusion may be inadequate, resulting in thickened and opaque nails, shiny and atrophic skin, decreased hair growth, dry or fissured heels, and loss of subcutaneous tissue in the digits. Check the patient's skin on a daily basis.

The most important part of the examination is palpation of the peripheral pulses. Absence of a normally palpable pulse is the most reliable sign of occlusive disease. Comparison of pulses in both extremities is helpful. Ascertain, also, whether the arterial wall is palpable, tortuous, or calcified. Auscultation over the main arteries is useful, as a bruit (sound produced by turbulent flow of blood through an irregular or stenotic lumen) often indicates an atheromatous plaque. A bruit over the right side of the neck is a possible indication of innominate artery involvement.

PSYCHOSOCIAL. Occlusive diseases are chronic or lead to chronic illness. They are usually slow in onset, and much irreversible vascular damage may have occurred before symptoms are severe enough to bring the patient for treatment. Treatment is often long and tedious and brings additional concerns regarding finances, curtailment of usual social outlets, and innumerable other problems. Assess the patient's ability to cope with a chronic illness.

DIAGNOSTIC HIGHLIGHTS

Test	Normal Result	Abnormality with Condition	Explanation
Ultrasound arteriography (Doppler ultrasonography)	Negative for presence of aneurysm or atherosclerosis or thrombus; normal blood flow velocity	Narrowed lumen, reduced blood velocity, or both	Reflects the velocity of blood flowing in the underlying vessel, structure, and size
Segmental arterial pressure monitoring	Blood pressure readings in thigh and calf are higher than in upper extremities	Blood pressure readings in thigh and calf are lower than in upper extremities with the presence of arterial disease	Simultaneous sphygmomanometer readings of systolic pressure placed on the extremities to measure pressure differences between upper and lower and between like extremities

Other Tests: Plethysmography; ophthalmodynamometry; digital vascular imaging; arteriogram; exercise testing

PRIMARY NURSING DIAGNOSES

Altered tissue perfusion (peripheral) related to decreased arterial flow.

OUTCOMES. Fluid balance; Muscle function; Tissue integrity: Peripheral

INTERVENTIONS. Circulatory care; Circulatory precautions; Fluid management; Medication management; Peripheral sensation management; Positioning; Pressure ulcer prevention; Skin surveillance; Embolus precautions; Exercise therapy

◻ PLANNING AND IMPLEMENTATION

Collaborative

SURGICAL. Surgery is indicated for patients who have advanced arterial disease or for those with severe pain that impairs activities. Surgical procedures include arterial bypass surgery, embolectomy, angioplasty, sympathectomy, and amputation.

If arteriosclerosis obliterans is rapidly progressing or has not responded to conservative management and intermittent claudication has become disabling, lower-extremity arterial bypass is performed. The femoropopliteal arterial segment is the most common site of occlusion. The diseased femoropopliteal segment can be bypassed with a synthetic prosthetic material (Teflon or Dacron) or an autogenous vein graft, such as with the saphenous vein, can be performed. Care following femoropopliteal bypass is the same as for other arterial surgery.

PERIOPERATIVE CARE. In the preoperative stage, assess the patient's circulatory status by observing skin color and temperature and checking peripheral pulses. Provide analgesia as needed. Use an infusion monitor or pump to administer heparin intravenously. Note any signs of cerebrovascular accident, such as periodic blindness or numbness in a limb.

PHARMACOLOGIC HIGHLIGHTS

Medication or Drug Class	Dosage	Description	Rationale
Anticoagulants	Varies by drug	Prolongs clotting time	Prevents extension of a clot and inhibiting further clot formation
Fibrinolytics	Varies by drug	Dissolves existing thrombi	Used when required to preserve organ and limb function.

Other Drugs: Intermittent claudication caused by chronic arterial occlusive disease may be treated with pentoxifylline (Trental), which can improve blood flow through the capillaries by increasing red blood cell flexibility. Antiplatelet agents: aspirin, dipyridamole, ticlopidine

Independent

PREVENTION AND TEACHING. Emphasize to the patient the need to quit smoking and limit caffeine intake. Recommend maintaining a warm environmental temperature of about 21°C (70°F) to prevent chilling. Teach the patient to avoid elevating the legs or using the knee gatch on the bed, to keep legs in a slightly dependent position for periods during the day, to avoid crossing the legs at the knees or ankles, and to wear support stockings. Explain why the patient needs to avoid pressure on the affected extremity and vigorous massage, and recommend the use of padding for ischemic areas.

Stress the importance of regular aerobic exercise to the patient. Explain that activity improves circulation through muscle contraction and relaxation. Exercise also stimulates collateral circulation that increases blood flow to the ischemic area. Recommend 30 to 40 minutes of activity with warm-up and cooldown activities on alternate days. Also suggest walking at a slow pace and performing ankle rotations, ankle pumps, and knee extensions daily. Recommend Buerger-Allen exercises, if indicated. If intermittent claudication is present, stress to the patient the importance of allowing adequate time for rest between exercise and of monitoring one's tolerance for exercise.

Provide good skin care, and teach the patient to monitor and protect the skin. Recommend the use of moisturizing lotion for dry areas, and demonstrate meticulous foot care. Advise the patient to wear cotton socks and comfortable, protective shoes at all times and to change socks daily. Advise the patient to seek professional advice for thickened or deformed nails, blisters, corns, and calluses. Stress the importance of avoiding the application of direct heat to the skin. The patient also needs to know that arterial disorders are usually chronic. Medical follow-up is necessary at the onset of skin breakdown such as abrasions, lesions, or ulcerations to prevent advanced disease with necrosis.

DOCUMENTATION GUIDELINES

- Physical findings: Presence of redness, pallor, skin temperature, peripheral pulses, trophic changes, asymmetrical changes in pulse quality, capillary blanch, condition of skin
- Neurologic deficits: Tenderness to touch, lameness, sensory or motor dysfunction
- Response to balanced activity: Lameness, pain, level of activity that produces pain
- Presence of complications: Infection, ulcers, gangrene, loss pulses
- Adherence to the rehabilitation program: Attitude toward exercise, changes in symptoms as response to exercise

DISCHARGE AND HOME HEALTHCARE GUIDELINES

PREVENTION. To prevent arterial occlusive disease from progressing, teach the patient to decrease as many risk factors as possible. Quitting cigarette smoking is of utmost importance and may be the most difficult lifestyle change. Behavior modification techniques and support groups may be of assistance with lifestyle changes.

MEDICATIONS. Be sure the patient understands all medications, including the dosage, route, action, adverse effects, and need for routine laboratory monitoring for anticoagulants.

ADHERENCE TO THE REHABILITATION PROGRAM. Ensure that the patient understands that the condition is chronic and not curable. Stress the importance of adhering to a balanced exercise program, using measures to prevent trauma and reduce stress. Include the patient's family in the plans.

Asthma

DRG Category: 096
Mean LOS: 5.2 days
Description: MEDICAL: Bronchitis and Asthma, Age > 17 with CC

Asthma is classified as an intermittent, reversible, obstructive disease of the lungs. It is a disease of the airways that is characterized by airway inflammation and hyperreactivity (increased responsiveness to a wide variety of triggers). Hyperreactivity leads to airway obstruction due to acute onset of muscle spasm in the smooth muscle of the tracheobronchial tree, thereby leading to a narrowed lumen. In addition to muscle spasm, there is swelling of the mucosa, which leads to edema. Lastly, the mucous glands increase in number, hypertrophy, and secrete thick mucus.

Asthma can be divided into two types: extrinsic and intrinsic. Extrinsic asthma results from an allergic response. An allergen (antigen) is introduced to the body, and sensitizing antibodies such as immunoglobulin E (IgE) are formed. IgE antibodies bind to tissue mast cells and basophils in the mucosa of the bronchioles, lung tissue, and nasopharynx. An antigen-antibody reaction releases primary mediator substances such as histamine and slow-reacting substance of anaphylaxis (SRS-A) and others. These mediators cause contraction of the smooth muscle and tissue edema. In addition, goblet cells secrete a thick mucus into the airways that causes obstruction. Intrinsic asthma results from all other causes except allergies, such as infections (especially viral), inhaled irritants, and other causes or etiologies. The parasympathetic nervous system becomes stimulated, which increases bronchomotor tone, resulting in bronchoconstriction.

CAUSES

The main triggers for asthma are allergies, viral infections, autonomic nervous system imbalances that can cause an increase in parasympathetic stimulation, medications, psychological factors, and exercise. Of asthmatic conditions in patients under 30 years old, 70% are caused by allergies. Three major indoor allergens are dust mites, cockroaches, and cats. In older patients the cause is almost always nonallergic types of irritants such as smog. Heredity plays a part in about one-third of the cases.

GENDER AND LIFE SPAN CONSIDERATIONS

Although the incidence of asthma is estimated at 1% to 5% in the general population, children have a higher incidence of 12%. Children make up about half of the people with asthma. Asthma is diagnosed more frequently in males under 14 years and over 45 years of age and in females between the ages of 15 and 45. Men are twice as likely as women to get asthma.

◻ ASSESSMENT

HISTORY. Because patients (especially children) with asthma have a history of allergies, obtain a thorough description of the response to allergens or other irritants. The patient may describe a sudden onset of symptoms after exposure, with a sense of suffocation. Symptoms include dyspnea, wheezing, and a cough (either dry or productive) and also chest tightness, restlessness, anxiety, and a prolonged expiratory phase. Ask if the patient has experienced a recent viral infection. Children with an impending asthma attack may have been vomiting because of the tendency to swallow coughed up mucus rather than expectorating it.

PHYSICAL EXAMINATION. The patient with an acute attack of asthma appears ill, with shortness of breath so severe that he or she can hardly speak. In acute airway obstruction, patients use their accessory muscles for breathing and are often profoundly diaphoretic. Some patients have an increased anteroposterior thoracic diameter. Children with asthma often prefer standing or sitting leaning forward to ease breathing. As airway obstruction becomes more serious, children may develop sternocleidomastoid contractions that indicate an increased expiratory effort, supraclavicular contractions that indicate an increased expiratory effort, and nasal flaring. If the patient has marked color changes such as pallor or cyanosis or becomes confused, restless, or lethargic, respiratory failure may be on the horizon. Percussion of the lungs usually produces hyperresonance, and palpation may reveal vocal fremitus. Auscultation reveals high-pitched inspiratory and expiratory wheezes, but with a major airway obstruction, breath sounds may be diminished. As the obstruction improves, breath sounds may actually worsen as they can be auscultated throughout the lung fields. Usually the patient also has a prolonged expiratory phase of respiration. A rapid heart rate, mild systolic hypertension, and a paradoxic pulse may also be present.

PSYCHOSOCIAL. The emergency situation and an unfamiliar environment can aggravate the symptoms of the disease, especially if this is the patient's first experience with the condition. If the patient is a child and the parent is anxious, the child's level of anxiety increases and the attack may worsen.

DIAGNOSTIC HIGHLIGHTS

Test	Normal Result	Abnormality with Condition	Explanation
Forced vital capacity (FVC): Maximum volume of air that can be forcefully expired after a maximal lung inspiration	4.0 L	50% of the predicted value	Airway obstruction decreases flow rates
Forced expiratory volume in 1 second (FEV$_1$): Volume of air expired in 1 second from the beginning of the FVC maneuver	3.0 L	25%–35% of the predicted value	Airway obstruction decreases flow rates; hospitalization is recommended if FVC is less than 1 L; FEV$_1$/FVC should be 80% normally, but in asthma it decreases to as low as 25%
Forced expiratory flow (FEF): Maximal	Varies by body size	25% of the predicted value	Predicts obstruction of smaller airways

flow rate attained during the middle (25%–75%) of FVC maneuver			
Residual volume (RV): Volume of air remaining in lungs at end of a maximal expiration	1.2 L	Increased up to 400% normal	Increased RV indicates obstruction; may remain increased for up to 3 weeks after the attack
Functional residual capacity (FRC): Volume of air remaining in lungs at end of a resting tidal volume	2.3 L	Increased up to 200%	Increased FRC indicates air trapping

Other Tests: Chest x ray, skin testing, pulse oximetry, arterial blood gases, serum IgE. Peak expiratory flow rates (PEFR; maximal flow rate attained during the FVC maneuver; decreased from baseline during periods of obstruction) may be used at home daily for patients who require daily medications.

PRIMARY NURSING DIAGNOSIS

Ineffective airway clearance related to obstruction from narrowed lumen and thick mucus

OUTCOMES. Respiratory status: Gas exchange; Respiratory status: Ventilation; Symptom control behavior; Treatment behavior: Illness or injury; Comfort level

INTERVENTIONS. Airway management; Anxiety reduction; Oxygen therapy; Airway suctioning; Airway insertion and stabilization; Cough enhancement; Mechanical ventilation; Positioning; Respiratory monitoring

☐ PLANNING AND IMPLEMENTATION

Collaborative

Patients often require intravenous fluid replacement. Unless contraindicated by a cardiac problem, 3000 to 4000 mL/day of fluid is usually administered intravenously, which helps loosen secretions and facilitates expectoration of the secretions. Low-flow oxygen therapy based on arterial blood gas results is often administered to treat hypoxemia. For the patient with increasing airway obstruction, endotracheal intubation and perhaps mechanical ventilation may be needed to maintain adequate airway and breathing. Close follow-up is needed when patients are discharged from the hospital because airway hyperactivity usually persists for 4 to 6 weeks after the event.

PHARMACOLOGIC HIGHLIGHTS

Medication or Drug Class	Dosage	Description	Rationale
Bronchodilators	Varies by	Inhaled beta$_2$ adrenergic	Reversal of airflow

	drug	agonists by metered-dose inhaler (MDI) such as albuterol	obstruction
Systemic corticosteroids	Varies by drug	Methylprednisolone IV; prednisone po	Decrease inflammatory response. Ideal dose is not defined well, but desired outcome is to speed recovery and limit symptoms

Other Drugs: Xanthines such as theophylline have been used successfully in treating chronic severe steroid-dependent asthmatics. Cromolyn sodium decreases bronchospasm, but it is not effective for acute bronchospasms and is used as a preventive measure.

Independent

Maintenance of airway, breathing, and circulation are the primary considerations during an acute attack. Patients should be on bed rest to minimize their oxygen consumption and to decrease the work of breathing. Note that patients usually assume a position to ease breathing; some patients breathe more easily while sitting in an upright position:do not impose bed rest on a patient who can only breathe in another position. Ask questions that can be answered by nodding or a brief one-word answer so the patient can conserve energy for breathing. If the patient is a child, allow the parents to stay with the child during acute attacks. Have the parents identify a security item that reassures the child, such as a special blanket or toy, and keep the item with the child at all times. Reinforce coping strategies to the parents, and allow them to express any feelings of guilt and helplessness.

For strategies to prevent future attacks, discuss triggers that can induce asthma attacks and ways to avoid them. If the attack is triggered by an allergen, explore with the patient or family the source and discuss possible strategies for eliminating it. Cold air and exercise may increase symptoms. Aspirin and nonsteroidal anti-inflammatory agents can cause sudden, severe airway obstruction.

Outline the signs and symptoms that require immediate attention. Instruct the patient to notify the physician should he or she develop a respiratory infection that could trigger an attack. Instruct patients regarding their medications, particularly metered-dose inhalers (MDIs), and the indications for use. It is important that the patient use the bronchodilator MDIs first, then use the steroid inhalers. Explain that patients on steroid inhalers need to rinse their mouths out after using them to avoid getting thrush.

DOCUMENTATION GUIDELINES

- Respiratory status: Patency of airway, auscultation of the lungs, presence or absence of adventitious breath sounds, respiratory rate and depth
- Response to medications, oxygen therapy, hydration, bed rest
- Presence of complications: Respiratory failure, ruptured bleb that may result in a pneumothorax

DISCHARGE AND HOME HEALTHCARE GUIDELINES

To prevent asthma attacks, teach patients the triggers that can precipitate an attack. Teach the patient and family the correct use of medications, including the dosage, route, action, and side effects. Provide instructions about the proper use of MDIs. In rare instances, asthma can lead to respiratory failure if patients are not treated immediately or are unresponsive to treatment (status asthmaticus). Explain that any dyspnea unrelieved by medications, and accompanied by wheezing and accessory muscle use, needs prompt attention from a healthcare provider.

Atelectasis

DRG Category: 101
Mean LOS: 4.6 days
Description: MEDICAL: Other Respiratory System Diagnoses with CC

Atelectasis is the collapse of lung tissue because of airway obstruction, an abnormal breathing pattern, or compression of the lung tissue. When the airway becomes completely obstructed, the gas distal to the obstruction becomes absorbed into the pulmonary circulation and the lung collapses. When gas is removed from portions of the lungs, unoxygenated blood passes unchanged through capillaries, and hypoxemia results.

Abnormal breathing patterns, such as hypoventilation and a slow respiratory rate, can also lead to atelectasis. In such cases, the lung does not fully expand, which causes the lower airways to collapse. Compression of the lung tissue from a tumor, pleural effusion, or pneumothorax can also result in atelectasis. Complications of atelectasis include hypoxemia, acute respiratory failure, and pneumonia.

CAUSES

Atelectasis occurs most frequently after surgery and is a major concern for acute care nurses. Patients with abdominal and/or thoracic surgery are the most susceptible, especially in the older age group. The duration of the surgery is also a risk factor. Patients in surgery for more than 4 hours have a 50% incidence of severe atelectasis, compared to a 19% incidence for those in surgery for 2 hours. Other causes of atelectasis are mucous plugs in patients who smoke heavily and inflammation from inflammatory lung disease. Atelectasis also occurs in patients with central nervous system depression following a drug overdose or a critical cerebral event such as a cerebrovascular accident.

GENDER AND LIFE SPAN CONSIDERATIONS

Premature infants with idiopathic respiratory distress syndrome develop atelectasis. Atelectasis, however, can occur at any age and equally in men and women. It can occur with a complete obstruction of the lung because of a foreign object, although foreign body aspiration is more common in children under age 4 than in adults. Generally, however, atelectasis occurs most often in the elderly because the aging lung is less compliant.

☐ ASSESSMENT

HISTORY. Assess the patient for such preoperative risk factors as obesity, preexisting respiratory problems, and smoking. Because surgical patients are at risk, be alert for components of the postoperative history that may contribute to atelectasis: a decrease in total lung volume because of pain and splinting, changes in breathing patterns from incisional discomfort or medications, advanced age, and a need for an increased fraction of inspired oxygen (FiO_2). Other factors include use of narcotic analgesics that depress the respiratory drive, immobility, a decrease in consciousness, muscular weakness, hypotension, sepsis, and use of a nasogastric tube.

PHYSICAL EXAMINATION. The patient may appear asymptomatic if only small areas of the lung are involved, or acutely ill with extreme shortness of breath and clinical signs of oxygen deficit such as confusion, agitation, rapid heart rate, and even combative behavior when large areas are affected. Suprasternal, substernal, and intercostal retractions may be present, depending on the severity of atelectasis. Percussion reveals a dullness over the affected lung area. When the patient's breath sounds are auscultated, you may hear decreased breath sounds or even find breath sounds to be absent. In addition, many patients have fine, late inspiratory crackles and coarse crackles or wheezes with airway obstruction.

PSYCHOSOCIAL. The patient with atelectasis may be very anxious if breathing becomes too difficult. If the atelectasis is a result of foreign body aspiration by a child, the parents may be upset and guilty. Determine the patient's and parents' abilities to cope with the stressful situation.

DIAGNOSTIC HIGHLIGHTS

Test	Normal Result	Abnormality with Condition	Explanation
Chest x ray	Clear lung fields	Areas of increased density at the site of alveolar collapse	Air-filled lungs are radiolucent (x rays pass through tissue, which appears as a dark area) but collapsed areas appear more dense. Findings may occur on the second day after the occurrence of atelectasis

Other Tests: Pulmonary function tests (PFTs); arterial blood gases (ABGs)

PRIMARY NURSING DIAGNOSIS

Ineffective airway clearance related to obstruction and lung collapse

OUTCOMES. Respiratory status: Gas exchange; Respiratory status: Ventilation; Symptom control behavior; Treatment behavior: Illness or injury; Comfort level

INTERVENTIONS. Airway management; Anxiety reduction; Oxygen therapy; Airway suctioning; Airway insertion and stabilization; Cough enhancement; Positioning; Respiratory monitoring

☐ PLANNING AND IMPLEMENTATION

Collaborative

Patients in pain, especially following abdominal and thoracic surgery, tend to breathe shallowly to decrease their discomfort. Pain medications allow them to breathe more deeply and expand their lungs. Use caution in overmedicating patients, however, because that will reduce respiratory excursion. In the immediate postoperative period, narcotic analgesia is often prescribed because it is readily reversible by naloxone (Narcan).

Incentive spirometry, chest percussion, and postural drainage may be prescribed by the physician to increase gas exchange and to decrease the risk of atelectasis. Oxygen may be delivered with humidification to improve clearance of mucus. If atelectasis persists, the physician may prescribe a mask with continuous positive airway pressure (CPAP). With the use of a CPAP mask, positive airway pressure is maintained throughout the respiratory cycle. In addition, CPAP prevents and reverses airway closure, thus expanding the lung volumes and reestablishing the functional residual capacity (FRC). If atelectasis persists and hypoxemia becomes life threatening, endotracheal intubation and mechanical ventilation with positive-pressure ventilation and positive end-expiratory pressure (PEEP) may be necessary, but these aggressive therapies are usually not needed.

PHARMACOLOGIC HIGHLIGHTS

Medication or Drug Class	Dosage	Description	Rationale
Bronchodilators	Varies with drug	Beta$_2$ agonists	Dilate bronchioles, stimulate cilia, facilitate in removal of secretions

Independent

Instruct the preoperative patient on coughing and deep-breathing exercises prior to surgery, before incisional pain makes learning difficult. Teach the patient breathing exercises, such as pursed-lip breathing and abdominal breathing to expand the lungs. As soon as the patient is awake and alert after surgery, with a patent airway and adequate breathing, encourage him or her to cough and breathe deeply to help expand the lung. If the patient has abdominal or thoracic incisions, use a pillow to splint the incision to reduce discomfort during breathing exercises. Encourage the patient to use the incentive spirometer at the bedside every 2 hours when he or she is awake.

Encourage the patient to ambulate as soon as possible to reduce complications of immobility, which cause retention of secretions and decreased lung volumes. Seating the patient upright allows the patient to breathe more deeply because the lungs can expand better. Turn patients on bed rest at least every 2 hours.

Encourage patients who can expectorate secretions to cough; place a paper bag on the side rails of the bed for sanitary tissue disposal. If the patient is not on fluid restriction, explain that he or she should drink at least 2 to 3 L of fluid a day to liquefy secretions. If the patient is unresponsive, suction the patient endotracheally to remove sputum and to stimulate coughing.

If a child has developed atelectasis because of foreign-body obstruction, teach the parents to maintain a safe environment. The most commonly aspirated objects are safety pins and hard foods such as corn, raisins, and peanuts. Parents should not allow children to run or walk while eating because activity predisposes the child to aspiration. Teach the patient and family to evaluate all toys for removable parts; explain that coins are commonly aspirated and should not be given to children. Explain to parents that they should not allow a young child to play with baby powder during diaper changes because if the top is altered and powder spills onto the child's face, the child can inhale it.

DOCUMENTATION GUIDELINES

- Physiologic response: Respiratory status of the patient, vital signs, breath sounds, presence of respiratory distress, arterial blood gases, or pulse oximetry results
- Response to pain medications, respiratory adjuncts
- Ability to cough and breathe deeply, mobilization of secretions

DISCHARGE AND HOME HEALTHCARE GUIDELINES

PREVENTION. To prevent atelectasis, instruct the patient prior to surgery about coughing, deep breathing, and early ambulation. Encourage the patient to request and take pain medications to assist with deep-breathing exercises. Explain that an adequate fluid intake is important to help loosen secretions and aid in their removal.

MEDICATIONS. Instruct patients regarding the use of any medications they are to take at home. Discuss the indications for use and any adverse effects. If patients are placed on antibiotics, instruct them to finish all of the antibiotics even if they feel better before the prescription is completed.

Atrial Dysrhythmias

DRG Category: 138
Mean LOS: 3.9 days
Description: MEDICAL: Cardiac Arrhythmia and Conduction Disorders with CC

A cardiac dysrhythmia is any disturbance in the normal rhythm of the electrical excitation of the heart. It can be the result of a primary cardiac disorder, a response to a systemic condition, or the result of an electrolyte imbalance or a drug toxicity. The severity of a dysrhythmia, depending on its hemodynamic effect on the cardiac output, varies based on the cause of the dysrhythmia and the myocardium's ability to adapt. An atrial dysrhythmia arises in the atria of the heart. If the dysrhythmia causes the patient to lose the "atrial kick" (the blood that is ejected into the ventricle during atrial systole), the patient may have more symptoms. The atrial kick provides approximately 35% of the total end-diastolic volume, which is an essential contribution to ventricular filling in individuals with heart disease. Atrial dysrhythmias that cause the loss of the atrial kick include atrial flutter and atrial fibrillation. Figure 1 illustrates types of atrial dysrhythmias in Lead II.

Sinus bradycardia, a heart rate less than 60 beats per minute, has a rhythm that is regular, with the electrical impulse originating in the sinoatrial (SA) node. There is a 1:1 ratio of P waves to QRS complexes, and the P wave and QRS complexes are of normal configuration. Sinus bradycardia is primarily caused by an excessive parasympathetic response. It can be a normal, asymptomatic occurrence in healthy individuals such as athletes or a desired medication effect with drugs such as digoxin and verapamil. Abnormal conditions such as pain, anxiety, increased intracranial pressure, or myocardial infarction can also cause sinus bradycardia. Because of its effects on cardiac output, sinus bradycardia can cause symptoms of dizziness, fatigue, palpitations, chest pain, and congestive heart failure.

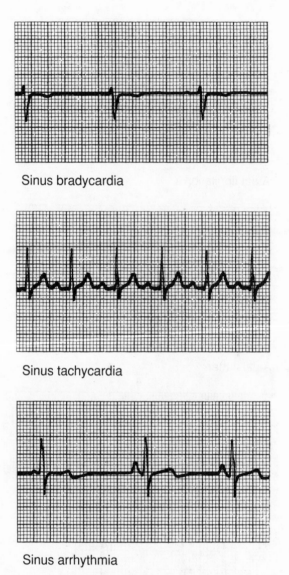

Sinus bradycardia

Sinus tachycardia

Sinus arrhythmia

Figure 1   Types of Atrial Dysrhythmias

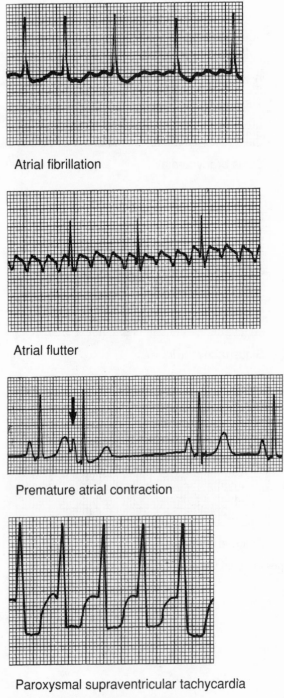

Atrial fibrillation

Atrial flutter

Premature atrial contraction

Paroxysmal supraventricular tachycardia

Figure 1 Types of Atrial Dysrhythmias (*continued*)

Sinus tachycardia, a heart rate greater than 100 beats but rarely more than 160 beats per minute, is a regular rhythm whose electrical impulse originates in the SA node. There is a 1:1 ratio of P waves to QRS complexes, and the P wave and QRS complexes are of normal configuration. Sinus tachycardia is generally the result of increased stimulation of the sympathetic nervous system and the resulting release of catecholamines. It can also be a normal response to an increased demand for oxygenation, as in exercise or fever, or in response to a decreased cardiac output, as in congestive heart failure or shock syndromes. It can also occur in response to stress; anxiety; or an intake of caffeine, nicotine, or anticholinergic medications.

Sinus arrhythmia, defined as a variable rate of impulse discharge from the SA node, occurs when the rhythm is irregular and usually corresponds to the respiratory pattern. The rhythm increases with inspiration and slows with expiration. There is a 1:1 ratio of P waves to QRS complexes, and the P wave and QRS complex are of normal configuration. Sinus arrhythmia can be a normal variation in children. The vagal effect of some medications and of SA nodal disease and conditions that affect vagal tone can also be a cause.

Atrial fibrillation, a rapid and disorganized atrial dysrhythmia, occurs at atrial rates of from 400 to 600 beats per minute. There are no clearly discernible P waves, but rather irregular fibrillatory waves. The QRS complex appears normal, but there is a variable, irregular ventricular response because of the atrioventricular (AV) node's ability to respond only partially to this rapid rate. Although atrial fibrillation can occur in healthy individuals, it is generally found in those patients with underlying cardiovascular diseases such as ischemic heart disease, mitral valve disease, congestive heart failure, and pericarditis.

Atrial flutter, defined as an abnormally fast, regular atrial rhythm that originates from an ectopic atrial focus, is usually in the range of 250 to 400 beats per minute. It is characterized by regular flutter or sawtooth-appearing waves. The QRS complex appears normal in configuration, and there is not a 1:1 ratio of the P to QRS complex because the ventricle cannot respond to the fast atrial rate. Atrial flutter is seldom seen in a healthy individual. Most frequently, atrial flutter is associated with ischemic myocardial disease, acute myocardial infarction, and rheumatic heart disease. The patient is usually asymptomatic because of a controlled ventricular response.

Premature atrial contractions (PACs), cardiac contractions initiated in the atria, occur earlier than expected. The underlying rhythm is regular, with the early beat producing a slight irregularity. There is usually a 1:1 ratio of P wave to QRS complex unless the P wave is blocked because of the refractory period of the AV node. The P wave of the premature beat may exhibit a slightly different configuration, since it does not originate in the SA node but, rather, from another area of the atrium. There may be a short "compensatory" pause after the ectopic (electrical stimulation of a cardiac contraction beginning at a point other than the sinoatrial [SA] node) beat. PACs can be a normal occurrence in all age groups, or they can be the result of ischemic heart disease, rheumatic heart disease, stimulant ingestion, or digitalis toxicity.

Paroxysmal supraventricular tachycardia (PSVT), the sudden onset of a rapid atrial and ventricular rate of from 160 to 250 beats per minute, occurs with a regular but aberrant P wave. The P waves are difficult to discern from the preceding T wave, but a P wave precedes each QRS. PSVT occurs when there is an intrinsic abnormality of the AV conduction or in conditions associated with stress, hypoxia, hypokalemia, hypertension, heart disease, or hyperthyroidism. It is also associated with digitalis toxicity, caffeine ingestion, and the use of central nervous system stimulants.

CAUSES

Each type of atrial dysrhythmia has specific causes, as listed previously.

GENDER AND LIFE SPAN CONSIDERATIONS

The normal aging process is associated with an increase in atrial tachydysrythmias and bradydysrythmias. They occur in both males and females; increasing incidence of cardiac diseases, atherosclerosis, and degenerative hypertrophy of the left ventricle that occurs with aging are all contributing factors.

☐ ASSESSMENT

HISTORY. Many patients with suspected cardiac dysrhythmias describe a history of symptoms, indicating periods of decreased cardiac output. Although many atrial dysrhythmias are asymptomatic, some patients report a history of dizziness, fatigue, activity intolerance, a "fluttering" in their chest, shortness of breath, and chest pain. In particular, question the patient about the onset, duration, and characteristics of the symptoms and the events that precipitated them. Obtain a complete history of all illnesses, dietary restrictions, and activity restrictions and a current medication history.

PHYSICAL EXAMINATION. Inspect the patient's skin for changes in color or the presence of edema. Auscultate the patient's heart rate and rhythm, and note the first and second heart sounds and any adventitious sounds. Auscultate the patient's blood pressure. Perform a full respiratory assessment, and note any adventitious breath sounds or labored breathing.

PSYCHOSOCIAL. Although not usually life threatening, any change in heart rhythm can provoke a great deal of anxiety and fear. Assess the ability of the patient and significant others to cope with this potential alteration.

DIAGNOSTIC HIGHLIGHTS

Test	Normal Result	Abnormality with Condition	Explanation
12-Lead electrocardiogram (ECG)	Regular sinus rhythm	See Figure 1, Types of Atrial Dysrhythmias	To detect specific conduction defects and to monitor the patient's cardiac response to electrolyte imbalances, drug effects, and toxicities

Other Tests: Use either pulse oximetry, ambulatory, or Holter monitoring to provide a 12- to 24-hour continuous recording of myocardial electrical activity as the patient performs normal daily activities.

PRIMARY NURSING DIAGNOSIS

Altered tissue perfusion (cardiopulmonary, cerebral, renal, peripheral) related to rapid heart rates or the loss of the atrial kick

OUTCOMES. Circulation status; Cardiac pump effectiveness; Tissue perfusion: Cardiopulmonary; Cerebral, Renal, Peripheral; Vital sign status

INTERVENTIONS. Circulatory care; Dysrhythmia management; Emergency care; Vital signs monitoring; Cardiac care; Cardiac precautions; Oxygen therapy; Fluid/electrolyte management; Fluid monitoring; Shock management: Volume; Medication administration; Resuscitation; Surveillance

☐ PLANNING AND IMPLEMENTATION

Collaborative

The dysrhythmia needs to be identified and appropriate treatment started. (See Table 9.) Trials of various medications or combinations of medications may be used to control the dysrhythmia if the patient is symptomatic. Low-flow oxygen by nasal cannula or mask is often prescribed for patients during tachycardic rhythms. Some patients may require cardioversion, a synchronized counter-shock for atrial dysrhythmias that are resistent to medical therapy.

TABLE 9 | **Treatment of Atrial Dysrythmias**

DYSRHYTHMIA	MANAGEMENT
Sinus tachycardia	· Treat the underlying cause of dysrhythmia
Sinus bradycardia	· Treat only if the patient is symptomatic
	· Determine the underlying cause
	· If appropriate, administer atropine
	· Consider isopreterenol or a pacemaker, if appropriate
Atrial flutter	· No treatment is needed in the aymptomatic patient
	· Treat symptomatic patients with cardioversion of rhythm to normal or controlled ventricular response
	· Give digitalis (unless the dysrhythmia is from digitalis toxicity); verapamil and quinidine sulfate may also be used
	· May need atrial pacing
Atrial fibrillation	· Convert rhythm to sinus rhythm or controlled ventricular rate to provide adequate cardiac output
	· Use cardioversion (generally successful in acute cases of atrial fibrillation)
	· Treat chronic atrial fibrillation with digitalis, quinidine sulfate, or propranolol; use anticoagulants to prevent thromboemboli formation
Paroxysmal supraventricular tachycardia	· Attempt noninvasive treatment with stimulation of vagal reflex by carotid massage or Valsalva's maneuver
	· Treat with adenosine when patient has symtpoms
	· May use other medications such as propranolol, quinidine sulfate, verapamil, or edrophonium
	· If the patient is unrepsonsive to medications, use cardioversion

PHARMACOLOGIC HIGHLIGHTS

Medication or Drug Class	Dosage	Description	Rationale
Beta adrenergic antagonists	Varies by drug	Blocks beta adrenergic receptors	May be used to slow the rate in sinus tachycardia if the patient has myocardial;

			ischemia; may also be used to control a rapid ventricular response in atrial fibrillation
Digitalis	Varies by drug	Increases strength of myocardial contraction, decreases heart rate, decreases speed of conduction	May be used for atrial fibrillation or flutter to control rate

Other Drugs: Calcium channel blockers; quinidine; anticoagulant therapy

Independent

Maintain the patient's airway, breathing, and circulation. To maximize oxygen available to the myocardium, encourage the patient to rest in bed until the symptoms are treated and subside. Remain with the patient to ensure rest and to allay anxiety. Discuss any potential precipitating factors with the patient. For some patients, strategies to reduce stress or lifestyle changes help to limit the incidence of dysrhythmias. Teach the patient to reduce the amount of caffeine intake in the diet. If appropriate, encourage the patient to become involved in an exercise program or a smoking cessation group. Provide emotional support and information about the dysrhythmia, the precipitating factors, and mechanisms to limit the dysrhythmia. If the patient is at risk for electrolyte imbalance, teach the patient any dietary considerations to prevent electrolyte depletion.

DOCUMENTATION GUIDELINES

- Cardiopulmonary assessment: Heart and lung sounds, cardiac rate and rhythm on the cardiac monitor, blood pressure, quality of the peripheral pulses, capillary refill, respiratory rate and rhythm
- Activity tolerance, ability to perform self-care
- Complications: Dizziness, syncope, hypotension, electrolyte imbalance, uncorrected cardiac dysrhythmias, ineffective patient or family coping

DISCHARGE AND HOME HEALTHCARE GUIDELINES

PATIENT TEACHING. Explain the importance of taking all medications as prescribed by the physician. If the patient needs periodic laboratory work to monitor the effects of the medications, discuss the frequency of the tests and where to have them drawn. Explain the actions, the route, the side effects, the dosage, and the frequency of the medication. Teach the patient how to take the pulse and recognize an irregular rhythm. Explain that the patient needs to notify the healthcare provider when symptoms such as irregular pulse, chest pain, shortness of breath, or dizziness occur. Emphasize the importance of stress reduction and smoking cessation.

Basal Cell Epithelioma

DRG Category: 283
Mean LOS: 4.8 days
Description: MEDICAL: Minor Skin Disorders with CC
DRG Category: 265
Mean LOS: 5.4 days
Description: SURGICAL: Skin Graft and/or Debride Except for Skin Ulcer or Cellulitis with CC

Basal cell epithelioma, a slow-growing skin tumor, commonly occurs from overexposure to the sun and accounts for approximately 80% of skin cancers. The physiologic changes that occur in skin cells arise from cancer-causing factors that lead to changes in undifferentiated basal cells. These cells become cancerous instead of differentiating into specialized cells such as sweat glands, sebum (a fatty secretion of the sebaceous glands of the skin), and hair. Basal cell epithelioma occurs on the skin in 94% of people who develop skin cancer. Over time, if left untreated, basal cell epitheliomas can become indurated and invasive, and this is followed by nodule formation and ulceration. (See Table 10.)

CAUSES

Basal cell epitheliomas are thought to be caused by a number of factors. Extended, long-term exposure to sunlight or radiation creates changes in pigmentation and DNA damage that may foster the development of skin cancers. Fair-skinned persons are more susceptible to basal cell epithelioma, which is the most common malignant tumor that affects fair-skinned European-Americans.

Burns and trauma can accelerate otherwise normal tissue growth or can exacerbate previously existing lesions. Arsenic ingestion is thought to be a contributing factor as well. Patients may ingest arsenic through well water, medications, insecticides, or exposure to an industrial mining site. Vaccination sites can create skin cell proliferation and permanent damage through scarring, and this creates a risk for development of basal cell epithelioma.

GENDER AND LIFE SPAN CONSIDERATIONS

Older individuals, over 40 years of age, with more years of exposure to risk factors are most susceptible to basal cell epitheliomas. People who work in the sun are particularly vulnerable. Exposure is more important than gender considerations in this disorder.

◻ ASSESSMENT

HISTORY. Elicit a history of skin problems, the length of time skin disorders have existed, daily routine skin care, and current medications. Ask the patient about exposure to sunlight; in particular, establish long-term patterns of exposure to sunlight, either at work or in recreational activities, and determine what form of sun protection the patient has customarily used. Record the patient's history of

TABLE 10 | **Kinds of Basal Cell Epitheliomas**

KIND	LOCATION	IDENTIFYING CHARACTERISTICS	COURSE	TREATMENT
Noduloulcerative	Face, eyelid margins, nasolabial skin folds	Small, pink, translucent papules with dilated vessels on a smooth surface	Can ulcerate and create an infective network in other tissues and structures	Curettage; electrodesication; penetrating radiation
Superficial	Chest, forearms and back	Threadlike borders surrounding irregularly shaped, flat, patchy areas; may be scaly, lightly pigmented with elevated borders	May become deeply invasive	Cryosurgery; excision of affected area; topical 5-fluorouracil
Sclerosing	Head and neck patches without any distinct surrounding border; yellow to white morphealike	Hardened and waxy	High rate or recurrence	Mohs surgery; excision; radiation

scars, vaccination sites, and burns. Establish a patient history of exposure to radiation or arsenic; be sure to ask about the patient's occupational history to discover if he or she has been at risk of ingesting arsenic at an industrial site.

PHYSICAL EXAMINATION. Observe the color, texture, turgor, and pigmentation of the patient's skin for deviations from normal skin parameters. Note in detail any lesions, nodules, or plaques.

PSYCHOSOCIAL. Patients with basal cell epitheliomas at the early stages can recover with minimal intervention, although some patients may experience distress over facial lesions that alter their appearance. Patients may have to deal with changes in activities that bring them into extended contact with environmental risk factors. Patients with more advanced basal cell epitheliomas or advanced age may have to cope with more aggressive and repeated treatments and surgery with some permanent disfigurement and poor prognosis.

DIAGNOSTIC HIGHLIGHTS

Test	Normal Result	Abnormality with Condition	Explanation
Lesion biopsy	Negative biopsy	Positive for basal cell epithelioma	Excisional biopsy may be treatment for small tumors; during excision, intra-operative frozen section analysis occurs to confirm negative margins of lesion

Other Tests: Basal cell epitheliomas are diagnosed by clinical appearance, histologic study, and biopsies.

PRIMARY NURSING DIAGNOSIS

Impaired skin integrity related to irritation and erosion; fluid volume deficit related to water loss

OUTCOMES. Wound healing: Primary intention; Tissue integrity; Knowledge: Treatment regime; Treatment behavior: Illness or injury

INTERVENTIONS. Incision site care; Medication administration: Topical; Skin care: Topical treatments; Skin surveillance; Wound care

☐ PLANNING AND IMPLEMENTATION

Collaborative

Curettage and electrodesiccation are used to dehydrate and cleanse the affected area by insertion of an active electrode into the tissue. Mohs surgery is microsurgery involving serial (step-by-step) removal of tissue. Topical chemotherapy with 5-fluorouracil interferes with the cells' ability to use essential metabolites. Chemotherapeutic agents destroy the life cycles of cells. Low-dose particulate–electromagnetic radiation to the specific carcinoma destroys the affected cells without destroying the normal cells. Chemosurgery consists of periodically applying fixative pastes such as zinc chloride and then removing fixed pathologic tissue until the tumor is completely removed.

PHARMACOLOGIC HIGHLIGHTS

Medication or Drug Class	Dosage	Description	Rationale
Liquid nitrogen	Varies by drug	Kills tumor cells	Destroys tumors less than 1 cm in diameter
Topical ointments	Varies by drug	Corticosteroid ointment, topical 5-fluorouracil.	Relieves local inflammation

Independent

Support the patient's body image and self-esteem by encouraging careful grooming. Explore ways of covering the lesion with clothing or flesh-colored dressings if the lesions are unsightly. Accept the patient's appearance and support a positive self-image by involving him or her in decision-making. Encourage the patient to verbalize fears and concerns; answer any questions, and offer reassurance as appropriate. Offer positive reinforcement for the patient's efforts to adapt to the condition, and remain with the patient during any episodes of increased anxiety or stress. Encourage the patient to interact with other patients who have experienced basal cell epithelioma.

Teach the patient to relieve local inflammation with cool compresses and topical ointments. Teach the patient with noduloulcerative basal cell epithelioma about correct facial hygiene techniques to prevent bleeding from ulcerations. Instruct the patient about lifestyle modifications, especially regarding exposure to sunlight, that can help in preventing recurrence of basal cell epithelioma.

Instruct the patient to eat small, high-protein meals frequently and to prepare meals in a blender or augment nutrition with liquid protein supplements if oral lesions make eating difficult.

DOCUMENTATION GUIDELINES

- Physical findings: Abnormal skin changes, wound healing, discomfort
- Response to medications and treatments
- Response to advanced treatment requiring further diagnostics and hospitalization
- Delayed healing and signs of complications (failure to heal)

DISCHARGE AND HOME HEALTHCARE GUIDELINES

PREVENTION. Teach the patient to avoid excessive or prolonged exposure to ultraviolet rays. Teach the patient how to protect skin surfaces at risk through appropriate attire and the use of sunscreen preparations. Suggest and support modifications of certain aspects of the patient's lifestyle.

AFTERCARE. Teach the patient proper care of the site(s) after procedures. Teach the patient what to expect from the healing process.

COMPLICATIONS. Teach the patient to watch for abnormal or recurrent postprocedural bleeding and the absence of a normal, healed appearance of the site(s), such as continued raw appearance, enlarged ulceration of site(s), drainage, and tenderness, as well as inflammation. Teach the patient the signs and symptoms that require calling the physician.

Benign Prostatic Hyperplasia (Hypertrophy)

DRG Category: 348
Mean LOS: 3.7 days
Description: MEDICAL: Benign Prostatic Hypertrophy with CC
DRG Category: 336
Mean LOS: 4.0 days
Description: SURGICAL: Transurethral Prostatectomy withCC

Benign prostatic hyperplasia or hypertrophy (BPH), one of the most common disorders of older men, is a nonmalignant enlargement of the prostate gland. It is the most common cause of obstruction of urine flow in men. The degree of enlargement determines whether or not bladder outflow obstruction occurs. As the urethra becomes obstructed, the muscle inside the bladder hypertrophies in an attempt to assist the bladder to force out the urine. BPH may also cause the formation of a diverticulum musculature that remains full of urine when the patient empties the bladder.

As the obstruction progresses, the bladder is unable to empty completely and urinary retention occurs. With marked bladder distension, overflow incontinence may occur with any increase in intra-abdominal pressure such as that which occurs with coughing and sneezing. Complications of BPH include urinary stasis, urinary tract infection, renal calculi, overflow incontinence, hypertrophy of the bladder muscle, bladder diverticuli, acute renal failure, hydronephrosis, and even chronic renal failure.

CAUSES

Because the condition occurs in older men, changes in hormone balances have been associated with the cause. Androgens (testosterone) and estrogen appear to contribute to the hyperplastic changes that occur. Other theories, such as those involving diet, heredity, race, and history of chronic inflammation, have been associated with BPH, but no definitive links have been made with these potential contributing factors.

GENDER AND LIFE SPAN CONSIDERATIONS

By the age of 50 years, 50% of men have some degree of prostate enlargement. Many of these men do not manifest any clinical symptoms in the early stages of hypertrophic changes. As men become older, the incidence of symptoms increases to more than 75% for those over 80 years of age. Of those men with symptoms, approximately 50% of men are symptomatic to a moderate degree and 25% of those have severe symptoms that require surgical interventions. With proper treatment and follow-up care, the normal life span for the patient can be achieved.

☐ ASSESSMENT

HISTORY. Generally, men with suspected BPH have a history of frequent urination, nocturia, straining to urinate, weak stream, and an incomplete emptying of the bladder. Distinguish between these obstructive symptoms and irritative symptoms such as dysuria, frequency, and urgency, which may indicate an infection or inflammatory process. A "voiding diary" can also be obtained to determine the frequency and nature of the complaints. In addition, ask the patient to complete the self-administered American Urology Association (AUA) Symptom Index (see Box 3), which consists of seven questions that relate to symptoms associated with BPH that the person is experiencing. Patients with scores of 0 to 7 have mild symptoms; scores of 8 to 19 indicate moderate symptoms, and scores of 20 to 35 indicate severe symptoms.

BOX 3 QUESTIONS ASKED ON AUA SYMPTOMS INDEX

- Over the last month, how often have you had a sensation of not emptying your bladder completely after urinating?
- Over the last month, how often have you had to urinate again in less than 2 hours after finishing voiding?
- Over the last month, how often have your stopped and started your stream again several times when you urinated?
- Over the last month, how often have you found it difficult to postpone urination?
- Over the last month, how often have you had a weak urinary stream?
- Over the last month, how often have you had to push or strain to begin urinating?
- Over the last month, how many times did you typically get up to urinate from the time you went to bed until the time you got up in the morning?

Adapted from the U.S. Department of Health and Human Services, 1994.

PHYSICAL EXAMINATION. Inspect and palpate the bladder for distension. A digital rectal exam (DRE) reveals a rubbery enlargement of the prostate, but the degree of enlargement does not consistently correlate with the degree of urinary obstruction. Some men have enlarged prostates that extend out into soft tissue without compressing the urethra. Determine the amount of pain and discomfort that is associated with the DRE.

PSYCHOSOCIAL. The patient who is experiencing BPH may voice concerns related to sexual functioning after treatment. The patient's degree of anxiety, as well as his ability to cope with the potential alterations in sexual function (a possible cessation of intercourse for several weeks, possibility of sterility or retrograde ejaculation) should also be determined to provide appropriate follow-up care.

DIAGNOSTIC HIGHLIGHTS

Test	Normal Result	Abnormality with Condition	Explanation
Urinalysis and culture	Minimal numbers of red and white blood cells; no bacteria; clear urine with no occult blood and no protein	Urinary tract infection may occur with the presence of bacteria and the abnormally increased numbers of red and white blood cells	Urinary retention may lead to infection

Uroflowmetry	Males 46–65 years of age have more than 200 mL of urine at a flow rate of 21 mL/ second	Flow rate is decreased	Prostate inflammation leads to a narrowed urethral channel and obstruction of urine outflow

Other Tests: Serum creatinine and blood urea nitrogen (BUN); prostate-specific antigen (PSA); postvoid residual volume (PRV); diagnostic ultrasound; cystourethroscopy

PRIMARY NURSING DIAGNOSIS

Urinary retention (acute or chronic) related to bladder obstruction

OUTCOMES. Urinary continence; Urinary elimination; Infection status; Knowledge: Disease Process, Medication, Treatment Regimen; Symptom control behavior

INTERVENTIONS. Urinary retention care; Bladder irrigation; Fluid management; Fluid monitoring; Urinary catheterization; Urinary elimination management; Tube care: Urinary

◻ PLANNING AND IMPLEMENTATION

Collaborative

SURGICAL. Those patients with the most severe cases, in which there is total urinary obstruction, chronic urinary retention, and recurrent urinary tract infection, usually require surgery. Transurethral resection of the prostate (TURP) is the most common surgical intervention. The procedure is performed by inserting a resectoscope through the urethra. Hypertrophic tissue is cut away, thereby relieving pressure on the urethra. Prostatectomy can be performed, in which the portion of the prostate gland causing the obstruction is removed.

The relatively newer surgical procedure called TUIP involves making an incision in the portion of the prostate attached to the bladder. The gland is split, reducing pressure on the urethra. TUIP is more helpful in men with smaller prostate glands that cause obstruction. Laser treatments can also be used.

POSTSURGICAL. Postsurgical care involves supportive care and maintenance of the indwelling catheter to ensure patency and adequacy of irrigation. Belladonna and opium suppositories may relieve bladder spasms. Stool softeners are used to prevent straining during defecation after surgery. Ongoing monitoring of the drainage from the catheter determines the color, consistency, and amount of urine flow. The urine should be clear yellow or slightly pink in color. If the patient develops frank hematuria or an abrupt change in urinary output, the surgeon should be notified immediately. The most critical complications that can occur are septic or hemorrhagic shock.

NONSURGICAL. In patients who are not candidates for surgery, a permanent indwelling catheter is inserted. If the catheter cannot be placed in the urethra because of obstruction, the patient may need a suprapubic cystostomy. Conservative therapy also includes prostatic massage, warm sitz baths, and a short-term fluid restriction to prevent bladder distension. Regular ejaculation may help decrease congestion of the prostate gland.

PHARMACOLOGIC HIGHLIGHTS

Medication or Drug Class	Dosage	Description	Rationale
Alpha-adrenergic blockers	Varies with drug	Prazosin hydrochloride; terazosin	Relaxes smooth muscles of the bladder
Finasteride	5 mg po qd	5-alpha reductase inhibitor	Shrinks prostate gland and improves urine flow

Independent

Patients with severe alterations in urinary elimination may require a catheter to assist with emptying the bladder. Never force a urinary catheter into the urethra. If there is resistance during insertion, stop the catheterization procedure and notify the physician. Monitor the patient for bleeding and discomfort during insertion. In addition, assess the patient for signs of shock from post-obstruction diuresis after catheter insertion. Ensure adequate fluid balance. Encourage the patient to drink at least 2 L of fluid per day to prevent stasis and infection from a decreased intake. Encourage the patient to avoid the following medications, which may worsen the symptoms: anticholinergics, decongestants (over-the-counter and prescribed), tranquilizers, alcohol, and antidepressants.

Evaluate the patient's and partner's feelings about the risk for sexual dysfunction. Retrograde ejaculation or sterility may occur after surgery. Explain alternative sexual practices, and answer the patient's questions. Some patients would prefer to talk to a person of the same gender when discussing sexual matters. Provide supportive care of the patient and significant others, and make referrals for sexual counseling if appropriate.

DOCUMENTATION GUIDELINES

- Presence of urinary discomfort, bleeding, frequency, retention, or difficulty initiating flow
- Presence of bladder distension, discomfort, and incontinence
- Intake and output; color of urine, presence of clots, quality of urine (clear versus cloudy)
- Presence of complications: Urinary retention, bleeding, infection
- Reaction to information regarding sexual function

DISCHARGE AND HOME HEALTHCARE GUIDELINES

PATIENT TEACHING. Instruct patients about the need to maintain a high fluid intake (at least 2 L per day) to ensure adequate urine output. Teach the patient to monitor urinary output for 4 to 6 weeks after surgery to ensure adequacy in volume of elimination combined with a decrease in volume of retention.

MEDICATIONS. Provide instructions about all medications used to relax the smooth muscles of the bladder or to shrink the prostate gland. Provide instructions on the correct dosage, route, action, side effects, and potential drug interactions and when to notify these to the physician.

PREVENTION. Instruct the patient to report any difficulties with urination to the physician immediately. Explain that BPH can recur and that he should notify the physician if symptoms of urgency, frequency, difficulty initiating stream, retention, nocturia, or bladder distension recur.

POSTOPERATIVE. Encourage the patient to discuss any sexual concerns he or his partner may have after surgery with the appropriate counselors. Reassure the patient that a session can be set up by the nurse or physician whenever one is indicated. Usually the physician recommends that the patient have no sexual intercourse or masturbation for several weeks after invasive procedures.

Bladder Cancer

DRG Category: 318
Mean LOS: 5.5 days
Description: MEDICAL: Kidney and Urinary Tract Neoplasm with CC
DRG Category: 303
Mean LOS: 9.7 days
Description: SURGICAL: Kidney, Ureter, and Major Bladder Procedures for Neoplasm

Cancer of the urinary bladder is the second most common genitourinary (GU) cancer after prostate cancer. It accounts for approximately 4% of all cancers and 2% of deaths from cancer in the United States. The majority of bladder tumors (90% to 95%) are transitional cell carcinomas arising in the epithelial layer of the bladder, although squamous cell (7%) or adenocarcinoma (2%) may occur. Most bladder tumors are multifocal, because the environment of the bladder allows for the continuous bathing of the mucosa with urine that contains tumor cells that can implant in several locations. The ureters, bladder neck, and prostate urethra may become obstructed. Direct extension can occur to the sigmoid colon, rectum, and, depending upon the sex of the patient, the prostate or uterus and vagina. Metastasis occasionally occurs to the bones, liver, and lungs.

Bladder cancer is staged based on the presence or absence of invasion and is graded (I to IV) based on the degree of differentiation of the cell, with grade I being the best differentiated and slowest growing. Both the stage and grade of the tumor are considered when planning treatment.

CAUSES

The cause of bladder cancer is not well understood; however, cigarette smoking and occupational exposure to aromatic amines (textile dyes, rubber, hair dyes, paint pigment) are established risk factors. Other associated factors include chronic bladder irritation and infection, vesical calculi, and exposure to cyclophosphamide (Cytoxan).

GENDER AND LIFE SPAN CONSIDERATIONS

Bladder cancer occurs most frequently in persons between 50 and 70 years of age. It is rare in persons under age 40, but the incidence in both younger men and women is increasing. Incidence is highest among European-American men, with a rate twice that of African-American men and four times that of European-American women. Younger men have reported less impotency following radical cystectomy than have older men. Persons living in urban areas are at higher risk for bladder cancer than persons living in rural areas.

□ ASSESSMENT

HISTORY. Gross, painless, intermittent hematuria is the most frequently reported symptom. Occult blood may be discovered during a routine urinalysis. Dysuria, urinary frequency, and urgency and burning on urination may be reported if there is infection present. The patient may not seek medical attention until urinary hesitance, decrease in caliber of the stream, and flank pain occur. Other symptoms may include suprapubic pain after voiding, bladder irritability, urinary frequency, dribbling, and nocturia.

PHYSICAL EXAMINATION. The physical examination is usually normal. A bladder tumor becomes palpable only after extensive invasion into surrounding structures.

PSYCHOSOCIAL. Diagnosis of cancer and treatment of cancer with radical cystectomy and creation of a urinary diversion system can threaten sexual functioning of both men and women. The procedure can cause impotence in men and psychological problems similar to those that accompany a hysterectomy and oophorectomy in women. Additionally, a portion of the vagina may be removed, thus affecting intercourse. The psychologic impact of a stoma and external urinary drainage system can cause changes in body image and libido.

DIAGNOSTIC HIGHLIGHTS

Test	Normal Result	Abnormality with Condition	Explanation
Serum carcinoembryonic antigen (CEA) level	< 2.5 ng/dL in nonsmokers; < 5.0 ng/mL in smokers	Approximately 50% of patients with late-stage bladder cancer have moderately elevated CEA levels	Useful in monitoring response to treatment and extent of disease
Urine cytology	Normal type and amount of squamous and epithelial cells of urinary tract	Abnormal cells (tumor and pretumor cells)	Evidence of urinary tract neoplasm

Other Tests: Intravenous pyelogram (IVP); ultrasonography; pelvic computed tomography (CT) scan; magnetic resonance imaging (MRI); bone scan; complete blood count (CBC)

PRIMARY NURSING DIAGNOSIS

Risk for altered urinary elimination related to the obstruction of urinary flow

OUTCOMES. Urinary continence; Urinary elimination; Knowledge: Disease process and Treatment regime; Self-care: Toileting; Self-esteem

INTERVENTIONS. Urinary elimination management; Urinary incontinence care; Teaching: Individual; Fluid monitoring; Urinary catheterization; Anxiety reduction; Infection control; Skin surveillance; Tube care: Urinary

□ PLANNING AND IMPLEMENTATION

Collaborative

Patients with higher-stage invasive disease are usually treated with radical curative surgery, whereas patients with lower-stage noninvasive disease can be controlled with more conservative measures. Papillary tumors, even when noninvasive, have a high rate of recurrence. Carcinoma in situ (CIS) is usually multifocal and also has a high rate of recurrence.

CONSERVATIVE. Superficial bladder tumors can be treated effectively with conservative measures that consist of surgical removal of the tumor by transurethral resection of the bladder (TURB) followed by electrical destruction or fulguration, intravesical instillation of chemotherapy or immunotherapy, and frequent follow-up cystoscopic examination. Superficial bladder tumors can also be destroyed with the neodymium:yttrium-aluminum-garnet (Nd:YAG) laser. Patients with multiple superficial bladder tumors receive intravesical instillation of chemotherapy or immunotherapy such as bacille Calmette-Guérin (BCG) in addition to TURB.

SURGICAL. Partial or segmental cystectomy may be recommended for patients with diffuse unresectable tumors or tumors that fail to respond to intravesical therapy. Because tumors are likely to continue to spread and metastasize to distant sites, procedures such as radical cystectomy with creation of a urinary diversion, external radiation therapy, or a combination of preoperative radiation therapy followed by radical cystectomy and urinary diversion are recommended.

The Bricker ileal conduit is the most popular method for creating the urinary diversion. In this procedure the ureters are implanted into an isolated segment of the terminal ileum. The proximal end of the ileal segment is closed, and a stoma is formed by bringing the distal end out through a hole in the abdominal wall. An external pouch for the collection of urine is worn continuously. Ureteral stents, which are left in place up to 3 weeks after surgery, may be placed during the procedure to promote the flow of urine.

POSTOPERATIVE. Postoperatively, direct nursing care toward providing comfort, preventing complications from major abdominal surgery, and promoting urinary drainage. Monitor the patient's vital signs, dressings, and drains for symptoms of hemorrhage and infection. Monitor the color of the stoma, as well as the amount and color of the urine in the collection pouch, every 4 hours. Urine should drain immediately. Some stomal edema is normal during the early postoperative period, but the flow of urine should not be obstructed.

RADIATION. External beam radiation therapy can be used as both adjuvant and definite treatment for bladder cancer. High-dose, short-course therapy consisting of 16 to 20 Gy can be delivered preoperatively to decrease the size of the tumor(s) and prevent spread during surgery. Radiation therapy with a curative intent may be a treatment option for patients who are opposed to a cystectomy and urinary diversion. Unfortunately, 50% of patients with invasive bladder cancer eventually relapse.

PHARMACOLOGIC HIGHLIGHTS

Medication or Drug Class	Dosage	Description	Rationale
Combination systemic chemotherapy	Varies with drug	Cisplatin, methotrexate, and vinblastine, with or without doxorubicin	Combination systemic chemotherapy may be effective in prolonging life but is rarely curative

Independent

For patients who require radical cystectomy with urinary diversion, offer support and reinforcement of the information. Be sure what to expect. Involve another family member in the preoperative education. If it is needed, arrange a preoperative visit by someone who has adjusted well to a similar diversion.

If any type of stoma is to be created, arrange for a preoperative visit from the enterostomal therapist. The enterostomal therapist can assist in the selection and marking of the stoma site (although the stoma site is somewhat contingent upon the type of urinary diversion to be performed) and can introduce the patient to the external urine collection pouch and related care. Suggest involvement with community associations such as the United Ostomy Association and the American Cancer Society.

POSTOPERATIVE. Encourage the patient to look at the stoma and take an active part in stoma care as soon as possible. Allow him or her to hold the equipment, observe the amount and characteristics of urine drainage, and empty the urine collection pouch. Implement care to maintain integrity of the skin around the stoma or urinary diversion that has been created. Empty the urinary drainage pouch when it is about one-third full to prevent the weight of the pouch from breaking the skin seal and leaking urine onto the skin. Depending on the type of urinary diversion created, begin teaching stoma care and care of the system 2 to 3 days after surgery.

Be sensitive to the patient's feelings about the potential for altered sexual functioning after radical cystectomy. Listen attentively, and answer any questions honestly. Encourage the patient and partner to explore alternative methods of sexual expression. Consider referral to a sex therapist. If appropriate, suggest that men investigate the possibility of a penile prosthesis with their physician.

DOCUMENTATION GUIDELINES

- Description of all dressings, wounds, and drainage collection devices
- Physical findings related to the pulmonary assessment, abdominal assessment, presence of edema, condition of extremities, bowel and bladder patterns of voiding
- Response to and side effects experienced related to intravesical instillations of chemotherapy or BCG; systemic chemotherapy
- Teaching performed, the patient's understanding of the content, the patient's ability to perform procedures demonstrated

DISCHARGE AND HOME HEALTHCARE GUIDELINES

PATIENT TEACHING. Following creation of an ileal conduit, teach the patient and significant others the care of the stoma and urinary drainage system. If needed, arrange for follow-up home nursing care or visits with an enterostomal therapist.

Teach the patient the specific procedure to catheterize the continent cutaneous pouch or reservoir. A simple stoma covering made from a feminine hygiene pad can be worn between catheterizations. Stress the need for the patient to wear a medical ID bracelet.

Following orthotopic bladder replacement, teach the patient how to irrigate the Foley catheter. Suggest the use of a leg bag during the day and a Foley drainage bag at night. Once the pouch has healed and the Foley catheter, ureteral stents, and pelvic drain have been removed, teach the patient to "push" or "bear down" with each voiding. Instruct the patient on methods for performing Kegel exercises during and between voidings to minimize incontinence. Suggest wearing incontinence pads until full control is achieved. Also instruct the patient on self-catheterization techniques in case the patient is unable to void. Instruct patients where to obtain ostomy pouches, catheters, and other supplies. Teach the patient how to clean and store catheters between use following the clean technique.

CARE OF SKIN IN EXTERNAL RADIATION FIELD. Encourage the patient to verbalize concerns about radiation therapy, and reassure the patient that he or she is not "radioactive." Instruct the patient to wash skin gently with mild soap, rinse with warm water, and pat the skin dry each day but not to wash off the ink marking that outlines the radiation field. Encourage the patient to avoid applying any lotions, perfumes, deodorants, or powder to the treatment area. Encourage the patient to wear nonrestrictive soft cotton clothing directly over the treatment area and to protect the skin from sunlight and extreme cold. Stress the need to maintain the schedule for follow-up visits and disease surveillance as recommended by the physician.

Blood Transfusion Reaction

DRG Category: 447
Mean LOS: 2.3 days
Description: MEDICAL: Allergic Reactions, Age > 17

Blood transfusion reactions are adverse responses to the infusion of any blood component, including red cells, white cells, platelets, plasma, cryoprecipitate, or factors. They may be classified as acute (within 24 hours of administration) or delayed (occurring days, weeks, months, or even years later). They range from mild urticarial reactions that may be treated easily to fatal hemolytic reactions. It is important to note that almost all fatal hemolytic reactions are attributable to human error. Blood transfusion reactions can be mediated by the immune system or by nonimmune factors. (See Table 11.)

The immune system recognizes red blood cells, platelets, white blood cells, or immunoglobulins as "non-self" because the donor's blood carries foreign proteins that are incompatible with the recipient's antibodies. Typing, screening, and matching of blood units before administration eliminates most incompatibilities, but all potential incompatibilities cannot be screened out in the match-

TABLE 11 | **Classification of Transfusion Reactions by Type**

TYPE	INCIDENCE (PER UNITS TRANSFUSED)	CAUSE	SIGNS AND SYMPTOMS
Allergic	1/100	Sensitivity to foreign proteins	Mild: Hives, urticaria, fever, flushing, itching
Acute nonhemolytic	1/200–1/100	Sensitization to donor white blood cells, platelets, plasma proteins	Fever, chills, headache, flushing, muscle aches, respiratory distress, cardiac dysrhythmias
Acute hemolytic	1/25,000; Fatal: 2/1,000,000	ABO incompatibility reaction to red blood cell antigens	Fever, chills, low back pain, flushing, tachycardia, hypotension, vascular collapse, shock, cardiac arrest
Anaphylactic	1/150,000	Administration of donor's IgA proteins to recipient with anit-IgA antibodies	Restlessness, urticaria, wheezing, shock, cardiac arrest
Delayed non-hemolytic		Exposure to infectious diseases	Patient develops symptoms of the disorder
	1/200	Viral hepatitis	
	1/14	Cyotmegalovirus conversion	
	1/50,000	HIV-1	
	1/40,000	Malaria	
	Rare	Graft-vs-host disease	
	Rare	Postransfusion purpura	
Circulatory overload	1/10,000	Infusion of blood at a rapid rate that leads to fluid volume excess	Pulmonary congestion, restlessness, cough, shortness of breath, hypertension, distended neck veins
Bacteremia		Infusion of blood contaminated with bacteria	Chills, fever, hypotension, vomiting, diarrhea, septic shock
	1/40,000	*Yersinia entercolitica*	
	1/360,000	Other bacteria	

ing process. Non-immune factors are usually related to improper storage. Complications to transfusion reactions include acute bronchospasm, respiratory failure, acute tubular necrosis, and acute renal failure. The most severe reactions can cause anaphylactic shock, vascular collapse, or disseminated intravascular coagulation. Also, current research shows that patients who receive transfusions have an increased risk of infection because the transfusion depresses the immune system for weeks and even months afterward.

CAUSES

The recipient's immune system responds to some transfusions by directing an immune response to the proteins in the donor's blood. Non-immune factors are involved when the blood or components are handled, stored, or administered improperly. The most dreaded reaction is the hemolytic reaction, which occurs when the donor's blood does not have ABO compatibility with the recipient's.

Individuals at greatest risk for transfusion reactions are those who receive massive blood transfusions. The transfusions may be administered over a short period of time, such as with trauma victims with severe blood loss or recipients of liver transplants. Individuals who receive a great number of transfusions throughout a more extended period of time, such as leukemia patients, are also at greater risk. Over time they develop more and more protective antibodies after each unit of blood is received. Eventually, they carry so many antibodies in their systems that they react much more readily than a person who is transfusion-naive.

GENDER AND LIFE SPAN CONSIDERATIONS

Infants and the elderly are more likely to experience problems of fluid overload with transfusion. The incidence of transfusion reactions does not appear to be based on gender.

☐ ASSESSMENT

HISTORY. Individuals who report a history of numerous allergies or previous transfusions should be monitored more carefully since they are at higher risk for reaction. A history of cardiovascular disease should be noted because those patients need to be monitored more carefully for fluid overload. Note also if a patient has a history of Raynaud's disease or a cold agglutinin problem, because, before being administered and with physician approval, blood needs to be warmed. Once the transfusion is in process, the patient may report any of the following signs of transfusion reaction: heat or pain at the site of transfusion, fever, chills, chest tightness, lower back pain, abdominal pain, nausea, difficulty breathing, itching, and a feeling of impending doom.

PHYSICAL EXAMINATION. A change in any vital sign can indicate the beginning of a transfusion reaction. Note if the urine becomes cloudy or reddish (hemolysis). Observe any change in skin color or the appearance of hives. Be alert for signs of edema, especially in the oropharynx and face. Auscultate the lungs before beginning the transfusion, and note any baseline adventitious sounds. Then monitor for crackles or wheezes if the patient shows any signs of fluid overload, and inspect the patient's neck veins for distension.

PSYCHOSOCIAL. Blood bank protocols have lowered the risk of human immunodeficiency virus (HIV) transmission from more than 25,000 cases before 1985 to a risk of 1 in 50,000 to approximately 1 in 500,000 currently. In spite of the decreased risk, many patients worry about contracting HIV when they need blood products. In reality, the risk of hepatitis B and C is much higher, with a transmission rate of approximately 1 in 100,000. If a blood transfusion reaction occurs, the fears and anxieties are compounded and may warrant specific interventions.

DIAGNOSTIC HIGHLIGHTS

In the event of a transfusion reaction, immediately stop the transfusion. Send the unit of blood, or empty bag and tubing if the infusion is complete, along with samples of the patient's blood and urine to the lab for analysis. Blood type and cross-matching are repeated to determine if mismatched blood was administered.

Test	Normal Result	Abnormality with Condition	Explanation
Free hemoglobin: urine and plasma	Negative in urine <3 mg/dL in blood	Free hemoglobin in urine and blood; hemoglobinuria occurs when more than 150 mg/dL of free hemoglobin is present in blood	Transfusion reaction leads to escape of hemoglobin from red blood cells during intravascular hemolysis

Other Tests: Blood culture to rule out bacterial infection; urinalysis for presence of protein; serum bilirubin; complete blood count; prothrombin time; partial thromboplastin time; fibrinogen

PRIMARY NURSING DIAGNOSIS

Risk for ineffective airway clearance related to airway swelling and obstruction

OUTCOMES. Respiratory status: Gas exchange; Respiratory status: Ventilation; Comfort level; Infection status; Knowledge: Treatment regime

INTERVENTIONS. Airway management; Airway insertion and stabilization; Airway suctioning; Anxiety reduction; Oxygen therapy; Respiratory monitoring

☐ PLANNING AND IMPLEMENTATION

Collaborative

PREVENTION. Typing, screening, and matching of blood units before administration eliminates most incompatibilities, but not all of them. If a transfusion reaction does occur, stop the transfusion immediately. The severity of the reaction is usually related to the amount of blood received. Begin an assessment to determine the severity and type of reaction. In minor reactions (urticaria or fever), the transfusion may be restarted after discussion with the physician and after giving the patient an antipyretic, antihistamine, or anti-inflammatory agent. Ongoing monitoring during the rest of the transfusion is essential. If the patient develops anaphylaxis, the patient's airway and breathing are maintained with oxygen supplement, intubation, and mechanical ventilation if needed.

PHARMACOLOGIC HIGHLIGHTS

With an acute hemolytic reaction there are three conditions to consider: renal failure, shock, and disseminated intravascular coagulation (DIC). To counteract shock and minimize renal failure, the physician prescribes aggressive normal saline or colloid intravenous infusion. Mannitol is often used to promote diuresis. Dopamine may be used if hypotension is a problem. Furosemide (Lasix) may be given to keep urine output at 50 to 100 mL per hour. For pyretic reactions, after the possibility of a hemolytic reaction is ruled out, an antipyretic such as acetaminophen may be given and the transfusion may be restarted with caution. For severe reactions see the table that follows.

Medication or Drug Class	Dosage	Description	Rationale
Epinephrine	0.1–0.25 mg of 1:10,000 concentration IV over 5–10 minutes	Sympathomimetic; catecholamine	Given for severe reactions for its pressor effect and bronchodilation.
Glucocorticoids	Varies by drug	Corticosteroid	Anti-inflammatory agents that limit laryngeal swelling

Independent

Adhere strictly to the policies regarding typing, cross-matching, and administering blood. Make sure that the recipient's blood sample is correctly labeled when it is sent to the laboratory. Check each unit before administration to make sure that it is not outdated, that the unit has been designated for the correct recipient, that the patient's medical records' number matches the number on the blood component, and that the blood type is appropriate for the patient. All patients should have their identification band checked by two people before the transfusion is begun. Notify the blood bank, and withhold the transfusion for even the smallest discrepancy when checking the blood with the patient identification. Maintain universal precautions when handling all blood products to protect yourself, and dispose of used containers appropriately in the hazardous waste disposal.

Begin the transfusion at a rate of 75 mL or less per hour. Remain with the patient for the first 15 minutes of the transfusion to monitor for signs of a hemolytic reaction. If the patient develops a reaction, stop the transfusion immediately; evaluate the adequacy of the patient's airway, breathing, and circulation; take the patient's vital signs; notify the physician and blood bank; and return the unused portion of the blood to the blood bank for analysis. If the patient develops chills, monitor the patient's temperature, and cover him or her with a blanket unless the temperature is above 102°F. Remain with the patient and explain that a reaction has occurred from the transfusion. If the patient has excessive fears or concerns about the risk of HIV or hepatitis infection, provide specific information to him or her and arrange for a consultation as needed with either a physician or a counselor.

DOCUMENTATION GUIDELINES

- Response to transfusion: Description of symptoms; severity of symptoms; adequacy of airway, breathing, and circulation; location and description of any skin changes, vital signs, including temperature; complaints of pain or itching
- Termination of transfusion: Amount infused; amount returned to blood bank; laboratory specimens sent; timing of reaction from start of transfusion

DISCHARGE AND HOME HEALTHCARE GUIDELINES

FOLLOW-UP. Teach the patient to report any signs and symptoms of a delayed reaction, such as fever, jaundice, pallor, or fatigue. Explain that these reactions can occur anytime from 3 days after the transfusion to several months later.

Explain that the patient should notify the primary healthcare provider if he or she develops any discomfort in the first few months after transfusion. Attributing these signs to specific diseases may make the patient unnecessarily anxious, but the patient should know to notify the healthcare provider for anorexia, malaise, nausea, vomiting, concentrated urine, and jaundice within 4 to 6 weeks after transfusion (hepatitis B); jaundice, lethargy, and irritability with a milder intensity than that of hepatitis B (hepatitis C); or flu-like symptoms (HIV infection).

Bone Cancer

DRG Category: 239
Mean LOS: 6.8 days
Description: MEDICAL: Pathologic Fractures and Musculoskeletal and Connective Tissue Malignancy

Bone cancers are sarcomas—that is, cancers of connective tissue. Primary bone cancers are relatively uncommon. Most (60% to 65%) tumors of the bone are secondary, or metastatic, ones from other primary tumors. Cancers originating in the osseus, cartilaginous (chrondrogenic), or membrane tissue are classified as bone cancer. Cancers originating from the bone marrow are usually classified as hematologic cancers. The most common type of primary bone cancer is osteosarcoma. (See Table 12.)

TABLE 12 | **Major Types of Primary Bone Cancer**

TYPE	AGES OF PEAK OCCURRENCE (YEARS)	MAJOR LOCATIONS IN THE BODY	AVERAGE NUMBER OF NEW CASES PER YEAR	TREATMENT IN ORDER OF IMPORTANCE
Osteogenic sarcoma or osteosarcoma	10–20	Bone of leg, arm hip	520	Surgery, radiation, chemotherapy
Chondrosarcoma	50–60	Cartilage of leg, hip, rib	428	Surgery, chemotherapy
Ewing's sarcoma	10–20	Bone of leg, hip, arm	234	Radiation, chemotherapy
Fibrosarcoma	30–40	Bone of leg, arm, hip	66	Surgery, radiation, chemotherapy
Chordoma	55–65	Spinal column or skull	56	Surgery, radiation
Parosteal osteosarcoma	30–40	Bone of arm or leg	26	Surgery, chemotherapy

An osteosarcoma arises from osteoblasts (bone-forming cells) and osteoclasts (bone-digesting cells) in the interior of the bone; it occurs most commonly in the femur but also in the tibia and humerus.

CAUSES

Evidence links the development of bone cancer with exposure to therapeutic radiation. A higher incidence has not occurred, however, in populations exposed to other radiation, such as survivors of the atomic bomb. There have been reports of siblings with bone cancer, suggesting genetic influences. Osteogenic sarcoma is most common after puberty, which suggests that hormonal fluctuations and spurts of growth may be involved. Bone cancers tend to be more common in adults who are affected by Paget's disease, hyperparathyroidism, and chronic osteomyelitis. The development of bone cancer has also been linked to trauma and sites of old bone infarcts or fractures.

GENDER AND LIFE SPAN CONSIDERATIONS

Primary cancers of the bone are more common in males and tend to occur in the late teen years or after age 60. Osteogenic sarcoma, or osteosarcoma, the most common kind of bone cancer, occurs mainly in teenagers. Metastatic bone cancer usually appears later in life since it accompanies other cancers, especially lung, breast, prostate, and thyroid cancer.

◻ ASSESSMENT

HISTORY. The focus of the assessment should be on gathering data that differentiate bone cancer from arthritic or traumatic pain. The patient usually reports the gradual onset of pain described as a dull ache. The patient often notices a swelling or the inability to move a joint as before. A distinctive trait of bone cancer pain is its tendency to be worse at night. Generally it is a localized, aching pain, but it may also be referred from the hip or spine. The sudden onset of pain does not rule out bone cancer, however, because a pathologic fracture may be present.

PHYSICAL EXAMINATION. Inspect for any unusual swellings or dilated surface vessels. The patient may walk with a limp or have weakness of the affected limb. If the tumor has progressed, you may note weight loss or cachexia, fever, and decreased mobility. Perform gentle range-of-motion exercises of all the extremities, and document any limitations in joint movement. Note any firm, nontender enlargements in the affected area when it is palpated. Consider, however, that bone tumors are not always visible or palpable. The tumor site may also be tender.

PSYCHOSOCIAL. Although some cancers can be cured with treatments that leave no visible signs, primary bone cancer often requires extensive surgical reconstruction or amputation of the affected limb as part of the treatment. Determine the patient's view of his or her body image and assess whether the impact of the treatment may lead to a body image disturbance.

DIAGNOSTIC HIGHLIGHTS

Test	Normal Result	Abnormality with Condition	Explanation
Serum alkaline phosphatase	4.5–13 units/dL	Elevated	Elevations occur with formation of new bone by increasing osteoblastic activity

X rays and computed tomography (CT)	No lesions	Visualization of lesions; malignant lesions often have poor margination, irregular new bone growth	Each tumor type has its own characteristic pattern; CT shows extent of soft tissue damage

Other Tests: In Ewing's sarcoma and metastatic bone lesions, increases occur in erythrocyte sedimentation rate as well as in leukocytosis and normocytic anemia. Bone biopsy, bone scan, serum calcium, magnetic resonance imaging (MRI).

PRIMARY NURSING DIAGNOSIS

Impaired physical mobility related to weakness, loss of limb, or pain

OUTCOMES. Ambulation: Walking; Joint movement: Active; Mobility level; Self-care: Activities of daily living; Transfer performance; Balance; Muscle function; Pain level

INTERVENTION. Exercise therapy: Ambulation and joint mobility; Positioning; Energy management; Exercise promotion; Self-care assistance; Teaching: Prescribed activity/exercise; Environmental management; Medication management; Pain management

☐ PLANNING AND IMPLEMENTATION

Collaborative

MEDICAL. Radiation has variable effectiveness in bone cancer. It is quite effective with Ewing's sarcoma, moderately effective with osteosarcoma, and relatively ineffective in chondrosarcoma. Even when a cure is not possible, radiation is often used to decrease pain and slow the disease process.

SURGICAL. Surgery may range from simple curettage (removal of necrotic tissue or tumor with a curet) when primary bone cancer is confined, to amputation or extensive resection such as a leg amputation with hemipelvectomy. Ongoing data are being collected that suggest that for many bone cancers limb-sparing treatment (surgical removal of only the tumor with chemotherapy and/or radiation) may provide the same cure rate as amputation. Pain is usually managed with narcotic analgesia in the immediate postoperative period. As the patient recovers, prosthetic devices are often fitted after amputations. The patient may have a prosthesis fitted immediately or a more traditional delayed fitting. Usually physical therapy works with the patient to help him or her learn ways to maintain mobility and the appropriate use of appliances and adjuncts.

PHARMACOLOGIC HIGHLIGHTS

Medication or Drug Class	Dosage	Description	Rationale
Chemotherapy	Varies by drug	Doxorubicin, cyclophosphamide, methotrexate with leucovorin.	Chemotherapy is often used preoperatively to reduce the size of the tumor, or post-

operatively to help eliminate the risk of micrometastasis.

Other Drugs: Immunotherapy, primarily interferon or tumor-specific transfer factor, remains investigational with bone cancer; analgesia.

Independent

Presurgical preparation is essential. Encourage the patient to eat foods high in protein and vitamins to foster wound healing. Begin teaching the exercises that, after surgery, prevent contractures and strengthen limbs to accept the adjustments in posturing and movement. With extensive resection, the patient is exposed to anesthesia for a longer period of time. Preparation for pulmonary toileting and methods to prevent venous stasis become even more important in those patients. When radiation or chemotherapy is used as well, begin preoperative teaching.

Start exercises within 24 hours after surgery to maintain muscle tone and prevent edema, joint contractures, and muscle atrophy. If a prosthesis is to be fitted after healing, take care to wrap the stump to promote proper shrinking and shaping without compromising the patient's circulation.

Whether the treatment is amputation, resection, chemotherapy, or radiation, the changes in the patient's body create severe emotional stress. Listen to the patient's concerns and support efforts to maintain grooming and hygiene. Provide opportunities for the patient to make treatment decisions and to maintain as much control over his or her environment as possible. If the patient develops a body image disturbance or ineffective coping, provide referrals for counseling or a support group when required. Acquaint the patient and family with the supports available through the American Cancer Society or hospice.

DOCUMENTATION GUIDELINES

- Appearance of the surgical incision site: Presence of inflammation, infection, or signs of healing
- Response to chemotherapy or radiation treatments
- Comprehension of treatment plan, including care of surgical site, purpose, and potential side effects of medical treatments
- Reaction to the loss or disfigurement and prognosis
- Readiness to adapt to a prosthetic device
- Presence of complications: Infection, bleeding, poor wound healing, ineffective coping by the patient or significant others

DISCHARGE AND HOME HEALTHCARE GUIDELINES

PREPARATION FOR PROSTHETIC. Teach the patient how to promote healing at the surgical site by keeping the incision clean, dry, and covered. Explain that the stump needs to be wrapped to promote shrinkage and proper shaping for the prosthesis. Teach exercises to maintain strength and range of motion and to prevent contractures. Explain the roles of the interdisciplinary team members in the patient's rehabilitation.

CONTINUING TREATMENT. If the patient receives outpatient chemotherapy or radiation, teach the patient the purpose, duration, and potential complications of those treatments.

Botulism

DRG Category: 423
Mean LOS: 7.1 days
Description: MEDICAL: Other Infectious and Parasitic Diseases Diagnoses

Botulism is a serious neurotoxic disorder that is caused by the gram-positive, spore-forming bacterium *Clostridium botulinum,* which is found in soil and in the gastrointestinal (GI) tract of birds, fish, and mammals. Although it is usually harmless in the spore state, the organism flourishes in warm anaerobic environments, causing germination with bacterial multiplication and toxin production. Botulism occurs when the bacterium is ingested into the GI tract or enters through an open wound. Once ingested or imbedded, the bacterium enters the vascular system. Toxins act at the neuromuscular junction by impairing the release of the neurotransmitter acetylcholine from the presynaptic membrane. Loss of acetylcholine causes paralysis of voluntary and involuntary muscles.

Botulism has a mortality rate as high as 25%, with death occurring as a result of respiratory failure during the first week. If onset is rapid (less than 24 hours) after ingestion of the bacterium, the course of the disease is more severe and potentially fatal. Paralytic ileus is another complication of botulism.

CAUSES

Food-borne botulism occurs when food contaminated with the toxin from the bacteria is ingested. It is caused by the consumption of improperly canned or stored food that is contaminated with spores. Infant botulism occurs when an infant ingests spores in honey or other foods that produce the toxin in the infant's GI tract. Wound botulism occurs from toxin produced in a wound contaminated with *C. botulinum.* Indeterminate botulism occurs in individuals over the age of 1 who have no recognizable source of the disease.

GENDER AND LIFE SPAN CONSIDERATIONS

Botulism has been observed in all age groups and equally in both genders; causative factors, however, may differ across the life span. *C. botulinum* is usually harmless to adults if ingested while in the spore state, but not so in infants.

☐ ASSESSMENT

HISTORY. Elicit a history from the patient or parents regarding food consumption for the last 12 to 96 hours. Note that the incubation period ranges between 12 and 36 hours but depends on the amount of toxin the person ingested. Encourage the patient not only to identify the type of food but also to explain the food preparation with particular attention to the level of heat to which the food was exposed during preparation. Ask the patient if he or she has experienced any puncture wounds recently, particularly while gardening or working with soil.

Patients may describe symptoms of botulism within 12 hours of exposure. Initially patients may describe nausea and vomiting, although often they remain alert and oriented without sensory or neurological deficits. Some patients report diarrhea or constipation, whereas others describe a very dry, sore throat; some may experience GI symptoms prior to neurological symptoms, or they may occur simultaneously. Patients also describe neuromuscular abnormalities. Symptoms usually occur in a descending order from the head to the toes. Ask the patient if he or she has experienced blurred vision, double vision, difficulty swallowing, difficulty speaking, or weakness of the arms and legs.

PHYSICAL EXAMINATION. On inspection, the patient is often awake and alert but may be drowsy, agitated, and anxious. Usually fever is absent.

Cranial nerve involvement occurs early in the disease course and leads to drooping eyelids, double vision, and extraocular muscle paralysis. Most patients lose their gag reflex, and fixed or dilated pupils occur in approximately 50% of patients as the disease progresses. Note if the patient has difficulty speaking. Inspect the symmetry of the facial expression. Evaluate the strength and motion of the extremities because weakness progresses to the neck, arms, thorax, and legs. Ask the patient to shrug his or her shoulders while you press gently on them to test for strength and symmetry. Check for respiratory depression and apnea. As the disorder progresses, respiratory muscle paralysis occurs from phrenic nerve involvement and the patient stops breathing.

PSYCHOSOCIAL. Because of the potential for lifestyle changes and the lengthy hospitalization, children with botulism are at risk for alterations in growth and development. Assess the growth and development level in all age groups.

DIAGNOSTIC HIGHLIGHTS

Test	Normal Result	Abnormality with Condition	Explanation
Serum or stool toxin level	Negative	Positive	*Clostridium botulinum* produces the toxin
Culture and sensitivity from gastric, wound, or stool specimen	Negative	Positive for *C. botulinum*	Bacteria that causes botulism

Note: Botulism is often diagnosed by history and physical examination.

PRIMARY NURSING DIAGNOSIS

Ineffective airway clearance related to respiratory muscle paralysis

OUTCOMES. Respiratory status: Gas exchange and ventilation; Safety status: Physical injury

INTERVENTIONS. Airway insertion; Airway management; Airway suctioning; Oral health promotion; Respiratory monitoring; Ventilation assistance

☐ PLANNING AND IMPLEMENTATION

Collaborative

Report cases of botulism toxicity so that others can be protected from the illness. When botulism poisoning from ingestion is suspected, the patient's stomach is lavaged to remove any unabsorbed toxin; a high colonic enema may also be administered for the same purpose. If impaired swallowing and chewing last longer than 72 hours, enteral feeding via a nasogastric (NG) or nasointestinal tube or total parenteral nutrition is instituted.

WOUND CARE. Infected wounds are explored and debrided. Usually the physician prescribes antibiotics such as penicillin to kill bacteria in the wound, although the treatment with antibiotics is controversial.

SUPPORTIVE CARE. If respiratory paralysis occurs, intubation or tracheostomy and mechanical ventilation are essential to maintain airway and breathing. At least every hour, monitor the patient's breath sounds, placement, and position of the endotracheal tube; the respiratory rate and lung expansion; and the type and characteristics of secretions. A Foley catheter is inserted to monitor urinary output and prevent bladder distension.

PHARMACOLOGIC HIGHLIGHTS

Medication or Drug Class	Dosage	Description	Rationale
Trivalent botulism antitoxin (TBA)	One vial IM, one vial IV	Equine antitoxin	Neutralizes absorbed toxin

Note: Dose is administered as soon as the diagnosis is suspected and before it is confirmed. If symptoms worsen during the next 4 hours, another vial is given intravenously. One more vial can be administered in 12 to 24 hours if indicated. Before administering the TBA, obtain a history of drug allergies from the patient. In addition, if the patient is allergic to horses, notify the physician immediately because TBA is prepared from equine (horse) serum. Have epinephrine available if the patient experiences an allergic reaction. Infants with botulism generally are not treated with medication, which has not been shown to be beneficial, but rather receive supportive care. Nonabsorbed toxin may be removed with cathartics.

Independent

Other family members who have been exposed to contaminated food should obtain health care immediately. Exposed family members should receive an immediate gastric lavage and a high colonic enema to purge their system of the toxin in the bowel if they were exposed.

Patients are not given food, fluids, or medications orally until their swallowing status is normal and they have an active gag reflex. Provide mouth care every 2 hours to improve comfort and to destroy oral flora. Because the patient has difficulty speaking, establish other routes for communication. Explain that the ability to speak returns as the condition resolves.

During periods of impaired mobility, turn patients every 2 hours, and monitor their skin for breakdown. Egg-crate mattresses or an air bed may be useful. At a minimum of every shift, perform active and/or passive range-of-motion exercises for immobile or bedridden patients. Position unconscious patients on their sides to prevent aspiration of stomach contents; tracheal suction and chest physiotherapy may be indicated to maintain pulmonary hygiene.

Offer clarification and support of the information regarding the diagnosis and prognosis to patients and families. Monitor the patient's and family's coping mechanisms to determine if effective coping mechanisms are in place.

DOCUMENTATION GUIDELINES

- Respiratory assessment: Rate and rhythm, lung expansion, breath sounds, color of skin and mucous membranes, oxygen saturation, patency and placement of artificial airways, response to mechanical ventilation
- Neurological assessment: Level of consciousness, strength and movement, status of cough and gag reflexes, cranial nerve function, ability to swallow
- Cardiovascular assessment: Heart rate and rhythm, blood pressure, peripheral pulses, color of complexion, skin temperature
- Response to medications, intubation, oxygen therapy, mechanical ventilation
- Condition of skin and mucous membranes
- GI assessment: Bowel sounds, presence of abdominal distension, volume and character of NG tube output, stool character, and bowel elimination patterns

DISCHARGE AND HOME HEALTHCARE GUIDELINES

PATIENT AND FAMILY TEACHING. Teach the family that botulism is a preventable disorder. Explain that patients should discard any canned food that has a broken seal or an expired date, or is swollen. Home-canned foods should be boiled, not warmed, before eating. Boiling for 20 minutes destroys botulism bacteria and spores. Instruct patients living in high altitudes to use a pressure cooker to boil foods adequately. Teach patients to use new cap seals with each canning session if they can at home. Teach the family to recognize the complications of botulism. If the patient survives the poisoning, teach patients and families that residual effects might be present for a year or more. Intensive, multidisciplinary rehabilitation and follow-up may be required to restore full function.

Brain Cancer

DRG Category: 010
Mean LOS: 6.7 days
Description: MEDICAL: Nervous System Neoplasms with CC
DRG Category: 001
Mean LOS: 9.6 days
Description: SURGICAL: Craniotomy Age >17 Except for Trauma

Primary brain cancers arise from several different tissues within the intracranial cavity and are fairly common in both children and adults. Although there are a wide variety of histologic types (see Table 13), a small number of tumor types account for most morbidity and mortality.

Primary brain tumors develop from various tissue types within the intracranial cavity. Tumors are customarily described as benign or malignant; however, all brain tumors may be considered malignant because without treatment the patient dies. Even tumors that are well contained may lead to serious consequences because they compress or invade neighboring structures within the enclosed skull. Brain tumors cause their symptoms directly by destroying neurons or indirectly by exerting pressure, displacing brain structures, and increasing intracranial pressure. Besides primary tumors arising from intracranial tissue, metastatic tumors

TABLE 13 | **Primary Intracranial Tumors**

TUMOR	PERCENTAGE OF CASES	MEAN AGE AT DIAGNOSIS	CLINICAL MANIFESTATIONS	TREATMENT AND PROGNOSIS
Glioblastoma multiform (spongioblastoma)	40	54	Twice as common in males. Increased ICP with nonspecific mental and behavioral changes at first. Later focal signs depending on location.	Surgery where possible. Poor response to radiation. Course is rapidly progressive with poor prognosis
Astrocytoma	16	37	Presentation similar to gliobastoma but slower. Headache, decreased motor strength and coordination; seizures or altered vital signs	By time of diagnosis, total excision is usually not possible unless there is a cerebellar lesion. Variable prognosis.
Medulloblastoma	<5	5	Seen frequently in children, males more than females. Nonspecific symptoms of increased ICP. Local signs vary with location.	Surgery combined with radiation and chemotherapy.
Ependymoma	<5	10	Similar to oligodendroglioma. Increased ICP hand hydrocephalus if tumor obstructs CSF pathway.	Surgical excision. Usually not radiosensitive.
Oligodendroglioma	<5	45	More common in middle-aged women. Slow growing with gradual development of symptoms. Decreased visual acuity and other visual disturbances.	Surgical excision, which is usually successful.
Meningioma	18	35	More common in females. Originates from dura or arachnoid. Compresses rather than invades structures. Headache, vomiting, seizures, mental and behavioral changes.	Surgery. May recur if excision is incomplete.

(continued)

TABLE 13 | **Primary Intracranial Tumors (*Continued*)**

TUMOR	PERCENTAGE OF CASES	MEAN AGE AT DIAGNOSIS	CLINICAL MANIFESTATIONS	TREATMENT AND PROGNOSIS
Schwannoma (acoustic neurinoma, neurilemma)	2	57	Higher incidence in women. Ipsilateral hearing loss is most common. Later may be accompanied by tinnitus, heacache, vertigo.	Excision by translabyrinth surgery, craniotomy, or both. Usually favorable outcome.
Pituitary adenoma	12	39	As tumor grows, it replaces endocrine gland cells, leading to endocrine symptoms such as hypopituitarism, Addisonian crisis, or diabetes insipidus. Conversly, they may produce excesses of the hormone. May also lead to visual symptoms, headaches, increased ICP.	Surgery (frontal or transphenoidal) or radiation for small tumors.
Lymphoma	2	46	Growing incidence, perhaps because of the growing incidence of immunosuppressed patients, such as those with acquired immunodeficiency syndrome and post-solid-organ or bone marrow transplant patients. May have no symptoms or focal ones.	Usually brain radiation. Chemotherapy may have an adjunctive role.

may also migrate to the area by hematogenous spread. Common sources for brain metastases are the lung, breast, and colon. Advances in diagnosis, surgical techniques, and adjunctive therapy have greatly improved the outlook for patients with brain cancer. About 50% are treatable with a hopeful prognosis.

CAUSES

Evidence suggests that therapeutic radiation for other purposes (e.g., leukemia) may predispose one to later development of a brain tumor. Brain tumors are also more common in the immunosuppressed population.

GENDER AND LIFE SPAN CONSIDERATIONS

Brain tumors may occur at any age and are fairly common in both children and adults, with about 100,000 symptomatic brain tumors, including metastatic brain tumors, diagnosed per year. They are common in children less than 1 year old, and then again between 2 and 13 years old. In children, primary tumors of the brain and spinal column are the second most common (after leukemias) type of childhood cancer—that is, the most common solid tumor. However, most central nervous system (CNS) tumors occur in patients over 45, with the peak incidence found after 70. More than 50% of those are metastatic rather than primary. Gender considerations depend on tumor type.

◻ ASSESSMENT

HISTORY. Symptoms produced by tumors vary by cell type and location and may cause generalized or focal symptoms. Although clearly every case of headache or dizziness is not a sign of brain tumor, it must always be considered. Any of the following indicate the possibility of a brain tumor: headache, progressive neurologic deficit, convulsions (focal or generalized), increased intracranial pressure (ICP), and organic mental changes.

The generalized symptoms are usually caused by increased ICP from the tumor, obstruction of the cerebrospinal fluid (CSF) pathways, or cerebral edema. Headache and vomiting are the most common first symptoms of increased ICP. Typically, headache is worse in the morning and may waken the patient from sleep. The patient or significant others may also report personality changes, increased fatigue, decreased endurance, visual disturbances, and a tendency toward social withdrawal. Generalized seizures are the presenting symptoms in 15% of adults and 30% of children.

Focal signs and symptoms result from local pressure or damage to limited parts of the brain and depend on the area of the brain affected. Tumors in the dominant hemisphere produce communication difficulties (aphasia); tumors near an optic tract will produce changes in visual fields. A lesion in the temporal lobe may lead to temporal lobe seizures that are exhibited by unexplained olfactory sensations, visual auras, or psychomotor seizures, all of which may be misdiagnosed as psychological problems or mental illness.

PHYSICAL EXAMINATION. Inspect the child suspected of a brain tumor before the sutures are closed; there may be head enlargement or bulging of the fontanelles from increased ICP. In rare cases, an adult with meningioma may have skull bulging. The appearance of the optic disc may change; if the tumor compresses the optic nerve, it will remain flat or atrophy. If ICP is increased, papilledema is possible. Perform a thorough neurologic examination to identify changes in vision, hearing, sensation, and movement. A tumor may exert local pressure causing apraxia (inability to use objects), paresthesia (numbness and tingling), paresis (partial or incomplete paralysis), or hyperreflexia.

PSYCHOSOCIAL. Assess for the presence of irritability and personality changes. Changes in a person's mental status and ability to perform various roles are extremely disturbing to patients and significant others. Families and patients often display profound grief, extreme anxiety, and disbelief upon receiving the diagnosis of a brain tumor.

DIAGNOSTIC HIGHLIGHTS

Test	Normal Result	Abnormality with Condition	Explanation
Computed tomography (CT) and magnetic resonance imaging (MRI)	No space occupying lesions	Locates size, location, and extent of tumor	Used for initial evaluation as well as response to treatment

Other Tests: Cerebral angiogram; electroencephalography; lumbar puncture; myelogram; brain scan; positron emission tomography.

PRIMARY NURSING DIAGNOSIS

Decreased intracranial adaptive capacity

OUTCOMES. Neurologic status; Neurological status: Consciousness; Fluid balance

INTERVENTIONS. Cerebral perfusion promotion; Cerebral edema management; Neurologic monitoring; Surveillance; Surveillance: Safety; Positioning: Neurologic; Vital signs monitoring; Medication management

☐ PLANNING AND IMPLEMENTATION

Collaborative

The type of treatment used for brain cancer depends on the type of tumor. (See Table 13.) The primary modes of treatment include surgery, radiotherapy, and pharmacologic therapy.

SURGICAL. Surgery remains the primary treatment modality. The goals of surgery are (1) total removal of the tumor, (2) subtotal removal to relieve symptoms, or (3) procedures to protect the brain from damage, for example, placement of a shunt to relieve hydrocephalus. Other modalities are used in combination. After the surgery, the patient needs careful monitoring for increased ICP. Notify the surgeon if the bone flap becomes elevated, which is a sign of increased ICP. The physician usually manages cerebral swelling and elevated ICP with fluid restriction (usually 1500 mL or less in 24 hours), steroids, and osmotic diuretics such as mannitol.

RADIATION. For tumors that are not accessible to surgical removal, radiation may be used. Locally contained tumors receive direct beam radiation focused on the lesion. For multiple lesions, especially metastatic brain lesions, whole-brain radiation therapy (WBRT) is used.

PHARMACOLOGIC HIGHLIGHTS

Medication or Drug Class	Dosage	Description	Rationale
Chemotherapy	Varies by drug	Some germ cell tumors respond well to a combination of vincristine, bleomycin, methotrexate, and cisplatin.	Chemotherapy plays a very minor role in treatment of brain metastases. The blood-brain barrier prevents delivery to the tumor of the cytotoxic agents in high concentrations.

Independent

The first priority is to ensure that the airway is patent. Keep equipment to manage the airway (endotracheal tube, laryngoscope, nasal and oral airway) within easy access of the patient. Make sure that working endotracheal suction is at the bedside. Note that an obstructed airway and increased levels of carbon dioxide contribute to increased ICP in patients with a space-occupying lesion. Keep the patient comfortable but not oversedated. If the patient is awake, encourage him or her to avoid Valsalva's maneuver and isometric muscle contractions when moving or sitting up in bed to limit the risk of increased ICP. Perform serial neurologic assessment to watch for sudden changes in mental status.. To reduce ICP and optimize lung expansion, place the patient in semi-Fowler position. Keep the head in good alignment with the body to prevent compression on the veins that allow for venous drainage of the head. Avoid hip flexion. Assist the patient to turn in bed and perform coughing, deep breathing, and leg exercises every 2 hours to prevent skin breakdown, as well as pulmonary and vascular stasis. As soon as allowed, help the patient get out of bed and ambulate in hallways three to four times each day. If the patient has sensory or motor deficits, work with the rehabilitation team to encourage activities of daily living and increased independence.

Patients who have been newly diagnosed with brain cancer are often in emotional shock, especially when the disease is diagnosed in the advanced stages or is inoperable. Encourage the patient and family to verbalize their feelings surrounding the diagnosis and impending death.

Assist family members in identifying the extent of home care that is realistically required by the patient. Arrange for visits by a home health agency. Suggest supportive counseling (hospice, grief counselor) and, if necessary, make the initial contact. Local units of the American Cancer Society offer assistance with home care supplies and support groups for patients and families. Instruct the patient to use the pain scale effectively and to request pain medication before the pain escalates to an intolerable level. Consider switching as-needed pain medication to an around-the-clock dosing schedule to keep pain under control.

DOCUMENTATION GUIDELINES

- Response to the diagnosis of cancer, the diagnostic tests, and recommended treatment regimen

- Physical responses: Patency of airway, neurologic assessments, vital signs, signs of increased ICP or seizure activity, description of all dressings and wounds, appearance of incision
- Response to and tolerance to therapy: Radiation, surgery, chemotherapy
- Presence of complications: Increased ICP, hemorrhage, infection, pulmonary congestion, activity intolerance, unrelieved discomfort
- Activity level, progress in rehabilitation if appropriate, ability to perform independent activities of daily living

DISCHARGE AND HOME HEALTHCARE GUIDELINES

FOLLOW-UP. Consult with occupational and physical therapists to develop an appropriate rehabilitation plan, if one is needed. Discuss aids for self-care and mobilization such as wheelchairs, bathroom rails, and speech aids and where and how they can be obtained. Evaluate the home situation before discharge to determine if wheelchair access is available if it is necessary.

Teach the patient and family strategies to avoid exposure to infection. If the patient develops an infection or notes increased bleeding, teach the patient to notify the primary healthcare provider immediately. Teach the patient and significant others the early signs of tumor recurrence so that they can notify the primary healthcare provider if they occur. Instruct the patient on care of the skin in the external radiation field.

Stress the need to maintain a schedule for follow-up visits as recommended by the physician.

MEDICATIONS. Explain the purpose, action, dosage, desired effects, and side effects of all medications prescribed by the physician.

Breast Cancer

DRG Category: 274
Mean LOS: 5.9 days
Description: MEDICAL: Malignant Breast Disorders with CC
DRG Category: 260
Mean LOS: 1.9 days
Description: SURGICAL: Subtotal Mastectomy for Malignancy without CC
DRG Category: 257
Mean LOS: 3.5 days
Description: SURGICAL: Total Mastectomy for Malignancy with CC

One in eight women in the United States will develop breast cancer in her lifetime, making it the most common cancer in women in this country. It is second to lung cancer in cause of cancer deaths in women. If it is found in early stages (in situ with no node involvement), the 10-year survival rate is 70% to 75% compared to 20% to 25% when the nodes are positive. Breast cancer can recur even 20 to 30 years after the first diagnosis.

Carcinoma of the breast stems from the epithelial tissues of the ducts and lobules. Breast cancer is classified as either noninvasive or invasive. Noninvasive carcinoma refers to cancer in the ducts of lobules and is also called carcinoma in situ (5% of breast cancers). Invasive carcinoma (also known as infiltrating carcinoma) occurs when the cancer cells invade the tissue beyond the ducts or lobules. The rate of cell division of the cancerous growth varies, but it is estimated that the time it takes for a tumor to be palpable will range from 5 to 9 years. When the cancer cells become invasive, they grow in an irregular or sunburst pattern that is palpated as a poorly defined lump or thickening. As the tumor continues to grow, fibrosis forms around the cancer, causing the Cooper's ligaments to shorten, which results in dimpling of the skin. Advanced tumors will interrupt the lymph drainage, resulting in skin edema and an "orange peel" (peau d'orange) appearance. Untreated cancer may erupt on the skin as an ulceration.

CAUSES

The origin of breast cancer is a complex interaction between the biologic and endocrine properties of the person and the environmental exposures that may precipitate mutation of cells to a malignancy. The greatest risk by far is family history of breast cancer.

Other risk factors include European ancestry, residence in North America or Europe, age of more than 40, personal history of breast cancer, history of benign breast disease, nulliparity or an age more than 30 years for the first-time pregnancy, menarche before 12, menopause after 55, and postmenopausal obesity. Recent studies support an association of breast cancer with moderate alcohol intake, high-fat diet, and prolonged hormonal replacement therapy. Other environmental factors include exposure to radiation (during childhood or significant chest radiation) or pesticide residues.

GENDER AND LIFE SPAN CONSIDERATIONS

Breast cancer is predominantly a disease of women over 40, with incidence rates increasing with age. Annual incidence of breast cancer is less than 60 per 100,000 below age 40; 100 per 100,000 by age 50; and nearly 200 per 100,000 at age 70. Only 1% of breast cancer affects men, and it usually occurs when they are over the age of 60. The case of the elderly with breast cancer is essentially the same as with younger patients.

☐ ASSESSMENT

HISTORY. Assess the patient's and family's previous medical history of breast cancer or other cancers. Obtain a detailed history of hormonal and reproductive sequences and medications (specifically hormonal supplements). Assess lifestyle variables such as diet, exercise, alcohol use, and occupational history. Determine how, when, and by whom the lump was found (breast self-examination [BSE], mammograph, accident). Ask how much time elapsed between finding the lump and seeking professional care in order to estimate the length of time the tumor has been present. Proceed with the systemic review with attention to areas where metastasis is common.

PHYSICAL EXAMINATION. Inspect the breast skin for signs of advanced disease: the presence of inflammation, dimpling, orange peel effect, distended vessels, and nipple changes or ulceration. Palpate both breasts to evaluate the tissues and identify the mass. Examine the axillary and supraclavicular areas for enlarged nodes. You may note the tumor is firm and immovable. Assess the patient for pain or tenderness at the tumor site.

PSYCHOSOCIAL. Patients present a wide range of responses: denial, fighting spirit, hopelessness, stoic acceptance, anxious preoccupation. Elicit a careful and ongoing assessment of the patient's feelings (anger, depression, anxiety, fear) and body image concerns. Identify the patient's perceptions of how breast cancer will affect her role relationships, lifestyle, femininity, and sexuality. Be sure to include the husband or significant other and children in the psychological assessment to learn of their emotional needs.

DIAGNOSTIC HIGHLIGHTS

General Comments: Often patients identify a lump when doing a monthly BSE.

Test	Normal Result	Abnormality with Condition	Explanation
Mammogram	No tumor noted	Radiodense or white mass is noted	Is an x ray of the breast; can only suggest a diagnosis of cancer
Ultrasound of the breast	No evidence of cyst or tumor	Appearance of a white lesion	Can differentiate between cystic and solid lesions
Stereotaxic biopsy or mammotomy probes	Benign	Malignant	Confirms the diagnosis

Other Tests: computed tomography (CT) scan; estrogen receptor (ER) assay and progesterone receptor (PR) assay; flow cytometry; DNA ploidy.

PRIMARY NURSING DIAGNOSIS

Body image disturbance related to significance of loss of part or all of the breast

OUTCOMES. Body image; Psychosocial adjustment: Life change; Acceptance: Health status

INTERVENTIONS. Body image enhancement; Support group; Support system enhancement; Wound care

◻ PLANNING AND IMPLEMENTATION

Collaborative

Treatment and prognosis for breast cancer are based on the stage of disease at diagnosis according to the TNM classification (T = tumor size, N = involvement of regional lymph nodes, M = metastasis). (See Table 14.) It is now recognized that treatment of breast cancer requires a multimodal approach. Surgery and radiation, either alone or in combination, control cancer in the breast and regional lymph nodes. Chemotherapy and hormonal therapy are intended to provide systemic control. Adjuvant therapy (pharmacologic treatment given to patients with no detectable cancer after surgery) is often recommended because cancer cells can break away from the primary breast tumor and begin to spread through the bloodstream, even in the early stages of disease. These cells cannot be felt or detected on x ray.

TABLE 14 | **TNM Classification: Staging for Breast Cancer**

STAGE	SIZE	INVOLVEMENT
Stage I	2 cm or less	No node involvement, no metastasis
Stage II	Up to 5 cm	May have axillary node involvement, no metastasis
Stage III	Varied (any size)	Extended to skin or chest wall, nodes involved (immovable axillary nodes)
Stage IV	Varied	Distant metastasis with ipsilateral supraclavicular nodes

SURGICAL. The goal of surgery is control of cancer in the breast and the axillary nodes. Most women have a choice of surgical procedures, but it depends on the clinical stage, tumor location, contraindications to radiation (pregnancy, collagen disease, prior radiation, multifocal tumors), and the presence of other health problems. Several types of surgical therapy are commonly available, as follow.

MODIFIED RADICAL MASTECTOMY (TOTAL MASTECTOMY). The most common surgical procedure for mastectomy removes the entire breast and some or all of the axillary nodes, as well as the lining over the pectoralis major muscle. At times, the pectoralis minor muscle is removed.

BREAST-PRESERVING SURGERIES. The breast-preserving surgeries combined with radiotherapy are recognized to be equivalent to modified radical mastectomy for stage I and II breast cancer for survival rates and local control.

Sentinel lymph node biopsy, a procedure using a radioactive tracer to determine which lymph nodes need to be removed during a mastectomy, is under investigation. This procedure will allow fewer lymph nodes to be removed, decreasing the uncomfortable side effect of lymphedema that can occur with surgery.

COMPLICATIONS OF SURGERY. The complications of breast surgery may be infection, seroma (fluid accumulation at the operative site), hematoma, limited range of motion (ROM), sensory changes, and lymphedema. A seroma is usually prevented with the placement of a gravity drainage device (Hemovac, Jackson-Pratt) in the site for up to 7 days postoperatively. Drains are usually removed when drainage has decreased to about 30 cc per day. ROM for the lower arm is begun within 24 hours postoperation, and full ROM and other shoulder exercises are ordered by the surgeon after the drains are removed. Sensory changes include numbness, weakness, skin sensitivity, itching, heaviness, or phantom sensations that may last a year.

RADIATION THERAPY. Radiotherapy is routinely given 2 to 4 weeks after breast-preserving surgery for stage I and II breast cancer. Sometimes, it is indicated after modified radical surgery if four or more nodes are positive. The incision needs to be healed, and ROM of the shoulder should be restored. Radiotherapy may consist of an external beam to the breast for 4 to 6 weeks or by an experimental method called brachytherapy (interstitial iridium-192 implants) directly to the tumor site, or both. Radiation can be given at the same time as chemotherapy.

CHEMOTHERAPY/HORMONAL THERAPY. Combination chemotherapy is recommended for pre- and postmenopausal patients with positive nodes. Hormonal therapy is used to change the levels of hormones that promote cancer growth and increase survival time in women with metastatic breast cancer. Tumors with a positive ER assay (tumors that need estrogen to grow) have a response rate to hormonal therapy of 65% compared to a 10% response rate with negative ER assay. PR assays that are also positive enhance endocrine therapy response even more. There is a 77% response rate if both ER and PR are positive, as compared to a 5% response rate if both are negative.

AUTOLOGOUS BONE MARROW TRANSPLANT (ABMT). Certain patients (with chemosensitive tumors) with stage III cancer are being treated with high-dose chemotherapy preceded by removal of the patient's bone marrow, which is then restored after chemotherapy.

RECONSTRUCTION. Approximately 30% of women who have mastectomies choose to have breast reconstruction. (See Table 15.)

TABLE 15 | **Types of Breast Reconstructive Surgery**

TYPE	DESCRIPTION
Saline-filled implants	A tissue expander is placed under the pectoralis muscle and expanded slowly over months with saline injections. The expander is removed and replaced with a permanent saline implant. The expander may be the adjustable type, serving a dual purpose of expanding and permanent implant.
Autologous tissue transfer	Surgical procedure uses the women's own tissue to form a breast mound. In two procedures (latissimus dorsi flap of the transverse rectus abdominus muscle [TRAM]), the surgeon tunnels a wedge of muscle, fascia, subcutaneous tissue, and skin to the mastectomy site. In free-flap reconstruction (free tissue transfer), the surgeon uses a microvascular technique to transfer a segment of skin and subcutaneous tissue with its vascular pedicle to the chest wall.

Almost all patients who have mastectomies are candidates. It can be immediate (at the time of mastectomy) or delayed for several years.

Postoperatively, use a flow sheet every hour and assess adequate blood supply to the flap and donor site by evaluating the following: color (to verify that it is the same as skin from the donor area [not opposite breast]); temperature (warm); tissue turgor (to verify that it is not tight or tense); capillary refill (well-perfused flap will blanch for 1 to 3 seconds); and anterior blood flow using ultrasonic or laser Doppler. Unusual pain or decreased volume of drainage may indicate vascular impairment to the flap. Early detection of impaired circulation can be treated with anticoagulants or antispasmodics and possibly prevent further surgical interventions. Provide emotional support for the patient who is distraught over her appearance to reassure her the breast will look more normal with healing. The nipple and areola can be added 6 to 9 months later.

PHARMACOLOGIC HIGHLIGHTS

Medication or Drug Class	Dosage	Description	Rationale
Cyclophosphamide + methotrexate +	Depends on drug, stage of cancer, and	Antineoplastics	Interfere with growth of cancer;

fluorouracil (CMF)	patient condition		often used in combination
Cyclophosphamide + doxorubicin (Adriamycin) + fluorouracil (CAF)			
Doxorubicin (Adriamycin) + cyclophoshpamide (AC) with or without paclitaxel (Taxol)			
Doxorubicin followed by CMF			
Tamoxifen citrate	10–20 mg bid po or 20 mg po q	Antiestrogen	Provides hormonal control of cancer growth; adjuvant treatment after a mastectomy
Toremifene (Fareston)	60 mg po q		
Anastrozole	1 mg po q		
Trastuzumab (Herceptin)	4 mg/kg loading dose; 2 mg/kg maintenance, IVPB	Recombinant DNA–derived humanized monoclonal antibody	Indicated only for HER2/neu receptive tumors; decreases breast cancer growth and stimulates immune system to more effectively attack the cancer
Acetaminophen; NSAIDs; opiods; combination of opiod and NSAIDs	Depends on the drug, and the patient's condition and tolerance	Analgesics	Choice of drug depends on the severity of the pain

Experimental Therapy: Biologic-response modifiers (interferon, interleukins, monoclonal antibodies), doxetaxel, capecitabine, vinorelbine, irinotecan and gemcitabine hydrochloride (an antineoplastic currently used to treat pancreatic cancer) individually, and in combination, are under investigation. Tamoxifen and raloxifene hydrochloride are also under investigation for prophylaxis of breast cancer in high-risk and post-menopausal women.

Independent

The focus of nursing care for a patient with a mastectomy during the 2- to 3-day hospital stay will be directed toward early surgical recovery. Teach pain management, mobility, adequate circulation, and self-care activities to prepare the patient for discharge. In the immediate postoperative period, keep the head of the bed elevated 30 degrees, with the affected arm elevated on a pillow to facilitate lymph drainage. Instruct the patient not to turn on the affected side. Place a sign at the head of the bed immediately after surgery with directions for no blood pressures, blood draws, injections, or intravenous lines on the arm of the operative side; this should help prevent circulatory impairment.

Emphasize the importance of ambulation and using the operative side within 24 hours. Initially, the arm will need to be supported when the patient is out of bed. As ambulation progresses, encourage the patient to hang her arm at her side normally, keeping her shoulders back to avoid the hunchback position and to prevent contractures. Within 24 hours, begin with exercises that do not stress the incision.

Teach the patient how to empty the drainage device (Hemovac or other), measure the drainage accurately, and observe for the color and consistency of the drainage. Create a flow sheet for record keeping in the hospital, and send it home with the patient to use until the drain is removed. At the dressing change, begin teaching the dressing change procedure and the indications of complications such as infection (purulent drainage, redness, pain), presence of fluid collection, or hematoma formation at the incision. Be sensitive to the patient's reactions upon seeing the incision for the first time with full realization that her breast is gone. Explain that phantom breast sensations and numbness at the operative site along the inner side of the armpit to the elbow are normal for several months because of interruptions of nerve endings.

Women may have feelings of loss not only of their breast but also of lifestyle, social interactions, sexuality, and even life itself. Patients often feel more comfortable expressing their feelings with nurses than with family members or the physician. Effective coping requires expression of feelings. Discuss the services and goals of Reach to Recovery (psychologic and physical support). If the patient is willing, arrange for an in-hospital visit or early home visit.

DOCUMENTATION GUIDELINES

- Response to surgical interventions: Condition of dressing and wound, stability of vital signs, recovery from anesthesia
- Presence of complications: Pain, edema, infection, seroma, limited ROM
- Knowledge of and intent to comply with adjuvant therapies
- Reaction to cancer and body changes
- Knowledge of and intent to comply with incision care, postoperative exercises, arm precautions, follow-up care, and early detection methods for recurrence

DISCHARGE AND HOME HEALTHCARE GUIDELINES

PATIENT TEACHING. The patient can expect to return home with dressings and wound drains. Instruct the patient to do the following: empty the drainage receptacle twice a day, record the amount on a flow sheet, and take this information along when keeping a doctor's appointment; report symptoms of infection or excess drainage on the dressing or the drainage device; sponge bathe until the sutures and drains are removed; continue with daily lower arm ROM exercises until the surgeon orders more strenuous exercises; avoid caffeinated foods and drinks, nicotine, and secondary smoke for 3 weeks postoperatively. Review pain medication instructions for frequency and precautions.

Teach precautions to prevent lymphedema after node dissection (written directions or pamphlet from American Cancer Society [ACS] is desirable for lifetime referral):
Request no blood pressure or blood samples from affected arm.

Do not carry packages, handbags, or luggage with the affected arm; avoid elastic cuffs.

Protect the hand and arm from burns, sticks, and cuts by wearing gloves to do gardening and housework, using a thimble to sew, applying sunscreen and insect repellent when out-of-doors.

Report swelling, pain, or heat in the affected arm immediately.

Put the arm above the head and pump the fist frequently throughout the day.

FOLLOW-UP. Prepare the patient and family for a variety of encounters with healthcare providers (radiologist, oncologist, phlebotomist). Try to provide a continuity between the providers (yourself, clinical nurse specialist, or nurse consultant system, if available) as a resource for the patient or family to call with questions.

Provide lists and information of local community resources and support groups for emotional support: Reach to Recovery, Y-ME, Wellness Center, Can Surmount, I Can Cope; a list of businesses that specialize in breast protheses; phone numbers for ACS and Cancer Information System.

Recurrence is a lifetime threat. Inform the patient that it is necessary to continue monthly BSE (even on the operative side) and annual mammogram and physician examinations of both the reconstructed and nonreconstructed breasts. Be certain the patient can demonstrate an accurate BSE.

Bronchiolitis (Respiratory Syncytial Viral Infection)

DRG Category: 80
Mean LOS: 4.7 days
Description: MEDICAL: Respiratory Infections and Inflammations, age 0–17

Bronchiolitis is a common disease of the lower respiratory tract that is most commonly caused by the respiratory syncytial virus (RSV). The infection, which causes inflammation leading to obstruction of the small respiratory airways, can range from a mild infection that lasts only a few days to a severe episode that causes severe respiratory distress. Older children and adults often experience a "mild" upper respiratory infection with RSV because they have larger airways and can tolerate the airway swelling with fewer symptoms than do infants. The virus leads to necrosis of the bronchiolar epithelium, hypersecretion of mucous, and infiltration and edema of the surrounding cells. These changes are further complicated by mucous plugs that obstruct the bronchioles and lead to collapse of the distal lung tissue.

The incubation period is approximately 4 days from the time of exposure to the time of the first manifestation of the illness. Infants shed the virus for up to 12 days, and the spread of infection occurs when large infected droplets (airborne or through direct contact with secretions) are inoculated in the nose or eyes of a susceptible person. In temperate climates, infants most often contract RSV during the winter months. Mortality of infants with a lower respiratory infection due to RSV is approximately 2%. Young premature infants have a poorer outcome. A significant number of infants who develop bronchiolitis have reactive airway disease later in life.

CAUSES

Bronchiolitis has a viral derivation; RSV is responsible for up to 75% of the cases, but other viruses such as parainfluenza virus (type 3), mycoplasma, or adenoviruses cause the remainder of illnesses. RSV is a medium-sized RNA virus that develops within the infected cell and reproduces by budding from the cell membrane. Generally the source of the RSV is an older family member with a mild upper respiratory infection.

GENDER AND LIFE SPAN CONSIDERATIONS

Bronchiolitis commonly occurs in the first 2 years of life. Severe infections are rare in children less than 6 weeks old because maternal antibodies have a protective effect during the first weeks of life. Bronchiolitis and pneumonia due to RSV are more common in boys than in girls (ratio 1.5 to 1).

☐ ASSESSMENT

HISTORY. Ask if any members of the household have had a cold or upper respiratory infection. The infant usually has a history of an upper respiratory infection and runny nose (rhinorrhea) that lasts for several days. Infants may have increasing restlessness or depressed sensorium. Infants often have a moderate fever of approximately 102°F, a decrease in appetite, poor feeding, and gradual development of respiratory distress. A cough usually appears after the first few days of symptoms. Some children wheeze audibly.

PHYSICAL EXAMINATION. The infant or child appears to be in acute respiratory distress with a rapid respiratory rate, air hunger, nasal flaring, hyperexpansion of the lungs, and even intercostal and subcostal retractions with cyanosis. When you auscultate the infant's chest, you will likely hear diffuse rhonchi, fine crackles, and wheezes. The liver and spleen are easily palpable because they are pushed down by the hyperinflated lungs. Signs of life-threatening respiratory distress include listlessness, central cyanosis, tachypnea at a respiratory rate of over 70 breaths a minute, and apnea. Usually the most critically ill infants have greatly hyperexpanded chests that are silent to air movement upon auscultation. Inspect the infant for a rash and conjunctivitis.

PSYCHOSOCIAL. The parents and child will be apprehensive. Assess the parents' ability to cope with the acute or emergency situation and intervene as appropriate. Note that many children are treated at home rather than in the hospital; your teaching plan may need to consider home rather than hospital management.

DIAGNOSTIC HIGHLIGHTS

General Comments: Diagnostic testing involves identifying the causative organism, determining oxygenation status, and ruling out masses as a cause of obstruction.

Test	Normal Result	Abnormality with Condition	Explanation
Pulse oximetry	≥95%	<95%	Low oxygen saturation is present if there is

			obstruction in the lung passages
Chest x ray	Normal lung structure	Air trapping or hyper-expansion, peribronchial thickening or interstitial pneumonia, segmental consolidation	Results of inflammation and mucous plugs

Other Tests: Complete blood count; arterial blood gases; differential, bacterial cultures; immunofluorescence analysis of nasal washings to detect RSV

PRIMARY NURSING DIAGNOSIS

Ineffective airway clearance related to bronchial infection and obstruction

OUTCOMES. Respiratory status: Airway patency; Respiratory status: Gas exchange; Respiratory status: Ventilation

INTERVENTIONS. Airway management; Respiratory monitoring; Vital signs monitoring; Anxiety reduction

◻ PLANNING AND IMPLEMENTATION

Collaborative

The aim of treatment is to maintain a patent airway and provide adequate respiratory exchange. Medical management includes cool, oxygenated mist for severely ill infants who require hospitalization and careful intravenous hydration. Tube feeding for hydration is preferable to intravenous therapy if suckling is difficult. Generally, antibiotics are not considered useful and lead to bacterial resistance. Antiviral drugs are used in the most severely ill infants.

Measures to ensure prevention are very important. During RSV season, high-risk infants should be separated from those with respiratory symptoms. Careful hand washing and isolation techniques are important for all healthcare personnel.

PHARMACOLOGIC HIGHLIGHTS

Medication or Drug Class	Dosage	Description	Rationale
Albuterol aerosol	Per nebulizer, varies dependent on size of child	Bronchodilator	Dilates the bronchioles, opening up respiratory passages; used only in those infants with wheezing who seem to benefit from the treatment
Ribavirin	190 μg/L; delivered at a rate of 12.5 L of mist per minute by small-particle aerosol for 20 of the 24 hours for 3–5 days	Antiviral	Halts the replication of the RSV virus by disrupting RNA and DNA synthesis
Antipyretics	Varies with drug	Acetaminophen	Reduces fever

Other Therapy: Corticosteroids are used only as a last resort; the use of bronchodilators is controversial.

Independent

Ongoing, continuous observation of the patency of the child's airway is essential to identify impending obstruction. Prop infants up on pillows or place them in an infant seat; older children should have the head of the bed elevated so that they are in Fowler's position. Usually seriously and critically ill infants are hospitalized because their care at home is difficult. Hospitalized infants are usually elevated to a sitting position at 30 to 40 degrees with the neck extended at the same 30- to 40-degree angle.

Children should be allowed to rest as much as possible to conserve their energy; organize your interventions to limit disturbances. Provide age-appropriate activities. Crying increases the child's difficulty in breathing and should be limited if possible by comfort measures and the presence of the parents; parents should be allowed to hold and comfort the child as much as possible. If the child is in a cool mist tent, parents may need to be enclosed with the child, or the child may need to be held by the parents with the mist directed toward them. Children sense anxiety from their parents; if you support the parents in dealing with their anxiety and fear, the children are less fearful. Careful explanation of all procedures and allowing the parents to participate in the care of the child as much as possible help relieve the anxiety of both child and parents.

Provide adequate hydration to liquefy secretions and to replace fluid loss from increased sensible loss (increased respirations and fever). The child might also have a decreased fluid intake during the illness. Apply lubricant or ointment around the child's mouth and lips to decrease the irritation from secretions and mouth breathing.

DOCUMENTATION GUIDELINES

- Respiratory status: Rate, quality, depth, ease, breath sounds
- Response to treatment: Cool mist oxygen tent, medications, positioning
- Infant's response to illness, feeding, rest, activity
- Parents' emotional responses

DISCHARGE AND HOME HEALTHCARE GUIDELINES

When the infant is ready for discharge, make sure the caregiver understands any medications that are required at home. Instruct the parents to recognize the signs of increasing respiratory obstruction, and advise them when to take the child to an emergency department. If the child is cared for at home, provide the following home care instructions:

Prop the infant in a sitting position to ease breathing, not in a flat position.

Do not use infant aspirin products because of the chance of Reye's syndrome.

Provide a cool mist humidifier.

Bronchitis

DRG Category: 096
Mean LOS: 5.2 days
Description: MEDICAL: Bronchitis and Asthma, Age > 17 with CC

Bronchitis, a form of chronic obstructive pulmonary disease, is an inflammation of the mucous membranes of the bronchi. It is a disease of the larger airways, unlike emphysema, which is a disease of the smaller airways. Inflammation of the airway mucosa leads to edema and the enlargement of the submucosal glands. Damage occurs to cilia and the epithelial cells of the respiratory tract. In addition, leukocytes and lymphocytes infiltrate the walls of the bronchi and lead to inflammation and airway narrowing. Hypersecretion of the submucosal glands leads to obstruction of the airways from excessive mucus. The most prominent symptom is sputum production.

Acute bronchitis has a short, severe course that subsides without long-term effects. Chronic bronchitis leads to excessive production of mucus sufficient to cause a cough for at least 3 months during the year for two consecutive years. Chronic bronchitis, which can often be reversed after the removal of the irritant, is complicated by respiratory tract infections and can lead to right-sided heart failure, pulmonary hypertension, and acute respiratory failure.

CAUSES

Acute bronchitis is usually caused by viruses. The primary cause of chronic bronchitis is smoking or exposure to some type of respiratory irritant. Established risk factors include a history of smoking, occupational exposures, air pollution, reduced lung function, and heredity. Children of parents who smoke are at higher risk for pulmonary infections that may lead to bronchitis.

GENDER AND LIFE SPAN CONSIDERATIONS

Acute bronchitis can occur at any age. Chronic bronchitis can appear between the ages of 25 to 45 years but is more commonly diagnosed between the ages of 40 to 55 years. Up to 20% of adult men in the United States have chronic bronchitis.

☐ ASSESSMENT

HISTORY. Patients with acute bronchitis usually have a self-limiting upper respiratory infection that is associated with chills, fever (100 °F to 102°F), malaise, substernal tightness and achiness, and cough. The patient describes a painful, dry cough that becomes productive with mucopurulent secretions for several days. The secretions generally clear as the inflammation subsides and the symptoms decrease.

Patients with chronic bronchitis usually have a history of smoking or occupational exposure to a respiratory irritant. Patients generally seek health care when they become short of breath, have a cough, or notice increased sputum production. The cough may initially be more common in the winter months and gradually develop into a constant problem regardless of the season. Ask patients if they have experienced fatigue or difficulty with activities of daily living because of shortness of breath. Question their sleep patterns and positions because patients often need to sleep sitting up so that they can breathe better. Request that they explain their eating patterns because often a patient with chronic bronchitis has a poor appetite with difficulty eating because of shortness of breath. A decrease in the patient's weight leads to a decrease in the mass of the diaphragm, which contributes to poor respiratory muscle function.

PHYSICAL EXAMINATION. Patients with acute bronchitis appear acutely ill. Generally they are febrile, mildly dehydrated, and somewhat short of breath. Patients with chronic bronchitis often appear short of breath, a condition that worsens as they speak. To help with breathing, they may use accessory muscles, such as the abdominal muscles, the sternocleidomastoids, and the intercostal muscles. Patients sometimes appear cyanotic. Some with advanced disease have a high $PaCO_2$ that leads to disorientation, headaches, and photophobia (eyes are sensitive to light). Expect copious amounts of mucus that is gray, yellow, or white. Chronic bronchitis may lead to signs of right-sided heart failure, such as peripheral edema and neck vein distension. When you auscultate the patient's lungs, you may hear scattered, fine or coarse crackles, and wheezing, and there may be a prolonged time for expiration.

PSYCHOSOCIAL. The patient with acute bronchitis has a self-limiting disease that lasts approximately 1 to 2 weeks. In contrast, a patient with chronic bronchitis is dealing with a chronic, progressive disease. As the disease progresses, patients become more and more dependent on others for assistance. They may feel isolated and depressed. Patients are limited in their mobility and frequently are homebound. Others are reluctant to go out if they are dependent on oxygen.

DIAGNOSTIC HIGHLIGHTS

Test	Normal Result	Abnormality with Condition	Explanation
Sputum culture and sensitivity	Negative	Presence of bacteria or other microorganisms may occur in chronic bronchitis	Common organisims are *Streptococcus pneumoniae, Haemophilus influenzae*

Other Tests: Chest x ray; arterial blood gas; pulmonary function tests. Monitor the patient's PaO_2 with a pulse oximeter to determine if the oxygen therapy is maintaining adequate oxygenation.

PRIMARY NURSING DIAGNOSIS

Impaired gas exchange related to obstructed airways

OUTCOMES. Respiratory status: Gas exchange; Respiratory status: Ventilation; Comfort level; Anxiety control

INTERVENTIONS. Airway management; Cough enhancement; Respiratory monitoring; Oxygen therapy; Laboratory data interpretation; Positioning; Smoking cessation assistance; Ventilation asssistance

◻ PLANNING AND IMPLEMENTATION

Collaborative

Most hospitalized patients with chronic bronchitis are on low-flow oxygen therapy. If patients retain carbon dioxide, a high level of oxygen shuts off their drive to breathe and they become apneic. Patients with chronic bronchitis may require chest physiotherapy (PT) to help mobilize their secretions. The physician may prescribe postural drainage, chest percussion, and chest vibration to the lobes that are involved, several times daily. Schedule the chest PT sessions so that they occur at least 1 hour before or 2 hours after meals to limit the risk of aspiration.

PHARMACOLOGIC HIGHLIGHTS

General Comments: An important effect of the xanthines is that they may assist with respiratory muscle strength by increasing the contractility of the diaphragm. Steroids are used more often with asthma but may occasionally be used in patients with bronchitis.

Medication or Drug Class	Dosage	Description	Rationale
Antibiotics	Varies with drug	Examples: Amoxicillin, doxycycline, azithromycin	Manage respiratory infections
Bronchodilators	Varies with drug	Ultrasonic or nebulized treatments of medications may be used to open large airways and facilitate clearance of mucus	Relax smooth muscles in the airways and reduce local congestion.

Other Drugs: Xanthines such as aminophylline and theophylline are administered to reduce mucosal edema and smooth-muscle spasms.

Independent

The patient with bronchitis is often short of breath and fatigued. Space the activities to allow frequent rest periods. These patients may be dependent upon others for some of their activities of daily living, especially if they are in the hospital for an exacerbation of their disease. Elevate the head of the bed to allow the patient to assume an easier position for breathing. Patients often assume a tripod position, that is, an upright position with arms resting on a table and shoulders hunched forward. Do not impose bed rest on a patient who is short of breath. Patients usually assume the position most advantageous for breathing and, if repositioned, may have worsening gas exchange and even a respiratory arrest. If the patient becomes extremely dyspneic and "air hungry," notify the physician immediately.

If the patient is not on fluid restriction, encourage him or her to drink at least 3 L of fluid a day. Provide frequent mouth care to improve the patient's comfort and to limit the risk of infection. If appropriate, teach a family member or significant other how to perform postural drainage and chest percussion. Encourage the patient to remain recumbent for 10 minutes before the session so that secretions are expectorated more easily after treatment.

DOCUMENTATION GUIDELINES

- Respiratory status of the patient: Respiratory rate, breath sounds, use of oxygen, color of nail beds and lips; note any respiratory distress
- Response to activity: Degree of shortness of breath with any exertion
- Response to medications, oxygen, and breathing treatments
- Need for assistance with activities of daily living
- Response to diet and increased caloric intake, daily weights

DISCHARGE AND HOME HEALTHCARE GUIDELINES

MEDICATIONS. Be sure that the patient understands all medications, including the dosage, route, action, and adverse effects. Patients on aminophylline should have blood levels drawn as ordered by the physician. Before being discharged from the hospital, the patient should demonstrate the proper use of metered-dose inhalers.

COMPLICATIONS. Instruct patients to notify their primary healthcare provider of any change in the color or consistency of their secretions. Green-colored secretions may indicate the presence of a respiratory infection. Patients should also report consistent, prolonged periods of dyspnea that are unrelieved by medications.

FOLLOW-UP. Consider that patients with severe disease may need assistance with activities of daily living after discharge. Note any referrals to social services. Send patients home with a diet, provided by the dietitian and reinforced by the nurse, which provides a high-caloric intake. Encourage the patient to cover the face with a scarf if he or she goes out of doors in the winter. If the patient continues to smoke, provide the name of a smoking cessation program or a support group. Encourage the patient to avoid irritants in the air.

Bulimia Nervosa

DRG Category: 432
Mean LOS: 4.6 days
Description: MEDICAL: Other Mental Disorder Diagnoses

Bulimia nervosa is an eating disorder that is characterized by repeated episodes of binge eating. During binges the individual rapidly consumes large amounts of high-caloric food (upward of 2000 to 5000 calories), usually in secrecy. The binge is followed by self-deprecating thoughts, guilt, and anxiety over fear of weight gain. Purging is used to relieve these fears. Most bulimic patients purge by inducing vomiting or using laxatives, but some use excessive exercise and diuretics. The individual is caught in a binge-purge cycle that can recur multiple times each day, several times a week, or at an interval of up to 2 weeks to months. Bulimic patients experience frequent weight fluctuations of 10 pounds or more but are usually able to maintain a near normal weight.

As anorexic patients mature, they may turn to bulimic behavior as a way of controlling food intake. In contrast to anorexic patients, bulimic individuals are aware that their behavior is abnormal but conceal their illness because of embarrassment. Bulimic patients typically have difficulty with direct expression of feelings, are prone to impulsive behavior, and may have problems with alcohol and other substance abuse. Because patients can maintain a near-normal weight and, if females, have regular menstrual periods, the problem may go undetected. Bulimic behaviors have been known to persist for decades.

Depending on the severity and duration of the condition, there are medical consequences. Chronic induced vomiting of stomach contents produces volume depletion and a hypochloremic alkalosis. Dizziness, syncope, thirst, orthostatic changes in vital signs, and dehydration occur in the volume-depleted patient. Renal compensation for the metabolic alkalosis and volume depletion leads to further electrolyte imbalances, which may predispose the patient to cardiac dysrhythmias, muscle cramps, and weakness. Discoloration of the teeth and dental caries are common because of chronic self-induced vomiting. Laxative abuse is a potentially dangerous form of purging, leading to volume depletion, increased colonic motility, abdominal cramping, and loss of electrolytes in a watery diarrhea. Irritation of intestinal mucosa or hemorrhoids from rapid and frequent stools may cause rectal bleeding. When laxative abuse stops, transient fluid retention, edema, and constipation are common.

CAUSES

The cause of bulimia nervosa is unknown, but it is generally considered to be psychological. The onset occurs in late adolescence when the individual has left or is preparing to leave home. Experts suggest that the stress and depression that accompany this transition lead to binging and purging as a way of coping with these changes. Obesity usually precedes the onset of bulimia, and strict dieting usually triggers the binge-purge cycling. Changes in neurotransmitter metabolism and response to antidepressants suggest a biochemical component to the condition. Cultural pressures toward thinness may also contribute to the onset of bulimia.

GENDER AND LIFE SPAN CONSIDERATIONS

Bulimic patients are usually women, and the onset usually occurs in late adolescence or the early 20s. The typical bulimic patient is a young, college-educated woman with high achievement at work and school. Experts estimate that 5% of young women are bulimic.

☐ ASSESSMENT

HISTORY. Bulimic patients often report a family history of affective disorders, especially depression. The patient may describe patterns of weight fluctuation and frequent dieting, along with a preoccupation with food; this cluster of characteristics may be the first signs of bulimia. Complaints such as hematemesis, heartburn, constipation, rectal bleeding, and fluid retention may be the initial reasons the patient seeks health care from a primary healthcare provider. Patients may also have evidence of esophageal tears or ruptures, such as pain during swallowing and substernal burning. If patients seek treatment for bulimia, they usually have exhausted a variety of ways to control their binging and purging behavior. A detailed history of dieting, laxative and diuretic use, and the frequency and pattern of binging and purging episodes is essential. You may need to make a direct inquiry about binging and purging patterns for those patients who are seeking help but are ashamed to volunteer the information. Assess which foods and situations are most likely to trigger a binge.

PHYSICAL EXAMINATION. Note a normal weight for the patient's age and height. In patients with chronic vomiting, you may notice parotid swelling, which gives the patient a characteristic "chipmunk" facial appearance. Assess the patient for signs of dehydration such as poor skin turgor, dry mucous membranes, and dry skin. Note dental discoloration and caries from excessive vomiting, scars on the back of the hand from chronic self-induced vomiting, and conjunctival hemorrhages. Poor abdominal muscle tone may be evidence of rapid weight fluctuations. Tearing or fissures of the rectum may be present on rectal examination because of frequent enemas. A neurological assessment is important to rule out possible signs of a brain tumor or seizure disorder. Chronic hypokalemia from laxative or diuretic abuse may lead to an irregular pulse or even cardiac arrest and sudden death.

PSYCHOSOCIAL. Assess the patient's current career goals, peer and intimate relationships, psychosexual development, self-esteem, and perception of body image. Pay particular attention to any signs of depression and suicidal ideation and behavior. Assess the patient's ability to express feelings and anger; determine the patient's methods for coping with anxiety, as well as impulse control. Assess the family's communication patterns, especially how the family deals with conflict and solves problems. Assess the degree to which the family supports the patient's growth toward independence and separation.

DIAGNOSTIC HIGHLIGHTS

General Comments: No laboratory test is able to diagnose bulimia nervosa, but supporting tests are used to follow the response to treatment and progression of the illness.

Test	Normal Result	Abnormality with Condition	Explanation
Complete blood count	Red blood cells (RBC) 4.0–5.5 million/μL; white blood cells (WBC) 4,500–11,000/μL; hemoglobin (Hg) 12–18 g/dL; hematocrit (Hct) 37–54%; reticulocyte count 0.5–2.5% of total RBCs; platelets 150,000–400,000/μL	Anemia; RBC < 4.0; Hct < 35%; Hg < 12 g/dL. Bleeding tendencies due to platelets < 150,000/μL	Caused by protracted undernutrition
Amylase	50–180 units/dL	Elevated	Elevated levels indicate patient is practicing vomiting behaviors; increases within 2 hours of vomiting and remains elevated for approximately a week
Albumin	3.5–5.0 grams/dL	Hypoalbuminemia; albumin < 3.5 grams/dL	Caused by protracted under-nutrition

Other Tests: Serum electrolytes may show hypokalemia, hypochloremia, hypomagnesemia, hypocalcemia, or hypoglycemia. Other laboratory tests include arterial blood gases (metabolic alkalosis); blood urea nitrogen (elevated); cholesterol (elevated); luteinizing hormone (decreased); testosterone (decreased); thyroxine (mildly decreased); electrocardiogram; chest x ray.

PRIMARY NURSING DIAGNOSIS

Altered nutrition: Less than body requirements related to recurrent vomiting after eating; excessive laxative and diuretic use; and preoccupation with weight, food, or diets

OUTCOMES. Nutritional status: Food and fluid intake; Nutrient intake; Body mass; Energy

INTERVENTIONS. Eating disorders management; Nutrition management; Nutritional counseling; Nutritional monitoring; Weight management

◻ PLANNING AND IMPLEMENTATION

Collaborative

Patients with bulimia generally do not need hospitalization unless they experience severe electrolyte imbalance, dehydration, or rectal bleeding. The bulimia is usually managed with individual and group therapy, family education and therapy, medication, and nutritional counseling. Work with the interdisciplinary team to coordinate efforts and refer the patient to the physician to evaluate the need for antidepressants and anti-anxiety medication.

Work with the patient to evaluate the effectiveness of antidepressant or anti-anxiety medications, as well as to explore ways to identify situations that precede depression and anxiety. Work with the dietitian to ensure that the patient is educated about appropriate nutrition and dietary intake. Encourage the patient to participate in individual, family, and group sessions to help the patient develop ways to express feelings, handle anger, enhance self-esteem, explore career choices, and develop sexual identity and assertiveness skills.

PHARMACOLOGIC HIGHLIGHTS

Medication or Drug Class	Dosage	Description	Rationale
Potassium supplements	20–40 mEq po	Electrolyte replacement	Replace potassium lost through vomiting

Other Drugs: Some experts recommend the use of monoamine oxidase inhibitors (tranylcypromine sulfate, phenelyzine sulfate). Drugs that facilitate serotonergic neurotransmission such as fluoxetine, sertraline hydrochloride, and paroxetine may be used. Other drugs may be used such as tricyclic antidepressants, nortriptyline hydrochloride, or desipramine hydrochloride.

Independent

Teach the patient to choose correct portion sizes. Encourage the patient to eat slowly and avoid performing other activities such as reading or watching television while eating. Most patients are encouraged not to use diet foods or drinks until a stable body weight is established. Encourage the patient to eat a low-sodium diet to prevent fluid retention. Fluid retention is common until the body readjusts its fluid balance; the patient may need support if she or he experiences edema of the fingers, ankles, and face. As he or she begins to eat and drink normally, support the patient if he or she becomes upset about weight gain and reassure the patient that the weight gain and swelling are temporary. Also encourage the patient to establish a normal exercise routine but to avoid extremes.

The goals of nursing interventions are to enhance self-esteem, facilitate growth in independence, manage separation from the family, develop sexual identity, and make career choices. Explore ways for the patient to identify and express feelings, manage anger and stress, develop assertive communication skills, and control impulses or delay gratification. Help the patient learn ways to cope with feelings of anxiety and depression, as opposed to binging and purging. Explore ways to reduce the patient's vomiting, laxative, and diuretic abuse. Some patients respond well to contracting or behavioral management to reduce these behaviors. Educate the family about appropriate nutrition. Explore ways the family can manage conflict, and support the patient's move toward independence.

DOCUMENTATION GUIDELINES

- Nutrition: Diet planning and food intake; frequency and duration of binge-purge episodes
- Volume depletion: Signs of dehydration; pertinent laboratory findings if available
- Response to care and teaching: Understanding of the disease process and the relationship of dehydration and self-induced vomiting, laxative abuse, and diuretic abuse; understanding of ways to identify and cope with anxiety, anger, depression, and own impulses and needs
- Family meeting: Family interactions and support of move toward independence

DISCHARGE AND HOME HEALTHCARE GUIDELINES

Teach the patient ways to avoid binge-purge episodes through a balanced diet. Discuss effective ways of coping with needs and feelings. Explore ways to identify and handle stress and anxiety. Teach the patient strategies to increase self-esteem. Explore ways to maintain increased independence and the patient's own choices.

Burns

DRG Category: 460
Mean LOS: 5.6 days
Description: MEDICAL: Nonextensive Burns
without Operating Room Procedure
DRG Category: 457
Mean LOS: 3.0 days
Description: MEDICAL: Extensive Burns without
Operating Room Procedure

Burns are the third leading cause of accidental death in the United States. Each year an estimated 2 million Americans experience burns severe enough to seek medical care. Approximately 50,000 of these patients are hospitalized, although 75% of those hospitalized have burns on less than 10% of their body surface area. The physiologic responses to moderate and major burns are outlined in Table 16.

TABLE 16 | **System Impact of Moderate or Major Burns**

SYSTEM	PHYSIOLOGIC CHANGES
Cardiovascular	Fluid shifts from the vascular to the interstitial space occur because of increased permeability related to the inflammatory response.
	Hypovolemic shock may result, or it may be overcorrected by overzealous fluid replacement, which can lead to hypervolemia
	Hypertension occurs in about 1/3 of all children with burns, possibly caused by stress.
Pulmonary	Pulmonary edema brought about by primary cellular damage or circumferential chest burns limiting chest excursion can occur.
	Byproducts of combustion may lead to carbon monoxide poisoning.
	Inhalation of noxious gases may cause primary pulmonary damage or airway edema and upper airway obstructions.
Genitourinary	Potential for renal shutdown brought about by hypovolemia or acute renal failure exists.
	Massive diuresis from fluid returning to the vascular space marks the end of the emergent phase.
	Patients may develop hemomyoglobinuria because of massive full-thickness burns or electric injury. These injuries cause the release of muscle protein (myoglobin) and hemoglobin, which can clog the renal tubules and cause acute renal failure.
Gastrointestinal	Paralytic ileus can result from hypovolemia and last 2 or 3 days. Children, in particular, are susceptible to Curling's ulcer, a stress ulcer, because of the overwhelming systemic injury.
Musculoskeletal	Potential exists for the development of compartment syndrome because of edema.
	Echaratomy (cutting of a thick burn) may be needed to improve circulation.
	Scarring and contractures are a potential problem if prevention is not started on admission.
Neurologic	Personality changes are common throughout recovery because of stress, electrolyte disturbance, hypoxemia, or medications.
	Children, in particular, are at risk for post-burn seizures during the acute phase.

CAUSES

Most burns result from preventable accidents. Thermal burns, which are the most common type, occur because of fires from motor vehicle crashes, accidents in residences, and arson or electrical malfunctions. Children may be burned when they play with matches or firecrackers or because of a kitchen accident. Chemical burns occur as a result of contact with, ingestion of, or inhalation of acids, alkalis, or vesicants (blistering gases). The percentage of burns actually caused by abuse is fairly small, but they are some of the most difficult to manage. Neglect or inadequate supervision of children is fairly common. Effective prevention and educational efforts such as smoke detectors, flame-retardant clothing, child-resistant cigarette lighters, and the Stop Drop and Roll program have decreased the number and severity of injuries.

GENDER AND LIFE SPAN CONSIDERATIONS

Preschool children account for over two-thirds of all fatalities. Clinicians use a special chart (Lund-Browder Chart) for children that provides a picture and a graph to account for the difference in body surface area by age. The younger child is the most common victim of burns that have been caused by liquids. Preschoolers, school-aged children, and teenagers are more frequently the victims of flame burns. Young children playing with lighters or matches are at risk, as are teenagers because of carelessness or risk-taking behaviors around fires. Toddlers incur electrical burns from biting electrical cords or putting objects in outlets. Most adults are victims of house fires or work-related accidents that involve chemicals or electricity. The elderly are also prone to scald injuries because their skin tends to be extremely thin and sensitive to heat.

Because of the severe impact of this injury, the very young and the very old are less able to respond to therapy and have a higher incidence of mortality. In addition, when a child experiences a burn, multiple surgeries are required to release contractures that occur as normal growth pulls at the scar tissue of their healed burns. Adolescents are particularly prone to psychological difficulties because of sensitivity regarding body image issues. No specific gender considerations exist in burns.

◻ ASSESSMENT

HISTORY. Obtain a complete description of the burn injury, including the time, the situation, the burning agent, and the actions of witnesses. The time of injury is extremely important since any delay in treatment may result in a minor or moderate burn becoming a major injury. Elicit specific information about the location of the accident, since closed-space injuries are related to smoke inhalation. If abuse is suspected, obtain a more in-depth history from a variety of people who are involved with the child. The injury may be suspect if there is a delay in seeking health care, if there are burns that are not consistent with the story, or if there are bruises at different stages of healing. Note whether the description of the injury changes or differs among family or household members.

PHYSICAL EXAMINATION. Although the wounds of a serious burn injury may be dramatic, a basic assessment of airway, breathing, and circulation (ABCs) takes first priority. Once the ABCs are stabilized, perform a complete examination of the burn wound to determine the severity of injury. The American Burn Association (ABA) establishes the severity of injury by calculating the total body surface area (TBSA) of partial and full-thickness injury along with the age of the patient and other special factors. (See Table 17.) Serial assessments of wound healing determine the patient's response to treatment. Ongoing monitoring throughout the acute and rehabilitative phases is essential for the burn patient. Fluid balance, daily weights, vital signs, and intake and output monitoring are essential to ensure that the patient is responding appropriately to treatment.

TABLE 17 | **Characteristics of Burns**

SUPERFICIAL (1ST DEGREE)	PARTIAL THICKNESS (2ND DEGREE)	FULL THICKNESS (3RD DEGREE)
Erythema, blanching on pressure, mild to moderate pain, no blister (typical of sunburn). Only structure involved—epidermis	Blisters, red, moist, shiny; severe pain because of exposed nerve endings. Epidermis and dermis involved; depth may vary.	Appears dry, waxy, and leathery. Thrombosed blood vessels visible, insensitive to pain because nerve destruction. Epidermis, dermis, and possibly, muscle, nerve, bone, or tendon involvement

PSYCHOSOCIAL ASSESSMENT. Even small burns temporarily change the appearance of the skin. Major burns will have a permanent effect on the family unit. A complete assessment of the family's psychological health before the injury is essential. Expect pre-existing issues to magnify during this crisis, and identify previous ways of coping in order to facilitate dealing with the crisis. Guilt, blame, anxiety, fear, and depression are commonly experienced emotions.

DIAGNOSTIC HIGHLIGHTS

Test	Normal Result	Abnormality with Condition	Explanation
Fiber-optic bronchoscopy	Normal larynx, trachea, and bronchi	Thermal injury and edema to oropharynx and glottis	Used to investigate suspected smoke inhalation and damage from noxious gases
Carboxyhemoglobin levels	8%–10% in smokers; < 8% in nonsmokers	> 10% indicates potential inhalation injury; > 30% is associated with mental status changes; > 60% is lethal	Carbon monoxide binds to hemoglobin with an affinity of 240 times greater than oxygen

Other Tests: Because burns are the result of trauma, there are no tests needed to make the diagnosis. Some of the more common tests to monitor the patient's response to injury and treatment are complete blood count, arterial blood gases, serum electrolytes, blood and wound cultures and sensitivities, chest x rays, urinalysis, and nutritional profiles.

PRIMARY NURSING DIAGNOSIS

Ineffective airway clearance related to airway edema

OUTCOMES. Respiratory status: Gas exchange; Respiratory status: Ventilation; Symptom control behavior; Treatment behavior: Illness or injury; Comfort level

INTERVENTIONS. Airway management; Anxiety reduction; Oxygen therapy; Airway suctioning; Airway insertion and stabilization; Cough enhancement; Mechanical ventilation; Positioning; Respiratory monitoring

◻ PLANNING AND IMPLEMENTATION

Collaborative

MINOR BURN CARE. Minor burn wounds are cared for by using the principles of comfort, cleanliness, and infection control. A gentle cleansing of the wound with soap and water 2 or 3 times a day, followed with a topical agent such as silver sulfadiazine or mafenide, prevents infection. Minor burns should heal in 7 to 10 days; however, if they take longer than 14 days, excision of the wound and a small graft may be needed. Oral analgesics may be prescribed to manage discomfort, and, as do all burn patients, the patient needs to receive tetanus toxoid to prevent infection.

MAJOR BURN CARE. For patients with a major injury, effective treatment is provided by a multidisciplinary team with special training in burn care. In addition to the physician and nurse, the team includes specialists in physical and occupational therapy, respiratory therapy, social work, nutrition, psychology, and child life for children. The course of recovery is divided into four phases: emergent-resuscitative, acute-wound coverage, convalescent-rehabilitative, and reorganization-reintegration.

The emergent-resuscitative phase lasts from 48 to 72 hours after injury or until diuresis takes place. In addition to managing the ABCs, the patient receives fluid resuscitation, maintenance of electrolytes, aggressive pain management, and early nutrition. Wound care consists of silver sulfadiazine or mafenide and surgical management as needed. To prevent infection, initial care includes debridement by washing the surface of the wounds with mild soap or aseptic solutions. Then the physician debrides devitalized tissue, and often the wound is covered with antibacterial agents such as silver sulfadiazine and occlusive cotton gauze.

The acute-wound coverage phase, which varies depending on the extent of injury, lasts until the wounds have been covered, through either the normal healing process or grafting. The risk for infection is high during this phase; the physician follows wound and blood cultures and prescribes antibiotics as needed. Wound management includes excision of devitalized tissue, surgical grafting of donor skin, or placement of synthetic membranes. Inpatient rehabilitation takes place during the convalescent-rehabilitative phase. Although principles of rehabilitation are included in the plan of care from the day of admission, during this time home exercises and wound care are taught. In addition, pressure appliances to reduce scarring, or braces to prevent contractures, are fitted. The reorganization phase is the long period of time that it may take after the injury for physical and emotional healing to take place.

PHARMACOLOGIC HIGHLIGHTS

Medication or Drug Class	Dosage	Description	Rationale
Topical antimicrobial agents	Silver sulfadiazine	Cream that lowers bacterial counts, minimizes water evaporation, and decreases heat loss	Anti-microbial agent that is not irritating and has the fewest adverse effects
	Mafenide acetate	Bacterial coverage for gram-negative and anaerobic coverage; deep eschar penetration	Painful but readily absorbed and can lead to metabolic acidosis

Independent

The nursing care of the patient with a burn is complex and collaborative, with overlapping interventions among the nurse, the physician, and a variety of therapists. However, independent nursing interventions are also an important focus for the nurse. The highest priority for the burn patient is to maintain the airway, breathing, and circulation. The airway can be maintained in some patients by an oral or nasal airway, or by the jaw lift-chin thrust maneuver. Patency of the airway is maintained by endotracheal suctioning, whose frequency is dictated by the character and amount of secretions. If the patient is apneic, maintain breathing with a manual resuscitator bag before intubation and mechanical ventilation.

If the patient is bleeding from burn sites, apply pressure until the bleeding can be controlled surgically. Remove all constricting clothing and jewelry to allow for adequate circulation to the extremities. Implement fluid resuscitation protocols as appropriate to support the patient's circulation. If any clothing is still smoldering and adhering to the patient, soak the area with normal saline solution and remove the material. Wound care includes collaborative management and other strategies. Cover wounds with clean, dry, sterile sheets. Do not cover large burn wounds with saline-soaked dressings, which lower the patient's temperature. If the patient has ineffective thermoregulation, use warming or cooling blankets as needed and control the room temperature to support the patient's optimum temperature. If the patient is hypothermic, limit traffic into the room to decrease drafts and keep the patient covered with sterile sheets. Help the patient manage pain and distress by providing careful explanations and teaching distraction and relaxation techniques.

As the wounds heal, use strategies such as tubbing, debridement, and dressing changes to limit infection, promote wound healing, and limit physical impairment. If impaired physical mobility is a risk, place the patient in antideformity positions at all times. Implement active and passive range of motion as needed. Get the patient out of bed on a regular basis to limit physical debilitation and decrease the risk of infection. Implement strategies to limit stress and anxiety.

DOCUMENTATION GUIDELINES

Emergent-Resuscitative Phase

• Flow sheet record of the critical physiologic aspects of this time period; depending on the patient's condition, documentation times may be established for 15-minute intervals or less for vital signs and fluid balance

- Flow sheet record of information related to the condition of the wound, wound care, and psychosocial issues

Acute-Wound Coverage Phase

- The condition of the wound, healing progress, graft condition, signs of infection, scar formation, and antideformity positioning are important documentation parameters
- Psychosocial issues and the family's involvement in care are also important information

Rehabilitative Phase

- Status of healing and the appearance of scars, as well as the patient's functional abilities
- Ability of the patient and family to perform the complex care required during the months to come

DISCHARGE AND HOME HEALTHCARE GUIDELINES

Patient teaching is individualized, but for most patients it includes information about each of the following.

WOUND MANAGEMENT. This includes infection control, basic cleanliness, and wound management.

SCAR MANAGEMENT. Functional abilities, including using pressure garments, exercises, and activities of daily living, must be assessed and taught.

NUTRITION. Nutritional guidelines are provided that maintain continued healing and respond to the metabolic demands that frequently last for some time after initial injury.

FOLLOW-UP. If respiratory involvement exists, include specific teaching related to the amount of damage and ongoing therapy. Teach various techniques for dealing with the reaction of society, classmates, or those in the workplace. Explain where and how to obtain resources (financial and emotional) for assisting the family and patient during the recovery process.

Calculi, Renal

DRG Category: 323
Mean LOS: 2.9 days
Description: MEDICAL: Urinary Stones with CC and/or ESW Lithotripsy

Renal calculi are stones that form in the kidneys from the crystallization of minerals and other substances that normally dissolve in the urine. Renal calculi vary in size, with 90% of them smaller than 5 mm in diameter; some, however, grow large enough to prevent the natural passage of urine through the ureter. Calculi may be solitary or multiple. Approximately 80% of these stones are comprised of calcium salts. Other types are the struvite stones (which contain magnesium, ammonium, and phosphate), uric acid stones, and cystine stones. If the calculi remain in the renal pelvis or enter the ureter, they can damage renal parenchyma (functional tissue). Larger calculi can cause pressure necrosis. In certain locations, calculi cause obstruction, lead to hydronephrosis, and tend to recur.

CAUSES

The precise cause of renal calculi is unknown, although they are associated with dehydration, urinary obstruction, calcium levels, and other factors. Patients who are dehydrated have decreased urine, with heavy concentrations of calculus-forming substances. Urinary obstruction leads to urinary stasis, a condition that contributes to calculus formation. Any condition that increases serum calcium levels and calcium excretion predisposes people to renal calculi. These conditions include an excessive intake of vitamin D or dietary calcium, hyperparathyroidism, heredity factors, and immobility. Metabolic conditions such as renal tubular acidosis, elevated serum uric acid levels, and urinary tract infections associated with alkaline urine have been linked with calculus formation. Cystine stones are associated with hereditary renal disease.

GENDER AND LIFE SPAN CONSIDERATIONS

Approximately 12% of the population develop a stone at some point in their lives. Calculi occur more often in men than in women, unless heredity is a factor, and occur most often between the ages of 30 to 50 years. Children rarely develop calculi.

☐ ASSESSMENT

HISTORY. Symptoms of renal calculi usually appear when a stone dislodges and begins to travel down the urinary tract and enters the ureter. Establish a history of pain, and determine the intensity, duration, and location of the pain. The location of the pain varies according to the placement of the stone. The pain usually begins in the flank area but later may radiate into the lower abdomen and the groin. Ask if the pain had a sudden onset. Patients may relate a recent history of hematuria, nausea, vomiting, and anorexia. In cases where a urinary tract infection is also present, the patient may report chills and fever. Determine the patient's history to identify risk factors.

PHYSICAL EXAMINATION. Inspection reveals a patient in intense pain who is unable to maintain a comfortable position. Assess the patient for bladder distension. Monitor the patient for signs of an infection such as fever, chills, and increased white blood cell counts. Assess the urine for hematuria. Auscultate the patient's abdomen for normal bowel sounds. Palpate the patient's flank area for tenderness. Percussion of the abdominal area is normal, but percussion of the costovertebral angle elicits severe pain.

PSYCHOSOCIAL. Patients with renal calculi may be extremely anxious because of the sudden onset of severe pain of unknown origin. Assess the level of the pain, as well as the patient's ability to cope. Since diet and lifestyle may contribute to the formation of calculi, the patient may face lifestyle changes. Assess the patient's ability to handle such changes.

DIAGNOSTIC HIGHLIGHTS

General Comments: The physician uses diagnostic tests to eliminate cholecystitis, peptic ulcers, appendicitis, and pancreatitis as the cause of the abdominal pain.

Test	Normal Result	Abnormality with Condition	Explanation
Kidney-ureter-bladder (KUB) and abdominal x rays	No renal stones	Presence of renal stones, most of which are radiopaque	Reveals most renal calculi except cystine and uric acid stones
Intravenous pyelography (IVP)	Normal anatomy of the kidney/ collection system	Obstructing stone	Performed when renal colic is severe and obstruction is suspected

Other Tests: Other supporting tests include kidney ultrasonograph, urinalysis, serum chloride and bicarbonate levels, urine culture and sensitivity, and serum calcium and phosphorus levels.

PRIMARY NURSING DIAGNOSIS

Altered urinary elimination related to the blockage of ureter with a calculus

OUTCOMES. Urinary elimination; Knowledge: Medication; Symptom severity; Treatment behavior: Illness or injury

INTERVENTIONS. Urinary elimination management; Medication prescribing; Fluid monitoring; Pain management; Infection control; Tube care: Urinary

☐ PLANNING AND IMPLEMENTATION

Collaborative

In about 80% of cases, renal calculi of 5 mm or less are treated conservatively with vigorous hydration, which results in the stone passing spontaneously. Increased fluid intake is ordered orally or intravenously (IV) to flush the stone through the urinary tract. Unless contraindicated, maintain hydration at 200 mL per hour of IV or orally. Strain the patient's urine to detect stones that are passed so they can be analyzed.

For calculi that are larger than 5 mm or that cannot be passed with conservative treatment, surgical removal is performed. Percutaneous ultrasonic lithotripsy or extracorporeal shock wave lithotripsy (ESWL) uses sound waves to shatter calculi for later removal by suction or natural passage. Calculi in the ureter may be removed with catheters and a cystoscope, while a flank or lower abdominal surgical approach may be needed to remove calculi from the kidney calyx or renal pelvis.

PHARMACOLOGIC HIGHLIGHTS

General Comments: If nausea and vomiting are present, administer antiemetics as ordered. Diuretics may be ordered to prevent urinary stasis.

Medication or Drug Class	Dosage	Description	Rationale
Analgesia	Varies with drug	Narcotics, nonsteroidal anti-inflammatory agents	To relax the ureter and facilitate passage of stone

Independent

Initially, the most important nursing interventions concentrate on pain management. Teach relaxation techniques, diversional activities, and position changes. Help promote the passage of renal calculi. Encourage the patient to walk, if possible. Offer the patient fruit juices to help acidify the urine. Teach the patient the importance of proper diet to help avoid a recurrence of the renal calculi.

To reduce anxiety, give the patient and family all pertinent information concerning the treatment plan and any diagnostic tests. Preoperatively, explain the procedure and what to expect afterward. For patients who are undergoing a flank or abdominal incision, teach deep breathing and coughing exercises. Give postoperative care and monitor for signs of infection or pneumonia. Do not irrigate urinary drainage systems without consulting with the physician.

DOCUMENTATION GUIDELINES

- Response to pain relief measures, degree of pain (location, frequency, duration)
- Record of intake and output, daily weights, vital signs
- Presence of complications: Infection, obstruction, hemorrhage, intractable pain
- Observation of color and consistency of urine, presence of stones

DISCHARGE AND HOME HEALTHCARE GUIDELINES

COMFORT MEASURES. Teach the patient to take analgesics as ordered and to use other appropriate comfort measures.

MEDICATION. Be sure the patient understands any medication prescribed, including dosage, route, action, and side effects. If the patient is placed on antibiotics, encourage him or her to complete the entire prescription.

PREVENTION. Instruct the patient to increase fluid intake to enhance the passage of the stone. Instruct the patient to strain all urine and, if a stone is obtained, emphasize the importance of returning the stone to the physician for analysis. If the patient has passed the stone and it has been analyzed, teach the necessary dietary changes, fluid intake requirements, and exercise regimen to prevent future stone formation. Patient should drink at least 2.5 liters a day of fluid to prevent recurrences.

COMPLICATIONS. Teach the patient to report any signs of complications, such as fever, chills, or hematuria, as well as any changes in urinary output patterns, to the primary caregiver.

Candidiasis (Moniliasis)

DRG Category: 283
Mean LOS: 4.8 days
Description: MEDICAL: Minor Skin Disorders with CC
DRG Category: 423
Mean LOS: 7.1 days
Description: MEDICAL: Other Infectious and Parasitic Diseases Diagnoses
DRG Category: 185
Mean LOS: 4.1 days
Description: MEDICAL: Dental and Oral Disorders Except Extractions and Restorations, Age > 17

Candidiasis is a yeast infection, an inflammatory reaction caused by Candida fungi. Infection occurs when Candida fungi penetrate the tissue, colonize, and release toxins that cause an acute inflammatory response. The infections are also termed moniliasis, which is defined as a yeast infection of the skin and mucous membranes. Infections are common in the mouth (thrush), esophagus, pulmonary system, vagina (moniliasis), and skin (diaper rash). Most typically, Candida infections occur in moist areas of the skin such as skin folds, around fingernails, and in mucous membranes, with the most common site being the vulvovaginal area. Candida may infest wounds, catheter sites, and intravenous sites. Infections may take 6 to 8 weeks to resolve. In immunosuppressed patients, candidiasis can become disseminated by entering the bloodstream and causing serious infections in other organs; such infections are difficult to eradicate. Candida albicans is the most common fungus that causes pathology in patients with the human immunodeficiency virus (HIV), and women with persistent and severe infections should have HIV testing.

CAUSES

The Candida fungus, which is not pathologic under normal conditions, is normally on the skin and in the gastrointestinal (GI) tract, the mouth, and the vagina. Candida causes infection when a body change permits its sudden proliferation. Changes that contribute to susceptibility to candidiasis include rising glucose levels caused by diabetes mellitus, lowered resistance caused by a disease such as carcinoma, an immunosuppressive drug such as corticosteroids, or radiation therapy. Other associated factors include aging, irritation from dentures, instrumentation (urinary or intravenous catheters), surgery, peritoneal dialysis, or the use of oral contraceptives. The most common factor remains the side effects caused by the use of broad-spectrum antibiotics.

GENDER AND LIFE SPAN CONSIDERATIONS

Candidiasis may occur at any age, under any condition, but it is more common in the genitourinary tract of women than in men. In infants, it can cause diaper rash; in females, it can cause vaginal infections. The elderly and patients with cancer and HIV infections are most susceptible to infection.

☐ ASSESSMENT

HISTORY. Question the patient carefully to elicit a history of risk factors or a history of repeated episodes of candidiasis. Factors such as cigarette smoking, tobacco chewing, or pipe smoking are often associated with Candida infections. Take a careful medication history, and pay particular attention to use of antibiotics, corticosteroids, or other immunosuppressive drugs. A reproductive history, including current pregnancy or oral contraceptive use, is important.

The patient may complain of a burning or painful sensation in the mouth or difficulty in swallowing. The patient may report regurgitation. Patients with vaginal infections will describe itchiness, irritation, and swelling of the labia. Patients may also describe a white, cheesy vaginal discharge.

PHYSICAL EXAMINATION. Inspect the patient's lips for color, texture, hydration, and lesions. Assess the patient's mouth thoroughly for bleeding, edema, white patches, nodules, or cysts. Inspect the mucosa; the roof and floor of the mouth; the tongue, including under the surface and the lateral borders; the gums; and the throat. Palpate any lesions or nodules. Inspect the patient's nail beds for swelling, redness, darkening, purulent discharge, or separation from the nails. Inspect the patient's skin for an erythematous, macular rash. Inspect the patient's vagina for vulval rash; erythema; inflammation; cheesy exudate; or lesions of the labia, vaginal walls, or the cervix. Palpate lesions for texture and tenderness.

Systemic infection causes symptoms that can include a high, spiking fever; lowered blood pressure; rashes; and chills. Pulmonary infection may produce a cough. Renal infection may produce painful or cloudy urination and blood or pus in the urine. If the infection occurs in the brain, symptoms can include headache and seizures. Eye infection can cause blurred vision, orbital or periorbital pain, scotoma (blind gap in visual field), and exudate. If the infection occurs in the endocardium, symptoms can include systolic or diastolic murmur or chest pain.

PSYCHOSOCIAL. Because of pain, severe oral cases may cause the patient to have difficulty eating and drinking, which may contribute to depression. Severe skin and vaginal infections can cause pain, itching, and unsightly lesions that may cause self-consciousness because of a change in body image. Because of painful symptoms, vaginal infection may affect sexual behavior.

DIAGNOSTIC HIGHLIGHTS

Test	Normal Result	Abnormality with Condition	Explanation
Potassium hydroxide (KOH) cultures of scrapings from skin, vagina, wound or cultures from sputum or blood	Negative	Positive	Opportunistic infection associated with antibiotic use, resulting in positive cultures

Other Tests: Diagnosis relies on signs and symptoms, supported by laboratory cultures.

PRIMARY NURSING DIAGNOSIS

Altered oral mucous membranes related to swelling and ulcers

OUTCOMES. Oral health; Tissue integrity: Skin and mucus membranes; Infection status; Nutritional status; Self-care: Oral hygiene

INTERVENTIONS. Oral health maintenance; Nutrition management; Oral health promotion; Oral health restoration; Pain management

◻ PLANNING AND IMPLEMENTATION

Collaborative

The first order of treatment is to improve any underlying condition that has triggered the onset of candidiasis—for example, discontinuing antibiotic therapy or catheterization or controlling diabetes. The other collaborative interventions are pharmacologic.

PHARMACOLOGIC HIGHLIGHTS

General Comments: Premedication with acetaminophen, antihistamines, or antiemetics can help reduce side effects of amphotericin B such as fever, anorexia, nausea, vomiting, or severe chills. Intravenous fluids or total parenteral nutrition therapy may be needed if the patient's fluid and nutritional intake is compromised. A topical anesthetic, such as lidocaine or xylocaine, may be provided at least 1 hour before meals to alleviate mouth pain.

Medication or Drug Class	Dosage	Description	Rationale
Antifungal agents	Varies by drug	Nystatin	Effective antifungal for superficial candidiasis; prescribed in ointments, creams, oral gels, or oral solutions
		Clotrimazole, fluconazole, and miconazole	Prescribed for mucous membrane or vaginal infections
		Amphotericin B, flucytosine, or miconazole.	Intravenous therapy may be prescribed for systemic infection

Independent

The most important nursing intervention for the patient with candidiasis is patient education about the infection and its treatment. Teach the patient to keep his or her skin dry and free of irritation and to use a clean towel and washcloth daily. Prescribed creams should be applied to the affected areas until the candidiasis is gone; for those patients with immunosuppression, the creams should be continued for 2 weeks after the symptoms disappear. Encourage the patient to use cold compresses and/or sitz baths to relieve itching. Instruct the patient to wash his or her hands thoroughly after touching infected areas to prevent the infection from spreading. Recommend cornstarch, nystatin powder, or dry padding to obese patients to help avoid irritation in skin folds. Educate the patient with a vaginal infection to avoid contamination with feces from the GI tract by wiping from front to back after defecation.

If the patient is having difficulty swallowing or chewing and this is adversely affecting his or her nutrition, encourage a soft diet, fluid intake, and small, frequent meals of high-calorie foods. Advise the patient to avoid spicy, hot, or acidic foods that might exacerbate lesions. Explain the need for mouth care before and after meals, recommending the use of a soft gauze pad, rather than a toothbrush, to clean the teeth, gums, and mucous membranes. Advise the patient to avoid mouthwashes with alcohol and to lubricate the lips.

DOCUMENTATION GUIDELINES

- Physical findings: Lesions, exudate, rashes, locations of skin irritation or breakdown
- Response to medications: Antifungals, analgesics
- Progressive wound healing
- Presence of complications, spreading, resistance, recurrence

DISCHARGE AND HOME HEALTHCARE GUIDELINES

PREVENTION. Teach the patient to keep his or her skin clean and dry, especially in skin folds. Teach the patient to allow the skin to be open to the air, to wear loose-fitting cotton clothing rather than tight-fitting clothing or synthetic fabrics. Teach the patient to maintain good oral care and to correct any ill-fitting dentures that may cause lesions. If the patient is diabetic, provide guidelines on how to maintain good control of blood sugar levels to decrease susceptibility to candidiasis. In recurrent vaginal infections, be sure the patient understands that her sexual partner may need to be treated.

MEDICATIONS. Teach the patient the action, dosage, route, and side effects of all medications.

COMPLICATIONS OF CANDIDIASIS. Patients should understand the symptoms of systemic infection caused by candidiasis, such as a high, spiking fever; chills; cloudy urine or urine with blood or pus; headache or seizures; blurred vision or eye pain. If these symptoms occur, the patient should inform the physician.

Cardiac Contusion (Myocardial Contusion)

DRG Category: 144
Mean LOS: 4.5 days
Description: MEDICAL: Other Circulatory System Diagnoses with CC

Cardiac (myocardial) contusion is a bruise or damage to the heart muscle. Damage to the heart ranges from limited areas of subepicardial petechiae or ecchymoses to full-thickness contusions with fragmentations and necrosis of cardiac muscle fibers. Cellular damage consists of extravasation of red blood cells into and between the myocardial muscle fibers and the selective necrosis of myocardial muscle fibers. Creatine phosphokinase (CPK) leaks out of the cells into the circulation. Complete healing occurs with little or no scar formation. When myocardial injury is extensive, the pathologic changes may resemble those seen in acute myocardial infarction, and the patient may experience some of the same complications associated with it, such as cardiac failure, cardiac dysrhythmias, aneurysm formation, or cardiac rupture.

CAUSES

Cardiac contusion can be caused by any direct traumatic injury to the chest. Most commonly, it is the result of a direct blow to the chest from a steering wheel injury in a motor vehicle crash, a sports accident, a fall from a high elevation, an assault, or an animal kick. Injury to the myocardium typically occurs as a result of acute compression of the heart between the sternum and the spine. The anterior wall of the right ventricle is most commonly involved because of its location directly behind the sternum.

GENDER AND LIFE SPAN CONSIDERATIONS

Cardiac contusion can occur at any age and in both sexes, although more males than females are involved in traumatic events. Anyone at high risk for traumatic injuries, such as children and young adults in the first four decades of life, is at high risk for myocardial contusion. Because their bones may be more brittle, elderly patients also have an increased risk; traumatic injury to the sternum is less tolerated in the elderly.

☐ ASSESSMENT

HISTORY. Elicit a thorough history of the injury event, including the time, place, and description. Determine the point of impact and any weapons (baseball bat, bricks, fist) used in an assault. Patients usually describe the most common symptom of cardiac contusion—that is, precordial pain resembling that of myocardial infarction. However, coronary vasodilators have little effect in relieving the pain. It is important to note that many patients may be asymptomatic for the first 24 to 48 hours after the chest trauma. In patients with multiple trauma, physical signs may be masked by associated injuries. Note the presence of blunt chest injuries, such as sternal, clavicular, or upper rib fractures; pulmonary contusion; hemothorax; or pneumothorax—all of which raise suspicion for the possibility of a myocardial injury.

PHYSICAL EXAMINATION. Generally, the physical signs of a cardiac contusion are few and nonspecific. Observe the chest wall for the presence of bruising, hematoma, swelling, or the imprint of a steering wheel if the patient has been driving a motor vehicle. Note the presence of pain (chest wall or musculoskeletal), dyspnea, tachycapnea, tachycardia, and diaphoresis. Be alert for the possibility of cardiac tamponade, active bleeding into the pericardial space that leads to myocardial compression, and cardiogenic shock. Note the presence of hypotension, muffled heart sounds, a paradoxic pulse, and shock from potential complications. (See Table 18.)

TABLE 18 | **Complications Associated with Myocardial Contusion**

COMPLICATION	SYMPTOMS
Atrial dysrhythmias: Sinus tachycardia, atrial fibrillation, premature atrial contractions	Palpitations, precordial pain, dizziness, faintness, confusion, loss of consciousness
Cardiac tamponade	Hypotention, pulsus paradoxus, muffled heart sounds, pericardial friction rub, anxiety, restlessness, tachypnea, weak to absent pulses, pallor, cyanosis
Congestive heart failure	Orthopnea, tachypnea, crackles, frothy cough, distended neck veins, anxiety, confusion
Pulmonary edema	Pallor, cyanosis, dyspnea
Ventricular aneurysm	Chest pain, dyspnea, orthopnea
Ventricular dysrhythmias: Premature ventricular contractions, ventricular fibrillation	Palpitations, precordial pain, dizziness, faintness, confusion, loss of consciousness

PSYCHOSOCIAL. The patient with a cardiac contusion usually has suffered an unexpected traumatic injury. He or she may have numerous other traumatic injuries that accompany the contused heart. Assess the patient's ability to cope with the unexpectedness of the traumatic event. Assess the patient's degree of anxiety regarding the traumatic event, injuries sustained, and the potential implications of the injuries. Note that trauma patients are often teenagers and young adults. During crises, the presence of their parents and peers is essential in their recovery but may challenge the nurse to provide a quiet and stress-free environment for patient recovery.

DIAGNOSTIC HIGHLIGHTS

Note: Cardiac contusion cannot be diagnosed by a specific serum laboratory test or diagnostic test. Several tests may help identify those patients at risk for complications and accompanying injury.

Test	Normal Result	Abnormality with Condition	Explanation
Echocardiogram	Normal size, shape, position, thickness and movement of structures	May identify injury to heart structures, such as echo-free zone anterior to right ventricular wall and posterior to left ventricular wall (cardiac tamponade), aneurysm, or valvular rupture	Records echoes created by deflection of short pulses of ultrasonic beam off structures; may be done as transesophageal procedure with transmitter inserted into esophagus (transesophageal echocardiogram, or TEE)
Electrocardiogram (ECG)	Normal PQRST pattern	ST segment depression, T wave inversion; may have transient ST elevation (less	Electrical conduction system adversely affected by myocardial ischemia due to injury; 65% of people with

		frequent); ECG may be normal	myocardial contusion have ECG changes
Creatine kinase isoenzyme (MB-CK)	< 5% of total CK	Elevated in some patients	Some patients with a cardiac contusion have actual tissue damage, and therefore would have enzyme elevation
Serum cardiac troponin I	< 0.6 μg/L	> 1.5 μg/L	Suggests myocardial damage and necrosis

Other Tests: Supporting tests include aspartate aminotransferase (AST; also known as serum glutamic-oxaloacetic transaminase [SGOT]), and lactic dehydrogenase (LDH), chest x ray, computer tomography (CT) scans.

PRIMARY NURSING DIAGNOSIS

Chest pain (acute) related to injury, swelling, bruising

OUTCOMES. Comfort level; Pain control behavior; Pain level; Well-being; Symptom severity

INTERVENTIONS. Analgesia administration; Pain management; Medication management; Distraction; Vital signs monitoring

☐ PLANNING AND IMPLEMENTATION

Collaborative

Management of patients with suspected or known cardiac contusion is similar to that of any myocardial ischemic problem. Strategies include oxygen therapy, cardiac and hemodynamic monitoring, analgesics, and, if necessary, antidysrhythmics and inotropic agents. Even in patients without obvious dysrhythmias, maintain intravenous access for treatment of complications that may be associated with myocardial contusion. Place the patient on continuous cardiac monitoring to assess for dysrhythmias. Perform serial monitoring of vital signs to determine if the patient's heart function is changing. If signs of falling cardiac output occur (confusion or decreased mental status, delayed capillary blanching, cool extremities, weak pulses, pulmonary congestion, increased heart rate, decreased urine output), the physician may insert a pulmonary artery catheter.

One of the more severe complications of myocardial contusion is pericardial tamponade, which can develop more than 1 week after the injury. Elective surgery for associated injuries (open reduction of fractures, repair of minor facial fractures) involving general anesthesia may be delayed, if possible, until cardiac function is stable. Delay allows for stabilization and healing of the contusion, which lowers intraoperative and postoperative risk for cardiac complications.

PHARMACOLOGIC HIGHLIGHTS

Medication or Drug Class	Dosage	Description	Rationale
Antidysrhythmics	Varies with drug	Lidocaine is the treatment of choice for ventricular tachycardia or fibrillation	Control dysrhythmias; drug depends on type of injury

		that persists after defibrillation; others are bretylium, magnesium sulfate, procainamide, atropine, adenosine, esmolol, propanalol, acebutolol	
Inotropic drugs	Varies with drug	Dopamine, dobutamine, amrinone, milrinone	Increase contractility if failure occurs

Other Drugs: Intravenous opiates such as morphine sulfate may be required in the acute phase for comfort and rest.

Independent

During recovery, nursing interventions focus on conserving the patient's energy. Activity restrictions, including bed rest, may be necessary for a short period of time (usually 48 to 72 hours) to decrease myocardial oxygen demands and to facilitate healing. Discuss the need for activity restriction with the patient and family.

The young adult trauma patient presents a challenge to the nursing staff. Provide age-appropriate diversionary activities to reduce anxiety. If the patient is a high school student, note that the hospital may be overwhelmed with peers from the local high school who are interested in visiting the patient, particularly if the injury was associated with a school event (prom, football game, party) and if the injury is life-threatening. Work with the parents and principal to arrange for a visitation schedule so that both the patient's and hospital's needs are met.

DOCUMENTATION GUIDELINES

- Detailed observations and assessments of physical findings related to traumatic injury: Skin integrity, swelling, fractures, alignment, mental status
- Detailed assessment findings of respiratory and cardiac systems: Heart and lung sounds, vital signs, signs of complications, cardiac rhythm

DISCHARGE AND HOME HEALTHCARE GUIDELINES

The patient may be sent home on oral analgesics and other medications to manage complications. Be sure the patient understands all medications, including the dosage, route, action, and adverse effects. Educate the patient about the symptoms of potential complications associated with cardiac contusions and instruct him or her to call the physician or go to the emergency department immediately if any of the associated symptoms occurs.

Cardiac Tamponade

DRG Category: 144
Mean LOS: 4.5 days
Description: MEDICAL: Other Circulatory System Diagnoses with CC

Acute cardiac tamponade is a sudden accumulation of fluid in the pericardial sac leading to an increase in the intrapericardial pressure. The pericardial sac surrounds the heart and normally contains only 10 to 20 mL of serous fluid. The sudden accumulation of more fluid (as little as 200 mL of fluid or blood) compresses the heart and coronary arteries, compromising diastolic filling and systolic emptying and diminishing oxygen supply. The end result is decreased oxygen delivery and poor tissue perfusion to all organs.

Acute cardiac tamponade is potentially life-threatening, needing emergency assessment and immediate interventions. Some patients develop a more slowly accumulating tamponade that collects over weeks and months. If the fibrous pericardium gradually has time to stretch, the pericardial space can accommodate as much as 1 to 2 L of fluid before the patient becomes acutely symptomatic. Complications include decreased ventricular filling, decreased cardiac output, cardiogenic shock, and death.

CAUSES

Cardiac tamponade may have any of a variety of etiologies. It can be caused by both blunt and penetrating traumatic injuries and also iatrogenic injuries, such as those associated with removal of epicardial pacing wires and complications after cardiac catheterization and insertion of central venous or pulmonary artery catheters.

Rupture of the ventricle after an acute myocardial infarction or bleeding after cardiac surgery can also lead to tamponade. Other causes include treatment with anticoagulants, viral infections, and disorders that cause pericardial irritation such as pericarditis, neoplasms, or myxedema, as well as collagen diseases such as rheumatoid arthritis or systemic lupus erythematosus.

GENDER AND LIFE SPAN CONSIDERATIONS

Although a patient of any age can develop a cardiac tamponade, the very young and the elderly have fewer reserves available to cope with such a severe condition. Because trauma is the leading cause of death for individuals in the first four decades of life, traumatic tamponade is more common in that age group, whereas the older adult is more likely to have an iatrogenic tamponade. Males have higher rates of unintentional injury than do females.

☐ ASSESSMENT

HISTORY. The patient's history may include surgery, trauma, cardiac biopsy, viral infection, insertion of a transvenous pacing wire or catheter, or myocardial infarction. Elicit a medication history to determine if the patient is taking anticoagulants or any medication that could cause tamponade as a drug reaction (procainamide, hydralazine, minoxidil, isoniazid, penicillin, methysergide, or daunorubicin). Ask if the patient has renal failure, which can lead to pericarditis and bleeding. Cardiac tamponade may be acute or accumulate over time, as in the case of myxedema, collagen diseases, and neoplasm. The patient may have a history of dyspnea and chest pain that ranges from mild to severe and increases on inspiration. There may be no symptoms at all before severe hemodynamic compromise.

PHYSICAL EXAMINATION. The patient who has acute, rapid bleeding with cardiac tamponade appears critically ill and in shock. Assess airway, breathing, and circulation, and intervene simultaneously. The patient is acutely hypovolemic (because of blood loss into the pericardial sac) and in cardiogenic shock and should be assessed and treated for those conditions as an emergency situation.

If the patient is more stable, when you auscultate the heart, you may hear a pericardial friction rub as a result of the two inflamed layers of the pericardium rubbing against each other. The heart sounds may be muffled because of the accumulation of fluid around the heart. If a central venous or pulmonary artery catheter is present, the right atrial mean pressure (RAP) rises to >12 mm Hg, and the pulmonary capillary wedge pressure equalizes with the RAP. Systolic blood pressure decreases as the pressure on the ventricles reduces diastolic filling and cardiac output. Pulsus paradoxus (>10 mm Hg fall in systolic blood pressure during inspiration) is an important finding in cardiac tamponade and is probably related to blood pooling in the pulmonary veins during inspiration. Other signs that may be present are related to the decreased cardiac output and poor tissue perfusion. Confusion and agitation, cyanosis, tachycardia, and decreased urine output may all occur as cardiac output is compromised and tissue perfusion becomes impaired.

Assessment of cardiovascular function should be performed hourly; check mental status, skin color, temperature and moisture, capillary refill, heart sounds, heart rate, arterial blood pressure, and jugular venous distension. Maintain the patient on continuous cardiac monitoring, and monitor for ST- and T-wave changes.

PSYCHOSOCIAL. Acute cardiac tamponade can be sudden, unexpected, and life-threatening, causing the patient to experience fear and anxiety. Assess the patient's degree of fear and anxiety, as well as his or her ability to cope with a sudden illness and threat to self. The patient's family or significant other(s) should be included in the assessment and plan of care. Half of all patients with traumatic injuries have either alcohol or other drugs present in their systems at the time of injury. Ask about the patient's drinking patterns and any substance use and abuse. Assess the risk for withdrawal from alcohol or other drugs during the hospitalization.

DIAGNOSTIC HIGHLIGHTS

Test	Normal Result	Abnormality with Condition	Explanation
Echocardiogram	Normal size, shape, position, thickness, and movement of structures	Echo-free zone anterior to right ventricular wall and posterior to the left ventricular wall; there may	Records echoes created by deflection of short pulses of ultrasonic beam off cardiac structures; may also be done as a transesophageal

also be a decrease in right ventricular chamber size and a right-to-left septal shift during inspiration	procedure with transmitter inserted into esophagus (transesophageal echocardiogram, or TEE)

Other Tests: Prolonged coagulation studies and/or a decreased hemoglobin and hematocrit if the patient has lost sufficient blood into the pericardium. Electrocardiogram (ECG) and chest x ray.

PRIMARY NURSING DIAGNOSIS

Decreased cardiac output related to decreased preload and contractility.

OUTCOMES. Circulation status; Cardiac pump effectiveness; Tissue perfusion: Abdominal organs and peripheral; Vital signs status; Fluid balance

INTERVENTIONS. Cardiac care: Acute, Fluid/electrolyte management, Fluid monitoring; Shock management: Volume, Medication administration, Circulatory care

□ PLANNING AND IMPLEMENTATION

Collaborative

The highest priority is to make sure the patient has adequate airway, breathing, and circulation (ABCs). If the patient suffers hypoxia as a result of decreased cardiac output and poor tissue perfusion, oxygen, intubation, and mechanical ventilation may be required. If the symptoms are progressing rapidly, the physician may elect to perform a pericardiocentesis to normalize pericardial pressure, allowing the heart and coronary arteries to fill normally, so that cardiac output and tissue perfusion are restored. Assist by elevating the head of the bed to a 60-degree angle to allow gravity to pull the fluid to the apex of the heart. Emergency equipment should be nearby because ventricular tachycardia, ventricular fibrillation, or laceration of a coronary artery or myocardium can cause shock and death. Pericardiocentesis usually causes a dramatic improvement in hemodynamic status. However, if the patient has had rapid bleeding into the pericardial space, clots may have formed that block the needle aspiration. A "false negative" pericardiocentesis is therefore possible and needs to be considered if symptoms continue.

The patient must be taken to surgery after this procedure to explore the pericardium and stop further bleeding. If the patient has developed sudden bradycardia (heart rate <50 beats per minute), severe hypotension (systolic blood pressure <70 mm Hg), or asystole, an emergency thoracotomy may be performed at the bedside to evacuate the pericardial sac, control the hemorrhage, and perform internal cardiac massage if needed. The patient may also require fluid resuscitation agents to enhance cardiac output.

PHARMACOLOGIC HIGHLIGHTS

Medication or Drug Class	Dosage	Description	Rationale
Sympathomemitic such as dopamine hydrocholoride	Varies by drug	Stimulates adrenergic receptors to increase myocardial contractility and peripheral resistance	Supports blood pressure and cardiac output in emergencies until bleeding is brought under control; only used if fluid resuscitation is initiated

Independent

The highest nursing priority is to maintain the patient's airway, breathing, and circulation. Emergency equipment should be readily available, should the patient require intubation and mechanical ventilation. Be prepared to administer fluids, including blood products, colloids or crystalloids, and pressor agents, through a large-bore catheter. Pressure and rapid volume warmer infusors should be used for patients who require massive fluid resuscitation. A number of nursing strategies increase the rate of fluid replacement. Fluid resuscitation is most efficient through a short, large-bore peripheral intravenous (IV) catheter in a large peripheral vein. The IV should have a short length of tubing from the bag or bottle to the IV site. If pressure is applied to the bag, fluid resuscitation occurs more rapidly.

Emotional support of the patient and family is also a key nursing intervention. If the patient is awake as you implement strategies to manage the ABCs, provide a running explanation of the procedures. If blood component therapy is essential, answer the patient's and family's questions about the risks of hepatitis and transmission of the human immunodeficiency virus (HIV).

DOCUMENTATION GUIDELINES

- Physical findings of cardiovascular and neurologic systems
- Adequacy of airway, breathing, and circulation; mental status; skin color; vital signs; moisture of mucous membranes; capillary refill; heart sounds; presence of pulsus paradoxus or jugular venous distension; hemodynamic parameters; intake and output
- Response to interventions
- Fluid resuscitation, inotropic agents, pericardiocentesis, surgery
- Presence of complications
- Asystole, ventricular tachycardia, ventricular fibrillation; recurrence of tamponade; infection; ongoing hemorrhage

DISCHARGE AND HOME HEALTHCARE GUIDELINES

MEDICATIONS. Be sure the patient understands all medications, including dosage, route, side effects, and any routine laboratory testing. The patient needs to understand to avoid over-the-counter medications that include aspirin or ibuprofen.

COMPLICATIONS. The patient needs to understand the possibility of recurrence and the symptoms to report to the physician. The patient and significant other(s) also need to understand that symptoms of inadequate tissue perfusion (change in mental status; cool, clammy, cyanotic skin; dyspnea; chest pain) warrant activation of the Emergency Medical System.

Cardiogenic Shock

DRG Category: 127
Mean LOS: 5.5 days
Description: MEDICAL: Heart Failure and Shock

Cardiogenic shock occurs when cardiac output is insufficient to meet the metabolic demands of the body, resulting in inadequate tissue perfusion. There are four stages of cardiogenic shock: initial, compensatory, progressive, and refractory.

During the initial stage, there is diminished cardiac output without any clinical symptoms. In the compensatory stage, the baroreceptors respond to the decreased cardiac output by stimulating the sympathetic nervous system to release catecholamines to improve myocardial contractility and vasoconstriction, leading to increased venous return and arterial blood pressure. Impaired renal perfusion activates the renin-angiotensin system, whose end product, angiotensin II, causes sodium and water retention as well as vasoconstriction. The progressive stage follows the compensatory stage if there is no intervention or if the intervention fails to reverse the inadequate tissue perfusion. Compensatory mechanisms, aimed at improving cardiac output and tissue perfusion, place an increased demand on an already compromised myocardium. As tissue perfusion remains inadequate, the cells begin anaerobic metabolism, leading to metabolic acidosis and fluid leakage out of the capillaries and into the interstitial spaces. A decrease in circulating volume and an increase in blood viscosity may cause clotting in the capillaries and tissue death.

As the body releases fibrinolytic agents to break down the clots, disseminated intravascular coagulation (DIC) may ensue. Lactic acidosis causes depression of the myocardium and a decrease in the vascular responsiveness to catecholamines, further reducing cardiac output. Blood pools and stagnates in the capillaries, and the continued increase in hydrostatic pressure causes fluid to leak into the interstitium. Severe cerebral ischemia causes depression of the vasomotor center and loss of sympathetic stimulation, resulting in blood pooling in the periphery, a decrease in preload, and further reduction in cardiac output. If there is no effective intervention at this point, the shock will progress to the refractory stage, when the chance of survival is extremely limited.

CAUSES

The most common cause of cardiogenic shock is acute myocardial infarction (MI) resulting in a loss of more than 40% of the functional myocardium. Cardiogenic shock occurs with 10% to 20% of all hospital admissions for acute MI and carries an 80% mortality rate. Other causes include papillary muscle rupture, left ventricular free wall rupture, acute ventricular septal defect, severe congestive heart failure, end-stage cardiomyopathy, severe valvular dysfunction, acute cardiac tamponade, cardiac contusion, massive pulmonary embolus, or overdose of drugs such as beta blockers or calcium channel blockers.

GENDER AND LIFE SPAN CONSIDERATIONS

Cardiogenic shock can occur at any age but is more common in the middle-aged and older adult. Anyone at risk for coronary artery disease, both men and women, is also at risk for cardiogenic shock as a result of an acute MI. The elderly are at greater risk because of their diminished ability to compensate for an inadequate cardiac output and tissue perfusion.

☐ ASSESSMENT

HISTORY. The patient is likely to have a history of symptoms of an acute MI, including crushing, viselike chest pain or heaviness that radiates to the arms, neck, or jaw, lasting more than 20 minutes and unrelieved by nitroglycerin and rest. Other MI symptoms include shortness of breath, nausea, anxiety, and a sense of impending doom. The patient may also have a history of symptoms of any of the other etiologies mentioned above.

PHYSICAL EXAMINATION. During the initial stage of shock, there are no clinical findings unless the cardiac output can be measured. When the patient has entered the compensatory stage, symptoms may include an altered level of consciousness; sinus tachycardia; the presence of an S3 or S4 gallop rhythm; jugular venous distension; hypotension; rapid, deep respirations; pulmonary crackles; venous oxygen saturation (SvO_2) less than 60%; cyanosis; urine output less than 20 mL/h; decreased urinary sodium; increased urinary osmolarity; peripheral edema; hyperglycemia; hypernatremia; cold, clammy skin; and decreased bowel sounds.

As the patient enters the progressive stage, the symptoms become more pronounced and resistant to treatment. The patient becomes mentally unresponsive; hypotension becomes worse, requiring high doses of positive inotropic agents; metabolic and respiratory acidosis become apparent; oliguria or anuria and anasarca may ensue; and symptoms of DIC may be present. When the shock reaches the refractory stage, multisystem organ failure is apparent, with the above symptoms unresponsive to treatment.

PSYCHOSOCIAL. The patient in cardiogenic shock is in a life-threatening situation. The chances for survival are small, and the patient may experience a sense of impending doom. The impaired tissue perfusion may lead to anxiety and fear. The patient and his or her family or significant other may be in crisis. Both the patient and family may be experiencing grief in response to the potential loss of life.

DIAGNOSTIC HIGHLIGHTS

Test	Normal Result	Abnormality with Condition	Explanation
Hemodynamic monitoring	Right atrial pressure (RA): 1–8 mm Hg; pulmonary artery occlusion pressure (PAO): 4–12 mm Hg; cardiac output (CO): 4–7 L per minute; systemic vascular resistance (SVR): 800–1200 dynes/s per cm^{-5}	RA: 6 mm Hg; PAO: > 18 mm Hg; CO: < 5 L per minute; SVR: > 1200 dynes/s per cm^{-5}	Elevated filling pressures in heart and low systolic blood pressure occur in the setting of low cardiac output; arterial constriction occurs as a compensatory mechanism. Hemodynamic monitoring with serial

measures of cardiac output is important in the diagnosis of cardiogenic shock.

Other Tests: Serum laboratory tests, urinalysis, hematologic and coagulation studies

PRIMARY NURSING DIAGNOSIS

Altered tissue perfusion (peripheral, cerebral, renal, and cardiopulmonary) related to inadequate cardiac output

OUTCOMES. Circulation status; Cardiac pump effectiveness; Tissue perfusion: Cardiopulmonary, Cerebral, Renal, Peripheral; Vital sign status

INTERVENTIONS. Circulatory care; Emergency care; Vital signs monitoring; Cardiac care; Cardiac precautions; Oxygen therapy; Fluid/electrolyte management; Fluid monitoring; Shock management: Volume, Medication administration, Resuscitation, Surveillance

☐ PLANNING AND IMPLEMENTATION

Collaborative

The primary goal in treating cardiogenic shock is improvement in tissue perfusion and oxygenation. To limit the infarct size and treat the dyspnea, pulmonary congestion, hypoxemia, and acidosis, the physician is likely to prescribe oxygen. If a previously normocapnic patient's $PaCO_2$ decreases below 50 mm Hg, then the patient may require endotracheal intubation and mechanical ventilation.

Although the patient needs an adequate blood pressure, afterload may also need to be decreased, which may be accomplished with the intra-aortic balloon pump (IABP). A left ventricular assist device (LVAD) may be used to replace the function of the patient's heart for several days to provide total rest for the heart. An LVAD diverts blood from the left atrium or left ventricle by means of a pressure gradient and moves it to the external pump, after which the blood is returned to the aorta during diastole. An LVAD can reduce the patient's right ventricular contraction. Monitor the patient's central venous pressure carefully.

PHARMACOLOGIC HIGHLIGHTS

General Comments: Improving cardiac output, which is necessary to improve tissue perfusion, can be accomplished in several ways. If the patient is able to maintain hemodynamic stability, the physician prescribes medications, namely diuretics and nitrates, to reduce preload. During the later phases of shock, the patient may be too hypotensive to tolerate the vasodilative effects of both diuretics and nitrates.

The patient needs improvement in myocardial contractility without adding significant workload on the heart. Dopamine may also be used in an attempt to improve contractility and cardiac output. Other vasoactive drugs, such as amrinone, may also be used. Vasopressors may be used in an attempt to increase the mean arterial blood pressure to a level that provides adequate tissue perfusion (greater than 70 mm Hg). Several agents that may be administered include dopamine, epinephrine, norepinephrine, and phenylephrine hydrochoride

Medication or Drug Class	Dosage	Description	Rationale
Dobutamine	2–40 μg/kg per minute (but usually in the range of 2–20 μg/kg per minute)	Sympathomimetic	Dobutamine improves heart contractility without much effect on heart rate; renal function may also improve through increased cardiac output and renal perfusion
Diuretics	Varies by drug	Loop diuretics, thiazide diuretics	Reduces venous return (preload)

Independent

Limiting myocardial oxygen consumption is a primary concern. Decreasing oxygen demand may limit ischemia, injury, and infarction. Restrict the patient's activity, and maintain the patient on bed rest. Address the patient's anxiety by explaining all procedures. Permit the family or significant others to remain with the patient as long as their presence does not cause added stress. Maintaining a calm and peaceful environment provides reassurance and reduces anxiety, which, in turn, will reduce myocardial oxygen consumption.

Restricted activity could lead to impaired skin integrity, necessitating frequent assessment and care of the skin. Adequate protein and calories are essential for the prevention or healing of impaired skin integrity and should be provided by oral, enteral, or parenteral means.

DOCUMENTATION GUIDELINES

- Physical findings: Cardiopulmonary, renal, neurologic, and integumentary systems; skin integrity
- Hemodynamic response to inotropic medications, diuretics, nitrates, IABP, and oxygen
- Presence of complications: Pulmonary congestion, respiratory distress, unrelieved chest pain, and skin breakdown
- Reaction to the crisis and prognosis

DISCHARGE AND HOME HEALTHCARE GUIDELINES

Teach the patient how to reduce controllable risk factors for heart disease. If the physician has referred the patient to a cardiac rehabilitation program, encourage attendance. Be sure the patient understands the medication prescribed.

RECURRENCE OF CHEST PAIN. Teach the patient to call 911 for any chest pain that is not relieved by rest and/or nitroglycerin. Instruct the patient not to ignore the pain or wait to call for assistance.

RECURRENCE OF HEART FAILURE. Teach the patient to restrict fluids to 2 to 2.5 L per day, or as prescribed by the physician, and observe sodium restrictions. The patient should report a weight gain of greater than 4 pounds in 2 days to the physician. Finally, teach the patient to monitor for increasing shortness of breath and edema and to report either of those signs or symptoms to the physician. If the patient experiences acute shortness of breath, he or she should call 911 or go to the emergency department immediately.

Cardiomyopathy

DRG Category: 144
Mean LOS: 4.5 days
Description: MEDICAL: Other Circulatory System Diagnosis with CC

Cardiomyopathy is a chronic or subacute disease process that involves the heart muscle and causes either systolic dysfunction or diastolic dysfunction, or both; it most commonly involves the endocardium and occasionally the pericardium. Cardiomyopathy is classified as primary when the cause is not known. Secondary cardiomyopathy is a result of some other primary disease process. Three common classifications of cardiomyopathy are dilated, hypertrophic, and restrictive cardiomyopathy. Dilated cardiomyopathy is the most common and is characterized by ventricular dilation, impaired systolic function, atrial enlargement, and stasis of blood in the left ventricle. This form of cardiomyopathy is progressive and leads to intractable congestive heart failure (CHF) and death in the majority of patients within 5 years.

Hypertrophic cardiomyopathy, also known as hypertrophic obstructive cardiomyopathy or idiopathic hypertrophic subaortic stenosis, consists of ventricular hypertrophy, rapid contraction of the left ventricle, and impaired relaxation. The process may go on for years with no or slowly progressive symptoms, or the first sign of the disease may be sudden cardiac death. Although the patient may live a "normal" life, deterioration usually occurs.

The third form of cardiomyopathy, restricted cardiomyopathy, is the least common form. Both ventricles become rigid, which distorts the filling phase of the heart. The contraction phase remains normal. The result is that ventricular walls become fibrotic, cardiac filling diminishes, and cardiac output decreases. Restricted cardiomyopathy has a poor prognosis; many patients die within 1 to 2 years after diagnosis.

CAUSES

The etiology of many cases remains a mystery. The major cause of dilated cardiomyopathy is excessive alcohol consumption. Cardiomyopathy may also be caused by amyloidosis, hemochromatosis, metastatic carcinoma affecting the myocardium, fibrosis secondary to radiation, hypertension, vitamin deficiencies, pregnancy, viral or bacterial infection, and immune disorders. Other risk factors include chemotherapy, myocarditis, infiltrative disorders, and hypersensitivity to penicillin, tetracycline, or sulfonamide drugs. It is suspected that hypertrophic cardiomyopathy may be transmitted genetically through an autosomal dominant trait, but the cause remains unknown.

GENDER AND LIFE SPAN CONSIDERATIONS

Cardiomyopathy may occur at any time from young adulthood to old age. Hypertrophic cardiomyopathy usually occurs in young adults with a family history of the disease. Dilated cardiomyopathy, which is twice as common among men as women, occurs most often in middle age.

☐ ASSESSMENT

HISTORY. To diagnose the specific form of cardiomyopathy, establish a history of signs, symptoms, and potential causes. (See Table 19.) Determine the patient's patterns of alcohol consumption. Inquire if the patient has been previously diagnosed with amyloidosis, vitamin deficiencies, hemochromatosis, metastatic carcinoma affecting the myocardium, myocarditis, an immune disorder, or an infiltrative disorder. Determine if the patient has had a recent viral or bacterial infection. Ask female patients if they are pregnant. Question the patient about any hypersensitive reactions to medications or any exposure to radiation.

TABLE 19 | **Signs and Symptoms of Cardiomyopathy**

TYPE	SIGNS AND SYMPTOMS
Dilated cardiomyopathy	Fatigue and generalized weakness
	Narrow pulse pressure; peripheral edema, and neck vein congestion
	Orthopnea, dyspnea on exertion, paroxysmal noctural dyspnea—signs of left-sided CHF
	Palpitations and chest pain
	Pulmonary congestion and pleural effusions
	Syncope
	Tachycardia
Hypertrophic cardiomyopathy	Angina and palpitations
	Dysrthythmia, possibly leading to sudden death.
	Loud systolic murmur caused by obstruction of outflow
	Orthopnea and dyspnea on exertion
	Pulmonary congestion
	Sudden loss of pulses
	Syncope
Restrictive cardiomyopathy	Bradycardia
	Dyspnea
	Fatigue and generalized weakness
	Peripheral edema, liver congestion, abdominal discomfort, and neck vein distention—signs of right sided CHF

PHYSICAL EXAMINATION. Assess the patient for signs and symptoms of congestive heart failure, which is the end result of cardiomyopathy. Check for altered mental status as a result of poor cerebral perfusion, and observe for anxiety or restlessness. Note if the patient's skin is cool or damp, and observe it for mottling, pallor, or cyanosis. Inspect the patient for peripheral edema, ascites, jugular venous distension and hepatojugular reflux. Palpate the patient's abdomen for signs of hepatomegaly. Assess the patient's breathing patterns for shortness of breath, dyspnea, tachypnea, or crackles. Note a decreased blood pressure and bounding or alternating strength of peripheral pulses. Auscultate for heart sounds, and note the presence of an S3 or S4 gallop, valvular murmurs associated with mitral or tricuspid regurgitation, or an outflow obstruction of hypertrophy, tachycardia, and dysrhythmias.

PSYCHOSOCIAL. The patient with cardiomyopathy may experience fear and anxiety as a result of living with a life-threatening, chronic disease process. These feelings may be exhibited by restlessness, insomnia, bouts of anger or withdrawal, or difficulty concentrating. Although some denial and depression are a normal part of the grieving process, if these conditions persist, patients may need assistance in moving on to accept their disease and prognosis.

DIAGNOSTIC HIGHLIGHTS

Test	Normal Result	Abnormality with Condition	Explanation
Cardiac catheterization	Normal right and left values	Right heart catheterization: elevated left and right ventricular end-diastolic and atrial pressures, and decreased cardiac output of the right heart Left heart catheterization: left ventriculogram may reveal decreased ventricular wall motion and/or mitral regurgitation	Impaired systolic and/or diastolic functioning of the heart

Other Tests: Supporting tests include sodium levels; blood urea nitrogen (BUN), potassium levels, and creatinine levels; chest x ray; electrocardiogram (ECG); if the patient has developed CHF as a result of the cardiomyopathy, the following tests might also be obtained: hematocrit, arterial blood gases (ABGs), and coagulation studies.

PRIMARY NURSING DIAGNOSIS

Decreased cardiac output related to reduced myocardial contractility

OUTCOMES. Circulation status; Cardiac pump effectiveness; Tissue perfusion: Cardiopulmonary, Cerebral, Renal, Peripheral; Vital sign status

INTERVENTIONS. Circulatory care; Emergency care; Vital signs monitoring; Cardiac care; Cardiac precautions; Oxygen therapy; Fluid/electrolyte management; Fluid monitoring; Shock management: Volume, Medication administration, Resuscitation, Surveillance

◻ PLANNING AND IMPLEMENTATION

Collaborative

The treatment for cardiomyopathy is palliative rather than curative. Control of the symptoms of CHF is the primary goal in treatment. Medical management may vary, depending on the type of cardiomyopathy present.

Surgical treatment most commonly consists of excision of part of the hypertrophied septum to reduce the outflow obstruction (septal myotomy-myectomy). The patient with restrictive cardiomyopathy usually undergoes surgery to implant a permanent cardiac pacemaker.

PHARMACOLOGIC HIGHLIGHTS

Medication or Drug Class	Dosage	Description	Rationale
Digoxin	0.25 mg qd	Direct action on cardiac muscle to increase contractility	Idiopathic dilated cardiomyopathy: improves contractility and slows the renin-angiotensin response.
Vasodilators	Varies by drug	Drugs such as nitrates and hydralazine dilate arteries	Reduce both preload and afterload by causing venous and arterial vasodilation

Other Medications: Angiotensin-converting enzyme inhibitors (ACEIs) may also be prescribed to inactivate the renin-angiotensin system, thereby decreasing vascular resistance and ventricular afterload. Beta-adrenergic antagonists have also been known to be beneficial in the treatment of dilated cardiomyopathy because of the resultant decrease in myocardial oxygen demand, improved ventricular filling, and inhibition of sympathetic vasoconstriction. Medical interventions for hypertrophic cardiomyopathy are aimed at decreasing the force of ventricular contraction and decreasing the outflow obstruction. Agents commonly used to achieve this goal include beta-adrenergic antagonists or calcium-channel blockers. Diuretic treatment is not indicated for hypertrophic cardiomyopathy because the outflow obstruction requires an adequate preload to maintain sufficient cardiac output. The longer filling time, optimal preload, and decrease in contractility diminish the outflow obstruction by the septum and mitral valve during systole. Calcium-channel blockers, most commonly verapamil, are used to promote relaxation of the ventricle, which also results in improved diastolic filling time.

Independent

Elevate the head of the patient's bed 30 to 45 degrees to help alleviate dyspnea. The elevation lowers pressure on the diaphragm, which is caused by the contents of the abdomen, and decreases venous return, thereby decreasing preload. If necessary, assist the patient with the activities of daily living. Although the patient requires frequent rest periods, maintain some level of activity. Prolonged periods of little or no activity can be very difficult to reverse.

Education of the patient and family is most important to prevent exacerbations and frequent hospital visits. CHF as a response to cardiomyopathy is a condition that is managed on an outpatient basis. Teach the patient and family how to prevent exacerbation and worsening of the condition. Explain the disease process clearly, using audiovisual aids whenever possible to help the patient understand the necessity of the prescribed medications, activity restrictions, diet, fluid restrictions, and lifestyle changes. Provide written material for the patient to take home and use as a reference; however, before giving the patient this material, be sure to assess his or her literacy level.

Teach the patient and family measures to prevent the condition from worsening. Patients and their families may be fearful and anxious, whether this is a new diagnosis or a progression of a chronic condition. The patient and family are required to make many lifestyle changes. Fear, anxiety, and grief can all stimulate the sympathetic nervous system, leading to catecholamine release and additional stress on an already-compromised heart. Helping the patient to work through these feelings may improve psychological well-being and cardiac output.

DOCUMENTATION GUIDELINES

- Physical findings: Vital signs; right atrial pressure, pulmonary artery pressure, pulmonary capillary wedge pressure, CO, systemic vascular resistance, pulmonary vascular resistance; skin temperature, color, dampness; presence or absence of jugular vein distension or hepatojugular reflux, ascites, edema, pulmonary crackles or wheezes, S3 or S4, or murmurs; intake and output; daily weight; mental status
- Laboratory results: Electrolyte, complete blood count, and ABG results
- Response to medications such as diuretics, nitrates, inotropes, and oxygen

DISCHARGE AND HOME HEALTHCARE GUIDELINES

PREVENTION. To prevent exacerbations, teach the patient and family to monitor for increased shortness of breath or edema and how to measure fluid intake and output and daily weights. Explain when to notify the physician of changes.

MEDICATIONS. Be sure the patient and family understand all medications, including effects, dosage, route, adverse effects, and the need for routine laboratory monitoring for drugs such as digoxin.

COMPLICATIONS. Instruct the patient to call for emergency assistance for acute shortness of breath or chest discomfort that is not alleviated with rest.

Carpal Tunnel Syndrome

DRG Category: 018
Mean LOS: 5.5 days
Description: MEDICAL: Cranial and Peripheral Nerve Disorders with CC
DRG Category: 006
Mean LOS: 2.2 days
Description: SURGICAL: Carpal Tunnel Release

Carpal tunnel syndrome (CTS), first described in 1854 as a complication of trauma and again in 1947 as an idiopathic syndrome, is part of a larger group of musculoskeletal alterations called upper extremity repetitive use syndrome, or cumulative trauma disorders. Cumulative trauma disorders involve injury to the tendon, tendon sheath, and related tissues (bones, muscles, and nerves) of the upper extremity. Carpal tunnel syndrome is the most common of the nerve entanglement syndromes.

Carpal tunnel syndrome occurs because of a compression of the median nerve as it passes through the wrist within the carpal tunnel, resulting in a slowing of nerve conduction velocity. The median nerve carries motor, sensory, and autonomic fibers to the hand and, when injured, results in an impairment of sensory and motor function.

CAUSES

Rheumatoid arthritis, flexor tenosynovitis, severe sprain of the wrist, or dislocation of the wrist are factors that predispose patients to CTS. Other factors include pregnancy, menopause, and hysterectomy. Diabetes mellitus, acromegaly, renal failure, hypothyroidism, tuberculosis, amyloidosis, and myxedema are also thought to be contributory factors, as well as aging and obesity.

Many researchers have reported an occupational link to the performance of certain jobs or ergonomic factors in the workplace. Jobs that require highly repetitive motions involving high hand force or awkward positions that deviate from normal wrist flexion, extension, or medial-lateral rotation positions are thought to cause CTS.

GENDER AND LIFE SPAN CONSIDERATIONS

CTS can occur in both sexes and at any age. However, the highest incidence appears to be in women between the ages of 30 and 49. One major study established a mean age for occupational CTS as 37, with women being twice as likely as men to develop CTS. The same study found that for nonoccupational CTS, the mean age was 51, with women three times as likely as men to develop CTS.

□ ASSESSMENT

HISTORY. Elicit a history of hand-related symptoms. Determine the patient's dominant hand, and ask if he or she has experienced attacks of painful tingling in the hand(s) at night sufficient to disturb sleep. Ask the patient if he or she has experienced accompanying daytime swelling and numbness of the hands or fingers. Elicit a history of aching, stiffness, and/or burning in the hand(s), fingers, or thumb(s).

Establish a history of contributing factors to CTS. Has the patient ever been diagnosed with rheumatoid arthritis, flexor tenosynovitis, diabetes mellitus, hypothyroidism, acromegaly, tuberculosis, amyloidosis, or myxedema? Ask if the patient has sprained or dislocated the wrist. Establish a history of pregnancies, menopause, and/or hysterectomy.

Establish an occupational history. Does the patient's work require use of the hands? Which hand is involved in repetitive movements or the use of tools?

PHYSICAL EXAMINATION. Examine the patient's hands and wrists. Check the nails for atrophy, and ask if the patient can clench the hands into fists. Note the patient's range of motion of the fingers and wrist, and the hand strength. Examine the patient for dry, shiny skin.

PSYCHOSOCIAL. Patients with CTS usually have had a progressive, long-term problem that interrupts their activities of daily living, along with their ability to perform occupational tasks. Anxiety is a common response. Assess the patient's coping, occupational status, and familial interactions. If an occupational change is necessary, assess the consequences for patient and family.

DIAGNOSTIC HIGHLIGHTS

Test	Normal Result	Abnormality with Condition	Explanation
Electromyography	Normal conduction	Detects median nerve motor conduction delay of more than 5 milliseconds.	The maximum latency difference (MLD) method, measured by centrimetric technique ("inching" up the arm) has a high predictive value
Tinel's sign	Negative test	Positive if gentle tapping over the median nerve at the wrist results in pain, tingling, or numbness in the median nerve distribution.	Compression of median nerve leads to positive test result
Finkelstein's test	Negative test	Positive if severe pain at radial styloid (process on distal end of the radium) results from flexing thumb against palm and finger flexed over thumb	Compression of median nerve leads to positive test result
Phalen's test	Negative test	Positive if unforced complete flexion of wrist for 60 seconds results in pain, tingling, or numbness over median nerve distribution	Compression of median nerve leads to positive test result

Other Tests: To diagnose CTS, the Occupational Safety and Health Administration (OSHA) requires at least one physical finding (positive Tinel, Finkelstein, or Phalen tests or swelling, redness, deformity, or loss of motion) or at least one subjective complaint (pain, numbness, tingling, aching, stiffness, or burning), resulting in medical treatment, lost work days, or transfer to another job. Nerve conduction studies, however, are considered the best means to determine the presence of CTS.

□ PLANNING AND IMPLEMENTATION

Collaborative

The most conservative treatment prescribed by physicians is splinting of the involved wrist and administering of medications. Physical therapy may be prescribed at any point in the treatment process to decrease swelling and promote healing. After 6 weeks of physical therapy, a vocational evaluation is performed to determine the patient's ability to return to his or her previous job. Vocational retraining may be recommended. If conservative treatment is not successful, the carpal ligament is released surgically to relieve compression of the median nerve. The surgeon may also perform neurolysis, freeing of the nerve fibers, if necessary.

PHARMACOLOGIC HIGHLIGHTS

Medication or Drug Class	Dosage	Description	Rationale
Nonsteroidal anti-inflammatory medications	Varies with drug	Includes a number of medications such as indomethacin (Indocin) or phenylbutazone	Reduce swelling

Other Medications: Steroid injections are also used to decrease the inflammation of the carpal ligament. Analgesics are administered as needed.

Independent

An important focus of nursing intervention is prevention of CTS. When discussing prevention, explain to the patient that people at risk should be rotated into other jobs that do not require similar tasks. Periodic rests should also be taken, accompanied by stretching of the wrist, hand, fingers, and thumbs. If the patient is to wear a splint, teach the proper techniques for applying the splint so that it is not too tight. Teach the patient how to remove the splint in order to exercise, and teach the patient how to perform daily, gentle range-of-motion exercises. If the patient is to wear a sling, instruct him or her to remove it several times daily to perform elbow and shoulder exercises. Advise the patient that occasional exercise in warm water is therapeutic. Encourage the patient to use the hands as much as possible. For patients whose hand use is impaired, assist with bathing and eating tasks. Encourage the patient to verbalize concerns about CTS. Answer questions, and arrange for consultations with a licensed physical therapist and a vocational rehabilitation counselor.

DOCUMENTATION GUIDELINES

- Physical findings: Hand, wrist, thumb, finger pain; numbness; tingling; burning
- Response to conservative or surgical treatment
- Attendance and response to physical therapy
- Ability to cope with immobility and inability to return to work

DISCHARGE AND HOME HEALTHCARE GUIDELINES

THERAPY. Be sure the patient understands and implements appropriate range-of-motion exercises. Emphasize the need to use the hands as often as possible and the value of warm water exercising.

EQUIPMENT. Teach the patient proper techniques for applying and removing splints and/or slings.

VOCATIONAL COUNSELING. Arrange for the patient to consult with a vocational rehabilitation counselor about returning to work and any modifications that must be made on the job.

Cataract

DRG Category: 039
Mean LOS: 1.5 days
Description: SURGICAL: Lens Procedure with or without Vitrectomy

Cataracts are the leading cause of preventable blindness among adults in the United States. A cataract is defined as opacity of the normally transparent lens that distorts the image projected on the retina. The lens opacity reduces visual acuity. As the eye ages, the lens loses water and increases in size and density, causing compression of lens fibers. A cataract then forms as oxygen uptake is reduced, water content decreases, calcium content increases, and soluble protein becomes insoluble. Over time, compression of lens fibers causes a painless, progressive loss of transparency that is often bilateral. The rate of cataract formation in each eye is seldom identical. Without surgery, a cataract can lead to blindness.

CAUSES

Cataracts have several causes and may be age-related, present at birth, or formed as a result of trauma or exposure to a toxic substance. The most common cataract is age-related (senile cataract). Traumatic cataracts develop after a foreign body injures the lens. Complicated cataracts develop as secondary effects in patients with metabolic disorders (e.g., diabetes mellitus), radiation damage (x ray or sunlight), or eye inflammation or disease (e.g., glaucoma, retinitis pigmentosa, detached retina, recurrent uveitis). Toxic cataracts result from drug or chemical toxicity. Congenital cataracts are caused by maternal infection (e.g., German measles, mumps, hepatitis) during the first trimester of pregnancy.

GENDER AND LIFE SPAN CONSIDERATIONS

Age-related cataracts begin to form at age 50 and are present in 18% of persons aged 65 to 75 and in 45% of persons aged 75 to 84. Some cataracts are present at birth. Cataracts occur in both men and women.

☐ ASSESSMENT

HISTORY. Changes in vision go unnoticed for a long time because of the slow progression. Patients frequently complain of problems with reading and night driving. Ask if the patient is color blind, has always worn glasses or contacts, has a history of cataracts, or is under the treatment of an eye doctor or optometrist. Generally, patients with cataracts report decreasing visual acuity with painless, increasingly blurred vision; visual distortion such as glare, dazzling effects, or dimness; or decrease in color perception and discoloration brought about by changes in lens color to yellow, amber, and finally to brown. The presence of other risk factors, such as trauma, radiation exposure, metabolic disorders, eye infection, and medication history, is important. Ascertain if the patient's mother contracted German measles, mumps, or hepatitis during pregnancy.

PHYSICAL EXAMINATION. Cataract formation causes blurred vision, a loss measured by use of the Snellen chart. Color perception of blue, green, and purple is reported as varying shades of gray. If the cataract is advanced, shining a penlight on the pupil reveals the white area behind the pupil. A dark area in the normally homogeneous red reflex confirms the diagnosis.

PSYCHOSOCIAL. Because the loss of vision is usually gradual, the patient may deny visual dysfunction until it affects the actions of daily life, reading, or driving. Anxiety and fear of losing one's eyesight are common emotional responses. Social isolation may also occur because visual difficulties impede easy movement away from the home and because of possible embarrassment caused by impaired vision.

DIAGNOSTIC HIGHLIGHTS

General Comments: No specific laboratory tests identify cataracts. Diagnosis is made by history, visual acuity test, and direct ophthalmoscopic exam.

Test	Normal Result	Abnormality with Condition	Explanation
Ophthalmoscopy or slit lamp examination	Normal conjunctiva, cornea, crystalline lens, iris, sclera	May reveal a dark area in the red reflex.	Microscopic instrument that allows detailed visualization of anterior segment of eye to identify lens opacities and other eye abnormalities

PRIMARY NURSING DIAGNOSIS

Sensory and perceptual alterations (visual) related to decreased visual acuity

OUTCOMES. Body image; Safety behavior: Personal; Safety behavior: Fall prevention; Safety behavior: Home physical environment; Anxiety control; Neurological status; Rest; Sleep

INTERVENTIONS. Communication enhancement: Visual deficit; Activity therapy; Cognitive stimulation; Environmental management; Fall prevention; Surveillance: Safety

☐ PLANNING AND IMPLEMENTATION

Collaborative

SURGICAL. There is no known medical treatment that cures, prevents, or reduces cataract formation. Surgical removal of the opacified lens is the only cure for cataracts. The lens can be removed when the visual deficit is 20/40. If cataracts occur bilaterally, the more advanced cataract is removed first. Extracapsular cataract extraction, the most common procedure, removes the anterior lens capsule and cortex, leaving the posterior capsule intact. A posterior chamber intraocular lens is implanted where the patient's own lens used to be. Intracapsular cataract extraction removes the entire lens within the intact capsule. An intraocular lens is implanted in either the anterior or posterior chamber, or the visual deficit is corrected with contact lenses or cataract glasses.

COMPLICATIONS. Complications may include retinal disorders, pupillary block, adhesions, acute glaucoma, macular edema, and retinal detachment. Following extracapsular cataract extraction, the posterior capsule may become opacified. This condition, called a secondary membrane or after-cataract, occurs when subcapsular lens epithelial cells regenerate lens fibers, which obstruct vision. After-cataract is treated by yttrium-aluminum-garnet (YAG) laser treatment to the affected tissue.

PHARMACOLOGIC HIGHLIGHTS

Medication or Drug Class	Dosage	Description	Rationale
Acetazolamide	250 mg po 1–4 times a day	Carbonic anhydrase inhibitor	Reduces intraocular pressure by inhibiting formation of hydrogen and bicarbonate ions
Phenylephrine	Topical ophthalmic use, 1–2 drops of 0.125% solution every 3–4 hours	Sympathomimetic	Causes abnormal dilation of the pupil, constriction of conjunctival arteries

Other Medications: Postoperatively, medications are prescribed to reduce infection (gentamicin or neomycin) and to reduce inflammation (dexamethasone), taking the form of eye drops. Acetaminophen is prescribed for mild discomfort; tropicamide is prescribed to induce ciliary paralysis.

Independent

If nursing care is provided in the patient's home, structure the environment with conducive lighting and reduce fall hazards. Suggest magnifying glasses and large-print books. Explain that sunglasses and soft lighting can reduce glare. Assist the patient with the actions of daily living as needed to remedy any self-care deficit. Encourage the patient to verbalize or keep a log on his or her fears and anxiety about visual loss or impending surgery. Help plan events to solve the problems with social isolation.

POSTOPERATIVE HOSPITAL CARE. Postoperative care includes covering the affected eye with an 8- to 24-hour patch and protective shield and positioning the patient supine or on the unoperated side. Apply cool compresses to reduce itching. Monitor and report any drainage, pain, or vital sign alteration. Teach the patient how to administer eye drops correctly, and caution the patient to notify the physician immediately upon experiencing eye pain. During recovery, teach the patient how to adjust home environments and daily activities to promote safety.

DOCUMENTATION GUIDELINES

- Presence of complications: Eye discharge, pain, vital sign alterations
- Response to eye medication
- Reaction to supine position

DISCHARGE AND HOME HEALTHCARE GUIDELINES

Be sure the patient understands all medications, including dosage, route, action, adverse effects, and need for postoperative evaluation, usually the next day, by the eye surgeon. Review installation technique of eye drops into the conjunctival sac. Teach the patient to avoid over-the-counter medications, particularly those with aspirin.

Instruct the patient to report any bleeding, yellow-green drainage, pain, visual losses, nausea, vomiting, tearing, photophobia, or seeing bright flashes of light. Instruct the patient to avoid activities that increase intraocular pressure such as bending at the waist, sleeping on the operative side, straining with bowel movements, lifting more than 15 pounds, sneezing, coughing, or vomiting. Instruct the patient to wear a shield over the operative eye at night to prevent accidental injury to the eye during sleep and to wear glasses during the day to prevent accidental injury to the eye while awake. Recommend that the patient avoid reading for some time after surgery to reduce eye strain and unnecessary movement so that maximal healing occurs.

Advise the patient not to shampoo for several days after surgery. The face should be held away from the shower head with the head tilted back so that water spray and soap avoid contact with the eye.

HOME HEALTH TEACHING. Vacuuming should be avoided because of the forward flexion and rapid, jerky movement required. Driving, sports, and machine operation can be resumed when permission is granted by the eye surgeon.

Clients fitted with cataract eye glasses need information about altered spatial perception. The eye glasses should be first used when the patient is seated, until the patient adjusts to the distortion. Instruct the client to look through the center of the corrective lenses and to turn the head, rather than only the eyes, when looking to the side. Clear vision is possible only through the center of the lens. Hand-eye coordination movements must be practiced with assistance and relearned because of the altered spatial perceptions.

Cephalopelvic Disproportion

DRG Category: 372
Mean LOS: 2.7 days
Description: MEDICAL: Vaginal Delivery with Complicating Diagnoses

Cephalopelvic disproportion (CPD) refers to the inability of the fetal head to pass through the maternal pelvis; it occurs in 1% to 3% of all primigravidas. In absolute CPD, the fetal head is too large for the maternal pelvis, so that vaginal birth cannot be safely achieved and cesarean delivery is required. In relative CPD, the fetus may be delivered vaginally if a favorable combination of other factors can be achieved: efficient uterine contractions; favorable fetal attitude, presentation, and position; maximization of maternal pelvic diameters; adequate molding of the fetal head; adequate expulsive efforts by the mother; and adequate stretching of maternal soft tissues.

CPD can lead to prolonged labor, with delayed engagement of the fetal head in the pelvis and increased risk of umbilical cord prolapse. Prolonged labor can place the mother at risk for dysfunctional uterine contractions, fluid and electrolyte imbalance, exhaustion, hypoglycemia, uterine rupture, need for operative delivery, and postpartum hemorrhage. Risks to the fetus include hypoxia, hypoglycemia, acidemia, and infection. Vaginal delivery may be difficult in these patients, with increased risk of maternal vaginal, cervical, and perineal lacerations; fractured sacrum or coccyx; fetal birth asphyxia; shoulder dystocia (difficult delivery because of fetal shoulder position); and traumatic birth injuries, especially cervical spine, nerve, clavicle, and cranial injuries. Some women who experience CPD that resulted in a cesarean delivery with one infant are able to deliver a subsequent infant vaginally.

CAUSES

The cause of CPD can be attributed to maternal and fetal factors. Maternal factors include inability of the pelvic soft tissues to stretch adequately and inadequate diameters of the maternal bony pelvis. Contractures of the maternal pelvis may occur in one or more diameters of the pelvic inlet, midpelvis, or pelvic outlet. Fetal macrosomia (fetal weight greater than 4000 grams), incomplete flexion of the fetal head onto the chest, occiput posterior or transverse fetal position, and inability of the fetal head to mold to the maternal pelvis all contribute to the syndrome.

GENDER AND LIFE SPAN CONSIDERATIONS

Any woman of childbearing age may experience CPD, although women who have already delivered one or more infants vaginally have less risk of CPD than those having their first vaginal delivery. Teenagers under the age of 18 have an increased risk of CPD because their pelvic growth may not be fully completed.

◻ ASSESSMENT

HISTORY. Patients may have a family history of fetal macrosomia or pelvic contractures. Any personal history of rickets, scoliosis, or pelvic fracture should also be noted. Gestational diabetes, which may contribute to fetal macrosomia, may be present. Ask the patient about her prior deliveries to ascertain whether she has delivered an infant vaginally before.

PHYSICAL EXAMINATION. Determine the pelvic type of the woman. Android and platypelloid pelvic classifications are not favorable for a vaginal birth; the gynecoid and anthropoid pelvis classifications are present in 75% of all women and are favorable for a vaginal birth. Perform an internal exam; the following findings indicate a contracted pelvis and a potential for CPD to occur if the woman becomes pregnant: ability to touch the sacral promontory with the index finger; significant convergence of the side walls; forward inclination of a straight sacrum; sharp ischial spines with a narrow interspinous diameter; and a narrow suprapubic arch.

If CPD is suspected during labor, physical assessment should include pelvic size and shape; fetal presentation, position, attitude, and presence of molding or caput succedaneum of the fetal head (swelling on the presenting part of the fetal head during labor); fetal activity level; maternal bladder distension and presence of stool in rectum; duration, frequency, and strength of contractions; effacement and dilation of the cervix; and descent of the fetal head in relation to the mother's ischial spines. Common assessment findings with CPD during labor include delayed engagement of the fetal head, a lack of progress in cervical effacement, and dilation in the presence of adequate uterine contractions. If fetal hypoxia or hypoglycemia occurs, loss of fetal heart rate variability, late decelerations, or fetal bradycardia may be seen on the electronic fetal monitor. Fetal scalp stimulation may fail to elicit heart rate acceleration, and fetal capillary blood pH obtained by scalp sampling may indicate acidosis.

PSYCHOSOCIAL. Assess the patient and partner (or other labor support people present) for ability to cope with the difficult labor and ability to maintain a positive self-concept and role performance. Assess the presence of anxiety or fear related to the mother's or baby's well-being or to medical interventions such as forceps or vacuum extractor use or cesarean delivery. Feelings of exhaustion, disappointment, or failure are common.

DIAGNOSTIC HIGHLIGHTS

General Comments: CPD cannot be diagnosed except in rare cases without allowing labor to proceed for several hours. In labor, the pubic symphysis and other pelvic joints gain mobility under the influence of high levels of relaxin and other hormones. Therefore, evidence of lack of progressive dilation and fetal descent in labor is usually considered more important than pelvic measurement in diagnosing CPD.

Test	Normal Result	Abnormality with Condition	Explanation
Clinical pelvimetry	Diagonal conjugate > 11.5 cm; outlet > 8 cm	Diagonal conjugate < 11.5 cm; outlet < 8 cm	An adequate pelvic inlet and outlet is needed for a vaginal delivery

PRIMARY NURSING DIAGNOSIS

Risk for injury of mother or fetus related to traumatic delivery

OUTCOMES. Risk control; Risk detection

INTERVENTIONS. Labor induction; Intrapartal care: High risk delivery; Electronic fetal monitoring: Intrapartum; Intrapartal care

☐ PLANNING AND IMPLEMENTATION

Collaborative

MEDICAL. Medical management of CPD can include the use of pitocin to induce or augment labor contractions, manual or forceps rotation of the fetus into an occiput anterior position, and vaginal delivery assisted by outlet forceps or vacuum extractor. The cutting of a midline or mediolateral episiotomy is often necessary. If shoulder dystocia occurs, the McRoberts maneuver (extreme flexion of the mother's legs at the hips) and firm suprapubic pressure may accomplish delivery. In some cases, intentional fracture of the infant's clavicle is used to accomplish delivery in the presence of severe shoulder dystocia. When vaginal delivery appears to be impossible or likely to be very traumatic, cesarean delivery is indicated.

Labor patients using analgesia or anesthesia require careful monitoring. For patients using narcotic analgesics, monitor the maternal pulse, blood pressure, and respirations. Watch for signs of respiratory depression. Since intravenous (IV) narcotics readily cross the placenta, observe the fetal heart rate; often a temporary loss of variability is seen. For patients using regional anesthesia, monitor maternal pulse, blood pressure, and respirations. Check the mother's blood pressure every 1 to 5 minutes for 15 minutes after the epidural or spinal bolus dosage. Watch for lowered blood pressure.

PHARMACOLOGIC HIGHLIGHTS

Medication or Drug Class	Dosage	Description	Rationale
Opiod analgesics; anesthetics	Varies with drug, usually given IVP or via epidural	Pain relievers	Labor is difficult and prolonged; often back pain is increased due to the position of the fetus; episiotomy repair, forcep or vacuum extraction requires anesthesia
Oxytocin (Pitocin)	Mix 10 units in 500 mL of IV solution, begin in fusion at 1 mU per minute; increase 1–2 mU per minute q 15–30 minutes until adequate labor is established	Oxytocic	Appropriate to induce labor, or to give the patient a trial labor; should be discontinued upon a definitive diagnosis of CPD, requiring a cesarean section

Independent

Have the laboring woman change positions frequently (approximately every half hour) to encourage movement of the fetal head into a favorable position for delivery. Sitting, squatting, positioning on hands and knees, or side lying (alternating sides) may be used. Avoid supine positioning. To encourage rotation of a fetus from a posterior position, suggest lying on the same side as the fetal limbs, or position the mother on her hands and knees. Pelvic rocking exercises may be helpful. Encourage periods of ambulation, as long as the membranes are not ruptured or the fetal head is well applied to the cervix.

Keeping the bladder and rectum empty allows maximum pelvic space for the descent of the fetal head. Fluid and caloric intake should be attended to during labor. In some delivery settings, however, patients may receive intravenous solutions for electrolyte, fluid, and/or glucose intake. In other settings, ice chips, clear liquids, or a light diet may be encouraged.

In the second stage of labor, instruct the laboring woman to use her diaphragm and abdominal muscles to bear down during contractions. Help her find a comfortable and effective position for pushing, such as supported squatting, semisitting, side lying, or sitting upright in bed or on a chair, birthing stool, or commode.

Provide encouragement of the patient's coping strategies and assistance with pain management. Nonpharmacologic aids that can be offered include breathing techniques, massage, sacral counterpressure, rocking chair, application of heat or cold, visualization or relaxation techniques, therapeutic touch, music, showering or bathing, companionship, and encouragement. Provide emotional support; families are often unprepared to deal with an unplanned, unwanted cesarean birth.

DOCUMENTATION GUIDELINES

- Progress in labor: Cervical effacement and dilation, station of fetal head, presence of molding or caput, contraction pattern
- Factors contributing to CPD: Pelvic size and shape; fetal presentation, position, and attitude; maternal position; bladder and bowel fullness; duration, frequency, and strength of contractions
- Indicators of fetal well-being: Fetal baseline heart rate, variability, presence of accelerations and decelerations; fetal activity level; response to scalp stimulation
- Indicators of maternal well-being: Tolerability of labor pain, effectiveness of coping strategies, presence of support people, indicators of psychological status, vital signs

DISCHARGE AND HOME HEALTHCARE GUIDELINES

BIRTH INJURIES. Be sure the patient understands the nature of and care of any birth injuries sustained by the infant. Ensure that plans for follow-up care can be carried out by the family.

POSTPARTUM SELF-CARE. Review use of any pain medication prescribed, as well as nonpharmacologic comfort measures for episiotomy, lacerations, and hemorrhoid care. Instruct the patient to report any increase in perineal or uterine pain, foul odor, fever or flulike symptoms, or vaginal bleeding that is heavier than a menstrual period.

Cerebral Aneurysm

DRG Category: 014
Mean LOS: 6.4 days
Description: MEDICAL: Specific Cerebrovascular, Except TIA
DRG Category: 001
DRG Category: 001
Mean LOS: 9.6 days
Description: SURGICAL: Craniotomy, Age > 17, Except for Trauma

Cerebral aneurysm is an outpouching of the wall of a cerebral artery that results from weakening of the wall of the vessel. Cerebral aneurysms have a variety of sizes, shapes, and causes. (See Table 20.) Most cerebral aneurysms are saccular or berrylike with a stem and a neck. The incidence of cerebral aneurysm has been estimated at 10 per 100,000 per population, with approximately 15% to 25% of patients having multiple aneurysms, often bilateral in the same location on both sides of the head. Clinical concern arises if an aneurysm ruptures or becomes large enough to exert pressure on surrounding structures. When the vessel wall becomes so thin that it can no longer withstand the surrounding arterial pressure, the cerebral aneurysm ruptures, causing direct hemorrhaging of arterial blood into the subarachnoid space (subarachnoid hemorrhage).

TABLE 20 | **Classification of Cerebral Aneurysms**

Size	Small, < 15 mm
	Large, 15–25 mm
	Giant, 25– 50 mm
	Supergiant, 50 mm
Shape	Berry: most common (95%); berry-shaped aneurysm with a neck or stem
	Sacular: any aneurysm with a sacular outpouching
	Fusiform: outpouching of an arterial wall, but with no stem
Etiology	Traumatic: aneurysm that results from traumatic head injury
	Charcot-Bouchard: microscopic aneurismal formation associated with hypertension; involves the basal ganglia and brainstem
	Dissecting: related to atherosclerosis, inflammation, or trauma; aneurysm in which the intimal layer is pulled away from the medial layer and blood is forced between the layers

Complications of a ruptured cerebral aneurysm can be fatal if bleeding is excessive. Subarachnoid hemorrhage can lead to cerebral vasospasm, cerebral infarction, and death. Rebleeding often occurs in the first 48 hours after the initial bleed but can occur any time within the first 6 months. Other complications include meningeal irritation and hydrocephalus.

CAUSES

Possible causes are congenital structural defects in the inner muscular or elastic layer of the vessel wall; incomplete involution of embryonic vessels; and secondary factors such as arterial hypertension, atherosclerotic changes, hemodynamic disturbances, and polycystic disease. Cerebral aneurysms also may be caused by shearing forces during traumatic head injuries.

GENDER AND LIFE SPAN CONSIDERATIONS

The peak incidence of cerebral aneurysm occurs between 35 and 60 years of age. Women in their late 40s through mid-50s are affected slightly more than men. Cerebral aneurysm rarely occurs in children and adolescents.

◻ ASSESSMENT

HISTORY. Prior to rupture, cerebral aneurysms are usually asymptomatic. The patient is usually seen initially after subarachnoid hemorrhage (SAH). Ask about one or more incidences of sudden headache with vomiting in the weeks preceding major SAH. Other relevant symptoms are a stiff neck, back or leg pain, or photophobia, as well as hearing noises or throbbing (bruits) in the head. "Warning leaks" of the aneurysm in which small amounts of blood ooze from the aneurysm into the subarachnoid space can cause such symptoms. These small "warning leaks" are rarely detected because the condition is not severe enough for the patient to seek medical attention.

Identify risk factors such as familial predisposition, hypertension, cigarette smoking, or use of over-the-counter medications (e.g., nasal sprays or antihistamines) that have vasoconstrictive properties. Ask about the patient's occupation, because if the patient's job involves strenuous activity, there may be a significant delay in going back to work or the need to change occupations entirely.

PHYSICAL EXAMINATION. In most patients the neurological examination does not point to the exact site of the aneurysm, but in many instances it can provide clues to the localization. Signs and symptoms can be divided into two phases: those presenting before rupture or bleeding and those presenting after rupture or bleeding. In the phase before rupture or bleeding, observe for oculomotor nerve (cranial nerve III) palsy—dilated pupil (loss of light reflex), possible drooping eyelids (ptosis), extraocular movement deficits with possible double vision—as well as pain above and behind the eye, localized headache, or extraocular movement deficits of the trochlear (IV) or abducens (VI) cranial nerves. Small, intermittent, aneurysmal leakage of blood may result in generalized headache, neck pain, upper back pain, nausea, and vomiting. Note if the patient appears confused or drowsy.

PSYCHOSOCIAL. The patient has to cope not only with an unexpected, sudden illness but also with the fear that the aneurysm may rupture at any time. Assess the patient's ability to cope with a sudden illness and the change in roles that a sudden illness demands. In addition, assess the patient's degree of anxiety about the illness and potential complications.

DIAGNOSTIC HIGHLIGHTS

Test	Normal Result	Abnormality with Condition	Explanation
Cerebral angiogram	Symmetrical, intact pattern of cerebral vessels	Pooling of contract medium, indicating bleeding or aneurysm	Radiographic views of cerebral circulation show interruptions to circulation or changes in vessel wall appearance
Computed tomography	Intact cerebral anatomy	Identification of size and location of site of hemorrhage	Shows anterior to posterior slices of the brain to highlight abnormalities

Other Tests: lumbar puncture (for patients not at risk for increased intracranial pressure [ICP]), skull x rays, and electrocephalography (EEG)

PRIMARY NURSING DIAGNOSIS

Alteration in tissue perfusion (cerebral) related to interruption in cerebral blood flow or increased ICP

OUTCOMES. Circulation status; Cognitive ability; Neurological status; Tissue perfusion: Peripheral; Communication: Expressive ability; Communication: Receptive ability

INTERVENTIONS. Cerebral perfusion promotion; Circulatory care; Intracranial pressure monitoring; Neurologic monitoring; Peripheral sensation management; Circulatory precautions; Hypovolemia management; Vital signs monitoring; Emergency care; Medication management

☐ PLANNING AND IMPLEMENTATION
Collaborative

The first priority is to evaluate and support airway, breathing, and circulation. For patients unable to maintain these functions independently, assist with endotracheal intubation, ventilation, and oxygenation, as prescribed. Monitor neurological status carefully every hour, and immediately notify the physician of any changes in the patient's condition.

Surgery is indicated to prevent rupture or rebleeding of the cerebral artery. The decision to operate depends on the clinical status of the patient, including the level of consciousness and severity of neurological dysfunction, the accessibility of the aneurysm to surgical intervention, and the presence of vasospasm. Surgical procedures used to treat cerebral aneurysms include direct clipping or ligation of the neck of the aneurysm to enable circulation to bypass the pathology. An inoperable cerebral aneurysm may be reinforced by applying to the aneurysmal sac such materials as acrylic resins or other plastics. Postoperatively, monitor the patient closely for signs and symptoms of increasing ICP or bleeding, such as headache, unequal pupils or pupil enlargement, onset or worsening of sensory or motor deficits, or speech alterations.

PHARMACOLOGIC HIGHLIGHTS

Medication or Drug Class	Dosage	Description	Rationale
Calcium channel blockers	Varies with drugs such as nimodipine, verapamil	Inhibits calcium entry across cell membranes in vascular smooth muscles	Prevent vasospasm and hypertension
Corticosteroids	Varies with drugs such as methylprednisolone, hydrocortisone	Inhibits inflammatory processes such as edema and capillary dilation	Reduce swelling

Other Medications: Hypotensive agents may be prescribed for patients with high blood pressure. Sedatives may be prescribed to promote rest and relaxation, and aminocaproic acid, a fibrinolytic inhibitor, may be given to minimize the risk of rebleeding by delaying blood clot lysis. The patient may receive colloids such as albumin or plasmanate to decrease blood viscosity and expand the intravascular volume.

Independent

The environment should be as quiet as possible, with minimal physiological and psychological stress. Maintain the patient on bed rest. Limit visitors to immediate family and significant others. Apply thigh-high elastic stockings and intermittent external compression boots. Discourage and control any measure that initiates Valsalva's maneuver, such as coughing, straining at stool, pushing up in bed with the elbows, turning with the mouth closed. Assist with hygienic care as necessary. If the patient has a facial weakness, assist him or her during meals.

Preoperatively, provide teaching and emotional support for the patient and family. Position the patient to maintain a patent airway by elevating the head of the bed 30 to 45 degrees to promote pulmonary drainage and limit upper airway obstruction. Suction the patient's mouth and, if needed, the nasopharynx and trachea. Before suctioning, oxygenate the patient well, and to minimize ICP increases, limit suctioning to 20 to 30 seconds at a time. If the patient has facial nerve palsy, apply artificial tears to both eyes. Take appropriate measures to prevent skin breakdown from immobility. Postoperatively, promote venous drainage by elevating the head of the bed 20 to 30 degrees. Emotional support of the patient and family is also important. The patient may be dealing with a neurological deficit, such as paralysis on one side of the body or loss of speech. If the patient cannot speak, establish a simple means of communication such as using a slate to write messages or using cards. Encourage the patient to verbalize fears of dependency and of becoming a burden.

DOCUMENTATION GUIDELINES

- Neurological findings: Level of consciousness; pupillary size, shape, and reaction to light; motor function of extremities; other cranial nerve deficits (blurred vision, extraocular movement deficits, ptosis, facial weakness); aphasia; headache and facial pain; and nuchal rigidity (stiff neck, pain in the neck or back, pain with flexion of the neck, photophobia); deterioration of neurological status
- Response to pain medications and comfort measures

DISCHARGE AND HOME HEALTHCARE GUIDELINES

Prepare the patient and family for the possible need for rehabilitation after the acute care phase of hospitalization. Instruct the patient to report any deterioration in neurological status to the physician. Stress the importance of follow-up visits with the physicians. Be sure the patient understands all medications, including dosage, route, action and adverse effects, and the need for routine lab monitoring if anticonvulsants have been prescribed.

Cerebral Concussion

DRG Category: 027
Mean LOS: 3.9 days
Description: MEDICAL: Traumatic Stupor and Coma, Coma > 1 hour
DRG Category: 028
Mean LOS: 5.5 days
Description: MEDICAL: Traumatic Stupor and Coma, Coma > 1 hour, Age > 17 with CC
DRG Category: 002
Mean LOS: 9.8 days
Description: SURGICAL: Craniotomy for Trauma, Age > 17

The word "concuss" means to shake violently. Cerebral concussion is defined as a transient, temporary, neurogenic dysfunction caused by mechanical force to the brain. Cerebral concussions are the most common form of head injury. Concussions are classified as mild or classic, based on the degree of symptoms, particularly those of unconsciousness and memory loss. Mild concussion is a temporary neurologic dysfunction without loss of consciousness or memory. Classic concussion includes temporary neurologic dysfunction with unconsciousness and memory loss. Recovery from concussion usually takes minutes to hours. Most concussion patients recover fully within 48 hours, but subtle residual impairment may occur.

In rare cases, a secondary injury caused by cerebral hypoxia and ischemia can lead to cerebral edema and increased intracranial pressure (ICP). Some patients develop a post-concussion syndrome (post-injury sequelae after a mild head injury). Symptoms may be experienced for several weeks and, in unusual circumstances, may last up to 1 year. In rare situations, patients who experience multiple concussions may suffer long-term brain damage. Complications of cerebral concussion include seizures or persistent vomiting. In rare instances, a concussion may lead to intracranial hemorrhage (subdural, parenchymal, or epidural).

CAUSES

The most widely accepted theory for concussion is that acceleration-deceleration forces cause the injury. Sudden and rapid acceleration of the head from a position of rest makes the head move in several directions. The brain, protected by cerebrospinal fluid (CSF) and cushioned by various brain attachments, moves more slowly than the skull. The lag between skull movement and brain movement causes stretching of veins connecting the subdural space (the space beneath the dura mater of the brain) to the surface of the brain, resulting in minor disruptions of the brain structures. Common causes of concussion are a fall, a motor vehicle crash, a sports-related injury, and a punch to the head.

GENDER AND LIFE SPAN CONSIDERATIONS

Cerebral concussions can be experienced by patients of all ages and both genders, but males are affected at higher rates than are females. Trauma, however, is the leading cause of death between the ages of 1 and 44. In addition, trauma is the leading cause of health-related problems in this age range. For those reasons, most instances of cerebral concussion occur in the first four decades of life.

◻ ASSESSMENT

HISTORY. If the patient cannot report a history, speak to the life squad, a witness, or a significant other to obtain a history. Determine if the patient became unconscious immediately and for how long—a few seconds, minutes, or an hour—at the time of the trauma. Find out if the patient experienced momentary loss of reflexes, arrest of respirations, and possible retrograde or antegrade amnesia. Elicit a history of headache, drowsiness, confusion, dizziness, irritability, giddiness, visual disturbances (seeing stars), and gait disturbances.

Mild cerebral concussions can cause headaches, dizziness, memory loss, momentary confusion, residual memory impairment, and retrograde amnesia; there is no loss of consciousness. Classic cerebral concussions cause a loss of consciousness lasting less than 24 hours; the patient usually experiences confusion, disorientation, and amnesia upon regaining consciousness. A postconcussive syndrome that may occur weeks and even months after injury may lead to headache, fatigue, inattention, dizziness, vertigo, and memory deficits.

PHYSICAL EXAMINATION. First evaluate the patient's airway, breathing, and circulation (ABCs). After stabilizing the patient's ABCs, perform a neurologic assessment, paying special attention to early signs of ICP: decreased level of consciousness, decreased strength and motion of extremities, reduced visual acuity, headache, and pupillary changes.

Check carefully for scalp lacerations. Check the patient's nose (rhinorrhea) and ears (otorrhea) for CSF leak, which is a sign of a basilar skull fracture (a linear fracture at the base of the brain). Be sure to evaluate the patient's pupillary light reflexes. An altered reflex may result from increasing cerebral edema, which may indicate a life-threatening increase in ICP. Pupil size is normally 1.5 to 6.0 mm. Several signs to look for include ipsilateral miosis (Horner's syndrome), in which one pupil is smaller than the other with a drooping eyelid; bilateral miosis, in which both pupils are pinpoint in size; ipsilateral mydriasis (Hutchinson's pupil), in which one of the pupils is much larger than the other and is unreactive to light; bilateral midposition, in which both pupils are 4 to 5 mm and remain dilated and nonreactive to light; bilateral mydriasis, in which both pupils are larger than 6 mm and are nonreactive to light.

Check the patient's vital signs, level of consciousness, and pupil size every 15 minutes for 4 hours. If the patient's condition worsens, he or she should be admitted for hospitalization. Continue neurologic assessment throughout the patient's hospital stay to detect subtle signs of deterioration. Observe the patient to ensure that no other focal lesion, such as a subdural hematoma, has been overlooked.

PSYCHOSOCIAL. The patient with a concussion has an unexpected, sudden illness. Assess the patient's ability to cope with the potential loss of memory and temporary neurologic dysfunction. In addition, assess the patient's degree of anxiety about the illness and potential complications. Determine the significant other's response to the injury. Expect parents of children who are injured to be anxious, fearful, and sometimes guilt-ridden.

DIAGNOSTIC HIGHLIGHTS

Test	Normal Result	Abnormality with Condition	Explanation
Computed tomography	Intact cerebral anatomy	Identification of size and location of site of injury	Shows anterior to posterior slices of the brain to highlight abnormalities

Other Tests: Skull x rays, cerebral spine x rays, and glucose test, using a reagent strip, of any drainage suspected to be cerebral spinal fluid.

PRIMARY NURSING DIAGNOSIS

Altered thought process related to cerebral tissue injury and swelling

OUTCOMES. Cognitive ability; Cognitive orientation; Concentration; Decision Making; Identity; Information processing; Memory; Neurologic status: Consciousness

INTERVENTIONS. Cerebral perfusion promotion; Environmental management; Surveillance; Cerebral edema management; Family support; Medication management

□ PLANNING AND IMPLEMENTATION

Collaborative

Patients with mild head injury often are examined in the emergency department and discharged home. Generally a family member is instructed to evaluate the patient routinely and to bring the patient back to the hospital if any further neurologic symptoms appear. Parents are often told to wake a child every hour for 24 hours to make sure that the patient does not have worsening neurologic signs and symptoms. Treatment generally consists of bed rest with the head of the bed elevated at least 30 degrees, observation, and pain relief.

PHARMACOLOGIC HIGHLIGHTS

General Comment: Narcotic analgesics and sedatives are contraindicated because they may mask neurologic changes that indicate a worsening condition.

Medication or Drug Class	Dosage	Description	Rationale
Acetaminophen	325–650 mg po q 4–6 hours	Nonnarcotic analgesic that is thought to inhibit prostaglandin synthesis in the central nervous system	Manages headache

Independent

Generally patients are not admitted to the hospital for a cerebral concussion. Make sure that before the patient goes home from the emergency department, the significant others are aware of all medications and possible complications that can occur after a minor head injury. Teach the patient and significant other(s) to recognize signs and symptoms of complications, including increased drowsiness, headache, irritability, or visual disturbances that indicate the need for re-evaluation at the hospital. Teach the patient that occasional vomiting after sustaining a cerebral concussion is normal. The patient should not go home alone, because ensuing complications are apt to include decreased awareness and confusion.

If the patient is admitted to the hospital, institute seizure precautions if necessary. Ensure that the patient rests by creating a calm, peaceful atmosphere and a quiet environment. Limit visitors to the immediate family or partner, and encourage the patient to rest for 24 hours without television or loud music.

DOCUMENTATION GUIDELINES

- Trauma history, description of the event, time elapsed since the event, whether or not the patient had a loss of consciousness and, if so, for how long
- Adequacy of airway, breathing, circulation; serial vital signs
- Appearance: Bruising or lacerations, drainage from the nose or ears
- Physical findings related to site of head injury: Neurologic assessment, presence of accompanying symptoms, presence of complications (decreased level of consciousness, unequal pupils, loss of strength and movement, confusion or agitation, nausea and vomiting)
- Patient's and family's understanding of and interest in patient teaching

DISCHARGE AND HOME HEALTHCARE GUIDELINES

MEDICATIONS. Instruct the patient or caregiver not to administer any analgesics stronger than acetaminophen. Explain that aspirin may increase the risk of bleeding.

COMPLICATIONS. Explain that a responsible caregiver should continue to observe the patient at home for developing complications. Instruct the caregiver to awaken the patient every 1 to 2 hours throughout the night to assess his or her condition. Explain that the caregiver should check the patient's orientation to place and person by asking "Where are you? Who are you? Who am I?" Teach the patient and caregiver to return to the hospital if the patient experiences persistent or worsening headache, blurred vision, personality changes, abnormal eye movements, a staggering gait, twitching, or constant vomiting. Teach the patient to recognize the symptoms of postconcussion syndrome, which may last for several weeks and include headache, dizziness, vertigo, anxiety, and fatigue.

PARENT TEACHING. When the patient is a child, teach the parent(s) that it is a common pattern for children to experience lethargy and somnolence a few hours after a concussion, even if they have manifested no ill effects at the time of the trauma. Such responses do not necessarily indicate serious injury. If the symptoms persist or worsen, explain that the parent(s) should notify the healthcare provider immediately.

Cerebrovascular Accident

DRG Category: 014
Mean LOS: 6.4 days
Description: MEDICAL: Specific Cerebrovascular Disorders Except TIA
DRG Category: 027
Mean LOS: 3.9 days
Description: MEDICAL: Traumatic Stupor and Coma, Coma > 1 hour
DRG Category: 002
Mean LOS: 9.8 days
Description: SURGICAL: Craniotomy for Trauma, Age > 17

Cerebrovascular accident (CVA), or "stroke," is the interruption of normal blood flow in one or more of the blood vessels that supply the brain. The tissues become ischemic, leading to hypoxia or anoxia with destruction or necrosis of the neurons, glia, and vasculature. CVA is the third leading cause of death in the United States and affects more than 500,000 Americans annually.

A CVA is an acute neurologic injury that occurs because of changes in the blood vessels of the brain. The changes can be intrinsic to the vessel (atherosclerosis, inflammation, arterial dissection, dilation of the vessel, weakening of the vessel, obstruction of the vessel) or extrinsic, such as when an embolism travels from the heart. Although reduced blood flow interferes with brain function, the brain can remain viable with decreased blood flow for long periods of time. However, total cessation of blood flow produces irreversible brain infarction within 3 minutes. Once the blood flow stops, toxins released by damaged neurons, cerebral edema, and alterations in local blood flow contribute to neuron dysfunction and death. Complications of CVA include unstable blood pressure, sensory and motor impairment, infection (encephalitis), pneumonia, contractures, and pulmonary emboli.

CAUSES

Thrombosis, embolism, and hemorrhage are the primary causes of CVA. In cerebral thrombosis, the most common cause of CVA, a blood clot obstructs a cerebral vessel. The most common vessels involved are the carotid arteries of the neck and the arteries in the vertebrobasilar system at the base of the brain near the circle of Willis. Cerebral thrombosis also contributes to transient ischemic attacks (TIAs), which are temporary episodes (10 to 30 minutes) of poor cerebral perfusion caused by partial occlusion of the arterial lumen. A thrombotic CVA that causes a slow evolution of symptoms over several hours is called a "stroke in evolution." When the condition stabilizes, it is called a "completed stroke."

In an embolic CVA, a clot is carried into the cerebral circulation, usually by the carotid arteries. Blockage of an intracerebral artery results in a localized cerebral infarction.

Hemorrhagic CVA results from hypertension, rupture of an aneurysm, arteriovenous malformations, or bleeding disorder. Risk factors thought to cause blood vessel changes that cause vessel walls to be more susceptible to rupture and hemorrhage include elevated low-density lipoprotein (LDL) and lowered high-density lipoprotein (HDL) levels, cigarette smoking, and a sedentary lifestyle.

GENDER AND LIFE SPAN CONSIDERATIONS

Five percent of the population in North America over the age of 65 are affected by stroke. CVA affects men slightly more often than women and is more common after the age of 50, although drug use is causing an increase in CVAs in younger people. African-Americans have a high rate of CVA because of their higher incidence of hypertension.

☐ ASSESSMENT

HISTORY. Determine if the patient is on any medications or abuses intravenous drugs. Elicit a history of neurologic deficits. (See Table 21.) Determine if the patient has experienced an inability to recognize familiar objects or persons through sensory stimuli (agnosia) or any memory loss (amnesia). Elicit a history of speech difficulties such as an inability to understand language or express language (aphasia), poorly articulated speech (dysarthria), or any other form of speech impairment (dysphasia). Determine if the patient has lost the ability to comprehend written words (alexia), read written words (dyslexia), or write (agraphia). Establish a history of visual difficulties such as double vision (diplopia), defective vision, or blindness in the right or left halves of the visual fields of both eyes (homonymous hemianopia), lack of depth perception, color blindness, blindness, blurring on the affected side, or drooping eyelids (ptosis).

TABLE 21 | **CVA Sites and Neurologic Deficits**

CVA SITE	SIGNS AND SYMPTOMS
Posterior cerebral artery	Visual field deficits, sensory impairments; reading difficulty (dyslexia); coma; cortical blindness resulting from ischemia in the occipital area; paralysis (rarely)
Vertebral or basilar artery	Numbness around the lips and mouth; dizziness; weakness on the affected side; vision deficits (color blindness; lack of depth perception; double vision [diplopia]); poor coordination; difficulty swallowing (dysphagia); slurred speech; amnesia; staggering gait (ataxia)
Internal carotid artery	Headache; weakness; paralysis; numbness; sensory changes; vision disturbances (blurring on the affected side or blindness); altered level of consciousness; bruits over the carotid artery; defective language function (aphasia); speech impairment (dysphasia); eyelid drooping (ptosis)
Middle cerebral artery	Defective language function (aphasia); speech impairment (dysphasia); reading difficulty (dyslexia); visual field deficits; hemiparesis on the affected side (more severe in the face and arm than in the leg)

Elicit a history of motor difficulties such as the inability to move the muscles (akinesia), inability to perform purposeful acts or manipulate objects (apraxia), poor coordination, impairment of voluntary movement (dyskinesia), muscular weakness or partial paralysis affecting one side of the body (hemiparesis), or paralysis of one side of the body (hemiplegia). Ask if the patient has experienced numbness and ascertain the specific location. Determine if the patient has experienced headaches. Establish a history of personality changes such as flat affect or distractibility.

PHYSICAL EXAMINATION. If the patient appears unconscious, quickly determine his or her airway status and level of consciousness. If the patient is conscious, he or she may be experiencing a TIA or a stroke in evolution. Determine the level of orientation; ability to respond to questions of intellectual functioning; and speech, hearing, and vision ability. Lightly touch the patient's skin on various parts of the body and ask the patient to identify the location. Apply firm pressure to various parts of the body and observe the patient's responses. Be sure to test skin sensations sensed in both hemispheres of the body and compare the responses.

Begin your assessment by determining the patient's understanding of your commands and the appropriateness of his or her verbal and nonverbal responses. In left-hemisphere CVA, there is likely to be loss of language ability, although memory may be intact. In right-hemisphere CVA, patients are often confused and disoriented, but the ability to speak remains. Determine the presence of hemiplegia or hemiparesis and the patient's muscle strength, gait, and balance. Assess the patient's cranial nerves (V, VII, IX, X, and XII) to determine the patient's tongue movement and ability to chew and swallow, as well as the presence of a gag reflex. Assess the patient for the presence of hemianopia by observing whether he or she sees objects on either side of the midvisual field. If the patient is disoriented or has lost the ability to understand language (receptive aphasia), assessing hemianopia is difficult. Try handing the patient a fork on the affected side, and ask the patient to tell you what it is you are holding or ask the patient to pick up the fork.

PSYCHOSOCIAL. During the early stages of their condition, many patients with CVA experience great despair and frustration trying to communicate their needs. The inability to communicate causes profound depression. Although patients may laugh or cry or display outbursts of anger and frustration at unusual times, it is impossible to know with any certainty if these responses are inappropriate for the patient.

DIAGNOSTIC HIGHLIGHTS

Test	Normal Result	Abnormality with Condition	Explanation
Computed tomography (CT)	Intact cerebral anatomy	Identification of size and location of site of hemorrhage or infarction	Shows anterior to posterior slices of the brain to highlight abnormalities

Other Tests: Magnetic resonance imaging (MRI) is more sensitive than CT if the stroke is small and/or in the brain stem. Continuous oximetry and electrocardiographic monitoring provides surveillance. Laboratory tests include complete blood count with differential, platelet count, PT, APTT, electrolytes, creatinine, glucose. Other diagnostic tests that help evaluate cerebral blood flow, identify abnormalities, or locate the CVA include positron emission tomography, cerebral blood flow studies, transcranial and carotid Doppler studies, transthoracic two-dimensional echocardiography to identify intracardiac sites for thrombi.

PRIMARY NURSING DIAGNOSIS

Sensory-perceptual alterations: Visual, auditory, kinesthetic, and tactile, as related to tissue injury

OUTCOMES. Cognitive orientation; Cognitive ability; Energy conservation; Neurologic status; Rest; Sleep; Body image; Anxiety control; Endurance

INTERVENTIONS. Cognitive stimulation; Feeding; Fluid monitoring; Neurologic monitoring; Environmental management; Exercise promotion; Exercise therapy; Surveillance: Safety; Reality orientation; Body mechanics promotion

◻ PLANNING AND IMPLEMENTATION

Collaborative

MEDICAL. Medical management for patients with CVAs typically includes support of vital functions and ongoing surveillance to identify early neurologic changes as the patient's condition evolves. Although the hallmark of stroke is the abrupt onset of neurologic symptoms and deficits due to the interruption of the vascular supply to a specific brain region, therapeutic intervention may save tissue that is at risk for infarction. Recombinant tissue-plasminogen activator (rt-PA) can improve outcome for some patients with acute nonhemorrhagic ischemic stroke if it is given within 3 hours of the onset of symptoms.

SURGICAL. When a CVA has occurred, the treatment consists of maintaining life, reducing intracranial pressure (ICP), limiting the extension of the CVA, and preventing complications. For patients who cannot maintain airway, breathing, and circulation independently, assist with endotracheal intubation, ventilation, and oxygenation as prescribed. In hemorrhagic CVA, surgery may be required to evacuate a hematoma or to stop bleeding. A ventricular shunt may be placed to drain cerebrospinal fluid.

Physical therapy is begun as soon as the patient's condition stabilizes. Flaccid muscles soon become spastic and subject to contractures. Use passive range-of-motion exercises on the affected side. Strengthening the unaffected side assists the patient in compensating for the losses of the opposite hemisphere. The physical therapist teaches the patient to transfer with the use of assistive devices, and the physical or occupational therapist teaches the patient how to perform self-care activity.

PHARMACOLOGIC HIGHLIGHTS

Medication or Drug Class	Dosage	Description	Rationale
Recombinant tissue-plasminogen activator (rt-PA) (alteplase, recombinant)	0.9 mg/kg up to a maximum of 90 mg with the first 10% given IV over 1 minute and the remainder given by infusion pump over 1 hour	Thrombolytic; activates the fibrinolytic system by directly cleaving the bond in plasminogen-producing plasmin; increases perfusion to ischemic areas.	Increases perfusion to at-risk tissue. Note that aspirin, heparin, and warfarin are not given during the first 24 hours

Pharmacologic Comments: Contraindications to rt-PA: duration of stroke for more than 3 hours, recent surgery, head injury or GI/urinary hemorrhage, seizure at stroke onset, bleeding disorder, hypertension. Some patients receive anticonvulsant agents to reduce the risk of seizures, stool softeners to decrease straining, corticosteroids to decrease cerebral edema, and analgesics to reduce headache. Cerebral edema may be reduced through dehydrating measures and the use of steroids and osmotics. For thromboembolic CVAs, pharmacologic agents such as anticoagulants are used to limit the extension of the CVA.

Independent

Position the patient to maintain a patent airway by elevating the head of the bed 30 degrees to promote pulmonary drainage and limit upper airway obstruction. Suction the patient's mouth and, if needed, the nasopharynx and trachea. Before suctioning, oxygenate the patient well; to minimize ICP increases, limit suctioning to 20 to 30 seconds at a time.

The patient with a CVA is at extremely high risk for complications caused by immobility. If appropriate, use compression boots to promote venous return and help prevent phlebitis. To reduce the risk of pulmonary infection, promote skin integrity, and prevent contractures, turn and reposition the patient every 2 hours. Keep the patient's joints in a functional position, and keep the affected hand elevated slightly on a pillow. Use a trochanter roll to prevent external rotation of the hip. Keep the patient safe by putting the bed in a low position and keeping the side rails up.

Prevent aspiration pneumonia by first determining the patient's ability to handle solids and liquids. Keep a suction machine nearby while feeding the patient. Some patients have difficulty with liquids, so thicken fluids with soft foods like cooked cereal, applesauce, soup, or mashed potatoes.

Make sure the patient has a bowel movement each morning after breakfast to stimulate normal peristalsis and prevent constipation. A catheter may be in place immediately after the CVA, but the goal is to have the patient gain control through a bladder training program. If the patient has expressive aphasia (inability to transform sounds into speech), give the patient ample time to respond to questions and be supportive if the patient becomes frustrated during speech. Be sure to accept any method of self-expression the patient uses, such as pointing, gesturing, or writing. Some patients find it easier to point to a picture that describes a word rather than trying to say the word.

Remember that the patient's family undergoes a struggle to deal with the patient's illness and needs support. If the patient or family seems to be coping poorly, arrange for a referral to a clinical nurse specialist, chaplain, or social worker. A magazine, *The Stroke Connection,* can be subscribed to by writing AHA Stroke Connection, 7272 Greenville Avenue, Dallas, TX 75231-44596.

DOCUMENTATION GUIDELINES

- Physical findings: Neurologic deficits, level of orientation, Glasgow Coma Scale, pupil responses, gait, range of motion, gag reflex, visual deficits
- Ability to communicate verbally and nonverbally
- Ability to perform self-care; bowel and bladder control
- Presence of complications, infections, contractures, skin breakdown
- Emotional response: Ability to cope, presence of depression, ability to socialize with others, anxiety and frustration over speech difficulties

DISCHARGE AND HOME HEALTHCARE GUIDELINES

Teach the family to check for skin breakdown and the development of contractures and to take appropriate preventative measures. Be sure the family performs frequent range-of-motion activities, as taught in the rehabilitation unit. Advise the family whom to call in an emergency. Be sure that the patient and family understand the importance of maintaining the mobility and self-care routine developed in the rehabilitation unit. Be sure that the social worker or rehabilitation personnel has provided the family with a list of resources for in-home care. Determine whether a home care agency will be providing in-home supervision and ongoing physical therapy support. Advise the family how to seek ongoing support for home maintenance.

Cervical Cancer

DRG Category: 366
Mean LOS: 5.9 days
Description: MEDICAL: Malignancy, Female Reproductive System with CC
DRG Category: 354
Mean LOS: 5.9 days
Description: SURGICAL: Uterine, Adnexa Procedure for Non-Ovarian/Adnexal Malignancy with CC

Cancer of the cervix is one type of primary uterine cancer (the other being uterine-endometrial cancer) and is predominately epidermoid. Invasive cervical cancer is the third most common female pelvic cancer.

Cervical cancer is of three types: dysplasia, carcinoma in situ (CIS), and invasive carcinoma. In dysplasia, the lower third of the epithelium contains abnormal cells with the earliest form of premalignant changes. These changes are considered preinvasive, and the atypical cells have some degree of surface maturation. CIS is carcinoma confined to the epithelium. The full thickness of the epithelium contains abnormally proliferating cells. Both dysplasia and CIS are considered preinvasive cancers and, with early detection, have a cure rate of 75% to 90%.

Invasive carcinoma occurs when cancer cells penetrate the basement membrane. Metastasis occurs through local invasion and by way of the lymphatic ducts. As many as 10 years can elapse between the preinvasive and invasive stages. A further 5 years can be added if one considers the precancerous changes that occur in atypical cells and dysplasia as the first step of malignancy.

CAUSES

Worldwide studies suggest that sexually transmitted human papillomaviruses (HPVs), type 16 or 18, are the primary cause of cervical cancer. Major risk factors associated with cancer of the cervix include early sexual activity, multiple sexual partners, or early first pregnancy; postnatal lacerations; multiparity; sexual partners with a history of penile or prostatic cancer; exposure to diethylstilbestrol (DES) in utero; and a history of cervicitis or sexually transmitted diseases.

GENDER AND LIFE SPAN CONSIDERATIONS

Although cervical cancer can occur from the late teens to old age, it occurs most commonly in women 35 to 55 years of age. Preinvasive cancer of the cervix is most commonly seen in the 25- to 40-year-old woman, whereas invasive cancer of the cervix is more common in the 40- to 60-year old. African-American women and women from lower socioeconomic groups are the highest risk groups for cervical cancer.

☐ ASSESSMENT

HISTORY. Because early cervical cancer is usually asymptomatic, establish a thorough history with particular attention to the presence of the risk factors and the woman's menstrual history. Establish a history of later symptoms of cervical cancer, including abnormal bleeding or spotting (between periods or after menopause); metrorrhagia (bleeding between normal menstrual periods) or increased frequency of menstrual bleeding; postcoital bleeding; leukorrhea in increasing amounts and changing over time from watery to dark and foul; and a history of chronic cervical infections. Determine if the patient has experienced weight gain or loss; abdominal or pelvic pain, often unilateral, radiating to the buttocks and legs; or other symptoms associated with neoplasms, such as fatigue.

PHYSICAL EXAMINATION. Conduct a pelvic examination. Observe the patient's external genitalia for signs of inflammation, bleeding, discharge, or local skin or epithelial changes. Observe the internal genitalia. The normal cervix is pink and nontender, has no lesions, and has a closed os. Cervical tissue with cervical cancer appears as a large reddish growth or deep ulcerating crater before any symptoms are experienced; lesions are firm and friable. The Pap smear is done before the bimanual examination. Palpate for motion tenderness of the cervix (Chandelier's sign); a positive Chandelier's sign (pain on movement) usually indicates an infection. Also examine the size, consistency (hardness may reflect invasion by neoplasm), shape, mobility (cervix should be freely movable), tenderness, and presence of masses of the uterus and adnexa. Conduct a rectal exam; palpate for abnormalities of contour, motility, and the placement of adjacent structures. Nodular thickenings of the uterosacral and cardinal ligaments may be felt.

PSYCHOSOCIAL. Uneasiness, embarrassment about a pelvic examination, or fear of the unknown may be issues for the patient. Determine the patient's level of knowledge about a pelvic exam and what she expects. Determine her recommended Pap test screening schedule, as well as how she obtains the results and their meaning.

If the patient requires follow-up to a positive Pap smear, assess her anxiety and coping mechanisms. Stressors may be fear of the unknown, of sexual dysfunction, of cancer, or of death, or she may have self-concept disturbances.

DIAGNOSTIC HIGHLIGHTS

Test	Normal Result	Abnormality with Condition	Explanation
Papanicolaou examination (Pap smear)	No abnormality or atypical cells noted	High class/grade cytologic results	Initial screening; indicates a need for further testing

Colposcopy followed by punch biopsy or cone biopsy	Benign results	Malignant cells	Vaginal vault and cul-de-sac are visualized; malignant diagnosis can be confirmed

Other Tests: chest x ray, cystoscopy, proctosigmoidoscopy, intravenous pyelogram, barium studies of lower bowel, ultrasound, computed tomography, magnetic resonance imaging, and lymphangiography

PRIMARY NURSING DIAGNOSIS

Pain (acute) related to postprocedure swelling and nerve damage

OUTCOMES. Pain control; Pain: Disruptive effects; Well-being

INTERVENTIONS. Analgesic administration; Pain management; Meditation; Transcutaneous electric nerve stimulation (TENS); Hypnosis; Heat/cold application

☐ PLANNING AND IMPLEMENTATION

Collaborative

Treatment depends on the stage of the cancer, the woman's age, and concern for future childbearing. Preinvasive lesions (CIS) can be treated by conization, cryosurgery, laser surgery, or simple hysterectomy (if the patient's reproductive capacity is not an issue). All conservative treatments require frequent follow-up by Pap tests and colposcopy because a greater level of risk is always present for the woman who has had CIS. A cone-shaped piece of tissue is removed from the cervix after epithelial involvement is clearly outlined as described with the cone biopsy. The cone includes all the abnormal and some normal tissue. Following this procedure, the woman can still have children. The major complication is postoperative bleeding.

CRYOSURGERY. Cryosurgery is performed 1 week after the patient's last menstrual period (thereby avoiding treatment in early pregnancy). The surgeon uses a probe to freeze abnormal tissue and a small amount of normal tissue. For laser surgery, a carbon dioxide laser is used. Healing takes place in 3 to 6 weeks, and recurrence rates are lower than with cryosurgery.

HYSTERECTOMY. A hysterectomy, removal of the cervix and uterus, is the definitive therapy for CIS. The risks of general anesthesia and abdominal surgery are present. Major risks are infection and hemorrhage.

INVASIVE CANCER. Invasive cancer (stages I to IV) can be treated with surgery, radiotherapy, or a combination of both. (See Table 22.) Pelvic exenteration can be done for recurrence and/or for advanced stage III or IV. Total exenteration entails the removal of the pelvic viscera, including the bladder, rectosigmoid, and all the reproductive organs. Irradiation of metastatic areas is done to provide local control and decrease symptoms.

TABLE 22 | **Treatment Alternatives for Invasive Cervical Cancer**

STAGE	TREATMENT ALTERNATIVE
I	May be managed conservatively (conization), with simple hysterectomy and close follow-up, or may be treated as stage II.
II	Surgery (total abdominal hysterectomy {TAH] or radical hysterectomy with bilateral pelvic lymphadenopathy) and radiotherapy are treatments of choice. Positive pelvic nodes usually receive full pelvic radiation postoperatively
III	Radiation alone
IV	Radiation alone or systemic or regional chemotherapy

RADIATION THERAPY. Radiation therapy may be internal (radium applications to the cervix), external, and interstitial (by the use of cesium). Radiation cystitis, procitis, and fistula formation (vesicovaginal) are major complications. Radiation sickness (nausea, vomiting, diarrhea, malaise, fever) may be a result of a systemic reaction to the breakdown and reabsorption of cell proteins. Internal radiation results in some cramping because of dilation of the cervix and in a foul-smelling vaginal discharge because of cell destruction. The patient who receives intracavity radiation is placed on bed rest and is only able to roll from side to side so as not to dislodge the implant. Vaginal packing, a urinary catheter, and pretreatment enemas plus a low-residue diet are designed to keep healthy tissue from the implant.

PHARMACOLOGIC HIGHLIGHTS

Medication or Drug Class	Dosage	Description	Rationale
Cisplatin	Depends on the patient condition, progress of the disease, and if other chemotherapeutic agents are given	Antineoplastic	Used to treat or stabilize the disease; 38% response rate documented; can also be used in combination with other chemotherapeutic agents
Acetaminophen; NSAIDs; opiods; combinations of opiod/NSAIDs	Depends on the drug and the patient's condition and tolerance	Analgesics	Analgesic chosen is determined by the severity of the patient's pain

Independent

Teaching about and providing access to regular Pap screening tests for high-risk and other women are the most important preventative interventions. The importance of regular pap smears cannot be understated because cervical CIS is 100% curable. Embarrassment, modesty, and cultural values may make seeking a gynecologic examination most difficult for some women. Provide clear explanations and respect the patient's modesty.

When a patient requires surgery, prepare her mentally and physically for the surgery and the postoperative period. Be certain to teach the patient about vaginal discharges that may follow a surgical procedure. Teach the patient that she will probably have to refrain from douching, using tampons, and coitus until healing occurs. Discuss any changes that may affect the patient's sexual function or elimination mechanisms. Explain to the patient that she will feel fatigued and that she should gradually increase activity, but should not do heavy lifting or strenuous or rough activity or sit for long periods. Encourage the patient to explore her feelings and concerns about the experience and its implications for her life and lifestyle. Provide the patient who has undergone a hysterectomy with information about what to expect.

If internal radiation is the treatment, the primary focus of the nursing interventions is to prepare the patient for the treatment, to promote her comfort, and to lessen her sense of isolation during the treatment. Explain to the patient and significant others the reason for the time-restricted visits while the insert is in place. Nursing care is of shorter duration and of essential nature only during this time; therefore, ensure that before the insertion of the implant, the patient has a bath and clean bed linen. Decrease the patient's feelings of isolation by providing diversionary activities and frequent interaction from a safe distance. If the patient has external radiation, teach her about how the treatment is given, how the skin is prepared, and how blood tests to monitor white blood cell count are done. Explain that her immunity to common colds and other illnesses is lessened, and teach the patient the proper use of antiemetics and antidiarrhetics.

DOCUMENTATION GUIDELINES

- Physical findings: Pain and discomfort; type, color, and amount of vaginal discharge; appearance of wounds or ulcers; urinary elimination; bowel movement
- Emotional response: Coping, fears, body image, response to examination, strategies to support modesty; partner's response to illness
- Response to treatment: Conization, cryosurgery, laser surgery, hysterectomy; presence of complications

DISCHARGE AND HOME HEALTHCARE GUIDELINES

MEDICATIONS. Be sure the patient and family understand any pain medication prescribed, including dosage, route, action, and side effects.

FOLLOW-UP. Make sure the patient knows all the postprocedure complications. Provide a phone number to call if any complications occur. Ensure that the patient understands the need for ongoing Pap smears if appropriate. Vaginal cytologic studies are recommended at 4-month intervals for 2 years, every 6 months for 3 years, and then annually.

Cervical Incompetence

DRG Category: 384
Mean LOS: 1.9 days
Description: MEDICAL AND SURGICAL: Other Antepartum Diagnoses without Medical Complications

Cervical incompetence is a condition in which the cervix spontaneously dilates during the second trimester, or early in the third trimester, of pregnancy, which results in expulsion of the uterine contents. Since this typically occurs in the fourth or fifth month of gestation before the point of fetal viability, the fetus dies unless dilation can be arrested. Incidence of an incompetent cervix has been estimated to be between 0.1% and 1.0% of all pregnancies. The incompetent cervix has abnormal musculature, with an increased proportion of smooth muscle tissue, and this results in a loss of sphincter tone. When the pressure of the expanding uterine contents becomes greater than the ability of the cervical sphincter to remain closed, the cervix suddenly relaxes, allowing effacement and dilation to proceed.

The cervical dilation that occurs with cervical incompetence is typically rapid, relatively painless, and accompanied by minimal bleeding. These features help distinguish the syndrome clinically from other causes of cervical dilation or bleeding, such as preterm labor, placental abruption, and placenta previa.

CAUSES

Congenital structural defects of the lower genital tract can cause cervical incompetence, depending on the nature and location of the defect. Such defects are more frequent in women who were exposed to diethylstilbestrol (DES) in utero. Another important cause of incompetent cervix is previous cervical trauma such as excessive mechanical dilation during previous obstetric procedures, removal of tissue during previous cervical biopsy, and improperly healed lacerations from previous deliveries. Hormonal factors can also contribute to cervical incompetence, particularly excessive levels of relaxin, which may cause loss of normal cervical resistance to dilation. Relaxin levels may be higher than usual during some multiple gestations, increasing the risk of cervical incompetence in these pregnancies.

GENDER AND LIFE SPAN CONSIDERATIONS

Any woman of childbearing age may experience cervical incompetence, although older childbearing women may be at greater risk because they are more likely to have experienced previous trauma to the cervix.

□ ASSESSMENT

HISTORY. Obtain a detailed obstetric and medical history. Ask about the date of the last menstrual period to determine the gestational age of the fetus. Inquire about risk factors that are related to cervical incompetence. Women experiencing cervical dilation because of cervical incompetence may have symptoms that range from feelings of low pelvic pressure or cramping to vaginal bleeding, loss of amniotic fluid, and spontaneous passage of the fetus and placenta. Patients who experience cervical incompetence frequently report a history of previous second-trimester pregnancy loss, induced abortion, dilation and curettage, cervical biopsy, or prenatal exposure to DES. A history of fertility problems may also be reported.

PHYSICAL EXAMINATION. Inspect the perineum for bleeding and fluid. Patients frequently have pink or dark red spotting, increased vaginal discharge, passage of the mucous plug, or leakage of amniotic fluid. Perform a sterile vaginal examination. The cervix is effaced and dilated, with progression in the absence of painful uterine contractions. A bulging amniotic sac or the fetal presenting part may be palpated through the cervix during the vaginal examination.

PSYCHOSOCIAL. The patient who experiences pregnancy loss because of an incompetent cervix is in a state of psychological crisis. If this is a first episode, the patient is likely to be bewildered because of the rapid progress of dilation and the unexpectedness of the loss. In patients who have experienced infertility or previous fetal loss, psychosocial reactions may be complicated by unresolved feelings or cumulative effects of grief experiences. Anger, fear, numbness, guilt, severe grief, and feelings of loss of control are common in both the pregnant woman and her significant others.

DIAGNOSTIC HIGHLIGHTS

General Comments: Diagnosis is clinically based on a history of habitual second trimester abortions, painless cervical dilation, and spontaneously ruptured membranes.

Test	Normal Result	Abnormality with condition	Explanation
Ultrasound (transvaginal)	Long, non-effaced, closed, internal cervical os	Cervix shortening; dilation of the internal os noted	Cervix will usually shorten or efface before dilation; the internal os dilates before the external os; thus serial imaging can alert one to cervical incompetence and potential loss

PRIMARY NURSING DIAGNOSIS

Anticipatory grieving related to an unexpected pregnancy outcome

OUTCOMES. Grief resolution

INTERVENTIONS. Grief work facilitation; Active listening; Presence; Truth telling; Support group

☐ PLANNING AND IMPLEMENTATION

Collaborative

Medical management depends on the degree of cervical dilation that has occurred at the time the patient is examined. If dilation is progressing rapidly or is complete, preparation is made for delivery of the fetus and placenta. As with any spontaneous abortion, careful evaluation of bleeding is required to detect hemorrhage. Dilation and curettage may be necessary to control bleeding if placental fragments are retained in the uterus.

In less advanced dilation, particularly if the membranes are not ruptured, the patient may be maintained on bed rest in Trendelenburg's position in an attempt to prolong the pregnancy. If cervical dilation is no greater than 3 cm, the membranes are intact, and bleeding and cramping are not present, a cerclage may be used. In this surgical procedure a purse-string suture is placed in the cervix at the level of the internal os to prevent dilation by mechanically closing the os. Either the Shirodkar or McDonald techniques can be used to create the cerclage. In any future pregnancies of women with a history of cervical incompetence, a cerclage may be placed prophylactically at 14 to 18 weeks' gestation. Local anesthesia is usually used during cerclage placement, although regional or light general anesthesia may occasionally be chosen. After a cerclage has been placed, assessment for signs of labor, rupture of membranes, maternal infection, and fetal well-being continues for the remainder of the pregnancy. The cerclage is removed at or near term, with vaginal delivery typically following shortly thereafter. Bleeding, uterine contractions, and ruptured membranes are all contraindications to placement of a cerclage.

Pharmacologic management of cervical incompetence is not indicated, until after the loss of the fetus and placenta have occurred.

PHARMACOLOGIC HIGHLIGHTS

Medication or Drug Class	Dosage	Description	Rationale
Oxytocin (Pitocin)	10–20 U IV after passage of tissue	Oxytocic	Stimulates uterine contractions to decrease postpartum bleeding
RhD immunoglobin (RhoGAM)	120 μg (prepared by blood bank)	Immune serum	Prevents Rh isoimmunizations in future pregnancies; given if mother is Rh negative and infant is Rh positive

Independent

Nursing care for patients with cervical incompetence centers on teaching, psychological support, and prevention of injury to the mother and fetus. Teach the woman about her condition and alert her to the potential for injury of the cervix if labor proceeds with a cerclage in place. Symptoms of labor, rupture of the membranes, and infection should be explained to the woman, with emphasis on the need to report such symptoms promptly if they occur. Consider the patient's support systems and coping mechanisms if the pregnancy is continuing. Determine if the patient has the social and financial resources to manage a difficult pregnancy, and make appropriate referrals if they are needed.

DOCUMENTATION GUIDELINES

- Continuation of pregnancy: Cervical dilation and effacement; station of fetal presenting part; intactness of membranes; absence of bleeding, contractions,

or foul discharge; maternal temperature; fetal heart tones and presence of fetal movement, if perceptible
- After spontaneous abortion: Pain; color, odor, and amount of bleeding; firmness and position of fundus; bladder function; vital signs
- Indicators of psychologic status: Affect, verbalizations of feelings, grieving behaviors, presence of support people, acceptance of anticipatory guidance and resource materials, effectiveness of coping strategies

DISCHARGE AND HOME HEALTHCARE GUIDELINES

FOLLOWING CERCLAGE PLACEMENT. Be sure that the patient understands the importance of immediately reporting any signs of labor or infection. If vaginal rest has been prescribed, teach the patient to avoid vaginal intercourse, orgasm, douching, or tampon use. If bed rest has been prescribed, assist the patient and family to develop strategies for maintaining bed rest at home. Ensure that the patient understands and can carry out plans for follow-up surveillance and care. Alert the patient of the signs and symptoms of preterm labor.

FOLLOWING DELIVERY OF VIABLE INFANT. Be sure that the woman understands the likelihood of repeated cervical incompetence and the possibility of prophylactic cerclage placement in future pregnancies.

FOLLOWING PREGNANCY LOSS. Teach the patient to report signs of infection or hemorrhage. Be sure that the patient understands the need for pelvic rest until the follow-up gynecologic appointment. Provide the patient and family with resources to support grieving, including anticipatory guidance, reading lists or materials, contact information for support groups, and referral to counseling, if desired.

Chlamydial Infections

DRG Category: 412
Mean LOS: 3.1 days
Description: MEDICAL: Viral Illness, Age > 17

Infection with *Chlamydia trachomatis* is the most common sexually transmitted infection (STI) in the United States today, with approximately 4 million cases reported annually. This statistic may actually be low because a comprehensive surveillance system to report chlamydial infections currently does not exist in this country. Because individuals with chlamydial infections are often asymptomatic, they transmit the disease but are unaware that they harbor the bacteria. Untreated infections in women can result in cervicitis, endometritis, acute salpingitis, bartholinitis, irregular menses, ectopic pregnancy, and pelvic inflammatory disease. Untreated infections in men can result in nongonococcal urethritis (NGU), epididymitis, or prostatitis. Infections in either gender can result in proctitis, lymphogranuloma venereum (LGV), and, potentially, infertility and sterility.

During pregnancy, *C. trachomatis* may be transmitted from mother to fetus, which may cause premature rupture of the membranes, premature labor, and increased fetal morbidity and mortality. Pregnant women who deliver vaginally or by cesarean section can transmit the bacteria to their infants. These newborns can develop otitis media, conjunctivitis, blindness, meningitis, gastroenteritis, respiratory infections, and pneumonia. Because mothers are often asymptomatic, medical personnel are unaware that the maternal–infant transmission has occurred until infants become very ill.

CAUSES

C. trachomatis is a gram-negative intracellular bacterium with several different immunotypes. It is transmitted through sexual intercourse and from mother to fetus during birth. The pathogen invades and reproduces inside of the cells that line the cervix, endometrium, fallopian tubes, and urethra. Symptoms can occur after a 1- to 2-week incubation period; however, overt symptoms often occur late in the disease.

GENDER AND LIFE SPAN CONSIDERATIONS

Although the occurrence of chlamydial infection is related more to sexual practices than to age, many women with chlamydial infection are young, under 24 years of age, and single. Indigent women with no prenatal care are a high-risk group. With more teens engaging in sexual activity, more adolescents of both genders are contracting infections. Depending on the population, 5% to 35% of pregnant women are infected with C. trachomatis.

❏ ASSESSMENT

HISTORY. Although sexual activity is potentially a sensitive topic, it is critical to obtain a detailed sexual and gynecologic history. Inquire about the number of partners, use of barrier protection and birth control measures, participation in oral or anal intercourse, and previous STIs. Most patients who present with C. trachomatis have a history of multiple sex partners and engaging in sexual intercourse without the use of barrier protection. Often patients are also positive for gonorrhea. Inquire if the patient has any thin or purulent discharge, burning or frequent urination, mucus-covered stools, lower abdominal pain, dyspareunia (painful sexual intercourse), headache, nausea, vomiting, chills, or bleeding after intercourse. Often patients are asymptomatic, and some may complain only of an increase in vaginal discharge. Male patients may report dysuria, urinary frequency, and pruritus. Ask the patient if he or she is experiencing any diarrhea, tenesmus, or pruritus, any of which indicates that the infection involves the rectum.

PHYSICAL EXAMINATION. For females, inspect the vagina, cervix, and labia and note any discharge. Gently touch the cervix; note any bleeding (friable cervix). Inspect males for purulent discharge at the urinary meatus. Scrotal swelling occurs if the organism has caused epididymitis. Inspect the anus for discharge and excoriation. If LGV is present, ulcerative lesions on the cervix, vagina, labia, anal/rectal area, or penis may occur. Enlarged lymph nodes also can be palpated in the groin. If these nodes rupture, they secrete a thick yellow granular substance.

PSYCHOSOCIAL. Assess the patient's knowledge of STIs and the implications. Assess the patient's ability to cope with having an STI. The diagnosis of an STI can be very upsetting to a male or female who believes he or she was involved in a monogamous relationship. Patients may feel embarrassed and guilty about their condition. Inquire about the patient's ability to obtain condoms. Identify all partners with whom the patient has been sexually active so that they can be examined and treated. Assess the patient's support system; this is especially important if the patient is pregnant.

DIAGNOSTIC HIGHLIGHTS

General Comments: Enzyme-linked immunosorbent assay (ELISA) and antigen detection by direct fluorescent antibody slide staining are less expensive tests to diagnose chlamydia; however, a tissue culture remains the gold standard. Testing, which is costly and sometimes inaccurate, is only recommended for those patients who are symptomatic or who are at risk for contracting a chlamydial infection. Because of fetal implications, most pregnant women are screened for chlamydia.

Test	Normal Result	Abnormality with Condition	Explanation
Cervical tissue culture (females); urethral tissue culture (males)	Negative culture	Positive culture	Growth of the organism confirms the diagnosis

Other Tests: Since symptoms of gonorrhea resemble a chlamydial infection, diagnosis is often made on the basis of a symptomatic patient with a negative gonorrhea culture.

PRIMARY NURSING DIAGNOSIS

Infection related to bacterial invasion

OUTCOMES. Risk control: Sexually transmitted diseases

INTERVENTIONS. Teaching: Safe sex; Medication management; Fertility preservation

□ PLANNING AND IMPLEMENTATION

Collaborative

Chlamydial infections can easily be cured with oral antibiotics, and patients are rarely hospitalized. Patients need to know to continue to take medication as ordered, even if the symptoms subside. Follow-up with both partners is recommended to assure that neither partner is still infected. Patients should abstain from sexual intercourse until they are infection-free.

PHARMACOLOGIC HIGHLIGHTS

Medication or Drug Class	Dosage	Description	Rationale
Doxycycline	100 mg po bid × 7 days	Broad spectrum antibiotic (tetracycline)	Effective in eliminating *C. trachomatis*

Tetracycline (men, non-pregnant women)	500 mg po qid × 7 days		
Azithromycin (all patients)	1 g, po single dose	Antibiotic (macrolide)	Safe for pregnant women to take, not as effective in eliminating *C. trachomatis* as doxycycline; amoxicillin preferred if nausea/ vomiting occurs with other meds
Erythromycin (pregnant women)	400–800 mg po qid × 7 days	Antibiotic (macrolide)	
Amoxicillin (pregnant women)	00 mg po tid 5× 7 days	Antibiotic (penicillin)	
Erythromycin (infants)	Ointment to conjunctiva sac after delivery	Anti-infective	Prophylaxis of neonatal conjuctivitis

Independent

Because patients are often asymptomatic, nurses need to identify those patients at risk for chlamydial infections and recommend screening. Prevention is an important nursing intervention. Teach patients that monogamous relationships with uninfected partners, use of mechanical barriers, and simultaneously treating the partner to prevent reinfection are ways to prevent transmission of *C. trachomatis*. Emphasize that it is possible for them to carry and transmit the bacteria, even if they are asymptomatic.

Since a chlamydial infection is easily cured by antibiotics, teach the patient about taking the medications properly. Instruct patients to take all medication until the course of treatment is finished, even if the symptoms subside. Explain that the patient should abstain from intercourse until all medication is gone to prevent reinfection. For discomfort, teach the patient about warm sitz baths and taking prescribed analgesics as ordered.

DOCUMENTATION GUIDELINES

- Screening done and results if available; note if a female patient is pregnant
- Physical signs and symptoms: Discharge (amount, color, odor, location), pain, bleeding, swelling, dysuria
- Patient's reaction to the diagnosis of an STI
- Patient's understanding of diagnosis, treatment, and prevention

DISCHARGE AND HOME HEALTHCARE GUIDELINES

MEDICATIONS. Be sure the patient understands the correct dosage, route, and time of the medication, as well as the importance of taking all prescribed medication, even if the symptoms resolve. Emphasize any dietary restrictions.

PREVENTION. Teach the patient about the importance of barrier contraception. Often patients on oral contraceptives do not realize that although they probably will not get pregnant, they are not protecting themselves from STIs. Emphasize the importance of follow-up visits to assure that the infection has resolved. Encourage the patient to enforce follow-up of all sexual partners and to refrain from intercourse during antibiotic therapy to prevent reinfection.

COMPLICATIONS. Teach the patient about potential long-term complications such as infertility and sterility if reinfection occurs.

Cholecystitis and Cholelithiasis

DRG Category: 493
Mean LOS: 4.3 days
Description: SURGICAL: Laparoscopic Cholecystectomy without C.D.E. with CC
DRG Category: 195
Mean LOS: 9.7 days
Description: SURGICAL: Cholecystectomy with C.D.E. with CC

Cholecystitis is an inflammation of the gallbladder wall; it may be either acute or chronic. It is almost always associated with cholelithiasis, or gallstones, which lodge in the gallbladder, cystic duct, or common bile duct. Silent gallstones are so common that most of the American public may have them at some time; only stones that are symptomatic require treatment.

Gallstones are most commonly made of either cholesterol or bilirubin and calcium. If gallstones obstruct the neck of the gallbladder or the cystic duct, the gallbladder can become infected with bacteria such as *Escherichia coli.* The primary agents, however, are not the bacteria but mediators such as members of the prostaglandin family. The gallbladder becomes enlarged up to two to three times normal, thus decreasing tissue perfusion. If the gallbladder becomes ischemic as well as infected, necrosis, perforation, and sepsis can follow.

CAUSES

Cholesterol is the major component of most gallstones in North America, leading to speculation that the high-fat diet common to many North Americans is the explanation for their increased frequency. Supporting theories that point to a high-fat diet note that acute attacks of cholelithiasis may be precipitated by fasting and sudden weight loss.

GENDER AND LIFE SPAN CONSIDERATIONS

The incidence of gallbladder disease increases with age. Most patients are middle-aged or older women, often ones who have borne several children and gained weight during the aging process. Since there is a tendency for it to be familial, some young people of both sexes with a familial history can be affected, as well as young women who have taken oral contraceptives.

☐ ASSESSMENT

HISTORY. Cholecystitis often begins as a mild intolerance to fatty food. The patient experiences discomfort after a meal, sometimes with nausea and vomiting, flatulence, and an elevated temperature. Over a period of several months or even years, symptoms progressively become more severe. Ask the patient about the pattern of attacks; some mistake severe gallbladder attacks for a heart attack until they recall similar, less severe episodes that have preceded it. An acute attack of cholecystitis is often associated with gallstones, or cholelithiasis. The classic symptom is pain in the right upper quadrant that may radiate to the right scapula, called biliary colic. Onset is usually sudden, with the duration from less than 1 to more than 6 hours. If the flow of bile has become obstructed, the patient may pass clay-colored stools and dark urine.

PHYSICAL EXAMINATION. The patient with an acute gallbladder attack appears acutely ill, is in a great deal of discomfort, and sometimes is jaundiced. A low-grade fever is often present, especially if the disease is chronic and the walls of the gallbladder have become infected. Right upper quadrant pain is intense in acute attacks and requires no physical examination. It is often followed by residual aching or soreness for up to 24 hours. A positive Murphy's sign, which is positive palpation of a distended gallbladder during inhalation, may confirm a diagnosis.

PSYCHOSOCIAL. The patient with an acute attack of cholelithiasis may be in extreme pain and very upset. The experience may be complicated by guilt if the patient has been advised by the physician in the past to cut down on fatty foods and lose weight. The attack may also be very frightening if it is confused with a heart attack.

DIAGNOSTIC HIGHLIGHTS

Test	Normal Result	Abnormality with Condition	Explanation
White blood cell count (WBC)	Adult males and females 4,500–11,000/µL	Infection and inflammation elevate the WBC count	Leukocytosis; WBCs range from 12,000 to 15,000/µL; if > 20,000, the condition may be associated with gangrene or perforation
Ultrasound scan	Normal gallbladder	Gallbladder wall thickening, pericholecystic fluid collections	Sensitive/specific test for cholethithisasis. Identifies presence of fluid collection.

Other Tests: Supporting tests include phosphatase, aspartate amino transferase (AST), lactate dehydrogenase (LDH), alkaline phosphatase, serum amylase, and serum bilirubin levels; oral cholecystogram (OCG), computed tomography (CT)

PRIMARY NURSING DIAGNOSIS

Pain (acute) related to obstruction and inflammation

OUTCOMES. Comfort level; Pain control behavior; Pain level; Symptom severity

INTERVENTIONS. Analgesic administration; Anxiety reduction; Environmental management: Comfort; Pain management; Medication management; Patient-controlled analgesia assistance

◻ PLANNING AND IMPLEMENTATION

Collaborative

MEDICAL. Medical management may include oral bile acid therapy.

SURGICAL. There are several surgical or procedural treatment options. The one seen most commonly today is a laparoscopic cholecystectomy, which is performed early (within 48 hours of acute onset of symptoms) in the course of the disease when there is minimum inflammation at the base of the gallbladder. The procedure is performed with the abdomen distended by an injection of carbon dioxide, which lifts the abdominal wall away from the viscera and prevents injury to the peritoneum and other organs. A laparoscopic cholecystectomy is done either as an outpatient procedure or with less than 24 hours of hospitalization. After the surgery, the patient may complain of pain from the presence of residual carbon dioxide in the abdomen.

The traditional open cholecystectomy is performed on patients with large stones, as well as with other abnormalities that need to be explored at the time of surgery. This procedure is particularly appropriate up to 72 hours after onset of acute cholecystitis. Timing of the operation is controversial. Early cholecystectomy has the advantage of resolving the acute condition early in its course. Delayed cholecystectomy can be performed after the patient recovers from initial symptoms and acute inflammation have subsided, generally 2 to 3 months after the acute event.

Extracorporeal shock wave lithotripsy similar to the type used to dissolve renal calculi is now also used for small stones. For those patients who are not good surgical candidates, both methods have the advantage of being noninvasive. However, they have the disadvantage of leaving in place a gallbladder that is diseased, with the same propensity to form stones as before treatment.

PHARMACOLOGIC HIGHLIGHTS

Medication or Drug Class	Dosage	Description	Rationale
Oral bile acid therapy; ursodeoxycholic acid	10–15 mg/kg per day for 6–12 months	Nonsurgical method to dissolve gall stones	Used for small stones (< 10 mm in diameter) in a functioning gallbladder in non-obese patients
Antibiotics	Varies with drug	Antibiotic regimen is focused on those appropriate for typical bowel flora (gram-negative rods and anaerobes): third-generation cephalosporin or aminoglycoside with metronidazole	Manage bacteria that are typical bowel flora
Demerol	25–100 mg IM, IV	Opiates relieve pain and promote spasms of the biliary duct	Pain is severe. Analgesia should be offered only after definitive diagnosis has occurred

Additional Pharmacologic Management: The pain is treated by both analgesics and anticholinergics during acute attacks. The anticholinergics relax the smooth muscle, preventing biliary contraction and pain. If inflammation of the gallbladder has led to gallstones and obstruction of bile flow, replacement of the fat-soluble vitamins is important to supplement the diet. Bile salts may be prescribed to aid digestion and vitamin absorption, as well as to increase the ratio of bile salts to cholesterol, aiding in the dissolution of some stones.

Independent

During an acute attack, remain with the patient to provide comfort, to monitor the result of interventions, and to allay anxiety. Explain all procedures in short and simple terms. Provide explanations to the family and significant others.

If the patient requires surgery, the nurse's first priority is the maintenance of airway, breathing, and circulation. Although most patients return from surgery or a procedure breathing on their own, if stridor or airway obstruction occurs, create airway patency with an oral or nasal airway and notify the surgeon immediately. If the patient's breathing is inadequate, maintain breathing with a manual resuscitator bag until the surgeon makes a further evaluation. The high incision makes deep breathing painful, leading to shallow respirations and impaired gas exchange. Splinting the incision while encouraging the patient to cough and breathe deeply help both pain and gas exchange. Elevate the head of the bed to reduce pressure on the diaphragm and abdomen.

Patients not undergoing surgery or a procedure need a thorough education. Explain the disease process, the possible complications, and all medications. Teach the patient to avoid high-fat foods, dairy products, and, if the patient is bothered by flatulence, gas-forming foods.

DOCUMENTATION GUIDELINES

- Physical response: Patency of airway; adequacy of breathing and circulation; vital signs; use of splinting or other measures to control pain while performing deep breathing
- Pain: Location, duration, quality, response to pain medications
- Type and amount of drainage from Penrose drain or T tube
- Condition of surgical incision and surrounding skin

DISCHARGE AND HOME HEALTHCARE GUIDELINES

After a laparoscopic cholecystectomy, provide discharge instructions to a family member or another responsible adult, as well as to the patient, because the patient goes home within 24 hours after surgery. Explain the possibility of abdominal and shoulder pain because of the instillation of carbon dioxide to prevent anxiety about a heart attack if the pain occurs. Teach the patient to avoid submerging the abdomen in the bathtub for the first 48 hours, to take the prescribed antibiotics to provide further assurance against infection, and to watch the incisions for signs of infection. Following a 3- to 5-day hospital stay for an open cholecystectomy, instruct the patient on the care of the abdomen wound, including changing the dressing and protection of any drains.

Reinforce pain control and deep-breathing exercises until the incision is completely healed. The patient may need instruction on control of elimination after this surgery. The continued use of opiate-type analgesics for 7 to 10 days may necessitate the use of laxatives or suppositories, which are generally prescribed by the physician before discharge. Explain that gradual resumption of both a normal diet and activity aid normal elimination. Instruct the patient to report to the physician if any new symptoms occur, such as the appearance of jaundice accompanied by pain, chills and fever, dark urine, or light-colored stools. Usually, the patient has no complications and is able to resume normal activity within a few weeks. Instruct the patient who has been treated nonsurgically with bile salts or extracorporeal shock wave lithotripsy about a low-fat diet to avoid recurrence of gallstones.

Chorioamnionitis

DRG Category: 373
Mean LOS: 1.9 days
Description: MEDICAL: Vaginal Delivery without Complicating Diseases
DRG Category: 370
Mean LOS: 4.9 days
Description: SURGICAL: Cesarean Section with CC

Chorioamnionitis is an infection of the chorion, amnion, and amniotic fluids that surround the fetus. Subsequently, the fetus also becomes infected. Chorioamnionitis, which can occur with subtle or acute signs and symptoms, can happen at any time during the prenatal or intrapartal period. It occurs in 1% of all pregnancies, most commonly after premature rupture of the membranes. Chorioamnionitis can also cause premature rupture of the membranes and preterm labor. If left untreated, it can lead to maternal sepsis or fetal demise.

The prognosis for the mother with chorioamnionitis is good. Once the baby is delivered, the source of infection is removed. Rarely does chorioamnionitis lead to septic shock. Occasionally pelvic inflammatory disease can develop if the infection is not totally resolved. The prognosis for the infant varies, depending on the degree of infection that is transmitted to the fetus. Occasionally no signs of infection develop for the infant, but this is not typical. Another factor involved in the infant's prognosis is prematurity; for the very premature infant, the risk of respiratory distress syndrome may be even greater than the risk of infection.

CAUSES

Chorioamnionitis is usually caused by bacteria that inhabit the genital tract. Less frequently, it can result from pathogens that cross over from the maternal circulation to the amniotic sac. Rarely is it caused by the descent of pathogens from the abdominal cavity through the fallopian tubes. Commonly identified pathogens that contribute to chorioamnionitis are *Escherichia coli, Streptococcus faecalis, Neisseria gonorrhea,* group A and B streptococci, *Chlamydia trachomatis,* and *Staphylococcus aureus.*

Predisposing factors that contribute to chorioamnionitis include poor maternal nutritional status, history of drug abuse, history of multiple sexual partners, premature or prolonged rupture of membranes, sexually transmitted infections (STIs), the placement of a cerclage (ligature around the cervix to treat cervical incompetence during pregnancy), chorionic villi sampling, intrauterine transfusion, amniocentesis, and repeated vaginal examinations during labor.

GENDER AND LIFE SPAN CONSIDERATIONS

Chorioamnionitis can occur with any pregnancy, regardless of the age of the mother.

☐ ASSESSMENT

HISTORY. Ask about the last menstrual period to determine the estimated date of delivery and the gestational age of the fetus. Inquire about any past history of vaginal infections or STIs. Question the patient as to the presence of any perineal pain, burning, malaise, or chills. Ask the patient if she is feeling contractions or if she has noted any leakage of the amniotic fluid. If the amniotic sac has ruptured, determine the time it occurred, the color of the fluid, and if the patient noted any odor. Also consider any prenatal tests or procedures, such as placement of a cerclage, chorionic villi sampling, intrauterine transfusions, or amniocentesis, that can predispose the patient to developing an intrauterine infection.

PHYSICAL EXAMINATION. Early clinical findings in patients with chorioamnionitis may be vague. Assess the patient's vital signs; patients with chorioamnionitis often display an elevated temperature and pulse. Palpate all quadrants of the abdomen for tenderness, noting the maternal response during examination of each quadrant. Foul odor of the vaginal discharge, color change of amniotic fluid from clear to light yellow to green, and an increase in the purulence of vaginal drainage are all consistent with chorioamnionitis.

Often preterm labor patients with undiagnosed chorioamnionitis have contractions that do not respond to routine treatments of intravenous hydration and tocolytic therapy. Evaluate the baseline fetal heart rate. Fetal tachycardia or decreased fetal heart rate or variability may be present with chorioamnionitis.

PSYCHOSOCIAL. Increased anxiety is usually present with patients who are experiencing preterm labor, premature rupture of membranes, or a history of a cerclage placement. Assess the patient's understanding of the situation, and encourage the patient to express her fears. Also include an assessment of the patient's social support and the response of significant others to the patient's condition.

DIAGNOSTIC HIGHLIGHTS

General Comments: Diagnosis may be difficult to establish early on because symptoms are vague. Examination of amniotic fluid is definitive.

Test	Normal Result	Abnormality with Condition	Explanation
Amniocentesis or endocervical culture	No growth	Growth of infecting organism	Culturing the amniotic fluid will reveal the presence of a causative organism, allowing for appropriate choice of antibiotic therapy

Other Tests: complete blood count (CBC) with differential, urinalysis

PRIMARY NURSING DIAGNOSIS

Infection related to microorganism invasion of sterile areas

OUTCOMES. Risk control

INTERVENTIONS. Medication management; Labor induction; Cesarean section care

◻ PLANNING AND IMPLEMENTATION

Collaborative

MEDICAL. The medical management of a patient diagnosed with chorioamnionitis is delivery of the infant, regardless of the gestational age. Tocolytic therapy is contraindicated if chorioamnionitis is present. Delivery benefits the mother by emptying the uterus of all infected material. Once delivered, the infant can then receive the necessary antibiotic therapy. Usually, spontaneous labor occurs because of the infection. If an adequate contraction pattern and progressive dilation of the cervix are not noted, contractions can be induced by oxytocin (Pitocin). Broad spectrum antibiotics administered during labor cross the placenta and achieve peak levels in the fetal circulation within an hour after parenteral administration to the mother. Cesarean section is typically avoided because of the increased risk of spreading the infection; however, if the fetus is showing signs of distress, a cesarean section is performed. If the fetus is preterm, arrange for a neonatologist or pediatrician to speak with the patient before delivery; notification of the nursery is also important. Immediately after delivery, cultures of the placenta and baby are obtained, and the newborn is monitored carefully for signs and symptoms of infection.

PHARMACOLOGIC HIGHLIGHTS

Medication or Drug Class	Dosage	Description	Rationale
Cefoxitin	Varies by drug and patient condition	Second-generation cephalosporin	Broad spectrum antibiotics are effective against gram-positive, gram-negative, aerobic, and anaerobic organisms; are less toxic; and cross the placenta to help the fetus
Mezlocillin		Extended spectrum antibiotics	
Ticarcillin; piperacillin		Penicillin	

Independent

Anticipatory guidance provided by the nurse is beneficial for the patient. Provide information about antibiotic therapy, procedures that occur during labor and delivery, and possible outcomes for the infant. Since the patient's anxiety level is elevated, you may need to repeat information several times. Allow the patient to express her fears. Answer the questions of the significant others and take time to listen to their concerns, as well.

Monitor the patient for signs of infection after delivery, including the mother's lochia, fundal height, vital signs, and incisional healing. The patient with an intrauterine infection is at a higher risk for a postpartum hemorrhage than are her noninfected counterparts. Careful and frequent assessments for vaginal bleeding and firmness of the fundus are critical. If the fundus is "boggy," massage the fundus until firm.

DOCUMENTATION GUIDELINES

If the Patient Is Undelivered

- Maternal vital signs; fetal heart rate pattern; uterine activity; maternal response to antibiotics; color, odor, and consistency of vaginal discharge

If the Patient Is Delivered

- Maternal and infant vital signs; amount and odor of lochia; involution of uterus; assessment of episiotomy or abdominal incision
- Amount of the infant's fluid intake and output, infant's response to antibiotics, daily weight of the baby

DISCHARGE AND HOME HEALTHCARE GUIDELINES

POSTPARTUM COMPLICATIONS. Instruct the patient to inform the physician if her temperature rises above 100.4°F. Increased vaginal bleeding, foul odor of the vaginal discharge, increased uterine tenderness, difficulty urinating, the appearance of hardened red areas in the breasts, pain in the calves of the legs, incisional pain, and redness or drainage from the incision are also reasons to notify the physician.

INFANT COMPLICATIONS. Instruct the patient to inform the pediatrician if the baby's rectal temperature is above 101°F. Decreased interest in feeding, increased jaundice, a red or draining umbilical cord or circumcision site, increased irritability, difficulty breathing, lack of a bowel movement in 2 days, and fewer than six wet diapers a day are also reasons to notify the pediatrician.

MEDICATIONS. Instruct the patient to take the entire prescription of antibiotics, even if symptoms subside. Encourage the patient to notify the physician if symptoms persist when the prescription has ended.

RESTRICTIONS. Instruct the patient to abstain from sexual intercourse until the 6-week follow-up visit. Teach the patient to resume activity gradually and to limit use of stairs for the first week. Explain that patients should not lift anything heavier than their infant for the first 2 weeks after delivery. Teach vaginally delivered patients to avoid driving for 1 week and cesarean patients to avoid driving until the pain ceases.

Chronic Fatigue Immune Dysfunction Syndrome

DRG Category: 463
Mean LOS: 4.5 days
Description: MEDICAL: Signs and Symptoms with CC

Chronic fatigue immune dysfunction syndrome (CFIDS) is a unique, controversial, and poorly understood chronic disease that has a sudden onset in most cases. It is a multiple symptom disease that affects the immune and neurologic systems and suggests chronic mononucleosis. Like many chronic illnesses, CFIDS is debilitating and is often accompanied by depression. CFIDS has been mentioned throughout history.

CAUSES

The cause of CFIDS is unknown. Current research is investigating whether the disease is a syndrome triggered by a virus with multiple contributing factors such as age, gender, toxic exposure, stress, and perhaps a precipitating event (recent trauma or surgery).

GENDER AND LIFE SPAN CONSIDERATIONS

CFIDS is more prevalent in females than in males, and it tends to affect persons between the ages of 25 and 50 years. However, it may be underdiagnosed in children and the elderly.

☐ ASSESSMENT

HISTORY. Establish a history of the sudden onset of flu-like symptoms accompanied by intense fatigue that does not resolve within 6 months. Determine if the patient has experienced any other symptoms of a neurological or psychological nature. Ask the patient if she or he has been exposed to a toxin or has recently experienced stress. Determine if the patient's occupation involves interaction with the public. It is important to remember that symptoms can vary widely with CFIDS.

PHYSICAL EXAMINATION. Assessment of the CFIDS patient may reveal flu-like symptoms such as sore throat, low-grade fever, chills, muscular pain, and swollen, painful lymph nodes. Neurologic assessment findings may include sensitivity to light, headache, inability to think clearly or concentrate, memory loss, sleep disorders, equilibrium problems, and depression.

PSYCHOSOCIAL. Patients with CFIDS are often depressed because of the stress of dealing with a chronic, debilitating illness that affects their total lifestyle. Anxiety and mood swings are common, and there are increased rates of divorce and suicide among these patients. Assess the effect of the disease on the patient's job and child-care responsibilities.

DIAGNOSTIC HIGHLIGHTS

There is no definitive method of diagnosing CFIDS. The Centers for Disease Control and Prevention (CDC) have set forth diagnostic criteria, however. (See Box 4.)

BOX 4   CDC CRITERIA FOR CFIDS

CDC definition of CFIDS stipulates that a patient must fulfill two major criteria, eight symptoms, or six symptoms and two physical signs.

Major Criteria

1. The patient has new-onset, persistent to relapsing, debilitating fatigue without a previous history of such symptoms. The fatigue does not resolve with bed rest and, for at least 6 months, is severe enough to reduce or impair average daily activity to a level less than 50% of what it was before the illness.
2. The fatigue is not explained by the presence of other evident medical or psychiatric illness.

Symptoms

1. Mild fever or chills
2. Sore throat
3. Painful adenopathy, posterior or anterior, cervical or axillary
4. Generalized muscle weakness
5. Myalgia
6. Prolonged generalized fatigue after previously tolerated levels of physical activity
7. Generalized headaches
8. Migratory arthralgia without swelling or redness
9. Neuropsychologic complaints
10. Sleep disturbance

Physical Signs

1. Low grade fever
2. Nonexudative pharyngitis
3. Palpable or tender anterior or posterior cervical or axillary lymph nodes

---

PRIMARY NURSING DIAGNOSIS

Activity intolerance related to muscle and joint pain, fatigue

OUTCOMES. Energy conservation; Coping; Knowledge: Disease process; Mood equilibrium; Symptom severity; Health beliefs: Perceived control

INTERVENTIONS. Energy management; Counseling; Exercise promotion; Hope instillation; Security management; Security enhancement; Presence

☐ PLANNING AND IMPLEMENTATION

Collaborative

Because there is currently no known cure, treatment of CFIDS is symptomatic. Some patients experience relief of the symptoms by avoiding environmental irritants and certain foods.

PHARMACOLOGIC HIGHLIGHTS

Medication or Drug Class	Dosage	Description	Rationale
Nonsteroidal anti-inflammatory drugs	Varies by drug	May reduce inflammation, thus reducing symptoms	Efficacy uncertain

Other Medications: Nonsedating antihistamines, antianxiety agents such as alprazolam, and tricyclic antidepressants may be helpful. Experimental treatments include the antiviral acyclovir and selected immunomodulating agents, such as intravenous gamma globulin, ampligen, transfer factor, and others.

Independent

It is important to set realistic goals when planning care with the CFIDS patient. Teach patients not to overexert themselves. It is believed that stress can prolong the disease or result in an exacerbation. Relaxation and stress-reducing techniques such as hypnosis, massage, biofeedback, and meditation may be useful if sleep patterns are altered. Explain that although the symptoms tend to wax and wane, they are often debilitating and may last for months or even years. The patient therefore needs to reduce his or her activities when symptoms are more pronounced but also needs to avoid bed rest, which has no proven therapeutic value for CFIDS patients. Encourage a graded exercise program, and provide an appropriate referral for continuing exercise. Stress the need to progress slowly with exercise to avoid overfatigue. Referring the patient and family to counseling and support groups may assist in developing appropriate coping skills for dealing with a chronic, debilitating illness.

DOCUMENTATION GUIDELINES
- Physical findings: Activity tolerance, pain, vital signs, range of motion
- Degree of discomfort: Location, frequency, duration, response to analgesia
- Response to medication therapy, rest, and relaxation
- Emotional response: Coping strategies, support from significant others, signs of depression or hopelessness

DISCHARGE AND HOME HEALTHCARE GUIDELINES

Instruct the patient to report any increase in physical symptoms or suicidal thoughts to the primary caregiver. Instruct the patient to obtain assistance as necessary to complete self-care activities and to meet family responsibilities. Teach the patient the proper route, dosage, and side effects to monitor with all medications. Make necessary plans for referrals and follow-up appointments.

Cirrhosis

DRG Category: 202
Mean LOS: 6.4 days
Description: MEDICAL: Cirrhosis and Alcoholic Hepatitis
DRG Category: 480
Mean LOS: 27.1 days
Description: SURGICAL: Liver Transplant

Cirrhosis is a chronic liver disease that is characterized by destruction of the functional liver cells, which leads to cellular death. Liver cells regenerate as fibrotic areas instead of functional cells, causing alterations in liver structure, function, blood circulation, and lymph damage. The major cellular changes include irreversible chronic injury of the functional liver tissue and the formation of regenerative nodules. These changes result in liver cell necrosis, collapse of liver support networks, distortion of the vascular bed, and nodular regeneration of the remaining liver cells.

The classification of cirrhosis is controversial at present. However, most types may be classified by a mixture of causes and cellular changes, defined as follows: alcoholic; cryptogenic and postviral or postnecrotic; biliary; cardiac; metabolic, inherited, and drug-related; and miscellaneous. The first three types are the most commonly seen, accounting for 55% to 90% of cases of cirrhosis. Although each of these types has a different etiology, the clinical findings, including portal vein hypertension and eventual liver failure, are much the same. (See Box 5.)

BOX 5   PATHOPHYSIOLOGY OF CIRRHOSIS: PROGRESSION OF EFFECTS

Effects of Occasional Drinking

- Several days after drinking synthesis of fatty acids and triglycerides increase.
- Fatty acid oxidation decreases.
- Formation and release of lipoproteins decreases.
- Fat appears in the liver.

Effects of Continual Drinking

- Liver cells enlarge because of accumulation of lipids.
- Enlarged liver cells rupture.
- Fatty contents from ruptured liver cells form fatty cysts.
- Cells between adjoining veins in the liver are linked by developing fibrosis.
- Continued scarring and necrosis lead to the liver shrinking.
- Liver function decreases or ceases.
- Obstructed flow of blood leads to increased pressure in the portal vein (portal hypertension).
- Blood backs up in the liver and spleen.
- Veins in the abdomen, rectum, and esophagus dilate.
- The congestion of blood in the liver leads to the leakage of plasma into the peritoneal cavity.
- The liver's production of albumin decreases.
- Decreased serum albumin levels allow more water to move into other body compartments.
- Renin and aldosterone production levels increase, leading to water and sodium retention.
- Ascites, the accumulation of fluid in the peritoneal cavity, results.

CAUSES

Liver cirrhosis is most commonly associated with alcohol abuse, malnutrition, and protein deficiency. Liver disease is also associated with biliary disease, chemical toxins, and infections, such as chronic active hepatitis. Alcoholic cirrhosis—also known as Laennec's, portal, nutritional, and fatty cirrhosis—is the most common form of cirrhosis in the western world, accounting for approximately 70% of cases of cirrhosis.

GENDER AND LIFE SPAN CONSIDERATIONS

Cirrhosis is most commonly seen in the middle-aged population; it is the fourth leading cause of death in the population that is 35 to 55 years of age. It is more common in males than in females. Although the cause is obscure, liver disease appears to be more prevalent in preterm infants who have minimum enteral feedings and who were begun on total parenteral nutrition (TPN) at an early age.

☐ ASSESSMENT

HISTORY. Determine if the patient has experienced personality changes such as agitation, forgetfulness, and disorientation. Inquire about fatigue, drowsiness, mild tremors, or flu-like symptoms. Ask about any past or present symptoms that may indicate cirrhosis, such as changes in bowel habits or menstrual irregularities. Elicit a history of easy bruising, nosebleeds, or bleeding gums. Determine the patient's drinking patterns and how long they have existed. Determine if the patient has had early-morning nausea and vomiting, anorexia, indigestion, weight loss, weakness, lethargy, epigastric discomfort, or altered bowel habits. Ask about any recent sexual dysfunction.

PHYSICAL EXAMINATION. Inspect for signs of muscle atrophy. Note whether the patient's abdomen is protruding. Assess the patient's skin, sclera, and mucous membranes, observing for poor skin turgor, signs of jaundice, bruising, spider angiomas, and palmar erythema (reddened palms). Observe the patient's trunk, and note the presence of gynecomastia (enlarged breasts). Observe the abdomen for distension, an everted umbilicus, and caput medusae (a plexus of dilated veins about the umbilicus); measure the abdominal girth.

When assessing the patient's upper extremities, test for asterixis (liver flap or flapping tremor). Have the patient stretch out his or her arm and hyperextend the wrist with the fingers separated, relaxed, and extended. The patient in stages II (impending) and III (stuperous) of hepatic encephalopathy may have a rapid, irregular flexion and extension (flapping) of the wrist. Note any tenderness or discomfort in the patient's abdomen. Palpate for hepatomegaly by gently rolling the fingers under the right costal margin. The liver is normally soft and usually can be felt under the costal margin. Percuss the patient's abdomen. Note a shifting dullness in the abdomen if ascites is present. Auscultate the abdomen and assess for hypoactive, hyperactive, or normal bowel sounds.

PSYCHOSOCIAL. Cirrhosis is a chronic disease that dictates lifestyle changes for the patient and significant others. Determine the patient's response to the diagnosis and his or her ability to cope with change. Identify the patient's past ability to cope with stressors, and determine if these mechanisms were successful.

DIAGNOSTIC HIGHLIGHTS

Test	Normal Result	Abnormality with Condition	Explanation
Percutaneous liver needle biopsy	Normal hepatocytes	Cellular degeneration	Distinguishes advanced liver disease from cirrhosis; excludes other forms of liver injury such as viral hepatitis
Liver enzymes: Aspartate aminotransferase (AST); alanine aminotransferase (ALT); lactate dehydrogenase (LDH)	AST: 8–20 units/L(u/L); ALT: Females 4–35 u/L; Males 7–46 u/L; DH: 45–90 u/L	Elevated	Liver cellular dysfunction leads to accumulation of enzymes

Other Tests: Other supporting tests include serum aklaline phosphate; total serum, serum bilirubin, indirect bilirubin, and urine bilirubin; serum ammonia; and serum albumin, serum total protein, and prothrombin.

PRIMARY NURSING DIAGNOSIS

Fluid volume excess related to retention

OUTCOMES. Fluid balance; Hydration; Nutrition management; Nutrition therapy; Knowledge: Treatment regime

INTERVENTIONS. Fluid/electrolyte management; Fluid monitoring; Medication administration

▢ PLANNING AND IMPLEMENTATION

Collaborative

MEDICAL. Patients are placed on a well-balanced, high-calorie (2500 to 3000 calories per day), moderate- to high-protein (75 g of high-quality protein per day), low-fat, low-sodium diet (200 to 1000 mg per day), with additional vitamins and folic acid. Accurate fluid intake and output are important to prevent fluid volume overload; for most patients, intake should be limited to 500 to 1000 mL per day. Frequently, vitamin K injections are ordered to improve blood clotting factors. If coagulopathies worsen, treatment may require whole blood or fresh-frozen plasma to maintain the hematocrit and hemoglobin. If alcohol is the primary etiologic factor in liver cirrhosis, strongly encourage the patient to cease drinking.

SURGICAL. Surgical intervention includes a LaVeen continuous peritoneal jugular shunt (peritoneovenous shunt), which may be inserted for intractable ascites. This procedure allows the continuous shunting of ascitic fluid from the abdominal cavity through a one-way valve into a silicone tube that empties into the superior vena cava. Paracentesis may be performed if conditions warrant. Indicators include a large volume of ascitic fluid that compromises the patient's respirations, causes abdominal discomfort, or poses a threat of rupturing an umbilical hernia.

Commonly seen in cirrhosis patients are esophageal varices due to portal vein hypertension. Varices can rupture as a result of anything that increases the abdominal venous pressure, such as coughing, sneezing, vomiting, or the Valsalva's maneuver. To remedy bleeding of esophageal varices, a Sengstaken-Blakemore tube can be placed. In cases of irreversible chronic liver disease, liver transplantation is an option; however, there are selection criteria. Candidates for liver transplantation fall into three categories: those with irreversible chronic liver disease; those with malignancies of the liver and biliary tree; and those with fulminant hepatic failure. Liver transplantation is considered an important therapeutic option for patients with end-stage liver disease, with 1-year and 5-year survival rates of 70% and 60%, respectively.

PHARMACOLOGIC HIGHLIGHTS

Medication or Drug Class	Dosage	Description	Rationale
Propylthiouracil (PTU)	50–150 mg per day maintenance	Anti-thyroid that inhibits synthesis of thyroid hormone	May reduce mortality if patient reduces alcohol intake

Other Medication: To remedy itching, an antihistamine can be administered. If a patient has nausea and vomiting, antiemetics may be prescribed. Use caution when administering antiemetics and acetaminophen to patients with liver damage because many medications are cleared through the liver.

Independent

Nursing considerations in the cirrhotic patient are to avoid infection and circulatory problems. Turn the patient and encourage coughing and deep breathing every 2 hours to prevent pneumonia. Because bleeding can occur, monitor the patient closely for signs of hypovolemia. Test any stool and emesis for blood. Follow closely any break in the patient's skin integrity for increased bleeding, and apply pressure to injection sites. Warn the patient against straining at stool, blowing his or her nose, or sneezing too vigorously. Suggest the patient use a soft toothbrush and an electric razor.

Because of fatigue, muscle atrophy, and wasting, the patient needs to rest. Plan activities to include regular rest periods. To prevent breakdown of the skin, place the patient on an egg-crate or air mattress. Avoid using soap to bathe the patient; use moisturizing agents or lubricating lotion. Use pressure-reducing mattresses or specialty beds to prevent skin breakdown. Apply lotion and massage areas of the skin that are potential breakdown sites.

Encourage the patient to verbalize questions, anxieties, and fears. In conversation, note any behavioral or personality changes, including increasing stupor, lethargy, or hallucinations. Arouse the patient periodically to determine his or her level of consciousness. Emotional and psychological support for the patient and family are important to eliminate anxiety and poor self-esteem. Involve the family members in the patient's care as a means of improving the patient's morale.

DOCUMENTATION GUIDELINES

- Physical findings: Bleeding, abdominal enlargement, weight gain or loss, fluid intake and output, easy respirations, breath sounds, heart sounds, level of

consciousness, gastrointestinal status (nausea, vomiting, anorexia, diarrhea), color of skin and sclera
- Laboratory results: White blood cell count, hemoglobin and hematocrit, albumin, serum electrolytes, ALT, AST
- Nutrition: Tolerance of diet, appetite, ability to maintain body weight
- Response to treatment: Medications, surgery, pericentesis

DISCHARGE AND HOME HEALTHCARE GUIDELINES

ALCOHOL ABUSE TREATMENT. Emphasize to the patient with alcoholic liver cirrhosis that continued alcohol use exacerbates the disease. Stress that alcoholic liver disease in its early stages is reversible when the patient abstains from alcohol. Encourage family involvement in alcohol abuse treatment. Assist the patient in obtaining counseling or support for his or her alcoholism.

FOLLOW-UP. Encourage the patient to seek frequent medical follow-up. Visits from a community health nurse to monitor the patient's progress and to help with any questions or problems at home are also helpful.

SUPPORT GROUPS. Refer the patient to an alcohol support group or liver transplant support group.

Cleft Lip;
Cleft Palate

DRG Category: 52
Mean LOS: 2.3 days
Description: SURGICAL: Cleft Lip and Palate Repair

Cleft lip and cleft palate are facial malformations of the upper lip or palate. They may appear separately or, more commonly, together. The malformation is a result of a failure of the maxillary and median nasal processes to fuse during the second month of embryonic development. Cleft lip may vary from a small notch to a complete cleft that extends into the base of the nose. When cleft palate occurs alone, it is midline, but when it occurs with cleft lip, it may extend into either side of the soft palate. Related complications of cleft lip and cleft palate include dental malformations, frequent otitis media leading to hearing impairment, speech difficulties, and social isolation due to poor self image and speech impairments.

The incidence of cleft lip with or without cleft palate is approximately 1 in 800 live births. The incidence of cleft palate alone is 1 in 2000 live births. Males are more likely to have cleft lip with or without cleft palate; females are more likely to have cleft palate alone. The incidence varies by race, with a higher rate among Japanese and a lower rate among African-Americans.

CAUSES

A genetic cause for cleft lip and palate is likely; however, environmental exposure to teratogens during critical embryonic development cannot be ruled out. Cleft lip with or without cleft palate is etiologically and genetically distinct from isolated cleft palate. Isolated cleft palate has a greater incidence of associated anomalies. There is a twofold increase in the occurrence of clefts with maternal smoking in early pregnancy.

GENDER AND LIFE SPAN CONSIDERATIONS

Surgical repair of a cleft lip is performed within the first month after birth. The repair improves the child's ability to suck. The optimal time to surgically correct a cleft palate is controversial. Times range from 28 days of life to 18 months. Most surgeons prefer to perform the surgery at an early age, before faulty speech habits develop. The more extensive the surgery required, the later the surgery may occur.

◻ ASSESSMENT

HISTORY. A family history of cleft lip or palate may or may not exist. Identical twins are more likely to share the disorder than are fraternal twins. Inquire about teratogen exposure during the first trimester of pregnancy.

PHYSICAL EXAMINATION. The cleft lip may vary from a small notch to a widespread open cleft and may be unilateral or bilateral. The cleft palate also varies in the extent of the malformation: it can involve only the uvula, extend into the soft and hard palate, or be unilateral, bilateral, or midline.

PSYCHOSOCIAL. Parents' and families' adjustments to an infant with cleft lip or palate may be difficult. The deformity is usually readily observable at birth and often totally unexpected. Support for the family is essential and includes explanations of the surgical procedures and long-term prognosis.

DIAGNOSTIC HIGHLIGHTS

There are no diagnostic tests for cleft lip or palate. Cleft lip is diagnosed by visual inspection. Cleft palate is diagnosed by palpating the palate with a gloved finger during the initial newborn assessment at birth. Inspect the palate during crying. It is possible today to diagnose the presence of cleft lip and palate in utero, with an ultrasound.

PRIMARY NURSING DIAGNOSIS

Altered nutrition: Less than body requirements related to inadequate intake

OUTCOMES. Nutritional status; Nutritional status: Food and fluid intake

INTERVENTIONS. Bottle feeding; Infant care

◻ PLANNING AND IMPLEMENTATION

Collaborative

SURGICAL. Cleft lip and palate are treated with a combination of surgery, speech therapy, and orthodontic work. Surgical repair of cleft lip (cheiloplasty) is usually uncomplicated with no long-term intervention, other than possible scar revision. Surgical repair of cleft palate (palatoplasty) is more extensive and may require more than one surgery. If the infant has horseshoe defect, surgery may be impossible. A contoured speech bulb attached to the back of a denture appliance to occlude the nasopharynx may help the child speak.

PHARMACOLOGIC HIGHLIGHTS

Medication or Drug Class	Dosage	Description	Rationale
Antibiotics	Depends on the drug and weight of the child		Prevent infection resulting from surgery
Analgesics	Depends on the drug and weight of the child		Relieve surgical pain

Experimental Treatment: Surgical repair of cleft lip in animals in utero demonstrated better healing of the lip than conventional means.

Independent

Because of the long-term, multidisciplinary nature of services needed for the child, assist the parents in accessing appropriate support within the health care system. Support the parents before and during the surgical procedure by identifying the positive features of the newborn. Call the infant by name. Current surgical practices provide excellent repairs with minimal scarring. Encourage parents to discuss their feelings about the child's appearance. Sharing pictures of children with successful cleft lip repairs may help the parents cope with their fears and anxieties.

Depending on the severity of the cleft, children with cleft lip and palate will have problems sucking. Work with the parents and experiment with devices that will improve nutrition, such as different kinds of nipples. The infant may feed better if the parents use a nipple with a flange that occludes the cleft or a large, soft nipple with large holes. Try holding the infant at different positions during feeding (for example at a 60 to 80 degree angle). Breastfeeding can be successfully carried out as long as the mother can maintain a seal during nursing. In some nursing pairs, the breast tissue may help form the seal. Otherwise, the mother can use the hand not holding the infant or she can use a molded nipple.

Parents should be allowed to verbalize fears and anxiety about the deformity. The first time parents see their baby, they may experience shock, disappointment, or guilt. If you help them see the baby's assets, you encourage bonding and acceptance. Allow ample time for the parents to hold the infant to promote bonding. Explain the surgical procedure and postoperative care to parents.

The postoperative management of an infant with a cleft lip focuses on protection of the operative site. Arm restraints prevent the child from rubbing the site and from self-injury. Hang baby toys within reach of the baby's restrained hands. Many infants are more comfortable in an infant seat rather than lying in a crib. In order to avoid facial contact with the sheets, do not place infants on their stomachs for sleep. Pacifiers are contraindicated, and feeding methods should be designed to reduce any tension on the suture line. Use a cotton-tipped applicator and a cleansing solution to clean the suture line. An antibiotic ointment may be prescribed. Pain should be controlled with analgesic medication and nonpharmacologic strategies such as holding and rocking.

The postoperative management of an infant with a cleft palate centers on prevention of injury to the operative site. Do not place sharp or potentially injurious objects in the child's mouth (spoons, forks, straws, etc.). Feeding may be done from the side, but self-feeding is prohibited. After feeding, make sure to cleanse the child's mouth with water or a cleansing solution.

DOCUMENTATION GUIDELINES

- Appearance of surgical site: Presence of redness, drainage, swelling; degree of approximation of wound edges
- Response to pain medication and other nonpharmacologic interventions
- Ability to feed and maintain weight

DISCHARGE AND HOME HEALTHCARE GUIDELINES

FEEDING. Teach the parents feeding techniques, how to observe for aspiration, and to bubble the infant frequently. After surgery, teach the parents to avoid putting objects into the infant's mouth.

PREVENTION OF INFECTION. Teach the parents to care for the incision and to assess the incision for infection. Explain the importance of keeping the infant's hands away from the face. Tell the parents that it is important to hold the infant and remove the restraints from time to time.

PAIN CONTROL. Teach the parents the signs of pain in an infant, and explore with them nonpharmacologic methods to relieve pain. Review with the parents the analgesic medication dosage, time, and route.

COMPLICATIONS. Instruct parents that the child may have more recurrent middle ear infections than other children. The child may also need orthodontic or speech therapy at some time because of the deformity of the mouth and palate.

Colorectal Cancer

DRG Category: 172
Mean LOS: 6.5 days
Description: MEDICAL: Digestive Malignancy with CC
DRG Category: 148
Mean LOS: 12.2 days
Description: SURGICAL: Major Small and Large Bowel Procedures with CC

Colorectal cancer accounts for about 15% of all malignancies and for about 11% of cancer mortality in both men and women living in the United States. It is the second most common cause of death from cancer among men and women, combined. In recent years, both the incidence and mortality rates have shown a decline, and this is attributed to improved primary and secondary prevention measures.

Of cancers of the colon, 65% occur in the rectum and in the sigmoid and descending colon, 25% occur in the cecum and ascending colon, and 10% occur in the transverse colon. Most colorectal tumors (95%) are adenocarcinomas and develop from an adenomatous polyp. Once malignant transformation within the polyp has occurred, the tumor usually grows into the lumen of the bowel, causing obstruction, and invades the deeper layers of the bowel wall. After penetrating the serosa and the mesenteric fat, the tumor may spread by direct extension to nearby organs and the omentum. Metastatic spread through the lymphatic and circulatory systems occurs most frequently to the liver, as well as the lung, bones, and brain.

CAUSES

Risk factors include a family history of colorectal cancer and a personal history of past colorectal cancer, ulcerative colitis, Crohn's disease, or adenomatous colon polyps. Persons with familial polyposis coli, an inherited disease that is characterized by multiple (>100) adenomatous polyps, possess a risk for colorectal cancer that approaches 100% by age 40.

It has been strongly suggested that diets high in fat and refined carbohydrates play a role in the development of colorectal cancer. High fat content results in increased amounts of fecal bile acid. It is hypothesized that intestinal bacteria react with the bile salts and facilitate carcinogenic changes. Additionally, fat and refined carbohydrates decrease the transit of food through the gastrointestinal (GI) tract and increase the exposure of the GI mucosa to carcinogenic substances that may be present.

GENDER AND LIFE SPAN CONSIDERATIONS

Colorectal cancer affects men and women fairly equally. The incidence of colorectal cancer is exceeded only by lung cancer in both men and women and by prostate cancer in men and breast cancer in women. There is a slight predominance of colon cancer in women and rectal cancer in men. The incidence increases after age 40 and begins to decline after age 75, although 90% of all newly diagnosed cancers are in people older than 50. Colorectal cancer can be diagnosed in individuals of any age, but malignancies that occur around age 20 to 30 are usually difficult to control and signify a poor prognosis.

☐ ASSESSMENT

HISTORY. Seek information about the patient's usual dietary intake, family history, and the presence of the other major risk factors for colorectal cancer. A change in bowel pattern (diarrhea or constipation) and the presence of blood in the stool are early symptoms and might cause the patient to seek medical attention. As the tumor progresses, symptoms develop that are related to the location of the tumor within the colon.

When the tumor is in the right colon, the patient may complain of vague cramping or aching abdominal pain and report symptoms of anorexia, nausea, vomiting, weight loss, and tarry-colored stools. A partial or complete bowel obstruction is often the first manifestation of a tumor in the transverse colon. Tumors in the left colon can cause a feeling of fullness or cramping, constipation or altered bowel habits, acute abdominal pain, bowel obstruction, and bright-red bloody stools. Additionally, rectal tumors can cause stools to be decreased in caliber, or "pencil-like." Depending on the tumor size, rectal fullness and a dull, aching perineal or sacral pain may be reported.

PHYSICAL EXAMINATION. Inspect, auscultate, and palpate the abdomen. Note the presence of any distension, ascites, visible masses, or enlarged veins (a late sign due to portal hypertension and metastatic liver involvement). Bowel sounds may be high-pitched, decreased, or absent in the presence of a bowel obstruction. An abdominal mass may be palpated when tumors of the ascending, transverse, and descending colon have become large. Note the size, location, shape, and tenderness related to any identified mass. Percuss the abdomen to determine the presence of liver enlargement and pain. A rectal tumor can be easily palpated as the physician performs a digital rectal exam.

PSYCHOSOCIAL. Individuals who observe healthy lifestyles may feel anger when the diagnosis is made. Treatment for colorectal cancer can result in a colostomy and impotence in men. Many persons have grave concerns about the possibility of these consequences. Assess the patient and his or her significant others' knowledge and feelings related to these issues.

DIAGNOSTIC HIGHLIGHTS

General Comment: Pathologic results from biopsied tissues provide the definitive diagnosis for cancer.

Test	Normal Result	Abnormality with Condition	Explanation
Hematest	Negative for blood in stool	Positive guaiac test for occult blood in the stool	An early sign of tumor development is blood in the stool
Endoscopy of the colon	Visualization of normal colon	Visualization of tumor and perform biopsy	Endoscopy allows for visualization and removal suspicious polyps or lesions
Serum carcinoembryonic antigen (CEA)	< 2.5 ng/mL (nonsmokers); < 5.0 ng/dL in smokers	Elevations are associated with tumor recurrence after resection; nonspecific elevations occur with cirrhosis, renal failure, pancreatitis, and ulcerative colitis	Glycoprotein is normally absent in normal adult colonic mucosa.

Other Tests: complete blood count (CBC), barium enema, computed tomography (CT) scan, magnetic resonance imaging (MRI), and abdominal x rays to determine abdominal obstruction.

PRIMARY NURSING DIAGNOSIS

Pain related to tissue injury from tumor invasion and the surgical incision

OUTCOMES. Comfort level; Pain control behavior; Pain level; Pain: Disruptive effects

INTERVENTIONS. Pain management; Analgesic administration; Anxiety reduction; Environmental management: Comfort; Patient-controlled anesthesia

□ PLANNING AND IMPLEMENTATION

Collaborative

Although treatment depends on individual patient characteristics, the location of the tumor, and the stage of disease at the time of diagnosis, surgery has been the primary treatment for colorectal cancers. Adjuvant chemotherapy and radiation therapy may be used to improve survival or control symptoms. The exact surgical procedure performed depends on the location of the tumor in the colon and the amount of tissue involved.

PREOPERATIVE. All patients who are undergoing bowel surgery require careful preoperative care in order to minimize the possibility of infection and promote the adjustment to bodily changes. If nutritional deficits are present, a low-residue diet high in calories, carbohydrates, and protein is given until serum electrolytes and protein levels return to normal. Total parenteral nutrition may be ordered. Twenty-four hours before the scheduled surgery, the physician usually orders a "bowel prep," which consists of a clear liquid diet, a regimen of cathartics and cleansing enema, and oral and intravenous antibiotics to minimize bacterial contamination during surgery.

POSTOPERATIVE. Postoperatively, direct nursing care toward providing comfort, preventing complications from major abdominal surgery, and promoting the return of bowel function. Monitor vital signs and drainage from wounds and drains for sign of hemorrhage and infection. A nasogastric (NG) tube connected to low intermittent or continuous suction is usually present for gastric decompression until bowel sounds return. Note the amount and color of the gastric drainage, as well as the presence of abdominal distension.

Patients who require a colostomy return from surgery with an ostomy pouch system in place, as well as a large abdominal dressing. Observe the condition of the stoma every 4 hours. A healthy stoma is beefy red and moist, whereas a dusky appearance could indicate stomal necrosis. A small amount of stomal bleeding is common, but any substantial bleeding should be reported to the surgeon. The colostomy usually begins to function 2 to 4 days after surgery. After surgery, adjuvant radiation therapy to the abdomen or pelvis is used when there is high risk for local recurrence. Adjuvant chemotherapy is used when there is high risk or evidence of metastatic disease. Radiation therapy and chemotherapy may be used as palliative measures to reduce pain, bleeding, or bowel obstruction in patients with advanced and metastatic disease.

PHARMACOLOGIC HIGHLIGHTS

Medication or Drug Class	Dosage	Description	Rationale
Narcotic analgesic	Varies with drug	Is often administered as patient-controlled anesthesia	Manages surgical pain or pain from metastasis

Independent

Encourage the patient to verbalize fears and clarify the physician's explanation of diagnostic results. Dispel any misconceptions about the need for a permanent colostomy, and clarify the purpose of a temporary colostomy, if suggested.

If a colostomy is to be performed, encourage the patient and his or her significant other to verbalize concerns about sexual functioning after surgery. Impotence is only a problem after abdominal perineal resection (APR) in men, but the presence of a stoma and a drainage pouch with fecal effluent can affect self-identity and sexual desires in both men and women.

After surgery, discuss methods to decrease the impact of the ostomy during intimate times. After surgery, help the patient avoid complications associated with bowel surgery. Assist the patient to turn in bed and perform coughing, deep-breathing, and leg exercises every 2 hours to prevent skin breakdown, as well as to avoid pulmonary and vascular stasis. Teach the patient to splint the abdominal incision with a pillow to minimize pain when turning or performing coughing and deep-breathing exercises. The patient who has had an APR may find the side-lying position in bed the most comfortable. Provide a soft or "waffle" pillow (not a rubber doughnut) for use in the sitting position. Change the perineal dressing frequently to prevent irritation to the surrounding skin.

Showing the patient pictures of an actual stoma can help reduce the "shock" of seeing the stoma for the first time. Allow him or her to hold the equipment, observe the amount and characteristics of effluent, and empty the ostomy pouch of contents or gas. Take care when emptying or changing the pouch system not to contaminate the abdominal incision with effluent. Teaching the patient about home care of an ostomy can begin on the second or third postoperative day. Have the patient and a family member demonstrate ostomy care correctly before hospital discharge. Be alert to signs that indicate the need for counseling, and suggest a referral if the patient is not adjusting well.

DOCUMENTATION GUIDELINES

- Response to diagnosis of colorectal cancer, diagnostic tests, and treatment regimen
- Description of all dressings, wounds, and drainage collection devices: Location of drains; color and amount of drainage; appearance of the incision; color of the ostomy stoma; presence, amount, and consistency of ostomy effluent

DISCHARGE AND HOME HEALTHCARE GUIDELINES

PATIENT TEACHING. Teach the patient the care related to the abdominal incision and any perineal wounds. Give instructions about when to notify the physician (if the wound separates or if any redness, bleeding, purulent drainage, unusual odor, or excessive pain is present). Advise the patient not to perform any heavy lifting (>10 lbs), pushing, or pulling for 6 weeks after surgery. If the patient has a perineal incision, instruct him or her not to sit for long periods of time and to use a soft or "waffle" pillow rather than a rubber ring whenever in the sitting position.

Teach the patient colostomy care and colostomy irrigation.

Give the following instructions for care of skin in the external radiation field: Tell the patient to wash the skin gently with mild soap, rinse with warm water, and pat the skin dry each day; not to wash off the dark ink marking that outlines the radiation field; to avoid applying any lotions, perfumes, deodorants, and powder to the treatment area; to wear nonrestrictive soft cotton clothing directly over the treatment area; and to protect skin from sunlight and extreme cold. Explain the purpose, action, dosage, and side effects of all medications prescribed by the physician.

FOLLOW-UP. Stress the need to maintain a schedule for follow-up visits recommended by the physician. Encourage patients with early-stage disease and complete healing of the bowel to eat a diet consisting of a low-fat and high-fiber content with cruciferous vegetables (brussels sprouts, cauliflower, broccoli, cabbage).

Most colorectal tumors grow undetected as symptoms slowly develop. Survival rates are best when the disease is discovered in the early stages and when the patient is asymptomatic. Unfortunately, 50% of patients have positive lymph node involvement at the time of diagnosis. Participation in procedures for the early detection of colorectal cancer needs to be encouraged.

Suggest follow-up involvement with community resources such as the United Ostomy Association and the American Cancer Society.

Coronary Artery Disease (Arteriosclerosis)

DRG Category: 132
Mean LOS: 3.6 days
Definition: MEDICAL: Atherosclerosis with CC
DRG Category: 125
DRG Category: 125
Mean LOS: 2.4 days
Definition: MEDICAL: Circulatory Disorders Except AMI, with Cardiac Catheter without Complex Diagnosis

Coronary artery disease (CAD) results when decreased blood flow through the coronary arteries causes inadequate delivery of oxygen and nutrients to the myocardium. The lumens of the coronary arteries become narrowed from either fatty fibrous plaques or calcium plaque deposits, thus reducing blood flow to the myocardium, which can lead to chest pain or even myocardial infarction (MI) and sudden cardiac death.

Plaque buildup in the coronary arteries is a result of arteriosclerosis, defined as thickening of the arterial walls' inner aspect and a loss of elasticity. Arterial walls may develop calcifications, which diminish the ability of the vessels to transport blood adequately. Atherosclerosis, the most common form of arteriosclerosis, produces yellowish plaques made up mostly of cholesterol and lipids that line the inner arterial wall. The process of atherosclerosis may be initiated by damage to the arterial endothelium. Plaque accumulation reduces the inner arterial lumen and leads to wall thickening, calcification, and reduced blood supply. Aging results in increased streaking of fatty substances and fibrous change in the arteries.

CAUSES

Atherosclerosis is the most common cause of CAD and is linked to many risk factors—primarily elevated serum cholesterol levels, elevated blood pressure, and cigarette smoking. Blood levels of cholesterol and low-density lipoproteins have been associated with increased risk of CAD. Hypertension places chronic stress on the blood vessels and may initiate plaque deposition. Because smoking increases myocardial oxygen requirements, blood pressure, and heart rate, cigarette smokers are twice as likely to have an MI and four times as likely to have sudden cardiac death. Other risk factors include heredity, obesity, lack of physical activity, stress, and diabetes mellitus.

GENDER AND LIFE SPAN CONSIDERATIONS

Of the 500,000 deaths from CAD in the United States annually, approximately 160,000 occur before the age of 65. More than one-half of these occur in women. For women in their mid to late 50s, CAD is a major cause of illness and death. Following age 80, the risk of CAD for women is equal to that of men. Of all deaths from cardiovascular problems in the elderly, 85% are related to CAD, although this prevalence is lower among elderly African-Americans. Many risk factors associated with CAD are found with increasing frequency among the elderly.

☐ ASSESSMENT

HISTORY. Patients with CAD describe symptoms of myocardial ischemia. A careful description of the pain, including location, severity, and precipitating factors, is essential. The most common symptom is angina, but some individuals remain asymptomatic. Cardiac pain is usually described as a diffuse aching pain or pressure that is relieved by rest or administration of nitroglycerin. The pain is usually substernal but may radiate to either arm, the neck, or between the shoulder blades. Often the pain is precipitated by extra physical or emotional demands. Atypical pain may originate in the elbow, jaw, or shoulder. The patient may have no pain sensation but may complain of being short of breath or having nausea, vomiting, lightheadedness, or sweating.

PHYSICAL EXAMINATION. Physical examination may reveal nothing abnormal. Labored breathing, pallor, and profuse sweating suggest that chest pain may be caused by MI. There may be evidence of flat or slightly raised yellowish tumors, most frequently found on the upper and lower lids (xanthelasma), or flat, slightly elevated, soft rounded plaque or nodules, usually on the eyelids (xanthoma). Auscultate the heart sounds carefully to identify accompanying cardiac problems such as valvular dysfunction or heart failure.

PSYCHOSOCIAL. Because the stress in one's life has long been associated with the development of CAD, problem solving to reduce stress is an important nursing function. Occupational stress or the obligations from multiple roles may vary for female and male patients. Individuals whose work involves heavy lifting may require vocational rehabilitation counseling in order to return to work. Continuation of a fulfilling sexual expression requires thoughtful assessment and teaching.

DIAGNOSTIC HIGHLIGHTS

Test	Normal Result	Abnormality with Condition	Explanation
Lipid profile	Range varies for age and gender; 140–200 mg/dL	Total cholesterol level above 200 mg/dL	Elevated levels are associated with CAD
Electrocardiogram (ECG)	Normal electrocardiographic representation with P, Q, R, S, and T waves	Q waves because of a prior MI; resting ST segment depression or elevation; T wave	Changes in the electrical activity of the heart are associated with cardiac ischemia,

inversion suggestive   injury, or necrosis of myocardial ischemia

Other Tests: Ambulatory ECG monitoring, exercise echocardiography, stress myocardial perfusion imaging, and cardiac catheterization. Exercise echocardiography is useful in establishing the diagnosis of CAD and allows some determination of risk in patients with angina.

PRIMARY NURSING DIAGNOSIS

Altered tissue perfusion (myocardial) related to narrowing of the coronary artery(ies) associated with atherosclerosis, spasm, and/or thrombosis

OUTCOMES. Cardiac pump effectiveness; circulation status; comfort level; pain control behavior; pain level; tissue perfusion: cardiac

INTERVENTIONS. Cardiac care; Cardiac precautions; Oxygen therapy; Pain management; Medication administration; Circulatory care; Positioning

❏ PLANNING AND IMPLEMENTATION

Collaborative

INVASIVE PROCEDURES. Several invasive but nonsurgical procedures can be used to manage CAD. Percutaneous transluminal coronary angioplasty (PTCA) is an invasive radiographic procedure that is performed under local anesthesia. A balloon-tipped coronary catheter is introduced into a coronary vessel and inflated and deflated in quick succession. The atheroma (fatty lesion) is compressed against the vessel wall, and the stenosis is dilated, which increases coronary blood flow. Clinical success has been reported at 85% to 95%. Other invasive procedures include arthrectomy, which is the removal of plaque by rotational or directional catheter. Ablation of plaque deposits by laser independently or in conjunction with PTCA can also be performed. Intravascular stents can be used to support arterial walls that have been damaged by dissection from another procedure.

CORONARY ARTERY BYPASS GRAFTING (CABG). A patent blood vessel from another part of the body is grafted to the affected coronary artery distal to the lesion. The new vessel bypasses the obstruction. Unfortunately, unless reduction of risks and modification of the lifestyle accompany this procedure, the grafted vessels will also eventually occlude. Vessels commonly used for grafting are the greater or lesser saphenous veins, basilic veins, and right and left internal mammary arteries.

Managing the patient after heart surgery involves complex collaborative strategies among the nurse, surgeon, and respiratory therapist. Usually a patient leaves the operating room with a systemic arterial and pulmonary artery catheter in place. Fluids and medications are administered according to the patient's hemodynamic response to the surgery. Monitoring for complications is also an essential role. Early complications from heart surgery include hypotension or hypertension (lowered or raised blood pressure), hemorrhage, dysrhythmias, decreased cardiac output, fluid and electrolyte imbalance, pericardial bleeding, fever or hypothermia, poor gas exchange, gastric distension, and changes in level of consciousness.

If the patient has a large amount of drainage from mediastinal tubes, the nurse may initiate autotransfusion. In the immediate postoperative period, patients will need airway management with an endotracheal tube and breathing support with mechanical ventilation. Some patients will also require temporary cardiac pacing through epicardial pacing wires that are inserted during the surgery. Patients will often need fluid therapy with blood, colloids, or crystalloids to replace lost fluids or bleeding.

PHARMACOLOGIC HIGHLIGHTS

Medication or Drug Class	Dosage	Description	Rationale
Nitrates and other antianginal agents	Varies by drug	Nitrates such as isosorbide and nitroglycerin, beta-adrenergic blockers such as atenolol and propranolol, and calcium channel blockers such as diltiazem, nifedipine, and verapamil	Increase coronary artery blood flow through vasodilation
Antilipemic agents	Varies by drug	Bile-sequestering agents (cholestyramine), folic acid derivatives (gemfibrozil), and cholesterol synthesis inhibitors (lovastatin)	Lower excessively high serum lipid levels

Other Drugs: Antihypertensives are also used since hypertension increases stress on damaged blood vessels. A direct vasodilating agent such as hydralazine or sodium nitroprusside may also be used. Angiotensin-converting enzyme inhibitors (ACEIs) are used to lower blood pressure.

Independent

During episodes of chest pain, encourage complete rest and allay the patient's anxiety by remaining close at hand. Monitor the blood pressure and heart rate, and initiate collaborative interventions such as administering nitroglycerin and oxygen. If the pain does not subside, notify the physician. When the episode is over, ask the patient to grade the severity of the pain (1 is low pain and 10 is severe pain), and document it in detail.

Explain strategies to reverse CAD through a program that includes a very low fat diet, aerobic exercise, and stress-reduction techniques. Information about resumption of sexual activity acceptable for the medical condition is helpful. Patient information literature is abundant and available from cardiac rehabilitation programs, as well as the American Heart Association. Although many patients will be admitted on the day of surgery, preoperative teaching about the intensive care unit environment, the procedure, postoperative coughing and breathing exercises, and postoperative expectations of care is essential. The surgery is a family crisis that may lead to a long recovery, patient dysfunction, and even death. The family needs emotional support and constant information about the patient's progress.

DOCUMENTATION GUIDELINES

- Episodes of angina describing character, location, and severity of pain; precipitating or mitigating factors; interventions; and evaluation
- Patient teaching about disease process and planned treatments, including medication regimen
- Perioperative hemodynamic response: Pulmonary and systemic arterial pressures, presence of pulses, capillary refill, urine output
- Pulmonary assessment: Breath sounds, ventilator settings, response to mechanical ventilation, secretions
- Complications: Bleeding, blood gas alterations, fluid volume deficit, hypotension, dysrhythmias, hypothermia
- Coping: Patient and family
- Mediastinal drainage and autotransfusion

DISCHARGE AND HOME HEALTHCARE GUIDELINES

PREVENTION. Review the risk factor and lifestyle modifications that are acceptable to the patient and his or her family members.

MEDICATIONS. Be certain that the patient and appropriate family members understand all medications, including the correct dosage, route, action, and adverse effects.

PERIOPERATIVE. *Care of incision:* Often the incision heals with no home healthcare, but the patient needs to know the signs of infection. *Activity Restrictions:* The activity recommendations will depend on the type and extent of the patient's underlying condition.

Cor Pulmonale

DRG Category: 144
Mean LOS: 4.5 days
Description: MEDICAL: Other Circulatory System Diagnoses with CC

Cor pulmonale is right-sided hypertrophy of the heart caused by pulmonary hypertension. Increases in pulmonary resistance cause the right side of the heart to work harder, which leads to hypertrophy of the right ventricle. An increase in pulmonary vascular resistance is the result of any or all of the following: anatomic reduction of the pulmonary vascular bed, pulmonary vasoconstriction, or abnormalities of ventilatory mechanics.

Anatomic reduction of the pulmonary vascular bed is related to alveolar wall damage that leads to loss of pulmonary capillaries or to stiffening of the vasculature as seen in pulmonary fibrosis. Constriction of the pulmonary vessels and hypertrophy of vessel tissue are caused by alveolar hypoxia and hypercapnia. Abnormalities of the ventilatory mechanics bring about compression of pulmonary capillaries. Cor pulmonale accounts for approximately 25% of all types of heart failure. Complications of cor pulmonale include biventricular heart failure, hepatomegaly, pleural effusion, and thromboembolism related to polycythemia.

CAUSES

Cor pulmonale is produced by a number of other pulmonary and pulmonary vascular disorders as well. In addition, respiratory insufficiency—such as chest wall disorders, upper airway obstruction, obesity hypoventilation syndrome, and chronic mountain sickness caused by living at high altitudes—can also lead to the disease. It can also develop from lung tissue loss after extensive lung surgery. A contributing factor is chronic hypoxia, which stimulates erythropoiesis, thus increasing blood viscosity. Cigarette smoking is also a risk factor.

GENDER AND LIFE SPAN CONSIDERATIONS

Middle-aged to elderly men are more likely to experience cor pulmonale, but incidence in women is increasing. In children, cor pulmonale is likely to be a complication of cystic fibrosis, hemosiderosis, upper airway obstruction, scleroderma, extensive bronchiectasis, neurological diseases that affect the respiratory muscles, or abnormalities of the respiratory control center.

◻ ASSESSMENT

HISTORY. Determine if the patient has experienced orthopnea, cough, fatigue, epigastric distress, anorexia, or weight gain or has a history of previously diagnosed lung disorders. Ask if the patient smokes cigarettes, noting the daily consumption and duration. Ask about the color and quantity of the mucus the patient expectorates. Determine the amount and type of dyspnea and if it is related only to exertion or is continuous.

PHYSICAL EXAMINATION. The patient may appear acutely ill with severe dyspnea at rest and visible peripheral edema. Observe if the patient has difficulty in maintaining breath while the history is taken. Evaluate the rate, type, and quality of respirations. Examine the underside of the patient's tongue, buccal mucosa, and conjunctiva for signs of central cyanosis, a finding in congestive heart failure. Oral mucous membranes in dark-skinned individuals are ashen when the patient is cyanotic. Observe the patient for dependent edema from the abdomen (ascites) and buttocks and down both legs.

Inspect the patient's chest and thorax for the general appearance and anteroposterior diameter. Look for the use of accessory muscles in breathing. If the patient can be supine, check for evidence of normal jugular vein protrusion. Place the patient in a semi-Fowler position with his or her head turned away from you. Use a light from the side, which casts shadows along the neck, and look for jugular vein distension and pulsation. Continue looking at the jugular veins, and determine the highest level of pulsation using your fingers to measure the number of fingerbreadths above the angle of Louis.

While the patient is in semi-Fowler position with the side lighting still in place, look for chest wall movement, visible pulsations, and exaggerated lifts and heaves in all areas of the precordium. Locate the point of maximum impulse (PMI) (at the fifth intercostal space, just medial of the midclavicular line) and take the apical pulse for a full minute. Listen for abnormal heart sounds. Hypertrophy of the right side of the heart causes a delayed conduction time and deviation of the heart from its axis, which can result in dysrhythmias. With the diaphragm of the stethoscope, auscultate heart sounds in the aortic, pulmonic, tricuspid, and mitral areas. In cor pulmonale, there is an accentuation of the pulmonic component of the second heart sound. The S_3 and S_4 sounds resemble a horse gallop. The presence of the fourth heart sound is found in cor pulmonale. Auscultate the patient's lungs, listening for normal and abnormal breath sounds. Listen for bibasilar rales and other adventitious sounds throughout the lung fields.

PSYCHOSOCIAL. The patient has had to live with the anxiety of shortness of breath for a long time. Chronic hypoxia can lead to restlessness and confusion, and the patient may seem irritated or angry during the physical examination.

DIAGNOSTIC HIGHLIGHTS

Test	Normal Result	Abnormality with Condition	Explanation
Chest x rays	Normal heart size and clear lungs	Enlarged right ventricle and pulmonary artery; may show pneumonia	Demonstrates right-sided hypertrophy of heart and possibly pulmonary infection with other underlying pulmonary abnormalities
Electrocardiogram (ECG)	Normal electrocardiographic wave form with P, Q, R, S, T waves	To reveal increased P-wave amplitude (P-pulmonale) in leads II, III, and a V_f seen in right-axis deviation and incomplete right bundle branch block.	Changes in cardiac conduction due to right-sided hypertrophy
Echocardiography	Normal heart size	To show ventricular hypertrophy, decreased contractility, and valvular disorders in both right and left ventricular failure.	Demonstrates heart hypertrophy and tricuspid valve malfunction if present

PRIMARY NURSING DIAGNOSIS

Decreased cardiac output related to an ineffective ventricular pump

OUTCOMES. Cardiac pump: Effectiveness; Circulation status; Tissue perfusion: Abdominal organs and peripheral; Vital sign status; Electrolyte and acid base balance; Endurance; Energy conservation; Fluid balance

INTERVENTIONS. Cardiac care; Circulatory care: Mechanical assist device; Fluid/electrolyte management; Medication administration; Medication management; Oxygen therapy; Vital signs monitoring

✷ PLANNING AND IMPLEMENTATION

Collaborative

The patient with an acute exacerbation of chronic obstructive pulmonary disease (COPD) requires mechanical ventilation and is usually admitted to an intensive care unit. Patients admitted with heart failure who require specialized treatment such as hemodynamic monitoring may also be admitted to a special care unit.

Specific medical treatment for cor pulmonale consists of reversing hypoxia with low-flow oxygen. In the case of acute cor pulmonale, associated with pulmonary emboli, higher concentrations of oxygen may be used. The physician seeks to correct fluid, electrolyte, and acid-base disturbances and may prescribe fluid and sodium restrictions to reduce plasma volume and the work of the heart. Phlebotomies may be used to reduce a patient's seriously elevated hemoglobin.

SUPPORTIVE CARE. Respiratory therapists provide bronchodilator therapy and may need to teach or reinforce the patient's use of breathing strategies. Therapists may also teach energy conservation. A dietitian confers with the patient and family about the need for low-sodium foods and small, nutritious servings. Specific nutritional deficiencies may need to be corrected as well. Fluids need to be limited to 1000 to 1500 mL per day to prevent fluid retention. Social service agencies will probably be needed for a consultation as well, since cor pulmonale creates long-term disability with the likelihood that the patient has not been employed for some time. Unless the patient is old enough to receive Medicare, hospitalization costs are a serious concern.

PHARMACOLOGIC HIGHLIGHTS

Medication or Drug Class	Dosage	Description	Rationale
Bronchodilators	Varies with drug	Beta$_2$ adrenergic agonists, anticholinergics	Relieve bronchospasm
Antibiotics	Varies with drug	Trimethoprim-sulfamethoxazole amoxicillin are examples	Manage respiratory infections

Other Medication: Depending on the specific findings, the physician may also order low-dose digitalis therapy, vasodilators, and antidysrhythmic drugs.

Independent

The patient requires bed rest and assistance with the activities of daily living if hypoxemia and hypercapnia are severe. Provide meticulous skin care. Reposition the bedridden patient frequently to prevent atelectasis. Reinforce proper breathing strategies for the patient: breathe in through the nose and out slowly through pursed lips, using abdominal muscles to squeeze out the air; inhale before beginning an activity and then exhale while doing the activity, such as walking or eating.

Nurses can teach patients to control their anxiety, which affects their breathlessness and fear. Teach the patient the use of relaxation techniques. Because patients are continually breathless, they become anxious if they feel rushed; focus on providing a calm approach. Help reduce the patient's fear of exertional dyspnea by providing thoughtful care that builds trust. Encourage the patient to progress in small increments.

Because of the exertion that talking requires, many patients with cor pulmonale may not be able to respond adequately in conversation. Try to understand the patient's reluctance to "tire out," and become familiar with reflective techniques that allow a patient to respond briefly. Integrate your teaching into the care to avoid the need to give the patient too much information to assimilate at the time of discharge.

DOCUMENTATION GUIDELINES

- Physical findings: Vein distension, presence of peripheral edema, cardiopulmonary assessment
- Responses to activity, treatments, and medications
- Understanding of and willingness to carry out prescribed therapy

DISCHARGE AND HOME HEALTHCARE GUIDELINES

COMPLICATIONS. Teach the patient and family the signs and symptoms of infection, such as increased sputum production, change in sputum color, increased coughing or wheezing, chest pain, fever, and tightness in the chest. Teach the patient how to recognize signs of edema. Make sure the patient knows to call the physician upon recognizing these signs.

MEDICATIONS. Be sure the patient understands any pain medication prescribed, including dosage, route, action, and side effects.

NUTRITION. Explain the importance of maintaining a low-sodium diet. Review nutrition counseling and the prescribed fluid intake.

ONGOING OXYGEN THERAPY. If the patient is going home with low-flow oxygen, ensure that an appropriate vendor is contacted. Determine whether a home care agency needs to evaluate the home for safety equipment and pollution factors.

Crohn's Disease

DRG Category: 179
Mean LOS: 6.4 days
Description: MEDICAL: Inflammatory Bowel Disease
DRG Category: 148
Mean LOS: 12.2 days
Description: SURGICAL: Major Small and Large Bowel Procedures with CC

Crohn's disease is a chronic, nonspecific inflammatory disease of the bowel that occurs most commonly in the terminal ileum, jejunum, and the colon, although it may affect any part of the gastrointestinal (GI) system from the mouth to the anus. Like ulcerative colitis, Crohn's disease is marked by remissions and exacerbations, but, unlike ulcerative colitis, it can affect any portion of the tubular GI tract.

The disease creates deep, longitudinal mucosal ulcerations and nodular submucosal thickenings called granulomas, which give the intestinal wall a cobblestone appearance and may alter its absorptive abilities. The inflamed and ulcerated areas occur only in segments of the bowel, and normal bowel tissue segments occur between the diseased segments. Eventually, thickening of the bowel wall, narrowing of the bowel lumen, and strictures of the bowel are common. Also, fistulae that connect to other tissue—such as the skin, bladder, rectum, and vagina—often occur.

CAUSES

Research has not established a specific cause for Crohn's disease. Infectious agents such as a virus or bacterium, an autoimmune reaction, environmental factors such as geographic location, and genetic factors are all being investigated. Researchers now believe that emotional stress and psychological changes are a result of the chronic and severe symptoms of Crohn's disease rather than a cause.

GENDER AND LIFE SPAN CONSIDERATIONS

Crohn's disease may occur at any age in both men and women, but it is generally first diagnosed between the ages of 15 and 30 years. Reports indicate that the number being diagnosed at 60 years of age and older is growing. Two factors that may predispose the elderly to Crohn's disease include an increased vulnerability to infection and a susceptibility to inadequate blood supply to the bowel because of the aging process.

◻ ASSESSMENT

HISTORY. Patients initially report insidious symptoms such as mild, non-bloody diarrhea (three to five semi-soft stools per day), fatigue, anorexia, and vague, intermittent abdominal pain. As the disease progresses, they complain of more severe, constant abdominal pain that typically localizes in the right lower quadrant, weight loss, more severe fatigue, and moderate fever. Some patients may also report skin breakdown in the perineal and rectal areas.

PHYSICAL EXAMINATION. Because Crohn's disease is a chronic disease that affects the GI system and causes anorexia and multiple episodes of diarrhea, common problems are malnutrition and dehydration. Inspect for hair loss, dry skin, dry and sticky mucous membranes, poor skin turgor, muscle weakness, and lethargy. Also, inspect the patient's perianal area for signs of fistula formation.

Palpate the patient's abdomen for pain, tenderness, or distension. Generally, pain localizes in the right lower quadrant, but note the location, intensity, type, and duration of discomfort. Auscultate the patient's abdomen for bowel sounds. Often, hyperactive sounds will be noted during an acute inflammatory episode.

PSYCHOSOCIAL. The effects of chronic illness and debilitating symptoms, along with frequent hospitalizations, often result in psychological problems and social isolation. Assess the coping mechanisms, as well as the patient's support system.

DIAGNOSTIC HIGHLIGHTS

Test	Normal Result	Abnormality with Condition	Explanation
Barium enema	Normal lower GI tract	To determine the location and extent of rectal involvement, including inflammation, strictures, perinanal disease, and fistulae	May help differentiate Crohn's disease from ulcerative colitis; should not be undertaken during acute episodes of illness
Sigmoidoscopy or colonoscopy	Normal GI tract on direct visualization	To detect location of illness, as well as early mucosal changes, inflammation, strictures, and fistulae	May help differentiate Crohn's disease from ulcerative colitis

Other Tests: Complete blood count (CBC), serum albumin, and stool specimens.

PRIMARY NURSING DIAGNOSIS

Alteration in nutrition: Less than body requirements related to anorexia, diarrhea, and decreased absorption of the intestines

OUTCOMES. Nutritional status: Food and fluid intake; Nutrient intake; Biochemical measures; Body mass; Energy; Bowel elimination; Endurance

INTERVENTIONS. Nutrition management; Nutrition therapy; Nutritional counseling and monitoring; Fluid and electrolyte management; Medication management; Enteral tube feeding; Intravenous therapy; Total parenteral nutrition administration

□ PLANNING AND IMPLEMENTATION

Collaborative

MEDICAL. Much of the medical management centers on medications. During acute exacerbations, bowel "rest" is important to promote healing; bowel rest can be achieved by placing the patient NPO with the administration of total parenteral nutrition to supply the required fluids, nutrients, and electrolytes. Once the acute episode has subsided and symptoms are relieved, a diet high in protein, vitamins, and calories is prescribed. In addition, a low-residue, milk-free diet is generally well tolerated.

SURGICAL. Surgery, though not a primary intervention, may be necessary for patients who develop complications such as bowel perforation, abscess, intestinal obstruction, fistulae, or hemorrhage and for those who do not respond to conservative management such as nutritional and drug therapy. Unfortunately, there is a 60% recurrence of the disease process after surgical intervention. Multiple resections also may lead to short bowel syndrome, defined as malabsorption of fluids, electrolytes, and nutrients, which leads to nutritional deficiencies. The syndrome occurs when less than 150 cm of functional small bowel remains.

PHARMACOLOGIC HIGHLIGHTS

Medication or Drug Class	Dosage	Description	Rationale
Mesalamine (5-ASA; see description) (Asacol, Pentasa)	800–1600 mg po tid	Anti-inflammatory agent, 5-aminosalicylic acid	5-ASA preparations like mesalamine have become treatment of choice; can be used in people who cannot tolerate sulfasalazine
Other anti-inflammatories	Varies with drug; sulfasalazine: 0.5–1.0 g po qid; prednisone: 10–40 mg po tid; methylprednisolone: 20–40 mg IV q 12 hours; hydrocortisone: 100 mg IV q 6 hours	sulfasalazine (Azulfidine) and corticosteroids	Slow the inflammatory process; sulfasalazine is not used in treatment of disease confined to small intestine; glucocorticoids such as prednisone are used in acute exacerbations. Agents are administered until clinical symptoms subside, at which time steroidal agents are tapered off
Anti-diarrheal agents	Varies with drug	Example: loperamide (Imodium)	Alleviate symptoms of abdominal cramping and diarrhea in patients with mild symptoms or post-resection diarrhea
Metronidazole (Flagyl)	250 mg po tid	Antibacterial agent	Effective in colon disease; treats infections with fistulae and perianal skin breakdown; beneficial in patients who have not responded to other agents
Immunosuppressive agents	Varies with drug	Azathioprine (Imuran) 6-mercaptopurine	Decrease inflammation and symptoms if steroids fail or decrease steroid requirements

Other Drug Therapy: Some patients who are suffering with severe abdominal pain may require narcotic analgesics such as meperidine (Demerol). Also, patients who develop deficiencies because of problems of malabsorption may require vitamin B12 injections monthly or iron replacement therapy. Other nutritional supplements include calcium, magnesium, folate, and other micronutrients.

Independent

Nursing care focuses on supporting the patient through acute episodes of inflammation and teaching measures to prevent future inflammatory attacks. Maintaining patient fluid and electrolyte balance is particularly important. Encourage the patient to drink 3000 mL of fluid per day, unless it is contraindicated. Implement measures to prevent skin breakdown in the perianal area.

Provide frequent rest periods. Maintain adequate nutritional status using calorie counts. Other measures include assisting the patient with frequent oral hygiene; providing small, frequent meals with rest periods interspersed throughout the day; monitoring intravenous fluids and total parenteral nutrition as prescribed; and noting the patient's serum albumin levels.

Encourage patients to express their feelings and refer them for more extensive counseling as needed. Also, discuss measures to diminish stressful life situations with the patient and family.

DOCUMENTATION GUIDELINES

- Evidence of stability of vital signs, hydration status, bowel sounds, and electrolytes
- Response to medications; tolerance of foods; ability to eat and select a well-balanced diet, and weight gains or losses
- Location, intensity, and frequency of pain; factors that relieve pain
- Number of diarrheal episodes and stool characteristics
- Presence of complications: Fistulae, skin breakdown, abscess formation, infection

DISCHARGE AND HOME HEALTHCARE GUIDELINES

Emphasize measures that will help prevent future inflammatory episodes, such as getting plenty of rest and relaxation, reducing stress, and maintaining proper diet (high protein, low residue). Teach the patient to recognize the signs of incipient inflammatory attacks. Explain all the prescribed medications, including the actions, side effects, dosages, and routes. Be certain the patient understands signs of possible complications, such as an abscess, fistula, hemorrhage, or infection, and the need to seek medical attention if any of them occurs. Caution the patient to be vigilant with skin care, especially in the perianal area. Instruct the patient to assess frequently for breakdown in this area and seek medical attention if it should occur.

Cushing's Syndrome

DRG Category: 300
Mean LOS: 6.3 days
Description: MEDICAL: Endocrine Disorders with CC

Cushing's syndrome is defined as the clinical effects of increased glucocorticoid hormone. It can be characterized by an excess production of glucocorticoids (primarily cortisol) by the cortex of the adrenal gland, but it is most commonly due to therapy with glucocorticoid drugs. Cortisol is an essential hormone for many body functions, including maintaining normal electrical excitation of the heart, blood glucose level, nerve cell conduction, and adequate circulatory volume, and for metabolizing proteins, fats, and carbohydrates.

Overproduction of glucocorticoids leads to a host of multisystem disorders in metabolism, water balance, wound healing, and response to infection. Complications affect almost every system of the body. Increased calcium resorption from bones may lead to osteoporosis and bone fractures. A blunted immune response causes a high risk for infection, as well as poor wound healing. Cushing's syndrome may also mask even life-threatening infections. Gastrointestinal (GI) irritation may lead to peptic ulcers, and both insulin resistance and glucose intolerance can cause hyperglycemia.

CAUSES

The causes are divided into three categories: iatrogenic, primary, and secondary. Iatrogenic causes are a result of excessive cortisol levels from chronic therapy with glucocorticoids. Approximately 25% of cases have a primary cause of excessive cortisol production from adrenal neoplasms such as adenomas or carcinomas. The tumors usually affect only one adrenal gland, and about 50% are malignant. Even with appropriate treatment, most patients with adrenal carcinoma die within 3 years because of metastases to the liver and lung. Secondary Cushing's syndrome is more common than primary, and bilateral adrenal hyperplasia is the most common secondary condition. It is caused by excessive production of adrenocorticotropic hormone (ACTH) from the anterior pituitary gland.

GENDER AND LIFE SPAN CONSIDERATIONS

Cushing's syndrome in infants usually results from adrenal carcinoma. Primary disease is often linked to a familial autoimmune disorder and is seen in children and young adults of both genders. Secondary disease is more common than primary disease in children older than 6 or 7 and, as in adults, is usually the result of overproduction of ACTH. In adults, secondary Cushing's syndrome that results from pituitary disease is most common in females aged 30 to 50 years. Secondary Cushing's syndrome that results from increased ACTH secretion is more common in males, possibly because of the higher incidence of bronchogenic carcinoma that is caused by smoking.

☐ ASSESSMENT

HISTORY. Ask if the patient has had recent changes in memory, attention span, or behavior. Discuss the patient's sleep–wake pattern, and evaluate the patient for sleep disturbances. Family members may comment on the patient's changed affect, short-term memory, emotional instability, and ability to concentrate.

Other signs include weakness, fatigue, back pain, general discomfort, difficulty completing activities of daily living, and changes in the urinary output. Be sure to question the patient about weight gain and changes in body proportions between the shoulders. Patients may also notice changes in their appetite and thirst. Other changes in appearance include hirsutism, oily skin, acne, purple striae, and poor wound healing. Women may have noted changes in menstruation, and both men and women may note changes in libido and in their feelings about themselves.

PHYSICAL EXAMINATION. Changes in fat metabolism lead to generalized obesity, a round ("moon") face, a hump in the interscapular area, and truncal obesity. Hyperpigmentation of skin and mucous membranes may be present as a result of increases in ACTH. Because of alterations in protein metabolism, loss of collagen support in the skin leaves the skin more fragile and easily bruised. Both males and females experience changes in secondary sexual characteristics and body hair distribution, along with an increase in acne. Some patients have peripheral edema from water and sodium retention. Muscle wasting, especially in extremities, leads to difficulty in getting up and down from a sitting position, difficulty in climbing stairs, or generalized weakness and fatigue. Note if the extremities are thin with atrophied muscles.

Auscultate the patient's blood pressure; most patients are hypertensive because of increased circulating volume or increased sensitivity of the arterioles to circulating catecholamines. Neck vein distension may be present.

PSYCHOSOCIAL. A diagnosis of Cushing's syndrome can be devastating. Determine the patient's response to the disease and the effect the disease has had on the patient's sexuality, body image, and relationships with others.

DIAGNOSTIC HIGHLIGHTS

General Comments: Abnormal blood chemistries are common, including hypokalemia, hypochloremia, and metabolic alkalosis because of increased excretion of potassium and chloride. Random cortical tests are not useful for diagnosis because of the wide range of normal values.

Test	Normal Result	Abnormality with Condition	Explanation
Overnight dexamethasone suppression test: 1 mg dexamethasone given po at 11 PM; plasma cortisol levels are measured at 8 AM the next morning	Plasma cortisol level (5 μg/dL	Elevated above 5 μg/dL	Failure to suppress normal cortisol response is diagnostic of Cushing's syndrome; abnormal results indicate need for low-dose dexamathasone suppression test
Low-dose dexamathasone suppression test; .5 mg dexamethasone given po q 6 hours for 48 hours	Urine cortisol (20 μg/dL for 24 hours	Elevated above 20 μg/dL for 24 hours	Failure to suppress normal cortisol response is diagnostic of Cushing's syndrome; testing should not be done during severe illness or depression, which may lead to false positive results; phenytoid therapy alters dexamethasone metabolism and may lead to false results

Other Tests: Complete blood count (CBC), serum ACTH, computed tomography (CT) scan, ultrasound, and angiogram

PRIMARY NURSING DIAGNOSIS

Fluid volume excess related to abnormal retention of sodium and water

OUTCOMES. Fluid balance; Hydration; Nutrition management; Nutrition therapy; Knowledge: Treatment regime

INTERVENTIONS. Fluid and electrolyte management; Fluid monitoring; Medication administration

☐ PLANNING AND IMPLEMENTATION

Collaborative

The main focus is to find the primary cause of the cortisol excess and remove it if possible. In the case of iatrogenic Cushing's syndrome, care is focused on alleviating as many of the signs and symptoms as possible when the therapy cannot be discontinued. If the patient has primary Cushing's syndrome from an adrenal tumor, the tumor is removed surgically. Even if the tumor is unilateral, the patient is treated for adrenal insufficiency after the surgery because the high levels of cortisol from the tumor may have caused the unaffected adrenal gland to atrophy. Patients with adrenal carcinoma are treated postoperatively with mitotane to treat metastases. Throughout the patient's recovery, fluid, electrolyte, and nutritional assessment and balance are essential.

For secondary Cushing's syndrome from a pituitary tumor, the preferred option is a transsphenoidal adenectomy, a procedure that explores the pituitary gland to find microadenomas. It is successful in from 20% to 70% of patients. A second option is the transsphenoidal hypophysectomy, a procedure that removes the entire pituitary gland and leads to a cure in 100% of the patients. It is usually used for more invasive tumors and requires lifelong hormone replacement (glucocorticoids, thyroid hormone, gonadal steroids, and antidiuretic hormone [ADH]). A third alternative is bilateral total adrenalectomy, which cures the signs and symptoms of excess cortisol but does not decrease ACTH secretion. The patient requires lifelong replacement therapy with glucocorticoids and mineralocorticoids. If the patient has secondary Cushing's syndrome because of ectopic production of ACTH from a non-endocrine tumor, the first concern is to remove the source of the ectopic secretion of ACTH. If this is not possible, mitotane (See Pharmacologic Highlights) decreases cortisol production in the adrenal gland but may cause damage to the gland and is used with caution. Radiation therapy is used when the patient has either no defined tumor or needs an adjunct to tumor removal.

POSTOPERATIVE. Patients with pituitary surgery need careful management of airway, breathing, and circulation. In the first postoperative hours, serial neurological examinations are important to identify the risk for increased intracranial pressure from edema. The incision is generally performed through the upper gum line; ask the surgeon about the procedure for oral hygiene. Nasal packing is removed after 2 days in most patients. At that time, observe for rhinorrhea and ask the patient to report a "runny" nose. Teach the patient to avoid coughing, sneezing, or blowing the nose immediately after surgery.

PHARMACOLOGIC HIGHLIGHTS

Medication or Drug Class	Dosage	Description	Rationale
Mitotane	2–16 g per day in divided doses po	Antineoplastic	Inhibits activity of adrenal cortex; used to treat inoperable adrenocortical carcinomas and Cushing's syndrome
Cyproheptadine	4 mg 2–3 times a day po	Antihistamine; serotonin antagonist	Inhibits the release of ACTH from pituitary gland; drug is considered last resort and often causes no improvement.

Other Drugs: Aminoglutethimide inhibits cholesterol synthesis, and metyrapone partially inhibits adrenal cortex steroid synthesis. These drugs may be used in conjunction with surgery or radiation if the tumor is not completely resectable or if complete remission is not expected.

Independent

An important goal is to limit the risk of infection for the patient. Note, document, and report any signs of skin or pulmonary infection. Restrict visitors with upper respiratory infections. Unless contraindicated after surgery, encourage the patient to cough and deep-breathe, turn in bed at least every 2 hours, and use good oral hygiene.

Focus on helping the patient deal with changes in body image, sexuality, and self-esteem. Let the patient know that many of the body changes are reversible with treatment; this information allows the patient to focus on setting goals. Include the patient's partner in all education. Patient and family teaching occurs throughout the patient's hospitalization and after discharge. Provide information about patient care and activity restrictions. Explanation of all diagnostic tests and their findings, as well as the treatment plan, are important. The patient and family often require time to consider treatment options. As time progresses, the patient and family need information about the disease process and lifelong management with medication and diet changes.

DOCUMENTATION GUIDELINES

- Physical response: Vital signs, neurological assessment, cardiopulmonary assessment, wound healing, signs of infection (fever, wound drainage, productive cough), important laboratory deviations (serious electrolyte imbalances, alterations in glucose levels)
- Nutrition: Daily weights, appetite, food tolerance, food preference, response to diet teaching, calorie count if indicated
- Emotional response: Concerns over body image, self-concept, mood, affect

DISCHARGE AND HOME HEALTHCARE GUIDELINES

Describe the pathophysiology of the disease. Identify factors that aggravate the disease (stress, changes in diet, injury), as well as the signs and symptoms. Explore complications of the disease, and ask whom to notify if they occur. Describe the treatment plan and expected effects, as well as possible complications. Describe all medications, including the name, dosage, action, side effects, route, and importance of lifelong dosing if indicated.

Cystic Fibrosis

DRG Category: 296
Mean LOS: 5.4 days
Description: MEDICAL: Nutritional and Miscellaneous Metabolic Disorders, Age > 17 with CC

Cystic fibrosis (CF) is a multisystem genetic disease of the exocrine glands—those glands with ducts such as the mucous, salivary, and sweat-producing glands. CF, originally called CF of the pancreas, is also associated with the glands of the respiratory system and the skin, and it has the potential for multiple organ involvement. The lungs are most frequently affected, but the gastrointestinal (GI) tract (including the small intestine and pancreatic and bile ducts) and eventually the reproductive organs are affected, as well.

CF leads to an increase in viscosity of bronchial and pancreatic secretions, which obstruct the glandular ducts. As thick secretions block the bronchioles and alveoli, the patient develops severe atelectasis (lung collapse) and emphysema. The GI effects of the disease lead to deficiency in the enzymes trypsin, amylase, and lipase. With enzyme deficiency, the conversion and absorption of fats and proteins are altered, and vitamins A, D, E, and K are not properly absorbed. Pancreatic changes include fibrosis, cyst formation, and the development of fatty deposits that lead to pancreatic insufficiency and decreased insulin production. Intelligence and cognitive function are typically not affected.

Complications of CF can be life-threatening. Respiratory complications include lung collapse, pneumothorax, airway collapse, and pneumonia. GI complications include dehydration, malnutrition, gastroesophageal reflux, and rectal prolapse.

CAUSES

The responsible gene, the CF transmembrane conductance regulator (CFTR), is mapped to chromosome 7. The underlying defect of this autosomal recessive condition involves a defective protein that interferes with chloride transport, which, in turn, makes the body's secretions very thick and tenacious. The ducts of the exocrine glands subsequently become obstructed.

GENDER AND LIFE SPAN CONSIDERATIONS

More than 25,000 Americans have CF, and 850 new cases are diagnosed annually in this country. CF is the most common fatal genetic disease of European-American children. Life expectancy has improved, however, and now many CF patients live until their late 20s or early 30s. Adolescence tends to exacerbate the symptoms, and it is often during this period that the number of hospitalizations to treat a pneumonia or "clean out" the lungs increases significantly. During adolescence the progression of the disease is manifested in delayed menses, delayed development of secondary sex characteristics, and decreased fertility as a result of the thickened cervical mucus in females. In the event the female patient does conceive, the pregnancy is even more difficult to maintain as a result of the stress on the already taxed respiratory and cardiac systems of the CF patient. Sterility is also likely in 99% of males, as the vas deferens is obstructed, preventing sperm from entering the semen. In about 3% of the cases, diabetes mellitus occurs and these children or young adults are insulin-dependent. There is no cure for CF.

□ ASSESSMENT

HISTORY. CF has a highly variable presentation and course, ranging from mild to severe. Parents often report that the child's skin has a characteristic taste of salt when they kiss the child. Hence, this classic early symptom is referred to as the "kiss of salt." In addition, during the first year or two of life, the child experiences repeated upper respiratory infections such as nasopharyngitis, croup, bronchiolitis, and pneumonia. Although the child has a voracious appetite, he or she does not gain weight and has steatorrhea (frequent foul-smelling, fatty stools). Moreover, the child may not achieve developmental milestones, particularly in the area of gross motor skills.

PHYSICAL EXAMINATION. The newborn may have a meconium ileus; this finding occurs in about 10% to 15% of the newly diagnosed cases. The infant or child may be classified as exhibiting organic failure to thrive and may fall below the 10th percentile. Early in the disease, the lungs have many adventitious breath sounds, such as rales, rhonchi, and wheezes. The anterior posterior to lateral diameter begins to increase as the disease progresses so that the child appears barrel-chested. Clubbing of the nails is indicative of advanced progression of the disease and may be noted in a toddler or a preschooler who has a severe form of the disease.

PSYCHOSOCIAL. Children or adolescents with CF deal with a chronic illness that makes them unique from their peers. They need to feel as if they have a degree of control in their lives; this need may be manifested in refusing to take their enzymes with their meals or their insulin if they become diabetic. Body image is especially critical because of their short stature and small body structure. Many adolescents are embarrassed and try to cover up a protuberant abdomen with baggy clothing and large shirts or to disguise the clubbing of their nails with dark nail polish. In addition, the patients often learn early to achieve a sense of competency by performing well in their academics or becoming computer "wizards," because they are unable to compete in sports.

DIAGNOSTIC HIGHLIGHTS

General Comments: Prenatal and genetic tests are performed to identify fetal disease and carrier status. Failure to thrive and frequent upper respiratory infections often lead to diagnostic testing to confirm the CF diagnosis.

Test	Normal Result	Abnormality with Condition	Explanation
Quantitative sweat electrolyte test (pilocarpine iontophoresis)	Cl, <40 mEq/L	>60 mEq/L (40–60 mEq/L is highly suggestive)	Almost all patients with CF have increased chloride and sodium in their sweat

	Na, <70 mEq/L	>90 mEq/L (70–90 mEq/L is highly suggestive)	
Deoxyribonucleic acid (DNA)	Delta 508 deletion not detected	Presence of Delta 508 deletion	This genetic alteration is found in 70% of all CF chromosomes

Other Tests: serum electrolytes, sputum analysis, chest x ray, arterial blood gases, and pulmonary function tests.

PRIMARY NURSING DIAGNOSIS

Ineffective airway clearance related to excess tenacious mucus

OUTCOMES. Respiratory status: Airway patency; Respiratory status: Gas exchange; Respiratory status: Ventilation; Infection control

INTERVENTIONS. Chest physiotherapy; Positioning; Airway management; Surveillance

☐ PLANNING AND IMPLEMENTATION

Collaborative

The major goals of treatment are to improve pulmonary, gastrointestinal, and pancreatic status. These goals are achieved through a combination of medications, nutrition, and exercise regimens. If antibiotics are given to prevent and treat pneumonia, the physician and pharmacist monitor therapeutic blood levels of the antibiotics to determine the peak and trough levels. To help prevent the recurrence of pneumonia, chest physiotherapy (CPT) is performed in the home or hospital four times a day before meals to avoid emesis or after an aerosol treatment. A ThAIRapy vest, a device that provides high-frequency chest wall oscillations to loosen secretions, may also be used.

Maintain calorie counts on daily meal plans; supplement nutritional needs with high-calorie feedings. A patient may also have nasogastric feedings to which pancreatic enzymes are added to ensure the digestion and absorption of fats, protein, and carbohydrates. The physician may also prescribe total parenteral nutrition and fat soluble vitamins (A, D, E, and K).

Regular exercise, including mobility and muscle-strengthening exercises should be encouraged on a regular basis. Exercise helps maintain physical wellness and supplements the patient's airway clearance strategies by helping to loosen pulmonary secretions.

Some patients develop right-sided heart failure, and if this occurs, most of them die within a year. They may require the use of home portable oxygen therapy and receive digoxin and/or diuretics. As the disease progresses toward the terminal phase, hemoptysis is present and cyanosis is markedly apparent.

PHARMACOLOGIC HIGHLIGHTS

Medication or Drug Class	Dosage	Description	Rationale
Ibuprofen	High doses	NSAID	Reduces inflammation that causes damage to lung tissue; slows lung deterioration
Trimethoprin sulfamethoxazole (Bactrim DS); t obramycin; clindamycin; piperacillin; other aerosol antibiotics	Depends on drug and patient	Antibiotic	Prevent and treat lung infections
Dornase alfa recombinant	2.5 mg inhaled once daily using a recommended nebulizer	Enzyme	Breaks down the DNA from neutrophils, loosening secretions
Pancrelipase; Lipase	0.7 g of powder with meals	Digestant	Aids in digestion of fats and proteins

Experimental Therapies: New peptide antibiotics (PA-1420, IB-357, IB-367, and SMAP-29) are being investigated as treatment for resistant bacteria. Gene and lung transplants are also being studied, and families should be informed of these options.

Independent

Educate to reinforce the importance of regular CPT and expectoration of the mucus. Encourage increased fluid intake to loosen the secretions, and provide frequent mouth care before meals. Teach the parents not to offer cough suppressants, which can lead to obstruction, lung collapse, and infection.

Support the child's or adolescent's body image concerns; compliment the patient on his or her strengths. Encourage the child to develop in as many areas as possible. Very often other CF patients become a significant support group as the child matures. The child is always dramatically affected when another peer with CF dies. Plan group discussions with the patients and have a psychiatric nurse clinical specialist serve as facilitator of this grief work for both patients and staff. In addition, siblings often worry that they may contract the disease or they may exhibit feelings of jealousy of the attention given to the sibling with CF. A referral to a social worker or the Cystic Fibrosis Foundation may be needed.

Counsel couples on the risk that subsequent pregnancies may result in a child with CF, since there is a one in four chance with any pregnancy that a child could have CF if both parents are carriers. Discuss the role of amniocentesis and the difficult issues surrounding terminating a pregnancy if CF is confirmed prenatally.

DOCUMENTATION GUIDELINES

- Physical response: Pulmonary assessment; color, odor, character of mucus; cardiac and GI assessment; pulse oximetry
- Nutritional data: Weight, use of enzymes, adherence to supplemental feedings

- Emotional response: Patient's feelings about dealing with a chronic illness, patient's body image, parents' coping ability, siblings' response

DISCHARGE AND HOME HEALTHCARE GUIDELINES

Teach the patient and family how to prevent future episodes of pneumonia through CPT, expectoration of sputum, and avoidance of peers with common colds and nasopharyngitis. Explain that medications need to be taken at the time of each meal, especially pancreatic enzymes and supplemental vitamins. Teach the parents protocols for home IV care, as needed. Teach parents when to contact the physician: when temperature is elevated over 100.5°F, sputum has color to it, or the child complains of increased lung congestion or abdominal pain. Also educate parents on the need to keep routine follow-up appointments for medication, laboratory, and general checkups. Teach the patient or parents proper insulin administration and the appropriate signs and symptoms of high and low glucose levels.

Cystitis

DRG Category: 320
Mean LOS: 5.9 days
Description: MEDICAL: Kidney and Urinary Tract Infections, Age > 17 with CC

Cystitis is an inflammation of the bladder wall, which may be acute or chronic. It is generally accepted to be an ascending infection, with entry of the pathogen via the urethral opening. Noninfectious cystitis is referred to as interstitial cystitis (IC), but this is a poorly understood disorder with an uncertain cause. In this condition, in spite of symptoms of cystitis, the urine is sterile. The person develops a decreased bladder capacity, possibly because of healing of bladder ulcers (called Hunner's ulcer) that leave behind scar tissue. If IC is associated with chemical agents that lead to bleeding, it is termed hemorrhagic cystitis; otherwise, IC may also be termed painful bladder disease (PBD).

Although cystitis occurs in both men and women, the incidence in women is significantly higher. Sexually active women have fifty times more cystitis than men in general. Females are more susceptible to cystitis because of their short urethra, which is 1 to 2 inches long, as compared to the male urethra, which is 7 to 8 inches in length. The placement of the female urethra, which is closer to the anus than is the male urethra, increases the risk of infection from bacteria in the stool.

CAUSES

The most common pathogen that leads to bladder infection is *Escherichia coli,* which accounts for about 80% of cases of cystitis. Predisposing factors are urethral damage from childbirth, catheterization, or surgery; decreased frequency of urination; other medical conditions such as diabetes mellitus; and, in women, frequent sexual activity and some forms of contraceptives (poorly fitting diaphragms, use of spermicides).

The cause of IC is unknown but has been linked to chemical agents such as some medications (cyclophosphamide) and radiation therapy. Some experts suggest that PBD is an autoimmune response.

GENDER AND LIFE SPAN CONSIDERATIONS

Cystitis is uncommon in young children and teenagers. Pregnancy increases the risk of infection because of hormonal changes in women and because the enlarging uterus restricts the flow of urine and creates urinary stasis and bacteria proliferation. Men, on the other hand, secrete prostatic fluid that serves as an antibacterial defense. As men age past 50, however, the prostate gland enlarges, which increases the risk for urinary retention and infection. As women age, vaginal flora and lubrication change; decreased lubrication increases the risk of urethral irritation in women during intercourse. By age 70, prevalence is similar for men and women.

IC occurs primarily in women. Although at one time IC was considered a disease of menopause, experts note that it is most common in middle-aged women.

◻ ASSESSMENT

HISTORY. Question the patient with cystitis about the presence of urinary symptoms, including frequency, urgency, pain, a sensation of incomplete emptying of the bladder, and possibly blood or pus in the urine. The patient may have a low-grade fever but generally does not have other systemic symptoms. Consider the patient's previous history of urinary infections, vaginal discharge, chronic conditions such as diabetes mellitus or neurologic problems, and recent sexual activity. Ask if the patient has experienced severe lower abdominal or pelvic pain, nocturia, urinary urgency, and excessive (up to 60 times a day) urinary frequency. Some women describe dyspareunia (painful sexual intercourse).

PHYSICAL EXAMINATION. Generally, the physical examination is unremarkable. Examine the patient to determine the presence of abdominal pain or costovertebral angle tenderness, which may indicate pyelonephritis. The examination should include surveillance for sexually transmitted diseases (STDs).

PSYCHOSOCIAL. Cystitis is typically an acute illness with rapid response to prescribed therapy. The patient usually does not experience a disruption of normal activity. Women with IC, however, need to learn to manage not only a chronic disease but also one that physicians may have either ignored, labeled as "psychosomatic," or related to hormonal changes that occur during menopause.

DIAGNOSTIC HIGHLIGHTS

Test	Normal Result	Abnormality with Condition	Explanation
Urine dip	Negative	Positive (purple shade)	Presence of leukocyte esterase indicates UTI; 90% accurate in detecting WBCs in the urine
Urine culture and sensitivity	<10,000 bacteria/mL	> 10,000 bacteria/mL or >100 in acutely symptomatic patients	Identifies causative organism; determines appropriate antibiotic

Urinalysis	WBC 0–4; RBC ≤2; nitrites-none; PH 4.6–8.0; crystals-none; Clear, aromatic	Increased WBC, RBC, pH, nitrites, crystals, cloudy, odor present	The presence of bacteria in the urine is indicated by several changes noted in a UA

Other Tests: In severe or recurrent cases of cystitis, an intravenous pyelogram, voiding cystourethrogram, retrograde pyelogram, or cystoscopy could be done to discover factors contributing to cystitis. Urodynamic evaluation, cystoscopy, and a bladder biopsy may be performed to diagnose IC.

PRIMARY NURSING DIAGNOSIS

Altered urinary elimination related to irritation of bladder mucosa

OUTCOMES. Urinary elimination; Knowledge: Medication, Symptom control

INTERVENTIONS. Medication prescribing; Urinary elimination management

☐ PLANNING AND IMPLEMENTATION

Collaborative

An acid-ash diet may be encouraged. A diet of meats, eggs, cheese, prunes, cranberries, plums, and whole grains can increase the acidity of the urine. Foods not allowed on this diet include carbonated beverages, anything containing baking soda or powder, fruits other than those previously stated, all vegetables except corn and lentils, and milk and milk products. The action of some medications used to treat urinary tract infections (UTI) is diminished by acidic urine (nitrofurantoin); thus review prescriptions before giving patients this diet.

Bacterial cystitis is usually treated with a 7- to 10-day course of antibiotics. Shortened and large single-dose regimens are currently under investigation. Most elderly patients need a full 7- to 10-day treatment, although caution is used in their management because of possible diminished renal capacity. Reinforce the need for patients to complete the therapy. Inform women of the possibility of developing a vaginal yeast infection during therapy, and review preventive measures.

PHARMACOLOGIC HIGHLIGHTS

General Comments: Antibiotics worsen the symptoms of patients with IC by irritating the bladder. The treatment of IC is controversial, and no single treatment is accepted as best. Commonly used medications include anti-inflammatories, antispasmodics, tricyclic antidepressants, and antihistamines, which are used with varying success. Other treatments include instillations of preparations such as sodium oxychlorosene (Clorpactin), silver nitrate, and dimethyl sulfoxide (DMSO) directly in the bladder to promote healing and relief of pain. Sodium pentosan polysulfate (Elmiron) is used orally to create a protective mucin layer in the bladder.

Medication or Drug Class	Dosage	Description	Rationale
Cephalexin monohydrate (Keflex)	250 mg–1g po q 6 hours	Antibiotic, first-generation cephalosporin	Bacteriocidal
Sulfisoxazole (Gantrisin)	Initially 2–4g po, then 1–2 g qid for 10–14 days	Anti-infective, sulfonamide	Bacteriocidal
Co-trimoxazole (Bactrim, Septra)	160 mg q 12 hours for 7–14 days	Anti-infective, sulfonamide	Bacteriocidal
Nitrofurantoin (Macrodantin)	50–100 mg po qid for 10–14 days	Urinary antiseptic	Bacteriocidal; concentrates in the urine and kidneys to kill bacteria
Phenazopyridine (Pyridium)	100–200 mg po tid until pain subsides	Urinary analgesic	Relieves pain

Independent

Encourage patients with infections to increase fluid intake to promote frequent urination. Recommend strategies to limit recurrence, such as increasing vitamin C intake, drinking cranberry juice, wiping from front to back after a bowel movement (women), avoiding tub and bubble baths, wearing cotton underwear, and avoiding tight clothing such as jeans.

Patients with IC present a challenge to the nurse because no clear treatment exists for the condition. Provide information about the condition, and validate that the symptoms are indeed shared by many other patients. Listen to the patient's feelings and provide her with a list of national and local resources that can provide further support.

DOCUMENTATION GUIDELINES

- Physical response: Pain, burning on urination, urinary frequency; vital signs; nocturia; color and odor of urine; patient history that may place the patient at risk
- Location, duration, frequency, and severity of pain; response to medications
- Absence of complications such as pyelonephritis

DISCHARGE AND HOME HEALTHCARE GUIDELINES

Explain the proposed therapy, including the medication name, dosage, route, and side effects. Explain the signs and symptoms of complications such as pyelonephritis and the need for follow-up before the patient leaves the setting. Explain the importance of completing the entire course of antibiotics even if symptoms decrease or disappear. Encourage the patient with gastrointestinal discomfort to continue taking the medications with a meal or milk unless contraindicated. Warn the patient that drugs with phenazopyridine turn the urine orange.

Cystocele; Rectocele

DRG Category: 369
Mean LOS: 2.9 days
Description: MEDICAL: Menstrual and Other Female Reproductive System Disorders
DRG Category: 356
Mean LOS: 3.2 days
Description: SURGICAL: Female Reproductive System Reconstructive Procedures

A cystocele is a structural problem of the genitourinary (GU) tract that occurs in women. The urinary bladder presses against a weakened anterior vaginal wall, thus causing the bladder to protrude into the vagina. The weakened vaginal wall is unable to support the weight of urine in the bladder, and this results in incomplete emptying of the bladder and cystitis.

A rectocele is a protrusion of the rectum through the posterior vaginal wall. The rectum presses against a weakened posterior vaginal wall, thus causing the rectal wall to bulge into the vagina. The pressure against the weakened wall is intensified each time the woman strains to have a bowel movement; feces push up against the vaginal wall and intensify the protrusion. Frequently a rectocele is associated with an enterocele, a herniation of the intestine through the cul-de-sac.

CAUSES

The primary cause of cystoceles and rectoceles is a weakened vaginal wall. Factors that contribute to this loss of pelvic muscle tone are repeated pregnancies, especially those spaced close together, congenital weaknesses, and unrepaired childbirth lacerations. Obesity, advanced age, chronic cough, constipation, and occupations that involve much standing and lifting are also contributing factors. Lack of estrogen after menopause frequently aggravates the condition.

GENDER AND LIFE SPAN CONSIDERATIONS

The disorders tend to occur in middle-aged and elderly women who have had children.

☐ ASSESSMENT

HISTORY. Patients with a cystocele often have a history of frequent and urgent urination, frequent urinary tract infections, difficulty emptying the bladder, and stress. Ask about the pattern and extent of incontinence: Does incontinence occur during times of stress, such as laughing and sneezing? Is it a constant, slow seepage? Is the amount such that the patient needs to use a peripad or adult diaper?

Patients with a rectocele have a history of constipation, hemorrhoids, pressure sensations, and difficulty controlling and evacuating the bowel. Obstetric history often reveals a forceps delivery. Some report that they are able to facilitate a bowel movement by applying digital pressure along the posterior vaginal wall when defecating to prevent the rectocele from protruding.

PHYSICAL EXAMINATION. Upon inspection, the bulging of the bladder and/or rectum may be visualized when the patient is asked to bear down. This bulge may also be palpated. In addition, inspect the patient for hemorrhoids.

PSYCHOSOCIAL. Assess feelings regarding stress incontinence and the patient's knowledge of the problem. Explore the effects on the patient's social life, ability to travel, ability to meet occupational demands, and sexual function.

DIAGNOSTIC HIGHLIGHTS

General Comments: No specific laboratory tests are indicated unless the patient has the symptoms of a urinary tract infection.

Test	Normal Result	Abnormality with Condition	Explanation
Bimanual exam	No bulging or protrusions felt along anterior or posterior vaginal walls	Bulging of anterior vaginal wall felt with cystocele; bulging of posterior vaginal wall felt with rectocele	Cystocles and rectoceles result in prominent protrusions into the vaginal canal

PRIMARY NURSING DIAGNOSIS

Altered urinary elimination

OUTCOMES. Urinary continence; Knowledge: Treatment regimen; Symptom control; Muscle function

INTERVENTIONS. Urinary incontinence care

☐ PLANNING AND IMPLEMENTATION

Collaborative

Mild symptoms of a cystocele may be relieved by Kegel exercises to strengthen the pelvic musculature. If the patient is postmenopausal, estrogen therapy may be initiated to prevent further atrophy of the vaginal wall. Sometimes the bladder can be supported by use of a pessary, a device worn in the vagina that exerts pressure on the bladder neck area to support the bladder. When the symptoms of cystoceles and rectoceles are severe, surgical intervention is indicated. For a cystocele, an anterior colporrhaphy (or anterior repair), which sutures the pubocervical fascia to support the bladder and urethra, is done. A posterior colporrhaphy (or posterior repair), which sutures the fascia and perineal muscles to support the perineum and rectum, is performed to correct a rectocele.

Preoperative care specifically for posterior repairs includes giving laxatives and enemas to reduce bowel contents. Postoperatively monitor the patient's vaginal discharge, which should be minimal, as well as the patient's pain level and response to analgesics. Sitz baths may be used for comfort. In an anterior repair, an indwelling urethral catheter is inserted and left in place for approximately 4 days. Encourage fluid intake to assure adequate urine formation. After a posterior repair, stool softeners and low-residue diets are often given to prevent strain on the incision when defecating.

PHARMACOLOGIC HIGHLIGHTS

Medication or Drug Class	Dosage	Description	Rationale
Stool softeners; laxatives	Varies with drug	Drug depends on patient and physician preference	Assist with bowel movement in patients with rectocele
Antibiotics	Varies with drug	Broad spectrum antibiotic	Prophylaxis for infection related to surgery
Non-salicylates; opiod analgesics	Varies with drug	Analgesics	Maintain comfort related to mild preoperative pain and more severe postoperative discomfort

Independent

Preventive measures include teaching the patient to do Kegel exercises 100 times a day for life to maintain the tone of the pubococcygeal muscle. If the patient has symptoms that are managed conservatively, teach the patient the use of a pessary—how to clean and store it; how to prevent infections—and to report any complications that may be associated with pessary use, including discomfort, leukorrhea, or vaginal irritation. Answer questions about treatment options, and explain the procedures and possible complications.

Listen to the patient's and her partner's concerns and assist them in decision making about care. For additional support, have the patient speak to others who have undergone similar treatments.

DOCUMENTATION GUIDELINES

- Level of comfort and response to pain medication
- Physical response: Fluid intake and output, urinary continence, ability to have a bowel movement, amount and type of vaginal discharge
- Presence of complications: Bleeding, inability to urinate after urethral catheter is removed, infection

DISCHARGE AND HOME HEALTHCARE GUIDELINES

MEDICATIONS. Instruct the patient on all medications, including the dosage, route, action, and adverse effects.

COMPLICATIONS OF SURGERY. Instruct the patient to notify the physician if signs of infection or increased vaginal bleeding are noted.

PATIENT TEACHING. Instruct the patient to avoid enemas, heavy lifting, prolonged standing, and sexual intercourse for approximately 6 weeks. Note that it is normal to have some loss of vaginal sensation for several months. Emphasize the importance of keeping follow-up visits.

Cytomegalovirus Infection

DRG Category: 421
Mean LOS: 4.0 days
Description: MEDICAL: Viral Illness, Age > 17

Cytomegalovirus (CMV) is a member of the herpes simplex virus group. The virus, transmitted by human contact, results in an infection so mild that it is usually overlooked because no symptoms are present. Approximately 80% of the general population experience a CMV infection by the time they reach middle age. Imunosuppressed patients, however, particularly patients who have received transplanted organs, are highly susceptible to CMV, with estimates as high as 90% of such patients contracting CMV infection. CMV infection is present in at least 80% of patients with AIDS, causing serious problems such as encephalitis, retinitis, pneumonia, and esophagitis in 30% of them.

The virus generally inhabits the salivary glands in a latent infection that is reactivated by pregnancy, blood transfusions, or immunosuppressive medications. Benign in people with normal immune systems, the virus can be devastating to an unborn fetus or a person with immunosuppression. The virus is spread throughout the body by the white blood cells (lymphocytes and mononuclear cells) to organs such as the liver, lungs, gastrointestinal (GI) tract, and central nervous system (CNS), leading to cellular inflammation and possibly organ dysfunction.

CAUSES

CMV is transmitted by contact with the fluids that contain the virus, such as saliva, urine, breast milk, cervical mucus, and semen. It can be transmitted during pregnancy from a primary or reactivated CMV infection. It can be transmitted during delivery from contact with cervical secretions or after delivery in the breast milk. The virus may be present for years after the primary infection.

GENDER AND LIFE SPAN CONSIDERATIONS

Fetuses and infants are at particular risk. Infection of the fetus by CMV may not be recognized until birth or several years after birth because pregnant women with CMV infections may not have clinical symptoms. Infants who have been infected with CMV during gestation may have intrauterine growth retardation, microcephaly (small head size), or hydrocephaly (increased cerebrospinal fluid in the brain). In adults, CMV may be serious and can cause blindness or a mononucleosis-type infection. CMV mononucleosis is the most common form of CMV infection, and it occurs at about 25 to 30 years of age. In adults with no immunosuppression difficulties, the risk of infection increases with age. Of adults over the age of 40, 50% have antibodies to CMV, but most do not have a history of infection.

◻ ASSESSMENT

HISTORY. Ask about immunosuppressive conditions such as recent traumatic injury that may have required multiple blood transfusions, organ transplantation, or HIV infection. The patient may describe a recent viral infection with symptoms such as sore throat, tiredness, joint and muscle aches, and headache. Some patients will remember an episode that lasted approximately 3 weeks with high fevers as the only symptom. In an immunosuppressed patient, there may be specific organ involvement, such as the lungs (dry cough, difficulty breathing), the GI tract (watery diarrhea, bloody diarrhea, nausea, vomiting, and cramping), and the CNS (blurred vision, headache, neck rigidity, tremors, lethargy, and even seizures and coma).

PHYSICAL EXAMINATION. Infants may show signs of delayed development and may show signs of jaundice, petechial rash, respiratory distress, and hearing loss.

With adults, assess all body systems, but the most severe signs and symptoms occur with CNS or liver involvement. Evaluate patients for signs of fever, pallor, changes in the lymph node tissue, and pharyngitis. Auscultate the patient's lungs to assess for crackles. Note decreased breath sounds, cough, shortness of breath, and symptoms of pneumonia.

Patients may also have mental status changes such as irritability, lethargy, and even seizures and coma. Patients may evidence hyperactive bowel sounds, tenderness to palpation of the stomach, and possible distension. Assess for neck rigidity, pupil changes, motor weakness, positive Babinski reflex, and tremors. Perform an eye exam to identify changes in the eye grounds, initially with small, white, cotton-wool spots with irregular borders on the retina that enlarge to fluffy white exudates and visible hemorrhages, causing vision loss progressing to blindness.

PSYCHOSOCIAL. Assess the patient's or his or her parents' ability to cope. The unborn child's mother and father will need counseling and support to deal with the possible effects of CMV on their unborn infant.

DIAGNOSTIC HIGHLIGHTS

General Comments: A viral culture is the most sensitive diagnostic laboratory procedure. Cultures however, take 3 to 7 days and cannot differentiate acute from chronic infection.

Test	Normal Result	Abnormality with Condition	Explanation
Culture of the urine, sputum, or mouth swab	Virus not isolated	Virus isolated	Presence of virus confirms the diagnosis
IgM antibodies	Antibodies not present	CMV antibodies present	Indicates a recent infection

Other Tests: Virus isolation of samples from cervix, semen, breast milk, white blood cells, and biopsy specimens.

PRIMARY NURSING DIAGNOSIS

Risk for infection (spread or reactivation) related to immune suppression

OUTCOMES. Risk control; Treatment behavior: Illness or injury; Risk detection

INTERVENTIONS. Infection protection; Medication prescribing

☐ PLANNING AND IMPLEMENTATION

Collaborative

INFANTS. Infants with congenital abnormalities require careful monitoring of growth and developmental patterns throughout infancy. Parents may need referrals for information on special education, physical therapy, and social services.

ADULTS. Treatment focuses on preventing complications and relieving symptoms; treatment varies depending on the type and degree of infection. Patients with a generalized infection receive antipyretics for fever and analgesics for aching and sore throat. Such patients need rest, good nutrition, and adequate fluid intake for chronic fatigue. Other, more severe infections, are usually treated with antiviral medications. The amount and duration of medication depend on the severity of the infection. Organ system complications are managed based on the symptoms.

PHARMACOLOGIC HIGHLIGHTS

Medication or Drug Class	Dosage	Description	Rationale
Ganciclovir	5 mg/kg q 12 hours of IV for 14– 21 days, then 5 mg/kg q day for 7 days, then 1000 mg po tid	Antiviral	Inhibits DNA production in CMV
Foscarnet	60 mg/kg q 8 hours or 90 mg/kg q 12 hours for 2–3 weeks, then 90–120 mg/kg per day of IV	Antiviral	Inhibits replication of virus

Independent

Important priorities are to maintain an adequate level of functioning, prevent complications, support the recuperative process, and provide information about the disease process, prognosis, and treatment. Patients, and caregivers in the case of infants, need to be educated about decreasing the risk of spreading CMV infection. Secretions, particularly in infants, are apt to contain the virus.

Families of infants with CMV infection will need emotional support. Answer questions about CMV infection, symptoms, complications, and treatment.

Teach adult patients about the CMV infection, the need for adequate rest, exercise, good nutrition, and fluid intake.

DOCUMENTATION GUIDELINES

- Physical changes, such as enlarged lymph nodes, GI symptoms, pulmonary symptoms, fundascopic abnormalities
- Response to medications and treatments
- Complications, resistance, recurrence of symptoms

DISCHARGE AND HOME HEALTHCARE GUIDELINES

PREVENTION. Teach the patient's caregiver to handle diapers carefully, washing hands to prevent the spread of CMV. In the hospital, universal precautions are needed for women of childbearing potential. Frequent fundascopic examinations are imperative in HIV-positive and AIDS patients. Female healthcare workers who are attempting pregnancy may wish to have CMV titers drawn to identify their risk for the disease. Pregnant women working in daycare centers or hospital nurseries need to avoid caring for infected infants and to use universal precautions.

MEDICATIONS. Teach the patient information about the prescribed dosage, route, action, and follow-up laboratory work needed for all medications. Teach the patient the appropriate use of antipyretics for fever and analgesics for pain and discomfort.

COMPLICATIONS. Inform the patient that signs of a relapse or complications may occur after an initial improvement. The patient should be instructed to report visual changes; changes in GI function, such as weight loss, nausea, vomiting, and anorexia; continued fever; and pulmonary symptoms (cough, shortness of breath, chest tightness). If these complications occur, teach the patient to seek medical attention.

Degenerative Joint Disease (DJD)

DRG Category: 244
Mean LOS: 4.9 days
Description: MEDICAL: Bone Disease and Specific Arthropathies with CC
DRG Category: 209
Mean LOS: 7.7 days
Description: SURGICAL: Major Joint and Limb Reattachment Procedure of Lower Extremity
DRG Category: 471
Mean LOS: 9.4 days
Description: SURGICAL: Bilateral or Multiple Major Joint Procedures of Lower Extremity

Degenerative joint disease (DJD), or osteoarthritis, is a nonsystemic, noninflammatory, progressive disorder of movable joints that is associated with aging and accumulated trauma. It is characterized by ulceration of articular cartilage that leaves the underlying bone exposed. Irritation of the perichondrium (membrane of fibrous connective tissue around the surface of cartilage) and periosteum (the fibrous membrane that forms the covering of bones except at their articular surfaces) causes proliferation of cells at the joint margins. Extensive hypertrophic changes produce bony outgrowths or spur formation that expand into the joint, causing considerable pain and limited joint movement when they rub against each other.

Primary DJD can occur unilaterally in one or more joints and is usually associated with wear and tear of the hand, wrist, hip, and knee joints. Secondary DJD is related to trauma in one or two joints, particularly the knees. The major weight-bearing, cervical spine, and distal interphalangeal joints are most often affected. The course of the disease is slow and progressive, without exacerbations and remissions. Patients may experience limitations that range from minor finger discomfort to severe disability of the hip or knee joints.

CAUSES

Specific causes of DJD are not known, although some predisposing factors have been identified. Aging, obesity, and familial tendencies are known risk factors. Other risk factors include joint injuries, bleeding into the joint, joint abnormalities, and excessive joint use, as in certain occupations such as high-impact sports, construction work, and dance.

GENDER AND LIFE SPAN CONSIDERATIONS

Symptoms of DJD generally begin after age 40 and are more common in women. Ninety percent of the population over 60 years of age has evidence of some joint degeneration.

☐ ASSESSMENT

HISTORY. Establish a history of deep, aching joint pain or "grating" joint pain during motion. Determine if the pain intensifies after activity and diminishes after rest and which joints are causing discomfort. Ask if the patient is taking medication for pain and, if so, how much and how often. Ask if the patient feels stiff upon awakening. Determine the relationship of the patient's stiffness to activity or inactivity. Ask if the joints ache during weather changes. Establish a history of altered gait contractures and limited movement. Determine whether the patient has had a severe injury in the past or has worked at an occupation that may have put stress on the weight-bearing joints, such as construction work or ballet dancing. Ascertain whether a family history of osteoarthritis exists.

PHYSICAL EXAMINATION. Observe the patient's standing posture and gait. Note any obvious curvature of the spine or shuffling gait, which are indicators of limited joint movement. Note if the patient uses a cane or walker. Determine the patient's ability to flex, hyperextend, and rotate the thoracic and lumbar spine. For a patient with lower back pain, place the patient in a supine position, raise the leg, and have the patient dorsiflex the foot. Intensified pain may indicate a herniated disk; if this occurs, defer the examination and report these findings to the physician. Otherwise, have the patient stand, stabilize the pelvis, and rotate the upper torso 30 degrees to the right and to the left. Support the patient if necessary, and ask her or him to bend over from the waist as far as is comfortable. Then ask the patient to bend backward from the waist. Ask the patient to stand up straight and bend to each side. Note the degree of movement the patient is capable of in each maneuver.

Determine the patient's ability to bend the hips. Do not perform this assessment if the patient has had a hip prosthesis. Ask the patient to stand and extend each leg backward with the knee held straight. Have the patient lie on the back and bring each knee up to the chest. Assess internal and external rotation by having the patient turn the bent knee inward and then outward. Have the patient straighten the leg and then adduct and abduct it. Again, note the degree of movement. Listen for crepitus, and observe for pain while the joint is moving.

If DJD is advanced, flexion and lateral deformities of the distal interphalangeal joints occur. Inspect any nodes for redness, swelling, and tenderness. Observe the patient's hands for deformities, nodules, erythema, swelling, and asymmetry of movement. Grasp the hands and feel for sponginess and warmth. Observe for muscle wasting of the fingers. Ask the patient to extend, dorsiflex, and flex the fingers. Assess for radial and ulnar deviation. Finally, have the patient adduct and abduct the fingers. Ask the patient about the degree of pain during each of these movements.

PSYCHOSOCIAL. If the patient has had the disease for some time, explore how it has affected her or his life and how well he or she is adapting to any lifestyle changes. Many elderly patients look forward to retirement and leisure and become depressed about the prospect of pain and limited movement. Trauma from occupational or accidental injuries leaves many individuals unable to work.

DIAGNOSTIC HIGHLIGHTS

Test	Normal Result	Abnormality with Condition	Explanation
X rays	Normal structure of bones and joints	Joint deformity with deterioration of articular cartilage and formation of reactive new bone at articular surface	Joint disease leads to tissue destruction, scarring, and laying of new bone

Other Tests: Serum calcium, serum albumin, ionized calcium, erythrocyte sedimentation rate, computed tomography (CT) scan, magnetic resonance imaging (MRI), bone scan

PRIMARY NURSING DIAGNOSIS

Pain (chronic) related to joint irritation and destruction

OUTCOMES. Comfort level; Pain control behavior; Pain level; Symptom control behavior; Symptom severity; Well-being

INTERVENTIONS. Pain management; Analgesic administration; Cutaneous stimulation; Heat or cold application; Touch; Exercise therapy; Progressive muscle relaxation

☐ PLANNING AND IMPLEMENTATION

Collaborative

MEDICAL. Initial medical treatment consists of prescribing pharmacologic therapy. An appropriate ongoing exercise program, which includes teaching proper body mechanics, is prescribed by the physical therapist. Therapy may include the use of moist heat in the form of soaks and whirlpools. Hot soaks and paraffin dips may be used to relieve hand pain, and a cervical collar and hand splints may be used for painful joints. A transcutaneous electric nerve stimulator (TENS) may be particularly helpful for vertebral pain relief. The physical therapist teaches the patient to use a walker and cane if indicated. Occasionally, the patient needs to learn to manage activities of daily living in the home with the help of assistive technical aids. If considerable help is required in learning these skills, the occupational therapist becomes part of the team effort.

SURGICAL. Surgical treatment may be undertaken to restore joint function when conservative treatment is ineffective. Patients who are in relatively good physical and mental condition may be candidates for joint reconstructive surgery (arthroplasty). Other surgical procedures include debridement, to remove loose debris within a joint, and osteotomy, which involves cutting the bone to realign the joint and shift the pressure points to a less denuded area of the joint. An osteotomy requires internal fixation with wires, screws, or plates, as well as limited joint movement with restricted weight bearing for a prescribed period of time. Fusion of certain joints (arthrodesis) may be done for the vertebrae and certain smaller joints when other types of procedures have not been successful in eliminating pain. Fusion eliminates movement in the joint and therefore is undertaken as a last resort. Patients who undergo knee replacement surgery are placed on a continuous passive motion machine, which is set to put the patient's leg through an increasing range of motion and thus prevent scar tissue.

PHARMACOLOGIC HIGHLIGHTS

Medication or Drug Class	Dosage	Description	Rationale
Salicylates and nonsteroidal anti-inflammatory drugs (NSAIDs)	Varies by drug	Ibuprofen, piroxicam, fenoprofen, phenylbutazone, indomethicin, propoxyphene, or naproxen, if the patient is intolerant to aspirin	Relieve pain and decrease inflammation
Prednisone	10–150 mg po qd	Corticosteroids	Decreases joint inflammation; used only for severe cases

Independent

Teach the patient assistive techniques to manage joint pain, such as meditation, biofeedback, and distraction. When the pain is reduced and mobility improves, encourage the patient to assume more responsibility for self-care. Recommend a firm mattress or bed board for lumbar and sacral spine pain. Apply moist heat pads to relieve hip pain, and assist with gentle range-of-motion exercises. A total or partial hip replacement requires limited joint movement and restricted weight bearing, depending on the type of prosthesis and surgical approach. Preventing dislocation of the hip prosthesis is extremely important. Keep the patient from lying on the affected side. Place three pillows between the patient's legs while he or she is sleeping and when you turn the patient. Avoid hip flexion. Keep the cradle boot in place, except for a brief period during a bath. Once the patient is allowed up, instruct him or her not to cross the legs while sitting and to avoid wearing shoes and stockings or bending over. After the recovery time is over, teach the patient to wear well-fitting supportive shoes and to replace worn-out heels.

Teach patients who have undergone knee replacement surgery to use a walker or crutches with limited weight bearing. Advise the patient to use special equipment in the home, such as grab bars, shower seats, and elevated toilet seats. Assist the patient in arranging for a home health nurse to visit and evaluate the patient's functioning in the home. Assist the patient in arranging ongoing physical therapy in the home. Assist the patient with activities of daily living, and teach strategies for managing self-care in the home. Teach the patient to carry out therapeutic regimens, including energy conservation. Suggest the use of a firm mattress and straight-back chairs with armrests. Show the patient how to avoid flexion contractures of the large muscle groups while sleeping and sitting. Teach the patient to avoid putting pillows under the legs while sitting and to avoid sitting in low chairs, which can cause hip flexion.

DOCUMENTATION GUIDELINES

- Physical findings: Deformed joints, swollen nodes, location and duration of pain, gait, range of motion
- Response to medication and treatments
- Ability to perform self-care, degree of mobility

DISCHARGE AND HOME MAINTENANCE GUIDELINES

Ensure that the patient understands the need to rest every hour, space work out over several days, and get at least 8 hours of sleep at night. Ensure that the patient knows whom to call in the event of sudden severe pain (as in a subluxation) or general worsening of the existing condition. Determine whether a home care agency needs to evaluate the home for safety equipment, such as rails and grab bars, and whether ongoing supervision is required. Instruct patients on salicylates that they may need periodic laboratory monitoring of liver and kidney functioning and that they should consider drug interactions. Review patient medication regimen for interactions with salicylates. Some drugs that potentially are affected by salicylates include anticoagulants, corticosteroids, NSAIDs, urine acidifiers, furosemide, para-aminobenzoic acid, certain antacids, phenobarbital, methotrexate, sulfonylureas, insulin, beta-adrenergic blockers, spironolactone, and nitroglycerin. Instruct the patient to watch out for the symptoms of bleeding, toxicity, or allergies and to report them to the primary caregiver. Instruct the patient not to take over-the-counter drugs or change the dosage of salicylates without consulting the primary caregiver. Advise the patient to take medications with food or after meals to avoid GI discomfort.

The Arthritis Foundation, which publishes information about arthritis, is engaged in a national education program about living with the condition. Help the patient get in touch with this organization by writing to Arthritis Foundation, 1314 Spring Street N.W., Atlanta, GA 30309.

Diabetes Insipidus

DRG Category: 300
Mean LOS: 6.3 days
Description: MEDICAL: Endocrine Disorders with CC

The disorder diabetes insipidus (DI) is characterized by excretion of large amounts of dilute urine. DI can be of central (neurogenic) or renal (nephrogenic) origin. In central DI, excess urine is caused by insufficient amounts of antidiuretic hormone (ADH, also known as plasma vasopressin). Renal DI occurs when the kidney has a decreased responsiveness to ADH.

Normally, body water balance is partially regulated by ADH, which is produced in the hypothalamus and is released from the posterior pituitary gland when body fluids become more concentrated than usual (serum osmolarity more than 283 mOsm/L). ADH causes water reabsorption in the distal portions of the nephron of the kidney by increasing the number of pores in the distal tubular system to allow for water reabsorption. ADH deficiency leads to little or no reabsorption; as a consequence, dilute urine formed in more proximal parts of the nephron is excreted essentially unchanged. The loss of solute-free water causes mild dehydration, a rise in plasma osmolality, and the stimulation of thirst.

Complications are most likely in patients with decreased mental alertness because their impairment makes it less likely they will drink in response to their stimulated thirst. The most serious complication of untreated DI is hypovolemia that may lead to hyperosmolarity, loss of consciousness, circulatory collapse, shock, and central nervous system (CNS) damage.

CAUSES

Causes of DI include trauma to or surgery of the pituitary gland, neoplasms, vascular changes such as stroke and aneurysm, infection, pregnancy, and unknown reasons. The brain swelling that accompanies anoxic brain death may also lead to DI. In addition, certain drugs (lithium, demeclocycline, methoxyflurane, or amphotericin) or metabolic conditions can induce DI. Approximately 50% of the patients who develop DI have a familial or idiopathic (from unknown causes) form. In addition, congenital DI in neonates occurs as a result of malformation of the CNS.

GENDER AND LIFE SPAN CONSIDERATIONS

DI may occur at any age and in both genders, depending on the underlying cause. Infants and the elderly exhibit more symptoms because they are less able to adjust to changes in fluid status. A temporary form of DI can occur during the fifth or sixth month of pregnancy but usually disappears spontaneously after delivery.

Primary neonatal DI occurs as result of a congenital defect in newborns. In children, DI is most frequently caused by tumors of the hypothalmus (craniopharyngiomas in particular). In children, a history of ocular abnormalities or growth failure can be suggestive of a midbrain tumor that leads to DI. Enuresis (involuntary discharge of urine after a child is toilet-trained), irritability, excessive thirst, and a preference for ice water in children are all signs of DI.

☐ ASSESSMENT

HISTORY. Generally patients with suspected DI complain of excessive urination (polyuria), excessive thirst (polydipsia), and nocturia (excessive urination at night). The onset is often abrupt. Daily urinary output is usually in the 4 to 15 L per day range but can be as high as 30 L per day. Assess the patient for a past history of known causative factors: recent surgery, head trauma, or medication use. The patient may also report a history of weight loss, lightheadedness, weakness, intolerance to activity, and constipation. Parents may notice that children are more irritable than usual and may have sleep disturbances and anorexia.

PHYSICAL EXAMINATION. DI is associated with few physical signs. Except in unusual cases, dehydration is not sufficient to be evident on the physical exam. Look for signs and symptoms of dehydration: decreased tear formation, dry lips and mouth, complaints of excessive thirst, skin tenting, and dizziness. In spite of signs of dehydration, urine is clear or pale yellow and in copious amounts. You may note tachycardia, orthostatic changes in blood pressure, and decreased muscle strength.

PSYCHOSOCIAL. Assess the patient's ability to cope with a chronic illness and the financial resources to manage a chronic illness.

DIAGNOSTIC HIGHLIGHTS

Test	Normal Result	Abnormality with Condition	Explanation
Urine osmolality (osmolality refers to a solution's concentration of solute particles per kilogram of solvent)	200–1200 mOsm/L	< 250 mOsm/L	Excretion of dilute urine in spite of dehydration and hypernatremia due to underproduction of ADH
Blood osmolality	275–285 mOsm/L	> 300 mOsm/L	Water loss in the urine and hypernatremia lead to hemoconcentration; levels above 320 mOsm/L are considered "panic levels" and require immediate intervention
Serum sodium	136–145 mEq/L	> 145 mEq/L	Water loss in the urine leads to hemoconcentration

Other Tests: Urine specific gravity and urine electrolytes

PRIMARY NURSING DIAGNOSIS

Alteration in urinary elimination related to polyuria

OUTCOMES. Urinary elimination; Urinary continence; Knowledge: Disease process, Medication, Treatment regimen, Neurological status, Symptom control behavior, Symptom severity

INTERVENTIONS. Fluid management; Fluid monitoring; Urinary elimination management; Medication prescribing

☐ PLANNING AND IMPLEMENTATION

Collaborative

The treatment of DI is primarily pharmacologic. In addition to medication, fluid replacement to maintain vascular volume is essential. Rapid correction of hypernatremia is potentially dangerous because of the possibility of a rapid shift of water into brain cells, which increases the risk of seizures or cerebral edema The water deficit is corrected gradually over 2 to 3 days with water by mouth or nasogastric tube or intravenously with half- or quarter-isotonic saline.

PHARMACOLOGIC HIGHLIGHTS

Medication or Drug Class	Dosage	Description	Rationale
Aqueous vasopressin*	5–10 units IV or SC 2–3 times a day	Hormone; vasopressor; antidiuretic	Supplement to provide hormone in ADH deficiency
Chlorpropamide (Diabinese)	250–500 mg daily	Sulfonylurea	Reduces urine output by 30%–70%
Thiazide diuretics	Varies by drug	Decreases ployures	Effective when the kidney does not respond to vasopressin-like substances

*Note that vasopressin tannate (suspended in oil) is an intramuscular preparation that is given as a 1- to 5-unit injection. The oil-based preparation may have a duration of action as long as 96 hours, whereas the aqueous form lasts from 3 to 6 hours. Desmopressin acetate (DDAVP), a synthetic analog of vasopressin, is given intranasally in a dosage of 10 to 25 units twice a day.

Independent

The most important nursing interventions focus on maintaining an adequate balance of fluid intake and output. Discuss dietary restriction of salt with the patient and family. The patient should also avoid coffee, tea, or other caffeinated substances since caffeine has exaggerated diuretic effects. The patient needs easy access to the bathroom, bedpan, or urinal. If the patient has muscle weakness or impaired mobility, make sure the pathway for ambulation to the bathroom is free from all obstructions to limit the risk of patient falls.

Monitor the response to all medications and treatments by measuring the urine specific gravity daily as part of assessment data. Normal specific gravity is greater than 1.010. To identify the intake and output balance, monitor and carefully record the oral fluid intake and urine volume over a 24-hour period.

Encourage the patient to wear a medical identification bracelet and to carry any medications at all times. Note that some medications needed for a chronic disease, such as DDAVP, are quite expensive. If the family does not have insurance coverage that includes medications, explore methods to obtain the needed medications. Refer the family to social service if necessary. Urge the patient and family to express their feelings about the patient's condition; if they are having difficulty in coping, arrange for a counseling session.

DOCUMENTATION GUIDELINES

- Physical response to treatment: Skin turgor, urinary output, color of urine
- Fluid balance: 24-hour intake and output, maintenance of body weight
- Urinary response to prescribed medications: Specific gravity
- Understanding of and interest in patient teaching
- Response (of patient and family) to chronic illness, if appropriate

DISCHARGE AND HOME HEALTHCARE GUIDELINES

PREVENTION. To prevent dehydration, teach the patient to use the thirst mechanism as a stimulus to drink oral fluids. To prevent polyuria, teach the patient to restrict salt and to avoid caffeine-containing products.

MEDICATIONS. Be sure the patient understands all medications, including the dosage, route, action, adverse effects, and the need for routine laboratory monitoring for DDAVP (plasma osmolarity). Ensure that the patient has access to the appropriate medications.

Diabetes Mellitus

DRG Category: 294
Mean LOS: 5.2 days
Description: MEDICAL: Diabetes, Age > 35

Diabetes mellitus (DM) is a chronic disorder of carbohydrate, protein, and fat metabolism in which there is a discrepancy between the amount of insulin required by the body and the amount of insulin available. DM affects over 10 million persons in the United States, and more than 35,000 people die from it each year. Diabetes mellitus is classified into several categories. (See Table 23.) The beta cells of the pancreas produce insulin and a protein called C-peptide, which are stored in the secretory granules of the beta cells and are released into the bloodstream as blood glucose levels increase. Insulin transports glucose and amino acids across the membranes of many body cells, particularly muscle and fat cells. It also increases the liver storage of glycogen, the chief carbohydrate storage material, and aids in the metabolism of triglycerides, nucleic acids, and proteins.

TABLE 23 | **Types of Diabetes Mellitus**

TYPE	DESCRIPTION
I	Patients are dependent on insulin for prevention of hyperglycemia or ketosis
	Referred to as insulin-dependent diabetes mellitus (IDDM)
	Approximately 10% to 20% of patients with DM have this type
	The most serious life-threatening problem is diabetic ketoacidosis
	Time of onset is usually under age 20 years
	Beta cells of pancreas have insulitis (pancreatic inflammatory response) with beta cell destruction

II	Patients are not dependent on insulin
	Patients have either insulin resistance or impaired insulin secretion
	Referred to as non-insulin-dependent diabetes mellitus (NIDDM)
	Most common type of DM: approximately 80%–90% of DM patients have this type
	The most serious problem is the development of hyperosmolar hyperglycemic nonketotic syndrome (HHNS)
	Time of onset is usually over age 30 years
	Beta cells have no insulitis; resistance to insulin occurs as the target cells
Gestational diabetes mellitus (GDM)	Patients develop glucose intolerance during pregnancy
Other types of diabetes	Diabetes develops secondary to other conditions, including pancreatic, hormonal, or endocrine disease and insulin resistance; or it is drug-induced
Malnutrition-related diabetes mellitus	Occurs in underdeveloped countries to individuals with a history of malnutrition

Long-term complications such as disease of the large and small blood vessels lead to cardiovascular disease (coronary artery disease, peripheral vascular disease, hypertension), retinopathy, and renal failure. Diabetic patients also have nerve damage (neuropathy) that can affect the peripheral nerves, resulting in numbness and pain of the hands or feet.

Because diabetic patients are hyperglycemic, they are at higher risk for infection because an elevated glucose encourages bacterial growth. The combination of peripheral neuropathies with numbness of the extremities, peripheral vascular disease leading to poor tissue perfusion, and the risk for infection makes the diabetic patient prone to feet and leg ulcers.

CAUSES

The cause of diabetes mellitus is not known, but genetic, autoimmune, viral, environmental, and socioeconomic factors have all been implicated in the development of the disease. Type I diabetes is most likely an autoimmune response in patients with genetic susceptibility. Following an environmental stimulus such as a virus or bacteria, antibodies attack the beta cells of the pancreas and cause insulitis—inflammation and destruction of the beta cells. It is thought that type II diabetes is caused by hereditary insulin resistance or abnormal insulin production. If insulin resistance is acquired rather than inherited, it is usually the result of obesity.

GENDER AND LIFE SPAN CONSIDERATIONS

Although diabetes mellitus can occur at any time and in both genders, the incidence increases with age, most commonly occuring in adults after age 30. Type I most commonly develops in childhood before age 20 but can occur at any age. Onset is often very abrupt. Because of the early age of onset, teenagers often deal with the long-term complications of the disease. Type II diabetes usually occurs after the age of 30, particularly with individuals who are overweight or have hereditary factors. Gestational diabetes mellitus (GDM), which is present during pregnancy, occurs in 3% of pregnant women, usually in those older than 30.

☐ ASSESSMENT

HISTORY. Establish a history of the patient's usual weight gains and losses; weight loss is common in Type I diabetes. Determine if the patient has been under stress. Ask females of childbearing age if they are pregnant. Establish a history of using medications that antagonize the effects of insulin.

Ask if the patient has experienced excessive thirst (polydipsia), excessive urination (polyuria), or excessive hunger (polyphagia). The most common symptom of DM is fatigue; determine if the patient has experienced fatigue out of the ordinary. Patients with Type II diabetes may not report these symptoms. However, ask whether the patient has experienced any recent itching or blurred vision or frequent infections, which are common complaints with Type II diabetes. Question if the patient has experienced any visual difficulties, kidney problems, or changes in circulation and sensation to the extremities such as numbness or tingling (paresthesia) or pruritus.

PHYSICAL EXAMINATION. Appearance may be entirely normal, or the patient with Type I diabetes may have weight loss, muscle wasting, and loss of subcutaneous fat. The patient with Type II diabetes, by contrast, may have thin limbs with fatty deposits around the face, neck, and abdomen. Observe the color of the skin, and note any changes in sensation of temperature, touch, and pain. Examine both feet closely, including the spaces between the toes, for signs of skin ulcers or infection. Assess the legs and feet to identify any unhealed wounds or ulcers. Check the temperature of the skin, which often feels cool, and the skin turgor, which is often poor.

When assessing vital signs, you may note hypertension, a common complication in diabetic patients. Palpate the peripheral pulses to determine their strength, regularity, and symmetry. During the neurological examination, use an ophthalmoscope to evaluate the patient for retinopathy or cataracts. Assess the patient for any signs and symptoms of hypoglycemia or hyperglycemia. (See Table 24.)

TABLE 24	**Signs, Symptoms, and Treatment of Hypoglycemia and Hyperglycemia**

HYPOGLYCEMIA

Cause: Usually secondary to excess insulin, exercise, or not enough food

Signs and Symtpoms:

Nervousness	Irritability
Diaphroesis (heavy sweating)	Hunger
Weakness	Tachycardia
Fatigue	Hypotension
Palpitations	Tachypnea
Tremors or shaking	Pallor
Blurred or double vision	Incoherent speech
Headache	Numbness of tongue and lips
Confusion	Coma
Seizures	

Treatment:
Provide rapidly absorbed source of glucose:
· Fruit juice or cola
· Graham crackers

- Sugar cubes, sugar packets
- Hard candy

As symptoms improve:
- Provide a meal or source of complex protein or carbohydrates

HYPERGLYCEMIA

Cause: Usually secondary to insufficient insulin, illness, or excess food

Signs and Symptoms:

Nausea	Confusion
Vomiting	Irritability
Anorexia	Fatigue
Abdominal cramping	Weakness
Thirst	Numbness
Lethargy	Tachycardia
Küssmall breathing	Hypotension
Increased temperature	Decreased level of consciousness
Flushed or dry skin	Coma
Poor skin turgor	Fruity breath
Dry mucous membranes	

Treatment (Requires Hospitalization):
- Restore fluid balance
- Replace electrolytes
- Lower blood glucose with regular insulin
- Monitor: Level of consciousness, vital signs, intake and output, and electrolytes
- Provide emotional support

PSYCHOSOCIAL. The need for daily management with medications, diet, and exercise repeatedly reminds the individual of the illness. In addition, the reality of a long-term illness may affect the individual's view of himself or herself, resulting in lower self-esteem. Young people with Type I diabetes may have trouble managing developmental tasks and a chronic disease simultaneously. Parents may become overprotective, and children may have delayed emotional maturation.

DIAGNOSTIC HIGHLIGHTS

Test	Normal Result	Abnormality with Condition	Explanation
Fasting (no food for at least 8 hours before measurement) plasma glucose	70–105 mg/dL	> 126 mg/dL	Insufficient insulin is available to transport insulin into body cells
Glucose tolerance test (2 hours after oral ingestion of 75 g of glucose; glucose is given after an overnight fast)	< 140 mg/dL	> 200 mg/dL; levels from 140 to 200 mg/dL indicate impaired glucose tolerance (IGT)	Insufficient insulin is available to transport insulin into body cells

Other Tests: Urinalysis (glycosuria)

PRIMARY NURSING DIAGNOSIS

Altered nutrition: Less than body requirements related to decreased oral intake, nausea, vomiting, and insulin deficiency

OUTCOMES. Nutritional status: Food and fluid intake; Nutrient intake; Biochemical measures; Body mass; Energy; Endurance

INTERVENTIONS. Nutrition management; Nutrition therapy; Nutritional counseling and monitoring; Fluid/electrolyte management; Medication management

PLANNING AND IMPLEMENTATION

Collaborative

There is no known cure for diabetes. Management of the disease focuses on control of the serum glucose level to prevent or delay the development of complications. Individuals with Type I diabetes require subcutaneous insulin administration. Insulin may be rapid, intermediate, or slow acting.

Patients with mild diabetes or those with Type II diabetes or GDM may be able to control the disease by diet management alone. A diabetic diet attempts to distribute nutrition and calories throughout the 24-hour period. Daily calories consist of approximately 50% carbohydrates and 30% fat, with the remaining calories consisting of protein. The total calories allowed for an individual within the 24-hour period are based on age, weight, activity level, and medications.

In addition to strict dietary adherence to control blood glucose, obese patients with Type II diabetes also need weight reduction. The dietitian selects an appropriate calorie allotment depending on the patient's age, body size, and activity level. A useful adjunct to the management of diabetes mellitus is exercise. Physical activity increases the cellular sensitivity to insulin, improves tolerance to glucose, and encourages weight loss. Exercise also increases the patient's sense of well-being concerning his or her health.

PHARMACOLOGIC HIGHLIGHTS

Medica tion or Drug Class	Dosage	Description	Rationale
Insulin	Varies with severity of disease; adjusted to maintain blood glucose of 80–140 mg/dL	Hormone; hypoglycemic	Hormonal supplement to replace deficient or absent levels of insulin
Anti-diabetics	Varies with drug	Four groups of medications besides insulin are available in the treatment of diabetes mellitus: sulfonylureas, alpha-glucosidase inhibitors, biguanides, thiazolinediones	Varies by drug. Sulfonylureas: stimulated release of insulin from beta cells of pancreas; alpha-glucosidase inhibitors: slow carbohydrate breakdown in small intestine; biguanides: decrease hepatic glucose output, enhance peripheral glucose uptake;

| thiazolinediones: decrease insulin resistance |

Independent

If the patient has recently been diagnosed with diabetes mellitus, explain the disease process, the goals of management, and strategies to limit complications. Use simple explanations, answer questions, and provide written information for the patient to refer to between teaching sessions. In addition to general information on the disease process and reinforcement of collaborative teaching about medications and nutrition, the patient needs specific information about foot care.

Explain that all cuts and blisters need to be cleaned and treated with an antiseptic preparation. If a cut or blister begins to appear infected (warmth, pain, swelling) or has drainage, encourage the patient to notify the primary healthcare provider immediately. Teach the patient to avoid constricting clothing such as constricting stockings, garters, girdles, or elastic slippers. If the patient needs to be on bed rest, encourage him or her to keep bed linens loose over the feet and legs. Instruct the patient to avoid very hot baths if peripheral neuropathy causes decreased temperature sensation.

If the patient is a child or teenager, recognize that a diagnosis of diabetes mellitus changes a family permanently. Parents usually expect their child to be healthy and often react with shock and disbelief. The impact on the child depends on the child's age. School-age children may be impressed with the new "condition" and may be challenged by the new skills it involves. Adolescents, in comparison, may feel unfairly victimized and respond by becoming depressed, resistant, uncooperative, or insecure. Work with the entire family to support their adaptation to the illness. Introduce the family to other families with the same problem. If the problems are abnormal, make a referral to a counselor.

DOCUMENTATION GUIDELINES

- Results of urine and blood tests for glucose
- Physical findings: Visual problems, skin problems or lesions, changes in sensation or circulation to the extremities
- Patient teaching, return demonstrations, patient's understanding of teaching
- Response to insulin

DISCHARGE AND HOME HEALTHCARE GUIDELINES

MEDICATIONS. Patients need to understand the purpose, dosage, route, and possible side effects of all prescribed medications. If the patient is to self-administer insulin, have the patient demonstrate the appropriate preparation and administration techniques.

PREVENTION. The patient and family require instruction in the following areas to minimize or prevent complications of diabetes mellitus.

DIET. Explain how to calculate the American Diabetic Association exchange list to develop a satisfactory diet within the prescribed calories. Emphasize the importance of adjusting diet during illness, growth periods, stress, and pregnancy.

Encourage patients to avoid alcohol and refined sugars and to distribute nutrients to maintain a balanced blood sugar throughout the 24-hour period.

INSULIN. Patients need to understand the type of insulin prescribed. Instructions should include onset, peak, and duration of action. Stress proper timing of meals and planning snacks for the time when insulin is at its peak, and recommend an evening snack for those on long-acting insulins. Reinforce that patients cannot miss a dosage and there may be a need for increasing dosages during times of stress or illness. Teaching regarding the proper preparation of insulin, how to administer, and the importance of rotating sites is necessary.

URINE AND BLOOD TESTING. Teach patients the appropriate technique for testing blood and urine and how to interpret the results. Patients need to know when to notify the physician and increase testing during times of illness.

SKIN CARE. Stress the importance of close attention to even minor skin injuries. Emphasize foot care, including the importance of properly fitting shoes with clean, non-constricting socks; daily washing and thorough drying of the feet; and inspection of the toes, with special attention paid to the areas between the toes. Encourage the patient to contact a podiatrist as needed. Because of sensory loss in the lower extremities, teach the patient to test the bath water to prevent skin trauma from water that is too hot and to avoid using heating pads.

CIRCULATION. Because of the atherosclerotic changes that occur with diabetes mellitus, encourage patients to stop smoking. In addition, teach patients to avoid crossing their legs when sitting and to begin a regular exercise program.

Diffuse Axonal Injury

DRG Category: 027
Mean LOS: 3.9 days
Description: MEDICAL: Traumatic Stupor and Coma, Coma > 1 Hour
DRG Category: 028
Mean LOS: 5.5 days
Description: MEDICAL: Traumatic Stupor and Coma, Coma < 1 Hour, Age > 17 with CC
DRG Category: 002
Mean LOS: 9.8 days
Description: SURGICAL: Craniotomy for Trauma, Age > 17

A diffuse axonal injury (DAI), the most severe of all brain injuries, occurs when nerve axons are stretched, sheared, or even torn apart. The severity and outcome of a DAI depend on the extent and degree of damage to brain structures and can be classified as mild, moderate, or severe DAI. All types of DAI are associated with an immediate and prolonged (more than 6 hours) coma. Mild DAI is associated with a coma that lasts from 6 to 24 hours and has a 15% mortality rate; 80% of patients experience a good recovery. Moderate DAI is associated with a coma that lasts 24 hours or more, decerebration (extension posturing), and decortication (flexion posturing). Approximately 25% of patients with moderate DAI die. Severe DAI, which has a mortality rate of 50%, occurs when there is an extensive disruption of axons in the white matter of the central nervous system (CNS). People who emerge from coma usually do so in the first 3 months after injury.

CAUSES

The predominant causes of injuries that lead to DAI are high-speed motor vehicle crashes (MVCs) and automobile-pedestrian crashes. The severity of the MVC is correlated with the severity of DAI.

GENDER AND LIFE SPAN CONSIDERATIONS

Traumatic injuries are the leading cause of death in Americans aged 1 through 44 years and the fourth leading cause of death for all age groups. Head injury, the leading cause of all trauma-related death, is associated with MVCs, which in the 15- to 24-year-old age group are three times more common with males than with females. European-Americans have a death rate that is 40% higher from MVCs than do African-Americans in the 15- to 34-year-old age group.

◻ ASSESSMENT

HISTORY. If the patient has been in an MVC, determine the speed and type of the vehicle, the patient's position in the vehicle, whether the patient was restrained, and whether the patient was thrown from the vehicle on impact. If the patient was injured in a motorcycle crash, determine if the patient was wearing a helmet. Determine if the patient experienced momentary loss of reflexes, momentary arrest of respiration, loss of consciousness, and the length of time the patient was unconscious. Determine if the patient has been experiencing excessive sweating (hyperhidrosis) or hypertension since the injury.

PHYSICAL EXAMINATION. The initial evaluation is centered on assessing the airway, breathing, circulation, and disability (neurological status). Exposure (undressing the patient completely) is incorporated as part of the primary survey. The secondary survey, a head-to-toe assessment, including vital signs, is then completed. Note a very high fever, hyperhidrosis, or hypertension. Observe posturing for flexion or extension.

The initial and ongoing neurological assessment includes monitoring of the vital signs, assessment of the level of consciousness, examination of pupil size and level of reactivity, and assessment of the Glasgow Coma Scale, which evaluates eye opening, best verbal response, and best motor response. Clinical findings may include a rapidly changing level of consciousness from confusion to coma, ipsilateral pupil dilation, hemiparesis, and abnormal posturing that includes flexion and extension. A neurological assessment is repeated at least hourly during the first 24 hours after the injury.

Examine the patient for signs of a basilar skull fracture: periorbital ecchymosis (raccoon's eyes), subscleral hemorrhage, retroauricular ecchymosis (Battle's sign), hemotympanum (blood behind the eardrum), and leakage of cerebrospinal fluid from ears (otorrhea) or nose (rhinorrhea). Gently palpate the entire scalp and facial bones, including the mandible and maxilla, for bony deformities or step-offs. Examine the oral pharynx for lacerations, and check for any loose or fractured teeth.

PSYCHOSOCIAL. DAI may alter an individual's ability to cope effectively. It may lead to significant cognitive and behavioral disabilities. Although it is not possible to assess the comatose patient's coping strategies, it is important to assist the family or significant others.

DIAGNOSTIC HIGHLIGHTS

Test	Normal Result	Abnormality with Condition	Explanation
Computed tomography (CT) scan	Normal brain and spinal cord	Cerebral edema, damage to brain structures	Identifies structural lesions in patients with head injuries.
Magnetic resonance imaging (MRI)	Normal brain and spinal cord	Cerebral edema, damage to brain structures	May be more valuable in diagnosing DAI than CT scanning.

Other Tests: Skull and cervical spine x rays, arterial blood gases, and complete blood count

PRIMARY NURSING DIAGNOSIS

Ineffective airway clearance related to hypoventilation or airway obstruction

OUTCOMES. Respiratory status: Gas exchange; Respiratory status: Ventilation; Comfort level

INTERVENTIONS. Airway management; Oxygen therapy; Airway suctioning; Airway insertion and stabilization; Anxiety reduction; Cough enhancement; Mechanical ventilation; Positioning; Respiratory monitoring

◻ PLANNING AND IMPLEMENTATION

Collaborative

Endotracheal intubation and mechanical ventilation are critical to ensure oxygenation and ventilation and to decrease the risk of pulmonary aspiration. A PaO_2 greater than 100 mm Hg and a $PaCO_2$ between 28 and 33 mm Hg may be maintained to decrease cerebral blood flow and intracranial swelling. Fluid administration guided by intracranial pressure (ICP), cerebral perfusion pressure (CPP; calculated number CPP = MAP − ICP; MAP is mean arterial pressure), arterial blood pressure, and saturation of mixed venous blood (SvO_2) is critical.

ICP monitoring may be used in patients with severe head injuries who have a high probability of developing intracranial hypertension. Some physicians use a Glasgow Coma Scale score of less than 7 as an indicator for monitoring ICP. The goal of this monitoring is to maintain the ICP at less than 10 mm Hg and the CPP at greater than 80 mm Hg. Management of intracranial hypertension can also be done by draining cerebrospinal fluid through a ventriculostomy.

Some patients may have episodes of agitation and pain, which can increase ICP. Sedatives and analgesics can be administered to control intermittent increases in ICP, with a resulting decrease in CPP. Additionally, some patients with severe head injuries may require chemical paralysis to improve oxygenation and ventilation. Other complications are also managed pharmacologically, such as seizures (by anticonvulsants), increased ICP (by barbiturate coma), infection (by antibiotics), and intracranial hypertension (by diuretics).

PHARMACOLOGIC HIGHLIGHTS

Medication or Drug Class	Dosage	Description	Rationale
Sedatives and chemical paralytics.	Varies by drug	Short acting: midazolam (Versed); propofol (Diprivan)	Control intermittent increases in ICP with a resultant decrease in CPP; improve oxygenation and ventilation
Analgesics	Varies by drug	Fentanyl (Sublimaze), morphine sulfate	Control intermittent increases in ICP with a resultant decrease in CPP

Independent

The highest priority is to maintain a patent airway, appropriate ventilation and oxygenation, and adequate circulation. Make sure the patient's endotracheal tube is anchored well. If the patient is at risk for self-extubation, maintain him or her in soft restraints. Note the lip level of the endotracheal tube to determine if tube movement occurs. Notify the physician if the patient's PaO_2 drops below 80 mm Hg, if $PaCO_2$ exceeds 40 mm Hg, or if severe hypocapnia ($PaCO_2$ less than 25 mm Hg) occurs.

Serial assessments of the patient's neurological responses are of the highest importance. When a patient's assessment changes, timely notification to the trauma surgeon or neurosurgeon can save a patient's life. The patient with DAI is dependent on nurses and therapists for maintaining muscle tone, joint function, bowel and bladder function, and skin integrity. Consult the rehabilitation department early in the hospitalization for evaluation and treatment. Frequent turning, positioning, and use of a pressure-release mattress help prevent alterations in skin integrity. Keep skin pressure points clean and dry.

Provide simple educational tools about head injuries. Referrals to clinical nurse specialists, pastoral care staff, and social workers are helpful in developing strategies to increase education and support. Establish a visiting schedule that meets the needs of the patient and family, while providing adequate time for patient care and rest. The mortality of patients with diffuse axonal injury ranges from 15% to 51%, with a wide variation in the level of cognitive functioning that the patient can reach through intensive rehabilitation. Education and support for the family are critical in assisting them in coping with severity of this injury.

DOCUMENTATION GUIDELINES

- Trauma history, description of the event, time elapsed since the event, whether or not the patient had a loss of consciousness, and if so, for how long
- Physical findings related to the site of head injury: Neurological assessment, presence of accompanying symptoms, presence of complications (decreased level of consciousness, unequal pupils, loss of strength and movement, confusion or agitation, nausea and vomiting), CPP, ICP, appearance, bruising or lacerations, drainage from the nose or ears

- Signs of complications: Seizure activity, infection (fever, purulent discharge from any wounds), aspiration pneumonia (shortness of breath, pulmonary congestion, fever, productive cough), increased ICP
- Response to medications used to control pain and increase ICP

DISCHARGE AND HOME HEALTHCARE GUIDELINES

Teach the patient and significant others the purpose, dosage, schedule, precautions, and potential side effects, interactions, and adverse reactions of all prescribed medications. Teach the patient and family the strategies required to prevent complications of immobility. Encourage participation in physical, occupational, and speech therapy. Verify that the patient and family have demonstrated safety in performing the activities of daily living.

Review with the patient and family all follow-up appointments that are necessary. If outpatient or home therapies are needed, review the arrangements. If appropriate, assist the patient and family in locating ongoing psychosocial support to cope with this injury.

Dislocation; Subluxation

Hip, Acquired DRG Category: 237
Mean LOS: 3.7 days
Description: MEDICAL: Sprain, Strain, and Dislocation of Hip, Pelvis, and Thigh
Hip, Acquired DRG Category: 210
Mean LOS: 9.0 days
Description: SURGICAL: Hip and Femur Procedures, Except Major Joint, Age > 17 with CC
Hip Acquired, DRG Category: 265
Mean LOS: 3.4 days
Description: MEDICAL: Other Musculoskeletal System and Connective Tissue Diagnoses
Hip, Congenital DRG Category: 212
Mean LOS: 3.6 days
Description: SURGICAL: Hip and Femur Procedures Except Major Joint, Age 0 to 17

Dislocation and subluxation are terms used to describe the anatomic displacement of a bone from its normal position in the joint. Dislocation is the complete separation of the bone from the articular surfaces of the joint, whereas subluxation is only a partial displacement in the joint. Both dislocations and subluxations refer to the position of the distal bone in relation to its proximal articulation. Although dislocation or subluxation can affect any joint, the most frequently occurring sites are the thumb, elbow, shoulder, and hip.

When dislocation or subluxation is a result of trauma, there are generally associated injuries to the blood vessels, nerves, ligaments, and soft tissues that surround the joint. In addition to the actual damage at the joint, tissue death from circulatory compromise to the distal extremity, or permanent nerve damage from edema, can occur. Avascular necrosis (death of bone cells because of inadequate blood supply) may occur if the bone is torn away from its normal position next to the vascular-rich bony surface.

CAUSES

Dislocations and subluxations can occur as a result of injury or developmental dysplasia of the hip (DDH), previously referred to as congenital hip dysplasia. Sports-related injuries, occupational injuries, and motor vehicle crashes are common causes. DDH can also lead to dislocations and subluxations, and there tends to be an increase in occurrence of DDH within families that have had other children with the condition. In addition, dislocation and subluxations may also be acquired as a result of chronic conditions such as rheumatoid arthritis.

GENDER AND LIFE SPAN CONSIDERATIONS

Trauma is the leading cause of death during the first four decades of life. In general, more men than women are injured in violent events. Traumatic dislocations occur most frequently in persons under 20 years of age as a result of their involvement in sports or risk-taking activities. The recurrence of a dislocation is very high in people who experience the first injury when they are under the age of 20. If the first injury occurs when the person is 30 or 40 years of age, the potential for a repeat dislocation decreases. Displacements as a result of chronic conditions are more prevalent with people of advanced age. DDH, as compared to unintentional injuries, is usually diagnosed in the newborn period or early childhood years.

☐ ASSESSMENT

HISTORY. When the condition is a result of injury, elicit complete details of the injury from the patient, significant others, or the life squad. Note the time of injury, as well as the description, angle of force, and the patient's immediate sensations. Always ask if the patient felt any numbness immediately after the injury. In an acquired dislocation or subluxation, note a complete history of recent alterations in mobility, pain, or any other changes. For traumatic or acquired displacements, it is important to obtain information about any previous dislocations of this joint or any other joint.

DDH can range from a minor instability to total dislocation. In moderate to severe DDH, diagnosis can be made at birth during the physical examination. However, for less severe conditions, symptoms may not occur until the child starts to crawl or walk. Elicit a developmental history from the parents covering the child's mobility.

PHYSICAL EXAMINATION. With traumatic or acquired dislocation, the immediate clinical manifestations may include severe pain, inability to move the extremity, a change in the length of the extremities, abnormal contour of the joint, and ecchymosis (bruising). The symptoms of subluxation are the same, but usually less severe. Make sure to remove all of the patient's clothing to observe skin surfaces. Assess joint range of motion unless there is suspected cervical spine injury. In that situation, defer motion until radiographs are completed. Palpate all extremities and note pain, crepitus, instability, and deformity.

Monitor the neurovascular status of the patient with a dislocation before and after reduction or other interventions. Impairment in circulation or neurological deficits may occur during injury, before the reduction, because of pressure from bleeding or edema and after the reduction or as a result of interventions. The impairment may occur at the joint, but it may also occur distal to the injury. Serial neurovascular assessment includes critical data related to the 5 P's: pain, pallor, paralysis, paresthesia, and pulselessness. Normal pulses do not rule out compartment syndrome.

Signs of congenital hip dislocation include asymmetry of gluteal and thigh folds, limited hip abduction, and apparent shortening of the femur with knees in flexion. If the child is beginning to walk, gait abnormalities occur. In the infant, a positive Ortolani-Barlow maneuver is an indication of dislocation. This maneuver involves placing the hands on the knees of the baby with fingers on the upper portion of the femur and abducting the hips while the infant lies on his or her back. Resistance to abduction, or the presence of a click as the femur slips out of the acetabulum, is considered a positive response.

PSYCHOSOCIAL. If the dislocation resulted from an injury, the sudden impact may have disrupted the individual's routines and created certain losses. If dislocation or subluxation is a result of a chronic disease process, the deficit may be a reminder of the deterioration of the body; depression may follow as a result of the decreased mobility or role change. With any congenital or developmental problem, parents may experience anxiety, guilt, or depression.

DIAGNOSTIC HIGHLIGHTS

Test	Normal Result	Abnormality with Condition	Explanation
Radiologic examination: chest, pelvis, lateral cervical (all cervical vertebrae including C7-T1 junction) spine x rays	Normal bone, joint, and soft tissue structure	Dislocations and subluxations; assessment of fractures or dislocations should include 2 views (90 degrees to each other, and of affected area with joints above and below)	If the patient is unconscious, spinal and pelvic injuries need to be ruled out

Other Tests: Supporting tests include computed tomography (CT) scan, magnetic resonance imaging (MRI), and ultrasound

PRIMARY NURSING DIAGNOSIS

Pain (acute) related to lack of the continuity of the bone to joint; edema and muscle spasms

OUTCOMES. Comfort level; Pain control behavior; Pain level; Symptom severity

INTERVENTIONS. Analgesic administration; Anxiety reduction; Environmental management: Comfort; Pain management; Medication management

☐ PLANNING AND IMPLEMENTATION

Collaborative

If the joint remains unreduced (to reduce is to restore the components of the joint to their usual relationships), the patient is at greater risk for avascular necrosis. The primary goal for therapeutic management is to realign the bones of the joint to their normal anatomic position. With injuries or chronic conditions, the physician will generally use a closed reduction (manually placing the bone into the joint) after giving the patient a sedative or a local or general anesthetic. The decision for a closed reduction depends on the person's age, condition, and severity of the injury. If the same joint has repeatedly become dislocated or if the condition is severe, an open reduction is required. This procedure requires general anesthesia or an anesthetic block and involves surgical intervention for repositioning the bones and repairing ligaments. Once the proper position has been achieved, the physician may use pins or screws to maintain alignment.

After the open or closed reduction is accomplished, the physician immobilizes the joint to allow for healing through slings, taping, splints, casts, or traction devices. Treatment of subluxation is similar to that of a dislocation, but subluxation generally requires less healing time. Patients require a carefully regulated exercise program to restore the joint to its original range of motion without causing another dislocation.

The goal for treating DDH is the same as other dislocations or subluxations. However, the age of the child and the developmental nature of the condition alter the intervention. Treatment approaches vary, according to the child's age. Infants under 3 months of age may simply require a triple diapering technique. This procedure abducts (by use of the thick diapers) positioning the femoral head into the acetabulum as the baby grows. Skin traction such as Bryant's or split Russell's may be used for the baby over 3 months of age. These procedures relocate the femur to the acetabulum while gently stretching the ligaments and muscles around the joint. For the 3- to 6-year-old patient, serial casting (the placement of several casts over time as the child grows or as realignment is required) or open reduction with casting may be needed.

PHARMACOLOGIC HIGHLIGHTS

Medication or Drug Class	Dosage	Description	Rationale
Analgesics and sedatives	Varies with drug	Analgesia: narcotics such as morphine or fentanyl (Sublimaze); sedation: midazolam (Versed)	To achieve easily arousable analgesia and sedation so that on-going assessments can occur

Note: The physician usually prescribes analgesics and muscle relaxants to control the pain and prevent muscle spasms. Frequently, the patient needs muscle relaxants so that the physician can manipulate the injured structures.

Independent

Before reduction of the joint, direct nursing care to relieve pain and protect the joint and extremity from further injury. Maintain proper positioning and alignment to limit further injury. Accompanying soft tissue injuries are treated by RICE therapy: rest, ice, compression bandage, and elevation with or without immobilization.

The patient and family need support to cope with a sudden injury. Allow time each day to listen to concerns, discuss the patient's progress, and explain upcoming procedures. Older patients may experience depression and loss if the injury has long-term implications about their self-care. Use social workers and advanced-practice nurses for consultation if the patient's anxiety or fear is abnormal. Immobilization involving the whole person rather than one extremity requires aggressive prevention of the hazards of immobility. Motivate and educate patients to help them prevent complications. Encourage a balanced diet which contains foods that promote healing, such as those that have protein and vitamin C. Stimulation of the affected area by isometric and isotonic exercises also helps promote healing.

DOCUMENTATION GUIDELINES

- Restrictions of movement before and after reduction, level of discomfort, pain relief, neurovascular assessment (pain, pallor, paresthesia, paralysis, pulselessness)
- Response to treatment (open or closed procedure)

DISCHARGE AND HOME HEALTHCARE GUIDELINES

Be certain that the patient and/or family understands the importance of the prescribed rehabilitation. For children, outline the appropriate activities to maintain growth and development. Demonstrate the adaptations required for patients with casts. Discuss the need to report any changes in pain, numbness, or other signs of neurovascular compromise. Make certain the patient or parents and family understand the signs and symptoms of suture line infections if open reduction has been accomplished and that odors or drainage from a cast should have immediate attention. If antibiotics have been ordered, stress the importance of completing the course as prescribed. Discuss the potential for repeat dislocations and the need for protection during sports or other activities.

Disseminated Intravascular Coagulation

DRG Category: 397
Mean LOS: 5.0 days
Description: MEDICAL: Coagulation Disorders

Disseminated intravascular coagulation (DIC) is a life-threatening hemostatic disarray in which bleeding and clotting occur simultaneously. It is also called consumptive coagulopathy and defibrination syndrome. The pathophysiology involves an overactivation of the clotting mechanisms with both enhanced fibrin production leading to small clots and fibrinolysis leading to enhanced bleeding. As its name implies, tiny clots accumulate in the microcirculation (capillaries) throughout the body, depleting the blood supply of its clotting factors. These microemboli interfere with blood flow and lead to ischemia and organ damage.

As the clots begin to lyse, fibrin degradation products (FDPs) (which have an anticoagulant property of their own) are released. The FDPs, along with decreased levels of clotting factors in the bloodstream, lead to massive bleeding internally from the brain, kidneys, adrenals, heart, and other organs, or from any wounds and old puncture sites.

CAUSES

DIC always occurs in response to another type of disease or trauma. DIC is usually acute, although it may be chronic in patients with cancer or more longstanding conditions. Conditions that may precede its development are cardiac and peripheral vascular disorders, transfusion reactions, sepsis, viremias, liver disease, leukemia, metastatic cancer, burn injuries, and obstetric complications (abruptio placentae, pregnancy-induced hypertension, saline abortion, amniotic fluid embolism, or a retained dead fetus). It is not known how these disorders trigger the onset of DIC, but they activate the intrinsic or extrinsic pathway of the coagulation cascade. Some experts suggest that these disorders cause a foreign protein to be released into the circulation and that the vascular endothelium is injured.

GENDER AND LIFE SPAN CONSIDERATIONS

DIC can occur any time during the life span. Women of childbearing age who develop pregnancy-induced hypertension and HELLP syndrome (hemolysis, elevated liver, low platelet) are potential candidates to develop DIC. Other high-risk patients are those with neoplasms (often the elderly), sepsis, or traumatic injuries (often young adult males) such as burns and crush injuries.

☐ ASSESSMENT

HISTORY. Obtain a history specific to the precipitating disorder. If the patient is alert, ask if he or she has any chest, joint, back, or muscle pain, which is often severe in DIC. Recognize that the patient may be confused and disoriented as a result of blood loss or the underlying condition, so that historic information may not be accurate.

PHYSICAL EXAMINATION. Assess the patient's skin for any petechiae, ecchymoses, hematoma formation, epistaxis, bleeding from wounds, vaginal bleeding in the labor or postpartum patient, hematuria, conjunctival hemorrhage, and hemoptysis. Bruising can occur anywhere in the body. Additionally, assess the patient's skin for bleeding or oozing at any intravenous (IV), intramuscular (IM), or epidural sites. Assess the patient's vital signs. If the patient is hypovolemic, expect to find a decreased blood pressure, rapid thready pulse, and increased respiratory rate. The patient may be restless, agitated, and confused. Measure the abdominal girth to obtain a baseline for further assessments. Note the presence of oliguria and compare current urine output to previous readings.

PSYCHOSOCIAL. Patients may feel a sense of "impending doom," and the family is probably fearful of losing a loved one. This situation is intensified if the patient is a young pregnant or newly delivered mother. Note that increased blood or bleeding is associated with death and dying for many people; the visible presence of multiple bleeding or oozing sites and the need for multiple transfusions may also be a source of anxiety.

DIAGNOSTIC HIGHLIGHTS

Test	Normal Result	Abnormality with Condition	Explanation
D-dimer	0–0.5 μg/dL	Elevated > 500 μg/dL indicates DIC	Fibrin degradation fragment; measured amount of clot breakdown products specific for cross-linked fragments derived from fibrin; in DIC extensive fibrinolysis occurs
Fibrin degradation products (FDPs)	< 8 μg/mL	Elevated > 40 μg/mL indicates DIC	7 split products are formed from splitting fibrin as a result of plasmin during dissolution of fibrin clots. FDP quantifies amount of split products present in blood. In DIC, extensive breakdown of clots occurs.
Fibrinogen	150–360 mg/dL	Decreased <150 mg/dL	Decreased levels of fibrinogen (factor I) occur due to depletion of clotting factors
Partial thromboplastin time (activated; APPT)	Varies by laboratory; generally 21–35 seconds	Prolonged; may be prolonged > 80 seconds	Indicates how long it takes for recalcified, citrated plasma to clot after partial thromboplastin is added; screens for deficiencies in all factors except VII and XIII; factors are depleted, causing prolonged APTT
Platelet count	190,000–405,000/mm	>100,000/mm^3	Platelets are consumed during clot formation
Prothrombin time (PT)	Varies by laboratory; generally 11–13 seconds	Prolonged > 15 seconds	Prothrombin is a vitamin K–dependent glycoprotein that is necessary for firm clot formation; converts to throbin in clotting cascade. In DIC clotting factors are depleted and PT is prolonged.

Other Tests: INR (International Normalized Ratio): Standardizes the PT ratio by allowing laboratories to compare values to an international standard provided by the World Health Organization. Formula is patient's PT in seconds/mean normal PT in seconds. In DIC, INR is elevated from a normal value of 1.3 to 1.6. Therapeutic range for INR is 2.0 to 3.0 for people on warfarin. Factors: Decrease in factors II, V, and VIII

PRIMARY NURSING DIAGNOSIS

Fluid volume deficit related to blood loss

OUTCOMES. Fluid balance; Circulation status; Cardiac pump effectiveness; Hydration

INTERVENTIONS. Bleeding reduction; Fluid resuscitation; Blood product administration; Intravenous therapy; Circulatory care; Shock management

□ PLANNING AND IMPLEMENTATION

Collaborative

Since DIC always occurs in association with another condition, medical treatment focuses on correcting the underlying disorder. In addition, the physician seeks to return the patient to normal hemostasis. Active bleeding is managed by blood component therapy. To ascertain the success of cell and factor replacement, constant surveillance of laboratory values is critical to determine which blood components should be administered. In general, packed red blood cells are used to improve oxygen delivery by increasing the hemoglobin content of the blood. Fresh-frozen plasma replaces many of the clotting factors, whereas cryoprecipitate is the best source of fibrinogen and factors V, VIII, and XIII. Platelet transfusion is used when the platelet count falls below $100,000/mm^3$.

If the patient is critically ill, the physician may place a pulmonary artery catheter (PAC) to monitor the patient's hemodynamic status. Note that increased bleeding tendencies make the insertion time of central access devices important; central catheters such as a PAC should be placed when the coagulation profile has been corrected with blood component therapy to prevent dangerous bleeding into the cardiopulmonary system.

If the patient is pregnant, fetal monitoring is continuous; notify the physician of late decelerations, decreased variability, or bradycardia. Keep the patient on her left side, and administer oxygen by mask at a rate of 10 L per minute. Turn and reposition the patient frequently and gently to avoid further bleeding. The goal is to keep the fetus oxygenated while stabilizing the mother so that a cesarean section can be done.

PHARMACOLOGIC HIGHLIGHTS

Medication or Drug Class	Dosage	Description	Rationale
Heparin	Varies with patient response, weight-based dosing is common, with a starting bolus of 80 units/kg and an infusion of 18 units/kg per hour. Then dosage is calculated based on APTT results	Anticoagulant	Controversial treatment; inhibits clot formation by inactivating thrombin and factors X and IX by antithrombin III
Analgesics	Varies with drug	Narcotics such as morphine and fentanyl	Relieve pain of hemarthrosis

Independent

When a bleeding disorder occurs in addition to another condition, the patient's and significant others' coping skills and resiliency may be at a low point. During this time, the patient and significant others need accurate information, honest reports about the patient's condition and prognosis, and an attentive nurse to listen to their concerns. Provide emotional support and educate them as to the interventions and expected outcomes. Help them understand the severity of the condition and the treatments; do not present false hopes. Offer to call a chaplain or religious counselor if needed.

The patient is usually maintained on complete bed rest. Pad the side rails to help prevent injury. Reposition the patient every 2 hours, and provide skin care. Gently touch the skin when repositioning and bathing; vigorous rubbing could dislodge a clot and initiate fresh bleeding. Crusted blood can be gently cleaned with a mixture of hydrogen peroxide and water and cotton. If the patient has experienced hemarthrosis (bleeding into the joints), the condition is very painful. Manipulate any joint gently and with great care to minimize discomfort and to limit further bleeding.

Communicate to all healthcare personnel coming in contact with the patient about his or her bleeding tendency. Place notations on the chart cover and at the head of the bed to alert caregivers to the patient's bleeding condition. Keep all venipunctures to a minimum, and hold pressure to any puncture site for at least 10 minutes.

DOCUMENTATION GUIDELINES

- Physical responses: Amount of blood loss, location of bleeding; fluid intake and output; condition of skin (oozing of puncture sites, bruising, petechiae); vital signs, including hemodynamic monitoring results if appropriate; patency of airway and adequacy of gas exchange
- Response to therapy: Fluid replacement; blood component therapy; heparin
- Laboratory findings: Coagulation profile
- Signs and symptoms of systems complications: Hemorrhage, hypovolemic shock, transfusion reaction
- Condition of newborn if recently delivered

DISCHARGE AND HOME HEALTHCARE GUIDELINES

Teach the patient and significant others about the disorder and that it is unlikely that it will recur in the future. If the patient required blood component therapy, provide information about the risk of hepatitis or HIV transmission. Check with the patient's obstetrician to determine if the patient can nurse the infant and resume unprotected sexual relations.

Provide discharge instructions related to the patient's primary diagnosis. Teach the patient to notify the physician of any uncontrollable bleeding or syncope.

Diverticular Disease

DRG Category: 182
Mean LOS: 4.3 days
Description: MEDICAL: Esophagitis, Gastrointestinal, and Miscellaneous Digestive Disorders, Age > 17 with CC
DRG Category: 148
Mean LOS: 12.2 days
Description: SURGICAL: Major Small and Large Bowel Procedures with CC

Diverticular disease has two clinical forms, diverticulosis and diverticulitis. People with diverticulosis have multiple, non-inflamed diverticula (outpouches of the intestinal mucosa through the circular smooth muscle of the bowel wall). Usually diverticulosis is asymptomatic and does not require treatment. Diverticulitis, in contrast, occurs when the diverticula become inflamed or microperforated. Diverticular disease usually occurs in the descending and sigmoid colon and is accompanied by signs of inflammation.

CAUSES

Patients generally have increased muscular contractions in the sigmoid colon that produce muscular thickness and increased intraluminal pressure. This increased pressure, accompanied by a weakness in the colon wall, causes diverticular formations. In addition, diet may be a contributing factor. A diet with insufficient fiber reduces fecal residue, narrows the bowel lumen, and leads to higher intra-abdominal pressure during defecation. Diverticulitis is caused when stool and bacteria are retained in the diverticular outpouches, leading to the formation of a hardened mass called a fecalith. The fecalith obstructs blood supply to the diverticular area, leading to inflammation, edema of tissues, and possible bowel perforation and peritonitis.

GENDER AND LIFE SPAN CONSIDERATIONS

Diverticular disease is rare in those under 40 years of age. When the disorder does occur before age 40, it can usually be attributed to a congenital predisposition. From 30% to 60% of people with diverticular disease are between 60 and 80 years old. As people age, structural changes in both genders occur in the muscular layers of the colon, which places the elderly at risk for the disease.

◻ ASSESSMENT

HISTORY. Patients with diverticulosis are generally asymptomatic but may report cramping abdominal pain in the left lower quadrant of the abdomen that is relieved with episodes of flatulence and a bowel movement. Occasional rectal bleeding may also be noted.

Patients with diverticulitis usually report cramping in the left lower quadrant with abdominal pain that radiates to the back. Other complaints frequently reported are episodes of constipation and diarrhea, low-grade fever, chills, weakness, fatigue, abdominal distension, flatulence, and anorexia. Patients may report that symptoms often follow and are accentuated by the ingestion of foods such as popcorn, celery, fresh vegetables, whole grains, and nuts. Symptoms are also aggravated during stressful times.

PHYSICAL EXAMINATION. Because diverticular disease is a chronic disorder that generally alters a patient's nutritional intake, inspect for malnutrition symptoms such as weight loss, lethargy, brittle nails, and hair loss. Assess vital signs, since temperature and pulse elevations are common. Palpate the patient's abdominal area for pain or tenderness over the left lower quadrant. Palpate for a mass in this area, which may indicate diverticular inflammation.

PSYCHOSOCIAL. Because emotional tension and stress commonly precipitate episodes of diverticulitis, determine the patient's current stressors and his or her coping mechanisms and what type of support system is available.

DIAGNOSTIC HIGHLIGHTS

Test	Normal Result	Abnormality with Condition	Explanation
Technetium 99 m sodium pertechnetate (gastric or Meckel's) scan	Normal gastric mucosa	May demonstrate diverticulum	Highlights the presence of mucosal abnormalities
Abdominal x rays	Normal abdomen	Identifies perforation of GI tract or left lower quadrant mass	May show signs of free air in the peritoneum if the GI tract has perforated.

Other Tests: Computed tomography (CT) scan, stool specimen, angiography if bleeding is occurring, and complete blood count. Barium enema usually fails to identify diverticulum.

PRIMARY NURSING DIAGNOSIS

Anxiety related to knowledge deficit of the disease process and treatment

OUTCOMES. Anxiety control; Coping; Acceptance: Health status; Symptom control behavior

INTERVENTIONS. Anxiety reduction; Calming technique; Coping enhancement; Presence; Distraction; Energy management; Teaching: Preoperative and procedure or treatment; Medication prescribing

▢ PLANNING AND IMPLEMENTATION

Collaborative

MEDICAL. For uncomplicated diverticulosis, a diet high in vegetable fiber is recommended. If constipation is a problem, bulk-forming laxatives and stool softeners are often prescribed to decrease stool transit time and minimize intraluminal pressure. For diverticulitis, care centers on "resting" the bowel until the inflammatory process subsides. Bed rest is recommended to decrease intestinal motility, and oral intake is restricted, with supplemental intravenous fluid administration followed by a liquid diet and eventually a bland, low-residue diet. After the inflammatory episode resolves, the patient is advanced to a high-fiber diet to prevent future acute inflammatory attacks.

SURGICAL. Surgical intervention may be required if the diverticular disease becomes symptomatic and is not relieved with conservative treatment. Surgery is mandatory if complications develop, such as hemorrhage, bowel obstruction, abscess, or bowel perforation. A colon resection with temporary colostomy placement may be necessary until the bowel heals.

PHARMACOLOGIC HIGHLIGHTS

Medication or Drug Class	Dosage	Description	Rationale
Anti-cholinergic drugs	Varies with drug	Diminishes colon spasms	Control pain by decreasing spasms
Oral antibiotics	Varies with drug	Kills invading bacteria	Control the spread of infection when a fever is present

Other Medications: Analgesics may also be ordered. Generally, meperidine (Demerol) is preferred, since morphine increases intracolonic pressure, thus creating more discomfort and possibly intestinal perforation.

Independent

For uncomplicated diverticulosis, nursing interventions focus on teaching measures to prevent acute inflammatory episodes. Explain the disease process and the strong connection between dietary intake and diverticular disease. Instruct the patient that a diet high in fiber—such as whole grains and cereals, fresh fruits, fresh vegetables, and potatoes—should be followed. Caution the patient to avoid foods with seeds or nuts, which may lodge in the diverticula and cause inflammation.

Teach the patient about prescribed medications. In addition, discuss measures to prevent constipation. Instruct the patient to avoid activities that increase intra-abdominal pressure, such as lifting, bending, coughing, and straining with bowel movements. Instruct the patient about relaxation techniques. Discuss symptoms that indicate an acute inflammation, which would require prompt medical attention.

For patients with diverticulitis, provide supportive care to promote bowel recovery and provide comfort. As the inflammation subsides, teach the patient measures to prevent inflammatory recurrences. Instruct the patient about the purpose of any diagnostic procedures ordered. Should surgery be required, instruct the patient preoperatively about the procedure and postoperative care, leg exercises, deep-breathing exercises, and ostomy care when appropriate. Postoperatively, meticulous wound care must be provided to prevent infection.

DOCUMENTATION GUIDELINES

- Presence of abdominal pain, nausea and vomiting, and diarrhea or constipation

- Patient's ability to cope with the stoma
- Appearance of abdominal wound and stoma
- Ability to manage a colostomy, if appropriate

DISCHARGE AND HOME HEALTHCARE GUIDELINES

Be sure the patient understands any prescribed medications, including purpose, dosage, route, and side effects. Explain the need to keep the wound clean and dry. Teach the patient any special care needed for the wound. Review stoma care with the patient. Teach the patient to observe the wound and report any increased swelling, redness, drainage, odor, separation of the wound edges, or duskiness of the stoma. Review with the patient measures for preventing inflammatory recurrences. Discuss the signs of diverticular inflammation, such as fever, acute abdominal pain, a change in bowel pattern, and rectal bleeding. Explain that such symptoms require prompt medical attention.

Dysfunctional Uterine Bleeding

DRG Category: 369
Mean LOS: 2.9 days
Description: MEDICAL: Menstrual and Other Female Reproductive System Disorders
DRG Category: 364
Mean LOS: 2.6 days
Description: SURGICAL: D & C, Conization Except for Malignancy

Dysfunctional uterine bleeding (DUB) is abnormal uterine bleeding in terms of amount, duration, or timing during the menstrual cycle, with no discernible organic cause. The normal menstrual cycle is dependent on the influence of four hormones: estrogen, which predominates during the proliferative phase (generally days 1 to 14); progesterone, which predominates during the secretory phase (generally days 15 to 28); and follicle stimulating hormone (FSH) and luteinizing hormone (LH), both of which stimulate the ovarian follicle to mature. Disrupting the balance of these four hormones usually results in anovulation and DUB. Complications of DUB include anemia, infection from prolonged use of tampons, and, in rare situations, hemorrhagic shock.

CAUSES

The cause of DUB is unknown. The term DUB indicates that abnormal bleeding is occurring without an organic cause. It is associated with polycystic ovarian disease and obesity; in both of these conditions, the endometrium is chronically stimulated by estrogen.

GENDER AND LIFE SPAN CONSIDERATIONS

DUB can occur from menarche to postmenopause. DUB occurs in teenagers as the result of anovulatory cycles that are related to the immaturity of the hypothalamic-pituitary-gonadal axis. DUB is most common in the perimenopausal woman as the result of changing hormonal levels. The older woman, approaching menopause, possibly suffers from DUB because of a decreased sensitivity of the ovary to follicle-stimulating and luteinizing hormones.

□ ASSESSMENT

HISTORY. Determine the duration of the present bleeding, the amount of blood loss, and the presence of associated symptoms such as cramping, nausea and vomiting, fever, abdominal pain, or passing of blood clots. Obtain a menstrual and obstetric history. Recent episodes of easy bruising or prolonged, heavy bleeding may indicate abnormal clotting times. The use of contraceptives, especially an intrauterine device (IUD) may contribute to abnormal uterine bleeding. Other possible causative factors, such as pregnancy, pelvic inflammatory disease, or other medical conditions, can be ruled out through a complete history.

PHYSICAL EXAMINATION. Most women have a normal physical examination. A complete examination is essential, however, to eliminate organic causes of bleeding. A pelvic speculum and bimanual examination should be done, with particular attention to the presence of cervical erosion, polyps, presumptive signs of pregnancy, masses, tenderness or guarding, or other signs of pathology that may cause abnormal uterine bleeding.

PSYCHOSOCIAL. For many women, DUB results in distress related to the uncertainty of the timing, duration, and amount of bleeding. A woman may feel that her usual activities need to be curtailed, a situation that may contribute to feelings of loss of control. Assess the woman's concerns and coping patterns to establish a framework for determining appropriate interventions.

DIAGNOSTIC HIGHLIGHTS

General Comments: Diagnosis of DUB is made by ruling out organic causes.

Test	Normal Result	Abnormality with Condition	Explanation
Endometrial biopsy	Presence of a "secretory-type" endometrium 3–5 days before normal menses; no pathological conditions	Hyperplastic proliferative polyps are found with DUB (polyps stimulate estrogen). With anovulation, no secretory changes are noted. Adenocarcinoma indicates uterine cancer	Other organic conditions must be ruled out before a diagnosis of DUB is made
Hysteroscopy	No pathology visualized	Polyps indicate DUB; other tumors or structural variations may be seen with other conditions	Direct visualization of the uterus is possible

Other Tests: Pelvic exam, uterine ultrasound, complete blood count, cultures for sexually transmitted infections

PRIMARY NURSING DIAGNOSIS

Fluid volume deficit related to blood loss

OUTCOMES. Fluid balance; Hydration; Circulation status

INTERVENTIONS. Bleeding reduction; Blood product administration; Intravenous therapy; Shock management

◻ PLANNING AND IMPLEMENTATION

Collaborative

The patient may be confronted with a prolonged evaluation and a variety of treatments before uterine bleeding resumes a more normal pattern or stops completely. Activities are not restricted and can be continued as the woman tolerates them. If infection or anemia is identified, appropriate pharmacologic therapy is initiated. Hormonal manipulation may be indicated, requiring careful dosing and attention to compliance with the treatment plan. Surgical management typically begins with dilation and curettage to remove excessive endometrial buildup, but may include intrauterine cryosurgery, laser ablation of the endometrium, or, as a last resort, a hysterectomy.

PHARMACOLOGIC HIGHLIGHTS

Medication or Drug Class	Dosage	Description	Rationale
Medroxyprogesterone acetate (MPA)	10 mg po daily, for 10 days (days 16–25 of the menstrual cycle	Synthetic progestin	Will transform proliferative endometrium into secretory endometrium
Conjugated estrogen (Premarin)	25 mg IV q 4 hours for 3 doses or until bleeding stops	Natural estrogen	Emergency treatment for severe bleeding, follow with progestins

Independent

Important interventions include strategies to assist the woman in maintaining normal activities during the evaluation. Instruct the woman about the signs and symptoms of toxic shock syndrome (fever, joint and muscle aches, malaise, weakness) if she continues to use tampons; more frequent than normal changes of the tampon may be indicated. The use of incontinence pads may be more beneficial than the standard feminine napkin in the presence of heavy bleeding.

Issues related to sexuality, especially if hysterectomy is indicated, require an accepting, open attitude of the nurse. The woman may feel her femininity is threatened but may have difficulty expressing these feelings. You may need to initiate discussions regarding the impact of evaluation and treatment on the woman. If appropriate, consider the effect on the woman's partner and include the partner in all discussions.

DOCUMENTATION GUIDELINES

- Findings on history and physical examination; complete blood count
- Records of the bleeding patterns kept by the woman
- Presence of symptoms from complications such as anemia

DISCHARGE AND HOME HEALTHCARE GUIDELINES

Provide a list of prescribed medications, if any, that includes the name, dosage, route, and side effects and the signs and symptoms of potential complications, including hypotensive episodes. Explain the need for careful monitoring and follow-up of the bleeding. Teach the patient to have appropriate laboratory follow-up of the complete blood count if indicated.

Ectopic Pregnancy

DRG Category: 378
Mean LOS: 2.6 days
Description: MEDICAL AND SURGICAL: Ectopic Pregnancy

An ectopic pregnancy is an implantation of the blastocyst (a solid mass of cells, formed by rapid mitotic division of the zygote, that eventually form the embryo) in a site other than the endometrial lining of the uterus. In more than 95% of ectopic pregnancies, this implantation occurs somewhere in the fallopian tubes, hence the term "tubal pregnancy." Other sites of potential implantation are the cervix, ovary, abdomen, and interstitial tissue of the uterus.

After the blastocyst implants in the tube, it begins to grow and can cause bleeding into the abdominal cavity. Eventually the ovum becomes too large, and the tube can rupture, thus causing further bleeding into the abdominal cavity. Ectopic pregnancies occur in approximately 1 in 200 pregnancies in European-Americans and in 1 in 120 pregnancies in non-European-Americans. It is the leading cause of maternal death from hemorrhage and accounts for 13% of all pregnancy-related deaths. Furthermore, an ectopic pregnancy reduces a woman's chance of future pregnancy because of tubal damage; approximately one-third of women who experience an ectopic pregnancy subsequently give birth to a live infant. Complications other than hemorrhage include peritonitis and infertility.

CAUSES

The major cause of ectopic pregnancy is tubal damage, which can result from pelvic inflammatory disease, previous pelvic or tubal surgery, or endometriosis. Other causes may be hormonal factors that impede ovum transport and mechanically stop the forward movement of the egg in the tube, congenital anomalies of the tube, and a blighted ovum. Pelvic infections and sexually transmitted diseases (STDs), specifically chlamydia and gonorrhea, are often involved.

GENDER AND LIFE SPAN CONSIDERATIONS

Ectopic pregnancy is most often seen in non-European-American women over the age of 35. It often occurs in teens who have engaged in high-risk sexual practices that have resulted in frequent pelvic infections.

□ ASSESSMENT

HISTORY. Elicit a history about the onset of menses, gynecologic disorders, pattern of sexual practices and birth control, and past pregnancies. Patients with an ectopic pregnancy often have some history of tubular damage as a result of infections or endometriosis. They may also have had tubal surgeries. Often patients describe a history of using an intrauterine device (IUD), and some may report a history of infertility. Question the patient about her last menstrual period to determine the onset, duration, amount of bleeding, and whether it was a "normal" period for her. This description is important because although amenorrhea may be present in many cases of ectopic pregnancy, uterine bleeding that occurs with ectopic pregnancy may be mistaken for a menstrual period. In addition to amenorrhea, the patient may exhibit other signs of pregnancy.

PHYSICAL EXAMINATION. Assess vaginal bleeding for the amount, color, and odor; if none is noted, bleeding may be concealed. Bleeding can occur as vaginal spotting, as a "slow leak," or as a massive hemorrhage, depending on the gestational age and whether the tube has ruptured. Usually the bleeding is slow, and the abdomen can become rigid and tender. Sometimes vaginal bleeding is present with the death of the embryo. If internal hemorrhage is profuse, the woman experiences signs and symptoms of hypovolemic shock (restlessness, agitation, confusion, cold and clammy skin, increased respirations and heart rate, delayed capillary blanching, hypotension).

Evaluate the patient's pain; it can range from a feeling of fullness in the rectal area and abdominal cramping to excruciating pain. Often the pain is one-sided and increases when the cervix is moved during a vaginal exam. Some women do not feel any pain until the tube is about to rupture, usually at the 3-month period of gestation. If the tube ruptures, the woman experiences sharp, one-sided, lower abdominal pain and syncope. The pain may radiate to the shoulders and neck and is aggravated by situations that cause increased abdominal pressure, such as lifting or having a bowel movement.

PSYCHOSOCIAL. Often the patient experiences anger, grief, guilt, and self-blame over the loss of the fetus. She may also be anxious about her ability to conceive in the future. Since much of her anxiety may stem from lack of information about her condition, assess her learning needs. Determine the ability of the father and other family members to cope and support the patient.

DIAGNOSTIC HIGHLIGHTS

General Comments: Diagnosis is based on a positive pregnancy and inability to visualize the embryo in the uterus.

Test	Normal Result	Abnormality with Condition	Explanation
Human chorionic gonadotropin (hCG)	Normally is not present in nonpregnant women	Elevated, but not as high as in a normal pregnancy	hCG doubles every 2 days during the first 40 days of pregnancy; failure to do so is evidence of abnormality
Transvaginal ultrasound	Intrauterine gestational sac	Unable to visualize intrauterine sac	This result, combined with a positive pregnancy

| is visualized | test (elevated hCG), confirms the diagnosis |

Other Tests: Laparoscopic examination of the abdominal cavity (only used in confusing cases), Rh antibody screen and blood type, complete blood count (CBC) and coagulation studies, and culdocentesis

PRIMARY NURSING DIAGNOSIS

Anticipatory grieving related to the loss of a pregnancy

OUTCOMES. Coping; Family coping; Grief resolution

INTERVENTIONS. Grief work facilitation; Perinatal death; Active listening; Presence

□ PLANNING AND IMPLEMENTATION

Collaborative

MEDICAL. Medical management of a tubal pregnancy depends on the patient's condition and whether the tube has ruptured. If the tube is intact, the gestation is less than 6 weeks, and the fertilized mass is less than 3.5 cm in diameter, methotrexate, a chemotherapeutic agent that inhibits cell division, may be ordered. If the tube is damaged or ruptured, surgical management is indicated.

SURGICAL. Laparoscopic laser surgery is usually performed, but if the tube has already ruptured, a laparotomy may be indicated. A salpingectomy (removal of the tube), salpingostomy (incision and evacuation of tubal contents), salpingotomy (incision and closure of the tube), or segmental resection and anastomosis can be performed. The goal is to salvage the tube, especially in women who desire future pregnancy.

Postoperative care includes monitoring vital signs and observing for other signs of shock. Monitor the fluid intake and output as well, and note the color and amount of vaginal bleeding. Observe the incision for any signs and symptoms of infection. Administer analgesics and assess the patient's level of pain relief from the medication.

PHARMACOLOGIC HIGHLIGHTS

Medication or Drug Class	Dosage	Description	Rationale
Methotrexate sodium (Folex)	15–30 mg/day IM for 5 days (may repeat with 1–2-week rest periods)	Antineoplastic	Inhibits the growth of the pregnancy by interfering with DNA, RNA, and protein synthesis
Analgesics	Varies by drug	Narcotics, NSAIDs; drug used depends on the level of pain	Relieve pain
RhoD immuno-globin (RhoGAM)	120–300 μg IM one time	Immune serum	Given only if mother is Rh- and father is Rh+; prevents the antigen-

> antibody response leading
> to Rh isoimmunization in
> future pregnancies

Independent

Provide emotional support, using therapeutic communication techniques to relieve the patient's anxiety. Emotional support of this patient is important because the termination of any pregnancy causes a host of psychological and physiologic changes. Inform the patient of perinatal grief support groups.

The patient may be concerned about infertility. Provide information, and clarify the physician's explanations if needed. If necessary, provide a referral for a clinical nurse specialist or counselor.

DOCUMENTATION GUIDELINES

- Physical responses: Amount and character of blood loss, vital signs, abdominal assessment (presence and description of pain, response to analgesics)
- Serial laboratory values: Hemoglobin and hematocrit, coagulation profile, white blood count; results of Rh test
- Response to treatments: Surgery, laparoscopy, fluid or blood replacement, medications
- Emotional status and coping abilities, partner's response
- Presence of complications: Hemorrhage, hypovolemic shock, infection.

DISCHARGE AND HOME HEALTHCARE GUIDELINES

PATIENT TEACHING. If the patient is receiving methotrexate on an outpatient basis, teach her that more severe pain may indicate treatment failure and that she needs to notify the physician. She may experience anorexia, nausea, and vomiting as side effects of methotrexate. She also needs to follow up with scheduled hCG testing.

If a salpingectomy was done, explain to the patient that becoming pregnant again may be difficult. Fertilization only takes place on the side of the remaining tube after ovulation of the ovary on the same side. If a tubal repair was done, the patient is at a higher risk for a subsequent ectopic pregnancy, as well as infertility. Educate the patient to recognize the signs and symptoms of ectopic pregnancy and to notify the doctor immediately if these should occur.

To prevent recurrence, advise the patient to engage in safe sexual practices. Teach her strategies to avoid STDs and pelvic infections that could cause further damage to the fallopian tubes.

POSTOPERATIVE INSTRUCTIONS. Give the patient the following instructions: Limit activity and get plenty of rest. Increase fluid intake. Keep the incision clean. Refrain from sexual intercourse for 2 weeks until the follow-up appointment with the physician occurs.

REFERRAL. If the patient is having difficulty dealing with the perinatal loss, referring her to a support group is appropriate. Often follow-up by the hospital perinatal grief counselor is done.

Emphysema

DRG Category: 088
Mean LOS: 5.6 days
Description: MEDICAL: Chronic Obstructive
Pulmonary Disease

Emphysema is a chronic obstructive pulmonary disease (COPD) that is characterized by abnormal, permanent enlargement of the air spaces past the terminal bronchioles, which results in the destruction of respiratory walls. The syndrome includes both chronic bronchitis and emphysema. COPD affects almost 15 million people and is the fourth leading cause of death overall in the United States. In emphysema, the affected terminal bronchioles contain mucous plugs that, when they are enlarged, eventually result in the loss of elasticity of the lung parenchyma, thus causing difficulty in the expiratory phase of respiration. The alveolar walls are destroyed by abnormal levels of enzymes (proteases) that break down respiratory walls. Gas exchange is impaired by the reduced surface area that results from the destruction of alveolar walls.

Four types of emphysema have been identified: paraseptal emphysema, which affects the periphery of the lobule; panacinar or panlobular emphysema, which affects the lower anterior segments or the entire lungs; centriacinar or centrilobular emphysema, the most common form, which destroys respiratory bronchioles and is associated with chronic bronchitis and cigarette smoking; and bronchiectasis or chronic necrotizing infection that leads to abnormal and permanent bronchial dilation, which occurs rarely. Complications from emphysema include cor pulmonale, respiratory failure, pneumothorax, and recurrent respiratory tract infections. Emphysema is the most common cause of death from respiratory disease in the United States.

CAUSES

The actual cause of emphysema is unknown. Risk factors for the development of emphysema include cigarette smoking, living or working in a highly polluted area, and a family history of pulmonary disease. Frequent childhood pulmonary infections have been identified as a cause of bronchiectasis.

GENDER AND LIFE SPAN CONSIDERATIONS

Symptoms of emphysema may begin in the third or fourth decade of life but usually become severe during the fifth decade or later. Emphysema occurs more often in males than in females.

☐ ASSESSMENT

HISTORY. Establish a history of dyspnea, determining if it has increased over time. Ask if the dyspnea is extreme during exertion and present even during rest. Determine if the patient has experienced anorexia, weight loss, and weakness. Ask if the patient has had a cough and, if so, for how long. Determine if there are signs of oxygen deficiency; ask significant others if the patient has been restless or confused or has experienced changes in mental status. Ask if the patient lives or works in a highly polluted area. Establish cigarette smoking habits, including how long, how many, and whether they are unfiltered. Elicit a history of family pulmonary disease or frequent childhood pulmonary infections.

PHYSICAL EXAMINATION. Inspect the patient for a decreased muscle mass and increased anteroposterior diameter (also known as barrel chest). Observe respirations for the use of accessory muscles, such as the sternocleidomastoid and pectoral muscles, as well as pursed-lip breathing during expiration. Assess the patient's respirations for rate, rhythm, and quality. Inspect the patient for neck vein distension or liver congestion. Note signs of oxygen deficiency, such as restlessness, changes in mental status, confusion, and tachycardia.

A cough may be present during the later stages of the disease; the small amount of sputum it produces is usually mucoid. Upon palpation, note decreased tactile fremitus. Percussion may elicit a diffusely hyperresonant sound. Auscultate for decreased or absent breath sounds, distant heart sounds, wheezes, and possibly crackles. Examine the patient for peripheral cyanosis or clubbing of the fingers.

PSYCHOSOCIAL. Patients with emphysema may be anxious or restless, depending on the degree of dyspnea they are experiencing. Emphysema may necessitate role or occupational changes that could lead to depression. Assess the patient's emotional, financial, and social resources to determine if they are available to the patient to help cope with a chronic disease.

DIAGNOSTIC HIGHLIGHTS

Test	Normal Result	Abnormality with Condition	Explanation
Forced vital capacity (FVC): Maximum volume of air that can be forcefully expired after a maximal lung inspiration	4.0 L	50% of the predicted value	Air trapping and obstruction with plugs decrease flow rates
Forced expiratory volume in 1 second (FEV_1): Volume of air expired in 1 second from the beginning of the FVC maneuver	3.0 liters or 84% of FVC	25%–35% of the predicted value	Air trapping and airway obstruction with plugs decrease flow rates
Forced expiratory flow (FEF): Maximal flow rate attained during middle (25%–75%) of FVC maneuver	Varies by body size	25% of the predicted value	Predicts airway trapping and obstruction of smaller airways
Residual volume (RV): Volume of air remaining in lungs at end of a maximal expiration	1.2 L	Increased up to 400% of normal	Increased RV indicates air trapping and obstruction

Functional residual capacity (FRC): Volume of air remaining in lungs at end of a resting tidal volume	2.3 L	Increased up to 200% of normal	Increased FRC indicates air trapping

Other Tests: Chest x ray, pulse oximetry, arterial blood gases, complete blood count, and electrocardiogram. Peak expiratory flow rates (PEFR; maximal flow rate attained during the FVC maneuver; decreased from baseline during periods of obstruction) may be used at home daily for patients who require daily medications

PRIMARY NURSING DIAGNOSIS

Impaired gas exchange related to destruction of alveolar walls

OUTCOMES. Respiratory status: Gas exchange; Respiratory status: Ventilation; Comfort level; Anxiety control

INTERVENTIONS. Airway management; Cough enhancement; Respiratory monitoring; Oxygen therapy; Laboratory data interpretation; Positioning; Smoking cessation assistance; Ventilation assistance

☐ PLANNING AND IMPLEMENTATION

Collaborative

Viral or bacterial infections may lead to bronchospasm or increased mucus secretions. Acute exacerbations are accompanied by dyspnea, fatigue, and even respiratory failure. Low-flow oxygen therapy based on arterial blood gas results is often administered to treat hypoxemia. For the patient with increasing airway obstruction and plugging, endotracheal intubation and perhaps mechanical ventilation may be needed to maintain adequate airway and breathing. Adequate hydration is also necessary to help liquefy secretions.

PHARMACOLOGIC HIGHLIGHTS

Medication or Drug Class	Dosage	Description	Rationale
Bronchodilators: beta$_2$ adrenergic agents	Varies by drug	Inhaled beta$_2$-adrenergic agonists by metered-dose inhaler (MDI) such as albuterol, metaproterenol, or terbutaline	Reversal of broncho-constriction
Bronchodilators: Anticholinergic agents	Varies by drug	Atropine sulfate, ipratropium bromide	Reversal of broncho-constriction
Systemic corticosteroids	Varies by drug	Methylprednisolone IV; prednisone po	Decrease inflammatory response and improve airflow in some patients for

a few days during acute exacerbations.

Other Drug Therapy: Bronchodilators, which are used for prevention and maintenance therapy, can be administered as aerosols or oral medications. Antibiotics are ordered if a secondary infection develops. As a preventive measure, influenza and pneumonia vaccines are administered.

Independent

Maintaining a patent airway is a priority. Use a humidifier at night to help the patient mobilize secretions in the morning. Encourage the patient to use controlled coughing to clear secretions that might have collected in the lungs during sleep. Instruct the patient to sit at the bedside or in a comfortable chair, hug a pillow, bend the head downward a little, take several deep breaths, and cough strongly.

Place patients who are experiencing dyspnea in a high Fowler position to improve lung expansion. Placing pillows on the overhead table and having the patient lean over in the orthopneic position may also be helpful. Teach the patient pursed-lip and diaphragmatic breathing. To avoid infection, screen visitors for contagious diseases and instruct the patient to avoid crowds.

Conserve the patient's energy in every possible way. Plan activities to allow for rest periods, eliminating nonessential procedures until the patient is stronger. It may be necessary to assist with the activities of daily living and to anticipate the patient's needs by having supplies within easy reach. Refer the patient to a pulmonary rehabilitation program if one is available in the community. Patient education is vital to long-term management. Teach the patient about the disease and its implications for lifestyle changes, such as avoidance of cigarette smoke and other irritants, activity alterations, and any necessary occupational changes. Provide information to the patient and family about medications and equipment.

DOCUMENTATION GUIDELINES

- Rate, quality, and depth of respirations; vital signs
- Physical findings: Dyspnea, cyanosis, decreased muscle mass, cough, increased anterioposterior chest diameter, and use of accessory muscles during respiration; characteristics of sputum
- Activity tolerance, ability to perform self-care
- Signs and symptoms of infection; response to pharmacologic therapy, response to oxygen therapy

DISCHARGE AND HOME HEALTHCARE GUIDELINES

Be sure the patient and family understand any medication prescribed, including dosage, route, action, and side effects. Instruct the patient to report any signs and symptoms of infection to the primary healthcare provider. Explain necessary dietary adjustments to the patient and family. Recommend eating small, frequent meals, including high-protein, high-density foods. Encourage the patient to plan rest periods around his or her activities, conserving as much energy as possible. Arrange for return demonstrations of equipment used by the patient and family. If the patient requires home oxygen therapy, refer the patient to the appropriate rental service, and explain the hazards of combustion and increasing the flow rate without consultation from the primary healthcare provider.

Encephalitis

DRG Category: 020
Mean LOS: 8.2 days
Description: MEDICAL: Nervous System In-
fection, Except Viral Meningitis

Encephalitis, or inflammation of the brain, usually occurs when the cerebral hemispheres, brainstem, or cerebellum is infected by a microorganism. Approximately 2000 cases of encephalitis are reported each year in the United States. Most forms have mortality rates of less than 10%, with the exception of eastern equine encephalitis, where mortality is as high as 50%.

Encephalitis has two forms: primary and postinfectious (or parainfectious). The primary form of the disease occurs when a virus invades and replicates within the brain. Postinfectious encephalitis describes brain inflammation that develops in combination with other viral illnesses or following the administration of vaccines such as measles, mumps, and rubella. In that case, encephalitis occurs because of a hypersensitivity reaction that leads to demyelination of nerves.

When the brain becomes inflamed, lymphocytes infiltrate brain tissue and the meninges of the brain. Cerebral edema results, and ultimately brain cells can degenerate, thus leading to widespread nerve cell destruction. Complications from encephalitis can be short term or lifelong. Bronchial pneumonia and respiratory tract infections may complicate the course of encephalitis. Patients may go into a coma and experience all the complications of immobility, such as contractures and pressure ulcers. Other complications include epilepsy, parkinsonism, behavioral and personality changes, and mental retardation. A comatose state may last for days, weeks, or months after the acute infectious state.

CAUSES

Most cases of encephalitis are related to viruses. In the United States, most cases of nonepidemic encephalitis are often caused by the LaCrosse virus and are most common in rural areas of the Midwest. Epidemics of both St. Louis encephalitis (found mostly in the East and Midwest) and western equine encephalitis (found across North America) have contributed a large number of the total cases since 1955. Many sources cite the St. Louis encephalitis virus as the most common form in this country, although many forms of the disease exist.

Encephalitis has been associated with many other diseases, including Creutzfeldt-Jakob disease, herpes simplex (specifically herpes simplex I), kuru, malaria, mononucleosis, rabies, trichinosis, and typhus.

GENDER AND LIFE SPAN CONSIDERATIONS

Encephalitis may occur at any age and in both genders. Encephalitis caused by herpes simplex I is most common in children and young adults. California encephalitis is most common in children from 5 to 10 years of age. Eastern equine encephalitis commonly occurs in children younger than 10 and in older adults, whereas western equine encephalitis occurs in infants under a year and in older adults. St. Louis encephalitis is seen most often in adults older than 35.

☐ ASSESSMENT

HISTORY. Obtain a history of recent illnesses,which may include an upper respiratory infection or a minor systemic illness that caused headache, muscle ache, malaise, sore throat, and runny nose. Note if the patient has other sites of infection, such as a recent skull fracture or head injury, middle ear infection, or sinus infection. Ask if the patient has had a recent immunization, exposure to mumps or herpes simplex virus, animal bites, recent travel, or exposure to epidemic outbreaks or mononucleosis. Ask if a child has been playing in a rural area where exposure to ticks or mosquitoes was possible.

Encephalitis typically has an abrupt onset. The patient, parents, or family may describe altered respiratory patterns, fever, headache, nuchal (neck) rigidity, and vomiting. Neurological symptoms generally follow 24 to 48 hours after the initial onset; often a seizure is the initial presenting symptom. The patient and family may describe other symptoms such as facial palsies, difficulty speaking, and decreased movement and sensation of the extremities.

PHYSICAL EXAMINATION. The patient appears acutely ill with an altered mental status that may range from mild confusion to delirium and coma. The patient may have tremors, cranial nerve palsies, and absent superficial or exaggerated deep tendon reflexes. There may be a decrease in sensation, along with weakness or even paralysis of the extremities. The patient may have no sense of taste or smell and may have difficulty speaking and swallowing. Heart and respiratory rates may be rapid. The patient's skin is often warm because of fever.

PSYCHOSOCIAL. Encephalitis can be life-threatening and lead to permanent disability; therefore, determine the patient's and family's ability to cope with sudden illness, anxiety, and stress, as well as disability. If the patient is a child, the parents may be excessively anxious. Analyze the family structure, the number of children, the financial resources, and the role of parental support systems to determine the extent of the problem.

DIAGNOSTIC HIGHLIGHTS

Test	Normal Result	Abnormality with Condition	Explanation
Lumbar puncture and cerebral spinal fluid (CSF) analysis	Pressure: 70–180 mm H_2O Glucose: 45–80 mg/dL Protein: 15–45 mg/mL	Slight to moderate increase in proteins and white blood cells in the cerebrospinal fluid (CSF); normal glucose level. CSF pressure is often normal or slightly increased. If the patient has herpes simplex virus, the CSF may contain red blood cells	Encephalitis is usually caused by viral infections rather than bacterial, hence the normal CSF glucose

Other Tests: Electroencephalogram (EEG), computed tomography (CT) scan, magnetic resonance imaging (MRI), CSF cultures, and radionuclide scans

PRIMARY NURSING DIAGNOSIS

Risk for ineffective airway clearance related to unresponsiveness and inability to clear secretions

OUTCOMES. Respiratory status: Gas exchange; Respiratory status: Ventilation; Symptom control behavior; Treatment behavior: Illness or injury; Comfort level

INTERVENTIONS. Airway management; Anxiety reduction; Oxygen therapy; Airway suctioning; Airway insertion and stabilization; Cough enhancement; Positioning; Respiratory monitoring

◻ PLANNING AND IMPLEMENTATION

Collaborative

To maintain a patent airway, many patients require endotracheal intubation, oxygen therapy, and mechanical ventilation if gas exchange is impaired. One of the most important roles of the nurse and physician is ongoing neurological assessment. Using serial assessments, the healthcare team documents changes in the patient's condition and initiates proper care immediately. Pupil size and reaction, level of consciousness, strength and motion of the extremities, and the patient's response to noxious stimuli are all essential for patient assessment and management.

PHARMACOLOGIC HIGHLIGHTS

Medication or Drug Class	Dosage	Description	Rationale
Anti-viral agents	Acyclovir 10 mg/dk q 8 hours; infuse IV over at least 1 hour; vidarabine (ARA-A) 15 mg/kg per day infused IV over 12 hours	Interferes with DNA synthesis and viral replication	Combat herpes simplex encephalitis

Independent

The maintenance of airway, breathing, and circulation is the foremost concern for the patient with encephalitis. If the patient is unable to clear secretions or maintain a patent airway as the disease progresses, notify the physician immediately, and prepare for endotracheal intubation. The family is likely to be anxious and need a great deal of support should intubation and mechanical ventilation be necessary. Once the airway is in place, maintaining an open airway with suctioning as needed is a primary nursing responsibility.

Always take into account patient safety, and weigh it against the possibility of the patient's further increase in intracranial pressure. Implement measures to limit the effects of immobility, such as skin care, range-of-motion exercises, and a turning and positioning schedule. Note the effect of position changes on intracranial pressure, and space activities as necessary.

The patient and significant others need assistance in learning about the disease process and treatments. The patient's behavioral and communication changes are often the most difficult to face and understand. Alterations can occur in thought processes when intracranial pressure begins to increase and the level of consciousness begins to decrease. Reorient the patient to time, place, and person as needed. Keep familiar objects or pictures around the patient. Allow visitation of significant others. Establish alternate means of communication if the patient is unable to maintain verbal contact (e.g., the patient who needs intubation).

DOCUMENTATION GUIDELINES

- Physical responses: Adequacy of airway, breathing, circulation; serial neurological assessments; signs of increased pressure; vital signs; seizures
- Ability to respond to environment, need for restraints

DISCHARGE AND HOME HEALTHCARE GUIDELINES

Although most patients recover fully before being discharged from the hospital, some have lifelong deficits following encephalitis. If the patient needs supportive care, teach the family, significant others, and caregivers how to plan and administer hygiene, nutrition, and medications. If arrangements need to be made for a nursing home or long-term facility, work with the family and social service to arrange for a careful transition.

Teach the patient and family about the disease process and signs of recurrence. Make sure that the patient and family know when the follow-up visit with the healthcare provider is scheduled. Teach the patient and family about the route, dosage, mechanism of action, and side effects of all medications. Provide written information so that the patient and family have a permanent record of the communication.

Endometriosis

DRG Category: 69
Mean LOS: 2.9 days
Description: MEDICAL: Menstrual and Other Female Reproductive System Disorders
DRG Category: 358
Mean LOS: 4.7 days
Description: SURGICAL: Uterine and Adnexa Procedures for Nonmalignancy with CC

Endometriosis is a benign growth of endometrial tissue that occurs atypically outside of the uterine cavity. Although endometriosis can grow anywhere in the body, it is found most commonly around the ovaries, cul-de-sac, cervix, uterosacral ligaments, rectovaginal septum, sigmoid colon, round ligaments, and pelvic peritoneum. During the reproductive years, the atypical endometrial tissue responds the same to hormonal stimulation as does the tissue within the uterus. Thus, the tissue grows during the proliferative and secretory phase of the woman's menstrual cycle and bleeds during or immediately after it. This bleeding drains into the peritoneal cavity and causes an inflammatory process with subsequent fibrosis and adhesions. Such scarring may lead to blockage or distortion of any of the surrounding organs.

The primary complication of endometriosis is infertility, which results from adhesions and scarring that are caused by bleeding from the atypical endometrial tissue. These adhesions may occur around the uterus and fix it into a retroverted position. They may also block the fallopian tubes or the fimbriated ends, thereby preventing the ovum from being carried into the uterus. Endometriosis can also lead to spontaneous abortion and anemia.

CAUSES

The cause of endometriosis is not known. The most predominant theory is the transplantation theory, which suggests that endometriosis results from a backflow of endometrial tissue from the uterus into the pelvic cavity during menstruation. This flow starts through the fallopian tubes and passes into the peritoneal cavity, where it implants to form atypical (ectopic) sites of endometrial tissue. There also may be a genetic predisposition for endometriosis. Women who have had mothers and sisters with this disease process have been found to be at higher risk of developing endometriosis.

GENDER AND LIFE SPAN CONSIDERATIONS

Endometriosis is estimated to occur in 7% of women of reproductive age in the United States; the highest incidence is in nulliparous Caucasian women. It can occur at any age after puberty, although it is most commonly found in women aged 30 to 40. There is a higher incidence of endometriosis in women who marry and bear children later in their lives. The course of the disease is individual and may worsen with each repeated cycle, or the woman may remain asymptomatic throughout her reproductive years. The symptoms and progression of the disease stop after menopause.

☐ ASSESSMENT

HISTORY. Elicit a complete history of the woman's menstrual, obstetric, sexual, and contraceptive practices. Endometriosis is difficult to diagnose because some of its symptoms are also manifestations of other pelvic conditions, such as pelvic inflammation, ovarian cysts, and ovarian cancers. A thorough description of the patient's symptoms becomes important, therefore, in the early diagnosis of the condition. Symptoms of endometriosis vary with the location of the ectopic tissue. Some women may even be asymptomatic during the entire course of the disease.

The symptoms may also change over time. The major symptom is dysmenorrhea (pain associated with menses) that is different from the normal uterine cramping during the woman's menstrual cycle. This cramping has been referred to as a deep-seated aching, pressing, or grinding in the lower abdomen, vagina, posterior pelvis, and/or back. It usually occurs 1 to 2 days before the onset of the menstrual cycle and lasts 2 to 3 days. Other possible symptoms are pain during a bowel movement around the time of menstruation, a heaviness noted in the pelvic region, abnormal vaginal bleeding, nausea, diarrhea, and pain during sexual intercourse (dyspareunia) or exercise.

PHYSICAL EXAMINATION. During a pelvic examination, the cervix may be laterally displaced to the left or right of the midline. Palpation of the abdomen may uncover nodules in the uterosacral ligament, with tenderness in the posterior fornix and restricted movement of the uterus. Palpation may also identify ovarian enlargement that was caused by the presence of ovarian cysts.

During acute flare-ups of the disease, an internal pelvic examination may cause the patient excruciating suprapubic and abdominal pain. The acute disease may be difficult to distinguish from appendicitis or other conditions that lead to an "acute abdomen." The patient may have a rigid abdomen, abdominal guarding, and a low-grade fever.

PSYCHOSOCIAL. Endometriosis is a chronic, long-term condition, with symptoms that occur every month for 2 to 3 days until menopause. Severe discomfort, interferences with activities of daily living or leisure activities, impaired sexual function, and the disappointments of infertility can contribute to depression in women with this chronic disease. Inquire about the level of partner support.

DIAGNOSTIC HIGHLIGHTS

General Comments: Endometriosis is often first diagnosed when the woman seeks help for infertility.

TEST	Normal Result	Abnormality with Condition	Explanation
Cancer-antigen 125 (CA-125)	0–35	Elevated	The elevation of this antigen correlates with the amount of disease present
Laparoscopy	No ectopic tissue visualized	Ectopic tissue is visualized	Presence of ectopic tissue confirms the diagnosis
Biopsy	N/A	Identifies the tissue as benign endometrial tissue	Rules out malignancy, confirming the diagnosis

PRIMARY NURSING DIAGNOSIS

Pain, chronic, related to cramping, internal bleeding, swelling, and inflammation during the menstrual cycle

OUTCOMES. Comfort level; Pain control; Depression control; Pain: Disruptive effects; Pain psychological response

INTERVENTIONS. Analgesic administration; Pain management; Heat/cold application, progressive muscle relaxation

◻ PLANNING AND IMPLEMENTATION

Collaborative

MEDICAL. Women who are nearing menopause are usually treated prophylactically until they enter menopause. If the woman is in no distress and is approaching menopause, no treatment will be necessary except observing the progression of the disease. By contrast, a younger woman who wishes to become pregnant may be treated more aggressively.

Some women may be instructed to get pregnant as quickly as possible if they wish to have children. Pregnancy and lactation suppress menstruation and result in shrinkage of the endometrial tissue implants. Relief from symptoms has been noted to persist years after the pregnancy.

SURGICAL. Surgery is performed conservatively, by laparoscopy or laparotomy using laser via the laparoscope. The goal is to remove as much of the ectopic endometrial tissue as possible and retain the woman's reproductive ability. In older women with severe symptoms who have completed childbearing, or as a last resort in childbearing-aged women, a hysterectomy may be the surgery of choice with or without a bilateral salpingo-oophorectomy.

PHARMACOLOGIC HIGHLIGHTS

Medication or Drug Class	Dosage	Description	Rationale
Oral contraceptives	1 tab per day	Hormonal therapy	Halts the spread and shrinks the endometrial implant, suppresses ovulation, prevents dysmenorrhea
Progestins (medroxyprogesterone acetate)	400 mg IM per month (maintenance)		
Danazol (Danocrine)	200–800 mg per day in 2 divided doses, for 3–9 months	Gonadotropin inhibitor; synthetic androgenic steroid similar to testosterone	Suppresses follicle stimulating hormone (FSH) and luteinizing hormone (LH), suppressing ovulation, thus resulting in atrophy of the endometrial tissue
Nafarelin (Synarel)	Metered nasal spray bid	Gonadotropin (Gn) releasing hormone agonist	Restricts the secretion of Gn hormones and the production of FSH, LH, and estrogen; produces a "pseudomenopause"
Leuprolide (Lupron)	3.75 mg IM daily/monthly (or 11.25 mg q 3 months)		
Goserelin (Zoladex)	Subcutaneous implant		
Acetaminophen, ASA, ibuprofen, various narcotics	Varies by drug	Over the counter and prescription pain-relieving drugs	Relieve discomfort, but do not affect the progress of the disease

Independent

Care focuses on strategies to relieve pain and discomfort, to support the patient during a stressful time, and to provide patient education. The pain of endometriosis can be mild or severe. Unless the patient has other underlying diseases, she will generally be managed on an outpatient basis until surgical intervention is needed. To relieve pain, instruct the woman that over the counter analgesics such as acetaminophen are preferable to nonsteroidal anti-inflammatory drugs (NSAIDs) and aspirin because of the latter's tendency to increase bleeding. Some patients obtain relief from cramping by lying on the side with the legs bent, taking warm baths, or using a heating device on the lower abdomen. Make sure that the patient uses heating devices on a low setting to prevent burns. Caution the patient with acute abdominal pain from unknown causes not to use a heating pad because of the risk of a perforated appendix.

Assess the woman's cultural and ethnic influences, which will play a part in her understanding and subsequent coping with endometriosis. Be emotionally supportive. Provide interested couples with information on the Endometriosis Association, Resolve (a support, education, research group for infertile couples), and newer techniques for infertility management. Encourage the couple to talk openly about the disease and its effects on their sexual compatibility, and urge the woman to tell her partner about any discomfort during sexual intercourse to minimize misunderstandings. Encourage the couple to try different positions during sexual intercourse to find those most comfortable for the woman.

DOCUMENTATION GUIDELINES

- Physical symptoms: Pain, cramping, abdominal guarding, degree of menstrual flow
- Response to interventions for relief of pain and treatment modalities
- Response of the partner to the disease process, possible changes in sexual practices, possibility of infertility
- Ability to carry out activities of daily living and other desired activities

DISCHARGE AND HOME HEALTHCARE GUIDELINES

MEDICATIONS. Ensure that the patient understands the dosage, route, action, and side effects before going home.

FOLLOW-UP. Encourage the patient to be alert to her emotions, behavior, physical symptoms, diet, and rest and exercise. Encourage the patient to maintain open communication with her significant other and her family to discuss concerns she may have about the disease process.

Epididymitis

DRG Category: 350
Mean LOS: 4.5 days
Description: MEDICAL: Inflammation of the Male Reproductive System

Epididymitis is an infection or inflammation of the epididymis—a coiled tube that is responsible for nutrition and maturation of the sperm. The epididymis carries sperm from the testicle to the urethra. Epididymitis, the most common intrascrotal infection, is usually unilateral. Epididymitis needs to be differentiated from testicular torsion, tumor, and trauma. If it is left untreated, epididymitis may lead to orchitis, an infection of the testicles, which may lead to sterility.

CAUSES

Infection that results in epididymitis is usually caused by either a sexually transmitted infection (STI) or another form of infection. STIs leading to epididymitis include infection by *Neisseria gonorrheae, Chlamydia trachomatis,* and syphilis. Epididymitis may be a complication of prostatitis or urethritis, or it may be associated with chronic urinary infection caused by *Escherichia coli, Pseudomonas,* or coliform pathogens. Strain or pressure during voiding may force urine that is harboring pathogens from the urethra or prostate through the vas deferens to the epididymis.

GENDER AND LIFE SPAN CONSIDERATIONS

Epididymitis commonly occurs in men 18 to 40 years of age, but rarely in those who have not reached puberty. In men under age 35, the most common cause is an STI. Generally, epididymitis in men over age 35 is from other bacterial causes.

◻ ASSESSMENT

HISTORY. Establish a history of sudden scrotal pain, redness, swelling, and extreme scrotal and groin tenderness. Determine if the patient has experienced fever, chills, or malaise. Ask the patient if he has experienced nausea and vomiting. Elicit a history of prostatitis, urethritis, or chronic urinary infections. Ask the patient if he has been diagnosed with tuberculosis. Determine if the patient has undergone a prostatectomy or has had a traumatic injury to the genitalia. Take a sexual history to determine if the patient has had unprotected sex with a partner who may have had an STI.

PHYSICAL EXAMINATION. Inspect the patient's scrotum, noting any marked edema or redness. Gently palpate the scrotum for tenderness or pain. Observe any urethral discharge. Observe the patient's gait; patients with epididymitis often assume a characteristic waddle to protect the groin and scrotum.

PSYCHOSOCIAL. The patient may be concerned about his sexuality. He may be fearful of becoming sterile or impotent and anxious about whether he can continue to have sexual relationships. The patient may express anger or feelings of victimization if the condition was caused by an STI.

DIAGNOSTIC HIGHLIGHTS

General Comments: Diagnosis is made based on visual symptoms and isolation of infective organsims.

Test	Normal Result	Abnormality with Condition	Explanation
Urinalysis	Clear, no pus	Pyuria; white blood cell count >10,000 mm³	A urinary tract infection can contribute to epididymitis
Urine culture and sensitivity tests	<10,000 bacteria/ml	>10,000 bacteria/mL; pathogen is identified	A urinary tract infection can contribute to epididymitis
Cultures for STIs	Negative culture	Positive for STI	An STI can lead to epididymitis
Prehn's sign	NA	Pain is relieved when the scrotum	Testicular torsion may be present if pain is not

is lifted onto the symphysis	relieved when the scrotum is lifted onto the symphysis

Other Tests: An ultrasound is done to rule out testicular torsion, which presents with similar symptoms, and is a medical emergency.

PRIMARY NURSING DIAGNOSIS

Pain (acute) related to swelling and inflammation of the scrotum

OUTCOMES. Pain level; Pain control; Pain: Disruptive effects

INTERVENTIONS. Analgesic administration; Medication administration; Heat/cold application; Positioning

▢ PLANNING AND IMPLEMENTATION

Collaborative

The goal of treatment is to combat infection and reduce pain and swelling. This is usually accomplished through the use of pharmacologic agents. The patient with epididymitis is usually on bed rest with bathroom privileges. Sexual activity is prohibited during the treatment process. If epididymitis is recurrent, an epididymectomy under local anesthesia or a vasectomy may be indicated, and this will result in sterility. If orchitis develops, it is treated with diethylstilbestrol (DES), which may relieve pain, fever, and swelling. Severe cases of orchitis may require surgery to drain the hydrocele and improve testicular circulation.

PHARMACOLOGIC HIGHLIGHTS

Medication or Drug Class	Dosage	Description	Rationale
Antibiotics	Dependson drug; usually given IV in the hospital and home	Antibiotic used is determined by its ability to eliminate the pathogen	Appropriate antibiotic is needed to eliminated infective organism
Antipyretics	Depends on drug	Preparation to reduce fever	Fever often is present with epididymitis
Analgesics	Depends on drug	Analgesic used depends on the severity of the pain	Decreases pain and discomfort

Independent

The most important interventions are pain control and emotional support. Lifting of the scrotum often relieves the pain in epididymitis; elevating the testicles on a towel eases tension on the spermatic cord and reduces pain. Ice packs to the scrotum also relieve pain, but a barrier between the scrotum and ice pack is necessary to prevent frostbite or the ascension of the testes into the abdominal cavity. Encourage oral fluids of up to 2 to 3 L per day. As the patient heals, he can resume walking, but he should wear an athletic supporter.

Encourage the patient to verbalize his fears and concerns. Answer questions nonjudgmentally. Point out that the patient's sexual partners are at risk if the condition was caused by an STI; urge the patient to notify his partners of his condition. The underlying STI is not restricted only to males and can be transmitted to female sexual partners. For patients who face the possibility of sterility, suggest professional counseling.

DOCUMENTATION GUIDELINES

- Physical findings: Swelling, redness, and tenderness of the scrotum; urethral discharge
- Color, odor, and consistency of urine
- Activity tolerance during ambulation
- Response to antibiotic therapy, analgesics, and other treatments
- Acceptance and understanding of sterility as a result of infection or epididymectomy

DISCHARGE AND HOME HEALTHCARE GUIDELINES

PREVENTION. Teach the patient to use a condom and spermicide for sexual encounters to prevent STIs. Encourage the patient to continue to increase fluid intake and to empty the bladder frequently.

POSTOPERATIVE TEACHING. If the patient had an epididymectomy, teach him to report incisional bleeding, unusual difficulty in starting the urine stream, blood in the urine, or increasing pain and swelling. Remind him of his postoperative appointment and that sexual activity is prohibited until after the postoperative checkup. Suggest the patient use an ice pack and athletic supporter to relieve minor discomfort from the surgery. Tepid sitz baths may also help relieve pain. Remind the patient to avoid strenuous activity and heavy lifting until he is seen by his physician.

COMPLICATIONS. Teach the patient to report problems of impotence to his physician immediately.

MEDICATIONS. Be sure the patient understands any medication prescribed, including dosage, route, action, and side effects. Emphasize the need to complete the course of antibiotic medications, even if symptoms have diminished.

Epidural Hematoma

DRG Category: 014
Mean LOS: 6.4 days
Description: MEDICAL: Specific Cerebrovascular Disorders Except TIA
DRG Category: 002
Mean LOS: 9.8 days
Description: SURGICAL: Craniotomy for Trauma, Age > 17

Epidural hematoma is a rapidly accumulating mass of blood, usually clotted, or a swelling confined to the space between the skull and the dura mater. It is usually found in the temporal area. It is categorized as a focal brain injury, and it accounts for approximately 50% of all head injuries and 60% of the mortality rate in head-injured patients. If an epidural hematoma expands rapidly, such as when the bleeding is arterial in origin, the injury is potentially fatal. The accumulation of blood rapidly displaces brain tissue and can result in cerebral herniation downward into the posterior fossa or toward the midline into the tentorial notch. If the hematoma is evacuated and bleeding is controlled promptly, the patient's prognosis is good. Mortality rates range from 5% to 30%.

Generally, head trauma involves both a primary injury and a secondary injury. The primary injury results from the initial impact, which causes immediate neurological damage and dysfunction. The secondary injury follows the initial trauma and probably stems from cerebral hypoxia and ischemia, which lead to cerebral edema, increased intracranial pressure (ICP), and brain herniation.

CAUSES

The injuries that cause the condition are a strong direct force to the head or an acceleration-deceleration force, which can occur in motor vehicle crashes (MVCs), automobile-pedestrian crashes, falls, and assaults. The injury causes a linear fracture of the temporal lobe in many patients. The bone fracture lacerates the middle meningeal artery or veins. Bleeding from these vessels leads to the accumulation of the hematoma within the extradural portion of the skull.

GENDER AND LIFE SPAN CONSIDERATIONS

Head injury is the leading cause of all trauma-related deaths. Most head injuries are associated with MVCs, which in the 15- to 24-year-old age group are three times more common in males than in females. European-Americans have a death rate that is 40% higher from MVCs than do African-Americans in the 15- to 34-year-old age group. Some experts suggest that the pediatric population may have improved neurological outcomes after head injuries than adults have.

◻ ASSESSMENT

HISTORY. Obtain a detailed description of the initial injury. Determine if the patient experienced momentary loss of reflexes or momentary arrest of respiration. Be sure to determine if the patient was unconscious at any time and, if so, for how long. Determine if the patient experienced nuchal rigidity, photophobia, nausea, vomiting, dizziness, convulsions, decreased respirations, or progressive insensitivity to pain (obtundity). Note that approximately one-third of patients with an epidural hematoma have initial unconsciousness followed by a period of lucidity and then subsequent unconsciousness. Some experienced clinicians suggest the initial period of unconsciousness is brought about by a concussion. The patient awakens, only to become unconscious again because of epidural bleeding.

PHYSICAL EXAMINATION. The initial evaluation is centered on assessing the airway, breathing, circulation, and disability (neurologic status). Exposure (undressing the patient completely) is incorporated as part of the primary survey. The secondary survey, a head-to-toe assessment including vital signs, is then completed.

The initial neurological assessment of the patient includes monitoring the vital signs, assessing the level of consciousness, examining pupil size and level of reactivity, and assessment using the Glasgow Coma Scale (GCS), which evaluates eye opening, best verbal response, and best motor response. The neurological signs and symptoms depend on the location, rapidity, and source of bleeding. More than half of patients develop symptoms within the first 6 hours. Common symptoms include pupil dilation, hemiparesis, and decerebrate posturing (extension). A neurological assessment is repeated at least hourly during the first 24 hours after the injury.

Examine the entire scalp and head for lacerations, abrasions, contusions, or bony abnormalities. Take care to maintain cervical spine immobilization during the examination. Patients may have associated cervical spine injuries or thoracic, abdominal, or extremity trauma. Examine the patient for signs of basilar skull fractures, such as periorbital ecchymosis (raccoon's eyes), subscleral hemorrhage, retroauricular ecchymosis (Battle's sign), hemotympanum (blood behind the eardrum), and leakage of cerebrospinal fluid from the ears (otorrhea) or nose (rhinorrhea). Gently palpate the facial bones, including the mandible and maxilla, for bony deformities or step-offs. Examine the oral pharynx for lacerations, and check for any loose or fractured teeth.

Ongoing assessments are important throughout the trauma resuscitation and during recovery. Assess the patient's fluid volume status, including hemodynamic, urinary, and central nervous system (CNS) parameters, on an hourly basis until the patient is stabilized. Notify the physician of any early indications that volume status is inadequate, such as delayed capillary refill, tachycardia, or a urinary output less than 0.5 mL/kg per hour. Monitoring urinary specific gravity, serum sodium, potassium, chloride, and osmolarity is helpful in assessing volume status. Infection surveillance is accomplished by assessing temperature curves, white blood cell counts, and the entrance sites of monitoring devices.

PSYCHOSOCIAL. Epidural hematoma is the result of a sudden, unexpected traumatic injury and may alter an individual's ability to cope effectively. The patient may be anxious during intervals of lucidity. Expect parents of children who are injured to feel anxious, fearful, and sometimes guilty. Note if the injury was related to alcohol consumption (approximately 40% to 60% of head injuries occur when the patient has been drinking), and elicit a drinking history from the patient or significant others. Assess the patient for signs of alcohol withdrawal 2 to 14 days after admission.

DIAGNOSTIC HIGHLIGHTS

Test	Normal Result	Abnormality with Condition	Explanation
Computed tomography (CT) scan	Normal brain structures	Structural abnormalities, including skull fractures, soft-tissue abnormalities, hemorrhage, cerebral edema, and shifting brain structures	Provides rapid, accurate diagnostic evaluation of asuspected epidural hematoma
Radiologic examination: skull, chest and cervical (all cervical vertebrae including C7-T1 junction) spine x rays with anteroposterior, lateral, and open-mouth view	Normal bone, joint, and soft tissue structure	Accompanying structural abnormalities	If the patient is unconscious, skull, chest and spinal injuries need to be ruled out

Other Tests: Transcranial Doppler ultrasound, and arterial blood gases

PRIMARY NURSING DIAGNOSIS

Ineffective airway clearance related to hypoventilation or airway obstruction

OUTCOMES. Respiratory status: Gas exchange; Respiratory status: Ventilation; Comfort level

INTERVENTIONS. Airway management; Oxygen therapy; Airway suctioning; Airway insertion and stabilization; Anxiety reduction; Cough enhancement; Mechanical ventilation; Positioning; Respiratory monitoring

◻ PLANNING AND IMPLEMENTATION

Collaborative

Endotracheal intubation and mechanical ventilation may be necessary to ensure oxygenation and ventilation and to decrease the risk of pulmonary aspiration. A PaO_2 greater than 100 mm Hg and $PaCO_2$ between 28 and 33 mm Hg can decrease cerebral blood flow and intracranial swelling.

Surgical evaluation of the clot, control of the hemorrhage, and resection of nonviable brain tissue may be warranted as soon as possible. A Jackson-Pratt drain may be used for 24 to 48 hours to drain the site. Complications include intracranial hypertension, reaccumulation of the clot, intracerebral hemorrhage, and the development of seizures. If surgical evacuation is not possible and the patient has a rapidly deteriorating status, the surgeon may place a burr hole on the same side as a dilated pupil or on the opposite side of motor deficits and the hematoma.

ICP monitoring may be used in patients who have a high probability of developing intracranial hypertension. The goal of this monitoring is to maintain the ICP at less than 10 mm Hg and the CPP at greater than 80 mm Hg. Intermittent or continuous draining of cerebrospinal fluid through a ventriculostomy can be used to reduce ICP.

PHARMACOLOGIC HIGHLIGHTS

Medication or Drug Class	Dosage	Description	Rationale
Sedatives, analgesics, anesthetics	Varies with drug	Midazolam (Versed); propofol (Diprivan); fentanyl (Sublimaze)	Control intermittent increases in ICP with a resultant decrease in CPP; the drugs are short-acting so that they can be temporarily stopped for intermittent neurological assessment
Chemical paralytic agents	Varies with drug	Mivacurium (Mivacron); atracurium (Tracrium); vecuronium (Norcuron)	Neuromuscular blocking agent to provide muscle relaxation is needed to improve oxygenation and ventilation; sedation must accompany paralysis

Other Pharmacological Treatment: Seizure activity can elevate ICP and increase oxygen demand. Phenytoin (Dilantin) may be used prophylactically, but the overall effectiveness has yet to be determined. Persistently elevated ICP, despite routine therapeutic interventions, may be managed by inducing a barbiturate coma to reduce the metabolic rate of brain tissue. Pentobarbital is commonly used. Before beginning this therapy, it is critical to determine adequate volume status to prevent hypotension and to ensure adequate tissue perfusion caused by the drug's depressant effect on myocardial contractility. Broad spectrum antibiotic therapy is used to treat meningitis until culture and sensitivity results are available. Commonly prescribed diuretics (furosemide and mannitol) may be used to assist in managing intracranial hypertension, although their use remains controversial.

Independent

The highest management priority is maintaining a patent airway, appropriate ventilation and oxygenation, and adequate circulation. Make sure the patient's endotracheal tube is anchored well. If the patient is at risk for self-extubation, use soft restraints. Note the lip level of the endotracheal tube to determine if tube movement occurs. Notify the physician if the patient's PaO_2 drops below 80 mm Hg, $PaCO_2$ exceeds 40 mm Hg, or severe hypocapnia ($PaCO_2 < 25$ mm Hg) occurs.

Avoid body temperature elevations and flexing, extending, or rotating the patient's neck to prevent a sudden increase in ICP. Maintain the patient in a normal body alignment to prevent obstruction of venous drainage. Maintain a quiet, restful environment with minimal stimulation. Time nursing care activities carefully to limit prolonged ICP elevations. When suctioning, hyperventilate the patient beforehand, and suction only as long as necessary. When turning the patient, prevent Valsalva's maneuver by using a draw sheet to pull the patient up in bed. Instruct the patient not to hold on to the side rails.

Provide support and encouragement to the patient and family. Provide educational tools, and teach the patient and family appropriate rehabilitative exercises. Provide diversionary activities appropriate to the patient's mental and physical abilities. Head injury support groups may be helpful. Referrals to clinical nurse specialists, pastoral care staff, and social workers are helpful in developing strategies for support and education.

DOCUMENTATION GUIDELINES

- Trauma history, description of the event, time elapsed since the event, whether or not the patient had a loss of consciousness and, if so, for how long
- Adequacy of airway, breathing, circulation; serial vital signs
- Appearance, bruising or lacerations, drainage from the nose or ears
- Physical findings related to the site of head injury: Neurological assessment, presence of accompanying symptoms, presence of complications (decreased level of consciousness, unequal pupils, loss of strength and movement, confusion or agitation, nausea and vomiting), CPP, ICP
- Signs of complications: Seizure activity, infection (fever, purulent discharge from any wounds), aspiration pneumonia (shortness of breath, pulmonary congestion, fever, productive cough), increased ICP
- Response to surgery: Stabilizations of vital signs, changes in neurological status
- Response to medications used to control pain and increase ICP

DISCHARGE AND HOME HEALTHCARE GUIDELINES

Review with the patient and family proper care techniques for wounds and lacerations. Discuss the recommended activity level, and explain rehabilitative exercises. Teach the patient and family to recognize symptoms of infection or a deteriorating level of consciousness, and stress the need to contact the physician if such signs or symptoms appear. Teach the patient the purpose, dosage, schedule, precautions, and potential side effects, interactions, and adverse reactions of all prescribed medications. Review with the patient and family all follow-up appointments that have been arranged. Review with the patient and family information regarding the use of safety restraints.

Epilepsy

DRG Category: 024
Mean LOS: 4.8 days
Description: MEDICAL: Seizure and Headache, Age > 17 with CC

Epilepsy is a paroxysmal neurological disorder and is characterized by recurrent episodes of convulsive movements or other motor activity, loss of consciousness, sensory disturbances, and other behavioral abnormalities. Because epilepsy occurs in more than 50 diseases, it is considered a syndrome rather than a disease.

Convulsive seizures are the most common forms of attacks of epilepsy. Seizures occur with abnormal electrical discharges from brain cells, and these discharges are caused by the movement of ions across the cell membrane. Although seizures are the dominant manifestation of epilepsy, patients can have a seizure and not have epilepsy. The current classification for seizures that is commonly used was redefined in the 1980s. (See Table 25). The characteristics of the seizure vary and depend on the focus or location of brain involvement. Seizures can vary from almost imperceptible alterations in the level of consciousness to a sudden loss of consciousness with tonic-clonic convulsions of all extremities accompanied by urinal and fecal incontinence and amnesia for the event.

TABLE 25 | **Classification of Seizures**

I. Partial (focal, local) seizures
   A. Simple partial seizures: No impairment of consciousness
   B. Complex partial seizures: Impaired consciousness, frequently include automatisms
   C. Partial seizures that secondarily generalize
II. Generalized seizures: All have impairment of consciousness
   A. Absence (previously known as petit mal) of "blank stare"; generally in children
   B. Myoclonic seizures: Short, abrupt muscular contractions
   C. Clonic seizures: Muscle contraction and relaxation
   D. Tonic seizures: Abrupt increase in muscle tone
   E. Tonic–Clonic seizures (previously known as grand mal): quick, bilateral, severe jerking movements
   F. Atonic seizures (drop attacks): Abrupt loss of muscle
III. Unclassified epileptic seizures: Inadequate or incomplete data to identify classification

Status epilepticus is defined as more than 30 minutes of unconsciousness with continuous or intermittent convulsive seizure activity. Usually status epilepticus results when more than six seizures occur in 24 hours or when the patient progresses from one seizure to the next without resolution of the postictal period. Pseudoseizures are the physical appearance of seizure activity without the cerebral electrical activity.

CAUSES

Seizures may be caused by primary central nervous system (CNS) disorders, metabolic or systemic disorders, or idiopathic origins. Primary CNS disorders include any potential mass effect (tumor, abscess, atrioventricular malformation [AVM], aneurysm, or hematoma) and all types of strokes, especially those that are embolic. Metabolic and systemic causes include acute overdose, acute drug withdrawal (especially CNS depressants, alcohol, benzodiazepines, and barbiturates), febrile states, hypoxia, hyperosmolarity, hypertensive encephalopathy, hyperthermia, and a multitude of electrolyte disturbances.

GENDER AND LIFE SPAN CONSIDERATIONS

Epilepsy occurs in all races, and it affects males and females equally. The incidence is approximately 1 in every 100 to 300 persons. Although epilepsy can occur in any age group, usually the onset is before the age of 20. Different age groups have distinct associated causes. In newborns up until 6 months of age, seizures are generally caused by birth trauma or metabolic disturbances, such as hypoxemia, hypoglycemia, and hypocalcemia. In children from 6 months to 5 years of age, etiology is related to febrile episodes or metabolic disturbances such as hyponatremia or hypernatremia, hypoglycemia, or hypocalcemia. In the 5- to 20-year-old group, seizures are primarily idiopathic (50%). In adults from 20 to 50 years of age, a new onset of seizures is almost exclusively caused by trauma or tumors. In older adults, seizures are generally caused by vascular disease and cardiac dysrhythmias.

☐ ASSESSMENT

HISTORY. Obtain a thorough history of past illnesses and surgeries. Lifestyle changes, medications or vaccinations, and history of past head injury may be significant. Obtain data about the age of onset and the frequency, duration, and severity of the seizures. Ask the patient if he or she experiences any type of aura or prodromal symptoms before the seizure or if there are any precipitating factors such as dizziness, palpitations, flashing lights, or fatigue. A history of seizure activity is crucial from both the patient and a significant other who has witnessed the activity. Elicit information about eye movements, body movements, level of consciousness, and presence of urinary or fecal incontinence. Ask the family to describe the patient's postictal state.

PHYSICAL EXAMINATION. A thorough neurological exam includes assessing changes in mental status, cranial nerve function, muscular tone and strength, sensations, reflexes, and gait. Describe in detail any seizure activity that may occur during the physical examination. Assess the initial manifestations, motor activity, pupil size, gaze, incontinence, and duration of the seizure. Assess what the patient is like in the postictal state. Since the patient may bite his or her tongue during the seizure, assess the patient for mouth and tongue injury.

PSYCHOSOCIAL. When it is poorly controlled, epilepsy may be seriously debilitating. Seizure activity in public is embarrassing and poorly understood by the public. Mobility is frequently disturbed because of the inability to drive. Attending school or going to work may be a serious trial to the poorly controlled epileptic.

DIAGNOSTIC HIGHLIGHTS

Test	Normal Result	Abnormality with Condition	Explanation
Electro-encephalogram (EEG)	Normal patterns of electrical activity	Abnormal patterns of electrical activity, reflecting seizure activity	Recording of electrical potentials based on distribution of waveforms generated by cerebral cortex of brain; waveforms demonstrate abnormal patterns during seizures; they are not useful in the acute management of status epilepticus

Other Tests: Computed tomography (CT) scans, magnetic resonance imaging (MRI), and skull x rays; serum laboratory data to explore possible causes include glucose; calcium; blood urea nitrogen (BUN); and electrolyte, toxic, and metabolic screens

PRIMARY NURSING DIAGNOSIS

Ineffective airway clearance related to clonic-tonic motor activity and tongue obstruction

OUTCOMES. Respiratory status: Gas exchange and ventilation; Safety status: Physical injury

INTERVENTIONS. Airway insertion; Airway management; Airway suctioning; Oral health promotion; Respiratory monitoring; Ventilation assistance

☐ PLANNING AND IMPLEMENTATION

Collaborative

MEDICAL. In general, the management of seizures is done pharmacologically. The patient with status epilepticus is considered a medical emergency. Airway management is critical, often endotracheal intubation is needed, and intravenous medications are administered. If there is a delay in treatment, or if the patient is unresponsive to treatment, irreversible brain damage, coma, or death can occur.

SURGICAL. Surgery, an extensive and expensive alternative, is considered as a last resort to control the seizures. Only 5% of all patients with epilepsy undergo surgery. Surgical removal of the epileptic focus is only appropriate for the patient who is uncontrolled with medication, has a single identifiable focus firing at least 80% of the seizure initiations, has no underlying medical problems, and has a focus lying in nonessential tissue.

PHARMACOLOGIC HIGHLIGHTS

Medication or Drug Class	Dosage	Description	Rationale
Anticonvulsants	Varies with drug	Multiple drug therapies are available: Phenytoin sodium (Dilantin), phenobarbitol, lorazepam (Ativan), diazepam (Valium).	Lorazepam (Ativan) or diazepam (Valium) may be used to stop seizures quickly. Phenytoin (Dilantin) is preferred maintenance anticonvulsant for status epilepticus. A newer drug, fosphenytoin, (Cerebyx) has been developed that is safer for parenteral administration. Phenobarbitol may be given if seizures occur after phenytoin loading.

Other: Thiamine 100 mg and 50 ml of 50% dextrose in water may be administered in an emergency to rule out seizures because of thiamine deficiency or hypoglycemia.

Other information about anticonvulsants: The primary treatment for epilepsy is one or more of the multitude of antiepileptic drugs (AED) or anticonvulsants. The choice of AED or combination of AEDs depends on seizure type, patient tolerance, and cost. Carbamazepine (Tegretol) is a widely used and cost-effective anticonvulsants. Valproic acid, primidone (Mysoline), clonazepam, and etho-suximide are prescribed, depending on the seizure type.

Independent

The most important nursing interventions are to maintain adequate airway, breathing, and circulation during the seizure, and to prevent injury. Have an oral airway and suction apparatus at the bedside at all times. A patient who begins a seizure should not be left alone. Use the call light to obtain assistance, and if the patient is upright, gently ease him or her to the floor. Position him or her to maintain the airway, but do not force anything into the patient's mouth if the teeth are clenched. If the patient's mouth is open, protect the patient's tongue by placing a soft cloth or a well-padded tongue blade between the teeth. Help the patient to a lying position, remove constricting clothing, and place a pillow or sheet under the patient's head to cushion him or her from injury. Clear the area of objects that are hard or sharp. Do not restrain the patient's movement during the seizure. Assist the patient with hygiene and linen changes, should incontinence occur during the seizure.

To lower the risk of injury, provide a safe environment at all times. Pad and raise the side rails, but do not use pillows for padding because of the possibility of suffocation. Take axillary rather than oral temperatures, and remove breakable objects such as water glasses from the area. The extent of seizure precautions should be consistent with the type of seizures. Good oral hygiene is important. Also observe for signs of infection if there is any damage to the tongue and oral mucosa.

Educate the patient and family about providing care during a seizure, the medication schedule and side effects, and the importance of regular follow-up. Involve the family as much as possible in patient care. Use patient and family teaching to dispel any myths and misconceptions about epilepsy. Assure the family that most patients can control the syndrome if they follow the prescribed routine. Since epilepsy can be a debilitating, restrictive disease, provide support and encouragement. Refer patients to national organizations (Epilepsy Foundation of America) and local support groups.

DOCUMENTATION GUIDELINES

- Seizure activity: Events preceding and following seizure, type, length, progression, airway maintenance, ability to follow commands, ability to respond verbally, and memory of events
- Complications: Airway compromise, extremity injury, tongue laceration, lowered self-esteem.
- Institution of safety precautions
- Response to AEDs: Drug levels and side effects, response to treatment
- Understanding of, and interest in, patient teaching

DISCHARGE AND HOME HEALTHCARE GUIDELINES

Be sure that the patient understands all medications, including the dosage, route, action, adverse effects, and need for routine laboratory monitoring of AEDs. Stress the need for taking medications as prescribed, even if seizure activity is under control. Ensure that the patient has basic epilepsy safety information, such as no tub baths, no swimming, and no driving without seizure control for at least 1 year. Family members should be able to verbalize what to do during a seizure. The patient should wear jewelry identifying him or her as having epilepsy.

HOME CARE. Emphasize the following management strategies:
- Maintain adequate rest and nutrition; check with a physician before dieting.
- Limit alcohol intake.
- Report infections promptly.
- Avoid trigger factors (flashing lights, hyperventilation, loud noises, video games, television).
- Brush the teeth regularly with a soft toothbrush.
- Avoid activities that precipitate seizure activity.
- Keep follow-up appointments.
- Lead as normal a life as possible.

Esophageal Cancer

DRG Category: 172
Mean LOS: 6.5 days
Description: MEDICAL: Digestive Malignancy with CC
DRG Category: 154
Mean LOS: 13.3 days
Description: SURGICAL: Stomach, Esophageal, and Duodenal Procedures, Age > 17 with CC

Carcinoma is the most common cause of obstruction of the esophagus. Approximately half of all esophageal cancers are squamous cell carcinomas, which usually occur in the middle and lower two-thirds of the esophagus. The remaining 50% are adenocarcinomas, which generally begin in glandular tissue of the esophagus. Adenocarcinomas are associated with Barrett's esophagus, a condition that occurs because of continued reflux of fluid from the stomach into the lower esophagus. Over time, reflux changes the cells at the end of the esophagus.

Esophageal tumors begin as benign growths and grow rapidly because there is no serosal layer to inhibit growth. Because of the vast lymphatic network of the esophagus, esophageal cancers spread rapidly, both locally to regional lymph nodes and distantly to the lungs and liver. Complications include pulmonary problems that result from fistulae and aspiration; invasion of the tumor into major vessels, thus causing a massive hemorrhage; and obstruction and compression of the other structures in the head and neck. Although survival rates are improving, esophageal cancer is usually diagnosed at a late stage, and most patients die within 6 months of diagnosis. Cancer of the esophagus accounts for approximately 4% of all cancer deaths in the United States; the 5-year survival rate is 9% to 13%, even with aggressive treatment.

CAUSES

Although its etiology is unknown, esophageal cancer occurs predominantly in people with a history of alcohol and tobacco use. Individuals who have achalasia, strictures, or hiatal hernias are also at increased risk. In parts of the world where it is most common (Japan, Russia, China, the Middle East, and South

Africa), the disease has been linked to nitrosamines and other contaminants in the soil. It has also been found to have a higher incidence in individuals whose diets are chronically deficient in fresh fruits, vegetables, vitamins, and proteins.

GENDER AND LIFE SPAN CONSIDERATIONS

Cancer of the esophagus usually occurs in men between the ages of 50 and 70 years. The disorder affects men in a 3:1 ratio to women. African-Americans are affected three times as often as European-Americans. It is also more common in Asian-American males than in the general population. Squamous cell carcinoma is more common in European-Americans, whereas adenocarcinomas are more common in African-Americans.

☐ ASSESSMENT

HISTORY. Obtain an accurate history of risk factors, including race, cultural background, use of cigarettes and alcohol, or any esophageal problems. Dysphagia, which is often the most common symptom, is usually experienced when at least 60% of the esophagus is occluded. Initially it is mild and intermittent, and it occurs only with solid foods. Patients may report a sensation that "food is sticking in their throat." Symptoms of the disease soon progress to the inability to swallow semisoft or liquid food, and the patient experiences a severe weight loss, as much as 40 to 50 pounds over 2 to 3 months. Eventually the patient is unable to swallow his or her own saliva. Also inquire about regurgitation, vomiting, chronic hiccups, odynophagia (painful swallowing), and dietary patterns.

PHYSICAL EXAMINATION. Observe the patient's ability to swallow food. Note any chronic coughing and increased oral secretions. Listen to the patient's voice: tumors in the upper esophagus can involve the larynx and cause hoarseness. Place the patient in the recumbent position; pain, hoarseness, coughing, and potential aspiration often occur in this position. Weigh the patient, and determine the patient's strength and motion of the extremities. Severe weight loss and weakness are common symptoms.

PSYCHOSOCIAL. The patient needs to make a psychological adjustment to the diagnosis of a chronic illness that is usually terminal. Evaluate the patient for evidence of altered mood (such as depression or anxiety), and assess the coping mechanisms and support systems.

DIAGNOSTIC HIGHLIGHTS

Test	Normal Result	Abnormality with Condition	Explanation
Barium swallow	Normal esophagus	Irregular areas in or narrowing of the esophagus	Locates and describes irregularities in the esophageal wall or fistulae
Endoscopy	Visualization of a normal esophagus and stomach	Direct visualization of tumor or fistula	Locates the tumor for a biopsy

Other Tests: Computed tomography (CT) scan, endoscopic ultrasound, thoracoscopy, laparoscopy, liver scan, bronchoscopy, and magnetic resonance imaging (MRI)

PRIMARY NURSING DIAGNOSIS

Altered nutrition: Less than body requirements related to dysphagia

OUTCOMES. Nutritional status: Food and fluid intake; Nutrient intake; Biochemical measures; Body mass; Energy; Endurance

INTERVENTIONS. Nutrition management; Nutrition therapy; Nutritional counseling and monitoring; Fluid/electrolyte management; Medication management

☐ PLANNING AND IMPLEMENTATION

Collaborative

Because esophageal cancer is often terminal, treatment is usually for palliative purposes and to relieve the effects of the tumor. Surgery, radiotherapy, and chemotherapy are all options for treating cancer of the esophagus, and they may be used alone or in combination. Two surgical procedures are commonly performed: esophagectomy (removal of all or part of the esophagus with a Dacron graft replacing the part that was removed) and esophagogastrectomy (resection of the lower part of the esophagus together with a proximal portion of the stomach, followed by anastomosis of the remaining portion of the esophagus and stomach). Postoperatively, monitor the nasogastric (NG) tube for patency. Expect some bloody drainage initially; within 24 to 48 hours, the drainage should change to a yellowish green. Do not irrigate or reposition the NG tube without a physician's order. Fluid and electrolyte balance should be monitored carefully, as well as intake and output. Monitor the patient who has had an anastomosis for signs and symptoms of leakage, which is most likely to occur 5 to 7 days postoperatively. These include low-grade fever, inflammation, accumulation of fluid, and early symptoms of shock (tachycardia, tachypnea).

Radiation reduces the size of the tumor and provides some relief to the patient. Usually external beam radiation therapy is used. Normal esophageal tissue is also affected by the radiation, which is given over a 6- to 8-week period to minimize the side effects. Side effects include edema, epithelial desquamation, esophagitis, odynophagia, anorexia, nausea, and vomiting. Although radiation by itself does not cure esophageal cancer, it eases symptoms such as pain, bleeding, and dysphagia.

PHARMACOLOGIC HIGHLIGHTS

Medication or Drug Class	Dosage	Description	Rationale
Chemotherapy	Varies by drug	Types of chemotherapy: 5-fluorouracil, cisplatin, bleomycin, mitomycin, doxorubicin, methotrexate, paclitaxel, vinorelbine, topotecan, irinotecan, mitoguazone	Kills cancer cells. Primary chemotherapy will not cure esosphageal cancer unless surgery and/or radiation is also used. Preoperatively, chemotherapy may be given to reduce tumor size. Approximately 10%–40% of patients will have a significant shrinking of the tumor from these drugs.

Independent

Carefully monitor the patient's nutritional intake, and involve the patient in planning the diet. Maintain a daily record of caloric intake and weight. Monitor the skin turgor and mucous membranes to detect dehydration. Keep the head of the bed elevated at least 30 degrees to prevent reflux and pulmonary aspiration. If the patient is having problems swallowing saliva, keep a suction catheter with an oral suction at the bedside at all times. Teach the patient how to clear his or her mouth with the oral suction.

When appropriate, discuss expected preoperative and postoperative procedures, including information about x rays, intravenous hydration (IVs), wound drains, NG tube and suctioning, and chest tubes. Immediately after surgery, implement strategies to prevent respiratory complications.

Provide emotional support. Focus on the patient's quality of life, and discuss realistic planning with the family. Involve the patient as much as possible in decisions concerning care. If the patient is terminally ill, encourage the significant others to involve the patient in discussions about funeral arrangements and terminal care such as hospice care. Provide a referral to the patient to the American Cancer Society, support groups, and hospice care as appropriate.

DOCUMENTATION GUIDELINES

- Physical assessment data: Ability to eat and swallow; patency of airway; regularity of breathing; temperature; daily weights; breath sounds; intake and output; calorie counts
- Chronologic record of symptoms and response to interventions
- The nature, location, duration, and intensity of pain; response to pain medication or other interventions

DISCHARGE AND HOME HEALTHCARE GUIDELINES

MEDICATIONS. The patient should be able to state the name, purpose, dosage, schedule, common side effects, and importance of taking her or his medications.

COMPLICATIONS. Teach the patient to report any dysphagia or odynophagia, which may indicate a regrowth of the tumor. Teach the patient to inspect the wound daily for redness, swelling, discharge, or odor, which indicate presence of infection.

HOME CARE. Teach family members to assist the patient with ambulation, splinting the incision, and chest physiotherapy. Educate caregivers on nutritional guidelines, food preparation, tube feedings, and parenteral nutrition, as appropriate. Inform the patient and family about the availability of high-caloric, high-protein, liquid supplements to maintain his or her weight.

RESOURCES. Provide patients with a list of resources for support after discharge: visiting nurses, American Cancer Society, hospice, support groups.

Esophageal Diverticula

DRG Category: 188
Mean LOS: 4.9 days
Description: MEDICAL: Other Digestive System Diagnoses, Age > 17 with CC
DRG Category: 154
Mean LOS: 13.3 days
Description: SURGICAL: Stomach, Esophageal, and Duodenal Procedures, Age > 17 with CC

Esophageal diverticula, or herniations of the esophageal musoca, are hollow outpouchings of the espahageal wall that occur in three main areas of the esophagus: proximally near the anatomic hypopharyngeal sphincter (Zenker's diverticulum, the most common location); near the midpoint of the esophagus (a midesophageal diverticulum); and just above the lower esophageal sphincter (an epiphrenic diverticulum, the least common location). Food, fluids, and secretions accumulate in these dilated outpouchings, creating discomfort. Aspiration pneumonia, bronchitis, bronchiectasis, and lung abscess may be the result of regurgitating contents of the esophageal diverticula. Esophageal diverticula may also lead to esophageal perforation.

CAUSES

Esophageal diverticula develop from weakened esophageal musculature (congenital and acquired), traumatic injury, and scar tissue associated with chronic inflammation. Developmental muscle weakness of the posterior pharynx above the border of the cricopharyngeal muscle leads to Zenker's diverticulum. Pressure caused by swallowing and contraction of the pharynx before the sphincter relaxes aggravates the muscle weakness and results in the development of diverticula. A response to scarring and pulling on esophageal walls by an external inflammatory process such as tuberculosis or by traction from old adhesions may lead to midesophageal diverticula. Other causes of esophageal diverticula include motor disturbances such as achalasia (absence of normal peristalsis in esophageal smooth muscle and elevated pressure at the physiologic cardiac sphincter), diffuse esophageal spasms, and reflux esophagitis.

GENDER AND LIFE SPAN CONSIDERATIONS

Infants and children have been known to have esophageal diverticula, although the disorder predominantly occurs in adults beyond midlife. It affects men three times as often as women. Epiphrenic diverticula usually occur in middle-aged men. Zenker's diverticulum occurs most often in men over the age of 60.

⬚ ASSESSMENT

HISTORY. Establish a recent history of weight loss, which is generally attributed to difficulty in eating. Determine if the patient has experienced subtle, gradually progressive esophageal dysphagia that primarily affected the swallowing of solid foods. Ask if the patient has experienced gagging, gurgling, or a sense of fullness in the throat as if something were "stuck." Inquire whether the patient has regurgitated food particles and saliva soon after eating. Determine if the patient has experienced an unpleasant taste and nocturnal coughing with regurgitation of retained secretions and undigested foods. Establish a history of heartburn following ingestion of coffee, alcohol, chocolate, citrus juices, or fatty foods, particularly when the patient was bending over or lying down within 2 hours of intake. These indicators suggest that the esophageal diverticula are secondary to achalasia.

PHYSICAL EXAMINATION. Assess the patient's appearance, noting apparent weight loss or the malnourished look that is associated with anorexia. Note halitosis, a common sign of esophageal diverticula. Inspect the patient's neck for visible signs of esophageal distension that has been caused by food trapped in the diverticula.

PSYCHOSOCIAL. The patient may experience self-imposed social isolation because of feelings of embarrassment. which are caused by noisy swallowing, unusual facial expressions during eating, or halitosis. The patient may become depressed because of the loss of pleasure and socialization connected with eating, along with grieving over the loss of dietary preferences. The patient's family may be anxious about the social effects of the patient's disease as well.

DIAGNOSTIC HIGHLIGHTS

Test	Normal Result	Abnormality with Condition	Explanation
Esophageal manometry	Multilumen esophageal catheter is introduced through the mouth, and pressures along the esophagus are measured during swallowing: normal contractions, swallowing, peristalsis	Abnormal contractions, swallowing, and peristalsis	Assesses and diagnoses dysphagia, esophageal reflux, spasm, and motility abnormalities, hiatal hernia
Barium swallow	Normal esophagus	Identifies irregular or abnormal areas of the esophagus	Locates and describes irregularities in the esophageal wall
Esophagoscopy	Visualization of a normal esophagus	Direct visualization of diverticula	Locates esophageal diverticula

PRIMARY NURSING DIAGNOSIS

Risk for aspiration related to regurgitation of food, fluid, or secretions that have accumulated in diverticula

OUTCOMES. Knowledge: Treatment procedures; Respiratory status: Ventilation; Neurological status; Nutritional status: Food and fluid intake; Oral health; Self-care: Eating

INTERVENTIONS. Airway suctioning; Surveillance; Respiratory monitoring; Feeding; Positioning

□ PLANNING AND IMPLEMENTATION

Collaborative

MEDICAL. When achalasia is implicated, pharmacologic therapy may be the first procedure. Assess the effects of treatments because the drugs may worsen the diverticula by relaxing an already weakened esophageal musculature.

SURGICAL. An esophagomyotomy (incision into the esophageal musculature) and diverticulectomy (surgical removal of the diverticulum) may be warranted, particularly for patients with Zenker's diverticulum. Postoperative care is determined by the incisional approach. With a cervical approach, a drain is commonly inserted in the neck to diminish edema at the incisional site. A chest incision (thoracic approach) requires care associated with a thoracotomy. Postoperative care is directed at monitoring the patency of the airway, maintaining pulmonary ventilation by chest drainage with chest tubes, monitoring neck drainage with either gravity drainage or low suction, and preventing aspiration.

PHARMACOLOGIC HIGHLIGHTS

Medication or Drug Class	Dosage	Description	Rationale
Smooth muscle relaxants	Varies with drug	Nitrates or calcium-channel	Relax the cardiac sphincter, preventing reflux blockers regurgitation of foods
Antacids	Varies with drug	Amphogel, Alternagel, Gelusil, Maalox, Mylanta	Neutralize gastric acid and reduce symptoms, especially with midesophageal or epiphrenic diverticula, because they usually do not produce complications

Independent

Care focuses on maintaining a patent airway, preventing aspiration of regurgitated food and mucus, providing emotional support, and providing adequate nutrition. Implement interventions to maintain airway patency if there is any suspicion it is at risk. Use the jaw thrust or chin lift, or insert an oral or nasal airway. Prevent aspiration of regurgitated food and mucus by positioning the patient carefully, with his or her head elevated or turned to one side. Recommend that the patient sleep with the head elevated (using pillows or bed blocks) to reduce esophageal reflux and nocturnal choking. Show the patient how to use massage to empty any visible outpouching to the neck to prevent aspiration during sleep.

Education, rather than medical or surgical intervention, may become the treatment of choice. Provide the patient with information on lifestyle changes to reduce symptoms. Teach appropriate nutrition. Advise the patient to explore textures and quantities of foods to determine which cause the least discomfort. Recommend that the patient consider semisoft and soft foods, and advise adding fiber to the diet to stimulate peristalsis of the gastrointestinal (GI) system, reducing lower GI tract pressure on the esophagus. Recommend food supplements between meals to prevent weight loss and malnourishment, and advise the patient to drink fluids intermittently with meals to aid in propulsion of the food bolus through the esophagus. Teach the patient to concentrate on the act of eating to maximize each phase of the process of ingesting food and fluids, moistening the mouth before eating to facilitate chewing and swallowing. Explain how to use Valsalva's maneuver to increase esophageal pressure, thus facilitating food bolus movement beyond the hypopharyngeal sphincter. Recommend that the patient sit upright when eating or drinking to facilitate gravitational flow through the esophagus, and advise remaining upright for at least 2 hours after eating.

Advise taking adequate fluids (greater than 15 mL) with medications to prevent chemical esophageal irritation. Recommend eliminating oral drugs immediately before bedtime to decrease the risk of deposits in diverticula that can create ulceration. Advise the patient to avoid food or fluids within 3 to 4 hours of bedtime to reduce nocturnal symptoms.

DOCUMENTATION GUIDELINES

- Physical findings: Rate and depth of respirations; breath sounds; presence of dysphagia, choking, or regurgitation
- Changes (improvement or lack of improvement) of symptoms
- Halitosis, dysphagia, regurgitation, gurgling with swallowing, coughing, persistence of a bad taste in the mouth
- Complications: Airway swelling, fever, productive cough, respiratory distress, weight loss, poor wound healing, wound infection

DISCHARGE AND HOME HEALTHCARE GUIDELINES

Teach the patient methods to reduce symptoms, prevent malnutrition and weight loss, and improve sleep and rest. Make sure the patient understands the dosage, route, action and purpose, side effects, and contraindications of the prescribed medications. Explain the potential for aspiration, respiratory impairment, weight loss or malnourishment, and sleep deprivation. Remind the patient to see the physician if symptoms of esophageal diverticula return or worsen.

Fat Embolism

DRG Category: 078
Mean LOS: 7.8 days
Description: MEDICAL: Pulmonary Embolism

An embolism is any undissolved mass that travels in the circulation and occludes a blood vessel. A fat embolism, which is an unusual complication from a traumatic injury, occurs when fat droplets enter the circulation and lodge in small vessels and capillaries, particularly in the lung and brain. Two theories exist that explain the pathophysiology of fat emboli: the mechanical theory and the biochemical theory. The mechanical theory states that trauma disrupts fat cells and tears veins in the bone marrow at the site of a fracture. Fat droplets enter the circulation because of increased pressure of the interstitium at the area of injury. The biochemical theory states that a stress-related release of cate-cholamines after trauma mobilizes fat molecules from a tissue. These molecules group into fat droplets and eventually obstruct the circulation. In addition, free fatty acids destroy pulmonary endothelium, increase capillary permeability in the lungs, and lead to pulmonary edema.

The result of either theory is the accumulation of fat droplets that are too large to pass easily through small capillaries, where they lodge and break apart into fatty acids, which are toxic to lung tissues, the capillary endothelium, and surfactant. Pulmonary hypertension, alveolar collapse, and even noncardiac pulmonary edema follow.

CAUSES

Fat embolism is associated with severe traumatic injury with accompanying long-bone (tibial or femoral) or pelvic fractures and generally occurs within 3 days of the fracture. It has also been reported in patients with severe burns, head injury, or a severely compromised circulation. Nontraumatic disease states that have occasionally been associated with fat embolism include acute pancreatitis, alcoholism, diabetes mellitus, and osteomyelitis. Procedures such as liposuc-tion, orthopedic surgery, joint replacement, abdominal surgery, and cardiac massage (closed chest) are also associated with fat embolism.

GENDER AND LIFE SPAN CONSIDERATIONS

Most patients who develop the disorder are under age 30 and have severe as-sociated injuries. Males are more likely than females to have a significant trau-matic injury.

☐ ASSESSMENT

HISTORY. Elicit a history of recent traumatic injury. In most patients, the injury is obvious because of the presence of casts or traction. Some patients exhibit changes in mental status such as restlessness, delirium, or drowsiness pro-gressing to coma and even seizures. Others complain of fever, anxiety, unex-plained discomfort, or respiratory distress (shortness of breath, cough).

Fat embolization may be classified into three distinct forms based on the pa-tient's progression of symptoms: subclinical, classic, and fulminant. Approxi-mately half of patients with uncomplicated fractures have subclinical fat emboli, which resolve spontaneously within a few days. Patients with the classic form gen-erally have a latent period of 1 to 2 days, followed by the development of symp-toms that include mental status changes, shortness of breath, fever, tachycardia, and petechiae. The fulminant form is characterized by an early onset of neurological and respiratory deterioration, as well as the onset of signs of right ventricular failure (distended neck veins, liver congestion, peripheral edema). A rapid onset of neurological deterioration in patients who sustained severe injuries and multiple fractures but who were initially conscious suggests a fat embolism.

PHYSICAL EXAMINATION. The patient with a life-threatening fat embolism appears acutely ill with shortness of breath, rapid heart rate, and fever. The neurological examination may reveal confusion, agitation, or even stuporousness. Some pa-tients may have a seizure. Note that neurological changes usually occur 6 to 12 hours before respiratory system changes and rarely without impending respi-ratory involvement.

Inspect the patient's skin for petechiae, a classic sign that appears 1 to 2 days after injury in more than half of patients with fat embolism. Petechiae are of short duration, last only 4 to 6 hours, and appear most commonly on the neck, upper trunk, conjunctivae, or retina. An ophthalmic examination may reveal fat globules in the retinal vessels. Approximately half of the patients who display neurological symptoms also develop microinfarcts of the retina. When you auscultate the patient's heart and lungs, you usually hear a rapid heart rate and rales, rhonchi, and possibly a pleural friction rub.

PSYCHOSOCIAL. Because fat embolism is a complication of other disease processes or traumatic injuries, the addition of another life-threatening complication could be the final breaking point for the family or significant others involved. Evaluate the patient's social network to determine what support is available during the acute illness.

DIAGNOSTIC HIGHLIGHTS

Test	Normal Result	Abnormality with Condition	Explanation
Platelet count	150,000–400,000 mm^3	Decreased < 15,000 mm^3	Platelets are used up in the clotting process
PaO$_2$	80–100 mm Hg	< 60 mm Hg	Hypoxemia occurs because of problems with ventilation perfusion due to obstruction of pulmonary circulation
Electrocardiogram (ECG)	Normal rate, rhythm, and P, Q. R. S, and T waves	Tachycardia, right bundle branch block, depressed ST segments	Obstruction of the pulmonary circulation leads to right heart strain

Other Tests: Increased serum lipase, fat in the urine, patchy infiltrates on chest x ray, and magnetic resonance imaging (MRI), pulse oximetry to detect arterial oxygen saturation

PRIMARY NURSING DIAGNOSIS

Ineffective airway clearance related to a decrease in mental status and accumulation of oral secretions

OUTCOMES. Respiratory status: Gas exchange; Respiratory status: Ventilation; Symptom control behavior; Treatment behavior: Illness or injury; Comfort level

INTERVENTIONS. Airway management; Anxiety reduction; Oxygen therapy; Airway suctioning; Airway insertion and stabilization; Cough enhancement; Mechanical ventilation; Positioning; Respiratory monitoring

□ PLANNING AND IMPLEMENTATION

Collaborative

SUPPORT FOR AIRWAY AND BREATHING. Management of the patient almost always requires support of the patient's airway and breathing with supplemental oxygen and possibly endotracheal intubation and mechanical ventilation. Patients who do not exhibit changes in mental status or pulmonary edema may benefit from supplemental oxygen by nasal cannula or facemask. Patients with a deteriorating mental status, dropping arterial oxygen saturations, and decreasing levels of PaO_2, less than 50 mm Hg, usually need positive pressure ventilation with positive end-expiratory pressure (PEEP) and possibly pressure control ventilation (PCV).

The nurse and trauma surgeon or orthopedist work together to prevent fat emboli whenever possible by encouraging adequate gas exchange; this entails clearing secretions and promoting good ventilation. Discuss the patient's activity restrictions with the physician. To limit the effects of immobilization, turn the patient frequently and, when he or she is ready, get the patient out of bed. If the injuries allow, encourage dangling or ambulation. Maintain the patient's hydration by intravenous or enteral fluids, as prescribed.

PHARMACOLOGIC. Diuretics may be needed if pulmonary edema develops. Many experts recommend prophylactic use of corticosteroids for patients at high risk for fat emboli, but they seem less effective after fat emboli develop. Some experts suggest that the introduction of steroids may help treat pulmonary manifestations by decreasing the inflammatory response of the pulmonary capillaries, as well as by stabilizing lysosomal and capillary membranes. Analgesics are also necessary to manage the pain of the traumatic injury.

The best treatment of fat emboli is preventing their occurrence. Surgical stabilization of extremity fractures to reduce bone movement probably minimizes the release of fatty products from the bone marrow. The location of the fracture determines whether the surgeon uses internal or external fixation techniques.

PHARMACOLOGIC HIGHLIGHTS

General Comments: Medications provide supportive management rather than curative measures.

Medication or Drug Class	Dosage	Description	Rationale
Corticosteroids	Varies with drug	Anti-inflammatories	Decrease inflammatory response of pulmonary capillaries; stabilize lysosomal and capillary membranes

Other Drugs: Diuretics may be needed if pulmonary edema develops. Analgesics are also necessary to manage the pain of the traumatic injury.

Independent

The highest priority is maintaining airway, breathing, and circulation. Ongoing monitoring of the cardiopulmonary system is essential, coupled with interventions such as suctioning, placement of an oral airway if appropriate, and immediate notification of the trauma service if the airway, breathing, or circulation becomes impaired.

The patient needs to be an active participant in his or her care. Before he or she undergoes activity or coughing and deep-breathing exercises, make sure that the patient's pain is controlled. In addition to administering prescribed medications, explore nonpharmacologic alternatives to pain management, such as diversionary activities and guided imagery.

The patient's and family's level of anxiety is apt to be exacerbated by the critical care environment. Explain all the equipment, and answer questions honestly and thoroughly. If the patient has to undergo endotracheal intubation, provide a method for communication such as a magic slate or point board. Work with the family to allow as much visitation as the patient's condition allows. Remember that although young people in their late teens often appear to be adult, they often regress during a serious illness and need a great deal of support from their parents and significant others.

DOCUMENTATION GUIDELINES

- Physical responses: Vital signs, cardiopulmonary assessment, neurological assessment, mental status, presence or absence of petechiae
- Emotional response: Coping strategies, mood, affect, flexibility, cooperation
- Presence of complications: Fever, infection, skin breakdown, loss of consciousness
- Ongoing monitoring: Pulse oximetry or ABG results that are abnormal, abnormal laboratory findings
- Response to treatment: Mechanical ventilation, response to fluid replacement and medications, response to supplemental oxygen

DISCHARGE AND HOME HEALTHCARE GUIDELINES

A patient who has recovered from the underlying disease process or injury is no longer at risk for developing fat embolism and can be discharged. Teach the patient about any medications and treatments needed before he or she leaves the hospital. Explain the disease process and how it occurred, and note that recurrence is doubtful unless the patient experiences another traumatic injury. Arrange for any follow-up care with the primary healthcare provider.

Fibrocystic Breast Condition

DRG Category: 276
Mean LOS: 4.0 days
Description: MEDICAL: Nonmalignant Breast Disorders

Fibrocystic breast condition (sometimes called fibrocystic complex) is the most common type of benign breast disorder. It was previously referred to as fibrocystic breast disease. Fibrocystic breast condition is a catch-all diagnosis that is used to describe the presence of multiple, often painful, benign breast nodules. These breast nodules vary in size and blend into surrounding breast tissue. However, the histologic changes responsible for the breast nodules could belong to one of several different categories.

The College of American Pathologists has categorized the types of fibrocystic breast condition according to the associated increased risk for subsequent invasive breast cancer and the particular histologic (microscopic) change that is present. These types include the following: no increased risk (nonproliferative changes, including microcysts, adenosis, mild hyperplasia, fibroadenoma, fibrosis, duct, apocrine metaplasia, and gross cysts); slightly increased risk (relative risk, 1.5 to 2; proliferative changes without atypia, including moderate hyperplasia and papilloma); moderately increased risk (relative risk, 4 to 5; proliferative changes with atypia or atypical hyperplasia); and significantly increased risk (relative risk, 8 to 10; ductal and lobular carcinoma in situ).

CAUSES

The monthly variations in the circulating levels of estrogen and progesterone are thought to account for most fibrocystic breast changes. Although the exact contribution of each hormone is not well understood, it is believed that an excess amount of estrogen over progesterone results in edema of the breast tissue. At the onset of menses, hormone levels decrease and the fluid responsible for the breast edema is removed by the lymphatic system. All the fluid in the breast may not be removed, and eventually the fluid accumulates in the small glands and ducts of the breast, allowing cyst formation.

GENDER AND LIFE SPAN CONSIDERATIONS

Fibrocystic changes that cause premenstrual pain, tenderness, and increased tissue density usually begin when a woman reaches her mid 20s to early 30s. Cysts occur most frequently in women in their 30s, 40s, and early 50s. Advanced stages can occur during the mid to late 40s. Symptoms should resolve and cysts should disappear once menopause is complete. However, symptoms may persist in women who are taking hormone replacement therapy for menopausal discomfort. Breast cysts are uncommon in women who are 5 years postmenopause and are not undergoing hormone replacement therapy. Therefore, the possibility of a more serious breast problem in any woman who is more than 5 years postmenopause and who presents with a breast mass should be carefully investigated.

◻ ASSESSMENT

HISTORY. Elicit a reproductive history. Women with a fibrocystic breast condition often have a history of spontaneous abortion, shortened menstrual cycles, early menarche, and late menopause. Patients are frequently nulliparous and have not taken oral contraceptives. Cyclic, premenstrual breast pain and tenderness that last about a week are the most common symptoms. With time, the severity of the breast pain increases, and onset occurs 2 to 3 weeks before menstruation. In advanced cases, the breast pain can be constant rather than cyclic.

Fibrocystic breast changes usually occur bilaterally and in the upper outer quadrant of the breast. A woman may appear with gross nodularity or with one or more defined lumps in the breast. The abnormality may be described as a hardness or a thickening in the breast. The areas are usually tender and change in size relative to the menstrual cycle (becoming more pronounced before menstruation and decreasing or disappearing by day 4 or 5 of the cycle). Approximately 50% of patients have repeated episodes of breast cysts.

PHYSICAL EXAMINATION. The breasts should be inspected in three positions: with the patient's arms at the her side, raised over her head, and on her hips. Instruct the patient to "press in" with her hands on the hips to contract the chest muscles. Compare her breasts for symmetry of color, shape, size, surface characteristics, and direction of nipple. Women with deep or superficial cysts or masses may have some distension of breast tissue in the affected area, but often no changes are noted on examination. Dimpling, retraction, scaling, and erosion of breast tissue indicate more serious breast conditions, and none of these disfigurations is usually found in fibrocystic breast condition.

Palpate the breasts in both the sitting and supine positions. Use the pads of the three middle fingers to palpate all breast tissue, including the tail of Spence, in a systematic fashion. Breast cysts are filled with fluid and feel smooth, mobile, firm, and regular in shape. Superficial cysts are often resilient, whereas deep cysts often feel like a hard lump. Cystic lesions vary from 1 to 4 cm in size, can appear quickly, are often bilateral, and occur in mirror-image locations.

To conclude palpation of the breasts, gently squeeze the nipple. About one-third of women with advanced fibrocystic change experience nipple discharge. Nipple discharge in benign conditions is characteristically straw yellowish, greenish, or bluish in color. A bloody nipple discharge often signals the presence of ductal ectasia or intraductal papillomatosis and should be further evaluated.

PSYCHOSOCIAL. Finding a lump or irregularity in the breast is distressing. The almost "overnight" appearance of cysts can make a woman doubt the validity of a recent negative physical examination or mammogram. Additionally, the pain associated with advanced fibrocystic changes can be debilitating. Assess the patient's prior experience with breast problems and her use of coping strategies.

DIAGNOSTIC HIGHLIGHTS

General Comments: Diagnostic testing is needed to rule out malignancy, as well as confirm the diagnosis. Some 80% of breast lumps are found to be benign.

Test	Normal Results	Abnormality with Condition	Explanation
Fine-needle aspiration (FNA)	Not applicable	Green, brown, or yellow fluid obtained	Confirms diagnosis; bloody fluid is suspicious and should be sent to pathology
Mammogram	No tumor noted	Well-rounded mass with a discrete border noted (cyst); vague asymmetric radiodensity (white)	Confirms diagnosis
Ultrasound	No abnormalities seen	Will show a fluid-filled mass, which is consistent with a cyst (not a solid mass, which is consistent with a malignant lump)	Confirms diagnosis
Biopsy	Benign	Benign	Is done if a lump remains after an FNA, to diagnose cancer

☐ PLANNING AND IMPLEMENTATION

Collaborative

The physician will attempt a fine-needle aspiration (FNA) of a breast mass that appears to be cystic. Once the fluid is removed, the cyst collapses and the pain is relieved. Medical therapies may be used in an effort to decrease breast nodularity and relieve breast pain and tenderness.

PRIMARY NURSING DIAGNOSIS

Pain (acute, chronic) that is related to edema, nerve irritation, and a pinching sensation in the breast

OUTCOMES. Comfort level; Pain control; Pain: Disruptive effects

INTERVENTIONS. Analgesic administration; Pain management

PHARMACOLOGIC HIGHLIGHTS

Medication or Drug Class	Dosage	Description	Rationale
Low-estrogen, high-progesterone oral contraceptives	Estrogen and progesterone dosages vary; 1 tab q day	Estrogen–progesterone combination	Successful in 60%–70% of young women; relieves pain during the first cycle and improves the condition in 6 months
Danazol (Danocrine)	50–200 mg po bid or tid, until desired response, then wean	Synthetic androgen (gonadotropin inhibitor)	Effective with 70%–90% of women with repeat episodes
Tamoxifen (Nolvadex)	10 mg po q day	Anti-estrogen	Prescribed for perimenopausal women

Controversial Therapy: The efficacy of vitamins E and A in reducing the symptoms of fibrocystic changes has been reported with conflicting results. Likewise, the benefit achieved by decreasing or eliminating the intake of methylxanthine (caffeine) has met with controversy.

PRIMARY NURSING DIAGNOSIS

Pain (acute, chronic) related to edema, nerve irritation, and pinching sensation in the breast

OUTCOMES. Comfort level; Pain control; Pain: Disruptive effects

INTERVENTIONS. Analgesic administration; Pain management

Independent

Women who are undergoing evaluation for a breast lump need support and understanding, especially if it is the patient's first experience with the condition.

Encourage the patient to express her feelings. Explain the purpose and procedure of diagnostic studies and surgical techniques (FNA, excisional biopsy). Encourage patients to request information as to the exact nature of a benign breast lump (such as whether it was nonproliferative or proliferative), and explain the actual risk for malignant breast disease that is associated with the various histologic changes.

Advise the patient to wear a brassiere that offers good support. Assess the amount of caffeine and salt present in the diet. Help the patient identify foods that are high in these substances and adopt measures to reduce their dietary intake.

DOCUMENTATION GUIDELINES

- Description of breast lump or any breast abnormality: Location, size, texture; color and amount of any nipple discharge
- Characteristics, location, intensity, duration of breast pain

DISCHARGE AND HOME HEALTHCARE GUIDELINES

CARE OF THE PUNCTURE SITE. Leave the Band-Aid in place for 24 hours; report any pain, warmth, severe ecchymosis, or drainage. Emphasize to patient that it is not uncommon for more cysts to form.

CARE OF INCISION. Leave the dressing in place until the sutures are removed; clean the site gently with soap and water once sutures are removed; teach the patient how to empty the drains if any are present.

MEDICATIONS. Explain the purpose, action, dosage, desired effects, and side effects of all medications that have been prescribed by the physician.

FOLLOW-UP VISITS. Women with gross cysts or solid masses in the breast are often seen every 6 months for repeat physical examinations.

EARLY DETECTION PROCEDURES. Assess the patient's knowledge and performance of breast self-examination (BSE); reinforce and teach BSE technique as indicated. Explain the importance of adhering to the follow-up visit schedule as recommended by the physician and to the American Cancer Society's recommendations for screening mammography: first screening by age 40; mammography repeated every 1 to 2 years from age 40 to 49; mammography repeated every year over age 50.

Gallbladder and Biliary Duct (Biliary System) Cancer

DRG Category: 203
Mean LOS: 6.3 days
Description: MEDICAL: Malignancy of Hepatobiliary System or Pancreas
DRG Category: 197
Mean LOS: 8.1 days
Description: SURGICAL: Cholecystectomy except by Laparoscope without C.D.E. with CC
DRG Category: 195
Mean LOS: 9.7 days
Description: SURGICAL: Cholecystectomy with C.D.E. with CC

Most cancers of the gallbladder and biliary tract are inoperable at the time of diagnosis. If the cancer has been found incidentally at the time of a cholecystectomy, longer survival may be possible. Gallbladder cancer and biliary duct cancer are relatively rare and account for fewer than 1% of all cancers. Most gallbladder and biliary duct cancers are adenocarcinomas, with a small number of squamous cell carcinomas. They most frequently occur at the bifurcation in the common bile duct.

Biliary system cancer is insidious and metastasizes via the lymphatic and blood systems and by direct extension to the liver, pancreas, stomach, and duodenum. Invasion of the gastrointestinal (GI) tract can cause complete obstruction of the extrahepatic bile ducts with intrahepatic biliary dilation and enlargement of the liver. If the tumor is restricted to one hepatic duct, biliary obstruction is incomplete and jaundice may not be present. Inflammatory disorders such as cholangitis (bile duct inflammation) and peritonitis often obscure an underlying malignancy. Infection often accompanies cancer of the gallbladder, and bile duct cancers are associated with ulcerative colitis. In most patients with gallbladder and biliary cancer, the disease progresses rapidly and patients usually survive little more than a year after diagnosis.

CAUSES

The cause of biliary system cancer is unknown, although a possibility is gallstones. Approximately 1% of all cholecystectomy specimens are found to be cancerous. Because of the risk of cancer, even for asymptomatic cholelithiasis, a cholecystectomy is recommended. Primary carcinoma of the gallbladder is rare and is usually associated with cholecystitis. Most biliary cancer is from metastasis, commonly from the head of the pancreas.

GENDER AND LIFE SPAN CONSIDERATIONS

Biliary system cancer occurs most commonly in individuals in their 70s and occurs three times more frequently in women than in men. It occurs rarely before the age of 40.

☐ ASSESSMENT

HISTORY. Some patients who do not have symptoms that can be traced back to the gallbladder may describe symptoms similar to those of cholelithiasis or cholecystitis because they result from obstructions and inflammation of the biliary tree. The most common symptom is intermittent to steady pain in the upper right abdomen. Mild pain in the epigastric area may also be reported.

Gastrointestinal symptoms are related to the blockage of bile. Patients may complain of anorexia, nausea, vomiting, belching, diarrhea, and weight loss. Diarrhea may be related to steatorrhea, and weight loss can be as much as 14 to 28 pounds. Because of frequent metastasis to the liver and pancreas, there may be clinical manifestations of cancer in those organs.

PHYSICAL EXAMINATION. Patients with extensive disease may appear thin and malnourished. Determine if the patient is jaundiced from an enlarging tumor that is pressing on the extrahepatic ducts, but note that jaundice may be delayed if only one main duct is involved. Inspect for skin irritation and skin trauma because of pruritus. If the tumor is of sufficient size, an abdominal mass may be palpated; this mass in the gallbladder area feels hard and is sometimes tender. Intrahepatic metastases are not usually palpable. If the abdomen is distended, individual organs may be difficult to palpate. The liver may be very large and smooth, 5 to 12 cm below the costal margin.

PSYCHOSOCIAL. Because the prognosis of biliary cancer is poor, determine how much the patient understands. Determine if the patient is moving through the stages of death and dying, and be accepting of the patient's attitude toward the diagnosis.

DIAGNOSTIC HIGHLIGHTS

Test	Normal Result	Abnormality with Condition	Explanation
Computed tomography (CT) scan	Normal gallbladder and duct system	Presence of tumor	Detects site and size of tumor
Ultrasonography	Normal gallbladder and duct system	Presense of tumor	Detects site and size of tumor

Other Tests: Serum bilirubin level, urinalysis, serum alkaline phosphatase levels, serum mitrochondrial antibody test, and liver biopsy. Radiologic studies include upper GI barium studies, endoscopic retrograde cholangiopancreatography (ERCP), cholangiography, and cholecystogram.

PRIMARY NURSING DIAGNOSIS

Pain (acute) related to obstruction of biliary tree

OUTCOMES. Comfort level; Pain control behavior; Pain level; Symptom severity

INTERVENTIONS. Analgesic administration; Anxiety reduction; Environmental management: Comfort; Pain management; Medication management; Patient-controlled analgesia assistance

☐ PLANNING AND IMPLEMENTATION
Collaborative

MEDICAL. Most medical treatment is aimed at supportive care, such as controlling the GI symptoms and the discomforts of jaundice.

SURGICAL. A cholecystectomy is done as soon as possible after the cancer is detected, although the cancer may have been found by doing the surgery for cholecystitis. Surgery may include removal of a section of the liver. Internal radiotherapy, using iridium-129 wire or radium needles, may be combined with biliary drainage. Chemotherapy has not been shown to be effective against this cancer. External radiation may be used palliatively for cancer of the bile duct but is not effective against gallbladder cancer. If the tumor is inoperable or increases in size after surgery and is occluding any of the bile ducts, palliative measures may be taken to allow the bile to flow into the duodenum. Drainage of the bile can be accomplished by an external system, similar to that of a T-tube, or an internal stent that drains directly into the duodenum. As an alternative to surgery, a stent made of specialized plastic or steel is placed either by endoscopy or percutaneously though the tumor to allow drainage of the trapped bile. Complications include cholangitis and obstruction and dislocation of the stent.

DIETARY. Dietary changes are similar to those needed by patients with cholelithiasis, except the emphasis is on gaining weight rather than on weight reduction. A diet balanced with high calories and protein and low fat helps control the GI symptoms. Each individual needs to determine what foods are best tolerated. Medications to control nausea may be needed before meals, and the patient usually needs a pain-control regimen.

PHARMACOLOGIC HIGHLIGHTS

Medication or Drug Class	Dosage	Description	Rationale
Narcotic analgesia	Varies with drug	Drugs such as morphine sulfate or Demerol may be used to control pain after surgery	Controls pain

Independent

The nurse has an important role in maximizing the patient's comfort. To augment the pain control obtained from analgesia, initiate nonpharmacologic strategies. Allow the patient to participate in the activities of daily living as much as possible. Assist with personal hygiene as much as needed, and include the significant others in learning the process. The itching associated with pruritus can be controlled by maintaining skin integrity, using soft, dry linens and cloths and warm water for bathing. Keep the area around all surgical incisions and drainage devices clean and dry. A large number of support groups exist to help patients and families manage cancer. Listen to the patient's concerns. Give the patient and family the number for the American Cancer Society and hospice care if appropriate.

DOCUMENTATION GUIDELINES

- Physical findings: Signs of blocked bile ducts (pain, nausea and vomiting, jaundice, brown urine, and gray or white stools); skin color and integrity; vital signs; signs of infection (fever, abdominal guarding, increasing white blood cell count)
- Pain control: Response to analgesics, response to nonpharmacologic strategies, location of pain, duration of pain, precipitating factors
- Postoperative assessment of incision, GI functioning, drainage devices (amount and color of drainage)
- Nutrition: Daily weights, appetite, food intake, tolerance to food, presence of nausea and vomiting

DISCHARGE AND HOME HEALTHCARE GUIDELINES

DRAINAGE SYSTEM. Whether the tube is internal or external, teach the patient the signs and symptoms of a blocked tube. If the drainage system is external, teach the patient how to care for the tube, including emptying of the bag, irrigating the tube, periodic clamping of the tube, and managing skin care around the tube.

COMPLICATIONS. Teach the patient to report signs of infection, excessive drainage, leakage, and obstruction to the physician. Provide the patient with a contact phone number.

PRURITUS. Teach the patient methods to control itching.

MEDICATIONS. Teach the patient about each medication, including the purpose and correct dosages, along with any potential side effects.

DIET. Explain the requirements for a low-fat, high-calorie, and high-protein diet.

Gastric Cancer

DRG Category: 172
Mean LOS: 6.5 days
Description: MEDICAL: Digestive Malignancy with CC
DRG Category: 154
Mean LOS: 13.3 days
Description: SURGICAL: Stomach, Esophageal, and Duodenal Procedures, Age > 17 with CC

Gastric cancer is a relatively uncommon malignancy, comprising approximately 2% of all cancers in the United States. Nearly 95% of gastric neoplasms are classified as adenocarcinomas. The most common sites for cancer in the stomach include the antrum, the pylorus, and along the area of lesser curvature. According to the Lauren classification, gastric adenocarcinomas are divided into two main histologic types: diffuse and intestinal. The diffuse type is ill-defined, infiltrates the gastric wall, and lacks a distinctive mass. The intestinal type, by contrast, is composed of neoplastic cells that cluster together, resembling glands; it is associated with a better prognosis, as are tumors along the area of lesser curvature. A poor prognosis is associated with tumors of the cardia or the fundus. Metastasis occurs via the lymphatics and the blood vessels by seeding of peritoneal surfaces or by direct extension of the tumor. Sites of metastasis are the liver, lungs, bone, adrenals, brain, ovaries, colon, and pancreas. Intestinal tumors are more likely to spread to the liver, whereas diffuse-type tumors are more likely to spread along peritoneal surfaces. Other complications include malnutrition, gastrointestinal (GI) obstruction, and iron-deficiency anemia.

CAUSES

Dietary factors linked to gastric cancer are associated with either gastric irritation or exposure to mutagenic or carcinogenic compounds. They include a high intake of salt, nitrite-preserved foods, starch, and fat, along with a low intake of fruits, vegetables, and animal proteins. Associated environmental factors include exposure to ionizing radiation and being employed in metal products or chemical industries. Physiologic factors are related to a rise in gastric pH or the formation of mutagenic or carcinogenic compounds. Other associated conditions include gastric ulcers, gastric polyps, pernicious anemia, intestinal metaplasia, achlorhydria, hypochlorhydria, gastric atrophy, *Helicobacter pylori* infection, chronic peptic ulcers, and atrophic gastritis. Similarly, patients who have undergone a partial gastrectomy for benign gastric disease are predisposed to developing gastric cancer. Genetic factors that are linked to an increased incidence of gastric cancer include a family history of stomach cancer and type A blood.

GENDER AND LIFE SPAN CONSIDERATIONS

Two-thirds of the patients with gastric cancer are older than 65 years of age. More men than women die of gastric cancer.

☐ ASSESSMENT

HISTORY. Gastric cancer may not produce symptoms until the disease is very advanced. About one-third of the patients report a long history of dyspepsia (painful digestion). The most common initial symptoms are mild epigastric discomfort, loss of appetite, nausea, and a sense of fullness or gas pains. Patients may also report experiencing unusual tiredness, abdominal pains, constipation, weight loss, and a bad taste in the mouth. Massive GI bleeding is unusual, although chronic bleeding may occur, which results in a positive occult blood test. Patients with advanced gastric cancer report the classic symptoms of anemia, such as fatigue and activity intolerance, as well as vomiting (coffee-ground or sometimes containing frank blood), anorexia, abdominal pain, dyspepsia, and dysphagia (difficulty swallowing).

PHYSICAL EXAMINATION. In the early stages of gastric cancer, the patient usually appears healthy. In later stages, patients may appear weak, pale, dyspneic, and fatigued from anemia; they are thin and seem to be malnourished. Only 37% of patients have a palpable abdominal mass. Observe for abdominal swelling and ascites, and palpate for hepatomegaly secondary to liver or peritoneal metastases. Some patients may have palpable lymph nodes, especially the supraclavicular and axillary nodes. Gastric cancer is frequently staged using the TNM classification system (T: primary tumor, N: lymph node, M: distant metastasis).

PSYCHOSOCIAL. Survival rates after treatment for gastric cancer remain discouraging (5-year survival rate is 21% for all gastric cancers), and patients with gastric cancer have special psychosocial concerns. Assess their support systems and their ability to cope with major lifestyle changes. As appropriate, assess their transition through the various stages of death and dying.

DIAGNOSTIC HIGHLIGHTS

General Comments: The presence of lactic acid and a high lactate dehydrogenase level in the gastric juice are suggestive of cancer. Often in patients with gastric cancer, plasma tumor markers are elevated. Positive fecal occult blood tests are associated with the chronic bleeding that is related to gastric cancer.

Test	Normal Result	Abnormality with Condition	Explanation
Upper GI series	Normal upper GI tract	Presence of cancer in the stomach	Identifies size and location of tumor
Endoscopy	Normal stomach	Visualization of cancer in the stomach	Visualizes tumor for biopsy

Other Tests: Cytology studies of the specimens obtained, computed tomography (CT) scan, abdominal ultrasonography, and laparoscopy.

PRIMARY NURSING DIAGNOSIS

Pain (acute) related to gastric erosion

OUTCOMES. Comfort level; Pain control behavior; Pain level; Symptom severity

INTERVENTIONS. Analgesic administration; Anxiety reduction; Environmental management: Comfort; Pain management; Medication management; Patient-controlled analgesia assistance

☐ PLANNING AND IMPLEMENTATION

Collaborative

Treatment includes surgery, chemotherapy, and radiation. Of patients with potentially curable gastric cancer, 80% die from a recurrence within 5 years of the initial treatment. If the cancer is resected before it has invaded the stomach wall, the 5-year survival rate is about 90%. A complete en bloc resection of an early, localized tumor is the only cure. Most patients undergo a subtotal gastrectomy, after which GI continuity can be restored by either a Billroth I (gastroduodenostomy) or a Billroth II (gastrojejunostomy) procedure. After such gastric surgery, patients are prone to vitamin B_{12} deficiency and megaloblastic anemia from lack of intrinsic factor; monthly vitamin B_{12} replacement is therefore necessary. For patients who undergo a Billroth I procedure, postprandial dumping syndrome is a problem. For patients who undergo a Billroth II procedure, postoperative intestinal obstruction is a concern.

For patients with advanced disease, palliative subtotal or total gastrectomies may be performed to alleviate gastric symptoms such as bleeding or obstruction. After surgery, chemotherapy or radiation, or both, may be provided.

PHARMACOLOGIC HIGHLIGHTS

Medication or Drug Class	Dosage	Description	Rationale
Chemotherapeutic agents	Varies with drug	Used as adjuvant (in addition to) or neoadjuvant (before surgery) often in combination: fluorouracil, doxorubicin, mitomycin, methyl-CCNU, cisplatin, methotrexate, leucovorin, etoposide	Treat cancer that has metastasized to organs beyond stomach; shrink tumors before surgery
Vitamins	Tablets come in various sizes	B vitamin complex	Combat vitamin B_{12} deficiency and megaloblastic anemia from lack of intrinsic factor
Narcotic analgesics	Varies with drug	Manage pain, side effects of treatment drugs such as morphine, meperidine	Increase patient comfort during end-stage disease

Other Medications: Antiemetics may be used to control nausea, which increases as the tumor enlarges. In the advanced stages, the physician may prescribe sedatives, narcotics, and tranquilizers to increase the patient's comfort. Antispasmodics and antacids may also help relieve GI discomfort.

Independent

PREOPERATIVE. Explain all preoperative and postoperative procedures. Preoperative needs include nutritional adequacy, intravenous fluids, and prophylactic bowel preparation. Inform the patient about the need for GI decompression via a tube for 1 to 3 weeks postoperatively. Explain the amount of pain that should be anticipated, and reassure the patient that analgesia provides relief. Teach coughing and deep-breathing exercises, and have the patient practice them.

POSTOPERATIVE. Maintain wound care; provide adequate fluid and nutrition; manage pain; and control symptoms. Monitor the patient for complications such as hemorrhage, intestinal obstruction, and infection. Teach wound care and the signs and symptoms of infection. Teach nonpharmacologic pain-management techniques. As indicated, teach the signs and symptoms of "dumping syndrome": epigastric fullness, nausea, vomiting, abdominal cramping, and diarrhea that occur within 30 minutes of eating. Teach patients that they may also experience sweating, dizziness, pallor, and palpitations related to the dumping syndrome. To relieve the symptoms, teach patients to avoid drinking fluids within one-half hour of meals and to eat small meals that consist of a low-carbohydrate content and a high-fat and high-protein content.

DOCUMENTATION GUIDELINES

- Physical findings related to gastric cancer: Epigastric discomfort, dyspepsia, anorexia, nausea, sense of fullness, gas pains, unusual tiredness, abdominal pains, constipation, weight loss, vomiting, hematemesis, blood in the stool, dysphagia, jaundice, ascites, bone pain
- GI decompression data: Irrigation and patency of tube, assessment of bowel sounds and passage of gas, complaints of nausea, amount and description of gastric fluid output
- Presence of postoperative complications: Hemorrhage, obstruction, anastomotic leaks, infection, peritonitis
- Presence of postoperative dumping syndrome and associated patient symptoms

DISCHARGE AND HOME HEALTHCARE GUIDELINES

Teach the patient the importance of compliance with palliative and follow-up care. Be sure the patient understands all medications, including the dosage, route, action, and adverse effects. Teach the patient the signs and symptoms of infection and how to care for the incision. Instruct the patient to notify the physician if signs of infection occur. Encourage the patient to seek psychosocial support through local support groups (e.g., I Can Cope), clergy, or counseling services. If appropriate, suggest hospice services. Teach the patient methods to enhance nutritional intake to maintain ideal body weight. Refer the patient to the dietitian for a consultation. Teach family members and friends prevention strategies. Strategies include increasing the intake of fresh fruits and vegetables that are high in vitamin C; maintaining adequate protein intake; and decreasing intake of salty, starchy, smoked, and nitrite-preserved foods.

Gastritis

DRG Category: 182
Mean LOS: 4.3 days
Description: MEDICAL: Esophagitis, Gastroenteritis, and Miscellaneous Digestion Disorders, Age > 17 with CC

Gastritis is any inflammatory process of the mucosal lining of the stomach. The inflammation may be contained within one region or be patchy in many areas. Gastric structure and function are altered in either the epithelial or the glandular components of the gastric mucosa. The inflammation is usually limited to the mucosa, but some forms involve the deeper layers of the gastric wall. Gastritis is classified into acute and chronic forms.

ACUTE. The most common form of acute gastritis is acute hemorrhagic gastritis, also called acute erosive gastritis. The gastric erosions are limited to the mucosa, which have edema and sites of bleeding. Erosions can be diffuse throughout the stomach or localized to the antrum.

CHRONIC. The three forms of chronic inflammation of the gastric mucosa are superficial gastritis, atrophic gastritis, and gastric atrophy. Superficial gastritis, the initial stage in the development of chronic gastritis, leads to red, edematous surface epithelium, small erosions, and decreased mucus content. The gastric glands remain normal. With atrophic gastritis, inflammation extends deeper into the gland area of the mucosa with loss of parietal and chief cells. Atrophic gastritis further develops into the final stage of chronic gastritis—gastric atrophy. In this stage there is a total loss of glandular structure.

Chronic gastritis has also been classified as type A and type B. Type A chronic gastritis, the less common form, involves the body of the stomach (fundus) rather than the antrum. Type B gastritis is a more common nonautoimmune inflammation of the lining of the stomach. It primarily involves the antrum but can affect the entire stomach as age increases. Patients with chronic gastritis have an increased risk (10%) for gastric cancer or may develop chronic iron deficiency. Untreated gastritis can also lead to hemorrhage and shock, gastric perforation, gastrointestinal (GI) obstruction, and peritonitis.

CAUSES

ACUTE GASTRITIS. Alcohol abuse or ingestion of aspirin or nonsteroidal anti-inflammatory drugs (NSAIDs) are the most common causes. Other causes are steroid or digitalis medications; ingestion of corrosive agents such as lye or drain cleaners; ingestion of excessive amounts of tea, coffee, mustard, cloves, paprika, or pepper; chemotherapy or radiation to the upper abdomen; severe stress that is related to critical illness; staphylococcus food poisoning; infections (candida, cytomegalovirus, herpesvirus) in immunosuppressed patients; and *Helicobacter pylori* in chronic gastritis).

CHRONIC GASTRITIS. Type A gastritis is considered primarily an autoimmune disorder. The primary cause of type B gastritis is *H. pylori,* which is found in nearly 100% of the cases of type B gastritis. In both acute and chronic type B gastritis, the normal gastric mucosal barrier is disrupted, which leads to mucosal injury.

GENDER AND LIFE SPAN CONSIDERATIONS

Acute gastritis occurs in men more than in women, whereas chronic gastritis occurs more frequently in women than in men. The incidence is highest in the ages between 50 and 70. Men and women who are heavy smokers and alcohol abusers are at particular risk. The incidence increases with age from 10% to 20% in persons in their 30s to over 45% in persons over 70 years of age.

◻ ASSESSMENT

HISTORY. Obtain a detailed history of past illnesses, as well as the onset, duration, and aggravating and relieving factors of any symptoms. Common symptoms include epigastric pain, changes in stool color, nausea and vomiting (emesis may be bright red, coffee ground, or bile colored), and appetite and weight changes. Assess the patient's usual daily diet, including alcohol, tea, and coffee ingestion. Obtain a complete medication profile that includes both prescribed and over the counter (OTC) drugs. Patients with gastritis may have only mild epigastric discomfort or intolerance for spicy or fatty foods. Patients with atrophic gastritis may be asymptomatic.

PHYSICAL EXAMINATION. The patient may appear normal or may seem to be in discomfort, with facial grimaces and restlessness. Inspect for signs of dehydration or upper GI bleeding, which may be the only sign of acute gastritis. Bleeding can range from a sudden hemorrhage to an insidious blood loss that can be detected only by stool guaiac testing for occult blood or an unexplained anemia. Pallor, tachycardia, and hypotension occur with dramatic GI bleeding accompanied by hematemesis and melena. Auscultate for decreased bowel sounds, which may or may not accompany gastritis. Palpate the abdomen to evaluate the patient for distension, tenderness, and guarding. Epigastric pain and abdominal tenderness are usually absent with patients who have GI bleeding. Gastritis that is caused by food poisoning and corrosive agents (ingestion of strong acids) results in epigastric pain, nausea, and vomiting.

PSYCHOSOCIAL. Assess the patient's and family's anxiety and ability to cope with the fears that are associated with hemorrhage. Assess the patient's understanding of disease management and his or her coping abilities to participate in lifestyle modifications.

DIAGNOSTIC HIGHLIGHTS

Test	Normal Result	Abnormality with Condition	Explanation
Esophagogastroduo-denoscopy (EGD) with biopsy	Visualization of normal stomach; biopsy results show normal cells	Visualization of inflamed gastric mucosa; biopsy results show the specific type of gastritis	Demonstrates location and depth of inflammation of stomach lining and rules out gastric cancer

Other Tests: Supporting tests include upper GI x rays, serum tests, and biopsy.

PRIMARY NURSING DIAGNOSIS

Altered nutrition: Less than body requirements related to decreased appetite, food intolerance, vomiting

OUTCOMES. Nutritional status: Food and fluid intake; Nutrient intake; Biochemical measures; Body mass; Energy; Endurance

INTERVENTIONS. Nutrition management; Nutrition therapy; Nutritional counseling and monitoring; Fluid/electrolyte management; Medication management

◻ PLANNING AND IMPLEMENTATION

Collaborative

The immediate treatment for acute gastritis is directed toward alleviating the symptoms and withdrawing the causative agents. The physician usually prescribes an H_2 antagonist. The medical goal is to maintain the pH of gastric contents above 4.0. Acute hemorrhagic gastritis may disappear within 48 hours because of rapid cell proliferation and restoration of gastric mucosa. If the bleeding is profuse and persistent, blood replacement is necessary. An infusion of vasopressin (Pitressin) or embolization of the left gastric artery is used to halt hemorrhage. Surgical intervention is not performed unless hemorrhage is uncontrollable. In this rare situation, vagotomy with pyloroplasty is usually performed.

There is no known treatment that will reverse the pathogenesis of chronic gastritis. Eradication of *H. pylori* bacteria halts active gastritis in approximately 92% of the cases unless there is permanent damage to the gastric epithelium. The medical regimen for eradicating *H. pylori* is a combination of bismuth salts and two antibiotics over a 2-week period. An important part of management of patients with chronic gastritis is long-term follow-up for early detection of gastric cancer. Patients who have either chronic type A or B gastritis may develop pernicious anemia; destruction of parietal cells in the fundus and body of the stomach leads to inadequate vitamin B_{12} absorption.

PHARMACOLOGIC HIGHLIGHTS

Medication or Drug Class	Dosage	Description	Rationale
H₂ receptor antagonist	Varies with drug	Ranitidine (Zantac); cimetidine (Tagamet); famotidine (Pepcid); nizatidine (Axid)	Blocks gastric secretion and maintains the pH of gastric contents above 4.0, thereby decreasing inflammation
Sulcrafate (Carafate)	1 gram qid	Mucosal barrier fortifier; antiulcer	Forms adhesive gel to protect damaged gastric mucosa
Vasopressin (Pitressin)	0.2–0.4 units per minute with progressive increases to 0.9 units per minute IV	Vasopressor, antidiuretic	Halts acute hemorrhage from gastritis

Other Drugs: Antacids used as buffering agents to neutralize gastric acid and maintain gastric pH above 4.0 include aluminum hydroxide with magnesium hydroxide (Maalox, Mylanta) or aluminum hydroxide (Amphojel); vitamin B_{12} prevents pernicious anemia. Drug therapy for *H. pylori* infection includes bismuth subsalicylates (Pepto-Bismol) with antibiotic combinations such as metronidazole (Flagyl) and tetracycline or ampicillin.

Independent

Encourage the patient to avoid aspirin and NSAIDs (indomethacin and ibuprofen) unless they have been prescribed. Reinforce the need to take these medications with food or to take enteric-coated aspirin. Other drugs that may contribute to gastric irritation include chemotherapeutic agents, corticosteroids, and erythromycin. Explain the importance of reading the labels of OTC drugs to identify those that contain aspirin. Instruct the patient about the action, dosage, and frequency of the medications (antacids, H₂ antagonists, antibiotic regimen) that are administered while the patient is in the hospital. Discuss the possible complications that can develop with acute or chronic gastritis (hemorrhage, pernicious anemia, iron-deficiency anemia, or gastric cancer). Explain the pathophysiology and treatment of each possible complication. Discuss how ingestion of caffeine and spicy foods results in irritation and inflammation of the mucosa of the stomach.

Be sure the patient understands how smoking and alcohol aggravate gastritis and that abstaining from both will facilitate healing and reduce recurrence.

Provide information about various smoking and alcohol rehabilitation programs available in the community. Explain the rationale for the need for support during this very difficult lifestyle change for permanent abstinence. Assist the patient in identifying his or her personal physical and emotional stressors. Review coping skills that the patient has used previously to change behaviors. Talk about how to adapt the environment to which the patient must return in order to meet the needs of lifestyle changes. Involve the family in assisting with the patient's needed changes. Assess the family's response and ability to cope.

DOCUMENTATION GUIDELINES

- Assessment findings: Epigastric discomfort, nausea, vomiting, hematemesis, melena, anemia, dehydration
- Response to medications: Antacids, H_2 antagonists, antibiotics
- Reaction to emotional and physical rest
- Presence of complications: Anemia, hemorrhage, pernicious anemia

DISCHARGE AND HOME HEALTHCARE GUIDELINES

Instruct the patient to avoid caffeine drinks, hot and spicy foods, identified aggravating foods, alcohol, smoking, salicylates, and NSAID OTC drugs. Provide a written list of symptoms of GI bleeding and pernicious anemia (weakness, sore tongue, numbness and tingling in the extremities, anorexia, weight loss, angina, shortness of breath, palpitations). Inform the patient of the need for lifetime vitamin B_{12} intramuscular injections if pernicious anemia develops. Reinforce the need for follow-up for early detection testing for gastric cancer. Review medication action, dosage, frequency, and side effects. Make referrals to smoking and alcohol cessation programs of the patient's choice. Reinforce relaxation exercises and stress management techniques.

Gastroenteritis

DRG Category: 182
Mean LOS: 4.3 days
Description: MEDICAL: Esophagitis, Gastroenteritis, and Miscellaneous Digestive Disorders, Age > 17 with CC

Gastroenteritis is an inflammation of the stomach and the small bowel. It is a self-limiting disease that is also called intestinal flu, traveler's diarrhea, viral enteritis, or food poisoning. The stomach and small bowel react to any of the causative agents with inflammation and increased gastrointestinal (GI) motility, thus leading to severe diarrhea. Gastroenteritis is a common disease throughout the world, and often outbreaks occur in epidemics, especially among people who are living in crowded conditions. It is also more common in autumn and winter than in the warmer seasons. Although it is a major cause of mortality and morbidity in underdeveloped countries, in the United States the condition is rarely life threatening. It does rank second to the common cold as a cause of sick days among American workers, however.

The viral or bacterial organisms enter the intestinal tract and cause inflammation to the intestinal lining and diarrhea by one of the following means: (1) enterotoxins are released from the organism and stimulate the intestinal mucosa to secrete increased amounts of water and electrolytes into the intestinal lumen; (2) the organisms either infiltrate the intestinal wall, causing cell destruction of the lining, or attach themselves to the epithelium, causing cell destruction of the intestinal villae.

CAUSES

The majority of organisms that cause intestinal infections are acquired through contaminated food and water. The major risk factor for gastroenteritis that is caused by food poisoning is improper handling and storage of food. Bacterial or viral food poisoning usually occurs within 16 hours after eating contaminated food.

Some infections are transmitted by person-to-person contact. Fecal-oral transmission is a result of poor hygiene. The viral forms are epidemic viral gastroenteritis and rotavirus gastroenteritis. The epidemic viral form, often called intestinal flu, is transmitted through the fecal-oral route in food and water; the incubation period ranges from 10 to 50 hours. Rotaviruses are transmitted via the fecal-oral or possibly fecal-respiratory routes; the incubation period is 24 to 72 hours.

There are three principal forms of bacterial gastroenteritis: *Campylobacter enteritis* (traveler's diarrhea), *Escherichia coli* diarrhea (also known as traveler's diarrhea), and shigellosis (bacillary dysentery). Factors that contribute to the host's susceptibility to the agent are an elevated pH with the use of antacids, decreased production of gastric acid, or excessive intake of high-fat foods, which protect the microbe from gastric acid. Also, slow small bowel motility increases the time the pathogen is in contact with the lumen of the bowel, which aids in the development and duration of symptoms. Normal intestinal flora protect a person from pathogenic organisms.

GENDER AND LIFE SPAN CONSIDERATIONS

Children under age 2 are more susceptible to infectious gastroenteritis because their immune system is not yet fully developed. Rotavirus gastroenteritis is usually confined to infants and children under 3 years of age. By age 3, most children develop antibodies against the rotaviruses. Both men and women with low levels of antibody can be infected, particularly family members of affected infants. Severe, prolonged diarrhea may be fatal in elderly persons and infants when severe fluid and electrolyte imbalance occurs. Infants become dehydrated very rapidly.

☐ ASSESSMENT

HISTORY. Diarrhea is the cardinal symptom of gastroenteritis, but the severity varies with the causative organism. Determine the frequency, color, consistency, and amount of bowel movements. The epidemic viral diarrhea lasts only 24 to 48 hours, whereas rotaviral infection may last up to 7 days. Campylobacter enteritis results in 20 to 30 foul-smelling stools per day for as long as a week. *E. coli* may cause blood and mucus in the stool, with a duration of 7 to 10 days. Diarrhea from shigellosis is greenish in color, may last from 2 to 20 days, and also contains blood and mucus. Nausea and vomiting usually are confined to the first 48 hours of illness. Ask if cramping, pain, nausea, or vomiting has accompanied the diarrhea.

Fever often occurs with bacterial intestinal infections. Flu symptoms (malaise, headache, myalgia [muscle achiness]) are associated with the epidemic viral gastroenteritis. Determine if other family members or coworkers have the same symptoms. It is important to determine if the gastroenteritis is communicable from contaminated food or water so that the community health department can be notified. Inquire about recent travel and food intake. Investigate what and where the patient has eaten in the last 2 days.

PHYSICAL EXAMINATION. The patient generally appears acutely ill, with dry skin and poor skin turgor. Inspect the mouth and note that the mucous membranes are usually dry, the tongue is furrowed, and salivation is decreased. Other signs include flattened neck veins, redness of the perianal area, and a decreased urine volume (less than 20 mL per hour or 480 mL in 24 hours) and increased urine concentration (a dark, concentrated color). When you perform auscultation, check for hyperactive bowel sounds. The patient may have abdominal distension with diarrheal stools that are liquid, green, foul-smelling, and bloody or mucus-filled.

PSYCHOSOCIAL. Identify the patient's perception of the threat of the symptoms. Assess for behaviors that may indicate anxiety, such as restlessness, irritability, and difficulty sleeping. Identify coping skills the patient is using, such as problem solving, anger, and daydreaming.

DIAGNOSTIC HIGHLIGHTS

Test	Normal Result	Abnormality with Condition	Explanation
Stool culture and Gram stain	Negative for pathogens; normal stool flora	Presence of enteric pathogens; enterotoxigenic *E. coli;* pus cells, white blood cells and shigella; white blood cells, red blood cells and campylobacter	Demonstrate presence of pathogens or the effect of pathogens

Other Tests: Blood chemistries to identify dehydration, electron microscopy and immunoassay for epidemic viral or rotavirus gastroenteritis.

PRIMARY NURSING DIAGNOSIS

Diarrhea related to increased intestinal motility

OUTCOMES. Bowel elimination; Electrolyte and acid/base balance; Fluid balance; Hydration; Infection status; Nutritional status: Food and fluid intake

INTERVENTIONS. Diarrhea management; Fluid/electrolyte management; Fluid monitoring; Perineal care; Skin surveillance; Medication management

❑ PLANNING AND IMPLEMENTATION

Collaborative

Many intestinal infections are short-lived (24 to 48 hours) and are adequately treated by resting the colon and with rehydration. The patient is instructed to take nothing by mouth until vomiting stops. Early fluid and electrolyte replacement is critical for debilitated, aged, and very young patients. Clear liquids are started slowly until tolerance is evaluated. Gatorade or other drinks with electrolytes are preferred to water. Oral rehydration therapy with products such as Resol may be used for elderly patients. The patient may advance to bland solids within 24 hours. When rapid dehydration occurs, the patient is admitted to the hospital for intravenous fluid replacement with solutions such as half-strength normal saline solution to prevent serious complications or possible death. Electrolytes such as potassium may be added to intravenous solutions, depending on the patient's blood chemistry results.

It is mandatory to notify the local health department for cases of shigellosis and in some areas mandatory to notify for *Campylobacter enteritis.* Check with the local and state health department guidelines for reporting gastroenteritis.

Antiemetics and anticholingerics are contraindicated because they slow the motility of the bowel, which interferes with evacuating the causative organism. The longer the infectious agent is in contact with the intestinal wall, the more severe the infection.

PHARMACOLOGIC HIGHLIGHTS

Medication or Drug Class	Dosage	Description	Rationale
Anti-diarrheal agents	Varies with drug	Kaolin-pectin (Kaopectate); bismuth subsalicylate (Pepto-Bismol)	Coat the intestinal wall and decrease intestinal secretions
Anti-infectives	Varies with drug	Trimethoprim-sulfamethoxazole (Bactrim, Septra)	Combat *Shigellosis enteritis*
Antibiotics	Varies with drug	Ampicillin; tetracycline hydrochloride	Combat infection if leukocytes are present in stools

Independent

Provide for periods of uninterrupted rest, which often helps decrease the patient's symptoms. The patient with gastroenteritis is anxious and weak from vomiting and diarrhea. Explain the rationale for the treatment regimen of having no oral intake, maintaining bed rest, and the administration of intravenous fluids. Measure all urine, emesis, and loose stools. Tell the patient to call for assistance to use the bathroom, and explain the use of the commode "hat" for the purpose of measuring output. Try to place the patient in a private room to decrease embarrassment about the frequent, foul-smelling stools and to limit cross-contamination. Encourage the patient to wash his or her hands carefully after each stool and after performing perianal care; make sure all staff use good hand-washing techniques and universal precautions when dealing with stool and vomitus to prevent disease transmission.

To prevent excoriation, provide skin protective agents and creams (petroleum jelly, zinc oxide) to apply around the anal region. Teach the patient to cleanse with water or barrier cleanser spray, wipe with cotton pads, and apply the cream after each bowel movement. Inspect the perineal area daily for further breakdown. Sitz baths for 10 minutes two to three times per day are helpful for perianal discomfort.

DOCUMENTATION GUIDELINES

- Frequency and characteristics of bowel movements: Number, presence of blood and mucus, color, consistency (formed, watery)
- Comfort: Presence of abdominal colicky pain, cramping
- Nutrition and fluid balance: Response to fluid and electrolyte replacement, intake and output, signs of dehydration, tolerance of fluids and food
- Complications: Increased abdominal discomfort or bleeding, uncorrected dehydration, skin breakdown
- Prevention: Understanding of measures to prevent transmission of infections

DISCHARGE AND HOME HEALTHCARE GUIDELINES

The primary goal of discharge teaching is to educate the patient and family about reducing the risk of transmitting the organisms that cause gastroenteritis. Demonstrate hand-washing techniques. Instruct the patient and family to use an antibacterial soap, such as liquid Dial, for hand washing after toileting. Stress the importance of daily bathing and meticulous personal hygiene with a focus on perianal cleansing. Frequent cleansing of the commode with an antibacterial cleanser is necessary to avoid exposure of stools to others. The patient should not handle food that will be eaten by others. Discuss the need for the patient to have his or her own toothpaste, towel, and washcloth and not to share dishes, utensils, or drinking glasses. Provide these instructions in written form; explain that they are to be carried out for at least 7 weeks—or for several months if the patient is diagnosed with shigellosis.

The patient may be discharged with a prescription for antibiotics or anti-infective agents. Teach the patient to continue the medications for the full length of therapy. Tell him or her to space the medication evenly around the clock; take with a full glass of water; and report symptoms of rash, fever, bleeding, bruising, or other new symptoms. Instruct the patient to report recurring symptoms of diarrhea, fever, vomiting, or any change in frequency and appearance of stool.

Gastroesophageal Reflux Disease (GERD)

DRG Category: 083
Mean LOS: 3 days
Description: MEDICAL: Esophagitis, Gastroenteritis, and Miscellaneous Digestive Disorders Age > 17 without CC
DRG Category: 155
Mean LOS: 3.3 days
Description: SURGICAL: Stomach, Esophageal, and Duodendal Procedures Age > 17 without CC

Gastroesophageal reflux disease (GERD) is a syndrome that is caused by esophageal reflux, or the backward flow of gastroesophageal contents into the esophagus. GERD occurs because of inappropriate relaxation of the lower esophageal sphincter (LES) in response to an unknown stimulus. Reflux occurs in most adults, but if it occurs regularly, the esophagus cannot resist the irritating effects of gastric acid and pepsin because the mucosal barrier of the esophagus breaks down. Without this protection, tissue injury, inflammation, hyperemia, and even erosion occur.

As healing occurs, the cells that replace the normal squamous cell epithelium may be more resistant to reflux but may also be a pre-malignant tissue that can lead to adenocarcinoma. Repeated exposure also may lead to fibrosis and scarring, which can cause esophageal stricture to occur. Stricture leads to difficulty in swallowing. Chronic reflux is often associated with hiatus hernia.

CAUSES

The causes of GERD are not well understood. Many patients with GERD have normal resting LES pressure and produce normal amounts of gastric acid. Possible explanations for GERD include delays in gastric emptying, changes in lower esophageal sphincter control with aging, and obesity. Environmental and physical factors that lower tone and contractility of the lower esophageal sphincter include diet (fatty foods, peppermint, alcohol, caffeine, chocolate) and drugs (nicotine, beta adrenergic blockers, nitrates, theophylline, anticholinergic drugs).

GENDER AND LIFE SPAN CONSIDERATIONS

GERD occurs at any age but is most common in people over 50 years of age. It occurs in both men and women, and it is a common disorder that affects as many as one-third of the total population.

☐ ASSESSMENT

HISTORY. Elicit a history of contributing factors, including the regular consumption of fatty foods, caffeinated beverages, chocolate, nicotine, alcohol, or peppermint. Take a drug history to determine if the patient has been taking drugs that may contribute to GERD: beta adrenergic blockers, calcium channel blockers, nitrates, theophylline, diazepam, anticholinergic drugs, estrogen and progesterone.

Little relationship appears to occur between the severity of symptoms and degree of esophagitis. Some patients have minimal evidence of esophagitis, whereas others with severe, chronic inflammation may have no symptoms until stricture occurs. Patients may describe the characteristic symptom of heartburn (also known as pyrosis or dyspepsia). The discomfort is often a sub- or retro-sternal pain that radiates upward to the neck, jaw, or back. Patients describe a worsening pain when they bend over, strain, or lie flat. With severe inflammation, discomfort occurs after each meal and lasts for up to 2 hours. Patients may describe coughing, hoarseness, or wheezing at night.

Patients may also report regurgitation, with a sensation of warm fluid traveling upward to the throat and leaving a bitter, sour taste in the mouth. Other symptoms may include difficulty swallowing (dysphagia) and painful swallowing (odynophagia) during eating, as well as eructation, flatulence, or bloating after eating.

PHYSICAL EXAMINATION. Generally the patient's physical appearance is unchanged by GERD. On rare occasions, some patients may experience unexplained weight loss.

PSYCHOSOCIAL. Psychosocial assessment should include assessment of the degree of stress the person experiences and the strategies he or she uses to cope with stress.

DIAGNOSTIC HIGHLIGHTS

Test	Normal Result	Abnormality with Condition	Explanation
Esophageal pH monitoring	> 5	< 5	Presence of gastric contents in the esophagus decreases pH
Esophageal manometry	Congruent esophageal pressures bilaterally; competent LES	Abnormal contractions and peristalsis; incompetentLES; low resting pressure of LES	Multilumen esophageal catheter introduced through mouth. Used to measure esophageal pressures during a variety of swallowing maneuvers

Other Tests: Endoscopy, barium swallow, scintigraphy, Bernstein's test (acidic solution infused into stomach causing heartburn in patients with GERD).

PRIMARY NURSING DIAGNOSIS

Pain related to esophageal reflux and esophageal inflammation

OUTCOMES. Comfort level; Pain control behavior; Pain level; Symptom control behavior; Symptom severity

INTERVENTIONS. Medication administration; Medication management; Pain management; Positioning; Environmental management: Comfort; Nutritional monitoring; Weight management

□ PLANNING AND IMPLEMENTATION

Collaborative

Although diet therapy alone can manage symptoms in some patients, most patients can have their GERD managed pharmacologically. Dietary modifications that may decrease symptoms include reducing intake of fatty foods, caffeinated beverages, chocolate, nicotine, alcohol, and peppermint. Reducing the intake of spicy and acidic foods lets esophageal healing occur during times of acute inflammation. Encourage the patient to eat five to six small meals during the day rather than large meals. Ingestion of large amounts of food increases gastric pressure and thereby increases esophageal reflux. Both weight loss and smoking cessation programs are also important for any patients who have problems with obesity and tobacco use.

Surgical procedures to relieve reflux are generally reserved for those otherwise healthy patients who have not responded to medications. Three major surgical procedures are used: Nissen fundoplication (surgeon wraps fundus of the stomach around esophagus to anchor the LES area below the diaphragm), Hill's repair (anchors gastroesophageal junction to the median arcuate ligament), and Belsey's repair (transthoracic approach with a fundic wrap around the distal esophagus).

PHARMACOLOGIC HIGHLIGHTS

Medication or Drug Class	Dosage	Description	Rationale
Antacids	Usually 30 mL between meals and as needed po	Aluminum or magnesium salts	Neutralize gastric acid and relieve heartburn
H_2 receptor antagonists or proton pump inhibitors	Varies with drug; routes vary	Decrease gastric acid production; cimetidine, ranitidine, famotidine, nizatidine, omeprazole, lansoprazole	Lower gastric acidity
Cisapride	10–20 mg po qid before meals and bedtime	GI stimulant	Increases LES pressure and improves esophageal clearance and gastric emptying
Metoclopramide	10 mg po tid before meals	GI stimulant	Improves gastric emptying and increases LES pressure
Sulcrafate	1 gram po qid	Antiulcer	Forms a protective adhesive gel over areas of injury or inflammation

Independent

Many patients experience nighttime reflux because of the recumbent position and infrequent swallowing. Changing the patient's position by elevating the head of the bed during sleep may mitigate symptoms. Place 6-inch blocks under the head of the bed or place a wedge under the mattress to enhance nocturnal acid clearance. Encourage the patient to avoid food for three hours before going to sleep, and advise the patient to eat slowly and chew food thoroughly.

Lifestyle changes to reduce intra-abdominal pressure may be helpful to relieve symptoms. Encourage the patient to avoid the following: restrictive clothing, lifting heavy objects, straining, working in a bent-over position, and stooping. Support the patient's efforts to stop smoking and lose weight. Make appropriate referrals to the dietician to provide the knowledge essential for weight control.

DOCUMENTATION GUIDELINES

- Discomfort: Timing, character, location, duration, precipitating factors
- Nutrition: Food and fluid intake; understanding of dietary restriction and weight reduction for each meal; daily weight measurement
- Medication management: Understanding drug therapy, response to medications
- Response to nighttime positioning: Progress of changing position of head of the bed at night, tolerance to position change

DISCHARGE AND HOME HEALTHCARE GUIDELINES

Teach the patient how to maintain adequate nutrition and hydration and to manage medications. Make sure that the patient and family understand all aspects of the treatment regimen. Review dietary limitations, recommendations to reduce weight and cut out tobacco, and dosage and side effects of all medications. Make sure the patient understands the need to change position at nighttime and that he or she has the supplies required to do so.

Glaucoma

DRG Category: 046
Mean LOS: 4.4 days
Description: MEDICAL: Other Disorders of the Eye, Age > 17 with CC
DRG Category: 042
Mean LOS: 1.7 days
Description: SURGICAL: Intraocular Procedures Except Retina, Iris, and Lens

Glaucoma is an acute or chronic condition in which there is an increase of intraocular pressure (IOP), which leads to damage of the retina and optic nerve, with resulting visual field loss. In the normal eye, IOP (10 to 21 mm Hg) exists as long as there is a balance between the production, circulation, and outflow of aqueous humor. Aqueous humor is produced in the posterior chamber ciliary processes and flows through the pupil into the anterior chamber. From the anterior chamber, it passes through the canal of Schlemm and out through the aqueous veins into the anterior ciliary veins.

Increased IOP compromises blood flow to the optic nerve and retina. Tissue damage occurs as a result of the deficient blood supply and progresses from the periphery toward the fovea centralis. If IOP is left untreated, blindness results.

CAUSES

Chronic open-angle glaucoma (primary open-angled) is the most common form of glaucoma, accounting for 90% of all glaucoma cases. It is caused by an over-production of aqueous humor or obstruction to its flow through the trabecular meshwork or the canal of Schlemm. The chamber angles between the iris and cornea remain open. IOP intensifies gradually because aqueous humor cannot leave the eye at the same rate that it is produced.

Acute glaucoma, also referred to as closed-angle glaucoma or narrow-angle glaucoma, is less common and, with its sudden onset, is treated as an emergency situation. Obstruction of the outflow of aqueous humor occurs by anterior displacement of the iris against the cornea, which narrows or obstructs the chamber angle. Attacks of acute glaucoma are caused by injury, pupil dilation, or stress. Secondary glaucoma occurs in other diseases of the eye when the circulation of aqueous humor is disrupted with either a decreased angle or increased intraocular volume. Uveitis, iritis, trauma, tumors, and postsurgical procedures on the eye are common causes of secondary glaucoma. Congenital glaucoma is caused by an autosomal recessive trait that results in dysfunctional development of the trabecular meshwork through which aqueous humor flows.

GENDER AND LIFE SPAN CONSIDERATIONS

Individuals over age 40 are at a higher risk of developing glaucoma. Approximately 2% of the U.S. population over age 40 and 10% of people over 80 have glaucoma. Glaucoma affects both men and women.

◻ ASSESSMENT

HISTORY. Ask the patient if he or she has had recent eye surgery, trauma, or infection. Use of antihistamines can precipitate closed-angle glaucoma because antihistamines cause pupils to dilate, and this may result in obstruction of fluid flow. Family visual history can help with a diagnosis of chronic open-angle glaucoma. Because open-angle glaucoma develops slowly, the visual history should focus on foggy vision, diminished accommodation, frequent changes in eyeglass prescription, mild eye pain, headache, visual field deficits, and halos around lights.

Gentle palpation of the covered eyeball reveals a firmer globe, which has been caused by the increased IOP. Blind spots and peripheral field losses are confirmed by a visual field examination. Inspect the patient's eyes for reddened sclera, turbid aqueous humor, and moderately dilated nonreactive pupils. Other symptoms include extreme unilateral eye pain, blurred vision, and possibly nausea and vomiting. Symptoms of congenital glaucoma include photophobia, cloudy corneas, excessive tearing, and muscle spasms around the orbital ridge (bleapharospasm).

Validate observations of anxiety, and explore coping strategies to deal with patient concerns. Grieving for the potential of vision loss or vision already lost follows the stages of denial, anger, bargaining, depression, and acceptance.

DIAGNOSTIC HIGHLIGHTS

Test	Normal Result	Abnormality with Condition	Explanation
Tonometry	12–20 mm Hg	Elevated: 22–28 mm Hg warning level; > 38 mm Hg major concern	Measures intraocular pressure using a tonometer (instrument that is pressed directly against the anesthetized eye); if a recording device is used (tonography), recorded slope indicates adequacy of drainage
Gonioscopy	Normal drainage angle in eye	Presence of adhesions, aberrant blood vessels, signs of injury	Visualization of entire 360° circumference of iridocorneal angle

Other Tests: Direct opthalmoscopic examination and visual field testing, perimetry, fundus photograph.

PRIMARY NURSING DIAGNOSIS

Sensory and perceptual alterations (visual) related to nerve fiber destruction caused by increased IOP

OUTCOME. Body image; Anxiety control; Neurological status; Safety behavior: Fall prevention and Personal; Safety status: Physical injury; Self-care: Activities of daily living

INTERVENTIONS. Activity therapy; Communication enhancement: Visual deficit; Environmental management; Fall prevention; Reality orientation; Surveillance: Safety; Eye care; Medication management

☐ PLANNING AND IMPLEMENTATION

Collaborative

Glaucoma is often treated medically. Surgery is required when medications are ineffective in reducing IOP. Argon laser trabeculoplasty is preferred because it has an 80% success rate in reducing IOP. Surgical filtering treatment produces a permanent fistula from the anterior chamber and the subconjunctival space. Filtering procedures include trabeculectomy, cyclodialysis, peripheral iridectomy, sclerectomy, and ocular implantation devices such as the Molento implant.

After surgical filtering, postoperative care includes dilation and topical steroids to rest the pupil. Postoperative care after peripheral iridectomy includes cycloplegic eyedrops only in the affected eye to relax the ciliary muscle and to decrease inflammation, thus preventing adhesions. When other surgical procedures have failed, cyclocryotherapy may be performed. Parts of the ciliary body are destroyed by the freezing effect of the probe, which reduces aqueous humor production.

PHARMACOLOGIC HIGHLIGHTS

Medication or Drug Class	Dosage	Description	Rationale
Miotic eyedrops	Varies with drug	Pilocarpine hydrochloride, echothiophate iodide, carbachol	Constrict pupil and contract ciliary muscle to promote outflow
Beta blockers	Varies with drug	Timolol, levobunolol	Reduce the production of aqueous humor
Carbonic anhydrase inhibitors	Varies with drug	Acetazolamide, methazolamide	Reduce the production of aqueous humor

Other Drugs: Epinephrine and dipivefrin hydrocholoride reduce aqueous humor production (not for use in closed angle glaucoma), osmotic agents such as oral glycerin or mannitol in emergencies to reduce IOP rapidly.

Independent

Blindness from glaucoma can frequently be prevented by early detection and lifelong treatment. Patients are informed that vision loss is permanent, but further vision loss may be prevented if IOP is controlled through medications or surgery.

To prevent injury that is related to reduced peripheral vision, arrange the environment to ensure safety. Place frequently used items where the patient can view them through central visual fields. Administer miotics, which cause pupillary constriction, blur vision for 1 to 2 hours after installation, and reduce adaptation to darkness. Miotics are often given four times a day to fit the patient's schedule, or have the physician order the gel form (pilocarpine HS gel), which can be given once a day at night. Some patients benefit by the use of Ocusert, a pilocarpine time-released wafer. The wafer is inserted weekly and is helpful to patients who cannot insert eyedrops.

To minimize self-care deficits, encourage independence with actions of daily living, and assist the patient as necessary. Encourage the patient to express anxiety, grieving, and concerns about glaucoma or blindness. Listen supportively, and explore coping strategies. Reinforce compliance with the recommended treatment plan and follow-up care.

DOCUMENTATION GUIDELINES

- Cupping and atrophy of the optic disk, palpation of the eyeball, peripheral field losses, reddened sclera, nonreactive pupils, turbid aqueous humor, pain, and nausea or vomiting
- Presence of surgical complications: Pain, nausea, infection, hemorrhage, profuse sweating, change in vital signs

DISCHARGE AND HOME HEALTHCARE GUIDELINES

To prevent increased IOP, teach the patient to avoid the following: bending at the waist, lifting heavy objects, coughing, vomiting, and straining to have a bowel movement. Note that following the medication schedule and routinely seeing the eye doctor can prevent further visual loss. Glaucoma requires strict, consistent treatment to prevent blindness.

Validate the patient's understanding of all medications, including dosage, route, action, and side effects. Be sure the patient has the dexterity to instill eyedrops correctly. Suggest a daily calendar log to record medication use. Written guidelines may be helpful. Review the date and time of the return visit to the eye surgeon after surgery. Instruct the patient to wear an eye shield over the operated eye at night and eyeglasses during the day to prevent accidental injury. Explain the need for the patient to call the eye doctor right away if any of the following symptoms occurs: pain in the eye, shortness of breath, nausea or vomiting, loss of vision, nonreactive pupils, reddened sclera, bleeding, discharge, or tingling in the hands or feet. Visiting nurses for home healthcare or social services can assist with rehabilitation or finances.

Glomerulonephritis, Acute

DRG Category: 331
Mean LOS: 5.1 days
Description: MEDICAL: Other Kidney and Urinary Tract Diagnoses, Age > 17 with CC

Acute glomerulonephritis (AGN) is an inflammatory disease of the specialized tuft of capillaries within the kidney called the glomerulus. In its several forms Ggomerulonephritis was the leading cause of chronic renal failure in the United States until the mid-1980s, but because of more aggressive treatment approaches, it is now third, after diabetes mellitus and hypertension. Glomerulonephritis continues to be a fairly common disorder worldwide, however. The inflammatory changes occur because of deposits of antigen-antibody complexes lodged within the glomerular membrane. Antigen-antibody complexes are formed within the circulation in response to an antigen or foreign protein. The antigen may be of external origin, such as a portion of the streptococcus bacterial cell wall, or of internal origin, such as the changes that occur in systemic diseases like systemic lupus erythematosus (SLE).

If the source of the causative antigen is temporary, such as a transient infection, the inflammatory changes subside and renal function usually returns to normal; if the source of antigen is long-term or permanent, the AGN may become chronic. During the acute phase of the disease process, major complications include hypertension, hypertensive encephalopathy, acute renal failure, cardiac failure, and seizures. Chronic glomerular nephritis leads to contracted, granular kidneys and end-stage renal disease.

CAUSES

Etiologic factors are unclear, but most experts identify an immunologic origin for the disease. AGN may occur as an isolated (primary) disorder, as a disorder associated with an infectious disease, or as a secondary disorder. Primary AGN occurs in mesangiocapillary glomerulonephritis and in IgA nephropathy. Infection-associated AGN follows an infection such as group A gb-hemolytic streptococcus (GABHS) infection. Nonstreptococcal postinfectious glomerulonephritis may occur after an attack of infective endocarditis, sepsis, pneumococcal pneumonia, viral hepatitis, mumps, or measles. Secondary AGN is associated with severe systemic diseases such as SLE, vasculitis, and Goodpasture's syndrome.

GENDER AND LIFE SPAN CONSIDERATIONS

AGN occurs primarily in the pediatric population after an infectious event, most commonly GABHS in boys from the age of 3 to 7. About 95% of children and 70% of adults have a full recovery in acute poststreptococcal glomerulonephritis. In both men and women, AGN may occur after an infection or with multisystem diseases such as SLE. Because adults may exhibit more signs of cardiovascular compromise than children do, treatment of the adult may require more support of the cardiovascular system through medications.

◻ ASSESSMENT

HISTORY. Question the patient or parents about an untreated respiratory tract infection that has occurred in the last 1 to 3 weeks. Ask the patient about the medical history to identify any multisystem diseases. Because patients often describe a history of weight gain and edema of the hands and face, ask the patient if his or her rings are tighter than usual. Some patients may also describe decreased urine volume, changes in urine color (dark, smoky), increased fatigue and activity intolerance, muscle and joint achiness, shortness of breath, and orthopnea. Elderly patients' symptoms may be more vague and nonspecific, such as achiness and nausea.

PHYSICAL EXAMINATION. Note any signs of fluid retention, such as edema in the face and hands. As you speak to the patient, you may notice dyspnea and labored breathing. Inspect the neck veins to determine if engorgement is present. The patient's urine output is usually decreased and is often dark or even coffee-colored. When you auscultate the patient's heart and lungs, you may hear basilar crackles and an S_3 heart sound. Most patients have an elevated arterial pressure. Weigh the patient each day, and monitor abdominal girth. Provide ongoing monitoring for visual changes, vomiting, adventitious breath sounds, abdominal distension, and seizure activity. These signs and symptoms indicate the potential onset of the complications and need to be reported to the physician.

PSYCHOSOCIAL. Patients and families may be anxious about changes in the patient's appearance, an uncertain prognosis, and the possibility of lifestyle changes. Older children and adults may be concerned about their appearance. Assess the patient's and family's coping mechanisms, support systems, and stress levels.

DIAGNOSTIC HIGHLIGHTS

Test	Normal Result	Abnormality with Condition	Explanation
Creatinine clearance	100–40 mL per minute	50 mL per minute	Damaged glomerulus no longer able to clear or filter normal amounts of creatinine from blood
Serum creatinine	0.5–1.2 mg/dL	< 2.0 mg/dL	Decreased ability of glomerulus to filter

Urinalysis	Minimal red blood cells; moderate clear protein casts; negative for protein	Red blood cells and red blood cell casts; elevated protein	creatinine leads to accumulation in the blood May also have renal tubular cells, white blood cells, increased white blood cell casts

Other Tests: Supporting tests include serum electrolytes, serum potassium, serum blood urea nitrogen, erythrocyte sedimentation rate (ESR), C-reactive protein (CRP), complement levels, cryoglobulins, serum mucoprotein levels, antistreptolysin O titers (ASO), and percutaneous renal biopsy.

PRIMARY NURSING DIAGNOSIS

Fluid volume excess related to glomerular inflammation and decreased renal filtration

OUTCOMES. Fluid balance; Hydration; Nutrition management; Nutrition therapy; Knowledge: Treatment regime

INTERVENTIONS. Fluid/electrolyte management; Fluid monitoring; Medication administration

◻ PLANNING AND IMPLEMENTATION

Collaborative

Most patients with AGN recover spontaneously. During the acute phase, when urine is grossly hematuric and blood pressure is elevated, the patient is placed on bed rest and symptoms are managed pharmacologically. A dietary consultation is necessary to implement dietary restrictions that can manage increased blood pressure, decreased urine output, and the presence of nitrogenous products in the urine. Usually sodium and fluid restriction is instituted to manage hypertension and edema. Depending on the course of their disease, some patients also need potassium and protein restrictions. If the patient is on fluid restriction, work with the patient and family to devise a schedule of fluid intake that maximizes patient preference and comfort.

PHARMACOLOGIC HIGHLIGHTS

Medication or Drug Class	Dosage	Description	Rationale
Antihypertensive and diuretics	Varies with drug	Antihypertensives: hydralazine; diuretics: furosemide	Manage hypertension and fluid overload

Other Drugs: Antibiotics may be administered for 7 to 10 days if the etiologic factor was an infectious agent such as streptococcus. Corticosteroids are controversial and considered by many experts to be of no value.

Independent

Focus on decreasing discomfort, reducing complications, and providing patient education. Work with the patient to develop a schedule for daily hygiene that limits fatigue and overexertion. Cluster care to provide for rest periods, and assist the patient with relaxation techniques. Assist children with the usual bedtime rituals. Increase activity gradually as symptoms subside.

While the patient is on bed rest, perform active or passive range-of-motion exercises each shift, and assist the patient to a new position every 2 hours. Monitor the patient's skin for breakdown. If the patient is recovering from an infection, prevent secondary infection. Take time to answer the patient's and parents' questions fully. If you note that the family is coping ineffectively with the illness or prognosis, make a referral to a clinical nurse specialist.

DOCUMENTATION GUIDELINES

- Cardiovascular responses: Blood pressure, pulse, presence of abnormal heart sounds; presence, location, and severity of edema; daily weights
- Renal responses: Character, amount, odor of urine
- Respiratory responses: Respiratory rate and effort, breath sounds
- Presence of complications: Fever, food intolerance, pulmonary congestion, shortness of breath, increasing peripheral edema, weight gain, skin breakdown, anuria
- Comfort: Type of discomfort, location and intensity, character, response to attempts to provide relief

DISCHARGE AND HOME HEALTHCARE GUIDELINES

Inform patients and families about the disease process, prognosis, and treatment plan. Discuss with them the possibility that abnormal urinary findings may persist for years after AGN has been diagnosed. Demonstrate all home care techniques, such as medication administration. Discuss the dosage, action, route, and side effects of all medications. If the patient is placed on antibiotics, encourage him or her to complete the entire prescription. Teach the patient and family to seek professional assistance for all infectious processes (particularly respiratory infections with sore throat and fever); monitor body weight and blood pressure at home or through a clinic; avoid contact with individuals with infectious processes. Discuss the need for ongoing laboratory monitoring of electrolytes and renal function tests during the months of convalescence, as recommended by the physician. Explain that after acute poststreptococcal glomerulonephritis, any gross hematuria that occurs when the patient has a viral infection needs to be reported to the physician.

Goiter

DRG Category: 300
Mean LOS: 6.3 days
Description: MEDICAL: Endocrine Disorders with CC

Goiter is the enlargement of the thyroid gland. It is usually a response to a thyroid hormone deficiency (primary hypothyroidism) that results in the hypersecretion of thyroid-stimulating hormone (TSH) from the anterior pituitary gland. Oversecretion leads to subsequent thyroid hypertrophy and hypervascularity. The body's response may compensate for thyroid hormone deficiency, leaving the patient asymptomatic. Goiter may also occur in conjunction with hyperthyroidism, known as Graves' disease. Finally, goiter may occur with the growth of thyroid tumors. Secondary hypothyroidism occurs with TSH deficiency in the pituitary gland and is not associated with goiter.

Most goiters are classified as simple (or nontoxic). They result from any enlargement of the thyroid gland that is not caused by an inflammation or a neoplasm. Simple goiters can be classified as sporadic or endemic and are not associated initially with either hyperthyroidism or hypothyroidism. Sporadic goiters occur after a person eats certain foods (peaches, strawberries, radishes, spinach, peas, cabbage, soybeans, or peanuts) or takes certain medications (iodides, lithium, propylthiouracil) that decrease thyroxine (T_4). Endemic goiters, in contrast, occur because of the patient's geographic location in areas where the soil is depleted of iodine. Endemic goiter that results from soil deficiencies is most likely to occur during autumn and winter.

Goiter becomes a problem only when the enlargement exerts pressure on other neck structures, such as the trachea, or when the enlargement is unsightly, causing the patient to become concerned.

CAUSES

The causes of goiter include iodine deficiency, benign or malignant tumors, and inflammation of the thyroid gland. The use of iodine food additives has greatly reduced the incidence of endemic goiter. Difficulty in determining the incidence of endemic goiter is complicated because many individuals with the condition experience no symptoms and are not diagnosed. Sporadic goiter, or goiter caused by interference with iodine metabolism, is affected by either hereditary factors or ingestion of foods or pharmacologic agents that inhibit T_4 production.

Goiter caused by thyroid nodules, a common condition, may also cause no symptoms. Although thyroid nodules or tumors may be either benign or malignant, more than 75% of thyroid nodules are benign.

GENDER AND LIFE SPAN CONSIDERATIONS

Although men younger than 20 or older than 70 have a higher risk for thyroid cancer than do other individuals, more women than men are affected with thyroid disease. Endemic goiter may be experienced by adolescents during growth spurts, but most thyroid dysfunction is found in women in their second to fifth decades. Additional thyroid hormone is required by the body during pregnancy and lactation, conditions that may result in the need for a higher index of suspicion of endemic goiter during these life stages. Elderly individuals who have depressive symptoms should also be assessed for uncompensated hypothyroidism.

◻ ASSESSMENT

HISTORY. Patients with suspected goiter most often complain of visible enlargement of the neck or difficulty in activities such as buttoning shirts with no accompanying weight gain to account for the problem. In advanced stages, they may complain of pressure on the neck or chest, difficulty in swallowing, or respiratory distress. Other symptoms may reflect either hypothyroidism or hyperthyroidism.

Obtain a drug history to determine past use of iodine-containing medications (including recent contrast media or oral contraceptives), which may falsely elevate serum thyroid function tests. Similarly, a severe illness, malnutrition, or the use of aspirin, corticosteroids, or phenytoin sodium may falsely depress serum thyroid function tests.

PHYSICAL EXAMINATION. The patient with a significantly enlarged goiter may have a visible thyroid gland on the anterior neck. Note that the gland rises with swallowing. When you palpate the gland, stand behind the patient and palpate the gland for tender areas, areas of irregularity, firmness, or any nodules. A normal lateral lobe is approximately the size of the distal phalanx (most remote bony segment) of the thumb. Remember that excessive palpation of the thyroid gland can precipitate thyroid storm (acute thyrotoxic crisis from an oversecretion of the thyroid hormones); therefore, palpate the gland gently and only when necessary. You may also hear a bruit over an enlarged thyroid gland when you auscultate over the lateral lobes. Some patients also have respiratory stridor from compression of the trachea. The patient may also have Pemberton's sign (dizziness, flushed face, fainting when the patient's arms are raised above the head) caused by compression from the goiter.

PSYCHOSOCIAL. While most types of thyroid dysfunction can be treated noninvasively, goiter that is caused by cancer may precipitate concern. Assess the patient's degree of anxiety about the illness and potential complications.

DIAGNOSTIC HIGHLIGHTS

Test	Normal Result	Abnormality with Condition	Explanation
Plasma thyroid-stimulating hormone (TSH) level	$< 10\ \mu U/mL$	$> 20\ \mu U/mL$ in primary hypothyroidism	TSH is overproduced to stimulate the poorly functioning thyroid gland
TSH stimulation test	>10% in radioactive iodine uptake	Primary hypothyroidism: no response; secondary hypothyroidism: normal response	Differentiates between primary and secondary hypothyroidism
Tri-iodothyronine (T_3) and thyroxine (T_4)	T_3: 110–230 ng/dL; T_4: 4.6–11 $\mu g/dL$	Hyperthyroid: increased;	Results depend on underlying disease

	hyperthyroid: decreased	process	

Other Tests: Supporting tests include thyroid scan, plasma T_4 index, thyroid antibody tests, and urinary iodine excretion.

☐ PLANNING AND IMPLEMENTATION

Collaborative

MEDICAL. The goal of medical management for the patient with a simple goiter is to reduce the size of the goiter by correcting the underlying cause. If the patient has decreased iodine stores, small doses of iodide (such as Lugol's solution) may correct the problem. If the patient is ingesting a known substance that leads to goiter, avoidance of the food or drug is necessary. Commonly, no specific cause of the goiter is found, and the patient is placed on thyroid-replacement therapy.

If the patient is elderly or has a long-standing goiter with many nodules, further testing is needed because levothyroxine may lead to thyrotoxic crisis; the patient may need radioiodine ablation therapy to destroy areas of hypersecretion. Surgical treatment is rarely indicated and is used only when symptoms of obstruction occur after a trial of medications. Patients with goiter and thyroid nodules may also need surgical exploration to determine if they have cancer.

PHARMACOLOGIC HIGHLIGHTS

Medication or Drug Class	Dosage	Description	Rationale
Thyroid replacements	Varies with drug	Levothyroxine, thyroxine	Suppress TSH formation and allow the thyroid to rest

PRIMARY NURSING DIAGNOSIS

Risk for ineffective airway clearance related to tracheal compression or obstruction

OUTCOMES. Respiratory status: Ventilation; Symptom control behavior; Medication management; Comfort level; Knowledge: Treatment regimen

INTERVENTIONS. Airway management; Anxiety reduction; Artificial airway management; Positioning; Respiratory monitoring; Surveillance; Ventilation monitoring

Independent

The first priority is to ensure an adequate airway and breathing. If you suspect that the patient's airway is compromised, keep an intubation tray and suction equipment at the bedside at all times. Pay particular attention to any sign of airway obstruction, such as stridor or dyspnea, and check on the patient frequently. Elevate the head of the patient's bed to high Fowler position during meals and for 30 minutes afterward to limit the risk of aspiration. If you suspect that the goiter is increasing in size, monitor the patient's neck circumference daily.

Care of the patient with goiter also focuses on the patient's anxiety and knowledge deficits. Whatever the cause of the goiter, the patient may be highly anxious about the medical diagnosis itself or the resulting symptoms. Make sure that patients have the information they need to understand the disease. If the goiter is unsightly, recommend that the patient choose clothing that neither restricts activity nor draws attention to the neck. If the patient's appearance is extremely distressing, refer the patient for appropriate counseling.

If patients need surgery for goiter removal, monitor them for acute airway obstruction and for thyrotoxic crisis, which is a potential complication of the surgery and leads to tachycardia, increased blood pressure, diaphoresis, and anxiety. Check both the incision and behind the neck for postoperative bleeding; notify the physician immediately if significant bleeding occurs. Each time you monitor the vital signs, assess the patient's vocal quality and compare it with the patient's preoperative speaking. Maintain the neck and head in good alignment, and support them during position changes to prevent traction on the sutures and damage to the operative site.

DOCUMENTATION GUIDELINES

- Physical findings: Respiratory status, postoperative wound healing, presence of dysphagia (difficulty swallowing), neck circumference
- Response to medications

DISCHARGE AND HOME HEALTHCARE GUIDELINES

Teach the patient to avoid medications and food that lead to endemic or sporadic goiter. Patients with endemic goiter should use iodized salt to supply at least 300 μg of iodine daily to prevent goiter. Be sure that the patient understands all medications, including the dosage, route, action, adverse effects, and the need for any laboratory monitoring of thyroid medications. Encourage the patient to take thyroid hormone supplements at the same time each day to maintain constant thyroid levels in the blood.

Have the patient immediately report to the physician any signs and symptoms of thyrotoxic crisis; these include rapid heart rate and palpitations, perspiration, shakiness and tremors, difficulty breathing, and nausea and vomiting. Teach the patient to report any increased neck swelling, difficulty in swallowing, or weight loss.

If the patient had surgery, teach him or her to change any dressings, to inspect the incision for redness, swelling, and discharge, and notify the physician about changes that indicate infection.

Gonorrhea

DRG Category: 350
Mean LOS: 4.5 days
Description: MEDICAL: Inflammation of the Male Reproductive System
DRG Category: 368
Mean LOS: 5.6 days
Description: MEDICAL: Infections, Female Reproductive System

Gonorrhea is one of the most common sexually transmitted infections (STIs) in the United States. The risk of developing the infection from intercourse with an infected partner is between 50% and 90% for females and is 20% for males. The risk for males increases three- to fourfold after four exposures. Two types of infection develop: local and systemic (disseminated). Local infection involves the mucosal surfaces of the genitourinary tract, rectum, pharynx, or eyes. Systemic infections occur because of bacteremia and can lead to multisystem involvement with connective tissues, the heart, and brain.

If left untreated, gonorrhea will involve the fallopian tubes, ovaries, and peritoneum, resulting in gonococcal pelvic inflammatory disease (PID) in women. Systemic complications of untreated, or undertreated, infections are disseminated gonococcal infections that lead to acute arthritis, tenosynovitis, dermatitis, polyarthritis, endocarditis, and meningitis. With adequate treatment, most people recover fully, but reinfection is common.

CAUSES

Gonorrhea is an STI caused by the bacterium *Neisseria gonorrhoeae,* an aerobic, pyrogenic, gram-negative diplococcus. An infant born to an infected mother can contract gonorrhea when it passes through the birth canal. Self-inoculation to the eyes can also occur if a person with gonorrhea touches his or her eyes with a contaminated hand. Risk factors include multiple sex partners, an unknown sex partner, and unprotected sexual contact.

GENDER AND LIFE SPAN CONSIDERATIONS

Gonorrhea is particularly prevalent in the young adult population between the ages of 15 and 29; the highest incidence of infection is in the 20- to 24-year-old age group.

☐ ASSESSMENT

HISTORY. Take a complete sexual history. To direct specimen collection, elicit information regarding sexual orientation and sexual practices (vaginal, oral, and anal). To determine treatment plans, inquire about medication allergies. Explore the patient's birth control practices and determine if the patient and partner regularly use condoms. Explore the number of sex partners, the incidence of unprotected sexual contacts, and the frequency of sex with unknown partners.

Men usually develop symptoms of urethritis 2 to 5 days after exposure, but symptoms may not appear until 3 weeks later. Usually the first symptom is a purulent yellow or greenish-yellow penile discharge. Additionally, dysuria, urinary frequency, and malaise may also be present. If the infection remains untreated after 10 to 14 days, it spreads from the anterior urethra to the posterior urethra, resulting in more intense dysuria, headaches, and lymphadenopathy. Untreated, the infection can result in prostatitis, epididymitis, and cystitis. With an anorectal infection, there is often a history of mucopurulent rectal discharge, rectal bleeding, rectal pain, and changes in bowel habits. Inspection will reveal erythema and discharge from the rectal and anal mucosa.

In women the incubation takes at least 2 weeks, although women are often asymptomatic. Symptoms include yellowish or greenish vaginal discharge, dysuria, urinary frequency, vaginal spotting between periods, heavy menses, backache, and abdominal and pelvic pain. In addition, there may be pruritus and burning of the vulva. If the infection is left untreated, it may ascend to the pelvic cavity, resulting in pelvic pain and fever. Frequently women have a gonococcal infection involving the rectum and anus, presumably from the spread of the exudate. Approximately one-third to one-half of all women who develop gonorrhea have a chlamydial infection as well.

PHYSICAL EXAMINATION. The patient may appear uncomfortable with symptoms of a local infection and may be mildly ill with a low-grade fever. When you inspect the female genitalia, you may note a greenish-yellow discharge from the Skene's or Bartholin's glands, along with a mucopurulent discharge at the cervical os. The vagina is engorged, red, and swollen. The cervix is usually friable and erythematic. Abdominal palpitation will reveal both lower-quadrant and rebound tenderness. Pelvic examinations will be painful, especially with cervical movement. The male's urethral meatus usually has purulent discharge. An anal infection in either gender leads to purulent discharge and bleeding from the rectum.

In newborns, gonorrheal conjunctivitis appears 1 to 12 days after birth. If conjunctivitis is left untreated, blindness results from corneal ulcerations. Symptoms include bilateral edema of the lid, followed by a profuse purulent discharge from the eye.

Examination of the patient with a systemic infection may reveal papillary skin lesions that appear as pustules or hemorrhages on the hands and feet. Joint motion causes the patient severe pain, and you may hear a cracking noise when joints are moved through their range of motion. In gonococcal arthritis, the joints are asymmetrically involved and only certain joints (knees, ankles, elbows) are usually affected.

PSYCHOSOCIAL. When taking a sexual history and counseling on sexual matters, be sensitive to the patient's need for privacy and yet be aware of the public health responsibility to report STIs. Urge the patient to notify all sexual partners of the infection promptly so that they can receive treatment. Because gonorrhea is an STI, sexual abuse should be considered when it is diagnosed in a child. Follow up immediately with appropriate referrals.

DIAGNOSTIC HIGHLIGHTS

General Comments: A simple tissue culture is the most accurate diagnostic method. Reculture 1 to 2 months later to detect both failures and reinfections; reinfection is more common than resistance to antibiotics.

Test	Normal Result	Abnormality with Condition	Explanation
GC culture	Negative culture	Positive culture	Growth of the organism confirms the diagnosis

PRIMARY NURSING DIAGNOSIS

Infection related to bacterial invasion

OUTCOMES. Risk control: Sexually transmitted diseases

INTERVENTIONS. Teaching: Safe sex; Medication management; Fertility preservation

☐ PLANNING AND IMPLEMENTATION

Collaborative

Treatment of gonorrhea is primarily pharmacologic, with antibiotic regimens. The Centers for Disease Control and Prevention (CDC) recommends that treatment for gonorrhea include concomitant therapy for chlamydia, because it is found in 20% to 40% of all patients with gonorrhea. Both partners should be treated at the same time and instructed to avoid sexual activity until negative cultures are obtained. If the male partner is symptomatic, the female should be treated even before culture results are obtained to prevent infertility. If a woman has an intrauterine device (IUD) in place, it may be removed.

PHARMACOLOGIC HIGHLIGHTS

Medication or Drug Class	Dosage	Description	Rationale
Ceftriaxone and doxycycline	125 mg IM × 1	Third-generation cephalosporin	Effective regimen recommended by the CDC; treats chlamydia also, because both STIs often present simultaneously
	100 mg po bid × 7 days	Broad spectrum antibiotic (tetracycline)	
Azithromycin	1 g po single dose	Macrolide antibiotic	Can be used as an alternative for doxycyline
Erythromycin	800 mg qid	Macrolide antibiotic	Used as an alternative for doxycycline for pregnant women
Quinolones	Varies by drug	Antibiotic	Can be substituted for ceftriaxone single dose
Erythromycin ointment (0.5%); tetracycline 1%	Apply to conjuctiva × 1 at delivery	Macrolide antibiotic	Opthalmic prophylaxis; prevents newborn blindness if maternal-newborn transmission occurred

Independent

In addition to explanations of all current treatments, teach patients strategies to prevent reinfection with gonorrhea because no natural immunity develops. Additional instruction focuses on transmission of gonorrhea and identification of symptoms of other STIs. Because of the confidential and private nature of the health history and health teaching, interact with the patient in a private location where you are unlikely to be interrupted. Many experts in STIs recommend that treatment be initiated before questioning the patient about all sexual contacts so that patients will not avoid treatment when they learn that STIs are reported to the Department of Public Health. Help the patient who has had multiple sexual partners compile a list so that the partners can be notified and treated. Note that this procedure is apt to be embarrassing and stressful for the patient, who will require support and a nonjudgmental approach from the nurse.

Instruct the patient about safe sexual practices. If the patient has several sexual partners, encourage him or her to receive regular checkups to screen for STIs. Remind patients that condoms are the only form of birth control known to decrease the chance of contracting an STI. Provide the patient and partner with the STI hotline number: 1-800-227-8922.

Comfort measures are important. Loose, absorbent undergarments that the patient changes frequently will decrease discomfort from the genitourinary mucous discharge. Discuss the importance of perineal or penile cleansing and good hand-washing techniques. Sitz baths may help decrease lower abdominal discomfort.

DOCUMENTATION GUIDELINES

- History: Onset of symptoms, risk factors
- Physical response: General symptoms; discomfort; type, color, odor, amount of discharge
- Response to treatment, lessening of symptoms

DISCHARGE AND HOME HEALTHCARE GUIDELINES

Explain that federal regulations require notification of all sexual partners so that they can seek treatment. Encourage the patient to refrain from all sexual activity (vaginal, anal, oral) until treatment is complete because of the high risk of reinfection. Explain that abstinence is the surest way to prevent STIs. If the partner's sexual history is unknown, or the partner is suspected of having an STD, suggest the use of condoms. Encourage patients to wash the genitalia with soap and water before and after intercourse and to avoid sharing washcloths or douching equipment.

Guillain-Barré Syndrome

DRG Category: 020
Mean LOS: 8.2 days
Description: MEDICAL: Nervous System Infection Except Viral Meningitis

Guillain-Barré syndrome (GBS; also known as acute idiopathic demyelinating polyneuropathy) is an acute, rapidly progressing form of polyneuritis that results in a temporary, flaccid paralysis lasting for 4 to 8 weeks. Motor, sensory, and autonomic functions may be involved. The syndrome is characterized by a diffuse inflammation or demyelination (or both) of the ascending or descending peripheral nerves that leads to a viral illness and then paralysis.

Although the syndrome is considered to be a medical emergency, over 80% of persons who are affected with GBS recover their functional abilities completely. The remaining individuals have some degree of neurological deficit after recovery from the disease, which results in a chronic disability. Fewer than 5% of patients with GBS die, and usually death is related to respiratory complications.

CAUSES

Although the exact cause of GBS is unknown, two-thirds of patients who develop it have had a viral infection 1 to 3 weeks before the development of symptoms. Common viruses associated with Guillain-Barré are Epstein-Barr virus and cytomegalovirus. Another 10% of patients have had recent surgical procedures during the 4 weeks before GBS developed. Other diseases that have been linked to the development of GBS are lymphoma, HIV disease, gastroenteritis, Hodgkin's disease, and lupus erythematosus. In some cases, GBS develops after immunization for influenza.

GENDER AND LIFE SPAN CONSIDERATIONS

The incidence of GBS is 1.9 per 100,000 persons, and it affects individuals of both genders and of all ages. Most commonly, it affects young and middle-aged adults 30 to 50 years of age.

☐ ASSESSMENT

HISTORY. Determine if the patient has had a recent viral illness or surgical procedure. Often the patient describes a minor upper respiratory or gastrointestinal febrile illness. Many, but not all, patients complain of paresthesia (numbness, prickling, tingling) early in the course of the illness. The patient or family generally seeks assistance when bilateral lower limb weakness begins to spread toward the trunk or has progressed to paralysis of the limbs. Urinary incontinence may be a problem initially, followed by difficulty in swallowing and speaking. Impairment of respiratory functions, the most life-threatening effect of GBS, does not occur until the paralysis has affected all of the peripheral areas and the trunk.

PHYSICAL EXAMINATION. The major neurological sign found in GBS is muscle weakness, but sensory loss, particularly in the legs and later in the arms, often occurs. Although the progression of symptoms is variable, the disease often progresses upward from the legs in 1 to 3 days. To follow the progression of symptoms, test for ascending sensory loss by gently using a pinprick upward from the level of T-12 on the vertebral column (level of the iliac crests) to the midscapular point (about T-6). Mark the patient's skin with a pen every 4 hours to document changes. Notify the physician immediately if the level reaches T-8 or higher, because muscles at that level are needed for breathing. Patients may also have ocular muscle paralysis, loss of position sense, and diminished or absent reflexes.

The function of cranial nerve VII (facial nerve) may be affected, especially in the later stages of the paralysis. To test for facial nerve weakness, inspect the patient's face at rest and during conversation. Have the patient raise both eyebrows, smile, frown, puff out the cheeks, and show both upper and lower teeth. If the facial nerve is involved, the patient may have problems talking, chewing, and swallowing.

Patients often have changes in their vital signs. Rapid or slow heart rates and a labile blood pressure may occur because of the effects on the vagus nerve (cranial nerve X), as well as profuse sweating and facial flushing. Patients require continuous cardiac monitoring to assess for dysrhythmias. Although respiratory function may be impaired in the later stages of paralysis, the nurse needs to assess the patency of the airway and adequacy of breathing in order to initiate prompt interventions when necessary.

PSYCHOSOCIAL. The patient is alert, but paralyzed, and this leads to considerable fear and anxiety both during the initial stages and throughout the course of the disease. As the paralysis ascends, the patient's level of anxiety will probably rise. The patient and significant others will need a great deal of emotional support to deal with the health crisis.

DIAGNOSTIC HIGHLIGHTS

Test	Normal Result	Abnormality with Condition	Explanation
Cerebrospinal fluid (CSF) assay	Protein: 15–45 mg/dL; glucose: 40–80 mg/dL; erythrocytes: 0–10/μL; leukocytes: 0–10/μL	Increase in CSF protein without an increase in cell count	High protein levels are often noted 1–2 weeks of illness; peak at 4–6 weeks

Other Tests: White blood cell counts showing mild leukocytosis, electromyography, pulmonary function tests, arterial and venous blood gases.

PRIMARY NURSING DIAGNOSIS

Ineffective airway clearance related to weakness, problems in swallowing, and respiratory muscle paralysis

OUTCOMES. Respiratory status: Gas exchange; Respiratory status: Ventilation; Symptom control behavior; Treatment behavior: Illness or injury; Comfort level

INTERVENTIONS. Airway management; Anxiety reduction; Oxygen therapy; Airway suctioning; Airway insertion and stabilization; Cough enhancement; Mechanical ventilation; Positioning; Respiratory monitoring

☐ PLANNING AND IMPLEMENTATION

Collaborative

During the acute phase of the illness, the patient may be in the intensive care unit, particularly to support pulmonary function with endotracheal intubation and mechanical ventilation. Sequential neurological, cardiopulmonary, and hemodynamic assessments are needed. Some patients have chest physiotherapy ordered, and all require aggressive pulmonary toileting to maintain a patent endotracheal or tracheostomy tube. Most patients need a Foley catheter to manage urinary function. Compression boots limit the risk of thromboembolic complications.

Plasmapheresis (plasma exchange) may be completed during the early stages (first few days) of the syndrome; research suggests that the procedure may reduce the circulating antibodies and shorten the period of paralysis. Care of the patient who is having plasmapheresis includes monitoring the amount of plasma removed and reinfused and monitoring for any reactions to the fluid replacement. Transfusion reactions should not occur because the patient's own blood is being returned. Complications such as infection and hyptertension require pharmacologic management. Other patients may become hypotensive and require fluid boluses or vasopressors.

PHARMACOLOGIC HIGHLIGHTS

Medication or Drug Class	Dosage	Description	Rationale
Antihypertensives	Varies with drug	Nitroprusside (Nipride); propranolol (Inderal)	Control hypertensive episodes
Heparin	5000 units SQ q 8–12 hours	Anticoagulant	Prevents thromboembolism during periods of immobility
Antibiotics	Varies with drug	Chosen on the basis of cultures and sensitivities	Combat urinary or pulmonary infection

Additional Drug Therapies: Antacids and histamine blockers may be used to reduce the risk of gastrointestinal bleeding. Corticosteroids may be given early in the course of the disease, but their usefulness is unproved, and they are generally considered ineffective by most experts. Note that muscles are tender (particularly in the trunk, thighs, and shoulders) during range-of-motion and turning procedures. Analgesics may be needed for muscle stiffness, pain, and spasm.

Independent

The most important interventions center on maintaining a patent airway and adequate breathing. Teach deep-breathing and coughing techniques. Monitor the patient who is mechanically ventilated for airway obstruction. Use deep endotracheal suction to maintain a patent airway, but monitor the patient carefully for dysrhythmias and a dropping oxygen saturation. Because respiratory complications are seen in 35% to 40% of patients, preparation for intubation or eventually a tracheostomy is appropriate. A viable call system for the patient is vital, and the type will depend on the extent of the paralysis. Cardiac dysrhythmias also occur in GBS, so patients require continuous cardiac monitoring.

Provide passive range-of-motion exercises at least twice a day; turn the patient at least every 2 hours, and use splints and pillow supports to keep the limbs in functional positions. Control the environment to limit the risk of injury from falls. Inspect for integrity of the skin. Frequent eye care is necessary for the individual with cranial nerve VII involvement. Protect the cornea with eye shields (some eye specialists may recommend suturing the eyes closed) and provide eye lubricants. Give mouth care at least every 4 hours.

The patient's psychological state is most important. Use relaxation exercises, include the patient in decision making, and provide frequent explanations of care to decrease the patient's anxiety. Mood swings are to be expected. Encourage the patient to ventilate fears and anger related to the paralysis and the prognosis. If the patient cannot speak because of endotracheal intubation or paralysis, try to establish communication by having the patient blink once for "yes" and twice for "no."

DOCUMENTATION GUIDELINES

- Respiratory and cardiovascular functions: Patency of airway, description of breathing, vital sign changes with rest or activity
- Neurologic functions: Level of paralysis, level of motor and sensory function, level of consciousness
- Bowel and bladder functions: Frequency of voiding, consistency and number of stools
- Pain: Location, duration, precipitating factors, interventions that alleviate pain
- Activity: Strength and motion of extremities, presence of deformities or atrophy and strategies used to manage dysfunction, response to activity
- Skin: Areas of potential or actual breakdown, successful strategies to manage breakdown

DISCHARGE AND HOME HEALTHCARE GUIDELINES

Especially during the recovery period, teach the patient to avoid exposure to further upper respiratory infections. Encourage self-care, but stress the avoidance of fatigue and the importance of frequent planned rest periods. Continue ongoing rehabilitation with physical therapy sessions to teach walking with a cane or walker and to provide active and passive range-of-motion exercises. Teach strengthening exercises for the hands, such as modeling clay or squeezing balls. Teach the patient and family how to manage the transfer from the bed to a wheelchair and from a wheelchair to the toilet or bathtub.

Teach the patient to maintain a high-calorie, high-protein diet and to include at least 2000 mL of fluid intake per day. Avoid constipation by increasing fluids and dietary fiber and using stool softeners as required. Teach the patient to use warm baths to manage muscle pain and diversional activities to decrease boredom during the slow recovery period.

Gunshot Wound

DRG Category: 191
Mean LOS: 13.6 days
Description: SURGICAL: Pancreas, Liver, and Shunt Procedures with CC
DRG Category: 392
Mean LOS: 10.1 days
Description: SURGICAL: Splenectomy Age > 17
DRG Category: 101
Mean LOS: 4.6 days
Description: MEDICAL: Other Respiratory System Diagnoses with CC
DRG Category: 110
Mean LOS: 9.1 days
Description: SURGICAL: Major Cardiovascular Procedures with CC
DRG Category: 486
Mean LOS: 10.5 days
Description: SURGICAL: Other Operating Room Procedures for Multiple Significant Trauma

Penetrating trauma from a gunshot wound (GSW) can cause devastating injuries. The most commonly injured organs and tissues are the intestines, liver, vascular structures, spleen, and intrathoracic structures. Evaluating injuries is difficult; it is important to determine the type of weapon, energy dissipated from the weapon, firing range of the weapon at the time of injury, and characteristics of the injured tissue. GSWs can lead to the need for extensive debridement, resection, or amputation. Among the many complications are sepsis, exsanguination, and death.

CAUSES

The energy of the missile is dissipated into tissues of the body, causing destruction of vital and nonvital structures. When the missile enters the body, it creates a temporary cavity, which stretches, distorts, and compresses the surrounding anatomic structures. The cavity that is produced often has a greater diameter than the missile itself. In a situation called "blast effect" or "muzzle blast," damage occurs in structures outside the direct path of the missile. High-velocity missiles (bullets from shotguns, rifles, or high-caliber handguns) cause extensive cavitation and significant tissue destruction, while low-velocity missiles (bullets from low-caliber handguns) have limited cavitation potential with less tissue destruction. Another characteristic of missiles is the yaw, which is the amount of tumbling and movement of the nose of the missile that occurs. The more yaw, the greater the tissue damage.

GENDER AND LIFE SPAN CONSIDERATIONS

Penetrating injuries are on the increase across all ages of the life span, particularly among adolescents and young adults in their teens and twenties. GSWs are more common in males than in females.

◻ ASSESSMENT

HISTORY. Establish a history of the weapon, including the type, caliber, and range at which it was fired. Determine if the gunshot wound was self-inflicted, as well as the patient's hand dominance and tetanus immunization history.

PHYSICAL EXAMINATION. The initial evaluation is always focused on assessing the airway, breathing, circulation, disability (neurological status), and exposure (completely undressing the patient), which are done simultaneously by the trauma resuscitation team. The secondary survey is a head-to-toe assessment, including vital signs.

After completing the primary survey, begin the secondary survey with a complete head-to-toe assessment. Examine the patient's entire skin surface carefully for abrasions, open wounds, powder burns, and hematomas, paying special attention to skin folds, groin, and axillae. Assess the patient's abdomen, back, and extremities for lacerations, wounds, abrasions, and deformities. Some high-velocity weapons may cause extensive tissue destruction and fractures. Inspect the patient for both entry and exit wounds.

Perform a thorough fluid volume assessment on at least an hourly basis until the patient is stabilized. This assessment includes hemodynamic, urinary, and central nervous system parameters. Notify the physician of overt bleeding and of any early indications that hemorrhage is continuing; this includes delayed capillary refill, tachycardia, urinary output less than 0.5 mL/kg per hour, and alterations in mental status, including restlessness, agitation, and confusion, as well as decreases in alertness. Body weights are helpful in indicating fluid volume status; note that many of the critical care beds have incorporated bed scales.

PSYCHOSOCIAL. The violent and often unexplained nature of this type of trauma can lead to ineffective coping for both the patient and family. Determine if the patient is at risk from himself or herself or others by questioning the patient, significant others, or police. If the patient is on police hold, determine the patient's and family's response to the pending legal charges.

DIAGNOSTIC HIGHLIGHTS

Test	Normal Result	Abnormality with Condition	Explanation
Complete blood count	Red blood cells (RBCs): 4.0–6.2 million/μL; hemoglobin: 12–18 g/dL; hematocrit: 37–54%; white blood cells:	Decreased values reflective of the degree of hemorrhage	Determines the extent of blood loss; note that it takes 2 hours for hemorrhage to be reflected in a dropping hemoglobin and hematocrit after injury

	4,500–11,000/µL; platelets: 150,000–400,000/µL		
X rays of areas near the GSW; if head or neck injury is suspected or patient is unconscious, x rays of chest, pelvis, and lateral cervical spine are needed	No injury in bony structures	Damage to bones and joints in area of wound	If wound is near bony structures, entire surrounding area needs to be assessed for injury
Computed tomography (CT) scan	No injury to body structures	Damage to organ and supporting structures; collection of blood in tissues, location of foreign bodies (missiles)	May be used to identify abdominal, urologic, chest, and head injuries (actual and suspected); injuries to bony structure; trajectory of penetrating missile

Other Tests: Blood chemistries, antiography, endoscopy, indirect laryngoscopy, arterial blood gases, pulse oximetry, urinalysis, and excretory urography.

PRIMARY NURSING DIAGNOSIS

Ineffective airway clearance related to airway obstruction secondary to tissue trauma

OUTCOMES. Respiratory status: Ventilation; Respiratory status: Gas exchange; Symptom control behavior; Medication management; Comfort level; Knowledge: Treatment regimen

INTERVENTIONS. Airway insertion and stabilization; Airway management; Airway suctioning; Anxiety reduction; Artificial airway management; Mechanical ventilation; Oxygen therapy; Positioning; Respiratory monitoring; Surveillance; Ventilation monitoring; Vital signs monitoring

◻ PLANNING AND IMPLEMENTATION

Collaborative

Maintaining a patent airway, maintaining oxygenation and ventilation, and supporting the circulation are the first priorities. Assist with endotracheal intubation and mechanical ventilation. Maintain the PaO_2 at greater than 100 mm Hg and the $PaCO_2$ at 35 to 45 mm Hg. The patient may require placement of a tube thoracostomy to drain blood and relieve a pneumothorax.

Restoring fluid volume status is critical in maximizing tissue perfusion and oxygenation; the use of pressure infusers and rapid volume/warmer infusers for trauma patients requiring massive fluid replacement is essential. Administering warm blood products and crystalloids assists in maintaining normothermia. Be prepared to administer vasopressors after fluid volume status is stabilized. Patients who require massive fluid resuscitation are at risk for developing hypothermia, which exacerbates existing coagulopathy and compounds their hemodynamic instability. Paramount in managing patients is a rapid fluid resuscitation with blood, blood products, colloids, and crystalloids through a large-bore peripheral intravenous (IV) catheter or a large-bore trauma catheter.

Patients frequently require surgical exploration to identify specific injuries and control hemorrhage. After surgical exposure is obtained, any of the following may be required: assessment of structures, control of hemorrhage, debridement, resection, or amputation. If definitive surgical intervention is not possible because of the patient's instability, a temporizing method known as "damage control" may be instituted. Damage control consists of the placement of packing to achieve a temporary tamponade, correction of coagulopathy, and aggressive management of hypothermia. The patient is then transferred to the critical care unit for continued monitoring and stabilization. The "second look" surgical exploration is generally done in 24 hours for definitive surgical intervention.

PHARMACOLOGIC HIGHLIGHTS

Medication or Drug Class	Dosage	Description	Rationale
Antibiotics: prophylactic antibiotic use is controversial; surgeons follow culture results and institute antibiotics sensitive to the organism that was cultured	Varies with drug	Second-generation cephalosporins or cephamycin	Prevent gram-negative infections when there is traumatic violation of the GI tract
Heparin	5000 units SQ q 8–12 hours	Anticoagulant	Prevent thromboembolism during periods of immobility after hemorrhage is controlled; not generally administered in patients with neural injuries

Other: Many trauma surgeons may choose to administer a tetanus booster to patients with chest trauma whose immunization history indicates a need or whose history is unavailable.

Independent

In the emergency phase of treatment, maintain the patient in a supine position unless it is contraindicated because of other injuries. Ensure adequate airway and breathing in this position. Avoid Trendelenburg's position because it may have negative hemodynamic consequences, increase the risk of aspiration, and interfere with pulmonary excursion. If the patient can tolerate the position, elevate the head of the bed to limit the risk of aspiration and to improve gas exchange.

Wound care varies, depending on the severity of wounds, whether an open fracture is present, and what type of fixation device is applied. Wounds and any exposed soft tissue and bone are covered with wet, sterile saline dressings. Standard Betadine-soaked dressings may not be used because of the need to limit iodine absorption and skin irritation. To decrease the risk of infection of the patient, use a gown, mask, gloves, and hair covers in caring for patients with extensive wounds. Document the size, description, and healing of the wound each day, and notify the surgeon if there are signs of wound infection. Use universal precautions in handling all bloody drainage.

If another person has initiated the violence toward the patient, consider assigning him or her a pseudonym for all hospital records to prevent another assault. Do not provide any information about the patient over the phone unless you are sure of the caller's name and relationship to the patient. If you fear for the patient's safety, talk to hospital security about strategies to ensure the patient's safety. If the patient has a self-inflicted injury, make a referral to a clinical nurse specialist or discuss a psychiatric consultation with the surgeon. If the patient is self-destructive, initiate suicide precautions according to unit protocol.

If the patient is being held by police, remember that the patient receives competent and compassionate care even when under arrest. Determine from hospital policy the regulations about visitors if the patient is held by the police. Provide a supportive atmosphere to promote healing of the injury, but use care to avoid being drawn into the legal aspects of the patient's arrest.

DOCUMENTATION GUIDELINES

- Physical response: Location, size and appearance of wound; description of dressings and drainage on dressings; amount of bleeding from wound; description of accompanying injuries, breath sounds, heart sounds
- Response to treatment: Vital signs, pulse oximetry, urine output, mental status, patency of airway, adequacy of circulation
- Presence of complications: Infection, hemorrhage, organ dysfunction, poor wound healing
- Pain: Location, duration, precipitating factors, response to interventions
- Laboratory results: Electrolytes, measures of organ function, complete blood count, coagulation studies

DISCHARGE AND HOME HEALTHCARE GUIDELINES

PREVENTION. To prevent complications of wound infection and impaired wound healing, review wound care instructions with the patient and family. Verify that they can demonstrate proper care with understanding and accuracy.

MEDICATIONS. Verify that the patient understands all medications, including dosage, route, action, and adverse effects. Provide written instructions to the patient or family.

FOLLOW-UP. Review with the patient all follow-up appointments that are arranged. If home care is necessary, verify that appropriate arrangements have been completed. Make sure that patients with self-inflicted wounds have counseling and support before and after the discharge.

Heart Failure

DRG Category: 127
Mean LOS: 5.5 days
Description: MEDICAL: Heart Failure and Shock

Heart failure (HF) occurs when the heart is unable to pump sufficient blood to meet the metabolic needs of the body. The result of inadequate cardiac output is poor organ perfusion and vascular congestion in the pulmonary or systemic circulation. HF is the leading cardiac cause of death in hospitalized patients and is responsible for 33% of the patients who die after a myocardial infarction.

HF may be described as backward or forward failure, high- or low-output failure, or right- or left-sided failure. In backward failure, the ventricle fails to eject its contents, which results in pulmonary edema on the left side of the heart and systemic congestion on the right. In forward failure an inadequate cardiac output (CO) leads to decreased organ perfusion. High-output failure is the inability of the heart to meet the increased metabolic demands of the body despite a normal or high CO. Low-output failure occurs when the ventricle is unable to generate enough CO to meet the metabolic demands of the body. This type of failure consists of impaired peripheral circulation and compensatory vasoconstriction. Right-sided failure occurs when the right ventricle is unable to maintain an adequate cardiac output, and systemic congestion occurs. When the left ventricle is unable to produce a CO sufficient to prevent pulmonary congestion, left-sided failure occurs. Complications of HF include pulmonary edema, renal failure, cerebral insufficiency, myocardial infarction, and cardiac dysrhythmias.

CAUSES

HF may result from a number of causes that affect preload (venous return), afterload (impedance the heart has to overcome to eject its volume), or contractility. Elevated preload can be caused by incompetent valves, renal failure, volume overload, or a congenital left-to-right shunt. Elevated afterload occurs when the ventricles have to generate higher pressures in order to overcome impedance and eject their volume. This disorder may also be referred to as an abnormal pressure load. An elevation in afterload also may be caused by hypertension, valvular stenosis, or hypertrophic cardiomyopathy. Abnormal muscle conditions may diminish contractility and cause a decrease in the ability of the heart muscle to act as a pump. Some common causes of diminished contractility include cardiomyopathy, coronary artery disease, acute myocardial infarction, myocarditis, amyloidosis, sarcoidosis, hypocalcemia, hypomagnesemia, or iatrogenic myocardial damage caused by drugs (adriamycin or disopyramide) or radiation therapy for mediastinal tumors or Hodgkin's disease.

GENDER AND LIFE SPAN CONSIDERATIONS

Heart failure may occur at any age and in both genders as a result of congenital defects, hypertension, valve disease, coronary artery disease, or autoimmune disorders. Elderly people, however, are much more prone to the condition because of chronic hypertension, coronary artery disease, myocardial infarction, chronic ischemia, or valve disease, all of which occur more frequently in the elderly population.

☐ ASSESSMENT

HISTORY. Patients with HF typically have a history of a precipitating factor such as myocardial infarction, recent open heart surgery, dysrhythmias, or hypertension. Symptoms vary based on the type and severity of failure. Ask patients if they have experienced any of the following: anxiety, irritability, fatigue, weakness, lethargy, mild shortness of breath with exertion or at rest, orthopnea that requires two or more pillows to sleep, nocturnal dyspnea, cough with frothy sputum, nocturia, weight gain, anorexia, or nausea and vomiting. Take a complete medication history, and determine if the patient has been on any dietary restrictions. Determine if the patient regularly participates in a planned exercise program.

PHYSICAL EXAMINATION. Observe the patient for mental confusion, anxiety, or irritability caused by hypoxia. Pale or cyanotic, cool, clammy skin is a result of poor perfusion. In right-sided heart failure, the jugular veins may become engorged and distended. If the pulsations in the jugular veins are visible 4.5 cm or more above the sternal notch with the patient at a 45-degree angle, jugular venous distension is present. The liver may also become engorged, and pressure on the abdomen increases pressure in the jugular veins, causing a rise in the top of the blood column. This positive finding for HF is known as hepatojugular reflux (HJR). The patient may also have peripheral edema in the ankles and feet, in the sacral area, or throughout the body. Ascites may occur as a result of passive liver congestion.

With auscultation, inspiratory crackles or expiratory wheezes (a result of pulmonary edema in left-sided failure) are heard in the patient's lungs. The patient's vital signs may demonstrate tachypnea or tachycardia, which occur in an attempt to compensate for the hypoxia and decreased cardiac output. Gallop rhythms such as an S_3 or an S_4, while considered a normal finding in children and young adults, are considered pathologic in the presence of HF and occur as a result of early rapid ventricular filling and increased resistance to ventricular filling after atrial contraction, respectively. Murmurs may also be present if the origin of the failure is a stenotic or incompetent valve.

PSYCHOSOCIAL. Note that experts have found that the physiologic measures of heart failure (such as ejection fraction) do not always predict how active, vigorous, or positive a patient feels about his or her health; rather, a person's view of health is based on many factors such as social support, level of activity, and outlook on life.

DIAGNOSTIC HIGHLIGHTS

Test	Normal Result	Abnormality with Condition	Explanation
Echocardiography (ECHO)	Normal heart size, structure, and cardiac output	Depressed cardiac output, evidence of cardiomegaly	Measures chamber size, valvular structure and function, ventricular wall motion, and an estimated ejection fraction
Multigated blood pool imaging (MUGA)	Normal cardiac output and ejection fraction	Alterations in cardiac output and ejection fraction, often decreased	Assesses cardiac volume both during systole and diastole; data are used to determine ejection fraction;values are depressed in low-output failure

Electrocardiography: To reveal ventricular hypertrophy, ventricular dilatation, and axis deviation, although this test is not conclusive in itself and needs to be followed up with an ECHO.

Chest X Ray: May show cardiomegaly, pulmonary vascular congestion, alveolar or interstitial edema, or pleural effusions.

Other Tests: Serum electrolytes, blood urea nitrogen (BUN), liver enzymes, prothrombin time, colorflow mapping, and cardiac angiograms.

PRIMARY NURSING DIAGNOSIS

Decreased cardiac output related to an ineffective ventricular pump

OUTCOMES. Cardiac pump: Effectiveness; Circulation status; Tissue perfusion: Abdominal organs and peripheral; Vital sign status; Electrolyte and acid-base balance; Endurance; Energy conservation; Fluid balance

INTERVENTIONS. Cardiac care; Circulatory care: Mechanical assist device; Fluid/electrolyte management; Medication administration; Medication management; oxygen therapy; Vital signs monitoring

◻ PLANNING AND IMPLEMENTATION

Collaborative

MEDICAL. Initial management of the patient with heart failure depends on severity of heart failure, seriousness of symptoms, etiology, presence of other illnesses, and precipitating factors. Medication management is paramount in patients with heart failure. The general principles for management are treatment of any precipitating causes, control of fluid and sodium retention, increasing myocardial contractility, decreasing cardiac workload, and reducing pulmonary and systemic venous congestion. The physician may also prescribe fluid and sodium restriction in an attempt to reduce volume and thereby reduce preload.

SURGICAL. If the elevated preload is caused by valvular regurgitation, the patient may require corrective surgery. Corrective surgery may also be warranted if the elevated afterload is caused by a stenotic valve. Another measure that may be taken to reduce afterload is an intra-aortic balloon pump (IABP). This is generally used as a bridge to surgery or in cardiogenic shock after acute myocardial infarction. It involves a balloon catheter placed in the descending aorta that inflates during diastole and deflates during systole. The balloon augments filling of the coronary arteries during diastole and decreases afterload during systole. IABP is used with caution because there are several possible complications, including dissection of the aortoiliac arteries, ischemic changes in the legs, and migration of the balloon up or down the aorta.

OTHER MEASURES. Other measures the physician may use include supplemental oxygen, thrombolytic therapy, percutaneous transluminal coronary angioplasty, directional coronary atherectomy, placement of a coronary stent, or coronary artery bypass surgery to improve oxygen flow to the myocardium. Finally, a cardiac transplant may be considered if other measures fail, if all other organ systems are viable, if there is no history of other pulmonary diseases, and if the patient does not smoke or use alcohol, is generally under 60 years of age, and is psychologically stable.

PHARMACOLOGIC HIGHLIGHTS

Medication or Drug Class	Dosage	Description	Rationale
Vasodilators	Varies by drug	To decrease arterial and venous vasoconstriction due to activation of adrenergic and rennin-angiotensin systems; increases venous capacitance; drugs such as nitroglycerin and angiotensin-converting enzyme (ACE) inhibitors such as captopril, enalapril, lisinopril	Reduce vasoconstriction, thereby reducing afterload and enhancing myocardial performance and decreasing preload and ventricular filling pressures
Diuretics	Varies by drug	Increases excretion of sodim and water with drugs such as furosemide (Lasix) and metolazone (Zaroxalyn)	Used for patients with volume overload
Digoxin	0.125–0.375 mg po qd	Cardiotonic	Increases cardiac contractility and helps manage some atrial dysrhythmias; may increase myocardial oxygen demand

Dobutamine: Sympathomimetic, selective beta$_1$ stimulator that increases contractility, improves cardiac output, decreases pulmonary capillary wedge pressure (PCWP), and increases renal blood flow (as a result of improved CO).

Dopamine: Low doses to stimulate dopaminergic receptors, causing renal vasodilation and improved renal function.

Other Drugs: Antihypertensive agents (hydralazine, minoxidil) and, in severe cases of heart failure, nitroprusside may be used in an attempt to reduce afterload and improve cardiac output.

Independent

To conserve his or her energy and to maximize the oxygen that is available for body processes, encourage the patient to rest. Elevation of the head of the bed to 30 to 45 degrees may alleviate some of the dyspnea by lowering the pressure on the diaphragm that is caused by the contents of the abdomen and by decreasing venous return, thereby decreasing preload. The patient may need assistance with activities of daily living, even eating, if the heart failure is at end stage and the least bit of activity causes fatigue and shortness of breath. To assess the patient's response to activity, check the blood pressure and heart rate, as well as the patient's subjective response both before and after any increase in activity level. Prolonged periods of little or no activity can be very difficult to reverse; therefore, maintaining some level of activity is highly encouraged.

To control symptoms, provide ongoing monitoring throughout the acute phases of the patient's disease. Monitor the patient for signs and symptoms of fluid overload, impaired gas exchange, and activity intolerance. Routine assessment of the cardiovascular and pulmonary systems is imperative in the early detection of exacerbation. Monitor daily intake and output, as well as daily weight, and conduct cardiopulmonary assessment.

Education of the patient and family is important for preventing exacerbations and frequent hospital visits. HF is clearly a condition that can be managed on an outpatient basis. A clear explanation of the disease process helps the patient understand the need for the prescribed medications, activity restrictions, diet, fluid restrictions, and lifestyle changes. Written material should be provided for the patient to take home and use as a reference.

The patient may no longer be able to live alone or support himself or herself. Fear, anxiety, and grief can all stimulate the sympathetic nervous system, leading to catecholamine release and additional stress on an already compromised heart. Helping the patient work through and verbalize these feelings may improve psychological well-being and CO.

DOCUMENTATION GUIDELINES

- Physical findings indicative of HF: Mental confusion, pale, cyanotic, clammy skin, presence of jugular vein distension and HJR, ascites, edema, pulmonary crackles or wheezes, adventitious heart sounds
- Fluid intake and output, daily weights
- Response to medications such as diuretics, nitrates, dopamine, dobutamine, and oxygen
- Psychosocial response to illness

DISCHARGE AND HOME HEALTHCARE GUIDELINES

PREVENTION. To prevent exacerbations, teach the patient and family to monitor for an increase in shortness of breath or edema. Tell the patient to restrict fluid intake to 2 to 2.5 L per day and restrict sodium intake as prescribed. Teach the patient to monitor daily weights and report weight gain of more than 4 pounds in 2 days.

MEDICATIONS. Be sure the patient and family understand all medications, including effect, dosage, route, adverse effects, and the need for routine laboratory monitoring for drugs such as digoxin.

COMPLICATIONS OF HF. Tell the patient to call for emergency assistance for acute shortness of breath or chest discomfort that is not alleviated with rest.

Hemophilia

DRG Category: 397
Mean LOS: 5.0 days
Description: MEDICAL: Coagulation Disorders

Hemophilia refers to a group of congenital coagulation disorders that are characterized by a deficiency or malfunction of specific clotting factors. Hemophilia A, or classic hemophilia, is caused by a defect in factor VIII (antihemophilic factor). Hemophilia B, or Christmas disease, is caused by a defect in factor IX (plasma thromboplastin component, or Christmas factor). Hemophilia A is more common, occurring once per 5,000 live male births, compared to hemophilia B, which occurs once per 30,000 live male births. Hemophilia C, or factor XI (plasma thromboplastin antecedent) deficiency, is even more rare, accounting for less than 5% of hereditary coagulopathies.

Of patients who have hemophilia, 85% have hemophilia A, which is classified by levels of factor VIII. Severe hemophiliacs have less than 1% activity and have bleeding episodes that require factor VIII therapy several times per month. Moderate hemophiliacs have 1% to 5% activity and have varying need for factor VIII therapy, whereas mild hemophiliacs have greater than 5% activity and require intervention only after trauma or surgery.

Persons with hemophilia are able to form a platelet plug but are unable to form a stable clot. Clinical manifestations and complications of hemophilia are usually secondary to recurrent bleeding. Complications from subcutaneous and intramuscular hematomas are caused by compression of nerves or other structures, resulting in peripheral neuropathies, pain, compromised airway, muscle atrophy, ischemia, and gangrene. Hemarthrosis, or bleeding into the joint or synovial cavity, is a common complication that often results in joint deformities. Life-threatening hemorrhage may result from minor injuries.

CAUSES

All forms of hemophilia are the result of an X-linked recessive trait disorder. Approximately one-third of all hemophiliacs have no family history of bleeding disorders, which indicates that there may be factors other than heredity involved and that the illness is a result of a new mutation.

GENDER AND LIFE SPAN CONSIDERATIONS

Males who inherit the genetic trait have hemophilia. Most females with the defective gene do not develop clinical manifestations because they usually inherit a normal X chromosome from the other parent. Hemophilic males do not transmit the disease to their sons, because the Y chromosome is not affected. However, all daughters of afflicted males become carriers of the trait, because they inherit the defective X chromosome. Female carriers have a 50% chance of transmitting the trait to their offspring. Half of the daughters become carriers, and half of their sons have manifestations of hemophilia.

Bleeding abnormalities that are associated with hemophilia are usually noticed when the child becomes active and learns to walk, but mild cases may go undetected until adulthood. Bleeding episodes seem to decrease at or after adolescence, which may be because of the decreased risk of trauma, as well as stabilization of the disease process.

☐ ASSESSMENT

HISTORY. Question the patient, parents, or caregiver about any history of prolonged bleeding episodes, either spontaneous or following any injury in the patient or family. Determine the patient's age at diagnosis and the specific nature of the bleeding problem; in the case of a child, determine the family member's relationship to the patient.

PHYSICAL EXAMINATION. Note hematomas from subcutaneous and intramuscular bleeding. Tissue over the bleeding site is hard, raised, and dark purple. The hemorrhage extends from this center concentrically, with each successive outer circle becoming lighter in color. Intramuscular bleeding usually spreads within a single fascial space. Fever or pain may occur, with or without the skin discoloration.

Monitor the patient for frank or occult hematuria, melena, or hematemesis. Bleeding disproportionate to the extent of a traumatic injury is characteristic of hemophilia. Typically, the bleeding is an intermittent oozing type that develops over several hours or days after the injury or procedure. Wound healing is often delayed.

When the patient's extremities are moved, note joint pain and swelling caused by hemarthrosis, or spontaneous or trauma-induced bleeding into the joint or synovial cavity. Acute hemarthrosis is often preceded by a warm tingling sensation in the affected joint. If absorption of the blood from around the periarticular structures is incomplete, the remaining blood can cause chronic inflammation of the synovial membranes. Other long-term clinical sequelae of hemarthrosis include impaired joint mobility, bone deformity and demineralization, and stunted growth. Approximately 40% of hemophilia patients have splenomegaly; there have been some reported cases of spontaneous splenic rupture.

PSYCHOSOCIAL. Hemophilic patients and their families contend with the challenges of a chronic illness and the constant threat of life-threatening hemorrhage. Children often feel isolated from their peers because of the activity restrictions. Feelings of guilt are common among mothers of hemophilic children. Research studies have shown a positive correlation between children's adaptation to hemophilia and parental acceptance of the disease. Also, children who have a greater understanding of hemophilia and its treatment are less likely to experience psychological distress.

DIAGNOSTIC HIGHLIGHTS

Test	Normal Result	Abnormality with Condition	Explanation
Genetic testing	Normal factors VIII, IX, or XI genes	Mutation on factors VIII, IX, or XI genes	Identifies genetic alterations from normal
Assay of factors VIII, IX, XI	VIII: 50%–150% of normal control activity; IX: 50%–150%; XI: 65%–135%	< 5% normal control activity	Determines level of activity of essential factors needed for bloodclotting
Coagulation studies; activated partial thromboplastin time (APPT); prothrombin time (PT); bleeding time; platelet count	APPT: 21–35 seconds; PT: 11–13 seconds; bleeding time (Duke): 1–5 minutes; platelets: 190,000–405,000/mm³	Hemophilia A and B: prolonged APPT; normal bleeding time, platelet count, PT	Determine for clot formation. APPT measures the time for clot to form in a section of clotting cascade affected by factors VIII, IX, and XI

Other Tests: Thrombin time, x rays of hemarthrotic joints, computed tomography (CT) scan, and magnetic resonance imaging (MRI).

PRIMARY NURSING DIAGNOSIS

Risk for injury related to altered hemostasis and adverse effects of treatment

OUTCOMES. Risk control; Safety behavior: Fall prevention; Knowledge: Personal safety; Safety status: Physical injury; Knowledge: Medication; Safety behavior: Home physical environment

INTERVENTIONS. Bleeding precautions; Bleeding reduction; Fall prevention; Environmental management; Safety; Health education; Surveillance; Medication management

◻ PLANNING AND IMPLEMENTATION

Collaborative

Replacement therapy and drug therapy may be used prophylactically or to control mild or major bleeding episodes. Desmopressin will raise factor VIII levels two- to threefold. Factor VIII replacement therapy is indicated for active bleeding or preparation for multiple tooth extractions or major surgery. Cryoprecipitate contains high levels of factor VIII and fibrinogen. Purified plasma-derived factor VIII concentrates are derived from large pools of plasma donors. Recent methods of screening and heating of these concentrates have greatly diminished the risk of contamination with the human immunodeficiency virus (HIV) but have little effect on the risk of hepatitis transmission. High-potency factor VIII preparations (those that are highly purified) are considered to be virtually virus-free. Recombinant factor VIII contains less risk of viral transmission but has a relatively high cost. A rule of thumb is that for every 1 unit/kg infused, factor VIII levels will increase 2%. In an emergency, a 50 unit/kg IV bolus will increase levels to 100%.

Factor VIII, also found in fresh-frozen plasma (FFP), is usually reserved for hemophilia A patients who are actively bleeding. Bleeding episodes in hemophilia B can be treated with FFP or purified factor IX. Hemophilia C rarely requires intervention. Prophylactic replacement therapy for factor VIII or factor IX deficiency has been found to be beneficial in preventing spontaneous bleeding episodes and in minimizing bleeding complications such as joint disease. Any incidence of head trauma should receive immediate therapy that raises the factor VIII or IX levels to 100% normal before any diagnostic tests are performed. Intracranial hemorrhage is the most common cause of death in hemophiliacs; approximately 50% of these are associated with acute head injury.

PHARMACOLOGIC HIGHLIGHTS

Medication or Drug Class	Dosage	Description	Rationale
Desmopressin, 1-deamino-8-d-arginine vasopressin (DDAVP)	0.3 mcg/kg IV diluted in 50 mL normal saline solution; intranasal: 300 mcg, 1 spray in each nostril	Antidiuretic	Stimulates rapid release of von Willebrand factor (vWF) into the blood; treatment of choice in hemophilia A patients who do not have life-threatening bleeding problems; avoided with infants; does mot play a role in treatment for hemophilia B.

Other Drugs: Analgesia for hemarthrosis; avoid products containing aspirin and nonsteroidal anti-inflammatories

Independent

To prevent trauma that may precipitate bleeding episodes, avoid intramuscular injections and minimize the number of venipuncture attempts. Alert other health team members about the patient's high risk for bleeding. Avoid sources of mucosal irritation such as rectal temperatures, urinary catheters, and suppositories. Use only sponge sticks and nonalcoholic rinses for oral care. Assure that tourniquets or blood pressure cuffs are applied no longer than necessary. Perform nasopharyngeal or oropharyngeal suctioning very gently and only when needed. Prevent skin breakdown through the use of frequent turning and preventive skin care.

When bleeding occurs, apply firm, direct pressure for at least 5 minutes or until bleeding has stopped completely to sites of subcutaneous injections and venipuncture sites. Use sandbags and pressure dressings to maintain pressure on large puncture sites after hemostasis has been established. Initially, provide rest and elevation to a bleeding joint. Initiate mobilization within a few days after the bleeding is controlled to facilitate restoration of normal joint range of motion. Apply ice packs to control epistaxis, hematoma formation, and hemarthrosis.

Evaluate the family's current coping mechanisms and the level of anxiety. Encourage the patient and family members to verbalize their feelings openly and clearly with staff and with each other.

DOCUMENTATION GUIDELINES

- Bleeding episodes: Site, extent, duration, associated signs and symptoms, response to interventions
- Physical responses: Alteration in circulation, movement, or sensation; redness, warmth or swelling around joints; changes in vital signs, intake and output, cognition
- Pain: Location, precipitating factors, quality, intensity, associated signs and symptoms, factors that alleviate or exacerbate the pain
- Therapeutic and adverse effects of medical or surgical interventions

DISCHARGE AND HOME HEALTHCARE GUIDELINES

Teach the patient and family the early and late clinical manifestations of bleeding. Outline measures to prevent bleeding episodes, such as use of a soft-bristled toothbrush or sponge sticks, avoidance of activities that are likely to result in trauma, and avoidance of nonsteroidal anti-inflammatory drugs.

Emphasize the importance of carrying identifying medical information at all times. Teach the patient or caregiver to inform all healthcare providers about the patient's diagnosis. Describe immediate actions the patient or caregiver should take to control bleeding. List indicators of the need for medical assistance. Teach the patient or caregiver the purpose of each medication, the correct procedure for administration, and potential adverse effects. Provide the patient or family with a list of referrals for genetic counselors, social workers, vocational counselors, or psychologists to assist in the long-term adjustment as necessary.

Hemorrhoids

DRG Category: 188
Mean LOS: 4.9 days
Description: MEDICAL: Other Digestive System Diagnoses, Age > 17 with CC
DRG Category: 157
Mean LOS: 4.4 days
Description: SURGICAL: Anal and Stomal Procedures with CC

Hemorrhoids are a common, generally insignificant swelling and distention of veins in the anorectal region. They become significant when they bleed or cause pain or itching. Hemorrhoids are categorized as either internal or external. Internal hemorrhoids, produced by dilation and enlargement of the superior plexus, cannot be seen because they are above the anal sphincter, whereas external hemorrhoids, produced by dilation and enlargement of the inferior plexus, are below the anal sphincter and are apparent on inspection.

Hemorrhoids develop when increased intra-abdominal pressure produces increased systemic and portal venous pressure, thus causing increased pressure in the anorectal veins. The arterioles in the anorectal area send blood directly to the swollen anorectal veins, further increasing the pressure. Recurrent and repeated increased pressure causes the distended veins to separate from the surrounding smooth muscle and leads to their prolapse (enlarged internal hemorrhoids that actually protrude through the anus).

First-degree hemorrhoids protrude a short distance into the anal canal; second-degree hemorrhoids prolapse but reduce spontaneously; third-degree hemorrhoids require manual reduction, and fourth-degree hemorrhoids are not reducible. Complications of hemorrhoids include local infection, thrombosis, inflammation, and recurrent or, in rare cases, severe bleeding.

CAUSES

Some factors that are associated with hemorrhoids are occupations that require prolonged sitting or standing; heart failure; anorectal infections; anal intercourse; alcoholism; pregnancy; colorectal cancer; and hepatic disease such as cirrhosis, amoebic abscesses, or hepatitis. Straining because of constipation, diarrhea, coughing, sneezing, or vomiting and loss of muscle tone because of aging, rectal surgery, or episiotomy can also cause hemorrhoids.

GENDER AND LIFE SPAN CONSIDERATIONS

Hemorrhoids are more common in women during late pregnancy and immediately after delivery. Young people who are engaged in heavy weightlifting and exercise are prone to hemorrhoids, and college students who do not eat balanced diets are also at risk. The greatest incidence occurs in adults from 20 to 50 years of age. In later life, congestive heart failure and obesity contribute to the development of hemorrhoids.

☐ ASSESSMENT

HISTORY. Establish a history of anal itching, blood on the toilet tissue after a bowel movement, and anorectal pain or discomfort. Ask if the patient has experienced any mucous discharge. Determine if the patient can feel the external hemorrhoids. Elicit a history of risk factors and dietary patterns.

PHYSICAL EXAMINATION. Inspect the patient's anorectal area, noting external hemorrhoids. Internal hemorrhoids are discovered through digital rectal examination or anoscopy. Note any subcutaneous large, firm lumps in the anal area.

PRIMARY NURSING DIAGNOSIS

Pain (acute or chronic) related to rectal swelling and prolapse

OUTCOMES. Comfort level; Pain control behavior; Pain level; Symptom severity; Well-being

INTERVENTIONS. Analgesic administration; Anxiety reduction; Pain management; Medication management; Heat/cold application; Bowel management; Coping enhancement

DIAGNOSTIC HIGHLIGHTS

Test	Normal Result	Abnormality with Condition	Explanation
Proctoscopy: endoscopic exam of rectum and anal canal	Normal rectal lining: continuous reddish, free of lesions or inflammation	Visualization of internal hemorrhoids	Determines size and location of hemorrhoids

Other Tests: Barium enema, protoscopic ultrasound.

☐ PLANNING AND IMPLEMENTATION

Collaborative

Generally hemorrhoids can be managed pharmacologically. Conservative treatments include application of cold packs to the anal region, Sitz baths for 15 minutes twice a day, and local application of over the counter treatments such as witch hazel (Tucks) or dibucaine (Nupercainal) ointment. If conservative treatment does not alleviate symptoms in 3 to 5 days, more invasive management may be needed.

Invasive treatment may be indicated for thrombosis or severe symptoms. Sclerotherapy obliterates the vessels when the physician injects a sclerosing agent into the tissues around the hemorrhoids. With elastic band ligation, rubber bands are put on the hemorrhoids in an outpatient setting. The banded tissue sloughs. Successive visits may be necessary for many hemorrhoids. Although rubber band ligation has a high success rate, it may temporarily increase local pain and cause hemorrhage. In cryosurgery, the physician freezes the hemorrhoid with a probe to produce necrosis. Cryosurgery is only used for first- and second-degree hemorrhoids.

The most effective treatment is hemorrhoidectomy, the surgical removal of hemorrhoids, which is performed in an outpatient setting in 10% of patients. When the patient can resume oral feedings, administer a bulk medication such as psyllium. This medication is given about 1 hour after the evening meal to ensure a daily stool, which dilates the scar tissue and prevents anal stricture from developing. Postoperative care includes checking the dressing for excessive bleeding or drainage. The patient needs to void within the first 24 hours. If prescribed, spread petroleum jelly on the wound site and apply a wet dressing. Complications include urinary retention and hemorrhage.

PHARMACOLOGIC HIGHLIGHTS

Medication or Drug Class	Dosage	Description	Rationale
Docusate sodium (Colace)	100 mg bid po	Stool softener	Eases defecation
Anusol suppositories	1 bid pr	Analgesic, emollient	Relieve pain and itching
Hydrocortisone ointment or suppositories	Topical or pr as needed for brief courses of therapy	Corticosteroid	Relieve itching and swelling

Note: Laxatives are prohibited.

Independent

Most patients can be treated on an outpatient basis. Teach patients and families about over-the-counter local applications for comfort. Explain the importance of promoting regular bowel habits. Emphasize the need for increasing dietary fiber and fluid through a balanced diet high in whole grains, raw vegetables, and fresh fruit. Moderate exercise such as walking can also help regulate bowel function.

Postoperative actions include administering ice packs for pain control and positioning the patient for comfort. After the first 12-hour postoperative period, Sitz baths three or four times a day may be instituted to prevent recto-anal spasms and reduce swelling. Explain that the first postoperative bowel movement is painful and may require suitable narcotic intervention for comfort.

DOCUMENTATION GUIDELINES

- Physical findings: Rectal examination, urinary retention, bleeding, and mucous drainage
- Wound healing: Drainage, color, swelling
- Pain management: Pain (location, duration, frequency), response to interventions
- Postoperative bowel movements: Tolerance for first bowel movement

DISCHARGE AND HOME HEALTHCARE GUIDELINES

Teach the patient the importance of a high-fiber diet, increased fluid intake, mild exercise, and regular bowel movements. Be sure the patient schedules a follow-up visit to the physician. Teach the patient which analgesic applications for local pain may be used. If the patient has had surgery, teach him or her to recognize signs of urinary retention, such as bladder distension and hemorrhage, and to contact the physician at their appearance.

Hemothorax

DRG Category: 085
Mean LOS: 6.2 days
Description: MEDICAL: Pleural Effusion with CC
DRG Category: 094
Mean LOS: 6.5 days
Description: MEDICAL: Pneumothorax with CC
DRG Category: 075
Mean LOS: 9.9 days
Description: SURGICAL: Major Chest Procedures

Hemothorax, an accumulation of blood in the pleural space, affects oxygenation, ventilation, and hemodynamic stability. Oxygenation is affected because the accumulation of blood exerts pressure on pulmonary structures, leading to alveolar collapse, a decreased surface area for gas exchange, and impaired diffusion of oxygen from the alveolus to the blood. Ventilation is likewise impaired as the accumulating blood takes the place of gas in the lungs. Hemodynamic instability occurs as bleeding increases in the pleural space and vascular volume is depleted. Pneumothorax, or air in the pleural cavity, often accompanies hemothorax.

The hemorrhage can occur from pulmonary parenchymal lacerations, intercostal artery lacerations, or disruptions of the pulmonary or bronchial vasculature. Low pulmonary pressures and thromboplastin in the lungs may aid in spontaneously tamponading parenchymal lacerations. Complications of hemothorax include hypovolemic shock, exsanguination, organ failure, cardiopulmonary arrest, and death.

CAUSES

Hemothorax is generally caused by blunt trauma from motor vehicle crashes (MVCs), assaults, and falls or by penetrating trauma from knives or gunshot wounds. One of every four patients with chest trauma has a hemothorax. Other causes include thoracic surgery, pulmonary infarction, dissecting thoracic aneurysms, tumors, and anticoagulant therapy.

GENDER AND LIFE SPAN CONSIDERATIONS

Hemothorax from traumatic injury occurs in both pediatric and adult populations. Because trauma is the leading cause of death in the first four decades of life, hemothorax is most commonly seen in children and young adults. Because they often have fewer compensatory mechanisms to respond to the injury, elderly people with such an injury have higher rates of complications and death. More males than females have injuries each year.

◻ ASSESSMENT

HISTORY. Establish a history of the injury. If the patient has been shot, ask the paramedics for ballistic information, including the caliber of the weapon and the range at which the person was shot. If the patient was in an MVC, determine the type of vehicle (truck, motorcycle, car), the speed of the vehicle, the victim's location in the car (driver or passenger), and the use, if any, of safety restraints. Determine if the patient has had recent tetanus immunization. If the patient can communicate, determine the location of chest pain and whether the patient is experiencing shortness of breath. If there is no chest trauma, establish a history of other risk factors. Determine if the patient has undergone thoracic surgery or anticoagulant therapy. Establish a history of pulmonary infarction, dissecting thoracic aneurysm, or tumor.

PHYSICAL EXAMINATION. The initial evaluation focuses on assessing the adequacy of the patient's airway, breathing, and circulation, as well as neurological status. The patient should be completely undressed for a thorough visual assessment. The initial evaluation, or primary survey, is completed by the trauma resuscitation team and may occur simultaneously with life-saving interventions as needed.

The secondary survey, completed after life-threatening conditions are stabilized, includes serial vital signs and a complete head-to-toe assessment. Assess the patient for a patent airway. Note respiratory rate, breathing pattern, and lung sounds on an hourly basis. Observe the patient's breathing; the affected side of the chest may expand and stiffen while the unaffected side rises. Auscultate for lung sounds; the loss of breath sounds is evidence of a collapsed lung. Percuss the lungs; blood in the pleural space yields a dullness. Note signs of respiratory failure; the patient may appear anxious, restless, even stuporous, and cyanotic. If the patient has a chest tube, monitor its functioning, the amount of blood loss, the integrity of the system, and the presence of air leaks.

Examine the thorax area, including the anterior chest, posterior chest, and axillae, for contusions, abrasions, hematomas, and penetrating wounds. Note that even small penetrating wounds can be life threatening if vital structures are perforated. Observe carefully for pallor, blood pressure, and pulse rate, noting the early signs of shock or massive bleeding such as a falling pulse pressure, a rising pulse rate, and delayed capillary refill.

PSYCHOSOCIAL. The patient may be fearful or panic-stricken because of difficulties in breathing and intense pain. Ongoing assessment of coping strategies of patient and family assists in planning and evaluating interventions. Note that approximately half of all traumatic injuries are associated with alcohol and other drugs of abuse. Assess the patient's drinking and drug-taking patterns.

DIAGNOSTIC HIGHLIGHTS

Test	Normal Result	Abnormality with Condition	Explanation
Chest x ray	Air-filled lungs	Opacity at the area of bleeding and lung collapse; blunted costophrenic angle; may show widening of mediastinum and intercostal spaces	Determines the location and extent of lung collapse and fluid accumulation

		with depressed diaphragm	
Complete blood count	Red blood cells (RBCs): 4.0–6.2 million/μL; hemoglobin: 12–18 g/dL; hematocrit: 37%–54%; white blood cells: 4,500–11,000/μL; platelets: 150,000–400,000/μL	Decreased values reflective of the degree of hemorrhage	Determines the extent of blood loss: note that it takes 2 hours for hemorrhage to be reflected in a dropping hemoglobin and hematocrit after injury
Arterial blood gases	PaO_2: 80–100 mm Hg; $PaCO_2$: 35–45 mm Hg; SaO_2: 95%–100%; PH: 7.35– 7.45	Hypoxemia; PaO_2 < 80 mm Hg; SaO_2 < 95%; $PaCO_2$ > 45 mm Hg	Determine adequacy of oxygenation; accumulation of blood and air in functional tissue of lungs decreases gas exchange leading to hypotemia and hypercapnea.

Other Tests: Coagulation studies, electrocardiogram, thoracentesis, and cervical spine x rays.

❏ PLANNING AND IMPLEMENTATION

Collaborative

Treatment of a hemothorax focuses on stabilizing the patient's condition by maintaining airway and breathing, stopping the bleeding, emptying blood from the pleural cavity, and re-expanding the underlying lung. Mild cases of hemothorax may resolve in 10 days to 2 weeks, requiring only observation for further bleeding. More severe cases of hemothorax (hemorrhaging that arises from arterial sites or major hilar vessels) generally require aggressive surgical intervention. Autotransfusion, a system that allows blood removed from the pleural cavity to be returned to the patient intravenously, is useful in the initial management of the patient with hemothorax. Reinfusion of shed blood from the chest injury can be accomplished by a variety of techniques. Significant blood loss may lead to hypovolemic shock.

A tube thoracostomy is the treatment of choice for hemothorax; approximately 80% of penetrating and blunt trauma can be managed successfully with this procedure. A hemothorax with a volume of 500 to 1500 mL that does not continue to bleed can be managed with a chest tube alone. A massive hemothorax, with an initial volume of 1500 to 2000 mL or one that continues to bleed between 100 to 200 mL per hour after 6 hours is an indication for a formal thoracotomy. Placement of more than one chest tube may be necessary to drain a hemothorax adequately.

An emergency thoracotomy at the bedside may be necessary in the setting of a massive hemothorax with accompanying hemodynamic instability. The approach is a left anterolateral incision and is reserved for those patients who are in a life-threatening situation. A formal thoracotomy performed in the operating room is accomplished by a variety of incisions. Once exposure is obtained, lung parenchyma and vascular structures, including the great vessels, can be evaluated and repaired.

PRIMARY NURSING DIAGNOSIS

Ineffective airway clearance related to airway obstruction secondary to trauma and tissue damage

OUTCOMES. Respiratory status: Ventilation; Respiratory status: Gas exchange; Symptom control behavior; Comfort level; Infection status; Cognitive ability

INTERVENTIONS. Airway management; Airway insertion and stabilization; Airway suctioning; Artificial airway management; Oxygen therapy; Respiratory monitoring; Ventilatory assistance; Vital signs monitoring

PHARMACOLOGIC HIGHLIGHTS

Medication or Drug Class	Dosage	Description	Rationale
Antibiotics	Varies with drug	Physicians may follow cultures of wounds, urine, blood, and sputum rather than use prophylactic antibiotics	Protect from or combat bacterial infections.
Analgesics	Varies with drug	IV morphine sulfate provides pain control and can be reversed with naloxone if complications occur.	Reduce pain so that they increase mobility

Other Drugs: Patients with significant chest trauma causing a hemothorax may benefit by the placement of an epidural catheter for pain management. A tetanus booster is administered to patients with chest trauma whose immunization history indicates a need or whose history is unavailable.

Independent

The most critical nursing intervention is maintaining airway, breathing, and circulation. Have an intubation tray available in case endotracheal intubation and mechanical ventilation are necessary. Maintain a working endotracheal suction at the bedside as well. If the patient is hemodynamically stable, position the patient for full lung expansion, using the semi-Fowler position with the arms elevated on pillows. Because the cervical spine is at risk after injury, maintain body alignment and prevent flexion and extension by a cervical collar or by other strategies dictated by trauma service protocols.

If the patient is hemodynamically unstable, consider alternate positions but never place the adequacy of airway and breathing at risk. When the patient has inadequate circulation, consider placing the patient flat with the legs raised if airway and breathing are adequate (usually when the patient is intubated and on mechanical ventilation). Trendelenburg's position is not recommended because it may increase the systemic vascular resistance and decrease the cardiac output in some patients, interfere with chest excursion by pushing the abdominal contents upward, and increase the risk of aspiration.

Establish adequate communication. The patient is likely to be very anxious, even fearful, for several reasons. If the hemothorax is the result of a chest trauma, the injury itself is unexpected and possibly quite frightening. The patient is experiencing pain and may not be receiving sedatives or analgesics until the pulmonary status stabilizes. The patient may have low oxygen levels, which lead to restlessness and anxiety. Remain with the patient at all times and reassure him or her until airway, breathing, and circulation have been stabilized.

DOCUMENTATION GUIDELINES

- Physical findings: Patency of airway, presence of clear breath sounds, vital signs, level of consciousness, urinary output, capillary blanch, skin temperature
- Response to pain: Location, description, duration, response to interventions
- Response to treatment: Chest tube insertion—Type and amount of drainage, presence of air leak, presence or absence of crepitus, amount of suction, presence of clots, response to fluid resuscitation; response to surgical management
- Complications: Hemorrhage (ongoing bleeding), infection (fever, wound drainage), inadequate gas exchange (restlessness, dropping SaO_2)

DISCHARGE AND HOME HEALTHCARE GUIDELINES

Be sure the patient and family understand any pain medication prescribed, including dosage, route, action, and side effects. Review with the patient all follow-up appointments that are arranged. Follow-up often involves chest x rays and ABG analysis, as well as a physical examination. If the injury was alcohol-related, explore the patient's drinking pattern. If the injury was binge-related, explain the relationship between injury and alcohol by stating the facts without being judgmental. If you think that the patient is either a problem or dependent drinker, refer him or her to an advanced practice nurse or an alcohol counselor. Teach the patient when to notify the physician for complication such as signs of infection, an unhealed wound, or anxiety and inability to cope. Provide the patient with a phone number for a primary healthcare provider, trauma clinic, or advanced practice nurse.

Hepatitis

DRG Category: 205
Mean LOS: 6.1 days
Description: MEDICAL: Disorders of Liver Except Malignancy, Cirrhosis, Alcoholic Hepatitis with CC

Hepatitis is a widespread inflammation of the liver that results in degeneration and necrosis of liver cells. More than 70,000 cases of hepatitis are reported each year in the United States. In most cases, the damage is reversible after the acute phase; in some, however, massive necrosis can lead to liver failure and death.

Acute viral hepatitis is a major public health concern because it is highly communicable and is transmitted before the onset of symptoms in the infected host. In general, the majority of cases of hepatitis are self-limiting and resolve without complications. Hospitalization is required only when symptoms are severe, persistent, or debilitating. Approximately 20% of acute hepatitis B and 50% of hepatitis C cases progress to a chronic state. In Americans, 5% to 10% of patients with hepatitis have hepatitis B virus (HBV) infections. In third world countries, the rates are much higher.

The most serious complication of hepatitis is fulminant hepatitis, which occurs in approximately 1% of all patients and leads to liver failure and hepatic encephalopathy and in some to death within 2 weeks of onset. Other complications include a syndrome that resembles serum sickness (muscle and joint pain, rash, angioedema), as well as cirrhosis, pancreatitis, myocarditis, aplastic anemia, or peripheral neuropathy.

CAUSES

Hepatitis can be caused by bacteria, by hepatotoxic agents (drugs, alcohol, industrial chemicals), or, most commonly, by a virus. Five agents have been identified as the cause of acute viral hepatitis (see Table 26): hepatitis A virus (HAV), hepatitis B virus (HBV), hepatitis C virus (HCV), delta virus or hepatitis D virus (HDV), hepatitis E virus (HEV), and Non-A Non-B hepatitis.

TABLE 26 | **Causative Agents of Hepatitis**

VIRAL AGENT	ROUTE OF TRANSMISSION	CHARACTERISTICS AND RISK GROUPS	INCUBATION PERIOD	CARRIER/ CHRONIC HEPATITIS
Hepatitis A virus (HAV) (infectious hepatitis)	Fecal-oral route; blood; sexual contact	Military personnel, children in day care. Incidence is rising in male homosexuals and in those with human immunodeficiency (HIV) viral infections.	2–7 weeks (often 4 weeks)	No/No
Hepatitis B virus (HBV) (accounts for 5%–10% of posttransfusion hepatitis)	Blood; sexual contact; perinatal contact	IV drug abusers; Native Asians; healthcare workers; transfusion recipients; incidence is rising in those with HIV infections	2–5 months	Yes/Yes
Hepatitis C virus (HCV)	Blood; sexual contact; perinatal contact; unknown factors	IV drug abusers; healthcare workers; transfusion recipients	1 week to several months	Yes/Yes
Hepatitis D virus (HDV) (delta hepatitis)	Blood; sexual contact; perinatal contact	IV drug abusers; people with HBV	3 weeks to 3 months	Yes/Yes
Hepatitis E virus	Fecal-oral.	Most common in people who travel to India, Asia, Africa, Central America	14–60 days	No/No

| Non-A Non-B hepatitis | Blood; sexual contact; perinatal contact | IV drug abusers; healthcare workers; transfusion recipients | 14–180 days | Perhaps/ Yes |

GENDER AND LIFE SPAN CONSIDERATIONS

All age, sex, and socioeconomic groups can be affected by hepatitis.

▢ ASSESSMENT

HISTORY. Question the patient about potential sources of transmission and risks: a history of blood dyscrasias, multiple blood or blood product transfusions, alcohol or drug abuse (sharing of needles), exposure to hepatotoxic chemicals or medications, and travel to third world countries or areas where the sanitation is poor. Since HAV transmission occurs in association with day-care centers, among male homosexuals, and among household contacts of persons with acute cases, inquire into these areas. Also ask about recent meals because hepatitis A occasionally occurs from contaminated food or improper sewage treatment. Determine the patient's occupation; teratogen exposure may cause a nonviral hepatitis.

Patients in the prodromal (initial) phase may complain of nausea, vomiting, malaise, headache, fatigue, anorexia (a distaste for cigarettes in smokers is characteristic of early profound anorexia), and fever. Ask about any changes in the sense of taste or smell, recent weight loss, and the presence of urticaria or arthralgias, which can occur early in the disease process. Pruritus may be mild and transient and is caused by the accumulation of bile salt in the skin. In the icteric phase (3 to 10 days later), there may be right upper-quadrant pain and no flu-like symptoms.

PHYSICAL EXAMINATION. In the prodromal phase, inspect the skin for a rash. Fever is usually between 101° and 102°F. In the icteric phase, the urine often appears dark and concentrated. Observe stools for a pale, clay color. Inspect the skin, sclera, and mucous membranes for jaundice, which is caused by the poor ability of the damaged liver to remove bilirubin from the bloodstream. Jaundice peaks within 1 to 2 weeks and fades during the recovery phase over the next 2 to 4 weeks.

On palpation, the liver is usually enlarged and sometimes tender. The edges remain soft and smooth. In 15% to 20% of cases, mild splenomegaly is present. In uncomplicated cases, signs of chronic liver disease are not seen. In alcoholic hepatitis, inspect the skin for spider nevi.

Potential complications include bleeding and the possibility of progressive liver degeneration. Assess for petechiae, bruising, bleeding gums or nose, prolonged bleeding from puncture sites, and obvious or occult blood in body secretions and fluids. Note that restlessness and confusion, decreasing blood pressure and pulse, abnormal complete blood count, and platelet and coagulation tests may indicate increased bleeding. Monitor for worsening symptoms, edema, ascites, and encephalopathy. Because an early sign of hepatic encephalopathy is deterioration of the handwriting, have the patient write his or her name each shift and monitor the signature for changes.

PSYCHOSOCIAL. The patient with hepatitis has a communicable disease. Assess for knowledge of possible sources of transmission, including behavioral risk factors. Ask about the patient's living conditions to assess the risk of spread of hepatitis to the family and significant others. Determine the patient's ability to cope with a communicable disease, anxiety level, and support mechanisms. Some families have a magnified fear of contracting a communicable disease and may respond to the diagnosis with irrational fears and concerns.

DIAGNOSTIC HIGHLIGHTS

Test	Normal Result	Abnormality with Condition	Explanation
Viral hepatitis seriologies	Negative results	Acute HAV: Positive anti-HAV IgM Acute HBV: Anti-HBV IgM, HB surface antigen Acute HCV: Anti-HCV antibody, HCV RNA HDV: Anti HDV IgM, HDV antigen HEV: not available Non A Non B: all tests negative	Identify immune response to virus leads to markers such as immunoglobulins (IgG and IgM), antigens, antibodies
Liver function tests	Alanine aminotrans-ferase (ALT): 4–46 U/L; aspartate aminotransferase (AST): 8–20 U/L; alkaline phosphatase: 32–92 U/L	ALT elevated as high or higher than 1,000 U/L; AST elevated as high or higher than 1,000 U/L; alkaline phosphatase mildly elevated	Determine the extent of inflammation

Other Tests: Bilirubin, prothrombin time, complete blood count, albumin, and liver biopsy.

PRIMARY NURSING DIAGNOSIS

Altered nutrition: Less than body requirements related to decreased oral intake, nausea, vomiting, and anorexia

OUTCOMES. Nutritional status: Food and fluid intake; Nutritional status: Nutrient intake; Nutritional status: Energy; Endurance

INTERVENTIONS. Nutritional therapy; Fluid management; Nutritional counseling; Nutritional monitoring; Weight management; Medication management; Teaching: Prescribed diet

◻ PLANNING AND IMPLEMENTATION

Collaborative

Immune globulin (IG) can provide protection against clinically apparent HAV. IG should be given to household contacts of patients with HAV and to persons who plan to travel on prolonged visits to third world countries or other places where sanitation is poor. It may also be given to people with exposure to hepatitis C and E, but its effectiveness for these two types is uncertain. Hepatitis B immune globulin (HBIG) should be given to persons with exposure to hepatitis B surface antigen-positive blood, including accidental needle sticks. Vaccination against HBV is available and should be considered in high-risk groups, including medical and healthcare personnel.

Dietary management usually includes a high-caloric, high-protein, high-carbohydrate, low-fat diet as tolerated. If oral intake is limited or compromised, parenteral or enteral nutrition may be implemented. With fluid retention or encephalopathy, sodium or protein restriction (because of the buildup of ammonia in the blood) may be indicated. Alcoholic beverages should not be taken at all during recovery.

PHARMACOLOGIC HIGHLIGHTS

Medication or Drug Class	Dosage	Description	Rationale
Immune globulin, gamma globulin	0.02 mL/kg as a single dose IM after exposure	Immune serum	Provides passive immunity to those exposed to HAV, HBV, hepatitis B surface antigen
Vitamin K phytonadione (Aquamephyton)	2.5–10 mg po; 1–2 mg IV diluted and infused slowly	Nutritional supplement	Enhances hepatic formation of coagulation factors II, VII, IX, and X

Other Drugs: Antiemetics such as trimethobenzamide hydrochloride (Tigan) can be given 30 minutes before meals to decrease nausea and vomiting and to increase the likelihood of an adequate intake. Avoid prochlorperazine maleate (Compazine) because of the effects on the liver. Additionally, analgesics and antipruritics may be administered to assist with comfort. Dosages may be decreased because of the altered ability of the liver to clear certain medications.

Independent

Observe enteric precautions if the patient has hepatitis A or E and universal precautions for hepatitis B, C, or D. To maintain fluid and electrolyte balance, implement measures to reduce nausea and vomiting. Encourage the patient to eat, but avoid greasy foods. Avoid overmedication, which can decrease appetite. Encourage rest before meals. Assist in providing oral care and maintain a relaxed environment to enhance the palatability of the meal. Encourage fluids to at least 4000 mL per day unless there are fluid restrictions for other accompanying illnesses. Supplement dietary fluids with soft drinks, ice chips, and iced pops. Determine if the patient is maintaining body weight.

Provide pain relief measures such as heat, back rubs, positioning, relaxation techniques, and age-appropriate diversion. Relieve pruritus with skin care. Implement measures to improve activity tolerance; facilitate adequate rest periods by organizing nursing and multidisciplinary care activities, adjusting visitation schedules, and reducing environmental stimulation. Institute measures to promote safety. Measures to prevent bleeding include using the smallest-gauge needle possible for venipunctures or injections; applying gentle, prolonged pressure to puncture sites; avoiding overinflation of the blood pressure cuff; and avoiding risk for trauma and falls by limiting clutter in the room.

DOCUMENTATION GUIDELINES

- Findings of physical exam and ongoing assessments: Nausea, vomiting, anorexia, diarrhea, color of stools and urine, daily weights, vital signs, jaundice, pruritus, edema, ascites, pain, level of consciousness
- Response to medical and nursing interventions: Medications, comfort measures, diet, hydration
- Pain: Location, duration, precipitating factors, response to interventions
- Presence of complications: Bleeding, progressive liver degeneration, changes in mental status
- Protection of household: Isolation procedures, family prophylaxis

DISCHARGE AND HOME HEALTHCARE GUIDELINES

Provide instruction on the prevention of the spread of hepatitis to others. With hepatitis A, do the following for 1 to 2 weeks after the onset of jaundice. Use strict hand washing after bowel movements and before meals. Have separate toilet facilities if possible (if not, clean the seat with bleach after each use). Wash linens, towels, and undergarments separately from other items in hot, soapy water. Do not donate blood or work in food services until such work is cleared by a physician.

With hepatitis B, C, or D, do the following, as directed by a physician, until antigen-antibody tests are negative. Maintain strict hand washing after urination and defecation. Do not share personal items (toothbrush, razor, washcloth). Use disposable eating utensils or wash utensils separately in hot, soapy water. Do not share food or eating utensils. Do not share needles, and dispose of them properly after a single use. Avoid intimate sexual contact; when sex can be resumed, use a condom and avoid intercourse during menstruation. Do not donate blood. Instruct the patient to inform household members and sexual partners of the fact that he or she has developed hepatitis and to encourage them to notify a primary healthcare provider immediately to assess the risk of the disease.

To prevent complications, teach the patient to avoid alcohol for 6 months to 1 year, avoid illicit drugs and toxic chemicals, and take acetaminophen only when necessary and not beyond the recommended dosage. Note that in viral hepatitis, the patient has immunity only to the type of hepatitis he or she has had.

Herniated Disk

DRG Category: 243
Mean LOS: 4.9 days
Description: MEDICAL: Back Problems
DRG Category: 214
Mean LOS: 6.5 days
Description: SURGICAL: Back and Neck Procedures with CC

The intervertebral disk is a complex structure that is situated between vertebrae; it provides additional structural support to the spinal column and cushions the vertebrae. The outer layer of the disk contains numerous concentric rings of tough, fibrous connective tissue called the annulus fibrosus. The central portion of the disk consists of a softer, spongier material called the nucleus pulposus. If the annulus fibrosus weakens or tears, then the nucleus pulposus may "slip" or herniate outward, creating the condition known as a "slipped disk," or, more precisely, herniated nucleus pulposus. When the disk material herniates, it can compress the spinal cord or the nerve roots that come from the spinal cord. Of herniations, 90% usually occur in the lumbar and lumbosacral regions, 8% occur in the cervical area, and 1% to 2% occur in the thoracic area. The disk between the fifth and sixth cervical vertebrae is involved most frequently.

CAUSES

Disk herniation is often seen in individuals who have had previous episodes of back problems; however, a herniation may occur without such a history. Repeated episodes are thought to weaken the annulus fibrosus. Heavy physical labor, including repetitive bending, twisting, and lifting, is a risk factor for herniated disk, especially if combined with weak abdominal and back muscles or poor body mechanics. Advancing age produces desiccations of the disk and friability of the annulus, which can increase the likelihood of injury.

GENDER AND LIFE SPAN CONSIDERATIONS

Disk herniations most often occur in adults, with a mean age at surgery of 40 years. Both men and women are affected.

◻ ASSESSMENT

HISTORY. Establish a history of back pain, including a description of the location and intensity of the pain. Often the symptoms are of a gradually progressing nature over a period of days to weeks. The development and distribution of extremity pain help determine the level of the involved disk. Ask about weakness in the extremities, altered sensation, or muscle spasms; ask if pain intensifies during Valsalva's maneuver, coughing, sneezing, or bending. Establish a history of sensory and motor loss in the area that has been innervated by the compressed spinal nerve root.

PHYSICAL EXAMINATION. Document any gait abnormalities, such as a limp. Test the patient's deep tendon reflexes in the upper and lower extremities. Perform a sensory evaluation of the patient's sharp-dull and fine touch discrimination. Motor strength testing of the involved extremities is also important, again to determine the extent of injury to the spinal cord or nerve roots. Perform range-of-motion studies of either the cervical, thoracic, or lumbar regions. Conduct stretch tests for nerve root irritation, including the straight leg raise test; if the sciatic nerve is irritated, there will be pain in the involved leg. The Braggart's test, passive stretching of the foot in dorsiflexion, is positive if it elicits pain along the sciatic nerve distribution. The "bow string" sign is performed with the patient sitting and the knees flexed just beyond a 90 degree angle, the body bent slightly forward to increase the stretch on the sciatic nerve. A positive response occurs when gentle pressure with the examiner's finger into the popliteal space further stretches the sciatic nerve, producing more pain. Check the patient's peripheral vascular status, including peripheral pulses and skin temperatures, to rule out ischemic disease, another possible cause of leg pain and numbness.

PSYCHOSOCIAL. The individual may be unexpectedly debilitated. The assessment should include an evaluation of the patient's ability to deal with unexpected changes in lifestyle, roles, and income. Along with severe pain, an employed person may be facing a prolonged period of disability and reduced income.

DIAGNOSTIC HIGHLIGHTS

Test	Normal Result	Abnormality with Condition	Explanation
X rays	Normal bony skeleton	Changes in spinal structure and alignment	Indicate the extent of bony injury
Computed tomography (CT) scan	Normal bony skeleton and soft tissue	Changes in spinal structure and alignment, deterioration or herniation of soft tissues	Indicate the extent of bony and soft tissue injury and deterioration

Other Tests: Magnetic resonance imaging (MRI), myelography, electromyography.

PRIMARY NURSING DIAGNOSIS

Pain (acute) related to inflammation and compression

OUTCOMES. Comfort level; Pain control behavior; Pain level; Symptom severity

INTERVENTIONS. Analgesic administration; Anxiety reduction; Environmental management: Comfort; Pain management; Medication management

☐ PLANNING AND IMPLEMENTATION

Collaborative

MEDICAL. Pharmacological measures are often used to manage symptoms. Physical therapy includes various passive modalities of treatment, such as heat, ice, massage, ultrasound, and electrogalvanic stimulation, often directed by a physical therapist, and exercises to stretch and strengthen the spine and supporting musculature. Spinal adjustments performed by osteopathic or chiropractic physicians can also relieve symptoms. Chemonucleolysis may be used by injecting the enzyme chymopapain into the nucleus pulposus. Ask if the patient is allergic to meat tenderizers, since such an allergy contraindicates the use of chymopapain in the procedure.

SURGICAL. When the medical and pharmacologic treatments are not successful, or if the symptoms become debilitating, then surgery is considered. Surgery involves removal of the disk using a microscope. A microdiskectomy removes fragments of the nucleus pulpolsus. More common is a laminectomy, which removes the protruding disk and a portion of the lamina. A spinal fusion of the bony tissues may be performed if there is evidence that the disk herniation is accompanied by instability of the surrounding tissues. Surgical treatment is usually successful but may involve a prolonged recovery time, especially with more involved procedures.

Postoperatively, enforce bed rest and monitor dressings for excessive drainage. Position the patient depending on the type of surgery performed. Teach the patient who has undergone spinal fusion how to wear a brace. Teach the patient proper body mechanics. Encourage the patient to lie down when he or she is tired and to sleep on his or her side, using an extra firm mattress or bed board. Caution the patient to maintain proper weight, since obesity can cause lordosis. Ongoing assessments are important if the patient requires surgery. Monitor the patient for signs of weakness, pain, changes in circulation, and numbness in the extremities. Assess the cardiovascular status of the patient's legs by observing for color, temperature, and motion. Assess the degree of pain in terms of intensity, location, and character.

PHARMACOLOGIC HIGHLIGHTS

Medication or Drug Class	Dosage	Description	Rationale
Muscle relaxants	Varies with drug	Cyclobenzaprine hydrochloride (Flexeril)	To relieve muscular irritation

Other Drugs: Narcotic analgesics such as codeine and meperidine are used to control pain. Nonnarcotics (such as propoxyphene [Darvon]) may also be used. Acute inflammation is usually treated with either a steroid or nonsteroidal anti-inflammatory drugs (NSAIDs).

Independent

Place the patient in a semi-Fowler position or in a flat position with a pillow between the patient's legs for side-lying to help reduce the pain. Instruct the patient to roll to one side when sitting up to minimize pain during position changes. Perform active and passive range-of-motion exercises within the prescribed regimen. Keep a schedule of progress to encourage the patient when he or she becomes discouraged, and provide an estimate of when the patient will return to normal functioning. Allow the patient to direct or perform self-care. Provide meticulous skin care.

DOCUMENTATION GUIDELINES

- Physical findings: Neural and musculoskeletal system assessments, degree of pain, tolerance to activity; presence of postoperative complications (infection, pain, immobility, poor wound healing)
- Response to physical therapy: Work status of the patient, ability to cope with both immobility and inability to return to work

DISCHARGE AND HOME HEALTHCARE GUIDELINES

Teach the patient the mechanics of disk function and how herniation occurs. Instruct the patient in proper body mechanics, and advise avoiding high-torsion activities, such as twisting and heavy lifting. Discuss an exercise program with the patient as a maintenance program, following the 6-week physical therapy regimen. Be sure the patient understands any medication prescribed, including dosage, route, action, and side effects. Advise the patient against driving or operating heavy machinery if the medications are likely to impair judgment.

Herpes Simplex Virus

DRG Category: 283
Mean LOS: 4.8 days
Description: MEDICAL: Minor Skin Disorders with CC

There are two types of herpes simplex virus (HSV), type I and type II. HSV I causes infection above the waist, such as "cold sores" that occur on the mouth. This type may occur in the genital area as a result of oral-genital sexual practices. After the initial infection, the virus is dormant, but the patient is a carrier and likely to have recurrent infections. Events that trigger recurrences are sun exposure, fever, menses, stress, or lack of sleep.

HSV II causes lesions in the genital area. In the primary episode multiple, blisterlike, painful vesicles erupt on the vulva, perineum, cervix, or perianal area within 3 to 5 days after the initial exposure. The virus then becomes dormant and resides in the nerve ganglia of the affected area. Repeated outbreaks can happen at any time, but most patients have less severe regular recurrences that are more likely to occur during menses, pregnancy, or times of illness and stress.

Active HSV is associated with spontaneous abortion in the first trimester of pregnancy and an increased risk of preterm labor after 20 weeks' gestation. If a patient has active herpes around the time of the estimated date of delivery, cesarean section is the preferred method of delivery. Infected infants can develop the following signs and symptoms after an incubation period of 2 to 12 days: fever, hypothermia, jaundice, seizures, poor feeding, and vesicular skin lesions.

CAUSES

To cause an infection, HSV needs to come into direct contact with the genitals, mouth, eyes, open sores, or cracks in the skin. HSV II is sexually transmitted through contact with an infected person. Pregnant women can transmit the herpes virus to the fetus, especially during a primary outbreak. Transmission can occur when the membranes rupture or during a vaginal delivery, but transplacental transmission is extremely rare. Asymptomatic transmission is very uncommon.

GENDER AND LIFE SPAN CONSIDERATIONS

Because teenagers are engaging in sexual activity earlier than ever before, they have a higher risk today than in the past of contracting HSV; the number of adolescents with HSV is therefore increasing. Since there is no cure for herpes, recurrent outbreaks of HSV occur over a lifetime. Both men and women are affected by herpes simplex.

◻ ASSESSMENT

HISTORY. If the patient has an oral lesion, ask about a sore throat, increased salivation, anorexia, and mouth pain. During a primary episode, the patient may experience flu-like symptoms, such as fever, malaise, and enlarged lymph nodes. If the lesion is not a primary one, the patient usually does not have any systemic complaints but may complain of a tingling, itching, or painful sensation at the site of the lesion. If the patient has a genital lesion, obtain a detailed summary of his or her sexual activity, including number of partners, use of barrier protection and birth control measures, participation in oral or anal intercourse, and previous (if any) history of sexually transmitted diseases (STDs). Inquire about any burning with urination, dysuria, dyspareunia, pruritus, fever, chills, headache, and general malaise.

PHYSICAL EXAMINATION. Inspect the lips and the oral and pharyngeal mucosa for lesions and inflammation. The lesion may appear as a red, swollen vesicle, or if it has ruptured, it is ulcerlike with yellow crusting. Palpation of the lymph nodes in the neck may reveal cervical adenopathy. Take the patient's temperature. Inspect the genitalia for fluid-filled vesicles, or if the vesicles have ruptured, note an edematous, erythematous oozing ulcer with a yellow center. Examine the cervix by using a speculum, and inspect the walls of the vagina. Inspect the patient's perianal skin and the labia and vulva or penis and foreskin carefully to identify all lesions; note any abnormal discharge.

PSYCHOSOCIAL. Ask the patient about sexual practices, partners, and birth control methods. Assess the patient's knowledge of STDs and their implications. Assess the patient's ability to cope with having an STD. The diagnosis of an STD can be very upsetting to a man or woman who believes he or she was involved in a monogamous relationship. Tell patients that an outbreak of genital HSV may have had its origins even 20 to 30 years before the outbreak.

DIAGNOSTIC HIGHLIGHTS

Test	Normal Result	Abnormality with Condition	Explanation
Viral culture	Negative	Positive for HSV; differentiates between HSV I and HSV II	Demonstrates presence of viruses in an active lesion; cultures are most accurate in the first several days of ulceration

PRIMARY NURSING DIAGNOSIS

Anxiety related to a knowledge deficit of cause, treatment, and prevention of HSV

OUTCOMES. Anxiety control; Coping; Social interaction skills; Acceptance: Health status; Symptom control behavior

INTERVENTIONS. Anxiety reduction; Coping enhancement; Presence; Teaching: Individual; Counseling; Support group; Medication prescribing

☐ PLANNING AND IMPLEMENTATION

Collaborative

Since HSV is not curable, treatment focuses on relieving the symptoms. The drug of choice to treat a primary infection of HSV I and II is acyclovir.

PHARMACOLOGIC HIGHLIGHTS

Medication or Drug Class	Dosage	Description	Rationale
Acyclovir	200–800 mg po bid to qid depending on severity of symptoms and location of lesions; 5% acyclovir ointment	Antiviral	Treats primary HSV infection (contraindicated during pregnancy); daily dosage for primary episodes is slightly lower than that used for recurrent infections. Some physicians may order chronic suppressive drug therapy, where acyclovir is taken for up to 6 months

Other Drugs: Antipyretics, analgesics, viscous lidocaine.

Independent

Instruct the patient to take all medication ordered, even if symptoms recede before the medication is used up. For comfort during the outbreak, patients may take prescribed analgesics or use warm soaks with Epsom salts or sitz baths. Lesions can be cleaned with Betadine. Encourage patients to wear loose clothing and cotton underwear and to avoid ointments that contain cortisone and petroleum because they slow healing and promote the growth of the virus. Encourage exercise, good nutrition, and stress reduction to decrease the number of recurrent outbreaks. (See Box 6.)

BOX 6   LIVING WITH GENITAL HERPES: WHAT PATIENTS NEED TO KNOW

Background

Each patient's symptoms are different; lesions can resemble blisters, cuts in the skin, or spider bites on the buttocks; flu-like symptoms that accompany lesions also vary, as do the frequency and duration of outbreaks.

Transmission

- Patients are at the highest risk of transmitting HSV to their partner during the time an active lesion is present until complete healing takes place.
- Condoms are not a safe barrier for transmission if an active lesion is present.
- During the time when active lesions are present, engage in sexual activities that avoid contact with the lesions.
- When lesions are active, extreme caution needs to be taken to avoid transmission by contact with articles such as towels, washcloths, and razors. Good hand washing with soap and water helps prevent the spread of the virus.
- Prevent self-infection to other areas of the body by not touching the sores and using good hand washing.
- It is a myth that if one person has herpes, so does his or her partner.

Outbreaks

- Be aware of events that can trigger a repeated outbreak: pregancny, menses, stress, fever, infectious illness
- For more information, use the Herpes Resource Center Hotline: 1-415-328-7710.

Help the patient understand that this is a minor problem with which he or she will be inconvenienced from time to time. Adherence to strict guidelines when active lesions are present allows the patient to have a normal sexual relationship. Healthcare workers with active herpes are prohibited from working with immunosuppressed patients or in a nursery setting because of the complications that result in the neonate if HSV transmission occurs.

DOCUMENTATION GUIDELINES

- Appearance, location, and number of lesions; drainage from lesions
- Presence of flu-like symptoms that accompany outbreaks
- Patient's knowledge of cause, treatment, and prevention of HSV
- Patient's reaction to the diagnosis of an STD

DISCHARGE AND HOME HEALTHCARE GUIDELINES

Be sure the patient understands the correct dosage, route, and time of the medication, as well as the importance of taking all prescribed medication, even if the symptoms subside. Review events that trigger outbreaks; emphasize the importance of avoiding contact with the lesion in preventing transmission. Teach the female patient that a potential long-term complication is the development of cervical cancer; yearly Papanicolaou tests are critical.

Herpes Zoster (Shingles)

DRG Category: 272
Mean LOS: 6.3 days
Description: MEDICAL: Major Skin Disorders with CC

Herpes zoster, also known as shingles, is a common viral skin eruption that is estimated to affect 300,000 persons a year in the United States. The virus causes acute unilateral inflammation of a dorsal root ganglion. Each nerve innervates a particular skin area on the body called a dermatome, which bends around the body in a pattern that has been mapped corresponding to the vertebral source. Generally, herpes zoster eruptions occur in the thoracic region and less commonly affect a single cervical, facial (trigeminal nerve), lumbar, or sacral ganglion.

Most patients recover completely, but approximately 12% experience complications that include post-herpetic neuralgia, uveitis, motor deficits, infection, and systemic involvement such as meningoencephalitis, pneumonia, deafness, or widespread dissemination. In some patients the scars are permanent.

CAUSES

The varicella zoster virus (VZV), which causes chickenpox, remains dormant in a nerve ganglion and may be reactivated later in life. A decrease in cellular immunity may allow the latent virus to become active and spread along the nerve, resulting in clinical zoster. Conditions that are associated with reactivation include acute systemic illness, acquired immunodeficiency syndrome (AIDS), lymphoma, Hodgkin's disease, lupus erythematosus, and situations in conjunction with immunosuppressive therapy such as steroids or antineoplastic drugs.

GENDER AND LIFE SPAN CONSIDERATIONS

Herpes zoster can occur at any age, in both genders, although it is uncommon in healthy children or young adults. Prevalence doubles in patients over the age of 50. It is hypothesized that 50% of all people who live to the age of 85 will have an attack, and that 10% may suffer from more than one occurrence.

◻ ASSESSMENT

HISTORY. Generally patients will describe a history of itching, numbness, tingling, tenderness, and pain in the affected area for 1 to 2 days before skin lesions develop. The rash begins as maculopapules (discolored patches on the skin mixed with elevated red pimples) that rapidly develop into crops of vesicles (blisters) on an erythematous (diffuse redness) base. New lesions continue to appear for 3 to 5 days as the older lesions ulcerate and crust. Malaise, low-grade fever, and adenopathy may accompany the rash. The patient will report a history of chickenpox.

PHYSICAL EXAMINATION. Observe the rash, noting the color, temperature, and appearance of lesions and their location and distribution over the body. Note lesion grouping, and identify the type. The involved skin may reveal redness, warmth, swelling, vesicles, or crusted areas. This area is generally tender to touch. Determine if lesions are present in the patient's mouth.

The appearance of the lesions changes over time. The initial maculopapules and blisters may evolve in 10 days to scabbed dry blisters and in 2 weeks to small, red nodular skin lesions spread around the area of the dermatome. The patient usually experiences intermittent or continuous pain for up to 4 weeks, although, in rare situations, intractable neurological pain may persist for years.

PSYCHOSOCIAL. Assess the patient's ability to cope with a sudden, unexpected illness that is generally very painful. Assess the amount of pain and degree of relief obtained. Some patients with facial palsy or visible skin lesions may have an altered body image that may cause anxiety.

DIAGNOSTIC HIGHLIGHTS

Test	Normal Result	Abnormality with Condition	Explanation
Viral culture	Negative culture	Positive for herpes zoster	Demonstrates presence of viruses in an active lesion; cultures are most accurate in first several days of ulceration

PRIMARY NURSING DIAGNOSIS

Pain (acute or chronic) related to nerve root inflammation and skin lesions

OUTCOMES. Comfort level; Pain control behavior; Pain level; Symptom severity

INTERVENTIONS. Analgesic administration; Anxiety reduction; Environmental management: Comfort; Pain management; Medication management

☐ PLANNING AND IMPLEMENTATION

Collaborative

The goals of therapy are to dry the lesions, relieve pain, and prevent secondary complications. These goals are met primarily through pharmacologic therapy. A wet-to-dry compress application of a Burow's solution (aluminum acetate) three to four times a day will help dry the lesions.

PHARMACOLOGIC HIGHLIGHTS

General Comments: Antihistamines may help with itching. Pain relief may vary—from the use of mild analgesics (such as aspirin or acetaminophen) to mild opiates (such as codeine) if the pain is excruciating. Nighttime sedation also may be helpful. Topical lidocaine sprays can be used to provide analgesia. The use of systemic corticosteriods appears to decrease the severity of post-herpetic neuralgia pain. Early corticosteroid therapy for 7 to 10 days can both shorten the duration of pain and prevent its chronic reoccurrence.

Medication or Drug Class	Dosage	Description	Rationale
Valacyclovir (Valtrex)	1 g tid for 7 days	Anti-viral	Treats herpes zoster; most effective if given in the first 48 hours of onset of rash
Capaicin (zostrix)	Topical cream applied directly to area of discomfort tid to qid	Topical analgesic	Treats neuralgia after shingles; avoid contact with broken skin

Independent

Normally, the only patients treated in the hospital for a herpes zoster infection are those with a primary disease that leads to immunosuppression and can place them at risk for shingles. The most important nursing intervention focuses on prevention of complications. Monitor for signs and symptoms of infection. Since involvement of the ophthalmic branch of the trigeminal nerve may result in conjunctivitis and possible blindness, be alert for lesions in the eye, and refer the patient to an ophthalmologist. Patients with involvement of sacral dermatomes may have changes in patterns of urinary elimination from acute urinary retention. Monitor intake and output to identify this complication.

Pain may be reduced by splinting the affected area with a snug wrap of nonadherent dressings and covering with an elastic bandage. Manage malaise and elevated temperature with bed rest and a quiet environment. Encourage diversionary activities and teach relaxation techniques to help the patient manage pain without medication. If oral lesions are painful, encourage use of a soft toothbrush and swishing and rinsing every 2 hours with a mouthwash based on a normal saline solution. A soft diet may be necessary during periods of painful oral lesions.

Discuss communicability of the disease. Although herpes zoster is not itself infectious, the patient can transmit chickenpox to those who have not had it or to those people who are immunocompromised.

DOCUMENTATION GUIDELINES

- Physical findings of rash: Vesicles, redness, and location; degree of healing
- Response to pain medications, rest, relaxation
- Presence of complications: Infection, involvement of eyes, urinary retention, central nervous system symptoms

DISCHARGE AND HOME HEALTHCARE GUIDELINES

PREVENTION. Explain that there is no means for eliminating the varicella virus from the nerve ganglia. (A varicella vaccine, however, is currently under development and may help with prevention of primary chickenpox and therefore might help with decreasing the incidences of herpes zoster.)

MEDICATIONS. Be sure the patient understands all medications, including the dosage, route, action, and adverse effects.

COMPLICATIONS. Instruct the patient to report redness, swelling, or drainage of the rash to the primary healthcare provider.

Hodgkin's Disease

DRG Category: 403
Mean LOS: 7.4 days
Description: MEDICAL: Lymphoma and Non-Acute Leukemia with CC
DRG Category: 401
Mean LOS: 9.2 days
Description: SURGICAL: Lymphoma and Non-Acute Leukemia with Other O.R. Procedures with CC

Hodgkin's disease, a neoplastic disorder, is characterized by painless, progressive enlargement of the lymph nodes, spleen, and other lymphoid tissue. The enlargement is caused by a proliferation of lymphocytes, histiocytes, eosinophils, and Reed-Sternberg giant cells, the cells that characterize Hodgkin's disease; their presence classifies a lymphoma as Hodgkin's, and their absence classifies a lymphoma as non-Hodgkin's. Hodgkin's is a progressive and fatal disease if not treated but is one of the most curable neoplastic diseases with treatment. The 1-year survival rate with treatment is 93%, and the 5-year survival rate is 82%. At 15 years the overall survival rate is 63%.

CAUSES

The cause of Hodgkin's disease is unknown. Many researchers have suspected an infectious component. Some of the early symptoms include fever, chills, and leukocytosis, as if a viral infection were present. Gene fragments similar to those of a murine leukemia virus have been found in Hodgkin's tissue. In particular, higher than usual Epstein-Barr antibodies have been found in many Hodgkin's patients, and a small increase in Hodgkin's incidence has been found in people who have had the Epstein-Barr-induced disease, infectious mononucleosis.

Some people who have reduced immune systems, such as those with AIDS, and organ transplant patients, are also at a higher risk for Hodgkin's disease.

GENDER AND LIFE SPAN CONSIDERATIONS

Hodgkin's disease tends to strike in young adulthood from the ages of 15 to 38 and is more common in men than in women. There is also a bimodal incidence, with the first major peak being in young adults and the second peak later in life after age 50. Elderly people tend to have a more advanced disease at diagnosis and a worse prognosis for cure.

☐ ASSESSMENT

HISTORY. Many patients present with asymptomatic peripheral adenopathy. Because there are numerous causes for enlarged lymph nodes, it is important to elicit information about recent infections, allergic reactions, and other events. In Hodgkin's, the nodes tend to be cervical, supraclavicular, and mediastinal. About 40% of patients report fever, night sweats, and recent weight loss, collectively called B symptoms. Less commonly, they may report pruritus during any stage. (See Table 27.) Because the B symptoms are necessary for staging, it is important to elicit that information in the history.

TABLE 27 | **Staging for Hodgkin's Lymphoma**

STAGES AND SUBCLASSIFICATIONS	DESCRIPTION	5-YEAR SURVIVAL RATE BASED ON STAGE
Stage I	Localized to a single lymph node or nodal group	90%–95%
Stage II	More than one nodal group on the same side of the diaphragm	90%–95%
Stage III	More than one nodal group on both sides of the diaphragm	85%–90%
Stage IV	Spread to organs other than lymph nodes or spleen	Approximately 80%
Subclassification	A: Asymptomatic B: Fevers, weight loss, night sweats are present E: Extra-lymphatic involvement such as stomach, small intestine S: Spleen involvement	

PHYSICAL EXAMINATION. During advanced phases of the disease, the patient may have edema of the face and neck, weight loss, and jaundice. Palpate all lymph node chains, including the submental, infraclavicular, epitrochlear, iliac, femoral, and popliteal nodes. Involved nodes are characteristically painless, firm, rubbery in consistency (unlike the rock-hard nodes of carcinoma), freely movable, and of varying size. Palpate the liver and spleen, which may be enlarged.

PSYCHOSOCIAL. The diagnosis of a neoplastic disorder in young adulthood is a devastating event for the patient and significant others. Rather than pursuing educational goals, job obligations, social interactions, or parenting responsibilities, the young adult is suddenly managing a potentially terminal disease. Although the disease is treatable in most cases, the patient needs to manage short- and long-term complications of therapy that may profoundly alter the patient's body image. Infertility in young adults after treatment may affect the patient's view of himself or herself and the long-term potential for the desired role of parenthood.

DIAGNOSTIC HIGHLIGHTS

Test	Normal Result	Abnormality with Condition	Explanation
Lymph node biopsy or bone marrow biopsy	Normal cells	Positive for Hodgkin's lymphoma cells (Reed-Sternberg giant cells)	Determines extent of disease and allows for staging of disease; bone marrow biopsy is generally done only for patients with anemia or fever and night sweats
Computed tomography (CT) scan or magnetic resonance imaging (MRI) of chest, abdomen, and pelvis	Normal structures	Spread of Hodgkin's lymphoma into organs and body cavities	Assists with staging; common sites of extralymphatic involvement include spleen, stomach, small intestine; combined with lymphangiography, can predict nodal involvement in 90% of cases
Lymphangiography, a radiographic test of lymphatic vessels and nodes; radiopaque iodine contrast medium is injected into lymphatics of foot or hand	Normal lymphatic system	Identification of structural abnormalities or tumor involvement	Test has been replaced in many situations by CT scanning but may still be used for staging; not usually performed in children

Other Tests: Complete blood cell count, chest x ray, erythrocyte sedimentation rate; tests for liver and renal function, including lactate dehydrogenase, alkaline phosphatase, blood urea nitrogen, and creatinine.

PRIMARY NURSING DIAGNOSIS

Risk for infection related to impaired primary and secondary defenses

OUTCOMES. Immune status; Knowledge: Infection control; Risk control; Risk detection; Nutritional status; Tissue integrity: Skin and mucous membranes; Treatment behavior: Illness or injury

INTERVENTIONS. Infection control; Infection protection; Surveillance; Nutritional management; Medication management; Teaching: Disease process

◻ PLANNING AND IMPLEMENTATION

Collaborative

Treatment begins with accurate classification and staging. Clinical staging is determined by initial biopsy, history, physical examination, and radiologic findings. Pathologic staging involves a more extensive surgical assessment of possible sites for spread. Due to continued improvement in radiologic staging, a staging laparotomy (thorough abdominal exploration, splenectomy, liver biopsy, bone marrow biopsy, and multiple lymph node samplings) is performed infrequently.

In general, radiation is used for early, less extensive disease. A combination of radiation and chemotherapy is used for stages IIB, IIIA, and B. Combination chemotherapy with drugs such as doxorubicin, bleomych, vinblastin, and dacarbazine (ABUD) is used for stage IV (see Pharmacologic Highlights). External beam radiation is the most effective single agent in the treatment of Hodgkin's disease and may be given after 3 to 4 courses of chemotherapy. Stages I and IIA Hodgkin's disease are routinely treated with external-beam radiation therapy. Mantle therapy (radiation to the chest wall, mediastinum, axilla, and neck—the region known as the mantle field) is done for supradiaphragmatic sites. Radiation-protective shields are used to block irradiation to unaffected areas. These shields are custom fit for each patient, based on his or her physical configurations. Surgery is not used as a treatment modality in Hodgkin's except in the role of staging. A dietary consultation may be needed to help the patient maintain weight and to help support healing.

If the disease does not respond to standard treatment, bone marrow transplantation may be offered, either as part of a clinical trial or outside of a clinical trial. The patient's own bone marrow is removed and stored. Then very high doses of chemotherapy, sometimes in combination with radiation therapy, are administered to eradicate the cancer. High doses also destroy bone marrow. The stored marrow is administered intravenously to the patient, and bone marrow cells enter the bloodstream and return to the bone. The transplanted marrow produces new red and white blood cells. In another type of transplant, peripheral blood stem cell transplant (PBSCT), only the stem cells (immature cells from which all blood cells develop) are removed and the rest of the blood is returned to the body. Stem cells are then frozen until they are returned to the patient after treatment is finished.

PHARMACOLOGIC HIGHLIGHTS

General Comments: Typically, chemotherapy is given in six or more cycles of treatment. Common side effects are alopecia, nausea, vomiting, fatigue, myelosuppression, and stomatitis. Patients who are receiving chemotherapy are administered antinausea drugs, antiemetics, and pain medicines as needed to help control adverse experiences.

Medication or Drug Class	Dosage	Description	Rationale
Chemotherapy	Varies with drug	Three common examples are ABVD, COPP, and MOPP.	Chemotherapy is used for stage IVA and all stage B patients; 6 or more cycles are used to combat stage IV disease

Note: ABVD refers to doxorubicin (Adriamycin), bleomycin, vinblastine, and dacarbazine. COPP refers to cyclophosphamide, vincristine (Oncovin), procarbazine, and prednisone. MOPP refers to mechlorethamine (nitrogen mustard), vincristine (Oncovin), procarbazine, and prednisone.

Independent

The primary nursing roles are to maintain comfort, protect the patient from infection, provide teaching and support about the complications of the treatment, and give emotional support. During mantle irradiation, the patient may suffer from a variety of uncomfortable or painful conditions. Dry mouth, loss of taste, dysphagia, nausea, and vomiting can be managed with frequent mouth care. Manage skin irritation and redness. Encourage the patient to avoid applying lotions, perfumes, deodorants, and powder to the treatment area. Explain that the skin must be protected from sunlight and extreme cold. Before starting treatments, arrange for the patient to have a wig, scarf, or hat to cover any hair loss, which occurs primarily at the nape of the neck. Explain to the patient that pneumonitis and hypothyroidism may occur; explain the signs and symptoms of each and when to notify the physician. During inverted-Y irradiation, nausea, vomiting, anorexia, diarrhea, and malaise require nursing management.

If the patient develops bone marrow suppression during hospitalization, make sure that all staff and visitors use good hand-washing techniques. Do not assign a nurse who is caring for infected patients. Encourage staff and visitors with infections to avoid all contact with the patient. If the patient receives chemotherapy, the side effects are equally uncomfortable. In addition to many of the symptoms that occur in response to radiation therapy (gastrointestinal symptoms, oral lesions, hair loss, bone marrow depression), the patient may develop joint pain, fever, fluid retention, and a labile emotional state (euphoria or depression) that need specific interventions based on their incidence and severity.

The disease presents severe emotional stressors to the patient and his or her significant others. The complexity of the diagnostic and staging process may make the patient feel lost in a crowd of specialists. It is important for the nurse to provide supportive continuity. Patience and repeated explanations are needed. Provide the patient with information about support groups, and refer the patient to either a clinical nurse specialist, support groups associated with the American or Canadian Cancer Society, or counselors.

DOCUMENTATION GUIDELINES

- Response to staging: Emotional and physical response to diagnostic testing, healing of incisions, signs of ineffective coping, response to diagnosis, ability to participate in planning treatment options, response of significant others
- Response to treatment: Effects of chemotherapy or radiation therapy, or both; response to treatment of symptoms, presence of complications (weight loss, infection, skin irritation)
- Emotional state: Effectiveness of coping, presence of depression, interest in group support or counseling, referrals made

DISCHARGE AND HOME HEALTHCARE GUIDELINES

Although they are cured of the disease, patients who survive Hodgkin's disease continue to have immune defects that persist throughout life. Defects include transiently depressed antibody production, decreased polymorphonuclear chemotaxis, decreased antigen-induced T-cell proliferation, and changes in delayed hypersensitivity. Coupled with the sometimes lingering aftereffects of radiation and chemotherapy, the patient needs to maintain infection vigilance even after remission is obtained. Teach the patient lifelong strategies to avoid infection.

Patients may have other complications for up to 25 years after mantle radiation therapy, including hypothyroidism, Graves' disease, and thyroid cancer. Irradiation can also cause pulmonary and pericardial fibrosis and coronary artery changes, and it may increase the risk for the development of solid tumors such as lung cancer, breast cancer, and others. Explain the presenting symptoms of the disorder, provide written information for the patient, and encourage yearly physicals to maintain follow-up. Because infertility may be a complication of chemotherapy, men may want to think of sperm banking before treatments, although many have sperm dysfunction at diagnosis.

Hydronephrosis

DRG Category: 323
Mean LOS: 2.9 days
Description: MEDICAL: Urinary Stones with CC and/or ESW Lithotripsy
DRG Category: 304'
Mean LOS: 8.7 days
Description: Kidney, Ureter, and Major Bladder Procedures; Nonneoplastic with CC

Hydronephrosis is the distension of the pelvis and calyces of one or both kidneys, resulting in thinning of the renal tubules because of obstructed urinary flow. When the obstruction is a stone or kink in one of the ureters, only one kidney is damaged. The obstruction causes backup, resulting in increased pressure in the kidneys. If the pressure is low to moderate, the kidney may dilate with no obvious loss of function.

Over time, intermittent or continuous high pressure causes irreversible nephron destruction. If the patient has a chronic partial obstruction, the kidneys lose their ability to concentrate urine. The kidneys may lose renal mass and atrophy and have a lowered resistance to infection and pyelonephritis because of urinary stasis. If hydronephrosis is caused by an acute obstructive uropathy (any disease of the urinary tract), the patient may develop a paralytic ileus. If bilateral hydronephrosis is left untreated, renal failure can result.

CAUSES

Any type of urinary obstruction can lead to hydronephrosis. The most common types of obstruction are caused by prostate hypertrophy (enlargement), renal calculi that form in the renal pelvis or drop into the ureter, or urethral strictures. Causes that are more unusual include structure of the ureter or bladder outlet, tumors pressing on the ureter, congenital abnormalities, blood clots, and a neurogenic bladder.

GENDER AND LIFE SPAN CONSIDERATIONS

Hydronephrosis can occur in patients of either gender, regardless of age. Men, especially elderly men, with prostate difficulties have a higher risk of hydronephrosis. Urinary tract obstruction is rare in children.

☐ ASSESSMENT

HISTORY. Elicit a careful history about urinary patterns to determine a history of burning sensations or abnormal color. The patient may be completely anuric (no urine flow) or experience polyuria (large urine output) or nocturia (excessive urination at night) because of a partial urinary obstruction. Determine any recent history of mild or severe renal or flank pain that radiates to the groin. Ask about vomiting, nausea, or abdominal fullness. Ask a male patient if he has had prostate difficulties. Establish any history of blood clots, bladder problems, or prior urinary difficulties. Some patients will report very mild or even no symptoms.

PHYSICAL EXAMINATION. Inspect the flank area for asymmetry, which indicates the presence of a renal mass. Inspect the male urethra for stenosis, injury, or phimosis (narrowing so that the foreskin cannot be pushed back over the glans penis). A genitourinary (GU) exam is performed in the female patient to inspect and palpate for vaginal, uterine, and rectal lesions. When the flank area is palpated, you may feel a large fluctuating soft mass in the kidney area that represents the collection of urine in the renal pelvis. Palpate the abdomen to help identify tender areas. If the hydronephrosis is the result of bladder obstruction, markedly distended urinary bladder may be felt. Gentle pressure on the urinary bladder may result in leaking urine from the urethra because of bladder overflow. Rectal examination may reveal enlargement of the prostate or renal or pelvic masses.

PSYCHOSOCIAL. Although hydronephrosis is a treatable condition, the patient is likely to be upset and anxious. Many find GU examinations embarrassing. Urinary catheterization can also be a stressful event, particularly if it is performed by someone of the opposite gender. If the patient's renal condition has been permanently affected, determine the patient's ability to cope with a serious chronic condition.

DIAGNOSTIC HIGHLIGHTS

Test	Normal Result	Abnormality with Condition	Explanation
Serum creatinine	0.5–1.2 mg/dL	< 2.0 mg/dL if renal damage has occurred	Decreased ability of glomerulus to filter creatinine leads to accumulation in the blood
Blood urea nitrogen	5–20 mg/dL	May be elevated	Urinary tract obstruction with diffusion of urea nitrogen back into bloodstream through renal tubules may occur
Urinalysis and culture	Minimal numbers of red and white blood	Urinary tract infection may occur with	Urinary retention may lead to infection

cells; no bacteria; clear urine with no occult blood and no protein.	presence of bacteria and abnormally increased numbers of red and white blood cells; colony counts as low as 100 to 10,000 bacteria/mL may indicate infection; bacteriuria: more than one organism per oil-immersion field; pyuria- more than eight leukocytes per high-power field

Other Tests: Serum electrolytes, intravenous pyelogram (IVP; excretory urogram), retrograde pyelogram, renal sonogram.

PRIMARY NURSING DIAGNOSIS

Risk for infection related to urinary stasis and instrumentation

OUTCOMES. Knowledge: Infection control; Risk control; Risk detection; Nutritional status; Tissue integrity: Skin and mucous membranes; Treatment behavior: Illness or injury

INTERVENTIONS. Infection control; Tube care: Urinary; Infection protection; Surveillance; Nutritional management; Medication management; Teaching: Disease process

☐ PLANNING AND IMPLEMENTATION

Collaborative

Temporary urinary drainage may be achieved by a nephrostomy or ureterostomy. Other options are ureteral, urethral, or suprapubic catheterization. When no infection is present, immediate surgery is not necessary even if there is complete obstruction and anuria. Many surgeons will wait until acid-base, fluid, and electrolyte balances are restored before operating. Surgery includes options such as prostatectomy for benign prostatic hypertrophy, tumor removal, and dilation of urethral strictures.

When bilateral complete urinary obstruction is relieved, the patient usually has massive polyuria and excessive natriuresis (sodium loss in the urine). In general, the physician will prescribe the replacement of two-thirds of the loss of urinary volume per day to be replaced by salt-containing intravenous solutions. Further expansion of the extracellular volume may sustain the diuresis. With impaired renal function, a diet low in sodium, potassium, and protein is often prescribed. Preoperative diet restrictions are sometimes used to limit the progression of renal failure before surgical removal of the obstruction.

The urinary drainage system requires close monitoring. Check the color, consistency, odor, and amount of urine hourly and as needed. Inspect the tube insertion site for signs of infection (purulent drainage, swelling, redness) and bleeding. If the tube is obstructed, follow the appropriate protocol for either irrigation or physician notification. Clamp the drainage tube only after specific discussion with the physician.

PHARMACOLOGIC HIGHLIGHTS

Medication or Drug Class	Dosage	Description	Rationale
Antibiotics	Varies with drug	Anti-infectives to manage bacterial infections. Examples: trimethoprim-sulfamethoxazole (Bactrim, Septra), ciprofloxacin hydrochloride (Cipro)	Treatmentbased on bacterial sensitivity, as well as the ability of the antibiotic to concentrate in yjr urinary system. Course of treatment is at least 1–4 weeks
Analgesics	Varies with drug	Acetaminophen; mild narcotics	Relieve pain

Independent

The patient requires careful fluid balance. Weigh the patient at the same time of day on the same scale with the same clothing. Elicit the patient's and family's support in maintaining an accurate record of fluid intake and output.

Pay particular attention to the patient's response to the illness. Respect the patient's privacy by isolating him or her from others during urinary drainage system insertion and insertion site care. Provide an honest appraisal of the patient's condition, and answer all questions. Note that both men and women link urinary functioning to sexual functioning. Be open to and supportive of the patient's fears of sexual dysfunction and provide accurate information.

Provide meticulous skin care. Request a consultation from the enterostomal nurse for unusual problems.

DOCUMENTATION GUIDELINES

- Physical changes: Abdominal pain, abdominal distension, bladder distension, signs of infection (painful urination, cloudy urine, fever, fatigue)
- Fluid balance: Daily weights, intake and output, description and appearance of urine
- Emotional response: Anxiety, coping, depression
- Presence of complications: Infection, urinary tract obstruction, electrolyte imbalance

DISCHARGE AND HOME HEALTHCARE GUIDELINES

PREVENTION. Teach the importance of adequate fluids. Explain the importance of notifying the physician at the first signs of inability to void or of urinary infection, such as burning or painful urination, cloudy urine, rusty or smoky urine, blood-tinged urine, foul odor, flank pain, or fever.

MEDICATIONS. Be sure the patient, family, or other caregiver understands all medications, including the dosage, route, action, and adverse effects. Encourage the patient to take the entire course of antibiotics as prescribed.

CARE OF INDWELLING CATHETERS. Teach the patient, family, or other caregiver how to drain a Foley catheter or nephrostomy tube and to examine the insertion site for infection. Encourage older male patients with a family history of benign prostatic hypertrophy or prostatitis to have annual medical checkups.

Hypercalcemia

DRG Category: 296
Mean LOS: 5.4 days
Description: MEDICAL: Nutritional and Miscellaneous Metabolic Disorders, Age > 17 with CC

Hypercalcemia occurs with a serum calcium level above 10.5 mg/dL in the bloodstream. It develops when an influx of calcium into the circulation overwhelms the calcium regulatory hormones (parathyroid hormone [PTH] and metabolites of vitamin D) and renal calciuric mechanisms or when there is a primary abnormality of one or both of these hormones.

Calcium is vital to the body for the formation of bones and teeth, blood coagulation, nerve impulse transmission, cell permeability, and normal muscle contraction. Although 99% of the body's calcium is found in the bones, three forms of serum calcium exist: free or ionized calcium, calcium bound to protein (primarily albumin), and calcium complexed with citrate or other organic ions. Ionized calcium is resorbed into bone, absorbed from the gastrointestinal (GI) mucosa, and excreted in urine and feces as regulated by the parathyroid glands. When extracellular calcium levels rise, a sedative effect occurs within the body, causing the neuromuscular excitability of cardiac and smooth muscles to decrease and impairing renal function. The calcium precipitates to a salt, causing calculi to form, and this leads to diuresis and volume depletion.

At levels above 13 mg/dL, renal failure and soft-tissue calcification may occur. Hypercalcemic crisis exists when the serum level reaches 15 mg/dL. Serious cardiac dysrhythmias and hypokalemia can result as the body wastes potassium in preference to calcium. Hypercalcemia at this level can cause coma and cardiac arrest. It is considered to be a serious electrolyte imbalance, with a mortality rate as high as 50% when not treated quickly.

CAUSES

More than 90% of cases of hypercalcemia result from primary hyperparathyroidism or malignancy. Malignancies likely to cause hypercalcemia include squamous cell carcinoma of the lung; cancer of the breast, ovaries, prostate, bladder, kidney, neck, and head; leukemia; lymphoma; and multiple myeloma. These conditions raise serum calcium levels by destroying bone or by releasing PTH or a PTH-like substance (osteoclastic-activating factor), or prostaglandins. Other causes of hypercalcemia are vitamin D toxicity, the use of thiazide diuretics or lithium, sarcoidosis, immobilization, renal failure, excessive administration of calcium during cardiopulmonary arrest, and metabolic acidosis.

GENDER AND LIFE SPAN CONSIDERATIONS

Hypercalcemia can occur in any age group and in both sexes. In infants, it can be caused by ingestion of large amounts of chicken liver or vitamin D or vitamin A supplements. Children and adolescents who consume large amounts of calcium-rich foods and drinks may develop hypercalcemia. Paget's disease, which causes increased bone turnover, leads to hypercalcemia in elderly people who are immobilized. Primary hyperparathyroidism causes most cases of hypercalcemia in people who are ambulatory and is more common in elderly women than in elderly men. Nearly 85% of cases result from an adenoma of a single parathyroid gland.

☐ ASSESSMENT

HISTORY. Determine a history of risk factors, with a particular focus on medications. Establish a history of anorexia, nausea, vomiting, constipation, polyuria, or polydipsia. Ask about muscular weakness or digital and perioral paresthesia (tingling) and muscle cramps. Ask family members if the patient has manifested personality changes.

PHYSICAL EXAMINATION. The signs and symptoms are directly related to the serum calcium level. In some patients, hypercalcemia is discovered upon routine physical examination. Evaluate the patient's neuromuscular status for muscle weakness, hypoflexia, and decreased muscle tone. Observe for signs of confusion. Hypercalcemia slows GI transit time; therefore, assess the patient for abdominal distension, hypoactive bowel sounds, and paralytic ileus. Strain the urine for renal calculi. Assess for fluid volume deficit by checking skin turgor and mucous membranes. Auscultate the apical pulse to determine heart irregularities.

PSYCHOSOCIAL. Increased calcium in the cerebrinospinal fluid may result in behavior changes. The symptoms can range from slight personality changes to the manifestations of psychosis. They may include mental confusion, impaired memory, slurred speech, or hallucinations. Assess the patient's mental status and the family's response to alterations in it.

DIAGNOSTIC HIGHLIGHTS

Test	Normal Result	Abnormality with Condition	Explanation
Serum calcium: total calcium including free ionized calcium and calcium bound with protein or organic ions	8.6–10.3 mg/dL	> 10.5 mg/dL	Accumulation of calcium above normal levels in the extracellular fluid compartment; clinical manifestations generally occur when calcium levels are above 12 mg/dL and tend to be more severe if hypercalcemia develops rapidly
Serum ionized calcium: unbound calcium; level unaffected by albumin level	4.5–5.1 mg/dL	> 5.5 mg/dL	Ionized calcium is approximately 46%–50% of circulating calcium and is the form of calcium available for enzymatic

			reactions and neuromuscular function; levels increase and decrease with blood pH levels; for every 0.1 pH decrease ionized calcium increases 1.5%–2.5%
Serum parathyroid hormone level	10–65 pg/mL	Elevated in more than 90% of people with primary hyperparathy- roidism	Determines presence of hyperparathyroidism

Other Tests: Electrocardiogram (shortened QT interval), urine calcium clearance.

PRIMARY NURSING DIAGNOSIS

Risk for injury related to bone demineralization and confusion

OUTCOMES. Fluid balance; Electrolyte/acid-base balance; Risk control; Safety behavior: Fall prevention; Knowledge: Personal safety; Safety status: Fall occurrence and physical injury; Symptom control behavior; Knowledge: Medications; Mobility level; Neurological status: Consciousness

INTERVENTIONS. Electrolyte management: Hypercalcemia; Medication management; Medication administration; Fall prevention; Environmental management: Safety; Fluid/electrolyte monitoring; Fluid/electrolyte management; Neurologic monitoring; Exercise promotion

☐ PLANNING AND IMPLEMENTATION

Collaborative

The goals of treatment are to reduce the serum calcium level and to identify and correct the underlying cause. Conservative measures include administering fluids to restore volume and enhance renal excretion of calcium; prescribing a low-calcium diet; eliminating calcium-containing medications (calcium supplements, calcium-containing antacids) or medications that impair calcium excretion (thiazide diuretics, lithium); and, when possible, keeping active.

In severe cases of hypercalcemia, administer large volumes of normal saline (0.9% NaCl) at a rate of 300 to 500 mL per hour until the extracellular volume is restored (usually 3 to 4 L in the first 24 hours), at which time the rate is slowed and the infusion is maintained to promote renal calcium excretion. The physician may prescribe furosemide with the saline infusion, which helps prevent fluid volume overload. Monitor for signs of congestive heart failure in patients who are receiving 0.9% NaCl solution diuresis therapy. If hypercalcemia is the result of a malignancy, then surgery, chemotherapy, or radiation may be used.

PHARMACOLOGIC HIGHLIGHTS

Medication or Drug Class	Dosage	Description	Rationale
Furosemide (Lasix)	20–40 mg IV bid qid	Loop diuretic	Used with saline diuresis when clinical evidence of heart failure occurs
Pamidronate	60 mg in 500 mL of 0.9% saline infused as single dose over 4 hours; for severe hypercalcemia (>13.5 mg/dL) dose may be increased to 90 mg in 1000 ml 0.9% saline over 24 hours	Hypocalcemic; biphosphonate	Reduces calcium levels by decreasing phosphate release from bone and increasing calcium excretion by kidneys; response begins in 2 days with peak response in 7 days
Calcitonin	4–8 IU/kg IM or sq q 6–12 hours	Calcium regulator	Inhibits bone resorption and increase renal calcium excretion; lowers calcium 1–3 mg/dL within several hours, but hypocalcemic effect wanes after several days
Mithramycin	25 μg/kg in 500 mL D5W	Bone resorption inhibitor	Inhibits the action of PTH on the osteoclasts, resulting in decreased bone demineralization and serum calcium levels; second-line agent in malignant hypercalcemia

Other Drugs: Bulk laxatives and stool softeners; loop rather than thiazide diuretics; glucocorticoids such as prednisone (inhibit serum calcium by inhibiting cytokine release, inhibiting intestinal calcium absorption, and increasing urinary calcium excretion).

Independent

Encourage sufficient fluid intake. Encourage ambulation as soon as possible and as frequently as allowed, being sure to handle the patient carefully to prevent fractures. Reposition bedridden patients frequently, and encourage range-of-motion exercises to promote circulation and prevent urinary stasis, as well as calcium loss from bone. Choose fluids containing sodium, unless contraindicated. Discourage a high intake of calcium-rich foods and fluids, and provide adequate bulk in the diet to help prevent constipation. If confusion or other mental symptoms occur, institute safety precautions as necessary. Orient the patient frequently, and design a safe environment to prevent falls.

DOCUMENTATION GUIDELINES

- Current mental status
- Physical findings: Skin turgor and appearance of mucous membranes, presence or absence of bowel sounds, presence or absence of renal calculi
- Response to pain medications
- Tolerance of activity

DISCHARGE AND HOME HEALTHCARE GUIDELINES

Encourage ambulation and a fluid intake of 3 to 4 L of fluid per day, including acid-ash juices (e.g., cranberry juice). Explain the importance of avoiding excessive amounts of calcium-rich foods and calcium-containing medications. Caution the patient against taking large doses of vitamin D. Be sure the patient understands any medication prescribed, including dosage, route, action, and side effects. Remind the patient to report to the physician the appearance of any symptoms of flank pain, hematuria, palpitations, or irregular pulse.

Hyperchloremia

DRG Category: 296
Mean LOS: 5.4 days
Description: MEDICAL: Nutritional and Miscellaneous Metabolic Disorders, Age > 17 without CC

Serum chloride excess, hyperchloremia, occurs when the serum chloride level is greater than 108 mEq/L. Normal serum chloride level is 95 to 108 mEq/L. Chloride is the major anion in extracellular fluid (ECF). Chloride is regulated in the body primarily through its relationship with sodium. Serum levels of both sodium and chloride often parallel each other.

Chloride performs a number of essential physiologic functions. One is to join with hydrogen to form hydrochloric acid (HCl), which aids in digestion and activates enzymes, such as salivary amylase. Chloride also plays a role in maintaining the serum osmolarity and the body's water balance. The normal serum osmolarity ranges from 280 to 295 mOsm/L. Hyperchloremia, like hypernatremia, causes an increase in the serum osmolarity (the proportion of sodium and chloride ions to water in the ECF). Chloride influences the acid-base balance as well. To maintain acid-base balance, the kidneys excrete chloride or bicarbonate. Each sodium ion that is reabsorbed in the renal tubules reabsorbs either a chloride or a bicarbonate ion, depending on the acid-base balance of the ECF. In metabolic acidosis the kidney excretes chloride in exchange for bicarbonate.

CAUSES

The most common cause of hyperchloremia is body fluid loss, or dehydration, which leads to renal retention of water. Other causes are changes in hormones, trauma, and acid-base imbalances (hyperchloremic acidosis). Excessive levels of adrenal cortical hormones can cause excess sodium levels, and thereby chloride, in the body. In head-injured patients, sodium is frequently retained and thus chloride is also retained. Additionally, hyperchloremia can be caused by any condition that allows for excessive chloride intake or absorption.

GENDER AND LIFE SPAN CONSIDERATIONS

Infants, young children, and elderly people of both sexes are at particular risk since they are prone to dehydration.

☐ ASSESSMENT

HISTORY. Ask the patient about factors that could cause hyperchloremia, such as severe dehydration, a recent head injury, or taking adrenal corticosteroids. Be aware that thought processes may be affected, so that self-reported information may not be totally accurate. Ask about all of the patient's medications, past illnesses and surgeries, and any recent signs and symptoms that deviate from past health patterns.

PHYSICAL EXAMINATION. Physical findings depend on the source of the chloride imbalance. Assess the patient's respiratory status. If the hyperchloremia is associated with metabolic acidosis, the patient may have rapid, deep respirations. Dyspnea and pitting edema may be present with excess ECF volume. Tachycardia and hypertension may also be noted. Perform a thorough neurological assessment and note that patients may experience weakness, cognitive changes, and, if the condition is severe, mental status deterioration and loss of consciousness. Since most patients who have hyperchloremia also have hypernatremia, assess for signs and symptoms that are associated with this imbalance, including restlessness, agitation, irritability, muscle twitching, hyperreflexia, and seizures.

PSYCHOSOCIAL. Assess the patient's and family's knowledge and understanding of dehydration to prevent future episodes. In the trauma patient, assess the patient's and family's ability to cope with a head injury, and assist him or her to understand the effects of head injury on fluid and electrolyte regulation. Patients on steroids often have to deal with many changes, such as fluid retention. Assess the patient's knowledge regarding steroid use.

DIAGNOSTIC HIGHLIGHTS

Test	Normal Result	Abnormality with Condition	Explanation
Serum chloride	95–108 mEq/L	> 108 mEq/L	Reflects an excess of chloride
Serum osmolarity	280–295 mOsm/L	> 295 mOsm/L	Reflects increased concentration of particles in extracellular fluid

Other Tests: Serum bicarbonate.

PRIMARY NURSING DIAGNOSIS

Fluid volume deficit related to water loss and dehydration

OUTCOMES. Fluid balance; Electrolyte and acid-base balance; Hydration; Nutritional status: Food and fluid intake; Knowledge: Treatment regimen; Knowledge: Medication

INTERVENTIONS. Electrolyte management; Intravenous therapy; Electrolyte monitoring; Surveillance; Venous access device maintenance; Medication management; Nutrition management

☐ PLANNING AND IMPLEMENTATION

Collaborative

Report any serum chloride levels greater than 108 mEq/L, and observe the patient for increases in serum potassium and sodium levels. Note any decrease in serum bicarbonate level, which indicates metabolic acidosis.

Severe hyperchloremia secondary to hypernatremia because of dehydration may require an intravenous (IV) solution of hypotonic saline, such as 0.45% sodium chloride (one-half normal saline). Infuse the solution cautiously because rapid infusion can cause a rapid shift of water into the cerebral cells, creating cerebral edema and the risk of death. Patients with hyperchloremia from metabolic acidosis may receive IV sodium bicarbonate; monitor them closely for overcorrection (metabolic alkalosis and respiratory depression). Dietary changes are seldom necessary; however, for severe conditions, a low-sodium diet prevents further accumulation of chloride and sodium.

PHARMACOLOGIC HIGHLIGHTS

Medication or Drug Class	Dosage	Description	Rationale
Sodium bicarbonate	IV 2–5 mEq/kg over 4–8 hours	Alkalinizing agent	Corrects metabolic acidosis; dosage is guided by laboratory values

Independent

Maintain safety measures for patients who develop neuromuscular weakness or lethargy. If the patient's mental status is affected, initiate strategies to maintain an adequate airway, breathing, and circulation. Guard the patient's airway by positioning the patient on his or her side, and keep the patient's mouth free of secretions. If you suspect airway compromise, insert an oral or nasal airway; if airway compromise is accompanied by impaired breathing, notify the physician immediately and prepare for endotracheal intubation.

DOCUMENTATION GUIDELINES

- Laboratory findings: Serum electrolytes, osmolarity; daily flowsheet for easy day-to-day comparisons
- Physical responses: Respiratory status (rate, quality, depth, ease, breath sounds); vital signs with any tachycardia or hypertension; muscle strength, steadiness of gait, ability to perform activities of daily living; fluid balance, intake and output

- Nutrition: Tolerance for dietary restrictions, interest in and understanding of diet teaching

DISCHARGE AND HOME HEALTHCARE GUIDELINES

Educate about the effect of dehydration on chloride levels. Teach the patient to report any signs and symptoms of neuromuscular weakness or changes in body weight in 1 week to the primary healthcare provider. Teach the patient to maintain a healthy diet with all the components of adequate nutrition. Teach the patient the name, dosage, route, action, and side effects of all medications, particularly those that affect chloride and sodium balance in the body.

Hyperglycemia

DRG Category: 463
Mean LOS: 4.5 days
Description: MEDICAL: Signs and Symptoms with CC

Hyperglycemia exists when the blood glucose level is greater than 110 mg/dL. Normal blood glucose levels can be maintained between 70 and 110 mg/dL when there is an adequate balance between insulin supply and demand. In acutely ill individuals, hyperglycemia is usually not diagnosed until a random test of serum glucose level shows an increase above the 150 to 200 mg/dL range. Glucose is the most important carbohydrate in body metabolism. It is formed from the breakdown of polysaccharides, especially starch, and is absorbed from the intestines into the blood of the portal vein. As it passes through the liver, glucose is converted into glycogen for storage, but the body maintains a blood level for tissue needs.

Insulin is produced by the beta cells of the pancreas, which are stimulated to release it when the blood glucose level rises. Insulin transports glucose, amino acids, potassium, and phosphate across the cell membrane. Insufficient production or ineffective use of insulin causes an elevated blood glucose level (hyperglycemia), which promotes water movement into the bloodstream from the interstitial space and intracellular fluid compartments. As blood glucose levels increase, the renal threshold for glucose reabsorption is exceeded, and glycosuria (loss of glucose in the urine) occurs. Glucose in the urine acts as an osmotic diuretic, and the patient has an increased urinary output in response that can lead to a serious fluid volume deficit. As glucose levels climb, the blood becomes more viscous and the patient is also at risk for thromboembolic phenomena.

CAUSES

The two primary causes of hyperglycemia are diabetes mellitus and hyperosmolar nonketotic syndrome (HNKS). Other conditions that can lead to hyperglycemia include glucocorticoid imbalances (Cushing's syndrome), increased epinephrine levels during times of extreme stress (multiple trauma, surgery), excess growth hormone secretion, excessive ingestion or administration of glucose by total parenteral nutrition or enteral feedings, and pregnancy.

GENDER AND LIFE SPAN CONSIDERATIONS

Children and young adults of both sexes who are at risk for insulin-dependent diabetes mellitus are between the ages of 6 months and 30 years, whereas adults older than 35 are more at risk for non-insulin-dependent diabetes mellitus. Elderly people are at highest risk for HNKS.

▢ ASSESSMENT

HISTORY. Ascertain if the patient has any disorders that are risk factors for hyperglycemia. Elicit a complete medication history, focusing on whether the patient has ever taken insulin or oral antidiabetic medications. Ask about polyuria (excessive urination) and polydypsia (excessive thirst). Because it is common to have large amounts of dilute urine, ask if the patient has noted a larger urinary output than usual and if the color was light yellow or clear.

PHYSICAL EXAMINATION. The patient may not have any symptoms unless the blood glucose level has increased high enough to cause fluid volume deficit and dehydration. Perform a complete head-to-toe assessment, including a neurological examination. Patients with severe hyperglycemia also have an increased serum osmolarity (higher concentration of particles than water in the blood); when it goes above 300 mOsm/L, osmolarity causes decreased mental status. Assess the patient's level of consciousness and the cough and gag reflexes.

Inspect for signs of dehydration: dry mucous membranes, poor skin turgor, and dry scaly skin. Press gently on the patient's eyeballs; they may feel soft rather than firm. The patient's vital signs may reveal hypotension from fluid loss and tachycardia. If the dehydration has occurred for several days, the patient may have warm skin and an elevated temperature. In spite of the state of dehydration, the urine may not appear concentrated.

PSYCHOSOCIAL ASSESSMENT. Ask about the home environment, occupation, knowledge level, financial situation, and support systems, which may provide information that can be used to prevent future episodes. Determine the patient's and significant other's social, economic, and interpersonal resources to help manage a potentially chronic condition such as diabetes mellitus.

DIAGNOSTIC HIGHLIGHTS

Test	Normal Result	Abnormality with Condition	Explanation
Serum glucose level (fasting)	65–110 mg/dL	> 110 mg/dL	Elevation of glucose resulting from insulin deficit, insulin resistance, or pancreatic disease; fasting serum glucose of > 126 mg/dL is an indication of possible diabetes mellitus
Serum osmolarity	280–295 mOsm/L	> 295 mOsm/L	Reflects increased concentration of particles in extracellular fluid

Other Tests: Complete blood count, sodium bicarbonate, blood urea nitrogen, urine glucose and acetone.

PRIMARY NURSING DIAGNOSIS

Fluid volume deficit related to excess urinary output

OUTCOMES. Fluid balance; Nutritional status: Food and fluid intake; Circulation status; Hydration; Knowledge: Medication

INTERVENTIONS. Medication management; Hyperglycemia management; Nutrition management; Electrolyte management; Electrolyte monitoring; Fluid resuscitation; Intravenous therapy

☐ PLANNING AND IMPLEMENTATION

Collaborative

In patients with extreme physiologic stress, such as thermal injuries, multiple trauma, or shock, a serum glucose of approximately 200 to 250 mg/dL is expected, considering the release of epinephrine that accompanies the stress response. No treatment is needed because the healthcare team usually prefers the patient to be mildly hyperglycemic rather than hypoglycemic, which can have detrimental effects on the patient's outcome.

If the serum glucose level is above 250 mg/dL and the fluid balance is adequate, insulin is usually prescribed either as a subcutaneous (SQ) injection or as an intravenous (IV) push injection. Often patients are placed on a "sliding scale" of insulin every 6 hours. If a patient has an elevated serum glucose along with a fluid volume deficit, the fluid volume deficit is corrected first, often with normal saline solution (0.9% sodium chloride), before the glucose excess. If glucose is reduced on a fluid volume–depleted patient before volume resuscitation, the vascular volume decreases and the patient can develop hypovolemic shock.

If the patient has hyperglycemia because of diabetes mellitus or HNKS, management is based on the severity of his or her symptoms. Because HNKS is associated with extraordinarily high levels of glucose (some reports describe levels higher than 1000 mg/dL), the patient usually requires volume resuscitation followed by an insulin infusion. Often patients receive intermittent SQ or IV doses of insulin as well. This should be done cautiously, however, because if the serum glucose level is reduced too rapidly, fluid shifts into the central nervous system, leading to cerebral edema and death. No matter what the diagnosis, once the glucose level and the patient are stabilized, a full workup to determine the cause and long-term treatment is needed to prevent recurrences of hyperglycemia.

PHARMACOLOGIC HIGHLIGHTS

Medication or Drug Class	Dosage	Description	Rationale
Insulin	Varies with severity of disease; adjusted to maintain blood glucose of 80–140 mg/dL	Hormone; hypoglycemic	Replaces deficient or absent levels of insulin

Independent

The first priority is to maintain adequate fluid balance. The action of glucose as an osmotic diuretic places the patient at risk for severe fluid volume deficits. If he or she is awake, encourage the patient to drink water and sugar-free drinks without caffeine. Because patients are usually tachycardic, caffeinated beverages are contraindicated. Because severe hyperglycemia is accompanied by increased serum osmolarity and accompanying decreases in mental status, fluid replacement is accomplished by the IV route in most cases. If rapid fluid resuscitation is needed, use a large-gauge peripheral IV site with a short length to provide for rapid fluid replacement. Keep the tubing as short as possible from the IV bag or bottle, and avoid long loops of tubing at a level below the patient's heart. Monitor for signs of underhydration (mental status that remains depressed, dry mucous membranes, soft eyeballs) and overhydration (pulmonary congestion, neck vein distension, shortness of breath, frothy sputum, cough).

Patients with the most severe cases of hyperglycemia have a risk of ineffective airway clearance because of decreased mental status and airway obstruction by the tongue. Have airway equipment near the patient's bedside at all times, including an oral and nasal airway, an endotracheal tube, and a laryngoscope. If the patient develops snoring, slow respirations, or apnea, maintain the patient's airway and breathing with a manual resuscitator bag and notify the physician immediately.

If the patient has hyperglycemia because of diabetes mellitus or HNKS, provide appropriate patient teaching. Discuss the administration of insulin; a consistent and appropriate technique of insulin administration is critical for optimal blood glucose control. Whenever possible, have the patient administer his or her own insulin. Encourage exercise. Instruct the patient about self-monitoring to recognize the signs and symptoms of hyperglycemia and hypoglycemia. Teach the patient and significant others how to prevent skin and lower-extremity infection, ulcers, and poor wound healing.

DOCUMENTATION GUIDELINES

- Fluid balance and nutrition: Intake and output, color of urine, amount and type of volume resuscitation, "sliding scale" and response to insulin, signs of hypoglycemia or hyperglycemia, daily weights, signs of dehydration or rehydration
- Effectiveness of diet, medications, and activity on blood glucose
- Patient's understanding of teaching: Pathophysiology of underlying disorder, nutrition education, insulin and technique of administration, oral hypoglycemic medication, exercise program, self-monitoring of blood glucose (if appropriate), prevention of complications
- Complications such as skin lesions, hypoglycemic reactions

DISCHARGE AND HOME HEALTHCARE GUIDELINES

Teach the patient strategies for managing the disorder. Provide a written list of all medications, including dosage, route, time, and side effects. If appropriate, give the patient a phone number to call if he or she has any problems with self-administration of insulin or self-monitoring of blood glucose. Provide the patient with a list of referrals, such as an outpatient diabetic clinic or community contacts, for follow-up care and information. Provide a list of equipment and materials needed for home care. Give the patient any pamphlets or written materials about the management of hyperglycemia.

Hyperkalemia

DRG Category: 296
Mean LOS: 5.4 days
Description: MEDICAL: Nutritional and Miscellaneous Metabolic Disorders, Age > 17 with CC

Normal serum levels of potassium range from 3.5 to 5.0 mEq/L. Hyperkalemia, defined as a potassium level greater than 5.0 mEq/L, is usually associated with impaired renal function, but it may also be produced by treatments for other disorders. Increased potassium intake, reduction in potassium excretion, and shift of potassium out of the cells all may result in hyperkalemia. Because potassium plays a key role in cardiac function, a high serum potassium level is of great concern. It is sometimes the first symptom of cardiac arrest.

Potassium functions as the major intracellular cation and balances sodium in the ECF to maintain electroneutrality in the body. It is excreted by the kidneys: the normal ratio is approximately 40 mEq of potassium in 1 L of urine. Potassium is not stored in the body and needs to be replenished daily through dietary sources. It is also exchanged for hydrogen when changes in the body's pH call for a need for cation exchange. This situation occurs in metabolic alkalosis or other alterations that lead to increased cellular uptake of potassium, including insulin excess and renal failure. Potassium is regulated by two stimuli, aldosterone and hyperkalemia. Aldosterone is secreted in response to high renin and angiotensin II or hyperkalemia. The plasma level of potassium, when high, also increases renal potassium loss.

CAUSES

Factors that result in decreased potassium excretion include oliguric renal failure, potassium-sparing diuretics (such as spironolactone), multiple transfusions or transfusions of stored blood, decrease in adrenal steroids, and nonsteroidal anti-inflammatory medications. Too much potassium is taken into the body by overuse of oral potassium supplements, inappropriate intravenous (IV) administration of potassium, or excessive use of potassium-based salt substitutes.

Transcellular shift of potassium from within the cells to the extracellular fluid can also lead to hyperkalemia. This situation occurs in tumor lysis syndrome, rhabdomyolysis, metabolic acidosis, and insulin deficiency with hyperglycemia. Other causes include severe digitalis toxicity and the use of beta-adrenergic blockers and the drugs heparin, captopril, and lithium. Hyperkalemia can also be produced by adrenocorticol insufficiency and hypoaldosteronism.

GENDER AND LIFE SPAN CONSIDERATIONS

Hyperkalemia can occur at any age and across both genders. It may be more common in the elderly population because renal failure and potassium replacement therapy are more common in this group.

☐ ASSESSMENT

HISTORY. Take a thorough history of medications and dietary patterns to determine if excess potassium is a result of excess ingestion. Because hyperkalemia is a side effect of a disease process (as in renal failure) or a treatment (as in overuse of potassium supplements), a careful history of all past and present illnesses is important. The symptoms of potassium excess include nausea and diarrhea because of hyperactivity of the gastrointestinal (GI) smooth muscle. Patients often experience muscle weakness, which may extend to paralysis if severe. A complaint of general weakness is an early sign of hyperkalemia. A history of heart irregularities, dizziness, and postural hypotension may be reported.

PHYSICAL EXAMINATION. The most common effects of hyperkalemia are cardiac and are reflected in the electrocardiogram (ECG) tracings. Heart sounds may reveal a slowed overall rate with or without irregular or extra beats.

Neuromuscular effects are primarily on the peripheral nervous system, leading to significant muscular weakness that progresses upward from legs to trunk. The muscles of respiration may be affected, as well as those that produce voice. Paresthesia of the face, feet, hands, and tongue may occur. General anxiety and irritability may also be present, and the patient may have a low urinary output.

PSYCHOSOCIAL. Feelings of physical weakness can increase the sense of powerlessness. The patient may experience feelings of irritability, restlessness, and confusion. In addition, if the condition is caused by nonadherence to a medication regimen, the patient may feel personally responsible for the problem.

DIAGNOSTIC HIGHLIGHTS

Test	Normal Result	Abnormality with Condition	Explanation
Serum potassium	3.5–5.0 mEq/L	> 5.0 mEq/L	Potassium excess is reflected in serum and extracellular fluid compartment
Electrocardiogram (ECG)	Normal PQRST pattern	Early: Increased T wave amplitude or peaked T waves Middle: Prolonged PR interval and QRS duration, atrioventricular conduction delay, loss of P waves Late: Progressive widening on QRS complex and merging with T wave to produce sine wave pattern	Cardiac toxicity does not correlate well with degree of hyperkalemia; depolarization is prolonged, and bradycardia may occur along with atrioventricular block

PRIMARY NURSING DIAGNOSIS

Decreased cardiac output related to ineffective cardiac pumping and cardiac arrest

OUTCOMES. Electrolyte and acid-base balance; Cardiac pump effectiveness; Circulatory status; Tissue perfusion: Abdominal organs and peripheral; Vital signs status

INTERVENTIONS. Electrolyte management: Hyperkalemia; Medication management; Medication administration; Fluid/electrolyte management; Cardiac care: Acute; Code management; Airway management; Dysrhythmia management

☐ PLANNING AND IMPLEMENTATION

Collaborative

If hyperkalemia is not severe, it can often be remedied by simply eliminating potassium supplements or potassium-sparing diuretics and drugs that lead to the disorder.

In more serious situations, pharmacologic therapy is important. Be aware of concerns related to sodium retention when using sodium polystyrene sulfonate. Monitor the patient's response to the medication; if no stools result, notify the physician. Emergency management of hyperkalemia is threefold with administration of IV calcium gluconate, glucose, and insulin. Excess potassium can also be removed by dialysis. This approach is reserved for situations in which less aggressive techniques have proved ineffective. Hemodialysis takes longer to initiate but is more effective than peritoneal dialysis.

PHARMACOLOGIC HIGHLIGHTS

Medication or Drug Class	Dosage	Description	Rationale
Calcium gluconate	10 mg of a 10% solution IV over 2–3 minutes	Electrolyte replacement	Decreases membrane excitability; one dose lasts 30–60 minutes; dose may be repeated after 5–10 minutes if no change in ECG occurs
Insulin	10–20 units of regular insulin IV	Hormone	Lowers serum potassium by enabling more potassium to enter the cell
Glucose	25–50 grams IV	Sugar	Protects the patient from a hypoglycemic reaction
Sodium polystyrene sulfonate (Kayexalate)	Orally or by enema: 15 g per 60 mL in 20–100 mL sorbitol to facilitate passage of resin through intestinal tract	Cation exchange resin: 0.5–1.0 mEq/L of potassium is removed with each enema, but an equivalent amount of sodium is retained	Exchanges sodium for potassium in the GI tract, leading to the elimination of potassium

Other: As an emergency measure, sodium bicarbonate delivered IV (one ampule of a 7.5% $NaHCO_3$ solution) increases pH and causes potassium to shift into the cells; it is particularly effective in treating metabolic acidosis.

Independent

Provide clear explanations and allow the patient to express concerns throughout the treatment course. Involve family members and the support system in teaching. Patients who are experiencing hyperkalemia should avoid foods high in potassium. These include potatoes, beet greens, bananas, orange juice, dried fruit, coffee, tea, and chocolate. Draw blood samples to ensure accurate potassium-level measurement. Do not draw a sample from above an IV site where potassium is infusing, make certain the sample gets to the lab quickly, do not leave a tourniquet on for prolonged periods, and do not have the patient repeatedly clench and relax his or her fist.

DOCUMENTATION GUIDELINES

- Cardiac and musculoskeletal assessment: Cardiac rhythm changes and resolution of changes
- Patient's understanding of potassium use if the cause of hyperkalemia is related to mismanagement of medication

DISCHARGE AND HOME HEALTHCARE GUIDELINES

PREVENTION. Assess the patient's understanding of the relationship between dietary intake of potassium-containing foods and supplements and hyperkalemia. Discuss strategies to improve or eliminate those factors that are leading to elevated potassium levels. Have the patient describe the changes in diet or home care that are necessary to prevent recurrence. For example, what could be done to assure potassium supplements are taken as prescribed?

MEDICATIONS. Evaluate the patient's understanding of the appropriate use of potassium supplements and salt substitutes.

Hyperlipoproteinemia

DRG Category: 299
Mean LOS: 4.3 days
Description: MEDICAL: Inborn Errors of Metabolism

Hyperlipoproteinemia is a condition of increased lipids (fats) in the blood that has been caused by an increased rate of synthesis or a decreased rate of lipoprotein breakdown. Because lipoproteins transport triglycerides and cholesterol in the plasma, an increased level may cause pancreatitis and atherosclerosis.

Lipids are a mixed group of biochemical substances that are manufactured by the body or are derived from metabolism of ingested substances. The plasma lipids (cholesterols, triglycerides, phospholipids, and free fatty acids) are derived from dietary sources and lipid synthesis. Cholesterol and triglycerides are implicated in atherogenesis.

Hyperlipidemia, an elevation of serum cholesterol or triglycerides, can be primary or secondary to another underlying condition. Lipoprotein elevation, or hyperlipoproteinemia, is described by five specific types: Types I, II, III, IV, and V. (See Table 28.)

TABLE 28 | **Types of Hyperlipoproteinemia**

TYPE	DEFINITION AND CAUSE	ASSESSMENT
I	Fat-induced hyperlidemia or idiopathic familial hyperlididemia, which is a rare condition caused by deficient or abnormal lipase; rare genetic disorder that is present in infancy	Recurrent attacks of severe abdominal pain after fat intake; malaise; anorexia
II	Familial hyperbetalipoproteinemia and essential familial hypercholesterolemia because of deficient cell surface receptors	Chest pain from prematurely accelerated coronary artery disease; tendinous xanthomas (firm masses) on Achilles' tendons, tendons of hands and feet; juvenile corneal arcus (grayish ring around the cornea of the eye)
III	Familial broad-beta disease xanthoma tuberosum caused by a deficient low-density lipoprotein receptor	Chest pain from early progression of atherosclerosis; xamthomas over elbows, knees, palms, and fingertips
IV	Endogenonous hypertriglyceridemia and hyperbetalipoproteinemia with an idiopathic cause; often associated with obesity and diabetes	Chest pain from early progression of coronary artery disease; obesity, hypertension
V	Mixed hypertriglyceridemia from defective triglyceride clearance; often secondary to other disorders such as renal disease or obesity	Abdominal pain from pancreatitits; visual changes; xanthomas on arms and legs; enlarged liver and spleen

CAUSES

Primary hyperlipoproteinemia results from rare genetic disorders. Secondary hyperlipoproteinemia occurs as a manifestation of other diseases, which include hypothyroidism, nephrotic syndrome, diabetes mellitus, alcoholism, glycogen storage disease (type 1), Cushing's syndrome, acromegaly, anorexia, renal disease, liver diseases, immunologic disorders, stress, and the use of oral contraceptives or glucocorticoids.

GENDER AND LIFE SPAN CONSIDERATIONS

Type I disease is a rare disorder that is present at birth. Type II disease usually causes symptoms in young adults in their 20s, but may begin as early as 10 years of age. Symptoms from type III disease usually occur during the teenage years or early 20s. Type IV disease, more common than the other forms of hyperlipoproteinemia, occurs primarily in middle-aged men. Type V disease occurs in late adolescence or in the early 20s.

☐ ASSESSMENT

HISTORY. Take a thorough history of existing illnesses because secondary hyperlipoproteinemia is related to a number of other conditions. Ask the patient if he or she has a history of renal or liver disease, diabetes mellitus, other endocrine diseases, or immune disorders.

Ask if the patient is taking corticosteroids or oral contraceptives, and determine the extent of the patient's alcohol use. Because hyperlipoproteinemia is sometimes treated with a range of bile acid sequestrant medications, which can affect the absorption of other medications, ask if the patient is taking any of the following: warfarin, thiazides, thyroxine, beta-adrenergic blockers, fat-soluble vitamins, folic acid, diuretics, or digitoxin.

Symptoms of hyperlipoproteinemia vary, depending on which of the five types the patient has. Ask about recurrent bouts of severe abdominal pain, usually preceded by fat intake, or if the patient has experienced malaise, anorexia, or fever.

PHYSICAL EXAMINATION. Observe general appearance for signs of obesity, which may be an exacerbating factor for hyperlipoproteinemia. Inspection may reveal papular or eruptive deposits of fat (xanthomas) over pressure points and extensor surfaces; likely locations include the Achilles' tendons, hand and foot tendons, elbows, knees, and hands and fingertips (where you may observe orange or yellow discolorations of the palmar and digital creases). Ophthalmoscopic examination typically reveals reddish-white retinal vessels. In some forms of hyperlipoproteinemia, an opaque ring surrounding the corneal periphery (juvenile corneal arcus) is visible. Palpate the abdomen for spasm, rigidity, rebound tenderness, liver or spleen tenderness, and hepatosplenomegaly. Check for signs of hypertension and hyperuricemia.

PSYCHOSOCIAL. Hyperlipoproteinemia is not an abrupt illness; it develops over years. The patient may have developed coping mechanisms during that time, but the patient may be anxious because of accelerated symptoms of atherosclerosis and coronary artery disease. The patient may have experienced the premature death of parents from this disorder and have long-lasting fears about his or her own early death. Body image disturbance may also occur because of obesity or the presence of unsightly xanthomas.

DIAGNOSTIC HIGHLIGHTS

Test	Normal Result	Abnormality with Condition	Explanation
Total cholesterol	Varies with age, ethnicity, and gender; desirable is < 200 mg/dL	Borderline high 200–239 mg/dL; high > 239 mg/dL	Used for screening and initial classification of risk of coronary heart disease; elevations determine hyperlipidemia.
Low-density lipoprotein cholesterol (LDL-C)	Optimal < 100 mg/dL; desirable level is < 130 mg/dL	Borderline high risk 130–159 mg/dL; high risk > 159 mg/dL	Elevated levels are associated with increased risk for coronary heart disease
High-density lipoprotein cholesterol (HDL-C); fasting level is essential	> 35 mg/dL	< 35 mg/dL	Considered a major risk factor for coronary heart disease; high HDL-C (> 60 mg/dL) is considered protective
Triglycerides	< 200 mg/dL	Borderline high risk 200–400 mg/dL; high risk 400–1000 mg/dL; very high risk >1000 mg/dL hyperlipidemia.	Used for screening and initial classification of risk of coronary heart disease; elevations determine

Other Tests: ECG, genetic testing

PRIMARY NURSING DIAGNOSIS

Altered nutrition: More than body requirements related to lipoprotein accumulation and accelerated blockage of the coronary arteries

OUTCOMES. Nutritional status: Food and fluid intake, Nutrient intake, and Body mass; Knowledge: Medication, Diet; Disease process; Health behaviors; Treatment regimen

INTERVENTIONS. Teaching: Prescribed diet; Weight management; Medication management; Nutritional monitoring; Nutritional therapy; Nutritional counseling; Exercise promotion; Mutual goal setting; Teaching: Individual

☐ PLANNING AND IMPLEMENTATION

Collaborative

The primary treatment is dietary management, weight reduction, increased physical activity, and the restriction of saturated animal fat and cholesterol intake. Adding polyunsaturated vegetable oils to the diet helps reduce LDL-C concentration. Secondary treatment is aimed at reducing or eliminating aggravating factors, such as alcoholism, diabetes mellitus, or hypothyroidism. To reduce risk factors that contribute to atherosclerosis, the regimen includes treating hypertension, implementing an exercise program, controlling blood sugar, and stopping smoking. For type V hyperlipoproteinemia, female patients are taken off oral contraceptives. Medications also may be prescribed to lower the plasma concentration of lipoproteins, either by decreasing their production or by increasing their removal from plasma.

In rare instances, for patients who cannot tolerate medication therapy, surgical creation of an ileal bypass may be necessary to accelerate the loss of bile acids in the stool and lower plasma cholesterol levels. For children with severe disease, surgery to create a portacaval shunt may be performed as a last resort to decrease plasma cholesterol levels. Plasma exchanges may also be used to reduce cholesterol levels.

PHARMACOLOGIC HIGHLIGHTS

Medication or Drug Class	Dosage	Description	Rationale
Drugs that lower LDL-C	Varies with drug	Bile acid sequestrant resins (cholestyramine, colestopol); nicotinic acid (niacin); HMG-CoA reductase inhibitors (statins such as levostatin, pravastatin, simvastatin, fluvastatin, atorvastatin); estrogen in postmenopausal women	Lower the plasma concentration of lipoproteins, either by decreasing their production or by increasing their removal from plasma
Drugs that lower triglycerides	Varies with drug	Nicotinin acid (niacin), fibric acid derivatives (gemfibrozil), and HMG-CoA reductase inhibitors (statins such as	Lower the plasma concentration of lipoproteins, either by decreasing their

		simvastatin and atorvastatin in particular)	production or by increasing their removal from plasma
Drugs that increase HDL-C	Varies with drug	Nicotinic acid (niacin), estrogen in postmenopausal women	Lower the plasma concentration of lipoproteins, either by decreasing their production or by increasing their removal from plasma

Independent

Teach the patient about ways to manage diet to control the disorder. Urge the patient to adhere to a 1000 to 1500 calorie per day diet and avoid excess sugar intake. Explain the components of the lipid profile and their ramifications and discuss various means of lowering VLDL and LDL levels and increasing HDL levels.

Explain the prescribed medication regimen, by providing verbal and written information to the patient or significant others. Refer to effective programs or support groups for controlling cigarette and alcohol use. Teach alternate methods of contraception to the female patient who can no longer use oral contraceptives.

A patient faces significant health threats unless he or she makes permanent lifestyle changes. Encourage him or her to verbalize fears, such as those concerning coronary artery disease. Offer support and provide clear explanations for the patient's questions about the lifestyle changes and consequences.

DOCUMENTATION GUIDELINES

- Physical findings: Xanthomas, organ enlargement, abdominal pain or distension, chest pain
- Response to pain-management strategies

DISCHARGE AND HOME HEALTHCARE GUIDELINES

PREVENTION. Teach the patient the importance of dietary and lifestyle changes. Refer the patient to a dietician if appropriate.

MEDICATIONS. Be sure the patient understands all medications, including the dosage, route, action, adverse effects, and the need for routine laboratory monitoring for lipid profiles.

COMPLICATIONS. Teach the patient to report to his or her physician the occurrence of signs and symptoms of coronary artery disease, such as chest pain, shortness of breath, and changes in mental status. Teach the patient the need for follow-up serum cholesterol and serum triglyceride tests. Instruct the patient to maintain a stable body weight and to adhere to any dietary restrictions before undergoing cholesterol tests. Most tests require the patient to fast for 12 hours before the test.

Hypermagnesemia

DRG Category: 296
Mean LOS: 5.4 days
Description: MEDICAL: Nutritional and Miscellaneous Metabolic Disorders, Age > 17 with CC

Hypermagnesemia occurs when the serum magnesium concentration is greater than 2.7 mg/dL (2.3 mEq/L). The normal serum magnesium level is 1.7 to 2.7 mg/dL (1.4 to 2.3 mEq/L). Magnesium, like calcium, is bound to albumin in plasma, although approximately 25% of serum magnesium is bound to albumin as compared to 50% of bound calcium. An average-sized adult has approximately 25 g of magnesium in his or her body. About half of the body's total magnesium is found in the bones, 1% is located in the extracellular compartment, and the remainder is found within the cells.

Magnesium plays an important role in neuromuscular function. It also has a role in several enzyme systems, particularly the metabolism of carbohydrates and proteins, as well as maintenance of normal ionic balance (it triggers the sodium-potassium pump), osmotic pressure, myocardial functioning, and bone metabolism. Because the kidneys are able to excrete large amounts of magnesium (more than 5000 mg per day), either the patient has to ingest extraordinary amounts of magnesium or the glomerular filtration of the kidneys needs to be very depressed for the patient to develop hypermagnesemia. Complications include complete heart block, cardiac arrest, and respiratory paralysis.

CAUSES

Hypermagnesemia, although rare, usually occurs in patients with chronic renal disease who consume excessive quantities of magnesium, commonly in the form of magnesium-containing laxatives or antacids. Obstetric patients who are treated with parenteral magnesium for pre-eclampsia or patients with acute adrenocortical insufficiency (Addison's disease) may also develop hypermagnesemia. Both hypothermia and shock can also lead to a high serum magnesium level.

GENDER AND LIFE SPAN CONSIDERATIONS

Hypermagnesemia may occur at any age and in both sexes, but it is seen much more frequently in the older patient with chronic renal failure. Children may develop this condition if they have renal failure or consume significant quantities of medications that contain magnesium.

☐ ASSESSMENT

HISTORY. The patient's chief complaint may be muscle weakness and fatigue. Precipitating factors may include renal failure, laxative or antacid abuse, adrenal insufficiency, diabetes, or acidosis. Medication history may include magnesium-containing laxatives such as milk of magnesia, antacids that contain magnesium hydroxide, or parenteral administration of magnesium sulfate. Ask the patient to describe any symptoms, which may range from none to full cardiopulmonary arrest. The patient may experience nausea and vomiting, flushed skin, or diaphoresis; changes in the cardiac rhythm lead to palpitations or dizziness, depression, lethargy, thirst, muscle weakness, or even paralysis.

PHYSICAL EXAMINATION. Generally, patients do not develop signs and symptoms until the serum magnesium reaches more than 4 mEq/L. Assess the vital signs, which may show tachycardia, bradycardia, or hypotension. The patient may be disoriented, confused, or even unresponsive. When strength and movement are assessed, you may find the patient has lost deep tendon reflexes, has muscle weakness, and may even have some paralysis. Cardiopulmonary arrest may occur when the respiratory muscles are paralyzed as a result of a magnesium level in excess of 10 mEq/L or as a consequence of depressed myocardial contractility.

PSYCHOSOCIAL. The patient with hypermagnesemia usually has chronic renal failure. Assess the patient's ability to cope with a chronic disease, as well as an acute complication. The patient may have had to cope with a change in lifestyle and roles that may be compromised by the sudden and potentially life-threatening complication of hypermagnesemia. The patient's degree of anxiety about the illness should also be assessed.

DIAGNOSTIC HIGHLIGHTS

Test	Normal Result	Abnormality with Condition	Explanation
Serum magnesium	1.7–2.7 mg/dL	> 2.7 mg/dL	Excess of magnesium ions
Electrocardiogram (ECG)	Normal PQRST pattern	Early: Bradycardia, prolonged PR, QRS, and QT intervals; late: complete heart block, asystole	Magnesium excess leads to alterations in generation and conduction of the action potential

PRIMARY NURSING DIAGNOSIS

Risk for injury related to neurosensory alterations secondary to hypermagnesemia

OUTCOMES. Cardiac pump effectiveness; Circulation status; Electrolyte and acid-base balance; Knowledge: Medication; Respiratory status: Ventilation and gas exchange

INTERVENTIONS. Artificial airway management; Resuscitation; Electrolyte management: Hypermagnesemia; Cardiac care: Acute; Code management; Emergency care; Oxygen therapy; Medication administration; Medication management

☐ PLANNING AND IMPLEMENTATION

Collaborative

The physician discontinues all medications that contain magnesium. The patient may be given calcium gluconate in emergencies to antagonize the effects of magnesium. If the patient does not have severe renal failure, 1000 ml 0.9% saline with 2 g of calcium gluconate may be infused to increase magnesium excretion at a rate of 150 to 200 ml per hour. In patients with inadequate renal function, the physician may prescribe dialysis with magnesium-free dialysate. Prompt supportive therapy is essential, such as mechanical ventilation if the patient has respiratory failure or a temporary pacemaker if the patient has symptomatic bradycardia.

During treatment, monitor the serum magnesium in patients at risk for hypermagnesemia. Monitor vital signs, urine output, and the neuromuscular status, including level of consciousness, orientation, and muscle strength and function. Assess the patellar (knee-jerk) reflex in patients with a magnesium level above 5 mEq/L: with the patient lying flat or sitting on the side of the bed, support the knee and tap the patellar tendon firmly just below the patella. A normal response is extension of the knee. An absent reflex may indicate a magnesium level over 7 mEq/L and should be reported to the physician.

PHARMACOLOGIC HIGHLIGHTS

Medication or Drug Class	Dosage	Description	Rationale
Calcium gluconate 10%	10–20 mL IV (1–2 g) over 10 minutes	Electrolyte replacement; nutritional supplement	Antagonizes the effects of magnesium and counteracts neuromuscular effects; effect is temporary

Independent

Maintain the patient's airway, breathing, and circulation until the magnesium levels return to normal. Have emergency airway equipment and a manual resuscitator bag at the patient's bedside at all times. Keep a working endotracheal suction present. Maintain patient safety measures. Reassure the patient and significant others that the patient's neuromuscular status will return to baseline with treatment.

Educate the patient with chronic renal failure to review all over the counter medications with the physician and pharmacist before use. These medications include vitamin supplements that contain minerals because these usually contain magnesium. Provide a list of common magnesium-containing medications that the patient should avoid.

DOCUMENTATION GUIDELINES

- Serum magnesium level
- Vital signs; oxygen saturation; cardiac rhythm, ECG strip and interpretation
- Mental and neuromuscular status, including patellar reflex if appropriate
- Response to treatment: IV fluids, diuretics, dialysis, calcium gluconate

DISCHARGE AND HOME HEALTHCARE GUIDELINES

PREVENTION. To prevent a recurrence of hypermagnesemia, teach the patient to avoid sources of magnesium such as laxatives, antacids, and vitamin-mineral supplements and to consult with the pharmacist or physician before using any over the counter-medications. The patient should also be taught the signs and symptoms of hypermagnesemia (changes in level of consciousness, neuromuscular weakness, nausea and vomiting) and instructed to notify the physician if these return.

COMPLICATIONS OF NEUROMUSCULAR WEAKNESS. If the patient suffered from prolonged neuromuscular symptoms, he or she may have developed muscle weakness as a result of disease. Teach safety measures to the patient and significant others, including the use of any assistive devices (cane or walker) and seeking assistance when ambulating. The patient should also be taught muscle-strengthening exercises and may need a home care evaluation before being discharged.

Hypernatremia

DRG Category: 296
Mean LOS: 5.4 days

Description: MEDICAL: Nutritional and Miscellaneous Metabolic Disorders, Age > 17 with CC

Hypernatremia is a condition in which the serum sodium concentration is greater than 145 mEq/L (normal range is 136 to 145 mEq/L). Sodium is the most abundant cation in the body; a 70-kg person has approximately 4200 mEq of sodium. About 30% of the total body sodium, called silent sodium, is bound with bone and other tissues; the remaining 70%, called the exchangeable sodium, is dissolved in the extracellular fluid (ECF) compartment or in the compartments in communication with the ECF compartment. Sodium has five essential functions: it maintains the osmolarity of the ECF; it maintains ECF volume and water distribution; it affects the concentration, excretion, and absorption of other electrolytes, particularly potassium and chloride; it combines with other ions to maintain acid-base balance; it is essential for impulse transmission of nerve and muscle fibers.

Hypernatremia usually occurs when there is an excess of sodium in relation to water in the ECF compartment, resulting in hyperosmolarity of the ECF, which produces a shift in water from the cells to the ECF. The result is cellular dehydration. Three different manifestations of hypernatremia have been described, based on the ratio of total body water (TBW) to total body sodium: hypovolemic hypernatremia, hypervolemic hypernatremia, and euvolemic hypernatremia. (See Table 29.)

TABLE 29 | **Types and Causes of Hypernatremia**

TYPE OF HYPERNATREMIA	FLUID VOLUME AND SODIUM (NA) STATUS	CAUSES
Hypovolemic (most common)	Total body water (TBW) decreases in a greater proportion that Na is lost	Nonrenal: Fever, vomiting, diarrhea, exercise, heat exposure, severe burns, insensible loss from mechanical ventilation, profuse diaphoresis Renal: Diuresis, severe hyperglycemia, increased production of urea (high protein diet), IV administration of mannitol

| Hypervolemic (least common) | TBW is normal with increased Na | Overadministration of saline solutions, particularly in patients with diabetes ketoacidosis and osmotic diuresis; overadministration of hypertonic salt solutions; overingestion of salt |
| Euvolemic | TBW is decreased relative to a normal total body Na | Acute diabetes insipidus; hypodipsia in infants, elderly persons, and debilitated adults |

CAUSES

The cause of hypernatremia is associated with the ratio of TBW to total body sodium. In hypernatremia, there is often an excess of sodium relative to TBW. Causes of hypernatremia are explained in Table 29.

GENDER AND LIFE SPAN CONSIDERATIONS

Hypernatremia is most likely to occur in infants, elderly people, or debilitated patients. It is mostly linked to inadequate fluid intake. The total body sodium level does not vary significantly depending on the person's gender or age once childhood is over.

◘ ASSESSMENT

HISTORY. Inquire about the patent's daily fluid and salt intake. Patients with hypernatremia often report a decrease in fluid intake and possibly a high salt intake. Since polyuria moving to oliguria is an early sign of hypernatremia, ask about daily urine output and if the urine appears concentrated. Question the patient about fever, diarrhea, and vomiting, which might contribute to dehydration. If hypernatremia is severe, the patient may be confused. Ask the family if the patient has been lethargic, disoriented, or agitated. These changes in mental status, along with occurrence of a seizure, indicate severe hypernatremia.

PHYSICAL EXAMINATION. Assess the patient's vital signs; fever, tachycardia, decreased blood pressure, and orthostatic hypotension are characteristic of hypernatremia. Assess the skin and mucous membranes for signs of dehydration. With pronounced hypernatremia, expect poor skin turgor; flushed skin color; dry mucous membranes; and a rough, dry tongue. With more severe hypernatremia, assess the patient for muscle twitching, hyperreflexia, tremors, seizures, and rigid paralysis.

PSYCHOSOCIAL. Assess the patient's ability to obtain adequate fluid intake. The patient's lethargic state contributes to the poor fluid intake. Assess the quality and support of the caregivers regarding their ability to provide for the patient's fluid intake. Since in severe hypernatremia the symptoms are primarily neurological, assess the patient's level of orientation and his or her ability to communicate needs. Assess the safety needs of the patient, especially for the disoriented elderly or debilitated patient. Note that central nervous system symptoms are particularly upsetting for the patient and family and may create anxiety over the patient's long-term prognosis.

DIAGNOSTIC HIGHLIGHTS

Test	Normal Result	Abnormality with Condition	Explanation
Serum sodium	136–145 mEq/L	> 145 mEq/L	Imbalance between sodium and water lead to excess sodium
Blood urea nitrogen (BUN)	5–20 mg/dL	May be elevated	Conditions that lead to dehydration and fluid loss may elevate BUN because of decreased renal blood flow and abnormal absorption of urea back into the blood
Serum chloride	95–108 mEq/L	> 108 mEq/L	Reflects an excess of chloride
Serum osmolarity	280–295 mOsm/L	> 295 mOsm/L	Water loss in the urine and hypernatremia lead to hemoconcentration; levels above 320 mOsm/L are considered "panic levels" and require immediate intervention
Urine osmolality	200–1200 mOsm/L	Varies depending on cause; often > 800 mOsm/L	Used to diagnose nature of hypernatremia; osmolality refers to a solution's concentration of solute particles per kilogram of solvent; usual renal response to hypernatremia is excretion of maximally concentrated urine (< 500 mL/day) with an osmolarity > 800 mOsm/L

Other Tests: Complete blood count, protein level, urine specific gravity

PRIMARY NURSING DIAGNOSIS

Fluid volume deficit related to fluid loss, inadequate fluid intake, or fluid shifts to the extravascular space

OUTCOMES. Electrolyte and acid-base balance; Hydration; Fluid balance; Nutritional status: Food and fluid intake; Knowledge: Health behaviors; Urinary elimination

INTERVENTIONS. Electrolyte management: Hypernatremia; Fluid management; Fluid monitoring; Intravenous insertion; Intravenous therapy: Venous access devices maintenance

▢ PLANNING AND IMPLEMENTATION

Collaborative

The goal is to decrease the total body sodium and replace the fluid loss. Encourage liquids; if the patient cannot tolerate fluids, an intravenous (IV) hypotonic electrolyte solution (0.2% or 0.45% sodium chloride) or salt-free solution is usually ordered. Sometimes these two types of solutions are alternated to prevent hyponatremia. If 5% dextrose in water is ordered, monitor the urine output because this solution encourages diuresis, which can aggravate the hypernatremic condition. Maintain intake and output records and weigh the patient each day to monitor the fluid volume status.

Monitor the patient's serum sodium levels daily as well to determine the effectiveness of IV fluids. Administer the water replacement slowly as prescribed to reduce the serum sodium levels not more than 2 mEq/L per hour. If hypernatremia is corrected too quickly, the ECF shifts into the cells, resulting in cerebral edema and neurological problems. Monitor the patient for signs and symptoms of cerebral edema: headache, lethargy, nausea, vomiting, widening pulse pressure, and decreased pulse rate. Sometimes diuretic therapy is indicated to increase sodium excretion, along with a decrease of oral sodium intake in the diet. No pharmacologic management is usually required other than intravenous therapy.

Independent

Offer fluids and water frequently to patients with hypernatremia. Avoid caffeinated fluids and alcohol because they can increase the serum sodium level by causing water diuresis. Notify the physician of any changes in mental status, such as agitation, confusion, and disorientation. If the patient is at risk for seizures, initiate seizure precautions.

Give oral care every 2 hours; avoid using lemon glycerin swabs and alcoholic mouthwashes because they have a drying effect and can cause discomfort. Monitor the condition of the skin, and assist with position changes frequently. Determine the patient's ability to ambulate safely. If the patient is confused and disoriented, maintain the bed in the lowest position and maintain safety measures.

DOCUMENTATION GUIDELINES

- Intake and output, daily weights, urine specific gravity
- Vital signs: Presence of fever, tachycardia, low blood pressure, orthostatic changes
- Mental status: Orientation to person, place, and time; observations of confusion or agitation; ability to drink oral fluids; presence of gag reflex
- Condition of oral mucosa and skin
- Response to treatments: Oral and parenteral fluids, sodium restrictions, diuretics

DISCHARGE AND HOME HEALTHCARE GUIDELINES

Teach the patient and his or her caregivers the importance of an adequate fluid intake and normal sodium intake. Discuss the foods that are appropriate for a low-sodium diet, if indicated. Advise the patient or significant others to avoid over the counter medications that are high in sodium. Teach the patient about the early signs of hypernatremia: polyuria, nausea, vomiting, and orthostatic hypotension. Explain that as hypernatremia becomes severe, the patient or family will note changes in the patient's mental status. Encourage the patient or significant others to notify the primary healthcare provider if any of these signs and symptoms occur.

Hyperparathyroidism

DRG Category: 300
Mean LOS: 6.3 days
Description: MEDICAL: Endocrine Disorders with CC
DRG Category: 289
Mean LOS: 3.2 days
Description: SURGICAL: Parathyroid Procedures

Hyperparathyroidism refers to the clinical condition that is associated with oversecretion of parathyroid hormone (PTH). Primary hyperparathyroidism, the most common form, is a gland dysfunction that originates in the parathyroid gland. Secondary hyperparathyroidism, in contrast, refers to a parathyroid gland dysfunction that is a response to a disorder elsewhere in the body, such as chronic renal failure. PTH is produced by the parathyroid glands, which are four small endocrine glands that are located on the posterior surface of the thyroid gland. The primary function of PTH is to regulate calcium and phosphorus balance by affecting gastrointestinal (GI) absorption of calcium, bone resorption (removal of bone tissue by absorption) of calcium, and renal regulation of both calcium and phosphorus. Calcium and phosphorus have a reciprocal relationship in the body; high levels of calcium lead to low levels of phosphorus.

Hypercalcemia, the identifiable result of hyperparathyroidism, also leads to the most important clinical complications. The body is able to compensate for slowly increasing calcium levels but eventually becomes overcome with calcium excess and phosphorus deficiency. Since the bones hold the majority of the body's calcium, extracellular hypercalcemia is a result of demineralization of the bones. The calcium in the bones is replaced by cysts and fibrous tissue, thus leading to severe osteoporosis (reduction of bone mass per volume) and osteopenia (diminished bone tissue). Increased levels of extracellular calcium may be deposited in the soft tissues of the body and the kidney and lead to renal calculi, renal insufficiency, urinary tract infections, and eventually renal failure. Hypercalcemia can also trigger the increased secretion of gastrin, which leads to peptic ulcer disease. Other GI dysfunctions that may result include cholelithiasis and pancreatitis.

CAUSES

Primary hyperparathyroidism, which leads to the enlargement of at least one of the parathyroid glands, occurs in more than 85% of the cases because of a single benign adenoma (neoplasm of glandular epithelium). Other causes include genetic disorders and endocrine cancers such as pancreatic or pituitary cancers. Patients who have had head or neck radiation are also at increased risk. Secondary hyperparathyroidism occurs when a source for hypocalcemia occurs outside the parathyroid gland, thus stimulating the parathyroid glands to overproduce PTH. These conditions include chronic renal failure, rickets, vitamin D deficiency, and laxative abuse.

GENDER AND LIFE SPAN CONSIDERATIONS

Primary hyperparathyroidism affects women more than men and is more frequent in individuals older than 50 years. Postmenopausal women between the ages of 35 and 65 and elderly women are especially at risk. Regular screening of calcium levels as part of an annual physical examination is very important for all people older than 50.

◻ ASSESSMENT

HISTORY. Many patients are asymptomatic. Early symptoms are polyuria (large amounts of urine), anorexia, and constipation, as well as weakness, fatigue, drowsiness, and lethargy. As the hypercalcemia increases, abdominal pain (from peptic ulcer disease), nausea, and vomiting are typical. The patient may report generalized bone pain and may have had recent fractures from what appeared to be little cause.

PHYSICAL EXAMINATION. Little definitive data can be obtained in a physical examination. Hypertension is common, and if the patient is on digitalis, there may be a significantly lowered pulse rate, which signals increased sensitivity to the drug. Muscle atrophy and depressed tendon reflexes are late signs of hypercalcemia. The patient may have marked muscle weakness and atrophy (particularly in the legs) and skeletal deformities. If the central nervous system is affected, there will be changes in mental status, such as confusion, disorientation, and even coma. Palpation of even grossly enlarged parathyroid glands is generally impossible because of their location.

PSYCHOSOCIAL. The hypercalcemic patient or the significant others may note memory changes, confusion, irritability, and symptoms of depression or paranoia (or both). The psychological clinical manifestations may range from mild to acute psychosis, or possibly paranoid hallucinations. The patient and significant others may be understandably upset or anxious about the changes in the patient's behavior.

DIAGNOSTIC HIGHLIGHTS

Test	Normal Result	Abnormality with Condition	Explanation
Serum calcium: total calcium, including free ionized calcium and calcium bound with protein or organic ions	8.6–10.3 mg/dL	> 10.5 mg/dL; critical value is > 14 mg/dL	Accumulation of calcium above normal levels in the extracellular fluid compartment; clinical manifestations generally occur when calcium levels are above 12 mg/dL and tend to be more severe if hypercalcemia develops rapidly
Serum ionized calcium: unbound calcium; level	4.5–5.1 mg/dL	> 5.5 mg/dL	Ionized calcium is approximately 46%–50% of circulating calcium

unaffected by albumin level			and is the form of calcium available for enzymatic reactions and neuromuscular function; levels increase and decrease with blood pH levels; for every 0.1 pH decrease, ionized calcium increases 1.5%–2.5%.
Serum parathyroid hormone level	10–65 pg/mL	Elevated in more than 90% of people with primary hyperparathyroidism	Determines presence of hyperparathyroidism

Other Tests: Supporting tests include x rays, electrocardiogram (ECG), ultrasound, and magnetic resonance imaging (MRI).

PRIMARY NURSING DIAGNOSIS

Activity intolerance related to fatigue, muscle weakness, and bone pain

OUTCOMES. Energy conservation; Knowledge: Disease process, Diet, Medication, and Prescribed activity; Nutritional status: Energy; Pain level; Symptom severity

INTERVENTIONS. Electrolyte management: Hypercalcemia; Fluid management; Medication management; Exercise promotion; Fall prevention; Surveillance

☐ PLANNING AND IMPLEMENTATION

Collaborative

Surgical removal of the parathyroid glands is the only definitive treatment and is the treatment of choice for primary hyperparathyroidism. Indications for surgery include symptoms resulting from hypercalcemia, nephrolithiasis, reduced bone mass, serum calcium level in excess of 12 mg/dL, age younger than 50 years, and infeasibility of long-term follow-up. If hyperplasia (proliferation of normal cells) of the glands is excessive, all but one-half of one gland is removed because only a small amount of glandular tissue is necessary to maintain appropriate levels of PTH. The individual who has had all four glands removed will quickly become hypoparathyroid and must be treated accordingly. To prevent postoperative deficits of calcium, magnesium, and phosphorus, the patient may need either intravenous (IV) or oral supplements. Bone pain may subside as soon as 3 days after surgery, but renal dysfunction may be irreversible.

Nonsurgical management includes medications to assist in the excretion of calcium by the kidneys. Medical therapy, however, has not been shown to affect the clinical outcome of primary hyperparathyroidism. Postmenopausal women with primary hyperparathyroidism may receive estrogen replacement therapy. The patient may be placed on a low–vitamin D diet that is high in calories, but calcium restrictions are generally not beneficial. To increase calcium excretion, the patient needs a large fluid intake, at least 2 to 3 L per day, and 8 to 10 g of salt per day. Foods high in fiber will assist the patient to have normal bowel function.

Secondary hyperparathyroidism is managed by treating the underlying cause; either vitamin D therapy, prednisone, or aluminum hydroxide may be used, depending on the underlying cause of the disorder.

PHARMACOLOGIC HIGHLIGHTS

Medication or Drug Class	Dosage	Description	Rationale
Conjugated estrogen (Premarin)	0.3.–1.25 mg po qd, 21 days on, 7 days off	Estrogen; hormone	Decreases the sensitivity of bones to increased PTH, thereby increasing bone calcium
Predinosone	20–50 mg po bid	Glucocorticoids	Manages secondary hyperparathyroidism in the management of some cancers that lead to hypercalcemia

Independent

Generally, increase the patient's mobility, protect the patient from injury, monitor for possible complications, and provide patient education. Provide comfort measures for bone and joint pain. Increased activity limits further bone demineralization. Moderate weight-bearing activities are more beneficial to the patient than either range-of-motion exercises in bed or chair rest. Patients with hyperparathyroidism may be weak and at risk for falls and trauma. If the patient is hospitalized, maintain safety measures.

If the patient is recovering from a parathyroidectomy, the most life-threatening complication is airway compromise, either from swelling or from acute hypocalcemia. Keep emergency intubation and tracheostomy equipment in a readily available location. Notify the surgeon immediately if the patient develops respiratory distress, stridor, neck swelling, or hoarseness because of laryngeal nerve damage. Maintain the patient in a semi-Fowler position to decrease postoperative edema. If the patient develops tingling in the hands and around the mouth, notify the surgeon and obtain serum calcium levels if prescribed to determine if tetany is beginning.

As with many endocrine disorders, the patient may be frustrated with the clinical manifestations of the disease and require frequent reassurance. Reassure the patient that most of the symptoms will reverse with the return of normal calcium levels. Assist the patient in identifying stressors and methods of coping with the stressors.

DOCUMENTATION GUIDELINES

- Physical findings: Signs and symptoms of calcium imbalance, bone deformity, patency of airway
- Prevention of complications: Postoperative swelling, postoperative wound healing
- Response to mobility: Level of activity tolerance, response to activity, energy level, pain level

DISCHARGE AND HOME HEALTHCARE GUIDELINES

Teach the patient about the disease process and the signs and symptoms of calcium imbalance. Stress that the symptoms require immediate medical attention. Describe any dietary considerations, including a diet low in calcium with limitation and avoidance of milk products. If the patient is on potassium-depleting diuretics, note that a diet high in potassium-rich foods (apricots, fresh vegetables, citrus fruits) is necessary if no potassium supplements are prescribed. In addition, a diet with adequate fiber and fluid will aid normal bowel function. Teach the action, dosage, route, and side effects of all medications.

If the patient has a surgical incision, describe incisional care and arrange for a follow-up visit with the surgeon. Instruct the patient on the appropriate activity level. Note that recalcification of the bones will take some time. If the patient maintains mobility, recalcification will be increased. Suggest that the patient avoid bed rest; encourage the patient to space activity throughout the day and use the energy levels as a guide to activity. Remind the patient to avoid contact sports or other activities that place him or her at risk for falls or fractures.

Hyperphosphatemia

DRG Category: 299
Mean LOS: 4.3 days
Description: MEDICAL: Inborn Errors of Metabolism

Phosphorus is one of the primary intracellular ions in the body. It is found as both organic phosphorus and inorganic phosphorus salts. Phosphate plays a critical role in all of the body's tissues. It is an important structural element in the bones and is essential to the function of muscle, red blood cells, and the nervous system. It is responsible for bone growth and interacts with hemoglobin in the red blood cells, thus promoting oxygen release to the body's tissues. Phosphate is responsible for promotion of white blood cell phagocytic action and is important in platelet structure and function. It also acts as a buffering agent for urine. In one of its most important roles, phosphate is critical for the production of adenosine triphosphate (ATP), the chief energy source of the body. Approximately 85% of body phosphorus is in bone, and most of the remainder is intracellular; only 1% is in the extracellular fluid. Normal serum phosphate levels are 2.5 to 4.5 mg/dL, whereas intracellular phosphorus levels are as high as 300 mg/dL.

Phosphorus is absorbed primarily in the jejunum from foods such as red meats, fish, poultry, eggs, and milk products. Phosphate is regulated by the kidneys; 90% of phosphate excretion occurs by the renal route and 10% by the fecal route. Phosphate is also regulated by vitamin D and by parathyroid hormone. Phosphorus levels are inversely related to calcium levels. Hyperphosphatemia occurs when serum phosphorus levels exceed 4.5 mg/dL.

CAUSES

The primary cause of hyperphosphatemia is decreased phosphorus excretion because of renal insufficiency or renal failure (acute or chronic). Decreased phosphate excretion also occurs with hypoparathyroidism. Decreased parathyroid activity leads to decreased calcium concentration and increased phosphorus concentration. Increased serum phosphorus absorption may also occur with increased intake of vitamin D or excessive quantities of milk. An increased intake of phosphorus or phosphorus-containing medications, such as enemas, laxatives, or antacids, can cause substantial absorption of phosphorus. Blood transfusions may also cause increased levels of phosphorus because phosphate leaks from the blood cells during storage. Phosphates may be released in excessive quantities in patients who are receiving chemotherapy for neoplastic diseases. Muscle necrosis because of trauma, viral infections, or heat stroke may also cause hyperphosphatemia because muscle tissues store the bulk of soft tissue phosphates.

GENDER AND LIFE SPAN CONSIDERATIONS

Serum levels of phosphate are normally higher (3.5–5.5 mg/dL) in children because of the increased rate of skeletal growth. Infants who are fed cow's milk or formula may develop hyperphosphatemia because cow's milk contains more (940 mg/L) phosphorus compared to human milk (150 mg/L). The most common cause, renal failure, occurs across the life span and in both sexes.

☐ ASSESSMENT

HISTORY. Generally, patients with increased serum phosphorus levels exhibit signs and symptoms associated with hypocalcemia. Ask about a current history of chronic laxative or enema use, excess antacid use, and increased intake of foods containing large amounts of phosphorus (dried beans and peas, eggs, fish, meats, milk, nuts). Note if the patient has been admitted for massive burns or trauma, acute pancreatitis, acute or chronic renal failure, neoplastic disorders, or hypoparathyroidism.

Tetany, increased neural excitability, may develop. Determine if the patient has experienced tingling in the fingertips or around the mouth. As tetany progresses, tingling may progress up the limbs and around the face and increase in intensity from tingling to numbness followed by pain accompanied by muscle spasm. Tetany is more common in patients who have taken an increased phosphorus load by diet or through medication. It is less likely in the renal patient because calcium ionization is increased in the presence of acidosis.

PHYSICAL EXAMINATION. An elevated serum phosphorus level causes few signs or symptoms. Long-term consequences may involve soft tissue calcification for the patient with chronic renal failure resulting from precipitation of calcium phosphates in nonosseous sites, often the kidney, liver, and lungs. Other nonosseous sites may include arteries, joints, skin, or the corneas. Tetany may account for the majority of signs and symptoms because of hypocalcemia. Check for Trousseau's (development of carpal spasm when a blood pressure cuff is inflated above systolic pressure for 3 minutes) and Chvostek's (twitching facial muscles when the facial nerve is tapped anterior to the ear) signs.

PSYCHOSOCIAL. Hyperphosphatemia is most often associated with other chronic problems, such as renal failure, hypoparathyroidism, or chemotherapy for neoplastic diseases. Assess the patient's ability to cope with a serious disease and evaluate the patient's social network for available support and coping abilities.

DIAGNOSTIC HIGHLIGHTS

Test	Normal Result	Abnormality with Condition	Explanation
Serum phosphorus	2.5–4.5 mg/dL	> 4.5 mg/dL (adults); > 5.5 mg/dL (children)	Reflects phosphorus excess
Serum calcium*	8.6–10.3 mg/dL	< 8.5 mg/dL	Reflects calcium deficit
Serum ionized calcium (free calcium)	4.5–5.1 mg/dL	< 4.5 mg/dL	Reflects ionized calcium (46%–50% of circulating calcium)

Other Tests: ECG, blood urea nitrogen, creatinine

PRIMARY NURSING DIAGNOSIS

Alteration in nutrition: More than body requirements related to increased vitamin D or phosphorus intake

OUTCOMES. Nutritional status: Food and fluid intake; Nutrient intake; Knowledge: Medication, Treatment regimen

INTERVENTIONS: Electrolyte management: Hyperphosphatemia; Fluid balance; Electrolyte management: Hypocalcemia; Medication administration; Medication management; Surveillance

☐ PLANNING AND IMPLEMENTATION

Collaborative

Medical treatment is aimed at managing the underlying disease process. If the hyperphosphatemia is caused by excessive phosphate administration in medications, elimination or substitution of the products remedies the problem. In some cases, pharmacologic agents, such as aluminum hydroxide, are used. In some instances hemodialysis is needed to control the excess phosphate levels. Because hyperphosphatemia can impair kidney function, the physician monitors the patient's renal function carefully.

Adequate levels of phosphorus are easily maintained by a normal diet because phosphorus is abundant in many foods, including red meat, poultry, eggs, vegetables, hard cheese, cream, nuts, cereals such as bran or oatmeal, dried fruits, and desserts made with milk. These foods may need to be restricted in the diet when patients have increased levels of phosphorus because of chronic diseases. Because the most common dietary factor causing hyperphosphatemia is vitamin D, it is often temporarily eliminated from the diet. A referral to a dietitian can help the patient with menu alternatives.

PHARMACOLOGIC HIGHLIGHTS

Medication or Drug Class	Dosage	Description	Rationale
Phosphate binding agents	Varies with drug	Aluminum hydroxide (Amphojel) or	To cause phosphate binding in the

| Aluminum carbonate (Basaljel) | gastrointestinal tract, thereby decreasing serum phosphate levels |

Other: Calcium supplements to prevent tetany

Independent

Identify patients at risk for hyperphosphatemia. If those patients develop any signs of tetany (tingling sensations, numbness, or muscle spasms and cramps), notify the physician immediately because airway compromise from laryngospasm is a potential complication.

Teach patients at risk for phosphorus imbalances to use care in choosing over-the-counter medications such as antacids, laxatives, and enemas. Patients should learn to read medication ingredients and check with the healthcare provider about any questions regarding the phosphorus content of medications. Make sure that the patient understands the mechanism of action of phosphate binders. Stress the need to take phosphate binders with or after meals to maximize their effectiveness. Explain that phosphate-binding medications may lead to constipation. Encourage the patient to use bulk-building supplements or stool softeners if constipation occurs.

DOCUMENTATION GUIDELINES

- Physical response: Signs of tetany (tingling sensations, numbness, muscle spasms, or cramps)
- Phosphate levels
- Emotional response to chronic illness

DISCHARGE AND HOME HEALTHCARE GUIDELINES

Teach the patient to avoid the use of over-the-counter medications that contain phosphorus, such as certain enemas, antacids, or laxatives. Instruct the patient to avoid foods high in phosphorus and vitamin D. Teach the patient to recognize signs of low calcium. Notify the patient of the next appointment with the healthcare provider.

Hypertension

DRG Category: 134
Mean LOS: 3.5 days
Description: MEDICAL: Hypertension

Hypertension is a persistent or intermittent elevation of systolic arterial blood pressure above 140 mm Hg or diastolic pressure above 90 mm Hg. Over 60 million Americans have hypertension, which results in significant economic and personal costs, including disability and an increased mortality rate. African-Americans and elderly people are most prone to the disorder and its sequelae.

Hypertension is classified by three types: primary (essential) accounts for over 90% of cases and is often referred to as idiopathic, since the underlying cause is not known. This type has an insidious onset with few, if any, symptoms, so it is often not recognized until complications have occurred. Secondary hypertension results from a number of conditions that impair blood pressure regulation. A severe or accelerating form of hypertension, malignant hypertension, results from either type and can cause blood pressures as high as 240/150 mm Hg, possibly leading to coma and death. This condition is a medical emergency. Untreated, hypertension can cause major complications. It contributes to the development of atherosclerosis and increases the workload of the heart, thereby reducing perfusion to major organs and possibly resulting in transient ischemic attacks (TIAs), strokes, myocardial infarction, left ventricular hypertrophy, congestive heart failure, and renal failure. Damage to small arteries in the eye can lead to blindness.

CAUSES

The cause of primary hypertension is not known; however, it is known that the disease is associated with risk factors such as genetic predisposition, stress, obesity, and a high-sodium diet. Secondary hypertension results from underlying disorders that impair blood pressure regulation, particularly renal, endocrine, vascular, and neurological disorders; hypertensive disease of pregnancy (formerly known as toxemia); and use of estrogen-containing oral contraceptives.

The cause of malignant hypertension is also not known, but it may be associated with dilation of cerebral arteries and generalized arteriolar fibrinoid necrosis, which increases intracerebral blood flow, resulting in encephalopathy.

GENDER AND LIFE SPAN CONSIDERATIONS

Approximately two-thirds of Americans over age 65 have systolic hypertension, usually related to underlying atherosclerosis and stress. Younger individuals may also be affected, depending on the number of risk factors present. Malignant hypertension affects men more often than women, with the average age at diagnosis being 40 years of age.

☐ ASSESSMENT

HISTORY. Elicit a history of previously elevated blood pressure, elevated cholesterol counts, a family history of hypertension, and the presence of risk factors. Ask if the patient is experiencing stress at work or at home. Ask the patient about early signs and symptoms, such as malaise, fatigue, general weakness, or a vague sense of discomfort. Establish any history of headache, lightheadedness, dizziness, nosebleeds, ringing in the ears, or blurred vision. Ask about medications such as steroids, oral contraceptives, or cold medications. Symptoms may occur when the mean arterial pressure exceeds 150 mm Hg. Ask if the patient has experienced any loss of vision, shortness of breath, chest pain, confusion, increased irritability, seizures, transient paralysis or stupor, sleepiness, visual disturbances, severe headaches, or vomiting.

PHYSICAL EXAMINATION. The patient may appear symptom-free in early stages, although flushing of the face may be present. In later stages, a fundoscopic examination of the retina may reveal hemorrhage, fluid accumulation, and narrowed arterioles. Palpate peripheral pulses; note pulsus alternans (alternating strength of the pulse) and bounding arterial pulses. An atrial gallop (S4 heart sound) on auscultation is suggestive of hypertension.

Using a correctly sized blood pressure cuff, measure blood pressure in both arms three times 3 to 5 minutes apart while the patient is at rest in the sitting, standing, and lying positions. Three readings above 140/90 mm Hg indicate hypertension. (See Table 30.) Hypertension should not be diagnosed on the basis of one reading unless it is greater than 210/120 mm Hg. Hypertension can be classified by stage: Stage 1 (mild) hypertensive patients have a systolic pressure of 140 to 159 mm Hg and a diastolic pressure of 90 to 99 mm Hg. Stage 2 (moderate) patients have a systolic of 160 to 179 and a diastolic of 100 to 109. Stage 3 (severe) patients have a systolic of 180 to 209 and a diastolic of 110 to 119. Stage 4 (very severe) patients have a systolic of ≥ 210 and a diastolic of ≥ 120.

TABLE 30 | **Classification of Hypertension**

CATEGORY	SYSTOLIC (MM HG)		DIASTOLIC (MM HG)	RECOMMENDED FOLLOW-UP
Optimal	<120	and	<80	Recheck in 2 years
Normal	<130	and	<85	Recheck in 2 years
High normal	130–139	or	85–89	Recheck in 1 year
Hypertension				
Stage I	140–159	or	90–99	Confirm within 2 months
Stage II	160–179	or	100–109	Evaluate or refer promptly for additional care within 1 month
Stage III	>179	or	>110	Evaluate or refer promptly for additional care within 1 week

Note: Based on an average of two or more readings taken on two or more occasions, adults 18 or older
Source: http://www.americanheart.org/Heart_and_Stroke_A_Z_Guide/bplev.html (accessed September 3, 2001.

PSYCHOSOCIAL. When symptoms are exacerbated, the patient may become anxious or fearful. Since hypertension can result in changes in lifestyle and perception of body image, assess the patient's coping mechanisms.

DIAGNOSTIC HIGHLIGHTS

Test	Normal Result	Abnormality with Condition	Explanation
Blood urea nitrogen	5–20 mg/dL	May be elevated	Determines if renal dysfunction or fluid imbalances are present as a complication of hypertension
Serum creatinine	0.5–1.2 mg/dL	< 2.0 mg/dL	Determines if renal dysfunction is present as a complication of hypertension
Total cholesterol	Individual variations; desirable is < 200 mg/dL	Borderline high 200–239 mg/dL; high > 239 mg/dL	Used for screening to determine risk of coronary heart disease; assesses for hyperlipidemia.

| Triglycerides | < 200 mg/dL | Borderline high: 200–400 mg/dL; high: 400–1000 mg/dL; very high: >1000 mg/dL | Used for screening and initial classification of risk of coronary heart disease; elevations determine hyperlipidemia. |
| Electrocardiogram | Normal PQRST pattern | ECG may be normal or show signs of left ventricular hypertrophy: conduction delays, ST-T changes | Electrical conduction system may be altered by hypertrophied left ventricle |

Other Tests: Urinalysis, chest x ray, complete blood count, plasma glucose, serum potassium and calcium, uric acid

PRIMARY NURSING DIAGNOSIS

Knowledge deficit related to chronic disease management

OUTCOMES. Knowledge: Diet, Disease process, Health behaviors, Medication, Prescribed activity, Treatment regime

INTERVENTIONS: Health education; Teaching: Diet, Disease process, Health behaviors, Medication, Prescribed activity, Treatment regimen

☐ PLANNING AND IMPLEMENTATION

Collaborative

The long-term goal of care is to limit organ damage. For Stage 1 (mild) and Stage 2 (moderate) hypertension, a trial of nonpharmacologic management is usually initiated. Conservative medical management stresses diet, exercise, and changes in lifestyles. Since weight loss can result in a drop of 10 mm Hg in both systolic and diastolic blood pressure, patients are encouraged to reach a weight within 15% of their ideal body weight. Patients are placed on a low-sodium, low-cholesterol diet; reducing sodium intake by 2 g a day can lower systolic readings by 2.2 mm Hg. Advise patients to cease smoking and to reduce alcohol intake to one glass of wine or beer per day. Recommend an aerobic exercise regimen that builds up to 20 to 30 minutes three times a week. When these changes are not effective, drug therapy, along with these recommendations, becomes necessary.

If the blood pressure fails to respond to conservative management, the physician initiates pharmacologic management. Treatment for Stages 3 and 4 hypertension are similar to Stages 1 and 2, with shorter periods of follow-up. Patients with blood pressure greater than 180/110 mm Hg need to be treated with medication. If hypertensive crisis occurs (accelerated malignant hypertension, intracranial hemorrhage, aortic dissection, progressive renal failure, or eclampsia), the physician prescribes IV antihypertensives to be given with an infusion device. Maintain continuous noninvasive blood pressure monitoring if the patient does not have an intra-arterial catheter for invasive blood pressure monitoring.

PHARMACOLOGIC HIGHLIGHTS

Medication or Drug Class	Dosage	Description	Rationale
Beta-adrenergic antagonists	Varies with drug	Commonly used: atenolol, 50 mg po qd; metoprolol, 50 mg po bid; nadolol, 40 mg po qd; propranolol, 40 mg po bid; timolol, 10 mg po bid	Inhibit effects of catecholamines that decrease renin and cause resetting of baroreceptors to accept a lower level of blood pressure
Alpha- and beta-adrenergic antagonists	Varies with drug	Labetalol, 100 mg po bid; carvedilol, 6.25 mg po bid	Antagonize the effects of catecholamines at beta receptors and peripheral alpha$_1$ receptors
Centrally acting adrenergic agents	Varies with drug	Clonidine, guanfacine, methyldopa	Decrease peripheral venous tone and reduce systemic vascular resistance
Diuretics	Varies with drug	Thiazides; loop; potassium-sparing	Cause urinary sodium loss with subsequent intravascular volume loss; cause mild vasodilation
ACE (angiotensin-converting enzyme) inhibitors	Varies with drug	Captopril, enalapril, lisinopril, ramipril	Block production of angiotensin II by inhibiting ACE, thereby leading to vasodilation
Calcium channel blockers	Varies with drug	Diltiazem, nifedipine, verapamil, isradipine, nicardipine	Cause arateriolar vasodilation by blocking calcium channels
Intravenous (IV) antihypertensives	Varies with drug	Sodium nitroprusside, (IV infusion), diazoxide (IV bolus), labetalol (IV bolus), esmolol (IV bolus), nitrogycerin (IV infusion)	Manage hypertensive crisis with a variety of mechanisms of actions

Independent

Teach the patient the pathophysiology of hypertension. Explain the actions, dosages, and adverse effects of prescribed antihypertensive medications, and discuss risk factors that can cause organ damage. Review dietary restrictions. Stress the importance of reading food labels and avoiding prepared foods with high sodium content. Foods with sodium listed among the top five ingredients are not recommended. Recommend that canned meats and vegetables be rinsed for 1 minute to remove most of the sodium. Explain the need to decrease the intake of saturated fats and cholesterol. Encourage patients on potassium-losing medications to eat foods rich in potassium. Patients taking potassium-sparing diuretics should avoid excessive use of salt substitutes, since they may be high in potassium.

Teach the patient the need for regular aerobic exercise and stress reduction. Demonstrate relaxation techniques. Teach the patient the correct use of a self-monitoring blood pressure cuff. Advise the patient to record the reading at least twice weekly in a journal and to bring the journal with him or her when visiting the physician. Explain the need to take the blood pressure at approximately the same time and following a similar type of activity. Also encourage the patient to keep a record of the medications prescribed and their efficacy. Suggest that the patient establish a daily routine for taking antihypertensive medications, and remind him or her to avoid vasoconstricting over the counter cold and sinus medications.

DOCUMENTATION GUIDELINES

- Physical findings: Blood pressure readings, presence of headache, mental status, daily weights
- Response to diet therapy and exercise
- Response to medications
- Presence of complications
- Side effects of medications, noncompliance
- Ability to deal with stress and a chronic condition

DISCHARGE AND HOME HEALTHCARE GUIDELINES

Make sure that the patient understands the need to control risk factors through medication therapy, dietary modifications, exercise guidelines, stress reduction methods, and follow-up care. Have the patient demonstrate an understanding of how to take medicine, how often, and the potential side effects. Emphasize the need for frequent monitoring of blood pressure and laboratory work. Explain which signs and symptoms indicate a need to contact the physician. These symptoms include headache, blurred vision, dizziness, sleepiness, confusion, and changes in sexual performance. If the patient experiences altered sexual performance after starting a medication, encourage him or her to notify the physician immediately to have the medication changed rather than just stopping it without consultation.

Hypocalcemia

DRG Category: 296
Mean LOS: 5.4 days
Description: MEDICAL: Nutritional and Miscellaneous Metabolic Disorder, Age > 17 with CC

Hypocalcemia refers to a diminished calcium level, below 8.5 mg/dL, in the bloodstream. Calcium is vital to the body for the formation of bones and teeth, blood coagulation, nerve impulse transmission, cell permeability, and normal muscle contraction. Although nearly all of the body's calcium is found in the bones, three forms of calcium exist in the serum: free or ionized calcium, calcium bound to protein, and calcium complexed with citrate or other organic ions. Ionized calcium is resorbed into bone, absorbed from the gastrointestinal mucosa, and excreted in urine and feces as regulated by the parathyroid glands. Parathyroid hormone (PTH) is necessary for calcium absorption and normal serum calcium levels.

When calcium levels drop, neuromuscular excitability occurs in smooth, skeletal, and cardiac muscle, thus causing the muscles to twitch. The result can lead to cardiac dysrhythmias. Hypocalcemia can also cause increased capillary permeability, pathologic fractures, and decreased blood coagulation. Most severe cases result in tetany, which if left untreated, leads to carpopedal and laryngeal spasm, seizures, and respiratory arrest.

CAUSES

The most frequent cause of hypocalcemia is a low albumin level, but if serum ionized (free) calcium is normal, then no disorder of calcium metabolism is present and no treatment is needed. Causes of low ionized calcium, which is needed for enzymatic reactions and neuromuscular function, include renal failure, hypoparathyroidism, severe hypomagnesemia, hypermagnesemia, and acute pancreatitis. It is also associated with thyroidectomy and radical neck dissection when there is postoperative ischemia to the parathyroids.

Low serum calcium levels can also occur after small bowel resection, partial gastrectomy with gastrojejunostomy, and Crohn's disease. Severe diarrhea or laxative abuse may also cause hypocalcemia; when intestinal surfaces are lost, less calcium is absorbed. A transient low calcium level can result from massive administration of citrated blood. Some drugs that can result in hypocalcemia include loop diuretics, phenytoin, phosphates, caffeine, alcohol, antimicrobials (pentamidine, ketoconazole, aminoglycosides), anti-neoplastic agents (cisplatin, cytosine arabinoside), and corticosteroids.

GENDER AND LIFE SPAN CONSIDERATIONS

Hypocalcemia can occur at any age and in both sexes, but infants, children, and the elderly are at high risk. In infants, it occurs when cow's milk formula with a high concentration of phosphate is given. The large bone turnover during growth spurts accounts for hypocalcemia in children, especially if their calcium intake is deficient. Osteoporosis in the elderly is associated with a lifetime low intake of calcium, which leads to a total body calcium deficit.

◻ ASSESSMENT

HISTORY. Ask about a prior diagnosis of hypoparathyroidism, pancreatic insufficiency, or hypomagnesemia. Elicit a history of severe infections or burns. Ask if the patient has been under treatment for acidosis, which might lead to alkalosis. Determine if the patient has an inadequate intake of calcium, vitamin D, or both. Investigate causes of vitamin D or magnesium deficiency, such as a gastrointestinal disease that is associated with malabsorption, poor diet, gastrectomy, intestinal resection or bypass, or hepatobiliary disease. Ask about medication use that is associated with disordered calcium metabolism, such as phenytoin or plicamycin.

Inquire about anxiety, irritability, twitching around the mouth, laryngospasm, or convulsions, all central nervous system signs and symptoms of hypocalcemia. Establish a history of tingling or numbness in the fingers (paresthesia), tetany or painful tonic muscle spasms, abdominal cramps, muscle cramps, or spasmodic contractions. Ask the patient about gastrointestinal symptoms such as diarrhea.

PHYSICAL EXAMINATION. Assess airway, breathing, and circulation (ABCs). Hypocalcemia can lead to laryngospasm, dyspnea, and heart failure. Auscultate for heart sounds. The patient may have dysrhythmias, especially heart block and ventricular fibrillation. Tetany, increased neural excitability, accounts for the majority of signs and symptoms of hypocalcemia. Check for Trousseau's sign (development of carpal spasm when a blood pressure cuff is inflated above systolic pressure for 3 minutes) and Chvostek's sign (twitching facial muscles when the facial nerve is tapped anterior to the ear).

Inspect the patient's skin to see if it is dry, coarse, or scaly, which are signs of hypocalcemia. Note any exacerbation of eczema or psoriasis along with hair loss or brittle nails. Check for dental abnormalities. Inspect the patient's eyes for cataracts of the cortical portion of the lens, which may develop within a year after the onset of hypocalcemia.

PSYCHOSOCIAL. Severe hypocalcemia may produce mental changes. Assess for depression, impaired memory, and confusion. As the condition continues, delirium and hallucinations may be present. In severe cases of hypocalcemia, psychosis or dementia may develop. Electrolyte disturbances that affect a patient's personality often increase the patient's and family's anxiety. Assess the patient's and family's coping mechanisms.

DIAGNOSTIC HIGHLIGHTS

Test	Normal Result	Abnormality with Condition	Explanation
Serum calcium: total calcium, including free ionized calcium and calcium bound with protein or organic ions	8.6–10.3 mg/dL	< 8.5 mg/dL	Deficit of calcium below normal levels in the extracellular fluid compartment
Serum ionized calcium: unbound calcium; level unaffected by albumin level	4.5>–5.1 mg/dL	< 4.5 mg/dL	Ionized calcium is approximately 46%–50% of circulating calcium and is the form of calcium available for enzymatic reactions and neuromuscular function; levels increase and decrease with blood pH levels; for every 0.1 pH decrease, ionized calcium increases 1.5%–2.5%. If ionized calcium cannot be measured, total serum calcium can be corrected by adding 0.8 mg/dL to the total calcium level for every 1 g/dL decrease of serum albumin below 4 g/dL; the corrected value determines whether true hypocalcemia is present
Serum parathyroid hormone level	10–65 mg/mL pg	Elevated in disorders other than hypopara-	Determines presence or absence of hypoparathyroidism;

	thyroidism and magnesium deficiency	determines the cause of hypocalcemia

Other Tests: Electrocardiogram (prolonged QT interval; in patients taking digitalis preparations, hypocalcemia potentiates digitalis toxicity), phosphorus (elevated in hypocalcemia resulting from most causes, though in hypocalcemia from vitamin D deficiency, it is usually low), magnesium, creatinine, urine calcium. Note that alkalosis augments calcium binding to albumin and increases the severity of symptoms of hypocalcemia.

PRIMARY NURSING DIAGNOSIS

Risk for ineffective airway clearance related to laryngospasm

OUTCOMES. Respiratory status: Gas exchange; Respiratory status: Ventilation; Symptom control behavior; Treatment behavior: Illness or injury; Comfort level

INTERVENTIONS. Electrolyte management: Hypocalcemia; Airway management; Anxiety reduction; Oxygen therapy; Airway suctioning; Airway insertion and stabilization; Cough enhancement; Mechanical ventilation; Positioning; Respiratory monitoring

PLANNING AND IMPLEMENTATION

Collaborative

If the patient has an airway obstruction, endotracheal intubation and mechanical ventilation may be needed to manage laryngospasm. Hypocalcemia is treated pharmacologically. Acute hypocalcemia with tetany is a medical emergency that requires parenteral calcium supplements. Be aware of factors related to the administration of calcium replacement. A too-rapid infusion rate can lead to bradycardia and cardiac arrest; therefore, place patients who are receiving a continuous calcium infusion on a cardiac monitor, and place the infusion on a controlled infusion device. The infusion rate should be adjusted to avoid recurrent symptomatic hypocalcemia and to maintain serum calcium levels between 8 and 9 mg/dL. Monitor the patient's serum calcium levels every 12 to 24 hours, and ximmediately report a calcium deficit less than 8.5 mg/dL. When giving calcium supplements, frequently check pH levels because an alkaline state (pH < 7.45) inhibits calcium ionization and decreases the free calcium available for physiologic reactions.

Chronic hypocalcemia can be treated in part by a high dietary intake of calcium. If the deficiency is caused by hypoparathyroidism, however, teach the patient to avoid foods high in phosphate. Vitamin D supplements are prescribed to facilitate gastrointestinal calcium absorption.

PHARMACOLOGIC HIGHLIGHTS

Medication or Drug Class	Dosage	Description	Rationale
Calcium supplements	Varies by drug	Electrolyte supplement. Emergency supplementation:	Correct deficiency

| | | Calcium gluconate 2 g IV over 10 minutes followed by an infusion of 6 gs in 500 mL D5W over 4–6 hours; oral calcium gluconate, calcium lactate, or calcium chloride. Asymptomatic hypocalcemia can be alleviated with oral calcium citrate, acetate, or carbonate | |
| Magnesium sulfate | 1 g in 50 mL over 1 hr IV | Electrolyte supplement | Corrects magnesium deficiency; magnesium deficiency needs to be corrected in order to correct calcium deficiency |

Independent

If the patient has an altered mental status, institute the appropriate safety measures. Provide a quiet, stress-free environment for patients with tetany. Institute seizure precautions for patients with severe hypocalcemia. If tetany is a possibility, maintain an oral or nasal airway and intubation equipment at the bedside. Initiate patient teaching to prevent future episodes of hypocalcemia.

DOCUMENTATION GUIDELINES

* Maintenance of a patent airway, normal breathing, and adequate circulation
* Presence or absence of increased neuromuscular activity: Seizures, Trousseau's sign, Chvostek's sign, numbness, tingling
* Response to calcium therapy

DISCHARGE AND HOME HEALTHCARE GUIDELINES

Instruct the patient about foods rich in calcium, vitamin D, and protein. Emphasize the effect of drugs on serum calcium levels. High intakes of alcohol and caffeine decrease calcium absorption, as does moderate cigarette smoking. Patients with a tendency to develop renal calculi should be told to consult their physician before increasing their calcium intake. When hypocalcemia is caused by hypoparathyroidism, milk and milk products are omitted from the patient's diet to decrease phosphorus intake.

Be sure the patient understands any calcium supplements prescribed, including dosages, route, action, and side effects. Advise the patient that calcium may cause constipation, and review methods to maintain bowel elimination. Hypercalcemia may develop as a consequence of the treatment for hypocalcemia. Teach the patient the signs and symptoms of increased serum calcium levels and the need to call the physician if they develop.

Hypochloremia

DRG Category: 296
Mean LOS: 5.4 days
Description: MEDICAL: Nutrition and Miscellaneous Metabolic Disorders, Age > 17 with CC

Hypochloremia refers to a serum chloride level below 95 mEq/L. Normal serum chloride level is 95 to 108 mEq/L. Chloride is the major anion in the extracellular fluid (ECF). The intracellular level of chloride is only about 1 mEq/L. Chloride is regulated in the body primarily through its relationship with sodium. Serum levels of both sodium and chloride often parallel each other.

A main function of chloride in the body is to join with hydrogen to form hydrochloric acid (HCl). HCl aids in digestion and activates enzymes, such as salivary amylase. Chloride plays a role in maintaining the serum osmolarity and body water balance. The normal serum osmolarity ranges between 280 and 295 mOsm/L.

Chloride deficit leads to a number of physiologic alterations such as ECF volume contraction, potassium depletion, intracellular acidosis, and increased bicarbonate generation. Hypochloremia, similar to hyponatremia, also causes a decrease in the serum osmolarity. This decrease means that there is a decrease in sodium and chloride ions in proportion to water in the ECF. When there is a body water excess, chloride also may be decreased along with sodium, preventing reabsorption of body water by the kidneys.

CAUSES

The most common cause of hypochloremia is gastrointestinal (GI) abnormalities, including prolonged vomiting, naso-gastric suctioning, loss of potassium, and diarrhea. Loss of potassium, which occurs as a result of gastric suctioning and vomiting, further leads to hypochloremia because potassium frequently combines with chloride to form potassium chloride (KCl). Chloride is also lost through diarrhea, which has a high chloride content.

Other causes of hypochloremia are dietary changes, renal abnormalities, acid-base imbalances, and skin losses. Diets low in sodium can contribute to hypochloremia, as can medications such as thiazide and loop diuretics. Another common cause in hospitalized patients is the combination of stopping all oral intake during an illness and placing patients on intravenous (IV) fluid.

GENDER AND LIFE SPAN CONSIDERATIONS

Infants, children, and adults of both sexes are at risk for developing hypochloremia. Elderly patients are particularly at risk when they are placed on multiple medications or if they have persistent bouts of vomiting and diarrhea. Identify high-risk groups, such as those with GI abnormalities. Note that hospitalized patients across the lifespan are often at risk because of the treatments, such as naso-gastric suction, used to manage their illnesses.

☐ ASSESSMENT

HISTORY. Ask about any recent signs and symptoms that deviate from past health patterns that could cause hypochloremia, such as vomiting and diarrhea. Ask the patient to list all medications, especially diuretics, which contribute to chloride loss. Obtain a history of past illnesses and surgeries. If the patient is already hospitalized, review the records for prolonged dextrose administration and a history of gastric suctioning.

PHYSICAL EXAMINATION. Physical findings depend on the cause of the chloride deficit. Inspect the patient for tetany-like symptoms, such as tremors and twitching; these neuromuscular symptoms are present with hypochloremia associated with hyponatremia. If hypochloremia is caused by metabolic alkalosis secondary to the loss of gastric secretions, respiratory and neuromuscular symptoms appear. Assess the patient's respirations and note the depth and rate; the patient's breathing may become shallow and depressed with severe hypochloremia. If the chloride deficit is not corrected, eventually a decrease in blood pressure occurs.

PSYCHOSOCIAL. In most cases, hypochloremia is a result of gastrointestinal abnormalities. Assess the patient's tolerance and coping ability to handle the discomfort. If the patient is upset about changes in nerves and muscles, explain that the symptoms disappear when chloride is supplemented.

DIAGNOSTIC HIGHLIGHTS

Test	Normal Result	Abnormality with Condition	Explanation
Serum chloride	95–108 mEq/L	< 95 mEq/L	Reflects a deficit in chloride
Serum osmolarity	280–295 mOsm/L	< 280 mOsm/L	Reflects decrease in concentration of particles in extracellular fluid

Other Tests: Serum bicarbonate, serum sodium, urine electrolytes, urine osmolarity

PRIMARY NURSING DIAGNOSIS

Altered protection related to neuromuscular changes

OUTCOMES. Electrolyte and acid-base balance; Neurological status: Consciousness; Nutritional status; Fluid balance

INTERVENTIONS. Surveillance: Risk identification; Surveillance: Safety; Nutrition management; Teaching: Individual; Medication management; Fluid/electrolyte management

☐ PLANNING AND IMPLEMENTATION

Collaborative

Treatment of hypochloremia involves treating the underlying cause and replacing the chloride. Careful monitoring of fluid and electrolyte status is critical.

Monitor serum chloride levels and report any levels less than 95 mEq/L. Observe for decreases in serum potassium and sodium, and note any increase in serum bicarbonate, which indicates metabolic alkalosis. Maintain strict intake and output records, noting any excessive gastric secretion loss, emesis, and diarrhea. Weigh the patient at the same time each day.

In mild hypochloremia, replacement of chloride can be accomplished orally with salty broth. If the condition is severe, IV fluid replacement is necessary. If the patient is hypovolemic, administration of 0.9% sodium chloride increases fluid volume, as well as serum chloride levels. Ammonium chloride can also be given for replacement, and if metabolic alkalosis is present, potassium chloride is administered. Dietary changes are seldom necessary.

PHARMACOLOGIC HIGHLIGHTS

Medication or Drug Class	Dosage	Description	Rationale
Potassium chloride	Oral or IV: 10–40 mEq orally depending on severity of deficit; intravenous dosages should not exceed 20 mEq per hour, except in unusual situations	Electrolyte replacement	Replaces needed electrolytes, particularly in metabolic alkalosis

Independent

Institute safety measures for patients who develop neuromuscular symptoms, with particular attention to changes in level of consciousness and risks to airway patency. Have emergency equipment for airway and breathing maintenance available at all times. Educate those at risk in preventive measures. Teach patients the complications of medication therapy and how to maintain fluid and electrolyte balance nutritionally.

DOCUMENTATION GUIDELINES

- Laboratory findings: Serum electrolytes, osmolarity; daily flowsheet for easy day-to-day comparisons
- Physical responses: Respiratory status (rate, quality, depth, ease, breath sounds); vital signs; GI symptoms (nausea, vomiting, diarrhea); muscle strength, signs of muscle twitching, steadiness of gait, ability to perform activities of daily living; fluid balance, intake and output
- Condition of IV site, complications of IV therapy (infection, infiltration phlebitis)

DISCHARGE AND HOME HEALTHCARE GUIDELINES

Caregivers of the elderly and infants should be alerted to the effect of vomiting and diarrhea on chloride levels. Teach the patient to report any signs and symptoms of neuromuscular hyperactivity. Teach the patient to maintain a healthy diet with all the components of adequate nutrition. Teach the patient the name, dosage, route, action, and side effects of all medications, particularly those that affect chloride and sodium balance in the body.

Hypoglycemia

DRG Category: 296
Mean LOS: 5.4 days
Description: MEDICAL: Nutritional and Miscellaneous Metabolic Disorders, Age > 17 with CC

Hypoglycemia occurs when the blood glucose falls below 50 mg/dL. Normal blood glucose values range between 70 and 110 mg/dL. A series of complex physiological responses is set off when a patient develops a low level of blood glucose. The most dramatic is the sympathetic nervous system (SNS) or adrenergic response, which is primarily the result of epinephrine. Epinephrine stimulates the liver to convert glycogen into glucose to support the falling serum glucose. In addition, the reticular activating system creates a state of alertness and wakefulness (fight-or-flight reaction).

Cerebral dysfunction occurs when the central nervous system (CNS) is deprived of glucose for cellular needs. In contrast to muscle and fat cells in the body that can break down amino and fatty acids for energy, the brain cells depend on glucose for energy. When the liver's supply of glycogen is depleted and no replacement is available, brain damage results. Prolonged periods of hypoglycemia can lead to coma, permanent brain damage, and death.

CAUSES

Causes can best be understood by breaking them into the nondiabetic and diabetic categories. In the nondiabetic patient, there are three classifications of hypoglycemia: organic, iatrogenic, and reactive. Organic hypoglycemia is caused by liver diseases such as hepatitis, cirrhosis, liver cancer, and insulin-secreting tumors. Iatrogenic hypoglycemia is associated with consumption of alcohol and reactions to drugs such as beta-adrenergic blockers and sulfonylureas, the two most common for this problem. Reactive hypoglycemia is caused by an adrenergic response that is triggered within 5 minutes of meal consumption in susceptible individuals. Symptoms are transient. Reactive hypoglycemia occurs in approximately 75% of all spontaneous hypoglycemic reactions.

Hypoglycemia occurs more often in patients who are receiving insulin or oral hypoglycemic agents. Usually this reaction is the result of an imbalance between insulin/hypoglycemic agent intake in relation to exercise or food intake. In the patient with diabetes mellitus, hypoglycemia occurs usually for the following reasons: medication errors (too much insulin or hypoglycemic agent), diet changes (too little food intake or omission), and activity level (increase in activity in relation to medication and food intake). Other causes in the diabetic patient include alcohol consumption, drugs, emotional stress, and infections.

GENDER AND LIFE SPAN CONSIDERATIONS

The potential exists for all individuals to experience a hypoglycemic episode, regardless of age. Diabetic and elderly patients, however, are at higher risk.

◘ ASSESSMENT

HISTORY. General complaints include headaches, tiredness, palpitations, hunger, tremulousness, irritability, nervousness, dizziness, mental confusion, and blurred vision. Question the patient or significant others about the patient's medical history and any current medications. Ask about the possibility of medication errors and changes in diet and activity. Find out when the patient last ate and the content of the meal.

PHYSICAL EXAMINATION. The patient may be apprehensive, stare into space, and have trouble with speech or train of thought. Skin changes include pallor and diaphoresis. Trembling of the hands and seizures are possible. If the hypoglycemia has persisted, the patient may be unresponsive. As the hypoglycemia progresses, the patient becomes unconscious. Infants and children with hypoglycemia tend to have vague signs and symptoms, such as refusing to eat or nurse or a weak, high-pitched cry. As hypoglycemia progresses, children may appear to have poor muscle tone or have twitching, seizures, or coma.

PSYCHOSOCIAL. Ask about the home environment, occupation, knowledge level, financial situation, and support systems, which may provide information that can be used to prevent future episodes. Determine the patient's and significant others' social, economic, and interpersonal resources to help manage a potentially chronic condition such as reactive hypoglycemia or diabetes mellitus.

DIAGNOSTIC HIGHLIGHTS

Test	Normal Result	Abnormality with Condition	Explanation
Serum glucose level	65–110 mg/dL (fasting)	< 50 mg/dL	Deficiency of glucose

PRIMARY NURSING DIAGNOSIS

Altered nutrition: Less than body requirements related to glucose deficit or insulin excess

OUTCOMES. Nutritional status: Food and fluid intake; Nutritional status: Nutrient intake; Nutritional status: Energy; Endurance

INTERVENTIONS. Nutrition management; Nutritional counseling; Energy management; Hypoglycemia management; Intravenous therapy; Medication management; Teaching: Individual and prescribed diet

◘ PLANNING AND IMPLEMENTATION

Collaborative

The immediate management is to maintain a patent airway, regular breathing, and adequate circulation (ABCs) and to replace the glucose to restore the energy source for cells. If the patient is alert, has a patent airway, and can safely ingest oral carbohydrates, you may provide a cup of milk, fruit juice without additives, a granola bar, or cheese and crackers. Approximately 15 to 20 g of carbohydrates can be found in each of the following foods: 4 ounces of orange or grapefruit juice; 8 ounces of milk; three graham crackers; 2 teaspoons of honey; or seven lifesavers. Oral glucose and sugar-containing fluids are effective but may lead to hyperglycemia.

The unconscious, hospitalized patient with severe hypoglycemia or the patient with suspected medication overdose needs a source of intravenous glucose immediately. Occurring simultaneously with glucose administration, if needed, is management of the airway and breathing with endotracheal intubation and breathing with a manual resuscitator bag. Usually with restoration of airway, breathing, and serum glucose, the patient does not have circulatory instability, but the patient may receive IV fluid hydration and inotropic drugs to maintain circulation. If the patient is receiving insulin by continuous infusion either in a crystalloid or in total parenteral nutrition, the infusion is tapered or turned off, and the physician reevaluates the dose.

Once the patient regains consciousness, the oral intake of carbohydrates is increased to maintain the serum glucose. Whether in the hospital or at home, an aggressive search is conducted by the healthcare team to identify the precipitating cause of the hypoglycemic episode, and preventive strategies are instituted for the future.

PHARMACOLOGIC HIGHLIGHTS

Medication or Drug Class	Dosage	Description	Rationale
50% dextrose	IV 25–50 mL, followed by an infusion of dextrose 5% or 10% in water to maintain a blood glucose of 100 mg/dL	Sugar; antihypoglycemic	Supplies a source of carbohydrate that can be immediately converted to glucose
Glucagon	1 mg IM or SC	Antihypoglycemic; promotes hepatic glycogenolysis and gluconeogenesis, stimulates production of cyclic AMP; peak action occurs in 30 minutes and the effect lasts for 2 hours	Treats hypoglycemia if the person cannot maintain oral intake and if IV access is not available; note that the drug may cause vomiting

Independent

Never force an unconscious or semiconscious patient to drink liquids because of the risk of aspiration into the lungs. Continue to repeat the oral intake of carbohydrates until the blood glucose rises above 100 mg/dL, and administer the next meal as soon as possible. If the next scheduled meal is not ready for more than 30 minutes or longer, provide the patient with a combination of carbohydrate and protein, such as 1/2 cup milk, 1 ounce of cheese, and three saltine crackers.

Teach the patient and family prevention, detection, and treatment of hypoglycemia. Encourage a daily exercise, diet, and medication regimen on a consistent basis. Remind the patient to consume extra foods before increased exercise and to carry a rapid-absorbing carbohydrate at all times. Teach the patient and significant others to keep glucagon available in the home or at work or school. Instruct coworkers, teachers, and neighbors how to treat hypoglycemia.

DOCUMENTATION GUIDELINES

- Physical response: Patency of airway, regularity of breathing, adequacy of circulation; assessment of the CNS (level of consciousness, signs and symptoms of hypoglycemia; strength and motion of extremities; pupillary response; SNS response); response to therapeutic interventions
- Blood glucose level; trend of levels after interventions

DISCHARGE AND HOME HEALTHCARE GUIDELINES

Teach the patient and significant others about the signs and symptoms of hypoglycemia and how to manage them at home. Include the following: written materials to reinforce the assessment and management of hypoglycemia and instructions to the patient to carry a diabetic identification card or bracelet.

Discuss with the patient and family the reason for the hypoglycemic episode, and explore ways to prevent its recurrence. If appropriate, assess the patient's understanding of diabetes mellitus and the medications used to manage the disorder. Refer the patient to a dietitian if you note the need for more in-depth dietary consultation than you are able to provide.

Hypokalemia

DRG Category: 296
Mean LOS: 5.4 days
Description: MEDICAL: Nutritional and Miscellaneous Metabolic Disorders, Age > 17 with CC

Hypokalemia is defined as a serum potassium ion level below 3.5 mEq/L. It typically occurs when there is an increase in the potassium concentration gradient between the intracellular fluid (ICF) and extracellular fluid (ECF). Potassium functions as the major intracellular cation and balances sodium in the ECF to maintain electroneutrality in the body. It is excreted by the kidneys: approximately 40 mEq of potassium in 1 L of urine. Potassium is not stored in the body and needs to be replenished daily through dietary sources. It is also exchanged for hydrogen when changes in the body's pH call for a need for cation exchange. This situation occurs in metabolic alkalosis or other alterations that lead to increased cellular uptake of potassium, including insulin excess and renal failure. Potassium is regulated by two stimuli, aldosterone and hyperkalemia. Aldosterone is secreted in response to high renin and angiotensin II or hyperkalemia. The plasma level of potassium, when high, also increases renal potassium loss.

Because 98% of the body's potassium is intracellular, small variations in the potassium concentration gradient can cause major changes in cell membrane excitability. Hypokalemia is a relatively common electrolyte imbalance with potentially life-threatening consequences because symptoms can affect virtually all body systems. Complications of hypokalemia include paralytic ileus, cardiac dysrhythmias, shock, and sudden cardiac death.

CAUSES

Decreased potassium intake can be caused by decreased intake, transcellular shifts, nonrenal loss, and renal loss. Situations that lead to decreased intake include anorexia, fad diets, prolonged periods without oral intake (NPO), and prolonged intravenous therapy without potassium. Abnormal movement of potassium from extracellular fluid to intracellular fluid can be caused by alkalosis, hyperalimentation, hyperinsulinism, and transfusion of frozen red blood cells, which are low in potassium.

Increased non-renal loss occur from prolonged use of digitalis or corticosteroids; laxative abuse; excessive vomiting or diarrhea; excessive diaphoresis; excessive wound drainage (especially gastrointestinal); and prolonged nasogastric suctioning. Renal excretion can be caused by inappropriate or prolonged use of potassium-wasting diuretics, such as acetazolamide, ethacrynic acid, furosemide, bumetanide, and thiazides; diuresis phase after severe bodily burns; increased secretion of aldosterone as in Cushing's syndrome; and renal disease that has impaired reabsorption of potassium.

GENDER AND LIFE SPAN CONSIDERATIONS

Potassium imbalance may occur at any age and in both sexes. Elderly patients are at a particularly high risk because the concentrating ability of the kidney diminishes with age and excessive urinary potassium loss may occur. They also are more likely to take medications that place them at higher risk for potassium deficit.

☐ ASSESSMENT

HISTORY. Question the patient about dietary habits, recent illnesses, recent medical or surgical interventions, and medication use (prescribed or over-the-counter), especially the use of diuretics and corticosteroids. Patients with hypokalemia may complain of anorexia, nausea and vomiting, fatigue, drowsiness, lethargy, muscle weakness, and leg cramps. Knowledge of the patient's usual mental status and mood is helpful. Changes in cognitive ability, behavior, and level of consciousness are not uncommon in hypokalemic patients.

PHYSICAL EXAMINATION. Symptoms vary greatly from patient to patient but usually do not occur unless the potassium drops below 3 mEq/L. Assess the patient's level of consciousness and orientation. Hypokalemic patients may be confused, apathetic, anxious, irritable, or, in severe cases, even comatose. Assess the rate and depth of respirations and the color of nail beds and mucous membranes. Note cardiovascular changes, such as weak and thready peripheral pulses and heart rate variability. The apical pulse may be excessively slow or excessively rapid, depending on the type of dysrhythmia present. Check the patient's blood pressure when he or she is lying, sitting, and standing to assess for postural hypotension. These changes occur in early stages, and the patient's symptoms deteriorate to a generalized hypotensive state in advanced stages of hypokalemia. Note the presence of skeletal muscle weakness, as evidenced by bilateral weak hand grasps, inability to stand, hyporeflexia, and profound flaccid paralysis in severe hypokalemic states. Gastrointestinal function is altered during hypokalemia, and the patient may have abdominal distension and hypoactive bowel sounds.

PSYCHOSOCIAL. Although it is seldom long-term and easily can be corrected, hypokalemia can lead to life-threatening complications. Typically the patient is dealing not only with the hypokalemic state but also with the underlying cause of the hypokalemia. Assess the patient's ability to cope.

DIAGNOSTIC HIGHLIGHTS

Test	Normal Result	Abnormality with Condition	Explanation
Serum potassium	3.5–5.0 mEq/L	< 3.5 mEq/L	Potassium deficit is reflected in serum and extracellular fluid compartment
Electrocardiogram (ECG)	Normal PQRST pattern	Early: flat or inverted T wave, prominent U wave, ST segment depression, prolonged QU interval Late: prolonged PR interval, decreased voltage and widening of QRS interval, increased risk of ventricular dysrhythmias	Potassium deficit leads to changes in the generation and conduction of action potential

PRIMARY NURSING DIAGNOSIS

Altered nutrition: Less than body requirements related to decreased potassium intake, anorexia, nausea, vomiting

OUTCOMES. Nutritional status: Nutrient intake; Electrolyte and acid-base balance; Cardiac pump effectiveness; Knowledge: Medication and treatment procedures

INTERVENTIONS. Electrolyte management: Hypokalemia; Nutrition management; Nutrition monitoring; Vital signs monitoring; Medication management; Venous access devices maintenance; Teaching: Individual

◻ PLANNING AND IMPLEMENTATION

Collaborative

To prevent hypokalemia, most physicians closely monitor serum potassium levels and prescribe supplements to those patients who are in the high-risk categories. Most patients who develop hypokalemia are placed on either oral or parenteral potassium supplements. Potassium is not administered intramuscularly or subcutaneously because potassium is a profound tissue irritant. Parenteral potassium should be administered with extreme caution. Potassium solutions irritate veins and can cause a chemical phlebitis.

Foods high in potassium can help restore potassium levels, as well as prevent further potassium loss. Collaboration between the nurse and a registered dietitian can ensure accurate teaching on dietary maintenance of potassium levels. Common foods high in potassium are bananas, cantaloupe, raisins, skim milk, avocados, mushrooms, potatoes, spinach, and tomatoes.

PHARMACOLOGIC HIGHLIGHTS

General Comments: Administer IV solutions that contain potassium through a controller or pump device to regulate the rate. Mix oral potassium supplements in at least 4 ounces of fluid or food to prevent gastric irritation.

Medication or Drug Class	Dosage	Description	Rationale
Potassium chloride	Oral or IV: 10–40 mEq orally, depending on severity of deficit; intravenous dosages should not exceed 20 mEq per hour except in unusual situations	Electrolyte replacement	Replaces needed electrolytes. Dilute IV potassium solutions because rapid IV administration can be dangerous as rapid increases of serum potassium levels depress cardiac muscle contractility and can lead to life-threatening dysrhythmias

Independent

Interventions are focused on the prevention of potassium imbalances, restoration of normal potassium balance, and supportive care for altered body functions until the hypokalemia is resolved. Teach all patients who are placed on potassium-depleting medications to increase their dietary intake of potassium. Encourage the patient to eat bulk-forming foods and drink at least 2 L of fluid a day unless fluids are restricted because of other patient conditions. Evaluate the patient's knowledge of dietary sources of potassium, and teach the patient and family the needed information. Institute safety measures to prevent falls because of confusion, muscle weakness, or fatigue.

DOCUMENTATION GUIDELINES

- Physical findings associated with hypokalemia, including the current cardiac rate and rhythm on electrocardiogram, bowel function, and degree of muscle weakness
- Detailed description of the K+ supplement route and dosage administration
- Detailed description of the IV site and date of insertion
- Dietary intake, especially as related to foods high in potassium
- Presence of complications related to hypokalemia

DISCHARGE AND HOME HEALTHCARE GUIDELINES

Teach patients at risk, especially those on diuretics, measures to increase potassium in their diet. Teach signs and symptoms that may indicate the presence of hypokalemia: muscle weakness, leg cramps, slow or irregular heart rate, slight confusion or forgetfulness, inability to concentrate, abdominal distension, and nausea. These symptoms should be reported to the physician. Teach the patient how to take his or her pulse each morning and how to keep a daily record of the pulse rate. Remind the patient and family members to give oral K+ supplements in at least 4 ounces of fluid or food and not to take the supplement on an empty stomach. Instruct the patient to report any dizziness, extreme anxiousness or irritability, confusion, extreme muscle weakness, heart palpitations or irregularities, or difficulties in breathing to the primary healthcare provider.

Hypomagnesemia

DRG Category: 296
Mean LOS: 5.4 days
Description: MEDICAL: Nutritional and Miscellaneous Metabolic Disorders, Age > 17 with CC

Hypomagnesemia occurs when the serum magnesium concentration is less than 1.7 mg/dL (1.4 mEq/L). The normal serum magnesium level is 1.7 to 2.7 mg/dL (1.4 to 2.3 mEq/L). An average-sized adult has approximately 25 g of magnesium in his or her body. About 50% of the body's total magnesium is found in the bones, 1% is located in the extracellular compartment, and the remainder is found within the cells. The body's requirement is met by ingesting foods such as meat, milk, and chlorophyll-containing vegetables and fruits.

Magnesium is regulated by vitamin D–regulated gastrointestinal (GI) absorption and renal excretion. Magnesium plays an important role in neuromuscular function. It also has a role in several enzyme systems, particularly the metabolism of carbohydrates and proteins, as well as maintenance of normal ionic balance (it triggers the sodium-potassium pump), osmotic pressure, myocardial functioning, and bone metabolism. Deficits of magnesium lead to deficits in calcium, and the two electrolyte imbalances are difficult to differentiate. The hypocalcemia that accompanies hypomagnesemia cannot be corrected unless the magnesium is replaced. Hypomagnesemia is also a stimulus for renin release, which leads to aldosterone production, potassium wasting, and hypokalemia. Because magnesium regulates calcium entry into cells, consequences of magnesium deficiency include ventricular dysrhythmias, an enhanced digitalis toxicity, and sudden cardiac death. Deficits in potassium and calcium potentiate the dysrhymogenic effect of low magnesium.

CAUSES

The primary sources of magnesium deficit are reduced intestinal absorption and increased renal excretion. Sources of reduced GI absorption include losses from intestinal or biliary fistulae, prolonged nasogastric suction, diarrhea, malabsorption syndrome, and laxative abuse. Decreased oral intake of magnesium also decreases absorption and is caused by malnutrition, chronic alcoholism, starvation, and prolonged administration of magnesium-free parenteral fluids. Increased renal excretion of magnesium occurs because of prolonged diuretic use; the diuretic phase of acute renal failure; acute alcohol intoxication; hyperaldosteronism; syndrome of inappropriate antidiuretic hormone (SIADH); or medications such as cisplatin, digoxin, tobramycin, gentamicin, cyclosporine, and amphotericin. Other conditions that are associated with low magnesium include malignancies, diabetic ketoacidosis, hypocalcemia, hypoparathyroidism, acute and chronic pancreatitis, burns, multiple transfusions of stored blood, and toxemia of pregnancy.

GENDER AND LIFE SPAN CONSIDERATIONS

Anyone with a chronic illness that causes malabsorption or renal loss of magnesium is susceptible. Pregnant women with toxemia are particularly at risk, as are the elderly who are placed on diuretic therapy and people with cancer who are taking chemotherapy.

□ ASSESSMENT

HISTORY. The following conditions put a patient at risk: poor nutrition, diuretics or chemotherapy, pregnancy, old age, or a history of alcohol abuse. Ask about the patient's diet and drinking history, including the amount of alcohol intake on a usual day and an unusual day. Ask the patient to describe bowel patterns, and note if the patient has diarrhea or a history of an eating disorder with laxative abuse. Determine if the patient has experienced irregular heartbeats, lethargy, muscle weakness, tremors, mood alterations, anorexia, nausea, or dizziness.

PHYSICAL EXAMINATION. Observe any signs of muscular changes, such as tetany, spasticity, or tremors. Note the person's affect and mental status because hypomagnesemia can lead to seizures, mood changes, irritability, confusion, hallucinations, psychosis, and depression. The patient's vital signs may reflect hypotension and tachycardia. When you examine the patient's eyes, you may note nystagmus (involuntary cyclical movement of the eyeball) and positive Trousseau's and Chvostek's signs. Trousseau's sign is the development of carpal spasm when a blood pressure cuff is inflated above systolic pressure for 3 minutes; Chvostek's sign is twitching facial muscles when the facial nerve is tapped anterior to the ear.

PSYCHOSOCIAL. The patient may be confused, psychotic, or depressed, which can be relieved with magnesium replacement. If the patient has chronic alcoholism, symptoms may persist beyond treatment of the hypomagnesemia and should be addressed with appropriate consultation and possible rehabilitation. Assess the patient's and significant others' abilities to cope with this sudden illness and any changes in roles that may result.

DIAGNOSTIC HIGHLIGHTS

Test	Normal Result	Abnormality with Condition	Explanation
Serum magnesium	1.7–2.7 mg/dL	< 1.7 mg/dL	Deficit of magnesium ions
Serum calcium: total calcium, including free ionized calcium and bound calcium	8.6–10.3 mg/dL	< 8.5 mg/dL	Deficit of calcium below normal levels in the extracellular fluid compartment

| Serum ionized calcium: unbound calcium; level unaffected by albumin level | 4.5–5.1 mg/dL | < 4.5 mg/dL | Ionized calcium is approximately 46%–50% of circulating calcium; calcium available for enzymatic reactions and neuromuscular function |
| Electrocardiogram (ECG) | Normal PQRST pattern | Prolonged PR and QT intervals; patients on digitalis may have atrial and ventricular dsyrhythmias | Magnesium deficit leads to alterations in generation and conduction of the action potential |

Other Tests: Serum potassium level

PRIMARY NURSING DIAGNOSIS

Risk for injury related to muscle weakness, unstable gait

OUTCOMES. Cardiac pump effectiveness; Circulation status; Electrolyte and acid-base balance; Knowledge: Medication; Respiratory status: Ventilation and gas exchange

INTERVENTIONS. Electrolyte management: Hypomagnesemia; Intravenous therapy; Cardiac care: Acute; Emergency care; Medication administration; Medication management

☐ PLANNING AND IMPLEMENTATION

Collaborative

If the levels are severely low, the patient needs intravenous (IV) or intramuscular magnesium replacement with magnesium sulfate ($MgSO_4$). Calcium gluconate may be administered with IV magnesium replacement therapy to reduce the risk of sudden reversal to hypermagnesemia. If the patient does not suffer from chronic malabsorption requiring total parenteral nutrition, an increase in dietary intake of magnesium is prescribed. Foods high in magnesium include bananas, chocolate, green leafy vegetables, grapefruit, oranges, nuts, seafood, soy flour, and wheat bran.

Monitor for signs of hypermagnesemia during IV infusions. These symptoms include hypotension, labored respirations, and diminished or absent patellar reflex (knee jerk). If any of these symptoms occurs, stop the infusion and notify the physician immediately. If hypokalemia occurs simultaneously with hypomagnesemia, the magnesium level should be corrected first because magnesium is necessary for the movement of potassium into the cell. Be aware that hypomagnesemia may precipitate digitalis toxicity by enhancing the effects of digitalis, which places the patient at increased risk for digitalis-induced atrial and ventricular dysrhythmias and Mobitz type I AV block (Wenckebach). Alkalosis should be avoided or corrected because this condition may precipitate tetany.

PHARMACOLOGIC HIGHLIGHTS

Medication or Drug Class	Dosage	Description	Rationale
Magnesium supplements	Oral (for mild or chronic hypomagensium): 240 mg elemental magnesium po qd to bid; preparations such as magnesium oxide (Mag-Ox 400 and Uro-Mag) may be used; magnesium-containing antacids (preparations that contain aluminum hydroxide and magnesium hydroxide such as Mylanta or Maalox) may be prescribed if the problem was not caused by chronic GI loss (such as diarrhea) IV: 1–2 g magnesium sulfate IV over 15 minutes followed by an infusion of 6 g magnesium sulfate in at least 1 L of IV fluid over 24 hours	Electrolyte replacement	Replace magnesium

Independent

The patient's safety is of primary concern. Reorient the patient as necessary, and reassure both the patient and family that mood changes and the altered level of consciousness are temporary and improve when magnesium levels return to normal. If neurological and muscle status places the patient at risk for injury, evaluate the patient's environment to limit risks for trauma. Symptoms of hypomagnesemia are similar to those of delirium tremens (DTs) in chronic alcoholism; if you suspect the patient of developing either DTs or hypomagnesemia, discuss the symptoms with the physician and monitor the magnesium levels to determine the cause of the symptoms.

Maintain seizure precautions for patients with symptoms and keep environmental stimuli to a minimum. Encourage active range-of-motion (ROM) exercises or perform passive ROM exercises several times a day to help prevent complications of inactivity. Dysphagia may also occur in these patients, and their ability to swallow should be assessed before giving them food or liquids. Encourage the intake of magnesium-enriched foods in small, frequent meals if the patient is suffering from inadequate nutrition. Keep the environment as pleasant as possible. Include the patient and family in meal planning, and request a nutritional consultation if necessary.

DOCUMENTATION GUIDELINES

- Serum magnesium, potassium, and calcium levels; patency of the IV line
- Vital signs, cardiac rhythm, and ECG strip and interpretation
- Neurological assessment findings: Level of consciousness, orientation, muscle strength and sensation, presence of Chvostek's and Trousseau's signs
- Presence of complications: Respiratory distress, tetany, IV infiltration
- Response to treatment: Magnesium sulfate or magnesium-containing antacids, calcium gluconate

DISCHARGE AND HOME HEALTHCARE GUIDELINES

Teach the patient to eat foods high in magnesium and to eat several small meals. Tell him or her to use any prescribed antiemetics before eating if nausea, vomiting, or diarrhea is a problem. Teach the signs and symptoms of hypomagnesemia (changes in level of consciousness, neuromuscular weakness), and instruct the patient to notify the physician if these return.

Explain any oral magnesium supplements, including the dosage, action, adverse effects, and need for routine laboratory monitoring if hypmagnesemia is a chronic problem. Explain that many of the magnesium-containing antacids may cause diarrhea, and instruct the patient to notify the physician if this occurs. Teach the use of assistive devices (cane or walker). The patient should also be taught muscle-strengthening exercises and may need a home care evaluation before discharge.

Hyponatremia

DRG Category: 296
Mean LOS: 5.4 days
Description: MEDICAL: Nutritional and Miscellaneous Metabolic Disorders, Age > 17 with CC

Hyponatremia is defined as a serum sodium concentration less than 135 mEq/L (normal range is 136 to 145 mEq/L). Sodium is the most abundant cation in the body; a 70-kg person has approximately 4200 mEq of sodium in his or her body. Sodium has five essential functions: it maintains the osmolarity of the extracellular fluid (ECF); regulates ECF volume and water distribution; affects the concentration, excretion, and absorption of other electrolytes, particularly potassium and chloride; combines with other ions to maintain acid-base balance; and is essential for impulse transmission of nerve and muscle fibers.

Hyponatremia is the most common of all electrolyte disorders. As serum sodium decreases, water in the ECF moves into the cells. There is less sodium available to move across an excitable membrane, which results in delayed membrane depolarization. Central nervous system (CNS) cells are most likely to be affected by these changes. Four different manifestations of hyponatremia have been described based on the ratio of total body water (TBW) to total body sodium: hypovolemic hyponatremia, hypervolemic hyponatremia, euvolemic hyponatremia, and redistributive hyponatremia. (See Table 31.)

TABLE 31 | **Types and Causes of Hyponatremia**

TYPES OF HYPONATREMIA	FLUID VOLUME AND SODIUM (NA) STATUS	CAUSATIVE CLINICAL CONDITIONS
Hypovolemic	Na loss > TBW loss	Diuretic usage (especially thiazides), diabetic glycosuria, aldosterone deficiency, intrinsic renal disease, vomiting, diarrhea, excessive perspiration, hemorrhage, burns, fever
Hypervolemic	TBW increases at a greater rate than Na	Edematous disorders, congestive heart failure, hepatic cirrhosis, nephrotic syndrome, renal failure

| Euvolemic | TBW is moderately increased; Na is normal | Syndrome of inappropriate secretion of antidiuretic hormone; continuous antidiuretic hormone secretion because of pain, emotion, medication |
| Redistributive | No change in TBW or Na; water shifts between extracellular and intracellular compartments, relative to Na concentrations | Pseudohyponatremia, hyperglycemia, hyperlipidemia |

If the serum sodium decreases slowly, or if it is greater than 125 mEq/L, the patient may be symptom-free. If the serum sodium level drops below 115 mEq/L, cerebral edema and increased brain cell volume occur that could result in death. If it is left untreated, hyponatremia can lead to potassium, calcium, chloride, and bicarbonate electrolyte imbalances; shock; convulsions; coma; and death.

CAUSES

The cause of hyponatremia is associated with the ratio of TBW to total body sodium. In many cases of hyponatremia, there is an excess of TBW relative to sodium. Causes are listed in Table 31.

GENDER AND LIFE SPAN CONSIDERATIONS

Hyponatremia can occur in any age group and in both sexes. It is more common, however, in infants, young children, elderly people, and debilitated patients because these groups are more likely to experience variation in the TBW. Hyponatremia can occur in healthy individuals, such as athletes or outdoor laborers, as a result of sodium loss through excessive perspiration.

☐ ASSESSMENT

HISTORY. Obtain a medical history of any of the disorders that might predispose the patient to hyponatremia. Inquire if the patient is taking any prescribed or over-the-counter medications, because some drug interactions may alter sodium balance. Obtain a diet history to determine the normal sodium and fluid consumption patterns. Ask about nausea, vomiting, diarrhea, abdominal cramps, headache, or dizziness. Inquire about weight loss; mild hyponatremia can cause anorexia. Ask the patient and family if they have noted any change in mental status or behavior. Often the patient with hyponatremia experiences confusion, a flat affect, and personality changes.

PHYSICAL EXAMINATION. Assess the patient's vital signs. In hyponatremia, a low diastolic blood pressure, tachycardia, orthostatic hypotension, and a weak pulse may be noted. Inspect the skin and mucous membranes for dryness and a pale color. Note the skin turgor and peripheral vein refilling time. Assess the patient for decreased muscle strength and decreased deep tendon reflexes. Auscultate the lung fields bilaterally, and note that you may hear adventitious breath sounds with congestive heart failure. Auscultate the bowel sounds and note any hyperactivity that may accompany hyponatremia.

PSYCHOSOCIAL. Assess the patient for anxiety, hostility, and the level of orientation to reality. Discuss the family's ability to cope with changes in the patient's mental status and their ability to provide dietary supervision and care for the patient at home. Because symptoms are primarily neurological in severe hyponatremia, assess the patient's level of orientation and ability to communicate needs.

DIAGNOSTIC HIGHLIGHTS

Test	Normal Result	Abnormality with Condition	Explanation
Serum sodium	136–145 mEq/L	< 136 mEq/L	Imbalance between sodium and water leads to deficits in sodium
Serum osmolarity	280–295 mOsm/L	< 275 mOsm/L	Hyponatremia leads to hemodilution, showing a decrease in the ration of water to particles
Urine osmolality and specific gravity (SG)	200–1200 mOsm/L; SG = 1.016–1.022	Varies depending on cause; often < 100 mOsm/L with SG <1.003	Shows that urine is very dilute as kidneys excrete free water and retain as much sodium as possible

Other Tests: Complete blood count, serum chloride

PRIMARY NURSING DIAGNOSIS

Altered thought processes related to neurological dysfunction

OUTCOMES. Electrolyte and acid-base balance; Cognitive ability; Concentration; Neurological status: Consciousness; Fluid balance; Respiratory status: Gas exchange; Safety behavior

INTERVENTIONS. Electrolyte management: Hyponatremia; Cerebral perfusion promotion; Surveillance: Safety; Intravenous therapy; Fluid management; Fluid monitoring; Seizure precautions

☐ PLANNING AND IMPLEMENTATION

Collaborative

The course of treatment depends on the cause; the goal is to correct the TBW-to-sodium ratio. Hypovolemic hyponatremic patients should be treated with isotonic saline to correct the volume deficit. If hyponatremia is severe (serum sodium >115 mEq/L), an infusion of 3% to 5% sodium chloride solution may be administered slowly in small volumes. Monitor the patient carefully for signs and symptoms of circulatory overload (dyspnea, crackles, engorged veins). Fluid administration should be regulated with an intravenous (IV) controller to decrease the possibility of fluid overload. A diuretic may be given concurrently to avoid the occurrence of circulatory overload. Because IV hypertonic solutions are irritating to the vein, monitor the IV site closely. Monitor the effectiveness of fluid administration by following the serum sodium and osmolality levels, as well as daily weights and intake and output.

Hypervolemic or edematous patients are treated with a fluid restriction: 800 to 1000 mL of fluid is allowed per day. Euvolemic patients need only a water restriction without a sodium restriction. Endocrine abnormalities should be specifically addressed and treated, such as the syndrome of inappropriate antidiuretic hormone (SIADH), which is treated with a water restriction.

PHARMACOLOGIC HIGHLIGHTS

Medication or Drug Class	Dosage	Description	Rationale
3%–5% saline IV solutions	3% saline administered at a rate of 1–2 mL/kg per hour for the first 3–4 hours to target 120–125 mEq/L over 24–48 hours	Hypertonic saline	Correct the sodium deficit

Independent

If the patient is on a fluid restriction, offer cold liquids because they satisfy thirst better than hot liquids. If indicated, encourage the patient to drink liquids high in sodium, such as broth. Report the signs and symptoms of water intoxication (increased irritability, change in sensorium, headache, hyperreflexia) to the physician immediately. If the patient is confused, provide frequent orientation to person, place, and time. Because seizures are a possible consequence of hyponatremia, institute seizure precautions. Keep the side rails padded and raised and the bed in the low position.

Maintain a stable, safe environment. Avoid sensory overload and confusing stimuli that may contribute to the patient's confused or agitated state. Explain to family members the rationales for disturbances in the patient's thought processes, for the fluid restriction, and for the measurement of intake and output.

DOCUMENTATION GUIDELINES

- Fluid intake and output, daily weights, urine specific gravity, serum sodium level
- Vital signs: Presence of fever, tachycardia, low blood pressure, orthostatic changes
- Mental status: Orientation to person, place, and time; observations of confusion or agitation, ability to drink oral fluids, presence of gag reflex
- Response to treatments: Oral and parenteral fluids, dietary and fluid restrictions

DISCHARGE AND HOME HEALTHCARE GUIDELINES

Teach the patient and caregivers the importance of an adequate fluid intake and normal sodium intake and the food appropriate for a balanced sodium diet. If fluid restriction is indicated, tell the patient that using ice chips, iced pops, or lemon drops may reduce thirst. Teach the family that hyponatremia can recur with persistent vomiting or diarrhea because sodium is abundant in the gastrointestinal tract; this fact is especially important for infants, children, and elderly and debilitated patients.

Hypoparathyroidism

DRG Category: 300
Mean LOS: 6.3 days
Description: MEDICAL: Endocrine Disorders with CC

The parathyroid glands—four small endocrine glands located on the posterior surface of the thyroid gland—produce parathyroid hormone (PTH), which regulates calcium and phosphorus balance by affecting gastrointestinal (GI) absorption of calcium, bone resorption (removal of bone tissue by absorption) of calcium, and renal regulation of both calcium and phosphorus. Calcium and phosphorus have a reciprocal relationship in the body; high levels of calcium lead to low levels of phosphorus. Hypoparathyroidism is a rare clinical syndrome and is associated with a deficiency or absence of PTH or a decreased peripheral action of PTH.

Although both hypocalcemia and hyperphosphatemia result from hypoparathyroidism, hypocalcemia accounts for the majority of clinical manifestations. The human body is able to compensate for low or moderate hypocalcemia. The seriousness of the disease is variable with the degree of hypocalcemia and the speed with which it develops. Acute hypoparathyroidism follows swiftly after trauma or removal of the parathyroid glands. The acute form, as with most hormone deficiencies, can result in life-threatening conditions: tetany, hypocalcemic seizures, and respiratory obstruction caused by laryngospasm. Autoimmune hypoparathyroidism develops more slowly. Most clinical manifestations are reversible with treatment; those that are a result of calcification deposits associated with chronic hypoparathyroidism (such as cataracts) and parkinsonian symptoms are not.

CAUSES

Hypoparathyroidism can be classified as idiopathic, acquired, or reversible. Idiopathic hypoparathyroidism has an unknown cause with an unspecified origin. Acquired hypoparathyroidism is irreversible and is most commonly caused by damage to or removal of the parathyroid gland therapeutically. Acquired hypoparathyroidism may also occur as an iatrogenic complication during thyroid or other neck surgery. Reversible hypoparathyroidism occurs in children before the age of 16 as a result of a rare autoimmune disease. It has also been known to occur as a rare side effect of ^{131}I treatment for Graves' disease or with metastases of malignant tumors. Other causes of reversible hypoparathyroidism include hypomagnesemia (which impairs PTH synthesis) and delayed maturation of the parathyroid glands.

GENDER AND LIFE SPAN CONSIDERATIONS

The disease may occur at any age and across both sexes. No specific life span considerations exist.

◻ ASSESSMENT

HISTORY. History may reveal damage to the parathyroid glands during some form of neck surgery. The patient may report many GI symptoms, including abdominal pain, nausea and vomiting, diarrhea, and anorexia. Signs of hypocalcemia—such as paresthesia (numbness and tingling in the extremities), increased anxiety, headaches, irritability, and sometimes depression—may be reported. Some patients complain of difficulty swallowing or throat tightness. Others report difficulty with balancing and a history of falls or injuries.

PHYSICAL EXAMINATION. Note dry skin, thin hair with patchy areas of hair loss, ridged fingernails, and teeth in poor condition. The patient may speak with a hoarse voice or have unexplained wheezing. The patient may have neuromuscular irritability with involuntary tremors and muscle spasms. Check for Trousseau's (development of carpal spasm when a blood pressure cuff is inflated above systolic pressure for 3 minutes) and Chvostek's signs (twitching facial muscles when the facial nerve is tapped anterior to the ear).

PSYCHOSOCIAL. Patients may have altered behavior, exhibiting irritability, depression, and anxiety. The patient and significant others may describe an inability to cope with the physical manifestations of the disease and the stressors of daily life.

DIAGNOSTIC HIGHLIGHTS

Test	Normal Result	Abnormality with Condition	Explanation
Serum parathyroid hormone level	10–65 pg/mL	< 10 pg/dL	Determines presence of hypoparathyroidism
Serum calcium: total calcium, including free ionized calcium and calcium bound with protein or organic ions	8.6–10.3 mg/dL	< 8.5 mg/dL	Deficit of calcium below normal levels in the extracellular fluid compartment
Serum ionized calcium: unbound calcium; level unaffected by albumin level	4.5–5.1 mg/dL	< 4.5 mg/dL	Ionized calcium is approximately 46%–50% of circulating calcium and is the form of calcium available for enzymatic reactions and neuromuscular function

Other Tests: Electrocardiogram (prolonged QT interval; in patients taking digitalis preparations, hypocalcemia potentiates digitalis toxicity), phosphorus (elevated in hypocalcemia resulting from most causes, though in hypocalcemia from vitamin D deficiency, it is usually low), magnesium, creatinine, urine calcium. Note that alkalosis augments calcium binding to albumin and increases the severity of symptoms of hypocalcemia.

PRIMARY NURSING DIAGNOSIS

Risk for ineffective airway clearance related to laryngospasm

OUTCOMES. Respiratory status: Gas exchange; Respiratory status: Ventilation; Symptom control behavior; Treatment behavior: Illness or injury; Comfort level

INTERVENTIONS. Electrolyte management: Hypocalcemia; Airway management; Anxiety reduction; Oxygen therapy; Airway suctioning; Airway insertion and stabilization; Cough enhancement; Mechanical ventilation; Positioning; Respiratory monitoring

☐ PLANNING AND IMPLEMENTATION

Collaborative

The treatment is to increase the ingestion and absorption of calcium. When the patient is acutely hypocalcemic, generally calcium chloride or gluconate is rapidly administered IV. Give oral calcium supplements with meals but not with foods that interfere with calcium absorption, such as chocolate. Vitamin D supplements are usually given to increase the absorption of calcium. The individual with hypoparathyroidism needs a diet that is rich in calcium, low in phosphorus, and that includes a high fluid and fiber content.

During the acute phase of hypocalcemia, monitor the ECG patterns for conduction block, the patient's respiratory status for dyspnea and stridor, and the central nervous system for seizure activity. Alkalosis worsens the symptoms of hypocalcemia because more free calcium binds with proteins when the blood pH increases. Strategies that increase carbon dioxide retention, such as breathing into a paper bag or sedating the patient, can control muscle spasm and other symptoms of tetany until the calcium level is corrected.

PHARMACOLOGIC HIGHLIGHTS

Medication or Drug Class	Dosage	Description	Rationale
Calcium supplements	Varies by drug	Electrolyte supplement. Emergency supplementation: calcium gluconate 2 g IV over 10 minutes followed by an infusion of 6 grams in 500 mL D5W over 4–6 hours; oral calcium gluconate, calcium lactate, or calcium chloride. Asymptomatic hypocalcemia can be alleviated with oral calcium citrate, acetate, or carbonate	Correct deficiency: IV calcium is given cautiously to patients who are receiving epinephrine or digitalis; note that calcium can be irritating to veins when given by the intravenous route
Phosphate binders	Varies by drug	Aluminum hydroxide, aluminum carbonate	Assist in the excretion of phosphates; as phosphate levels decrease, calcium levels increase

Independent

The primary nursing goal is the prevention of hypocalcemia in the high-risk population: those patients with recent neck surgery. In addition to a careful ongoing assessment for the symptoms of hypocalcemia, the patient should have a calm environment. Tell the patient to notify you immediately if he or she has difficulty swallowing or has tightness in the throat. To prepare for emergency airway obstruction from tetany, have intubation or tracheostomy equipment available, as well as IV calcium supplements.

Once the acute phase is over, and the patient has been switched to oral medications and foods, begin patient teaching about a diet high in calcium and medications. The neuromuscular irritability and weakness place the patient at increased risk for falls. Evaluate the patient's ability to ambulate, and remove any obstructions in the patient's room. Assist the patient to identify both stressors and coping mechanisms to deal with the stressors. In particular, the patient needs to learn to avoid stressors such as fatigue and infection. Encourage the patient to ventilate feelings of anger or fear.

DOCUMENTATION GUIDELINES

- Physical findings: Signs and symptoms of calcium imbalance, bone deformity, patency of airway
- Response to mobility: Level of activity tolerance, response to activity, ability to maintain a safe environment

DISCHARGE AND HOME HEALTHCARE GUIDELINES

Encourage the patient to maintain a balance between dietary and pharmacologic calcium. Dietary calcium should be increased and phosphorus decreased. Fluid and fiber should be increased. Milk, milk products, meat, poultry, fish, egg yolks, and cereals, although high in calcium, should be limited because of their phosphorus content. Chocolate is known to interfere with calcium absorption.

Remind the patient to take medications exactly as prescribed and not to substitute over the counter medications for prescribed calcium. Vitamin D supplements are frequently prescribed as well, sometimes in large doses. The patient may take a phosphate binder before or after meals. Some patients may also be placed on thiazide diuretics to control serum calcium. Remind women of childbearing age that pregnancy will significantly alter their calcium needs. Teach the patient about the disease process and the signs and symptoms of calcium imbalance. Stress which symptoms require immediate medical attention, and teach the patient the necessity of ongoing medical follow-up and the need to wear a Medic Alert bracelet.

Hypophosphatemia

DRG Category: 299
Mean LOS: 4.3 days
Description: MEDICAL: Inborn Errors of Metabolism

Phosphorus is a major anion in the intracellular fluid that is measured in the serum; normal serum phosphorus levels range between 1.7 and 2.6 mEq/L (2.5 and 4.5 mg/dL). In children, the serum phosphorus level is higher, at 4.0 to 7.0 mg/dL. Hypophosphatemia occurs when the serum phosphorus levels fall below 1.7 mEq/L (2.5 mg/dL). The possible complications of hypophosphatemia are grave and include dysrhythmias, heart failure, shock, destruction of striated muscles, seizures, and coma.

Approximately 85% of body phosphorus is in bone, and most of the remainder is intracellular. Only 1% is in the extracellular fluid. Phosphorus serves many functions in the body, such as maintenance of the normal nerve and muscle activity; formation and strength of bones and teeth; maintenance of cell membrane structure and function; metabolism of carbohydrates, proteins, and fats; maintenance of oxygen delivery to the tissue; maintenance of acid-base balance; and activation of the B complex vitamins. Phosphorus is excreted by the kidneys (90%) and gastrointestinal (GI) tract (10%). Regulation of phosphorus is controlled by parathyroid hormone (PTH). PTH stimulates a vitamin D derivative (calcitriol) to increase phosphorus absorption by the GI tract. PTH acts on the renal tubules to increase phosphate excretion.

CAUSES

The many causes of hypophosphatemia include dietary changes, GI abnormalities, drug interactions, hormonal changes, and cellular changes. Changes in the diet as a result of malnutrition or alcoholism can significantly reduce the serum phosphorus levels. Inadequate amounts of phosphorus in total parental nutrition may also lead to hypophosphatemia. GI problems that result in a phosphorus deficit include vomiting, chronic diarrhea, and intestinal malabsorption because of vitamin D deficiency. Two types of medications that most commonly decrease serum phosphorus are aluminum-containing antacids and diuretics. Aluminum binds with phosphorus in the GI tract, and most diuretics promote urinary excretion of phosphorus. Infusion of glucose also leads to phosphate depletion, as do increased levels of PTH, which increase the urinary excretion of phosphorus. Cellular changes in several disorders, such as diabetic ketoacidosis (DKA), burns, and acid-base disorders, lead to hypophosphatemia.

GENDER AND LIFE SPAN CONSIDERATIONS

Hypophosphatemia can occur at any age and across both sexes. Identifying high-risk groups—such as individuals with alcoholism, diabetes, malnourishment, or parathyroid disease—is critical.

☐ ASSESSMENT

HISTORY. Ask patients about their diet and if they have had any nausea, vomiting, diarrhea, or loss of appetite. Inquire about medications, especially aluminum-containing antacids and diuretics. Determine if the patient is a diabetic or has a history of alcoholism, hyperparathyroidism, or a serious recent burn.

PHYSICAL EXAMINATION. Symptoms do not usually occur unless there is total body depletion of phosphorus or the serum level drops below 1 mg/dL. With acute hypophosphatemia, the patient appears apprehensive. Ask if the patient has any chest pain, muscle pain, or paresthesia. With chronic hypophosphatemia, an accurate history may be difficult to obtain because often there is memory loss. The patient may report a history of anorexia, muscle and bone pain, and paresthesia.

Hypophosphatemia generally creates neuromuscular, cardiopulmonary, hematologic, and GI abnormalities. Perform a thorough neuromuscular assessment; assess the patient's hand grasp and leg strength, and note tremors of the extremities. Assess the deep tendon reflexes; often hyporeflexia is found. Neurological deficits include paresthesia, dysarthria, confusion, stupor, seizures, and coma. The patient's voice may be weak and shaky. Assess the patient's ability to swallow and the gag reflex. Auscultate the heart; the pulse may be weak and irregular. Assess the respiratory status, and note if the respirations are rapid and shallow because of impaired diaphragmatic function. Weigh the patient and assess for signs and symptoms of malnutrition, such as pallor, dull hair, poor skin turgor, weight loss, and fatigue.

PSYCHOSOCIAL The patient with hypophosphatemia may be anxious and concerned about the muscular weakness, paresthesia, and ability to perform activities of daily living. Assess coping skills and family support and ability to assist with care.

DIAGNOSTIC HIGHLIGHTS

Test	Normal Result	Abnormality with Condition	Explanation
Serum phosphorus	2.5–4.5 mg/dL	Moderate: 1.0–2.5 mg/dL; severe: < 1mg/dL	Reflects phosphorus deficit
Urine phosphorus	400–1300 mg/day	> 100 mg/day when patient is hypophosphatemic	Reflects excessive renal loss of phosphorus

Other Tests: ECG, serum total calcium, serum ionized calcium, parathyroid hormone level, urine amino acids, blood urea nitrogen, creatinine, serum Vitamin D assays

PRIMARY NURSING DIAGNOSIS

Altered nutrition: Less than body requirements related to alcoholism, dietary changes, GI abnormalities

OUTCOMES. Nutritional status; Nutritional status: Nutrient intake; Electrolyte and acid-base balance; Cardiac pump effectiveness; Knowledge: Medication and treatment procedures

INTERVENTIONS. Electrolyte management: Hypophosphatemia; Nutrition management; Nutrition monitoring; Vital signs monitoring; Medication management; Venous access devices maintenance; Teaching: Individual

□ PLANNING AND IMPLEMENTATION

Collaborative

The most important goals are to replace the phosphorus and to correct the underlying cause of the phosphorus deficit. Phosphorus is replaced either by dietary intake or oral administration of phosphate salt tablets or capsules. If hyperphosphatemia inadvertently occurs, hypocalcemia is also likely. Assess for tetany, and be sure that the patient has an open airway, adequate breathing, normal circulation, and an adequate urine output. Routine serum phosphate and calcium levels are ordered to determine the effectiveness of the replacement. Monitor the IV site for infiltration because potassium phosphate can cause tissue sloughing and necrosis.

PHARMACOLOGIC HIGHLIGHTS

Medication or Drug Class	Dosage	Description	Rationale
Phosphate supplements	Oral: 0.5–1.0 g elemental phosphorus po bid-tid IV: phosphate infusion IV over 6 hours	Oral: Neutra-Phos (250 mg phosphorus and 7 mEq each of sodium and potassium); Neutra-Phos K (250 mg phosphorus and 14 mEq sodium; IV: Potassium phosphate and sodium phosphate, 2.5–5.0 mg/kg in 500 mL 0.45% saline solution	Replace phosphorus; often capsules are preferred because the tablet form may cause nausea; if the deficit is severe, IV infusion of potassium phosphate is needed

Other Drugs: Analgesics may be ordered for bone pain. Monitor the effectiveness of the pain medications. Avoid administering antacids that contain aluminum. If the patient develops alcohol withdrawal, the treatment of choice is the benzodiazepine class of medications.

Independent

Maintain an open airway and adequate breathing. Keep an artificial airway, manual resuscitator bag, and suction at the bedside at all times. If you hear stridor or see respiratory distress, notify the physician immediately, insert an oral or nasal airway if appropriate, and keep the airway clear with oral or nasal suction. If the patient is unresponsive, use the jaw lift or chin thrust to maintain the airway until a decision is made whether to intubate the patient.

Maintain a safe environment. The patient may need assistance with ambulation and activities of daily living. Orient the patient as needed. Encourage patient involvement in self-care as much as possible. If the patient develops signs of alcohol withdrawal (restlessness, insomnia, thirst, and tremors progressing to fever, hallucinations, and combative and irrational behavior), notify the physician and decrease stimulation as much as possible. Place the patient in a quiet, darkened room with a cool temperature. Provide frequent sips of water and fruit juices, but avoid fluids with caffeine. Place the patient in a room where he or she can be monitored frequently to decrease the risk of injury.

DOCUMENTATION GUIDELINES

- Laboratory: Maintain a flowsheet on serum electrolytes for easy day-to-day comparisons
- Physical responses: Adequacy of airway, breathing, and circulation; vital signs, noting any respiratory difficulties such as rapid, shallow breathing patterns; cardiac rhythm; intake and output; presence of any neuromuscular twitching, tetany, or seizure activity; ability to swallow; presence or absence of gag reflex
- Any signs of alcohol withdrawal; management of the symptoms; response to treatment
- Duration, intensity, location, and frequency of pain; effectiveness of analgesics

DISCHARGE AND HOME HEALTHCARE GUIDELINES

Instruct the patient on all medications regarding dosage, route, action, and adverse effects. Instruct the patient to avoid antacids that contain aluminum and about the higher risk for recurrence if he or she is taking diuretics. Instruct the patient to eat foods high in phosphorus, such as meats (kidney, liver, and turkey), milk, whole-grain cereals, dried fruits, seeds, and nuts. Many carbonated drinks are high in phosphate as well. Discuss with the patient how to prevent reoccurrence of hypophosphatemia.

Hypothyroidism

DRG Category: 300
Mean LOS: 6.3 days
Description: MEDICAL: Endocrine Disorders with CC

Hypothyroidism occurs when the thyroid gland produces a deficient amount of the thyroid hormones, thus resulting in a lowered basal metabolism. Many individuals with mild hypothyroidism are frequently undiagnosed, but the hormone disturbance may contribute to an acceleration of atherosclerosis or complications of medical treatment, such as intraoperative hypotension and cardiac complications after surgery. In severe hypothyroidism, a hydrophilic ("water-loving") mucopolysaccharide is deposited throughout the body, causing nonpitting edema (myxedema) and thickening of the facial features. The most severe level of the disease is myxedema coma, a life-threatening state that is characterized by cardiovascular collapse, severe electrolyte imbalances, respiratory depression, and cerebral hypoxia.

Hypothyroidism is generally classified as cretinism, juvenile hypothyroidism, and adult hypothyroidism. Cretinism is a state of severe hypothyroidism found in infants. When infants do not produce normal amounts of thyroid hormones, their skeletal maturation and central nervous system development are altered, resulting in retardation of physical growth or mental growth, or both. Juvenile hypothyroidism is most often caused by chronic autoimmune thyroiditis and affects the growth and sexual maturation of the child. Signs and symptoms are similar to adult hypothyroidism, and the treatment reverses most of the clinical manifestations of the disease.

Complications of the disease affect every organ system. Cardiovascular depression can lead to poor peripheral perfusion, congestive heart failure, and an enlarged heart. Intestinal obstruction, anemia, deafness, psychiatric problems, carpal tunnel syndrome, and impaired fertility are a few of the systemic complications.

CAUSES

Hypothyroidism can be a primary disorder that results from disease in the thyroid gland itself or a secondary or tertiary disorder. In most cases, hypothyroidism occurs as a primary disorder and results from the loss of thyroid tissue, which leads to inadequate production of thyroid hormones (primary hypothyroidism). It is most frequently autoimmune in origin but can also be related to iodine deficiency. Secondary hypothyroidism, which occurs in only 5% of cases, is caused by a failure of the pituitary gland to stimulate the thyroid gland or a failure of the target tissues to respond to the thyroid hormones. Tertiary hypothyroidism is caused by failure of the hypothalamus to produce thyroid-releasing factor.

The most common cause of goitrous hypothyroidism in North America is Hashimoto's disease, which causes defective iodine binding and defective thyroid hormone production. Hashimoto's disease is common in the same family and is considered an autoimmune disorder.

GENDER AND LIFE SPAN CONSIDERATIONS

Hypothyroidism is most frequently found in women between 30 and 50 years of age, although also it may affect infants, the elderly of both genders, and men. Some women experience transient hypothyroidism with pregnancy; generally, they may experience it again with subsequent pregnancies. Because patients with myxedema may have confusing signs and symptoms that mimic the aging process, it is often undiagnosed in elderly patients, which can lead to potentially serious side effects from medications such as sedatives, opiates, and anesthetics.

☐ ASSESSMENT

HISTORY. The patient may describe a history of constipation, fatigue even with little activity, weight gain with decreased food intake, aches and stiffness, generalized weakness, slowing of intellectual functions, impaired memory, and loss of initiative. Often patients describe cold intolerance and, if hypothyroidism is accompanied by goiter, discomfort with clothes or jewelry that is close fitting around the neck. The patient may complain of hair loss or slow growing of hair and nails. Women may note heavy, irregular menstrual periods, and men may describe impotence. Both may experience decreased libido.

Determine if the patient's diet is deficient in iodine. Some foods (cabbage, spinach, radishes) and medications (antithyroids, lithium carbonate) can cause hypothyroidism in a person predisposed to the disease. In addition, medications such as digoxin and insulin are potentiated by the hypothyroid state.

PHYSICAL EXAMINATION. The patient has signs of a slowed metabolism and a slow tendon-reflex relaxation. Note a slow speech pattern, flat affect, and difficulty in forming replies to interview questions. The patient may have a dry, thick tongue and hoarseness; dry, flaky skin with a pale or yellowish tint; and edema of the hands and feet. Fingernails and toenails may appear thick, grooved, and brittle. The patient's face may have a distinctive appearance, with thick features, a mask-like appearance, edema around the eyes, drooping eyelids, and abbreviated eyebrows. The patient's hair is often thin and dry; patchy hair loss is common.

On palpation, the skin feels cool, rough, and "doughy." You may not be able to feel the thyroid tissue unless the patient has a goiter. Weak peripheral pulses, distant heart sounds, and hypotension are common findings. The patient has either decreased or absent bowel sounds and may have abdominal distension. Other findings include hypothermia, shortness of breath, and either depressive or agitated mood states. Rare findings include hypoventilation, pericardial or pleural effusions, deafness, and carpal tunnel syndrome.

PSYCHOSOCIAL. The patient's behavior may be depressed, agitated, disoriented, or even paranoid. You may notice intellectual slowing and impaired interactions with others; family members may be upset about the change in behavior.

DIAGNOSTIC HIGHLIGHTS

Test	Normal Result	Abnormality with Condition	Explanation
Thyroid stimulating hormone (TSH) assay	< 10 μU/mL	> 20 μU/mL	Normal value excludes primary hypothyroidism and a markedly elevated value confirms the diagnosis
Thyroxine (T$_4$) radioimmunoassay	5.0–12.0 μg/dL	Decreased	Reflects overproduction of thyroid hormones; monitors response to therapy
Tri-iodothyronine (T$_3$) radioimmunoassay	80–230 ng/dL	Decreased	Reflects overproduction of thyroid hormones
Electrocardiogram (ECG)	Normal PQRST pattern	Low voltage, T wave abnormalities	Determines electrical impulse generation and conduction

Other Tests: 24-hour radioactive iodine uptake

PRIMARY NURSING DIAGNOSIS

Activity intolerance related to weakness and apathy

OUTCOMES. Energy conservation; Endurance; Self-care: Activities of daily living; Ambulation: Walking; Circulation status; Immobility consequences: Physiological; Mobility level; Nutritional status: Energy; Symptom severity

INTERVENTIONS. Energy management; Exercise promotion; Exercise therapy: Ambulation; Nutritional management; Medication management; Surveillance; Vital signs monitoring

◻ PLANNING AND IMPLEMENTATION

Collaborative

Most patients are diagnosed and treated on an outpatient basis. The goal of treatment is to return the patient to the euthyroid (normal) state and to prevent complications. The treatment of choice is to provide thyroid hormone supplements to correct hormonal deficiencies. Treatment of the elderly patient is approached more cautiously because of higher risk for cardiac complications and toxic effects. The medication should not be given if the pulse rate is greater than 100. The treatment is considered to be lifelong, requiring ongoing medical assessment of thyroid function. Polypharmacy is a significant concern for the hypothyroid patient. Several classifications of drugs are affected by the addition of thyroid supplements, including beta blockers, oral anticoagulants, bronchodilators, digitalis preparations, tricyclic antidepressants, and cholesterol-lowering agents.

Because significant cardiovascular disease often accompanies hypothyroidism, the patient is at risk for cardiac complications if the metabolic rate is increased too quickly. Therefore, the patient needs to be monitored for cardiovascular compromise (palpitations, chest pain, shortness of breath, rapid heart rate) during early thyroid therapy. The diet for the hypothyroid patient is generally low in calories, high in fiber, and high in protein. As the metabolic rate rises, the caloric content can be increased. The patient's intolerance to cold may extend to cold foods, making meal planning more difficult.

PHARMACOLOGIC HIGHLIGHTS

Medication or Drug Class	Dosage	Description	Rationale
Thyroxine	100–125 μg po qd	Hormone replacement	Returns the patient to the euthyroid (normal) state

Independent

Monitor the patient carefully for cardiac complications (chest pain, shortness of breath, palpitations, rapid pulse); check vital signs frequently, and monitor the patient's intake and output. Monitor the patient's weight at least twice a week.

The patient with myxedema is generally weak and therefore progressively immobile. Hypothyroidism exposes the patient to the risk of skin breakdown. One goal is to increase the patient's mobility while accommodating his or her extreme weakness with frequent rest periods. Provide meticulous skin care.

Another patient concern is the intolerance to cold. Caution the patient against using electric blankets or other electric heating devices because the combination of vasodilation, decreased sensation, and decreased alertness may result in unrecognized burns. Use of layered clothing and extra bedclothes is helpful to increase comfort. Patients tolerate warm liquids better than cold. Decreased mental acuity, significant weakness, and slower reflexes make the individual at risk for many injuries.

Patients may have difficulty interacting with significant others who have not understood or accepted the changes in their loved one. As their condition improves, patients and families may feel guilty that they did not notice the changes until they were severe. The return to the euthyroid state takes some time. Patients need frequent reassurance that the treatment is appropriate. Patient learning may be difficult for the hypometabolic patient; you can facilitate understanding that most of the physical manifestations are abnormal and reversible.

DOCUMENTATION GUIDELINES

- Physical findings: Cardiovascular status, bowel activity, edema, condition of skin, and activity tolerance
- Response to medications, skin care regimen, nutrition
- Psychosocial response to changes in bodily function, including mental acuity

DISCHARGE AND HOME HEALTHCARE GUIDELINES

Explain all medications, including dosage, potential side effects, and drug interactions. Instruct the patient to check the pulse at least twice a week and to stop the thyroid supplement and notify the physician if the pulse is greater than 100. Explain that the healthcare professional should be notified about the condition. Explain that ongoing medical assessment is required to check thyroid function and that the medications may lead to hyperthyroidism despite the patient's underlying hypothyroidism.

Teach the patient about the thyroid gland and hypothyroidism, as well as complications such as heart disease and edema. Teach the patient that new cardiac or hyperthyroidism symptoms need to be reported immediately. Explain that the caloric and fiber requirements vary. The patient should report any abnormal weight gain or loss or change in bowel elimination.

Hypovolemic/ Hemorrhagic Shock

DRG Category: 296
Mean LOS: 5.4 days
Description: MEDICAL: Nutritional and Miscellaneous Metabolic Disorders, Age > 17 with CC

Hypovolemic shock results from a decreased effective circulating volume of water, plasma, or whole blood. A significant loss of greater than 30% results in a decrease in venous return, which, in turn, diminishes cardiac output and decreases perfusion to vital organs and causes the symptoms that are associated with shock. When there is insufficient oxygen available to the cells, metabolism shifts from aerobic to anaerobic pathways. In this process, lactic acid accumulates in the tissues, and the patient develops metabolic acidosis. In addition, the tissues do not receive adequate glucose, and they cannot accomplish the removal of carbon dioxide. This disruption in normal tissue metabolism results initially in cellular destruction and, if left uncorrected, death. Significant hypovolemic shock (< 40% loss of circulating volume) lasting several hours or more is associated with a fatal outcome.

The American College of Surgeons separates hypovolemic/hemorrhagic shock into four classifications: Stage I occurs when up to 15% of the circulating volume, or approximately 750 mL of blood, is lost. These patients often exhibit few symptoms because compensatory mechanisms support bodily functions. Stage II occurs when 15% to 30%, or up to 1500 mL of blood, of the circulating volume is lost. These patients have subtle signs of shock, but vital signs usually remain normal. Stage III occurs when 30% to 40% of the circulating volume, or from 1500 to 2000 mL of blood, is lost. This patient looks acutely ill. The most severe form of hypovolemic/hemorrhagic shock is stage IV. This patient has lost more than 40% of circulating volume, or at least 2000 mL of blood, and is at risk for exsanguination. Complications of hypovolemic shock include adult respiratory distress syndrome, sepsis, acute renal failure, disseminated intravascular coagulation, cerebrovascular accident, and multiple organ dysfunction syndrome.

CAUSES

The loss of circulating volume can result from a number of conditions. Hemorrhage caused by active blood loss that results from trauma is a frequent source of hypovolemia. Active bleeding or rupture of internal organs, such as the bowel or the fallopian tube when caused by an ectopic pregnancy, can quickly result in hypovolemia even without obvious bleeding. Profound decreases in circulating fluid volume can be caused by the plasma shifts seen in burns and ascites. Other sources of hypovolemia include decreases in fluid intake (dehydration) and increases in fluid output (vomiting, diarrhea, excessive nasogastric drainage, draining wounds, and diaphoresis). Excessive diuresis from diuretic overuse, diabetic ketoacidosis, and diabetes insipidus can also cause hypovolemia.

GENDER AND LIFE SPAN CONSIDERATIONS

Hypovolemic shock can occur at any age and in both sexes. Chronic illness can alter an individual's compensatory abilities in the setting of hypovolemia. The most common cause of hypovolemic shock in children and elders is dehydration. In comparison, although trauma can occur at any age, in young adults the major cause of hypovolemic shock is hemorrhage from multiple trauma.

☐ ASSESSMENT

HISTORY. If the patient is actively bleeding or is severely compromised, the history, assessment, and early management merge together into the primary survey. The primary survey is a rapid (30 to 60 seconds) head-to-toe assessment that encompasses the emergency management of threats to airway, breathing, and circulation (ABCs) or life. If the patient's condition is stable enough to warrant a separate history, ask questions about allergies, current medications, preexisting medical conditions, and the factors that surround the hypovolemic/hemorrhagic condition.

Generally, patients who are experiencing hypovolemia because of trauma have either obvious bleeding or a history of injury to a vascularized area. Elicit information from the patient, emergency medical personnel, or the family as to how much blood was lost or how long the bleeding has continued. In the case of traumatic blood loss, it is important to remember that the most obvious injury site may not be the cause of the evolving hypovolemic shock.

Explore the possibility of a mechanism of injury, such as a burn or crush injury, leading to plasma fluid shifts extravascularly. Likewise, a history of either recent alterations in fluid volume intake or excessive loss—as in vomiting, diarrhea, excessive diaphoresis, or diuresis—is a potential indicator. In addition, obtain a subjective history of thirst, lethargy, and decreased urinary output.

PHYSICAL EXAMINATION. The patient may appear either stable and alert or critically ill, depending on the phase of hypovolemic shock. If the patient can maintain the ABCs, assess the patient's level of consciousness. Restlessness, anxiety, agitation, and confusion may be indicators of diminished cerebral perfusion and are among the early signs of hypovolemic shock. Other early indicators include a decreased urinary output of less than 30 mL per hour, delayed capillary blanching, and signs of sympathetic nervous system stimulation (tachycardia, piloerection [gooseflesh]). Monitor vital signs, including heart and respiratory rate, blood pressure, and temperature. Changes in blood pressure (particularly hypotension) are a late rather than an early sign; pulse pressure, however, does initially widen and then narrow in the first two stages of shock. Orthostatic blood pressure changes also indicate hypovolemia. Inspect the patient's neck veins and palpate them for the quality of carotid pulse and neck vein appearance. Inspect the patient's abdomen for possible sites of fluid loss or compartmenting.

Percuss the chest and lung fields for the presence of fluid. Auscultate the patient's bilateral breathing, and note the patient's respiratory effort. Auscultate the patient's heart, and note any new murmurs or other adventitious heart sounds. When you auscultate the patient's abdomen, note the absence of bowel sounds, which may indicate a paralytic ileus, internal gastrointestinal bleeding, or peritonitis. If bowel sounds are hypoactive, bleeding may be causing blood to shunt to other more vital organs. Palpate the patient's peripheral pulses and note signs of decreased blood flow and inadequate tissue perfusion (cold, clammy skin; weak, rapid pulses; delayed capillary refill), but remember that these signs are late indicators of hypovolemic shock and may not be present until the patient reaches stage III.

PSYCHOSOCIAL. If the patient has a decreased level of consciousness, attempt to identify a family member or significant other to discuss the patient's psychosocial history. Expect family members to be frightened, anxious, and in need of support. Of particular concern are the parents of young trauma patients who have to deal with a sudden, life-threatening event that may lead to the death of a child. Spouses of critically injured patients deal with role reversals, economic crises, and the fear of loss. Expect the family and partner of critically injured patients to express a range of emotions from fear and anxiety to grief and guilt.

DIAGNOSTIC HIGHLIGHTS

General Comments: No one specific diagnostic test identifies the degree of hypovolemic shock state. Several laboratory indicators do provide valuable information on the status of the patient, however. These include arterial blood gases (ABGs), hemodynamic parameters (cardiac output and cardiac index, oxygen delivery, oxygen consumption, central venous pressure, pulmonary capillary wedge pressure, and systemic vascular resistance), blood lactate level, hemoglobin, and hematocrit.

PRIMARY NURSING DIAGNOSIS

Fluid volume deficit related to active bleeding or fluid loss

OUTCOMES. Fluid balance; Circulation status; Cardiac pump effectiveness; Hydration

INTERVENTIONS. Bleeding reduction; Fluid resuscitation; Blood product administration; Intravenous therapy; Circulatory care; Shock management

☐ PLANNING AND IMPLEMENTATION

Collaborative

The initial care of the patient with hypovolemic shock follows the ABCs of resuscitation. Measures to ensure adequate oxygenation and tissue perfusion include establishing an effective airway and a supplemental oxygen source, controlling the source of blood loss, and replacing intravascular volume. The American College of Surgeons recommends crystalloid fluids such as normal saline solution or lactated Ringer's solution for stages I and II and crystalloids plus blood products for stages III and IV. Although vasopressors, such as norepinephrine or dopamine, do increase blood pressure in the setting of hypovolemic shock, they should never be started if there is insufficient intravascular fluid or if tissues remain underperfused despite an adequate blood pressure.

The objective of fluid replacement is to provide for adequate cardiac output to perfuse the tissues. Generally, any fluid transiently improves perfusion, but only red blood cells (RBCs) can carry enough oxygen to maintain cellular function. Three mL of crystalloid solutions should be infused for every 1 mL of blood loss. It is currently recommended to use caution in replacing fluids after trauma because the low flow state may protect the patient from further bleeding until the traumatic injury is repaired. After repair, fluid resuscitation can be used aggressively. RBCs or whole blood should be considered when fluid resuscitation with crystalloids is not successful. RBCs are preferred because they contain an increased percentage of hemoglobin per volume. Type-specific blood is preferred, although O-negative can be used if type-specific blood is not immediately available.

Independent

After initial stabilization of airway and breathing, the most important nursing intervention is to ensure timely fluid replacement. Fluid resuscitation is most efficient through a short, large-bore peripheral intravenous (IV) catheter in a large peripheral vein. The IV line should have a short length of tubing from the bag or bottle to the IV site. If pressure is applied to the bag, fluid resuscitation occurs more rapidly. If fluids can be warmed before infusion, the patient has a lower risk of hypothermia.

Positioning the patient can also increase perfusion throughout the body; place the patient in a modified Trendelenburg's position to facilitate venous return and to prevent excessive abdominal viscera shift and restriction of the diaphragm that occurs with the head-down position.

Patients and their families are often frightened and anxious. If the patient is awake, provide a running explanation of the procedures to reassure him or her. Hold the patient's hand to offer reassurance when possible. Explain the treatment alternatives to the family and keep them updated as to the patient's response to therapy. If blood component therapy is essential, answer the patient's and family's questions about the risks involved.

DOCUMENTATION GUIDELINES

- Adequacy of airway: Patency of airway, ease of respiration, chest expansion, respiratory rate, presence of stridor or wheezes
- Cardiovascular assessment: Capillary blanch, quality of peripheral pulses, presence of gooseflesh, changes in vital signs (blood pressure and heart rate), skin color, cardiac rhythm, signs of uncorrected bleeding
- Body temperature
- Fluid balance: Intake and output, patency of IV lines, speed of fluid resuscitation

DISCHARGE AND HOME HEALTHCARE GUIDELINES

Provide a complete explanation of all emergency treatments, and answer the patient's and family's questions. Explain the possibility of complications to recovery, such as poor wound healing, infection, and anemia. Explain the risks of blood transfusion, and answer any questions about exposure to blood-borne infections. As required, provide information about any follow-up laboratory procedures that might be needed after the patient is discharged.

Idiopathic Thrombocytopenia Purpura

DRG Category: 397
Mean LOS: 5.7 days
Description: MEDICAL: Coagulation Disorders

Idiopathic thrombocytopenia purpura (ITP) is an acquired hemorrhagic disorder that is characterized by an increased destruction of platelets because of antiplatelet antibodies. The antibodies attach to the platelets, reduce their life span, and lead to a platelet count below 100,000 mm^3 but occasionally as low as 5,000 mm^3. ITP can be divided into two categories: acute and chronic. Acute ITP is generally a self-limiting childhood disorder, whereas chronic ITP predominantly affects adults and is characterized by thrombocytopenia of more than 6 months.

The most life-threatening complication of ITP is intracerebral hemorrhage, which is most likely to occur if the platelet count falls below 1,000 mm^3. Hemorrhage into the kidneys, abdominal cavity, or retroperitoneal space is also possible. Prognosis for acute ITP is excellent, with nearly 80% of patients recovering without treatment. Prognosis for chronic ITP is good, with remissions lasting weeks or even years.

CAUSES

Acute ITP is thought to be a response to a viral infection. Generally, a viral infection, such as rubella or chickenpox, occurs 2 to 21 days before the onset of the disease. Acute ITP may occur after live vaccine immunizations and is most prevalent during the winter and spring months when the incidence of infection is high. It is also associated with human immunodeficiency virus (HIV). Chronic ITP generally has no underlying viral association and is often linked to immunologic disorders, such as lupus erythematosus, or to drug reactions.

GENDER AND LIFE SPAN CONSIDERATIONS

Acute ITP affects children of both sexes between the ages of 2 and 9 years. Almost 50% of those children recover in 1 month, and 93% recover completely by 1 year. More than 80% of acute ITP patients recover, regardless of treatment, but 10% to 20% progress to chronic ITP. ITP can also occur during pregnancy, and 5% to 20% of the neonates born to these mothers will have severe thrombocytopenia and are at risk of intracranial hemorrhage during vaginal birth. Chronic ITP occurs mainly between the ages of 20 and 50 years and affects women almost three times as often as men.

◻ ASSESSMENT

HISTORY. Ask if the patient has recently had rubella or chickenpox or a viral infection with symptoms such as upper respiratory or gastrointestinal (GI) symptoms. Ask if the patient was recently immunized with a live vaccine. Check for a history of systemic lupus erythematosus; easy bruising; or bleeding from the nose, gums, or GI or urinary tract. Because the symptoms of chronic ITP are usually insidious, patients may not have noticed an increase in symptoms. With a female patient, ask for the date of the last menstrual period, whether recent menses lasted longer and were heavier than usual, or whether she is pregnant. Ask if the patient has had HIV testing.

PHYSICAL EXAMINATION. Physical examination of patients with acute ITP reveals diffuse petechiae (red to purple dots on the skin, 1 to 3 mm in size) or bruises on the skin and in oral mucosa. Chronic ITP patients may have no obvious petechiae. Other clinical features of ITP include ecchymoses (areas of purple to purplish-blue, fading to green, yellow, and brown with time), which can occur anywhere on the body from even minor trauma. In both types of ITP, the spleen and liver are often slightly palpable, with lymph node swelling. Ongoing assessment throughout patient management is essential to evaluate for signs of life-threatening bleeding.

PSYCHOSOCIAL. Children with acute ITP are usually brought to the pediatrician by highly anxious parents, who are concerned with the sudden appearance of easy bruising petechiae and occasionally bleeding gums and nosebleeds. Because these symptoms are so commonly associated with leukemia, parents and children need swift diagnosis and reassurance. Pregnant women are concerned about their own health, as well as the health of the fetus.

DIAGNOSTIC HIGHLIGHTS

Test	Normal Result	Abnormality with Condition	Explanation
Platelet count	190,000–405,000/mm^3	>100,000/mm^3	Platelets are consumed during clot formation; degree of platelet suppression predicts the severity of symptoms: 30,000–50,000 mm^3, bruising with minor trauma; 15,000–30,000 mm^3, spontaneous bruising, petechiae particularly on the arms and legs; > 15,000 mm^3, spontaneous bruising, mucosal bleeding, nosebleeds, bloody urine or stool, intracranial bleeding

Other Tests: Complete blood count and coagulation profiles, blood smear studies, bone marrow aspiration, HIV testing

PRIMARY NURSING DIAGNOSIS

Risk of injury related to increased bleeding tendency

OUTCOMES. Risk control; Safety behavior: Fall prevention; Knowledge: Personal safety; Safety status: Physical injury; Knowledge: Medication; Safety behavior: Home physical environment

INTERVENTIONS. Bleeding precautions; Bleeding reduction; Fall prevention; Environmental management; Safety; Health education; Surveillance; Medication management

◘ PLANNING AND IMPLEMENTATION

Collaborative

Treatment for ITP is primarily pharmacological. Because the risk of hemorrhage occurs early in the course of acute ITP, therapy is focused on a rapid, sustained elevation in platelet counts. Children with non-life-threatening bleeding are not generally given transfused platelets because the antiplatelet antibody found in their serum is directed against both autologous and transfused platelets.

If the patient fails to respond within 1 to 4 months or needs a high steroid dosage, splenectomy is usually considered. Splenectomy is effective because the spleen is a major site of antibody production and platelet destruction; research suggests that splenectomy is successful 85% of the time. In the face of life-threatening bleeding, such as intracranial or massive GI hemorrhages, a splenectomy is indicated.

PHARMACOLOGIC HIGHLIGHTS

Medication or Drug Class	Dosage	Description	Rationale
Intravenous immune globulin (IVIG)	1 g/kg IV qd for 2 days	Immune serum	Increases antibody titer and antigen-antibody reaction; provides passive immunity against infection and induces rapid but short-term increases, in platelet count
Glucocorticoids	Varies with drug	Prednisone 1–2 mg/kg po qd; methylprednisolone 1–2 g IV for 3 days	Decrease inflammatory response; glucocorticoids are highly controversial therapy for children. Chronic ITP requires a slow steroid taper over several months

Other Therapy: Alternative treatments include immunosuppression agents such as cyclophosphamide (Cytoxan) and vincristine sulfate. Plasmapheresis has been attempted with limited success.

Independent

Many children are managed as outpatients with frequent outpatient visits for therapeutics and platelet counts. If the platelet count is less than 15,000 mm^3, the condition may be considered serious enough to warrant hospitalization. Institute safety precautions to prevent injury and the resultant bleeding and to assist with ambulation. Protect areas of hematoma, petechiae, and ecchymoses from further injury. Avoid intramuscular injections, but if they are essential, apply pressure for at least 10 minutes **after the intramuscular injection** and for 20 minutes after venipuncture. Avoid nasotracheal suctioning, if possible, to prevent bleeding. If a child is being managed as an outpatient, discuss the home environment with the parents or caregivers. Encourage the parents to set up one or two rooms at home (such as the child's bedroom and the family room) as a protected environment. Pad all hard surfaces and corners with pillows and blankets and remove obstructions, furniture, and loose rugs.

Teach the patient and significant others about the nature of this disorder and necessary self-assessments and self-care activities. Teach the patient to report any signs of petechiae and ecchymoses formation, bruising, bleeding gums, and other signs of frank bleeding. Encourage the patient to stand unclothed in front of a mirror once a day to check for areas of bruising. Headaches and any change in level of consciousness may indicate cerebral bleeding and therefore need to be reported to the healthcare workers immediately. Teach the signs and symptoms of blood loss, such as pallor or fatigue. Demonstrate correct mouth care for the patient and significant others by using a soft toothbrush to avoid mouth injury. Recommend electric shavers for both men and women. Teach the patient to use care when taking a rectal temperature to prevent rectal perforation. Recommend care when clipping fingernails or toenails. If any bleeding does occur, instruct the patient to apply pressure to the area for up to 15 minutes or to seek help. Teach the patient to avoid aspirin, ibuprofen in any form, and other drugs that impair coagulation, with particular attention to over the counter remedies.

Provide a private, quiet environment to discuss the patient's or parents' concerns. The period of diagnosis is an anxious one, and parents need a great deal of emotional support. If the child is managed at home, parents need an opportunity to express their fears.

DOCUMENTATION GUIDELINES

- Physical findings of skin and mucous membranes: Presence of petechiae, ecchymoses, blood blisters, hematoma, bleeding
- Reaction to rest and activity
- Presence of complications: Bleeding, petechiae, ecchymoses, headache, increased bruising

DISCHARGE AND HOME HEALTHCARE GUIDELINES

To prevent bleeding episodes, the patient should avoid both physical activity that may lead to injury and medications that have anticoagulant properties. Instruct the patient or caregiver when to notify the physician and how to monitor for bleeding in the stool, urine, and sputum. Remind the patient or caregiver to notify any medical personnel of bleeding tendencies. If the patient is a school-age child, encourage the parents to notify the school of the diagnosis, treatment, and complications.

Explain all discharge medications, including dosage, route, action, adverse effects, and need for routine laboratory monitoring. If the patient is being discharged on a tapering corticosteroid dosage, be sure the patient or caregiver understands the schedule. If the patient had a central line placed for intravenous therapy, be sure the patient or caregiver has been properly trained in care, dressing changes, and sterile techniques. Teach the patient that antacids and oral drugs taken with meals can reduce gastric irritation. Weight gain, anxiety, and mood alterations are frequent side effects of steroid therapy. Parents and families need to be encouraged to lift activity restrictions when the child's platelet count returns to a safe range.

Infective Endocarditis

DRG Category: 135
Mean LOS: 4.3 days
Description: MEDICAL: Cardiac Congenital Valvular Disorders, Age > 17 with CC
DRG Category: 105
Mean LOS: 11.0 days
Description: SURGICAL: Cardiac Valve Procedures without Cardiac Catheter
DRG Category: 104
Mean LOS: 15.2 days
Description: SURGICAL: Cardiac Valve Procedures with Cardiac Catheter

Infective endocarditis is an inflammatory process that typically affects a deformed or previously damaged valve, which is usually the focus of the infection. Typically, endocarditis occurs when an invading organism enters the bloodstream and attaches to the leaflets of the valves or the endocardium. Bacteria multiply and sometimes form a projection of tissue that includes bacteria, fibrin, red blood cells, and white blood cells on the valves of the heart. This clump of material, called vegetation, may eventually cover the entire valve surface, leading to ulceration and tissue necrosis. Vegetation may even extend to the chordae tendineae, causing them to rupture and the valve to become incompetent. Most commonly, the mitral or aortic valve is involved. The tricuspid valve is mainly involved in intravenous drug abusers but is otherwise rarely infected. Infections of the pulmonary valve are rare.

Infective endocarditis can occur as an acute or subacute condition. Generally, acute infective endocarditis is a rapidly progressing infection, whereas subacute infective endocarditis progresses more slowly. Acute endocarditis usually occurs on a normal heart valve and is rapidly destructive and fatal in 6 weeks if it is left untreated. Subacute endocarditis usually occurs in a heart already damaged by congenital or acquired heart disease, on damaged valves, and takes up to a year to cause death if it is left untreated.

CAUSES

The etiology of acute infective endocarditis is predominantly bacterial. The two most common causes of bacterial endocarditis are staphylococcal and streptococcal infections. (See Box 7.) Subacute infective endocarditis occurs in people with acquired cardiac lesions. Possible ports of entry for the infecting organism include lesions or abscesses of the skin and genitourinary (GU) or gastrointestinal (GI) infections. Surgical or invasive procedures such as tooth extraction, tonsillectomy, bronchoscopy, endoscopy, cystoscopy, and prosthetic valve replacement also place the patient at risk.

BOX 7   CONDITIONS PREDISPOSING TO ENDOCARDITIS

- Rheumatic heart disease
- Congenital heart disease (patent ductus arteriosus, ventricular septal defect, bicuspid arotic valve, Fallot's tetratolgy)
- Prosthetic valve surgery
- Parenteral drug abuse
- Placement of intravascular foreign bodies (intravenous catheters, dialysis shunts, pacemakers, hyperalimentation catheters)
- Mitral valve prolapse
- Asymmetric septal hypertrophy
- Marfan's syndrome
- Previous episodes of endocarditis
- Skin, bone, and pulmonary infections

GENDER AND LIFE SPAN CONSIDERATIONS

The incidence of infective endocarditis in infancy and childhood is low. Nearly all children infected have identifiable predisposing lesions. Men over age 45 are at highest risk.

☐ ASSESSMENT

HISTORY. A common finding of patients with pre-existing cardiac abnormalities is a recent history (3 to 6 months) of dental procedures. Question the patient about the type of procedure performed and if bleeding of the gums occurred.

Patients with infective endocarditis may have complaints of continuous fever (103° to 104°F) in acute infective endocarditis, whereas in the subacute form temperatures are generally in the range of 99° to 102°F. Other symptoms include chills (limited to acute infective endocarditis), fatigue, malaise, joint pain, weight loss, anorexia, and night sweats.

PHYSICAL EXAMINATION. The patient appears acutely ill. Observe for signs of temperature elevation, such as warm skin, dry mucous membranes, and alternating chills and diaphoresis. Inspect the conjunctivae, upper extremities, and mucous membranes of the mouth for the presence of petechiae, splinter hemorrhages in nail beds, Osler nodes (painful red nodes on pads of fingers and toes), and joint tenderness. Palpate the abdomen for splenomegaly, which is present in approximately 30% of patients with infective endocarditis. Auscultate the heart for the presence of tachycardia and murmurs. Approximately 95% of those with subacute infective endocarditis have a heart murmur (most commonly mitral and aortic regurgitation murmurs), which is typically absent in patients with acute infective endocarditis.

PSYCHOSOCIAL. Lengthy interventions such as prophylactic antibiotic treatment are generally required. Therefore, determine the patient's ability to understand the disease, as well as to comply with prescribed long-term treatments.

DIAGNOSTIC HIGHLIGHTS

General Comments: There are no specific serum laboratory tests or diagnostic procedures that conclusively identify infective endocarditis, although some are highly suggestive of its presence. Special cultures or serologic tests may detect nonbacterial infective endocarditis.

Test	Normal Result	Abnormality with Condition	Explanation
Blood cultures and sensitivities	Negative	Positive for microorganisms in 90% of patients	If patients have been on antibiotics, they are less likely to have positive cultures; three sets of blood culture should be taken from separate sites over at least a 1-hour period before antibiotics are begun.

Other Tests: Complete blood count, M-mode and two-dimensional echocardiography, and transesophageal echocardiogram (TEE)

PRIMARY NURSING DIAGNOSIS

Infection related to the causative organism (streptococci, pneumococci, staphylococci, gram-negative bacilli, fungi)

OUTCOMES. immune status; knowledge: infection control; risk control; risk detection; nutritional status; treatment behavior: illness or injury

INTERVENTIONS. Infection control; Infection protection; Medication prescribing; Nutritional management; Surveillance; Nutritional management; Infection control: Intra-operative

☐ PLANNING AND IMPLEMENTATION

Collaborative

For persons at high risk for contracting infective endocarditis, most physicians prescribe antibiotic therapy to prevent episodes of bacteremia before, during, and after invasive procedures. Procedures that are particularly associated with endocarditis are manipulation of the teeth and gums or GU and GI systems, and surgical procedures or biopsies that involve respiratory mucosa.

If the patient has developed endocarditis as a result of IV drug abuse, an addiction consultation is essential, with a possible referral to an appropriate treatment program. Surgical replacement of the infected valve is needed in those patients who have an infecting microorganism that does not respond to available antibiotic therapy and for patients who have developed infectious endocarditis in a prosthetic heart valve. (See **Coronary Artery Disease**, p. 265, for a full discussion of the collaborative and independent management of a patient following open heart surgery.)

PHARMACOLOGIC HIGHLIGHTS

Medication or Drug Class	Dosage	Description	Rationale
Penicillin G	2 million units IV q 4 hours for 4 weeks	Antibiotic	Treats penicillin-susceptible streptococcal infections in subacute bacterial endocarditis
Oxacillin;	2 g IV q 4 hours;	Antibiotic	Treats acute bacterial

| gentamycin or tobramycin | up to 5 mg/kg per day IV q 8 hours | | endocarditis; staphylococcus aureus and gram-negative bacilli are the most likely bacteria. |
| Acetaminophen (Tylenol) | 650 mg as needed q 4–6 hours | Nonnarcotic analgesic; antipyretic | Relieves joint and muscle achiness; controls fever |

Independent

During the acute phase of the disease, provide adequate rest by assisting the patient with daily hygiene. Provide a bedside commode to reduce the physiological stress that occurs with the use of a bedpan. Space all nursing care activities and diagnostic tests to provide the patient with adequate rest. During the first few days of hospital admission, encourage the family to limit visitation.

Emphasize patient education. Individualize a standardized plan of care, and adapt it to meet the patient's needs. Areas for discussion include the cause of the disease and its course, medication regimens, technique for administering antibiotics intravenously, and practices that help avoid and identify future infections.

If the patient is to continue parenteral antibiotic therapy at home, make sure that, before he or she is discharged from the hospital the patient has all the appropriate equipment and supplies that will be needed. Make a referral to a home health nurse as needed, and provide the patient and family with a list of information that describes when to notify the primary healthcare provider about complications.

DOCUMENTATION GUIDELINES

* Observations and physical findings regarding level of consciousness, degree of abdominal or chest pain, skin temperature, and color; presence of petechiae, splinter hemorrhages, Osler nodes, joint tenderness, abnormal vital signs, dyspnea, cough, and crackles or wheezing
* Presence and characteristics of heart murmurs
* Response to antibiotic therapy and antipyretics
* Presence of complications: Signs of right- or left-sided heart failure, arterial embolization

DISCHARGE AND HOME HEALTHCARE GUIDELINES

To prevent infective endocarditis, provide patients in the high-risk category with the needed information for early detection and prevention of the disease. Instruct recovering patients to inform their healthcare providers, including dentists, of their endocarditis history, since they may need future prophylactic antibiotic therapy to prevent subsequent episodes.

Be sure the patient understands all medications, including the dosage, route, action, and adverse effects. Encourage the patient to seek prompt medical attention if side effects occur. Make sure the patient or significant others can demonstrate the appropriate method of antibiotic administration. Instruct the patient on proper intravenous catheter site care, as well as the signs of infiltration. Encourage good oral hygiene, and advise the patient to use a soft toothbrush and to brush at least twice a day. Teach patients to avoid irrigation devices and flossing. Teach the patient to monitor and record the temperature daily at the same time. Encourage the patient to take antipyretics according to physician orders. Instruct the patient to report signs of heart failure and embolization, as well as continued fever, chills, fatigue, malaise, or weight loss.

Influenza

DRG Category: 068
Mean LOS: 4.4 days
Description: MEDICAL: Otitis Media and Upper Respiratory Infection, Age > 17 with CC

Influenza (flu) is an acute, highly contagious viral respiratory infection that is caused by one of three types of myxovirus influenzae. Influenza occurs all over the world and is more common during winter months. The incubation period is 24 to 48 hours. Symptoms appear approximately 72 hours after contact with the virus, and the infected person remains contagious for 3 days. Influenza is usually a self-limited disease that lasts from 2 to 7 days. The disease also spreads rapidly through populations, creating epidemics and pandemics.

Complications of influenza include pneumonia, myositis, exacerbation of chronic obstructive pulmonary disease (COPD), and Reye's syndrome. In rare cases, influenza can lead to encephalitis, transverse myelitis, myocarditis, or pericarditis.

CAUSES

Infection with a specific strain of virus produces immunity only to that specific virus strain. Therefore, each year an influenza vaccine is developed to provide immunity against influenza virus strains that are projected to be prevalent for that season. Elderly persons, those with chronic diseases, and healthcare workers are advised to get influenza vaccinations annually in October or November.

GENDER AND LIFE SPAN CONSIDERATIONS

The incidence of influenza cases is highest in school-age children and generally decreases with age, probably because of immunity established by repeated infections as people age. During an outbreak of the disease, however, elderly persons and those disabled by chronic illnesses are most likely to develop severe complications. Males and females are equally susceptible.

□ ASSESSMENT

HISTORY. Determine if the patient has had contact with an infected person within the past 72 hours. Ask about immunization. Establish a history of fever and chills, hoarseness, laryngitis, sore throat, rhinitis, or rhinorrhea. Elicit a history of myalgia (particularly in the back and limbs), anorexia, malaise, headache, or photophobia. Ask if the patient has a nonproductive cough; in children, the cough is likely to be croupy. Determine if the patient has experienced gastrointestinal symptoms, such as vomiting and diarrhea.

PHYSICAL EXAMINATION. Observe the patient for a flushed face and conjunctivitis. When you inspect the patient's throat, you may note redness of the soft palate, tonsils, and pharynx. Palpate for enlargement of the anterior cervical lymph nodes. The patient's temperature usually ranges from 102° to 103°F and often rises suddenly on the first day before falling and rising again on the third day of illness. Check if influenza has produced respiratory complications. Note the patient's rate of respirations, which may be increased. Auscultate the patient's lungs for rales.

PSYCHOSOCIAL. The patient who feels very ill and is unable to continue with normal activities should be assured that the illness is self-limiting and that improvement occurs with rest and time.

DIAGNOSTIC HIGHLIGHTS

General Comments: No specific diagnostic tests are used because diagnosis is made by the history of symptoms and onset. If the patient has symptoms of a bacterial infection that complicates influenza, cultures and sensitivities may be required.

PRIMARY NURSING DIAGNOSIS

Infection related to the presence of virus in mucus secretions

OUTCOMES. Immune status; Knowledge: Infection control; Risk control; Risk detection; Nutrition status; Treatment behavior: Illness or injury; Hydration; Knowledge: Infection control

INTERVENTIONS. Infection control; Infection protection; Surveillance; Fluid/ electrolyte management; Medication management; Temperature regulation

□ PLANNING AND IMPLEMENTATION

Collaborative

Medical treatment does not cure influenza but is aimed at controlling the symptoms and preventing complications. Bed rest and increased intake of fluids are prescribed for patients in the acute stage of infection. For persons who are not immunized but are exposed to the virus, amantadine may prevent active infection. Amantadine is usually prescribed for outbreaks of influenza A within a closed population, such as a nursing home.

PHARMACOLOGIC HIGHLIGHTS

General Comments: Phenylephrine and antitussive agents such as terpin hydrate with codeine are often prescribed to relieve nasal congestion and coughing. In patients with influenza that is complicated by pneumonia, antibiotics may be administered to treat a bacterial superinfection.

Medication or Drug Class	Dosage	Description	Rationale
Antipyretics	Varies with drug	Aspirin, acetaminophen	Control fever and discomfort; generally aspirin is avoided to

			reduce the risk of Reyes syndrome
Amantadine	100–200 mg po qd, bid for several days	Antiviral	Provides antiviral action against influenza (prophylaxis and symptomatic); usually prescribed for outbreaks of influenza A within a closed population, such as a nursing home

Independent

The most important nursing intervention is prevention. Encourage all patients over 65 years or those with chronic conditions to receive annual influenza vaccinations. Teach the patient about potential side effects of vaccination, such as fever, malaise, discomfort at the injection site, and, in rare instances, Guillain-Barré syndrome. Note that influenza vaccine is not recommended for pregnant women unless they are highly susceptible to influenza.

Instruct patients and families to cover the mouths and noses when coughing, to dispose of used tissues appropriately, and to wash their hands after patient contact to prevent the virus from spreading. Limit visitors when necessary. Encourage a fluid intake of 3000 mL per day for adults. Explain that warm baths or the use of a heating pad may relieve myalgia. Provide cool, humidified air; maintain bed rest; and monitor vital signs to detect any change in the rhythm or quality of respirations.

DOCUMENTATION GUIDELINES

- Physical findings: Elevated temperature; erythema of pharynx; enlarged lymph nodes; change in skin color, amount and characteristics of sputum, fluid intake and output
- Presence of chest pain or difficulty in breathing
- Response to bed rest; complications of bed rest; tolerance to activity
- Response to patient teaching regarding immunization, hand washing, and disposal of infected articles

DISCHARGE AND HOME HEALTHCARE GUIDELINES

PREVENTION. To prevent complications, emphasize to the patient the need to maintain bed rest and high fluid intake for 2 to 3 days after the temperature returns to normal.

MEDICATIONS. Instruct the patient and family about the dosage, route, action, and side effects of all medications.

COMPLICATIONS. Instruct the patient and family to report any chest pain, ear pain, or change in respirations to the physician.

Inguinal Hernia

DRG Category: 188
Mean LOS: 4.9 days
Description: MEDICAL: Other Digestive System Diagnoses, Age > 17 with CC
DRG Category: 16
Mean LOS: 3.2 days
Description: SURGICAL: Inguinal and Femoral Hernia Procedures, Age > 17 with CC

A hernia is a protrusion or projection of an organ or organ part through the wall of the cavity that normally contains it. An inguinal hernia occurs when either the omentum, the large or small intestine, or the bladder protrudes into the inguinal canal. In an indirect inguinal hernia, the sac protrudes through the internal inguinal ring into the inguinal canal and in males may descend into the scrotum. In a direct inguinal hernia, the hernial sac projects through a weakness in the abdominal wall in the area of the rectus abdominal muscle and inguinal ligament.

Inguinal hernias make up approximately 80% of all hernias. Repair of this defect is the most frequently performed procedure by both pediatric and adult surgeons. Hernias are classified into three types: reducible, which can be easily manipulated back into place manually; irreducible or incarcerated, which cannot usually be reduced manually because adhesions form in the hernial sac; and strangulated, in which part of the herniated intestine becomes twisted or edematous, possibly resulting in intestinal obstruction and necrosis.

CAUSES

An inguinal hernia is the result of either a congenital weakening of the abdominal wall (when the processus vaginalis fails to atrophy and close) or weakened abdominal muscles because of pregnancy, excess weight, or previous abdominal surgeries. In addition, if intra-abdominal pressure builds up, such as related to heavy lifting or straining to defecate, a hernia may occur. Other causes include aging and trauma.

GENDER AND LIFE SPAN CONSIDERATIONS

A hernia may be detected in both children and adults. Low-birth-weight and male infants are at higher risk (8:1) for this defect than are female infants or full-term infants. Indirect hernias can develop at any age but are most common in infants under 1 year and are more common in males than in females.

☐ ASSESSMENT

HISTORY. An infant or a child may be relatively symptom-free until he or she cries, coughs, or strains to defecate, at which time the parents note painless swelling in the inguinal area. The adult patient may complain of pain or note bruising in the area after a period of exercise. More commonly, the patient complains of a slight bulge along the inguinal area, which is especially apparent when the patient coughs or strains. The swelling may subside on its own when the patient assumes a recumbent position or if slight manual pressure is applied externally to the area. Some patients describe a steady, aching pain, which worsens with tension and improves with hernia reduction.

PHYSICAL EXAMINATION. On inspection, the patient has a visible swelling or bulge when asked to cough or bear down. If the hernia disappears when the patient lies down, the hernia is usually reducible. In addition, have the patient perform a Valsalva's maneuver to inspect the hernia's size. Before palpation, auscultate the patient's bowel; absent bowel sounds suggests incarceration or strangulation.

You may be able to palpate a slight bulge or mass during this time and when the examiner slides the little finger 4 to 5 cm into the external canal that is located at the base of the scrotum. If you feel pressure against your fingertip when you have the patient cough, an indirect hernia may exist; if you feel pressure against the side of your finger, a direct hernia may exist. Palpate the scrotum to determine if either a hydrocele or cryptorchidism (undescended testes) is present.

PSYCHOSOCIAL. A delay in seeking health care may result in strangulation of the intestines and require emergency surgery. In the adult population, surgical intervention to correct the defect takes the patient away from home and the work setting and causes anxiety.

DIAGNOSTIC HIGHLIGHTS

General Comments: No specific laboratory tests are useful for the diagnosis of an inguinal hernia. Diagnosis is made on the basis of a physical examination.

PRIMARY NURSING DIAGNOSIS

Pain related to swelling and pressure

OUTCOMES. Pain: Disruptive effects; Pain level

INTERVENTIONS. Analgesic administration; Pain management

☐ PLANNING AND IMPLEMENTATION

Collaborative

If the patient has a reducible hernia, the protrusion may be moved back into place and a truss for temporary relief can be applied. A truss is a thick pad with an attached belt that is placed over the hernia to keep it in place. Although a truss is palliative rather than curative, it can be used successfully in elderly or debilitated adult patients who are poor surgical risks or who do not desire surgery.

Collaboration with the surgical team is necessary to prepare the patient and family for surgery. If the hernia is incarcerated, manual reduction may be attempted by putting the patient in Trendelenburg's position with ice applied to the affected side. Manual pressure is applied to reduce the hernia. Surgery then may occur within 24 to 48 hours. The surgeon replaces hernial contents into the abdominal cavity and seals the opening in a herniorrhaphy procedure. In a hernioplasty, the surgeon reinforces the weakened area with mesh or fascia.

Intravenous fluids are administered to prevent dehydration, especially for the newborn who is prone to fluid shifts. The patient should be able to tolerate small oral feedings before discharge and should be able to urinate spontaneously. Postoperatively, inspect for signs and symptoms of possible peritonitis, manage nasogastric suction, and monitor the patient for the return of bowel sounds. As with any postoperative patient, monitor the patient for respiratory complications such as atelectasis or pneumonia; encourage the patient to use an incentive spirometer or assist the patient to turn, cough, and deep breathe every 2 hours.

PHARMACOLOGIC HIGHLIGHTS

Medication or Drug Class	Dosage	Description	Rationale
Antibiotics	Varies with drug	Broad spectrum	Prevent infection postoperatively
Analgesics	Varies with drug	NSAIDs; narcotics	Relieve discomfort caused by hernial pressure, or postoperatively

Independent

The nurse explains what to expect before, during, and after the surgery. Parents, especially those of a newborn, are anxious because their child requires general anesthesia for the procedure. If possible, use preoperative teaching tools such as pamphlets and videotapes to reinforce the information. Allow as much time as is needed to answer questions and explain procedures.

The nurse also instructs patients and parents on the care of the incision. Often the incision is simply covered with collodion (a viscous liquid that, when applied, dries to form a thin transparent film) and should be kept clean and dry. Encourage the patient to defer bathing and showering and instead to use sponge baths until he or she is seen by the surgeon at a follow-up visit. Explain how to monitor the incision for signs of infection. Infants or young children who are wearing diapers should have frequent diaper changes, or the diapers should be turned down from the incision so as not to contaminate the incision with urine. Teach the patient or parents about the possibility of some scrotal swelling or hematoma; both should subside over time.

If the patient does not have surgery, teach the signs of a strangulated or incarcerated hernia: severe pain, nausea, vomiting, diarrhea, high fever, and bloody stools. Explain that if these symptoms occur, the patient must notify the primary healthcare provider immediately. If the patient uses a truss, he or she should use it only after a hernia has been reduced. Assist the patient with the truss, preferably in the morning before the patient arises. Encourage the patient to bathe daily and to apply a thin film of powder or cornstarch to prevent skin irritation.

DOCUMENTATION GUIDELINES

- Physical responses: Description of the hernia or incisional site, vital signs, gastrointestinal functioning, breath sounds
- Response to pain management; location, type, and duration of pain

DISCHARGE AND HOME HEALTHCARE GUIDELINES

Teach the patient signs and symptoms of infection: poor wound healing, wound drainage, continued incisional pain, incisional swelling and redness, cough, fever, and mucus production. Explain the importance of completion of all antibiotics. Explain the mechanism of action, side effects, and dosage recommendations of all analgesics. Caution the patient against lifting and straining. Explain that he or she can resume normal activities 2 to 4 weeks after surgery.

Intestinal Obstruction

DRG Category: 180
Mean LOS: 5.2 days
Description: MEDICAL: Gastrointestinal Obstruction with CC
DRG Category: 148
Mean LOS: 12.2 days
Mean LOS: 12.2 days
Description: SURGICAL: Major Small and Large Bowel Procedure with CC

Intestinal obstruction occurs when a blockage obstructs the normal flow of contents through the intestinal tract. Obstruction of the intestine causes the bowel to become vulnerable to ischemia. The intestinal mucosal barrier can be damaged, thus allowing intestinal bacteria to invade the intestinal wall and causing fluid exudation, which leads to hypovolemia and dehydration. About 7 L of fluid per day are secreted into the small intestine and stomach and usually reabsorbed. During obstruction, however, fluid accumulates, causing abdominal distension and pressure on the mucosal wall, which can lead to peritonitis and perforation. Obstructions can be partial or complete.

Complications of intestinal obstruction include bacteremia, secondary infection, or metabolic alkalosis or acidosis. If it is left untreated, a complete intestinal obstruction can cause death within a few hours from hypovolemic or septic shock and vascular collapse.

CAUSES

The two major types of intestinal obstruction are mechanical and neurogenic (or nonmechanical). Neurogenic obstruction occurs primarily after manipulation of the bowel during surgery or with peritoneal irritation, pain of thoracolumbar origin, or intestinal ischemia. It is also caused by the effect of trauma or toxins on the nerves that regulate peristalsis, electrolyte imbalances, and neurogenic abnormalities such as spinal cord lesions. Mechanical obstruction of the bowel is caused by physical blockage of the intestine. Examples of mechanical obstruction include adhesions and strangulated hernias (usually associated with the small intestine); volvulus (twisting of the intestine) of the cecum or sigmoid; intussusception (telescoping of the bowel); strictures; fecal or barium impaction; carcinomas (usually associated with the large intestine); or foreign bodies such as gallstones, worms, and fruit pits.

GENDER AND LIFE SPAN CONSIDERATIONS

Intestinal obstructions can occur at any age and in both sexes but are more common in patients who have undergone major abdominal surgery or have congenital abnormalities of the bowel. When it occurs in a child, the obstruction is most likely to be an intussusception.

□ ASSESSMENT

HISTORY. Establish any predisposing factors: surgery, especially abdominal surgery; radiation therapy; gallstones; Crohn's disease; diverticular disease; ulcerative colitis; or a family history of colorectal cancer. Ask if the patient has had hiccups, which is often a symptom of intestinal obstruction.

To establish the diagnosis of small bowel obstruction, ask about vomiting fecal contents, wavelike abdominal pain, or abdominal distension. Elicit a history of intense thirst, generalized malaise, or aching. A paralytic ileus usually causes a distended abdomen, with or without pain, but usually without cramping. To establish the diagnosis of large bowel obstruction, which has a slower onset of symptoms, ask about recent constipation with a history of spasmodic abdominal pain several days afterward. Establish a history of hypogastric pain and nausea. Ask if the patient has been vomiting. To establish neurogenic obstruction, ask about abdominal pain. Neurogenic obstruction characteristically produces diffuse abdominal discomfort rather than colicky pain. Establish a history of vomiting; ask the patient to describe the vomitus, which may consist of gastric and bile contents but rarely fecal contents.

PHYSICAL EXAMINATION. Inspect the patient's abdomen for distension. Observe the patient's abdomen for signs of visible peristalsis or loops of large bowel. Measure the patient's abdominal girths every 4 hours to observe the progress of an obstruction. Auscultate the patient's abdomen for bowel sounds in all four quadrants; you may hear rushes or borborygmus (rumbling noises in the bowels). Always auscultate the abdomen for up to 5 minutes for bowel sounds before palpation. Lack of bowel sounds can indicate a paralytic ileus. High-pitched tingling sounds with rushes can indicate a mechanical obstruction. Palpate all four quadrants of the abdomen to determine areas of localized tenderness, guarding, and rebound tenderness.

Assess the patient for tachycardia, a narrowed pulse pressure, urine output less than 30 mL per hour, and delayed capillary blanching—all indicators of severe hypovolemia and impending shock. Assess for fever, which may indicate peritonitis. Inspect the patient's skin for loss of turgor and mucous membranes for dryness.

PSYCHOSOCIAL. The patient with an intestinal obstruction is acutely ill and may need emergency intervention. Assess the patient's level of anxiety and fear. Assess the patient's coping skills, support system, and the significant others' response to the illness.

DIAGNOSTIC HIGHLIGHTS

Test	Normal Result	Abnormality with Condition	Explanation
Abdominal x ray	Normal abdominal structures	Distended loops of bowel; may have a ladder-like pattern with air-fluid levels	Identifies blockage of lumen of bowel with distal passage of fluid and air (partial) or complete obstruction
Water-soluble contrast enema	Normal abdominal structures	Blockage of lumen of bowel	Identifies site and severity of colonic obstruction

Other Tests: Complete blood count, colonoscopy, sigmoidoscopy, abdominal computed tomography (CT) scan

PRIMARY NURSING DIAGNOSIS

Fluid volume deficit related to abnormal loss of gastrointestinal fluids

OUTCOMES. Fluid balance; Hydration; Nutritional status: Food and fluid intake; Bowel elimination; Knowledge: Disease process

INTERVENTIONS. Fluid management; Intravenous insertion and therapy; Surveillance; Venous access devices maintenance; Vital signs monitoring

☐ PLANNING AND IMPLEMENTATION

Collaborative

SURGICAL. Surgery is often indicated for a complete mechanical obstruction. The operative procedure varies with the location and type of obstruction. A strangulated bowel constitutes a surgical emergency. A bowel resection may be necessary in some obstructions.

Postoperative care includes monitoring the patient's cardiopulmonary response and identifying surgical complications. The highest priority is maintaining airway, breathing, and circulation. The patient may require endotracheal intubation and mechanical ventilation temporarily to manage airway and breathing. The circulation may need support from parenteral fluids, and total parenteral nutrition may be prescribed if the patient has protein deficits. Care for the surgical site, and notify the physician if you observe any signs of poor wound healing, bleeding, or infection.

MEDICAL. Medical management with intravenous fluids, electrolytes, and administration of blood or plasma may be required for patients whose obstruction is caused by infection or inflammation or by a partial obstruction. Insertion of a nasogastric (NG) tube, often ordered by the physician to rest and decompress the bowel, greatly decreases the abdominal distension and the patient's discomfort.

Analgesic medication may be ordered after the cause of the obstruction is known, but it may be withheld until the diagnosis of intestinal obstruction is confirmed so as to not mask pain, which is an important clinical indicator. Explore nonpharmacologic methods of pain relief. The physician may order oxygen. Usually until the patient is stabilized, his or her condition precludes any oral intake.

PHARMACOLOGIC HIGHLIGHTS

Medication or Drug Class	Dosage	Description	Rationale
Antibiotics	Varies with drug	Broad spectrum antibiotic coverage	Antibiotics may be prescribed when the obstruction is caused by an infectious process

Independent

Focus on increasing the patient's comfort and monitoring for complications. Elevate the head of the bed to assist with patient ventilation. Position the patient in the Fowler or semi-Fowler position to ease respiratory discomfort from a distended abdomen. Reposition the patient frequently.

Instruct the patient about the need to take nothing by mouth. Frequent mouth care and lubrication of the mucous membranes can assist with patient comfort. Patient teaching should include the indications and function of the NG tube. Discuss care planning with the patient and the family.

Teach the causes, types, signs, and symptoms of intestinal obstruction. Explain the diagnostic tests and treatments, preparing the patient for the possibility of surgery. Explain surgical and postoperative procedures. Note the patient's and significant others' responses to emergency surgery if needed, and provide additional support if the family or patient copes ineffectively.

DOCUMENTATION GUIDELINES

- Physical findings: Vital signs, abdominal assessments, pulmonary assessment, fluid volume status
- Response to pain medications, antibiotics, NG intubation, and suctioning
- Presence of complications (preoperative): Peritonitis, sepsis, respiratory insufficiency, hypovolemia, shock
- Presence of complications (postoperative): Poor wound healing, hemorrhage, or infection

DISCHARGE AND HOME HEALTHCARE GUIDELINES

Teach postoperative care to patients who have had surgery. Teach the patient how to plan a paced progression of activities. Teach the patient the dosages, routes, and side effects for all medications. Review drug and food interactions with the patient. Instruct the patient to report bowel elimination problems to the physician. Emphasize that in the case of recurrent abdominal pain, fever, or vomiting, the patient should go to the emergency department for evaluation.

Intracerebral Hematoma

DRG Category: 014
Mean LOS: 6.4 days
Description: MEDICAL: Specific Cerebrovascular Disorders Except TIA
DRG Category: 002
Mean LOS: 9.8 days
Description: SURGICAL: Craniotomy for Trauma, Age > 17

An intracerebral hematoma (ICH) is a well-defined collection of blood within the brain parenchyma (functional tissue). Most intracerebral hematomas are related to cerebral contusions; ICHs complicate head injury in 2% to 3% of all head-injured patients. Although they are more frequently associated with closed-head injuries, they can also occur as a result of an open or penetrating injury or a depressed skull fracture. Similar to cerebral contusions, ICHs tend to occur most commonly in the frontal and temporal lobes and are uncommon in the cerebellum. They can also occur deep within the hemispheres in the paraventricular, medial, or paracentral areas in association with the shearing strain on small vessels that occurs with diffuse axonal injuries.

The patient can experience deterioration in cerebral functioning at the time of injury or in the first 48 to 72 hours after injury. Late hemorrhage into a contused area is possible as long as 7 to 10 days after injury. ICHs result in a mortality rate between 25% and 72%. Complications include intracranial hypertension, brain herniation, and death.

CAUSES

Traumatic causes of ICH include depressed skull fractures, penetrating missile injuries (gunshot wounds or stab wounds), or a sudden acceleration-deceleration motion. Depressed skull fractures cause penetration of bone into cerebral tissue. A high-velocity penetration (bullet) can produce shock waves that are trasmitted throughout the brain, in addition to the injury caused by the bullet directly. A low-velocity penetrating injury (knife) may involve only focal damage and no loss of consciousness. Motor vehicle crashes cause rapid acceleration-deceleration injuries. In cases in which there is no apparent cause for spontaneous ICH, hypertension is the most frequently associated disease. Other potential causes of ICH include hemorrhage at the site of a brain tumor and cerebrovascular accidents.

GENDER AND LIFE SPAN CONSIDERATIONS

Head injury, the leading cause of all trauma-related deaths, is associated with MVCS. Males in the 15- to 24-year-old age group are three times more likely than females to be injured in a crash. Whites have a death rate 40% higher from MVC than do African-Americans in the 15- to 34-year-old age group. Falls are the most common cause of head injury in adults over the age of 65.

ICH can occur from nontraumatic causes as well. Strokes are the third leading cause of death in Americans. Although a stroke can occur at any age, 72% occur in people over 65 years of age. About 10,000 people develop intracranial tumors in the United States each year. The peak incidence occurs in childhood (3 to 12 years of age) and in older adults (50 to 70 years of age).

□ ASSESSMENT

HISTORY. Generally, patients suspected of ICH have a history of traumatic injury to the head. If no history of trauma exists, determine if the patient has a history of hypertension or stroke. In trauma patients, if the patient is not able to report a history, question the pre-hospital care provider, significant others, or witnesses about the situation surrounding the injury. If the patient was in an MVC, determine the speed and type of the vehicle, the patient's position in the vehicle, whether the patient was restrained, and if the patient was thrown from the vehicle on impact. If the patient was injured in a motorcycle crash, determine whether the patient was wearing a helmet. Determine if the patient experienced momentary loss of reflexes, momentary arrest of respirations, and possible retrograde or anterograde amnesia (loss of memory for events immediately before the injury or loss of memory for events after the injury). Elicit a history of headache, drowsiness, confusion, dizziness, irritability, giddiness, visual disturbances (seeing stars), and gait disturbances. In addition, others may describe symptoms related to increased intracranial pressure (ICP), such as increased drowsiness or irritability and pupillary dilation on the ipsilateral (same as injury) side.

PHYSICAL EXAMINATION. When you examine the patient, note that just as in cerebral contusions, small frontal lesions may be asymptomatic, whereas larger bilateral lesions may result in a frontal lobe syndrome of inappropriate behavior and cognitive deficits. Dominant hemispheric lesions are often associated with speech and motor deficits. Because many of the symptoms of alcohol intoxication mimic those of head injury, never assume that a decreased level of consciousness is caused by alcohol intoxication alone (even if you can smell the alcohol on the patient's breath or clothing) rather than a head injury.

First evaluate and stabilize the patient's airway, breathing, and circulation with particular attention to the intactness of the patient's cervical spine (do not flex or extend the neck until you know the patient has no cervical spine injury). Next, perform a neurological assessment, watching for early signs of increased ICP: decreased level of consciousness, decreased strength and motion of extremities, reduced visual acuity, headache, and pupillary changes.

During the complete head-to-toe assessment, be sure to evaluate the patient's head for external signs of injury. Check carefully for scalp lacerations. Check the patient for cerebrospinal fluid (CSF) leakage from the nose (obrhinorrhea) or ear (obotorrhea), which is a sign of a basilar skull fracture (a linear fracture at the base of the brain). Other signs of basilar skull fracture include raccoon's eyes (periorbital ecchymosis or bruising around the eyes) and Battle's sign (bleeding and swelling behind the ear).

Be sure to evaluate the patient's pupillary light reflexes. An abnormal pupil reflex may result from increasing cerebral edema, which may indicate a life-threatening increase in ICP. Pupil size is normally 1.5 to 6.0 mm. Several signs to look for include ipsilateral miosis (Horner's syndrome), in which one pupil is smaller than the other with a drooping eyelid; bilateral miosis, in which both pupils are pinpoint in size; ipsilateral mydriasis (Hutchinson's pupil), in which one of the pupils is much larger than the other and is unreactive to light; bilateral midposition, in which both pupils are 4 to 5 mm and remain dilated and nonreactive to light; and bilateral mydriasis, in which both pupils are larger than 6 mm and nonreactive to light. Note the shape of the pupil as well because an oval pupil may indicate increased ICP and possible brain herniation. In more seriously injured patients, invasive ICP monitoring with an intraventricular catheter may be initiated for serial assessment of the ICP. Normally, ICP is 4 to 10 mm Hg, with an upper limit of 15 mm Hg. ICP is considered moderately elevated at levels of 15 to 30 mm Hg and severely elevated at levels above 30 mm Hg.

PSYCHOSOCIAL. Assess the patient's and family's ability to cope with a sudden illness and the change in roles that a sudden illness demands. Expect parents of children who are injured to be anxious, fearful, and sometimes guilt-ridden. Note if the injury was related to alcohol (approximately 40% to 60% of head injuries occur when the patient has been drinking), and elicit a drinking history from the patient or significant others.

Note that during the patient's recovery subtle neurological deficits (such as subtle personality changes or inability to perform mathematical calculations) may exist long after hospital discharge that may interfere with the resumption of parenting, spousal, or occupational roles.

DIAGNOSTIC HIGHLIGHTS

Test	Normal Result	Abnormality with Condition	Explanation
Computed tomography (CT) scan	Intact cerebral anatomy	Identification of size and location of site of injury or bleeding	Shows anterior to posterior slices of the brain to highlight abnormalities

Other Tests: Skull x rays, magnetic resonance imaging (MRI), cervical spine x rays, and glucose test of any drainage suspected to be cerebral spinal fluid using a reagent strip

PRIMARY NURSING DIAGNOSIS

Altered thought process related to cerebral tissue injury and swelling

OUTCOMES. Cognitive ability; Cognitive orientation; Concentration; Decision making; Identity; Information processing; Memory; Neurological status: Consciousness

INTERVENTIONS. Cerebral perfusion promotion; Environmental management; Surveillance; Cerebral edema management; Family support; Medication management

☐ PLANNING AND IMPLEMENTATION

Collaborative

If a lesion identified by CT scan is causing a shift of intracranial contents or increased ICP, immediate surgical intervention is necessary. A craniotomy is performed to evacuate the ICH and ischemic tissue if the site is operable, or to release intracranial pressure if viable tissue will be preserved.

Ongoing monitoring and serial assessments are essential. Intracranial pressure monitoring and sequential CT scanning may be needed in critically ill patients, and serial neurological assessments are needed on all patients to determine if ICP is increasing. Because bleeding and swelling can progress over several days after injury, the patient is monitored for deterioration even up to 10 days after injury. During periods of frequent assessment, the patient should not be sedated for longer than 30 minutes at a time; longer-acting sedation may mask neurological changes and place the patient at risk for lack of detection.

PHARMACOLOGIC HIGHLIGHTS

Medication or Drug Class	Dosage	Description	Rationale
Fentanyl (Sublimaze)	0.05 mg IV as needed	Short-acting opioid analgesic	Provides short-term (30 minutes) pain control and sedation without long-lasting effects that may mask neurological changes

Other Drugs: Some patients develop seizures as a complication and need anticonvulsants. Drugs to reduce intracranial pressure, such as mannitol, may be used.

Independent

After making sure that the patient has adequate airway, breathing, and circulation, ongoing serial assessments of the patient's neurological responses are of highest priority. Timely notification of the trauma surgeon or neurosurgeon when a patient's assessment changes can save a patient's life. If the patient is intubated, make sure that the endotracheal tube is anchored well. If the patient is at risk for self-extubation, maintain him or her in soft restraints. Notify the physician if the patient's PaO_2 drops below 80 mm Hg, if $PaCO_2$ exceeds 40 mm Hg, or if severe hypocapnia ($PaCO_2 < 25$ mm Hg) occurs. Aspiration pneumonia is a risk and can occur even with endotracheal intubation. Elevate the head of the bed at 30 degrees to help prevent this complication.

Help control the patient's ICP. Maintain normothermia by avoiding body temperature elevations. Avoid flexing, extending, or rotating the patient's neck because these maneuvers limit venous drainage of the brain and thus raise ICP. Avoid hip flexion by maintaining the patient in a normal body alignment, limiting venous drainage. Maintain a quiet, restful environment with minimal stimulation; limit visitors as appropriate. Time nursing care activities carefully to limit prolonged ICP elevations. Use caution when suctioning the patient. Hyperventilate the patient beforehand, and suction only as long as necessary. When turning the patient, prevent Valsalva's maneuver by using a draw sheet to pull the patient up in bed. Instruct the patient not to hold on to the side rails.

Strategies to maximize the coping mechanisms of the patient and family are directed toward providing support and encouragement. Provide simple educational tools about head injuries. Teach the patient and family appropriate rehabilitative exercises, as appropriate. Help the patient cope with long stretches of immobility by providing diversionary activities that are appropriate to the patient's mental and physical abilities. Head injury support groups may be helpful. Referrals to clinical nurse specialists, pastoral care staff, and social workers are helpful in developing strategies for support and education.

Help the significant others and family face the fear of death, disability, and dependency; involve the patient and the family in all aspects of care.

DOCUMENTATION GUIDELINES

- Trauma history, description of the event, time elapsed since the event, whether the patient had a loss of consciousness and, if so, for how long
- Adequacy of airway, breathing, circulation; serial vital signs
- Appearance: Bruising or lacerations, drainage from the nose or ears
- Physical findings related to the site of head injury: Neurological assessment, presence of accompanying symptoms, presence of complications
- Signs of complications: Seizure activity, infection (fever, purulent discharge from any wounds), aspiration pneumonia (shortness of breath, pulmonary congestion, fever, productive cough), increased ICP
- Response to medications used to control pain and increased ICP

DISCHARGE AND HOME HEALTHCARE GUIDELINES

Be sure the patient understands all medications, including the dosage, route, action, adverse effects, and the need for routine laboratory monitoring for convulsants. Teach the patient and caregiver the signs and symptoms that necessitate a return to the hospital. Teach the patient to recognize the symptoms and signs of post-injury syndrome, which may last for several weeks. Explain that mild cognitive changes do not always resolve immediately. Provide the patient and significant others with information about the trauma clinic and the phone number of a clinical nurse specialist in case referrals are needed. Stress the importance of follow-up visits to the physician's office. If alcohol counseling is needed, provide a phone number and the name of a counselor. Prepare the patient and family for the possible need for rehabilitation after the acute care phase of hospitalization.

Intrauterine Fetal Demise

DRG Category: 373
Mean LOS: 1.9 days
Description: MEDICAL: Vaginal Delivery without Complicating Diagnoses
DRG Category: 372
Mean LOS: 2.7 days
Description: MEDICAL: Vaginal Delivery with Complicating Diagnoses

An intrauterine fetal demise (IUFD), or stillbirth, is defined as a death that occurs in utero or during delivery after the completion of the twentieth week of pregnancy, or the death of a fetus that weighs 350 g or more in utero or during delivery. The specific gestational age and weight that classify the fetus as an IUFD vary from state to state. Labor and delivery of the dead fetus usually occur spontaneously within 2 weeks. Patients are under tremendous psychological stress. Disseminated intravascular coagulation (DIC) is the main complication that can result. Thromboplastin released from the dead fetus is thought to mediate DIC.

CAUSES

Approximately 1%, or 30,000, pregnancies per year end in an IUFD. Potential causes of IUFD are the following: genetic anomalies that are incompatible with life, uteroplacental insufficiency, umbilical cord prolapse or other cord problems, maternal disease or infection, trauma, placenta previa, and abruptio placentae. Patients have the option of requesting an autopsy to determine the cause of death. If an autopsy is not performed, it may not be possible to determine the exact cause of fetal death.

GENDER AND LIFE SPAN CONSIDERATIONS

The likelihood of the occurrence of an IUFD decreases with good prenatal care. IUFD occurs more often in older women and is thought to be the reason for the increase in perinatal mortality in this age group. IUFD accounts for 50% of all perinatal deaths.

☐ ASSESSMENT

HISTORY. Obtain a thorough obstetric and medical history. Determine the gestational age of the fetus by asking the patient the date of her last menstrual period and using Nagele's rule. Inquire about any contractions, bleeding, or leakage of fluid. Ask about exposure to environmental teratogens or the use of recreational or prescription drugs. Ask the patient when she last felt the baby move. Also inquire about any cultural and religious preferences related to labor, delivery, postpartum care, autopsy, and receiving a blood transfusion.

PHYSICAL EXAMINATION. Attempt to auscultate a fetal heart rate with a Doppler or electronic fetal monitor. If no heart rate is heard, perform an ultrasound to be sure no heart rate is present. Determine McDonald's measurement and compare this to previous data; the measurement is usually less than that expected for the gestational age if an IUFD has occurred. Palpate the abdomen for rigidity, which is often present with abruptio placentae, or for change in shape, which is often present with uterine rupture. Inspect the perineum for bleeding, and note any foul odors. Perform a vaginal examination to check for a prolapsed cord, and note any cervical dilation and effacement. If possible, determine the fetal presenting part and the station. Check the patient's vital signs. A temperature higher than 100.4°F may indicate the presence of infection. Weigh the patient; some may experience a weight loss. Because DIC is a potential complication of IUFD, monitor the patient for the following signs and symptoms of DIC: bleeding from puncture sites, episiotomy, abdominal incision, or gums; hematuria; epistaxis; increased vaginal bleeding, bruising, and petechiae.

PSYCHOSOCIAL. Assess the patient's reaction and ability to cope with the fetal death and her anxiety about going through the labor process. Determine the meaning of the pregnancy for the patient. Observe the interaction between the patient and her significant other to assess potential support.

DIAGNOSTIC HIGHLIGHTS

General Comments: Abdominal ultrasound easily and accurately confirms the diagnosis of IUFD.

Test	Normal Result	Abnormality with Condition	Explanation
Ultrasound (abdominal)	Heart beat seen; fetal growth appropriate for gestational age	No heart beat seen; "fetal collapse" noted, smaller than expected for gestational age	Absence of heart beat and shriveled fetal appearance indicative of IUFD

Other Tests: If sepsis or DIC is a potential threat, coagulation studies (fibrinogen, fibrin split products, prothrombin time, partial thomboplastin time, D-dimer) are done serially.

PRIMARY NURSING DIAGNOSIS

Anticipatory grieving related to fetal loss

OUTCOMES. Grief resolution

INTERVENTIONS. Grief work facilitation: Perinatal death; Active listening; Presence; Truth telling; Support group

❑ PLANNING AND IMPLEMENTATION

Collaborative

The treatment involves inducing labor to deliver the fetus. The timing of the delivery varies. A 48-hour wait is recommended to give the patient time to gather support from her family and to fathom the reality of the situation. Other patients may prefer to let the labor start on its own, but this could take weeks. The danger with this conservative treatment is that the necrotic fetus can lead to either DIC or infection, or both, in the mother. A cesarean section is rarely done, unless the maternal condition necessitates an immediate delivery.

Induction of labor is often a 2-day process. Insertion of a Laminaria tent into the endocervical canal dilates the cervix. If necessary, the Laminaria can be held in place by a tampon. The risk of infection in the presence of a dead fetus needs to be considered. Prostaglandin E_2 gel or 20-mg suppositories are alternatives to Laminaria. By the second day, the cervix is usually ripe and an oxytocic induction of labor can begin. Labor contractions are very uncomfortable for the patient. Liberal dosages of analgesia or anesthesia may be given if the patient desires because their effects on the fetus do not need to be considered. Intravenous narcotics, an epidural, and sedatives may be ordered for relief of pain and anxiety.

If the patient has an epidural, turn her from side to side hourly to ensure an adequate distribution of anesthesia. Patients have limited mobility and require assistance in turning and positioning comfortably. Use pillows to support the back and abdomen and between the knees to maintain alignment. Check the blood pressure and pulse every 30 minutes. Most patients are unable to void and require a straight catheterization every 2 to 3 hours to keep the bladder empty. Maintain the infusion of intravenous fluids to prevent hypotension, which can result from regional anesthesia. Monitor the patient's pain relief and notify the nurse anesthetist or physician if the patient is uncomfortable.

PHARMACOLOGIC HIGHLIGHTS

Medication or Drug Class	Dosage	Description	Rationale
Dinoprostone (Prostaglandin, Cervidil, Prepidil gel)	20-mg suppository; 0.5-mg gel; 10-mg inserts	Prostaglandins	Ripens, softens, begins to dilate the cervix and prepare it for labor
Oxytocin (pitocin)	10 U in 500 cc of IV fluid; start at 1 mU per minute and increase 1–2 mU per minute q 30 minutes	Oxytocic	Induces labor contractions
Analgesia/Anesthesia	Varies by drug; medication given either IVP or via epidural catheter	Narcotic analgesics; anesthetics	Labor contractions are very uncomfortable and especially difficult to tolerate with a demise of the fetus
RhoD immunoglobin (RhoGAM)	120 μg prepared by blood bank	Immune serum	Prevents Rh isoimmunizations in future pregnancies;

given if mother is Rh negative and infant is Rh positive

Independent

If possible, admit the patient to a room that is isolated from the nursery, patients in labor, and crying of newborns. Often units have some small symbol (a small bear, a heart) to hang on the door that denotes the patient has an IUFD to alert any healthcare workers who come into contact with the patient to be sensitive.

The nurse is present through the entire labor and delivery and plays a key role in assisting the patient and family through the initial grieving process. During this shocking event, encourage the patient and significant others to verbalize their feelings. Discuss the grieving process and expected feelings; use therapeutic communication skills. Be aware of the content of your messages to the patient.

Involve the patient and significant other in all decisions and discussions related to the labor, delivery, and aftercare. Before the delivery, educate them about the labor process. Prepare them for the appearance of a dead fetus (maceration of the skin, discolorations, specific anomalies, and trauma that can occur during delivery). During delivery, have only the minimum number of staff needed to provide safe care. Keep the room quiet and dim to promote a calm and peaceful atmosphere. Honor the parents' desires for seeing, holding, and touching the newborn. Prepare a "memory box" that contains tangible items, such as footprints, handprints, pictures, a lock of hair, identification bands, and any other items used for the baby. After the patient delivers, monitor her vital signs, location and firmness of fundus, amount of vaginal bleeding, ability to void, presence of edema and hemorrhoids, comfort level, and ability to cope. Provide time for the patient and significant other to be alone with the infant.

Provide reading material for the parents on coping with a neonatal loss. Offer to notify clergy if the patient desires, and respect any religious requests. Although it may be difficult to discuss, offer information regarding funeral arrangements. Discuss an autopsy and explain the advantages of determining the exact cause of death. Refer the patient to a bereavement support group. Often, follow-up counseling is done by a hospital grief counselor or by the nurse who was present at the delivery.

DOCUMENTATION GUIDELINES

- Progress of cervical dilation, progress of labor; response to pain of contractions; time of delivery; condition of fetus; vital signs
- Signs of abnormal bleeding; amount and character of lochia
- Patient's and significant other's expressions of grief
- Patient's ability to cope with the fetal loss

DISCHARGE AND HOME HEALTHCARE GUIDELINES

Teach the patient to be aware of the signs and symptoms that could indicate postpartum complications: pain in the calf of the leg; increase in vaginal bleeding; foul odor of vaginal discharge; fever; burning with urination; persistent mood change; or a hard, reddened area on the breast. Explain that the patient should not have intercourse or drive a car until after the postpartum check. Encourage participation in a bereavement support group, even if the patient and significant other seem to be coping with the loss. They may be able to help other couples cope.

Intussusception

DRG Category: 181
Mean LOS: 3.4 days
Description: MEDICAL: GI Obstruction without CC

Intussusception occurs when a bowel segment invaginates or telescopes into an adjoining portion of bowel; as peristalsis continues, the segment is propelled farther into the bowel, and blood supply is restricted. Tissue ischemia leads to an edematous and friable bowel, causing bleeding and, if the condition is not corrected, tissue necrosis, intestinal gangrene, shock, intestinal perforation, and peritonitis. Intussusception is considered a pediatric emergency because it is one of the most common causes of bowel obstruction in children and can be fatal if it is not treated within 24 hours.

Children with cystic fibrosis, gastroenteritis, polyps, lymphosarcoma, and celiac disease are particularly susceptible. Intussusception is classified according to the portion of the bowel involved. The most common location for intussusception is at or near the ileocecal valve, but intussusception can occur in both the small and large bowels.

CAUSES

In 90% of patients, the cause of intussusception is unknown. In infants over 1 year, a "lead point" on the intestine may cue the investigation. "Lead points" may be Meckel's diverticulum, a polyp, hypertrophy of lymphatic tissue of the bowel associated with infection (Peyer patch), or bowel tumors. When intussusception occurs in adults, it is most commonly associated with benign or malignant tumors or polyps. Current theories also suggest that intussusception may be associated with viral infections, such as an upper respiratory infections.

GENDER AND LIFE SPAN CONSIDERATIONS

About half the cases occur in children in their first year of life, particularly between the ages of 3 and 12 months. The majority of the rest of the cases occur before the age of 2. Intussusception occurs more frequently in males than females. Once corrected, there are no lifetime complications of the condition that are known to occur.

◻ ASSESSMENT

HISTORY. The child, usually a healthy male with no previous illness, experiences severe, intermittent abdominal pain; children often draw their legs up to the abdomen, turn pale and clammy, and cry sharply. In addition, the child may vomit and appear restless. The attack is followed by a period of normal behavior and then developing symptoms (see below). Adults may report general, chronic, intermittent symptoms such as abdominal tenderness; vomiting; and changes in bowel habits such as diarrhea, bloody stools, or constipation.

PHYSICAL EXAMINATION. As the condition continues, the child may have bile-stained or fecal vomiting and may pass bloody stools. The stool is often called "currant jelly stool" because of the mucus and blood from the injured bowel. The child may show some guarding of the abdomen, and a sausage-like mass may be palpable in the abdomen. Location of the mass and the guarding vary, depending on the location of the intussusception. Bloody mucus may be found on rectal examination. Hyperperistaltic rushes may be heard on auscultation.

Adult patients may have a distended abdomen and often pain in the right lower quadrant of the abdomen. Extremely severe pain, abdominal distension, rapid heart rate, and diaphoresis may indicate that intussusception has led to strangulation of the bowel.

PSYCHOSOCIAL. The sudden onset of intussusception and the severity of the pain and symptoms can provoke anxiety in the parents and the child. Assess the parents' coping ability and their support systems. Note that because the child experiences an emergency condition, the child has not been prepared for hospitalization, separation from the parents and the home environment, and possible surgery.

DIAGNOSTIC HIGHLIGHTS

Test	Normal Result	Abnormality with Condition	Explanation
Abdominal x ray	Normal abdominal structures	Distended loops of bowel; may have a ladder-like pattern with air-fluid levels	Identifies blockage of lumen of bowel with distal passage of fluid and air (partial) or complete obstruction
Barium or air contrast enema	Normal abdominal structures	Blockage of lumen of bowel with a "coiled spring" sign	Identifies site and severity of intussusception; not performed if there exists a high risk for perforation. Before using a barium or air-contrast enema, place a nasogastric tube, administer intravenous fluids, and begin broad spectrum antibiotics

Other Tests: Complete blood count, colonoscopy, sigmoidoscopy, abdominal computed tomography (CT) scan

PRIMARY NURSING DIAGNOSIS

Pain (acute) related to inflammation

OUTCOMES. Comfort level; Pain control behavior; Pain level; Symptom severity

INTERVENTIONS. Analgesic administration; Anxiety reduction; Environmental management: Comfort; Pain management; Medication management; Patient-controlled analgesia assistance

☐ PLANNING AND IMPLEMENTATION

Collaborative

Reduction of the intussusception is accomplished by hydrostatic pressure or pneumatic reduction (barium enema), surgical manipulation, or surgical resection. If the symptoms are less than 24 hours old and there is no evidence of complete obstruction, peritonitis, or shock, a barium enema can be used to reduce the high intestinal pressure. This technique has a 90% success rate. The maximum safe intra-luminal air pressure for young infants is 80 mm Hg and 110 to 120 mm Hg for older children. If the procedure does not result in a change in the intussusception, the procedure is terminated and the patient is evaluated for surgery. If the patient is an adult, surgery is always the treatment of choice.

Surgical resection of the affected bowel segment is performed in several situations: if the manipulation is unsuccessful, if the bowel is strangulated, or if it has necrotic areas. Recurrence, usually within the first 36 to 48 hours after treatment, can occur with either the barium enema method or bowel manipulation in approximately 10% of patients who are treated nonoperatively. Parents need to understand that when the barium enema is attempted, the child is also prepared for the possibility of surgery. Preoperatively the child may have a nasogastric (NG) tube and intravenous lines for fluid replacement; the child also needs medications administered as needed for pain relief. Postoperative management contains the same three components: management of NG drainage and decompression, fluid replacement, and pain relief. Also monitor the child for signs of bleeding and infection. If the child had a successful reduction using the hydrostatic barium enema, the parents need to understand that feedings will be in small amounts and that stools will be grayish white until the barium is passed. Children are usually kept in the hospital until they have normal stools.

PHARMACOLOGIC HIGHLIGHTS

Medication or Drug Class	Dosage	Description	Rationale
Antibiotics	Varies with drug	Broad spectrum	To prevent peritonitis or postoperative infection

Other: Patient-controlled analgesia in adults

Independent

Because intussusception occurs in otherwise healthy infants and is an emergency situation, the nurse's role is to provide comfort for the child and the parents, provide explanations to the parents, and evaluate the success of the treatment. Because the child appears normal between attacks, you may sometimes have difficulty convincing parents of the potential severity of the condition. Make sure that you explain the condition carefully. Early intervention is crucial to prevent complications. When you suspect intussusception, carefully elicit information from the parents about the progression of the symptoms and the type, location, and duration of pain. Comfort measures are needed for the child both before and after surgery, but do not mask abdominal pain with analgesia until the firm diagnosis is made.

If the child has surgery, check the incision for signs of infection (swelling, drainage, separation) or bleeding. Splint the wound with pillows, and encourage coughing and deep breathing. If the child is old enough to follow directions, encourage deep breathing every hour. Elicit the parents' help in maintaining good pulmonary function after surgery.

DOCUMENTATION GUIDELINES

- Location of pain, its duration, and response to interventions
- Physical appearance and frequency of stool and vomitus
- If patient has surgery, appearance of wound or presence or absence of drainage
- Amount and type of food or formula eaten; tolerance to food and fluids
- Presence of complications: Infection, dehydration, poor wound healing

DISCHARGE AND HOME HEALTHCARE GUIDELINES

Parents should know the chance of recurrence, the time frame of the highest risk after the reduction, signs, and the action to take. If the child had surgery, parents should be prepared to care for the surgical incision. Parents should be informed of possible complications, such as infection and poor wound healing.

Provide a list of diet restrictions or recommendations. If the patient is discharged on antibiotics, make sure that the parents know to complete the entire prescription before discontinuing the medication.

Iron Deficiency Anemia

DRG Category: 395
Mean LOS: 4.3 days
Description: MEDICAL: Red Blood Cell Disorders, Age > 17

Iron deficiency anemia, a common disorder throughout the world, is a condition in which there is a decrease in normal body stores of iron and hemoglobin levels. Iron deficiency anemia is caused by inadequate intake of iron, inadequate storage of iron, excessive loss of iron, or some combination of these conditions. The red blood cells (RBCs), which become pale (hypochromic) and small (microcytic), have a decreased ability to transport oxygen in sufficient quantities to meet body needs. Anemia is defined as a decrease in circulating RBC mass; the usual criteria for anemia are hemoglobin of less than 12 g/dL and hematocrit less than 36% in women and hemoglobin less than 14 g/dL with a hematocrit less than 41% in men.

Generally, iron deficiency anemia is more common in people who are economically disadvantaged because of the high cost of a well-balanced diet with iron-rich foods. Complications from iron deficiency anemia include infection and pneumonia. For patients suffering from pica (the urge to eat clay and other inappropriate items), lead poisoning may result from increased intestinal absorption of lead. Although it is a rare condition, Plummer-Vinson syndrome (iron deficiency anemia associated with difficulty swallowing, enlarged spleen, and spooning of the nails) may occur in severe cases of iron deficiency anemia, especially in middle-aged women who have recently had their teeth extracted.

CAUSES

The most common causes of iron deficiency anemia are menstrual blood loss and the increased iron requirements of pregnancy. Pathologic bleeding, particularly gastrointestinal (GI) bleeding, is a common cause of iron depletion in men. Iron malabsorption can lead to iron deficiency anemia. Pathologic causes include GI ulcers, hiatal hernias, malabsorption syndromes such as celiac disease, chronic diverticulosis, varices, and tumors. Other causes include surgeries such as partial gastrectomy and the use of prosthetic heart valves or vena cava filters.

GENDER AND LIFE SPAN CONSIDERATIONS

Infants may develop iron deficiency anemia in situations of prolonged unsupplemented breastfeeding or bottle-feeding; breast milk has some iron, but cow's milk yields none. During periods of rapid growth in childhood, adolescence, and pregnancy, patients may ingest inadequate supplies of iron. Young women, in particular, are at risk as a result of heavy menses or unwise weight reduction plans. Elderly patients living on a poorly balanced diet and alcoholics who fail to eat a well-balanced diet may also ingest inadequate supplies of iron.

◻ ASSESSMENT

HISTORY. Inquire about recent weight loss, fatigue, weakness, dizziness, irritability, inability to concentrate, sensitivity to cold, heartburn, loss of appetite, diarrhea, or flatulence. Establish a history of difficulty in swallowing, which is a sign of long-term oxygen deficit, as esophageal webbing ensues. Elicit any history of neuromuscular effects, including vasomotor disturbances, tingling or numbness of the extremities, or pain along a nerve. Ask if the patient has experienced difficulty in breathing on exertion, rapid breathing, or palpitations. With infants and children, ask the parents to establish a history of growth patterns. With premenopausal women, ask about heavy bleeding during menses. Ask female patients for a pregnancy history.

Take a complete diet and illness history. Ask if the patient regularly eats foods that are rich in iron, such as whole grains, seafood, egg yolks, legumes, green leafy vegetables, dried fruits, red meats, and nuts; ask if he or she takes iron in vitamin supplements. Elicit the patient's history of alcohol use. With infants, ask if breastfeeding or bottle-feeding has been used and if any iron supplements have been added to the diet. Establish any history of frequent nosebleeds. With elderly patients, elicit a history of food preparation and diet planning to find out who takes responsibility for the patient's diet. Ask the patient if he or she has had recent cravings for strange food (especially clay, laundry starch, or ice).

PHYSICAL EXAMINATION. Inspect the patient's mouth for signs of inflammation (stomatitis) or eroded, tender, and swollen corners (angular stomatitis). Observe the tongue to see if it is inflamed and smooth because of atrophy of the papillae (glossitis). Note the color of the patient's skin to see if it is pale with poor turgor. Note the color of the patient's sclera, which may be pearly white to bluish. Inspect the patient's fingernails to check for brittleness; note the shape of the fingernails, which may be spoon-shaped with central depressions and raised borders. Check the patient's hair to see if it is brittle and easily broken. In later stages, ankle edema may be present. Note any breathlessness or rapid breathing. Auscultate for heart sounds, noting rapid heart rate or a functional systolic murmur.

PSYCHOSOCIAL. Patients may be anxious or fearful about symptoms that have made it difficult for them to function at their usual level of energy. Discomfort from oral mucosa symptoms may prove upsetting. A pregnant patient may have additional stress over the well-being of her baby. Some patients may be resistant to proposed changes that would disrupt long-held eating patterns. Patients may also be upset about body changes such as pallor and weight loss.

DIAGNOSTIC HIGHLIGHTS

Test	Normal Result	Abnormality with Condition	Explanation
Bone marrow biopsy	Normal cells	Cells show absent staining for iron	Cells are iron-deficient
Complete blood count	Red blood cells 4.0–5.5 million/ microliter	Decreased; normal unless infection is present	Cells are iron-deficient; as hematocrit falls below 30%, hypochromic microcytic cells appear, followed by a decrease in MCV
	White blood cells 4,500–11,000/ microliter	Decreased	
	Hemoglobin 12–18 g/dL	Decreased	
	Hematocrit 37–54%	Decreased	
	Mean cell volume (MCV) 82–93 micrometers^3	Decreased	
Serum ferritin	11–200 ng/dL	< 10 ng/dL in women; < 20 ng/dL in men	Cells are iron-deficient

Other Tests: Serum iron, total iron-binding capacity

PRIMARY NURSING DIAGNOSIS

Activity intolerance related to imbalance between oxygen supply and demand

OUTCOMES. Energy conservation; Endurance; Self-care: Activities of daily living; Ambulation: Walking; Circulation status; Immobility consequences: Physiological; Mobility level; Nutritional status: Energy; Symptom severity

INTERVENTIONS. Nutritional management; Medication management; Energy management; Exercise promotion; Exercise therapy: Ambulation; Surveillance; Vital signs monitoring

☐ PLANNING AND IMPLEMENTATION

Collaborative

The two primary goals of treatment are to diagnose and correct the underlying cause of the iron deficiency and to correct the iron deficit. Medication therapy involves administering supplemental iron, which often shows results in the form of increased patient energy within 48 hours. Blood transfusions are not recommended for iron supplementation and should not be used to treat iron deficiency anemia unless there is cerebrovascular or cardiopulmonary compromise. Dietary supplementation of iron-rich food is needed to complement therapy and serve as a preventive model against future recurrence of the anemia. Pregnant women may also need to take prenatal vitamins and iron supplements.

PHARMACOLOGIC HIGHLIGHTS

Medication or Drug Class	Dosage	Description	Rationale
Supplemental iron	Varies with drug		Increases iron stores
		Oral therapy: ferrous sulfate (Feosol); ferrous gluconate (Fergon)	Oral: oral preparations should be taken with water or a straw to avoid staining teeth. Oral iron supplements may cause gastric irritation; irritation may be reduced by administering the supplement with meals as long as eggs, dairy products, coffee, tea, and antacids are avoided. Foods containing ascorbic acid, however, aid absorption.
		Parenteral therapy: iron dextran (Imferon)	
		Intramuscular: iron	Parenteral Therapy: Iron dextran (Imferon) is the preferred medication for intramuscular injections. Pregnant and elderly patients with severe iron deficiency anemia may be given total-dose intravenous infusions of iron dextran in a sodium chloride solution, after a small test dose is given to gauge any allergic reaction.

Independent

Nursing interventions focus on preventing infections, promoting comfort, and teaching the patient. Patients with iron deficiency anemia are apt to have other nutritional deficiencies that place them at risk for infection. Use good hand-washing techniques, and encourage the patient to avoid contact with people with known upper respiratory infections. If the patient experiences discomfort from oral lesions, provide mouth care. To limit activity intolerance, allow rest periods between all activities. Before the patient's discharge, arrange for home health follow-up if needed.

Teach the patient and significant others the causal relationships between bleeding tendencies and poor diet in relation to this anemia. Discuss the need to pace activities and allow for periods of rest. Emphasize to the patient the need for a well-balanced diet rich in iron; provide a list of iron-rich foods. Explain that any excess in iron stores may cause toxicity. Teach the patient that certain foods and medications—such as milk and antacids—interfere with the absorption of iron. Explain that stools normally turn greenish to black in color with iron therapy and that constipation may occur. Iron-rich foods such as fresh vegetables and red meat tend to be expensive, so that budget planning activities or assistance in attaining food stamps or other assistive programs may be essential. A social service referral or arranging of home care needs may be necessary. Parents of infants may need follow-up home visits to ensure that the growth and development of the child are progressing normally.

DOCUMENTATION GUIDELINES

- Physical findings: Oral mucosa alterations; weight loss; skin turgor
- Response to activity; ability to maintain activities of daily living
- Laboratory results: Reduced level of hemoglobin, RBCs, hematocrit, MCV
- Response to iron supplement therapy, side effects

DISCHARGE AND HOME HEALTHCARE GUIDELINES

Teach the patient that a well-balanced diet rich in both iron and iron supplements is necessary to prevent a recurrence of the anemia, and provide a list of iron-rich foods. Advise continuation of iron supplementation therapy even after the patient begins to feel better. Teach the route, dosage, side effects, and indications for use of iron supplements. Infection is a possibility because of the patient's weakened condition. Therefore, stress the importance of meticulous wound care, good hand-washing techniques, and periodic dental checkups. Emphasize the need for the patient to report immediately to the physician any signs of infection, such as fever or chills.

Irritable Bowel Syndrome

DRG Category: 182
Mean LOS: 4.3 days
Description: MEDICAL: Esophagitis, Gastrointestinal and Miscellaneous Digestive Disorders, Age > 17 without CC

Irritable bowel syndrome (IBS), sometimes called spastic colon, is the most common digestive disorder in the United States. It is a poorly understood syndrome of diarrhea, constipation, flatus, and abdominal pain that causes a great deal of stress and embarrassment to its victims. People often suffer with it for years before seeking medical attention.

Although people with IBS have a gastrointestinal (GI) tract that appears normal, colonic smooth muscle function is often abnormal. The autonomic nervous system, which innervates the large bowel, fails to provide the normal contractions interspaced with relaxations that propel stool smoothly forward. Excessive spasm and peristalsis lead to constipation or diarrhea, or both. Generally patients with IBS have either diarrhea- or constipation-predominant syndrome. Although complications are unusual, they include diverticulitis, colon cancer, and chronic inflammatory bowel disease.

CAUSES

IBS is a disorder of GI motility. Its exact cause remains unknown, although there is a familial link in about one-third of cases. The disorder is more common in whites, especially Jews, than in other groups. It is not caused by nerves or poor diet. Both stress and intolerance for some foods, however, can precipitate attacks. Other triggers include some types of abdominal surgery, acute illness that has disrupted bowel function, prolonged use of antibiotics, exposure to toxins, and emotional trauma. Ingestion of caffeine, alcohol, and other gastric stimulants and lactose intolerance seem to play roles for many individuals. The course of the disease is usually specific to the patient, who can identify the individual precipitating factors for exacerbations.

GENDER AND LIFE SPAN CONSIDERATIONS

Most newly diagnosed patients are young women in their 20s or early 30s. The incidence of newly diagnosed IBS is rare over age 50. Fewer than one-third of the cases of IBS are in men.

◻ ASSESSMENT

HISTORY. Symptoms that are reported most often are pain in the left lower quadrant, abdominal distension, diarrhea, and constipation, especially alternating bouts of the two. The pain may increase after eating and be relieved after a bowel movement. Pain is often cramping in nature and may be accompanied by nausea, belching, flatus, bloating, and sometimes anorexia. As the disease progresses, the patient may suffer fatigue and anxiety related to the many attempts to control the symptoms and lead a normal life. For some individuals with this disorder, the lifestyle is dictated by the need to remain close to a bathroom, which limits both occupation and social life.

PHYSICAL EXAMINATION. With auscultation of the abdomen, normal bowel sounds may be heard, although they may be quiet during constipation. Tympanic sounds may be heard over loops of filled bowel. Although palpation often discloses a relaxed abdomen, it may reveal diffuse tenderness, which becomes worse if the sigmoid colon is palpable. The patient may have pain on rectal examination but does not usually experience rectal bleeding.

PSYCHOSOCIAL. Many patients have consulted physicians who fail to take IBS seriously, telling them to eat a high-fiber diet and relax. Unfortunately, a high-fiber diet, which is good for ordinary constipation, often makes the irritable bowel worse. As the person suffers more frequent bouts of diarrhea and constipation, any attempts to relax become futile. Anxiety over control of symptoms makes the symptoms of IBS worse, creating a vicious cycle that becomes hard to break. Depression over the inability to control one's bodily functions or lead a normal life sometimes becomes a serious problem.

DIAGNOSTIC HIGHLIGHTS

Test	Normal Result	Abnormality with Condition	Explanation
Flexible sigmoidoscopy	Visualization of normal sigmoid	Intense spastic contractions; mucosa	Flexible sigmoidoscopy in adults younger than 40;

or colonoscopy	and colon	appears normal (smooth and pink)	colonoscopy in adults older than 40 years
Barium enema	Normal abdominal structures	Colonic spasms may occur during procedure; may have a normal exam	Identifies colonic spasms and rules out other pathology

Other Tests: Complete blood count, serologic tests, serum albumin, stool for guaiac (occult blood), abdominal x ray

PRIMARY NURSING DIAGNOSIS

Pain (acute) related to abdominal cramping

OUTCOMES. Comfort level; Pain control behavior; Pain level; Symptom severity

INTERVENTIONS. Medication management; Anxiety reduction; Environmental management: Comfort; Pain management

☐ PLANNING AND IMPLEMENTATION

Collaborative

As the symptoms worsen during the stress of other physical illnesses or trauma, fluid volume deficit may become a serious problem. It is usually treated by hypotonic intravenous solutions such as half-strength normal saline, sometimes with a potassium supplement. The nurse monitors the patient's state of hydration and intake and output. If the diarrhea continues to be severe, anti-diarrheal and anti-anxiety agents may be prescribed for a short period. Diarrhea, constipation, and abdominal pain are treated by a combination of drugs, diet, and attempts to establish an exercise routine that promotes normal bowel function.

The diet used most often for changes in GI motility is high in fiber and bulk. Bran may be added to increase dietary bulk and control diarrhea. A high-fiber diet may control symptoms and establish regular bowel movements in some; for others, a low-fiber, low-fat diet may be more effective. Lactose or sorbitol intolerance may require treatment, and hypersensitivity to particular foods may be found by eliminating wheat, citrus foods, and fatty foods.

PHARMACOLOGIC HIGHLIGHTS

Medication or Drug Class	Dosage	Description	Rationale
Bulk-forming laxatives	Varies with drug	Psyllium hydrophilic mucilloid (Metamucil); calcium polycarbophil (Mitrolan)	Facilitate defecation and enhance comfort
Antidiarrheal agents	Varies with drug	Diphenoxylate hydrochloride with atropine sulfate (Lomotil); loperamide (Imodium)	Decrease cramping and diarrhea; used only during an acute episode because they have a narcotic base and could easily lead to dependency

| Antispasmodic agents | Varies with drug | Dicyclomine hydrochloride (Bentyl); propantheline bromide (Pro-Banthine) | Relieve abdominal cramping and spasms |

Independent

The patient with IBS needs encouragement to eat meals at regular intervals, to chew the food slowly to help promote normal bowel function, and to drink eight glasses of water daily. Diet should include 30 to 40 grams of fiber each day. Most of the fluid intake should be at times other than mealtime. Foods to avoid include alcohol, caffeine, and anything that may irritate the GI tract. For example, if milk or milk products cause cramping or discomfort, they should be avoided.

Incorporating regular exercise in the daily routine may be helpful in controlling GI motility, but strenuous exercise is not desirable. Reassure the patient that stress does not cause the illness, even though it may be a major factor in its severity. Refer patients to a counselor if anxiety and stress management might help manage the condition.

DOCUMENTATION GUIDELINES

- Physical response: Hydration, GI assessment, frequency and consistency of bowel movements, level of discomfort
- Emotional response: Level of stress, mood and affect, coping ability
- Response to medications
- Nutritional status: Tolerance to food, body weight, appetite

DISCHARGE AND HOME HEALTHCARE GUIDELINES

Help the patient set a long-term goal to regain control of elimination patterns with manageable short-term goals to reduce stress. Progressive muscle relaxation helps relieve the tension that often stimulates stress-related diarrhea. Explain that as the patient experiences less frequent diarrhea, he or she begins to relax even more. Teach the patient about the disease, the treatment, and how to control the symptoms. Explain that the prognosis for control of the disease depends largely on the establishment of normal bowel habits and a plan for stress management. Explain all medications, including the dosage, action, route, and possible side effects. Explore the patient's dietary patterns and provide a dietary consultation if it is appropriate.

Junctional Dysrhythmias

DRG Category: 138
Mean LOS: 3.9 days
Description: MEDICAL: Cardiac Arrhythmias and Conduction Disorders with CC

Cardiac rhythms that are generated from the area around the atrioventricular (AV) junction node are termed junctional dysrhythmias. For a variety of reasons, the area that surrounds the AV node may generate impulses and become the cardiac pacemaker. Impulses produced in the junction do not necessarily result in an atrial contraction that precedes the ventricular contraction. This lack of coordination leads to a loss of ventricular filling during the last part of diastole; this loss of what is termed the "atrial kick" may reduce cardiac output by about 20% to 25%.

The inherent rate of the junctional tissue is 40 to 60 beats per minute. When the junctional pacemaker paces at its inherent rate, it produces what is called a passive junctional rhythm or a junctional escape rhythm. When it paces between 60 and 100 beats per minute, the term accelerated junctional rhythm is used. Junctional tachycardia occurs when the junctional pacemaker paces the heart at a rate between 100 and 160 beats per minute. Isolated complexes that arise from the junctional tissue are called premature junctional complexes (PJCs) if they come earlier than the expected sinus beat or junctional escape beats if they come later.

CAUSES

Junctional tissue may take over as the heart's pacemaker if the sinus node fails to produce an impulse or if that impulse is blocked in its conduction through the AV node. Junctional escape rhythms may be caused by digitalis toxicity, acute infections, oxygen deficiency, inferior wall myocardial infarction, or stimulation of the vagus nerve.

If the junctional tissue becomes irritable or increasingly automatic, it may override the sinus node and pace at a faster rate. Nonparoxysmal junctional tachycardia is often the result of enhanced automaticity, usually called irritability, which can be the result of digitalis toxicity, damage to the AV junction after an inferior myocardial infarction or rheumatic fever, or excessive administration of catecholamines or caffeine. Paroxysmal junctional tachycardia (a rapid rhythm that starts and stops suddenly) is usually the result of a re-entry mechanism.

PJCs may be found in healthy individuals, or they may be the result of excessive intake of stimulants such as caffeine, tobacco, or sympathomimetic drugs. Digitalis toxicity or use of alcohol may also cause PJCs. Junctional escape beats occur after pauses in the heart's rhythm. When the sinus node fails to fire, the junctional pacemaker should take over impulse initiation.

GENDER AND LIFE SPAN CONSIDERATIONS

Because of the common causes of junctional dysrhythmias, they occur more often in the elderly patient with cardiac disease. They can occur in any age group, however.

◻ ASSESSMENT

HISTORY. Many patients with suspected cardiac dysrhythmias describe a history of symptoms that indicate periods of decreased cardiac output. Although some junctional dysrhythmias are asymptomatic, some patients report a history of dizziness, fatigue, activity intolerance, a "fluttering" in their chest, shortness of breath, and chest pain. In particular, question the patient about the onset, duration, and characteristics of the symptoms and the events that precipitated them. Obtain a complete history of all illnesses, dietary restrictions, and activity restrictions and a current medication history.

PHYSICAL EXAMINATION. Symptoms are usually rate dependent. A passive junctional rhythm (junctional escape rhythm) is a bradycardia. Rates between 40 and 60 beats per minute with a loss of the atrial component to ventricular filling can produce signs of low cardiac output, such as syncope or lightheadedness. A patient who is experiencing accelerated junctional rhythm with a rate between 60 and 100 is asymptomatic if his or her cardiac status can accommodate the 20% to 25% reduction in cardiac output from loss of atrial kick.

Isolated PJCs usually produce no symptoms other than some palpitations and the sensation of a "skipped beat." Junctional tachycardia produces symptoms common to other supraventricular tachycardias. A junctional tachycardia may produce signs of low cardiac output and poor coronary perfusion. Common symptoms include labored breathing, shortness of breath, chest pain, feeling lightheaded, lowered blood pressure, and fainting.

PSYCHOSOCIAL. Patient response may vary, depending on the origin of the dysrhythmia. Certainly when the heart is beating unusually fast or slow or when palpitations are noticed, the patient may become distressed. Any disturbance in the brain's sensory apparatus as produced by low cardiac output can intensify fear or anxiety.

DIAGNOSTIC HIGHLIGHTS

Test	Normal Result	Abnormality with Condition	Explanation
12-Lead electrocardiogram (ECG)	Regular sinus rhythm	Junctional escape: heart rate of 40–60 beats per minute with regular R to R interval; P wave may be inverted and precedes the QRS with a short PR interval	Detects specific conduction defects and monitors the patient's cardiac response to electrolyte imbalances, drug effects, and toxicities
		Premature junctional beats: early beat disrupts rhythm; P wave may be inverted and precedes the QRS with a short PR interval.	
		Junctional tachycardia: ventricular rate is 100–160 beats per minute and regular; P wave may be inverted and precedes the QRS with a short PR interval.	

Other Tests: Pulse oximetry, ambulatory or Holter monitoring: To provide a 12- to 24-hour continuous recording of myocardial electrical activity as the patient performs normal daily activities.

PRIMARY NURSING DIAGNOSIS

Altered tissue perfusion (cardiopulmonary, cerebral, renal, peripheral) related to rapid or slow heart rates

OUTCOMES. Circulation status; Cardiac pump effectiveness; Tissue perfusion: Cardiopulmonary, Cerebral, Renal, Peripheral; Vital sign status

INTERVENTIONS. Circulatory care; Dysrhythmia management; Emergency care; Vital signs monitoring; Cardiac care; Cardiac precautions; Oxygen therapy; Fluid/electrolyte management; Surveillance

☐ PLANNING AND IMPLEMENTATION

Collaborative

Treatment of junctional dysrhythmias usually depends on the heart rate. Unless the cardiac output is compromised, treatment may not be initiated. Infrequent PJCs may be tolerated as benign.

PJCs are treated by attempting to alleviate the cause. Stimulants such as caffeine, tobacco, and sympathomimetic drugs may be discontinued. If digitalis toxicity is the cause, digitalis may be withheld. If PJCs are frequent, they may be suppressed by administration of an antidysrhythmic such as quinidine sulfate. Infrequent PJCs may not be treated.

Junctional escape rhythm is a marked bradycardia that may be treated with atropine sulfate intravenously (IV) to increase the rate. In rare circumstances, a temporary cardiac pacemaker is necessary if the bradycardia does not respond to treatment.

An accelerated junctional rhythm, with a rate between 60 and 100 beats per minute, rarely compromises the cardiac output. The rhythm is usually just observed.

Paroxysmal junctional tachycardia is treated the same as any narrow QRS complex tachycardia. If the ventricular rate is faster than 150 beats per minute, cardioversion may be indicated. If the rate is less than 150, vagal maneuvers may be attempted. The drug of choice for emergency treatment is adenosine. The nurse has an important role in the collaborative management of the patient by administering medications as ordered or according to protocol in emergency situations.

PHARMACOLOGIC HIGHLIGHTS

Medication or Drug Class	Dosage	Description	Rationale
Antidysrhythmics	Varies with drug	Quinidine sulfate, phenytoin, lidocaine	Suppress frequent PJCs
Calcium channel blockers and beta adrenergic blockers	Varies with drug	Verapamil, diltiazem, propranolol, esmolol, sotalol	Treat junctional tachycardia
Adenosine	6 mg IV over 1–3 seconds; may repeat in 1–2 minutes	Antiarrhythmic	Suppresses paroxysmal junctional tachycardia

Other Drugs: Atropine sulfate, digitalis, dopamine, epinephrine. Other drugs used for continuing significant bradycardias no matter what the origin, particularly when accompanied by hypotension, are dopamine (5 to 20 μg/kg per minute of IV infusion) and epinephrine (2 to 10 μg/kg per minute of IV infusion).

Independent

The nurse's role is one of monitoring and support. Support the patient who is experiencing symptoms from any rhythm disturbance. Maintain the patient's airway, breathing, and circulation. To maximize oxygen available to the myocardium, encourage the patient to rest in bed until the symptoms are treated and subside. Remain with the patient to ensure rest and to allay anxiety. Discuss any potential precipitating factors with the patient. For some patients, strategies to reduce stress or lifestyle changes help limit the incidence of dysrhythmias. Teach the patient to reduce the amount of caffeine intake in the diet. If appropriate, encourage the patient to become involved in an exercise program or a smoking cessation group. Provide emotional support and information about the dysrhythmia, the precipitating factors, and mechanisms to limit the dysrhythmia. If the patient is at risk for electrolyte imbalance, teach the patient any dietary considerations to prevent electrolyte depletion.

DOCUMENTATION GUIDELINES

- Rhythm strips: Record and analyze according to hospital protocol, note the monitoring lead and document any change in leads
- Patient symptoms and vital signs with any change or new onset of dysrhythmia
- Patient's response to symptoms
- Patient's response to management

DISCHARGE AND HOME HEALTHCARE GUIDELINES

Make sure the patient understands the role of stimulants in generating dysrhythmias. Explain the importance of taking all medications before discharge. Explain the ordered dosage, route, action, and possible adverse effects. Teach the patient to monitor his or her pulse and to report to the physician any significant changes in rate or regularity.

Kidney Cancer

DRG Category: 318
Mean LOS: 5.2 days
Description: MEDICAL: Kidney and Urinary Tract Neoplasm with CC
DRG Category: 303
Mean LOS: 9.7 days
Description: SURGICAL: Kidney, Ureter, and Major Bladder Procedures for Neoplasm

Kidney cancer is rare, comprising about 3% of all adult cancers. Kidney cancers are classified by cell type. The three most commonly seen in the adult are renal cell carcinoma, transitional cell carcinoma, and sarcoma. Renal cell carcinoma arises in the renal tubules and accounts for approximately 85% of kidney cancers. The other types of kidney cancer, transitional cell carcinoma and sarcomas, comprise the remaining 15%. Most kidney cancers occur in one kidney only (unilateral) and are large and nodular. Renal metastases from other sites are unusual.

Approximately 30,000 new cases of kidney cancer occur each year (not including Wilms' tumor in children). The 5-year survival rate is 40% to 45%. Complications from kidney cancer include renal hemorrhage and metastases to the lungs, central nervous system, and gastrointestinal tract. If it is left untreated, kidney cancer causes death.

CAUSES

Although the exact cause remains unknown, several factors seem to predispose a person to kidney cancer. Smokers are twice as likely to develop kidney cancer as nonsmokers. A link also exists between kidney cancer and occupational exposure to cadmium (found in batteries) or asbestos.

GENDER AND LIFE SPAN CONSIDERATIONS

Kidney cancer occurs twice as frequently in men as in women, commonly after age 40 with a peak incidence between the ages of 50 and 60 years. Children and infants diagnosed with kidney cancer usually have Wilms' tumors or a tumor of the renal pelvis and, with prompt treatment, usually have a good prognosis.

☐ ASSESSMENT

HISTORY. Question the patient about the classic triad of symptoms: hematuria, pain, and an abdominal mass. The most common single symptom is painless hematuria, whereas an abdominal mass is usually a late finding. The patient may also report vague signs and symptoms, such as a dull aching pain in the flank area. One-third of all patients diagnosed have these symptoms. One-third of patients have no symptoms at all, and the diagnosis is made during a routine physical examination. The other third of patients are diagnosed after the cancer has produced symptoms that are related to distant metastases.

PHYSICAL EXAMINATION. It is not unusual for the patient to have a normal physical examination. Occasionally the patient appears weak, with an unintentional weight loss since the last examination. The patient may have hypertension. The placement of the kidneys, deep within the abdomen and protected by layers of fat, makes palpation of renal masses difficult. On occasion, palpation may reveal a smooth, firm abdominal mass.

PSYCHOSOCIAL. The patient may be preparing to retire or be retired when the diagnosis is made. Consider the patient's and significant others' ability to cope with a life-threatening illness at this life stage. The diagnosis may be met with anger. The patient diagnosed with kidney cancer is facing a possibly terminal diagnosis. Assess support systems and consider making appropriate referrals if needed.

DIAGNOSTIC HIGHLIGHTS

Test	Normal Result	Abnormality with Condition	Explanation
Kidney sonogram (ultrasound)	Bilateral kidneys are properly located and of normal size with smooth outer contours	Usually a unilateral tumor in one kidney	Serves as alternative to renal dye imaging tests for people with allergies; creates oscilloscopic picture from echoes of high-frequency sound waves that pass over the flank area
Abdominal computed tomography (CT) scan	Bilateral kidneys are properly located and of normal size with smooth outer contours	Usually a unilateral tumor in one kidney	Produces pictures of peritoneal and retro-peritoneal cavity, based on differing densities and composition of body tissues

Other Tests: Magnetic resonance imaging (MRI), arteriography, blood urea nitrogen, creatinine, urinalysis, and intravenous pyelogram (IVP). To determine if metastasis has occurred: bone scan, chest x ray

PRIMARY NURSING DIAGNOSIS

Altered urinary elimination related to renal tissue destruction

OUTCOMES. Urinary continence; Urinary elimination; Knowledge: Medication; Disease process; Treatment regime; Symptom severity

INTERVENTIONS. Urinary elimination: Management; Fluid management; Medication prescribing; Urinary catheterization; Anxiety reduction; Pain management

☐ PLANNING AND IMPLEMENTATION

Collaborative

Depending on the stage, surgical intervention and further staging is the primary treatment for renal cell cancer. A radical nephrectomy, sometimes with lymph node removal, offers the patient the best chance for cure. The procedure is the treatment of choice for localized cancer or in patients with tumor extension into the renal vein and vena cava. Surgical intervention is not curative for disseminated disease. Because of the proximity of the kidney to the diaphragm, the surgeon may explore the pleura on the surgical side. The patient could therefore return from surgery with a chest tube placed to remove blood and air from the pleural space.

Nephrectomies involve large blood vessels and place the patient at risk for postoperative hemorrhage. Frequent assessment and serial vital signs to monitor for shock are part of postoperative management. Patients undergoing a nephrectomy experience moderate to severe pain; for this reason, the anesthesiologist may place an epidural catheter during surgery for pain management with morphine sulfate or other appropriate analgesia. Monitor the patient's urinary output through the Foley catheter for adequate volume and color and consistency of urine; if the patient's urine output decreases below 40 mL per hour, notify the physician.

Depending on the final stage of the kidney cancer, the surgeon may refer the patient for follow-up care by an oncologist. Kidney cancer is resistant to radiation therapy, which is used in high doses only when metastases have occurred into areas such as the perinephric region and the lymph nodes. Chemotherapy and hormonal therapy do not affect tumor growth. Although several experimental or alternative medications are being tested, they usually have many side effects or are of limited usefulness.

PHARMACOLOGIC HIGHLIGHTS

Medication or Drug Class	Dosage	Description	Rationale
Narcotics	Varies with drug and situation	Patient-controlled analgesia; patient is placed on patient-controlled analgesia pump attached to the peripheral intravenous site	Manage pain

Independent

Two of the most important priorities are to enhance gas exchange and to maintain the patient's comfort. Institute pulmonary care on a routine basis. Patients with a smoking history may take longer to recover normal lung function after surgery. Encourage the patient to turn, cough, and breathe deeply at least every 2 hours. Show the patient how to use diaphragmatic breathing techniques and how to splint the incision. Teach the patient how to use an incentive spirometer to improve gas exchange. Ask the patient to describe the degree of pain on a scale of 1 to 10. Instruct the patient on nonpharmacologic methods for pain relief. If the patient is receiving analgesia that is insufficient to relieve the pain, notify the physician.

Patients and their significant others are dealing with stressors that cause extreme anxiety and fear. Spend time each day discussing their concerns, being honest about the patient's chances for recovery. If the patient experiences an unusual degree of spiritual distress, refer to a chaplain or clinical nurse specialist. The diagnosis of kidney cancer is life-threatening, and the patient may need to work through the issues associated with a serious disease.

DOCUMENTATION GUIDELINES

- Respiratory response: Patency of airway; adequacy of ventilation (rate, quality, and presence of adventitious breath sounds); maintenance of chest tube system (suction, presence of air leaks, amount and quality of drainage)
- Incisional care: Description of dressing; appearance of wound
- Degree of pain; response to interventions to lessen pain
- Presence of complications related to the surgical procedure
- Amount of urinary output, color of urine, and patency of Foley catheter

DISCHARGE AND HOME HEALTHCARE GUIDELINES

Be sure the patient understands what medications are to be taken at home, their effects, and dosages. Explain follow-up information, such as when the physician would like to see the patient. Provide a phone number with written discharge information, and arrange for a home visit from nurses if appropriate. Refer the patient and family to hospital and community services such as support groups and the American Cancer Society. Reinforce any postoperative restrictions. Explain when normal activity can be resumed. Make sure the patient understands the need to have ongoing monitoring of the disease. Annual chest x rays and routine IVPs are recommended to check for other tumors.

Laryngeal Cancer

DRG Category: 064
Mean LOS: 5.0 days
Description: MEDICAL: Ear, Nose, Mouth, and Throat Malignancy
DRG Category: 482
Mean LOS: 13.0 days
Description: SURGICAL: Tracheostomy for Face, Mouth, and Neck Diagnoses

Cancer of the larynx is the most common malignancy of the upper respiratory tract. About 95% of all laryngeal cancers are squamous cell carcinomas; adenocarcinomas and sarcomas account for the other 5%. The American Cancer Society predicts approximately 10,000 new cases of laryngeal cancer annually with approximately 4,000 deaths.

Most cases of laryngeal cancer are diagnosed before metastasis occurs. If it is confined to the glottis (the true vocal cords), laryngeal cancer usually grows slowly and metastasizes late because of the limited lymphatic drainage of the cords. Laryngeal cancer that involves the supraglottis (false vocal cords) and subglottis (a rare downward extension from the vocal cords) tends to metastasize early to the lymph nodes in the neck because of the rich lymphatic drainage of this area.

CAUSES

The cause of laryngeal cancer is unknown, but the two major predisposing factors are prolonged use of alcohol and tobacco. Each substance poses an independent risk, but their combined use causes a synergistic effect. Other risk factors include a familial tendency, a history of frequent laryngitis or vocal straining, and chronic inhalation of noxious fumes.

GENDER AND LIFE SPAN CONSIDERATIONS

Cancer of the larynx is more common in men than in women (5:1 ratio) because heretofore men have been more likely to smoke cigarettes and drink alcohol, but the incidence in women is rising as more women also smoke and drink. Cancer of the larynx occurs most frequently between the ages of 50 and 70. Women are more likely to get laryngeal cancer between the ages of 50 and 60 and men between the ages of 60 and 70.

☐ ASSESSMENT

HISTORY. Be aware as you interview the patient that hoarseness, shortness of breath, and pain may occur as the patient speaks. Obtain a thorough history of risk factors: alcohol or tobacco usage, voice abuse, frequent laryngitis, and family history of laryngeal cancer. Obtain detailed information about the patient's alcohol intake; ask about drinks per day, days of abstinence, and patterns of drinking. Ask the patient how many packs of cigarettes he or she has smoked per day for how many years.

Most patients describe hoarseness or throat irritation that lasts longer than 2 weeks. Ask about dysphagia, persistent cough, hemoptysis, weight loss, dyspnea, or pain that radiates to the ear, which are late symptoms of laryngeal cancer. Because of potential problems with alcohol and weight loss, inquire about the patient's nutritional intake and dietary habits.

PHYSICAL EXAMINATION. Inspect and palpate the neck for lumps and involved lymph nodes. A node may be tender before it is palpable. Inspect the mouth for sores and lumps. Palpate the base of the tongue to detect any nodules. Perform a cranial nerve assessment because some tumors spread along these nerves.

PSYCHOSOCIAL. The patient with laryngeal cancer is faced with a potentially terminal illness. The patient may experience guilt, denial, or shame because of the association with cigarette smoking and alcohol consumption. Efforts to cure patients of this disease often result in a loss of normal speech and permanent lifestyle changes. Patients may experience radical changes in both body image and role relationships (interpersonal, social, and work). Assess both the patient's and significant others' coping mechanisms and support system because extensive follow-up at home is necessary.

DIAGNOSTIC HIGHLIGHTS

Test	Normal Result	Abnormality with Condition	Explanation
Nasopharyngosocopy/ laryngoscopy	Normal structures with no evidence of cancer	Visible cancers of the oral cavity and nasopharynx	Special fiberoptic scopes and mirrors allow visual inspection of the mouth and behind nose

Panendoscopy	Normal structures with no evidence of cancer	Visible cancers of larynx, hypopharynx, esophagus, trachea, and bronchi	Special fiberoptic scopes and mirrors allow visual inspection of larynx, hypopharynx, esophagus, trachea, and bronchi
Barium swallow	Normal structures with no evidence of cancer	Locations and extent of cancers evident	X rays performed while the patient swallows a liquid that contains barium

Other Tests: Magnetic resonance imaging, computed tomography (CT) scan, chest x rays

PRIMARY NURSING DIAGNOSIS

Ineffective airway clearance related to obstruction, swelling, and accumulation of secretions

OUTCOMES. Respiratory status: Gas exchange and ventilation; Comfort level; Knowledge: Treatment regime

INTERVENTIONS. Airway insertion; Airway management; Airway suctioning; Oral health promotion; Respiratory monitoring; Ventilation assistance

☐ PLANNING AND IMPLEMENTATION

Collaborative

A multidisciplinary team of speech pathologists, social workers, dietitians, respiratory therapists, occupational therapists, and physical therapists provide preoperative evaluation and postoperative care. The goal is to eliminate the cancer and preserve the ability to speak. The two types of therapy commonly used are radiation therapy and surgery. Chemotherapy has not been found to be beneficial in treating this type of cancer and, if used, is always employed in conjunction with surgery or radiation. Chemotherapy may be useful in treating cancer that has metastasized beyond the head and neck, however, and it may be useful as a palliative for cancers that are too large to be surgically removed or for cancer that is not controlled by radiation therapy.

Treatment choice depends on cancer staging. Stage 0 cancer is treated either by surgical removal of the abnormal lining layer of the larynx or by laser beam vaporizing of the abnormal cell layer. Stages I and II are treated either surgically or with radiation therapy. A common course of radiation therapy consists of daily fractions or doses administered five days a week for seven weeks. Radiation therapy is frequently used as the primary treatment of laryngeal cancer, especially for patients with small cancers. Radiation successfully treats 80% to 90% of patients with stage I laryngeal cancer and 70% to 80% of patients with stage II laryngeal cancer. A partial laryngectomy is an alternative treatment; however, voice results are generally better with radiation.

Stage III and stage IV laryngeal cancer are generally treated with a combination of surgery and radiation, radiation and chemotherapy, or all three treatments. Almost always, a total laryngectomy is performed, although a very few laryngeal cancers may be treated by partial laryngectomy. The patient loses his or her voice and sense of smell; the patient breathes through a permanent tracheostomy stoma. A radical neck dissection is done, in conjunction with a partial or a total laryngectomy, to remove carcinoma that has metastasized to adjacent areas of the neck. The 5-year survival rate for stage III and stage IV cancers treated with surgery and radiation is 50% to 80%.

Preoperatively, the physician and speech therapist should discuss the anticipated effect of the surgical procedure on the patient's voice. Postoperatively the most immediate concern is maintaining a patent airway. Suctioning needs to be done gently so as not to penetrate the suture line. Suction the patient's laryngectomy tube and nose because the patient can no longer blow air through the nose. Observe the suture lines for intactness, hematoma, and signs of infection. Assess the skin flap for any signs of infection or necrosis, and notify the physician of any problems.

A new advance in restoring speech is a procedure called tracheoesophageal puncture (TEP), which is performed either at the time of the initial surgery or at a later date. Through the use of a small one-way shunt valve that is placed into a small puncture at the stoma site, patients can produce speech by covering the stoma with a finger and forcing air out of the mouth.

PHARMACOLOGIC HIGHLIGHTS

Medication or Drug Class	Dosage	Description	Rationale
Analgesics	Varies with drug	Morphine sulfate, fentanyl	Relieve pain

Other Drugs: Chemotherapy may be used in certain circumstances.

Independent

Spend time with the patient preoperatively exploring changes in the patient's body, such as the loss of smell and the inability to whistle, gargle, sip, use a straw, or blow the nose. Explain that the patient may need to breathe through a stoma in the neck, learn esophageal speech, or learn to use mechanical devices to speak. Encourage the expression of feelings about a diagnosis of cancer and offer to contact the appropriate clergy or clinical nurse specialist to counsel the patient.

Postoperatively, assess the patient's level of comfort. Reposition the patient carefully; after a total laryngectomy, support the back of the neck when moving the patient to prevent trauma. Provide frequent mouth care, cleansing the mouth with a soft toothbrush, toothette, or washcloth. After a partial laryngectomy, the patient should not use his or her voice for at least 2 days. The patient should have an alternate means of communication available at all times, and the nurse should encourage its use. After 2 to 3 days, encourage the patient to use a whisper until complete healing takes place. Because the functional impairments and disfigurement that result from this surgery are traumatic, close attention should be paid to the patient's emotional status.

As soon as possible after surgery, the patient with a total laryngectomy should start learning to care for the stoma, suction the airway, care for the incision, and self-administer the tube feedings (if the patient is to have tube feedings after discharge). Assist the patient in obtaining the equipment and supplies for home use. Discuss safety precautions for patients with a permanent stoma. If appropriate, refer the patient to smoking and alcohol cessation counseling.

DOCUMENTATION GUIDELINES

- Preoperative health and social history, physical assessment, drinking and smoking history
- Postoperative physical status: Incisions and drains, patency of airway, pulmonary secretions, nasogastric feedings, oral intake, integrity of the skin
- Pain: Location, duration, frequency, precipitating factors, response to analgesia
- Preoperative, postoperative, and discharge teaching
- Patient's ability to perform self-care: Secretion removal, laryngectomy tube and stoma care, incision care, tube feedings

DISCHARGE AND HOME HEALTHCARE GUIDELINES

Teach the patient the name, purpose, dosage, schedule, common side effects, and importance of taking all medications. Teach the patient signs and symptoms of potential complications and the appropriate actions to be taken. Complications include infection (symptoms: wound drainage, poor wound healing, fever, achiness, chills); airway obstruction and tracheostomy stenosis (symptoms: noisy respirations, difficulty breathing, restlessness, confusion, increased respiratory rate); vocal straining; fistula formation (symptoms: redness, swelling, secretions along a suture line); and ruptured carotid artery (symptoms: bleeding, hypotension).

Teach the patient the appropriate devices and techniques to ensure a patent airway and prevent complications. Explore methods of communication that work effectively. Encourage the patient to wear a Medic Alert bracelet or necklace, which identifies him or her as a mouth-breather. Provide the patient with a list of referrals and support groups, such as visiting nurses, American Cancer Society, American Speech-Learning-Hearing Association, International Association of Laryngectomees, and the Lost Cord Club.

Laryngotracheobron-chitis (Croup)

DRG Category: 071
Mean LOS: 3.5 days
Description: MEDICAL: Laryngotracheitis

Laryngotracheobronchitis (LTB) is an inflammation and obstruction of the larynx, trachea, and major bronchi of children. In small children, the air passages in the lungs are smaller than those of adults, making them more susceptible to obstruction by edema and spasm. Because of the respiratory distress it causes, LTB is one of the most frightening acute diseases of childhood. It is sometimes called croup, although croup can be more specifically described as one of three entities: LTB, laryngitis (inflammation of the larynx), or acute spasmodic laryngitis (obstructive narrowing of the larynx because of viral infection, genetic factors, or emotional distress). Acute spasmodic laryngitis is particularly common in children with allergies and those with a family history of croup. Acute LTB usually occurs in the fall or winter and is often mild, self-limiting, and followed by a complete recovery.

CAUSES

LTB is generally caused by a virus. Parainfluenza 1, 2, and 3 viruses, respiratory syncytial virus, mycoplasma pneumoniae, and rhinoviruses are the most common causes. The measles virus or bacterial infections such as pertussis and diphtheria are occasionally the cause. Epiglottitis, a life-threatening emergency caused by acute inflammation of the epiglottis and surrounding area, differs from LTB because it usually results from infection with the bacteria *Haemophilus influenzae* type B.

GENDER AND LIFE SPAN CONSIDERATIONS

Children susceptible to LTB are generally between the ages of 3 months and 4 years. The susceptibility decreases with age, although some children seem more prone to repeat episodes of LTB. Acute spasmodic laryngitis occurs in the same age group and peaks at age 18 months. As with many respiratory diseases, boys are affected more often than girls.

☐ ASSESSMENT

HISTORY. The child usually has a history of an upper respiratory infection and a runny nose (rhinorrhea). After several days of respiratory symptoms, such as cough and increased respiratory rate, the child develops a barking, seal-like cough; a hoarse cry; and inspiratory stridor. The symptoms tend to occur in the late evening and improve during the day. A child may have LTB more than once but will outgrow it as the size of the airways increases. The course of the infection lasts several days to several weeks, and the child may have a lingering, barking cough.

PHYSICAL EXAMINATION. The initial sign of LTB is increasing respiratory distress. The child may develop flaring of the nares, a prolonged expiratory phase, and use of accessory muscles. When you auscultate the child's lungs, the breath sounds may be diminished and you may hear inspiratory stridor. The child may have a mild fever. Increasing respiratory obstruction is indicated by any of the following: increasing stridor, suprasternal and intercostal retractions, respiratory rate above 60, tachycardia, cyanosis, pallor, and restlessness. In addition, each type of croup can have particular symptoms, as shown in the table. (See Table 32.)

TABLE 32 | **Forms of Laryngotreacheobronchitis**

FORMS OF CROUP	SYMPTOMS
LTB	Fever, breathing problems at night, inability to breathe out because of bronchial edema, decreased breath sounds, expiratory rhonchi, scattered crackles
Laryngitis	Mild respiratory distress in children, increased respiratory distress in infants. Sore throat and cough, inspiratory stridor, dyspnea. Late phases: severe dyspnea, fatigue, exhaustion

| Acute spasmodic laryngitis | Hoarseness, rhinorrhea, cough, noisy inspiratory phase that worsens at night, anxiety, labored breathing, cyanosis, rapid pulse; the most severe symptoms may occur on the first night, with lessening symptoms on each of the following nights |

PSYCHOSOCIAL. The parents and child will be apprehensive. Assess the parents' ability to cope with the emergency situation, and intervene as appropriate. Note that many children are treated at home rather than in the hospital; your teaching plan may need to consider home rather than hospital management.

DIAGNOSTIC HIGHLIGHTS

General Comments: Diagnostic testing involves identifying the causative organism, determining oxygenation status, and ruling out masses as a cause of obstruction.

Test	Normal Result	Abnormality with Condition	Explanation
Blood culture; throat culture	No growth; no organism identified	Causative organism identified	Distinguishes between bacterial and viral infections
Pulse oximetry	$\geq 95\%$	$< 95\%$	Low oxygen saturation is present if there is obstruction in the lung passages
X rays	Normal structure	Narrowing of the upper airway and edema in epiglottal and laryngeal areas	Narrowing and/or blocked airway is characteristic of LTB

PRIMARY NURSING DIAGNOSIS

Ineffective airway clearance related to tracheobronchial infection and obstruction

OUTCOMES. Respiratory status: Airway patency; Respiratory status: Gas exchange; Respiratory status: Ventilation

INTERVENTIONS. Airway management; Respiratory monitoring; Vital signs monitoring; Anxiety reduction

□ PLANNING AND IMPLEMENTATION

Collaborative

The aim of treatment is to maintain a patent airway and provide adequate repiratory exchange. Medical management includes bronchodilating medications, cool mist in a croup tent during sleep, and intravenous hydration if oral intake is inadequate. Oxygen may be used, but it masks cyanosis, which signals impending airway obstruction. Sedation is contraindicated because it may depress respirations or mask restlessness, which indicate a worsening condition. Sponge baths may be needed to control temperatures above 102°F. You may need to isolate the child if the physician suspects syncytial virus or parainfluenza infections.

An intubation or a tracheostomy is performed only if no other method of airway maintenance is available. Keep intubation and tracheostomy trays near the bedside at all times, for use in case of emergencies.

PHARMACOLOGIC HIGHLIGHTS

Medication or Drug Class	Dosage	Description	Rationale
Racemic epinephrine	Per nebulizer, varies dependent on size of child	Sympathomimetic	Dilates the bronchioles, opening up respiratory passages
Corticosteroids	Varies with drug	Anti-inflammatory	Decrease airway inflammation if epinephrine is not effective
Antipyretics	Varies with drug		Reduce fever often present in LTB
Antibiotics	Varies with drug	Type of antibiotic depends on the causative organism	Fight bacterial infections

Independent

Ongoing, continuous observation of the patency of the child's airway is essential to identify impending obstruction. Prop infants up on pillows or place them in an infant seat; older children should have the head of the bed elevated so that they are in Fowler's position. Sore throat pain can be decreased by soothing preparations such as iced pops or fruit sherbet. If the child has difficulty swallowing, avoid thick milkshakes.

Children should be allowed to rest as much as possible to conserve their energy; organize your interventions to limit disturbances. Provide age-appropriate activities. Crying increases the child's difficulty in breathing and should be limited if possible by comfort measures and the presence of the parents; parents should be allowed to hold and comfort the child as much as possible. If the child is in a cool mist tent, parents may need to be enclosed with the child, or the child may need to be held by the parents with the mist directed toward them. Children sense anxiety from their parents; if you support the parents in dealing with their anxiety and fear, the children are less fearful. Careful explanation of all procedures and allowing the parents to participate in the care of the child as much as possible help relieve the anxieties of both child and parents.

Provide adequate hydration to liquefy secretions and to replace fluid loss from increased sensible loss (increased respirations and fever). The child also might have a decreased fluid intake during the illness. Clear liquids should be offered frequently. Apply lubricant or ointment around the child's mouth and lips to decrease the irritation from secretions and mouth breathing.

DOCUMENTATION GUIDELINES

- Respiratory status: Rate, quality, depth, ease, breath sounds
- Response to treatment: Cool mist tent, bronchodilators, racemic epinephrine, fluid, and diet

- Child's emotional response
- Child's response to rest and activity

DISCHARGE AND HOME HEALTHCARE GUIDELINES

PREVENTION. Children may have recurring episodes of LTB; parental instruction on mechanisms to prevent airway obstruction is therefore important. Cool mist humidifiers may be used in the child's room during the fall and winter months. Teach the parents to clean the humidifier every week with a vinegar mixture run through the machine for 30 minutes. If the child has an upper respiratory infection, encourage the parents to maintain an open airway by using a croup tent that may be improvised by draping sheets over a crib and a cool mist humidifier. Another option is to take the child into a closed bathroom with the shower or tub running to create an environment that has high humidity.

MEDICATIONS. If antibiotics have been prescribed, tell the parents to make sure the child finishes the entire prescription.

COMPLICATIONS. Instruct the parents to recognize the signs of increasing respiratory obstruction, and advise them when to take the child to an emergency department. Remind the parents that ear infections or pneumonia may follow croup in 4 to 6 days. Immediate medical attention is needed if the child has an earache, productive cough, fever, or dyspnea.

HOME CARE. If the child is cared for at home, provide the following home care instructions:
Keep the child in bed or playing quietly to conserve energy.
Prop the child in a sitting position to ease breathing; don't let him or her stay in a flat position.
Do not use aspirin products because of the chance of Reye's syndrome.
Give plenty of fluids, such as sherbet, ginger ale left to stand so there are no bubbles, gelatin dissolved in water, and iced pops; withhold solid food until the child can breathe easily.
Provide a cool mist humidifier.

Legionnaires' Disease

DRG Category: 079
Mean LOS: 8.3 days
Description: MEDICAL: Respiratory Infections and Inflammations, Age > 17 with CC
DRG Category: 475
Mean LOS: 9.5 days
Description: MEDICAL: Respiratory System Diagnosis with Ventilator Support
DRG Category: 483
Mean LOS: 41.9 days
Description: SURGICAL: Tracheostomy Except for Face, Mouth, and Neck Diagnoses

Legionnaires' disease is an acute bronchopneumonia that was named because of a major outbreak at the 1976 American Legion Convention in Philadelphia, in which 221 American legionnaires contracted the disease and 34 persons died. Thereafter, outbreaks were noticed to occur in late summer and early fall. Outbreaks of legionnaires' disease may be epidemic or confined to a small number of cases.

Legionnaires' disease has an incubation period of 2 to 10 days and is characterized by patchy pulmonary infiltrates, lung consolidation, and flu-like symptoms. Pneumonia is the presenting clinical syndrome in more than 95% of cases. Legionnaires' disease is spread by direct alveolar infection with the gram-negative bacterium *Legionella pneumophila*. From the initial site, the infection spreads through the bronchi and through the blood and lymphatic systems. Bacteremia occurs in about 30% of the patients and is the source of nonrespiratory infections in most patients.

Complications are extensive and serious with legionnaires' disease. Hypoxemia and acute respiratory failure can result from the severe case of pneumonia. The disease can also cause hypotension and hyponatremia as a result of salt and water loss. Central nervous system involvement is seen in almost 30% of patients. Renal involvement, which ranges from interstitial nephritis to renal failure, may occur. Untreated immunosuppressed patients have a mortality rate of 80%; untreated patients with no immune system compromise have a mortality rate of 25%.

CAUSES

L. pneumophila is an aerobic, gram-negative bacillus that seems to be transmitted by air. It is usually classified as a saprophytic water bacterium because it is natural to bodies of water such as rivers, lakes, streams, and thermally polluted waters. Elevated temperatures (36° to 70°C) enhance growth of the bacterium. *L. pneumophila* is also found in habitats such as cooling towers, evaporative condensers, and water distribution centers, and it also has been found in soil samples and at excavation sites. Pathogenic microorganisms can enter the lung by aspiration, direct inhalation, or dissemination from another focus of infection.

GENDER AND LIFE SPAN CONSIDERATIONS

Legionnaires' disease is three times more common in men than in women; it is uncommon in children. At-risk groups include middle-aged or elderly people; patients with a chronic underlying disease such as chronic obstructive pulmonary disease, diabetes mellitus, or chronic renal failure; patients with immunosuppressive disorders such as lymphoma or patients who receive corticosteroids after organ transplantation; alcoholics; and cigarette smokers.

◻ ASSESSMENT

HISTORY. Ask about malaise, aching muscles, anorexia, headache, high fever, or recurrent chills. Establish a history of chest pain or coughing, which begins as a nonproductive cough but eventually becomes productive. Ask the patient about gastrointestinal symptoms such as diarrhea, nausea, and vomiting. Because the central nervous system is involved in about 30% of cases, ask the family or significant others if the patient has experienced recent confusion or decreased level of consciousness.

Determine if the patient has been close to a river, lake, or stream, which might have resulted in possible exposure to the bacteria. Establish a work history of employment at an excavation site or water distribution center, in a cooling tower, or near an evaporative condenser. Ask if the patient works or lives in a facility with central air conditioning or humidifiers. Ask if the patient has used a respiratory apparatus or a nasogastric tube in the recent past.

PHYSICAL EXAMINATION. The patient usually appears acutely ill, with a high fever. Note any neurological signs, such as altered level of consciousness, confusion, or coma. Inspect the patient's sputum, which may be grayish or rust-colored, nonpurulent, and, occasionally, blood-streaked. Note the respiratory rate, which may be rapid and accompanied by dyspnea.

Auscultate the breathing; fine or coarse crackles may be audible, depending on the stage of the disease process. Auscultate the blood pressure and heart rate; note that some patients develop severe hypotension and bradycardia. Percuss the chest for dullness over areas of secretions and consolidation or pleural effusions. Palpate the peripheral pulses to determine strength.

PSYCHOSOCIAL. A previously healthy person with a possible minor upper respiratory infection is at risk for life-threatening complications, such as multiple organ failure. Assess the patient's ability to cope with a sudden illness. Assess the patient's level of anxiety and fear.

DIAGNOSTIC HIGHLIGHTS

Test	Normal Result	Abnormality with Condition	Explanation
Sputum culture and sensitivity	Negative	Presence of *L. pneumophila*	Identify infecting organisms
Chest x ray	Air-filled lungs	Area of increased density of a lung segment, lobe, or entire lung	Locates the location and extent of infection

Other Tests: Urinalysis, direct fluorescent antibody studies, arterial blood gases, pulse oximetry, complete blood count, blood urea nitrogen, creatinine, serum electrolytes

PRIMARY NURSING DIAGNOSIS

Infection related to the presence of bacteria

OUTCOMES. Immune status; Risk control; Risk detection; Nutrition status; Treatment behavior: Illness or injury; Hydration; Knowledge: Infection control

INTERVENTIONS. Infection control; Infection protection; Surveillance; Fluid/electrolyte management; Medication management; Temperature regulation

◻ PLANNING AND IMPLEMENTATION

Collaborative

PHARMACOLOGIC. Antibiotics can be administered before test results are available. The drug of choice is erythromycin. Intravenous fluids and electrolyte therapy may be considered when the patient has fluid volume deficit. Careful monitoring of fluid balance is required because of the possible renal complications from interstitial nephritis or renal failure. If renal failure does ensue, the patient may require temporary renal dialysis.

Oxygen per cannula at 2 to 4 L per minute is effective with many patients, although in some patients with respiratory insufficiency it is necessary to proceed with intubation and assisted ventilation. Atelectasis may occur at any stage of the pneumonia. Pleural effusion may occur, which may require a diagnostic thoracentesis and a chest tube. The patient may need continuous pulse oximetry to monitor the response to mechanical ventilation and suctioning. Continuous cardiac monitoring and hourly urine outputs may be necessary to assess the patient's response to the disease.

PHARMACOLOGIC HIGHLIGHTS

Medication or Drug Class	Dosage	Description	Rationale
Erythromycin	250 mg po qid for a 3-week regimen; IV administration is often advisable for the first 3 days at a dose of 15–20 mg/kg per day in divided doses with a maximum of 4 g per day	Antibiotic	Halts division of bacteria, thereby limiting infection
Rifampin	600 mg per day, po or IV	Anti-tubercular	Manages severe disease, such as multilobar pneumonia, respiratory failure, endocarditis, or severe immunosuppression. If erythromycin is contraindicated because of allergy, rifampin may

> be used alone or combined with
> doxycycline or cotrimoxazole.

Other Treatment: Antipyretics

Independent

The most important intervention is improvement of airway patency. Retained secretions interfere with gas exchange and may cause slow resolution of the disease. Encourage a high level of fluid intake up to 3 L per day to assist in loosening pulmonary secretions and to replace fluid lost via fever and diaphoresis. Provide meticulous sterile technique during endotracheal suctioning of the patient. Chest physiotherapy may be prescribed to assist with loosening and mobilizing secretions.

To maintain the patient's comfort, keep the patient protected from drafts. Institute fever-reducing measures if necessary. To ease the patient's breathing, raise the head of the bed at least 45 degrees, and support the patient's arms with pillows. Provide mouth and skin care and emotional support. Include the patient and family in planning care, and allow them to make choices.

DOCUMENTATION GUIDELINES

- Physical findings: Vital signs, head-to-toe assessment, rate of breathing, breath sounds, description of sputum
- Response to treatments such as chest physiotherapy, oxygen, antipyretics, and fluid therapy
- Presence of complications: Hypotension, dehydration, chest pain, changes in patterns of urination, laboratory findings

DISCHARGE AND HOME HEALTHCARE GUIDELINES

Explain the medications to the patient, including the route, dosage, side effects, and need for taking all antibiotics until they are gone. Explain food and drug interactions. Provide information on smoking cessation programs. Note the source of the patient's legionnaires' disease; if the cause was from within a patient's home or workplace, recommend appropriate action to prevent recurrence and decrease chances of further outbreaks. Instruct the patient to contact the physician if he or she has a fever or worsening pleuritic pain. Stress the need to go immediately to the nearest emergency department if the patient becomes acutely short of breath.

Leukemia, Acute

DRG Category: 473
Mean LOS: 9.3 days
Description: MEDICAL: Acute Leukemia
without Major O. R. Procedure, Age > 17

Leukemias account for approximately 8% of all human cancers, and approximately half of these cases are classified as acute leukemia. Acute leukemia, a malignant disease of the blood-forming organs, results when white blood cell (WBC) precursors proliferate in the bone marrow and lymphatic tissues. The cells eventually spread to the peripheral blood and all body tissues. Leukemia is considered acute when it has a rapid onset and progression and when, if it is left untreated, it leads to 100% mortality within days or months.

There are two major forms of acute leukemia: lymphocytic leukemia and nonlymphocytic leukemia. Lymphocytic leukemia involves the lymphocytes (cells that are derived from the stem cells and circulate among the blood, lymph nodes, and lymphatic organs) and lymphoid organs; nonlymphocytic leukemia involves hematopoietic stem cells that differentiate into monocytes, granulocytes, red blood cells (RBCs), and platelets. Up to 90% of acute leukemias are a form of lymphocytic leukemia, acute lymphoblastic leukemia (ALL), which is characterized by the abnormal growth of lymphocyte precursors called lymphoblasts. Acute myelogenous leukemia (AML) (also known as acute nonlymphocytic leukemia, or ANLL) causes the rapid accumulation of megakaryocytes (precursors to platelets), monocytes, granulocytes, and RBCs. As the disease progresses, the patient may have central nervous system dysfunction with seizures, decreased mental status, or coma and renal insufficiency. Death occurs when the abnormal cells encroach on vital tissues and cause complications and organ dysfunction.

Estimates projected 30,800 new cases of leukemia in the year 2000, approximately 28,090 of them adult cases and 2,710 children. AML is the most common adult leukemia; 9,700 cases were anticipated with another 3,200 adults expected to develop ALL. Two out of three children who develop acute leukemia develop ALL as chronic leukemia is rare in children. Approximately 21,700 adults and children were expected to die of all forms of leukemia in 2000. Patients with AML or ALL can be kept in long-term remission or cured in approximately 20% to 30% of adults. Five-year survival rates for children with ALL are close to 80% and for children with AML close to 40%.

CAUSES

The exact cause of acute leukemia is unknown, but there are several risk factors. Overexposure to radiation even years before the development of the disease, particularly if the exposure is prolonged, is a major risk factor. Other risk factors include exposure to certain chemicals (benzene), medications (alkylating agents used to treat other cancers in particular), and viruses. Other related factors in children include genetic abnormalities such as Down syndrome, albinism, and congenital immunodeficiency syndrome. People who have been treated with chemotherapeutic agents for other forms of cancer have an increased risk for developing AML. Such cases generally develop with 9 years of chemotherapy.

GENDER AND LIFE SPAN CONSIDERATIONS

The peak age for children to develop ALL is between 2 and 3 years of age. AML is most common in the first two years of life and less so in older children; AML tends to increase in occurrence in the teen years. AML most often strikes older people; the average age of a patient with AML is 65. There is a 1 in 50,000 chance for a 50-year-old to develop AML, but the odds increase to a 1 in 7,000 chance for a 70-year-old. ALL is more common among children; the majority of patients are under 10 years of age. Males are more susceptible to AML than are females, and the disease is more common in European-Americans than in other Americans; more than twice as many European-Americans as African-Americans develop ALL. ALL is the most common type of childhood leukemia.

☐ ASSESSMENT

HISTORY. Question the patient (or the parents of the patient, as appropriate) about any exposure to radiation, chemicals, viruses, and medications, including chemotherapy for cancer. Determine the adult patient's occupation, and pay particular attention to radiation exposure of healthcare workers, workers in a power plant, or those serving in the military. Often the patient describes a sudden onset of high fever and signs of abnormal bleeding (increased bruising, bleeding after minor trauma, nosebleeds, bleeding gums, petechiae, and prolonged menses). Some patients report increased fatigue and malaise, weight loss, palpitations, night sweats, and chills. Parents of children with leukemia often report a series of recurrent pulmonary, urinary tract, and perirectal infections. Patients may also complain of abdominal or bone pain.

PHYSICAL EXAMINATION. The patient appears acutely ill, short of breath, and pale. Children are often febrile. When you inspect the lips and mouth, you may note bleeding gums and ulcerated areas of the mouth and throat. On palpation, you may feel lymph node swelling and enlargement of the liver and spleen. When you auscultate the patient's lungs, you may hear decreased breath sounds, shallow and rapid respirations, a rapid heart rate, and a systolic ejection murmur.

PSYCHOSOCIAL. When the diagnosis of acute leukemia is made, patients, parents, and significant others are shocked and fearful. If the patient is a child, determine the patient's stage of development and his or her relationship with parents, caregivers, or grandparents. If the patient is an adult, determine the patient's job, childcare, and financial responsibilities. Assess the patient's home situation to determine the possibility of home healthcare. Determine the support systems available to the patient, including emotional, religious, financial, and social support.

DIAGNOSTIC HIGHLIGHTS

Test	Normal Result	Abnormality with Condition	Explanation
Complete blood count	Red blood cells (RBCs) 4.0–5.5 million/μL; white blood cells 4,500–11,000/μL; hemoglobin (Hg)	Increased white blood cell counts (notably blast cells), lowered red cell blood count, insufficient	Changes in numbers of different blood cell types and how the cells look under a microscope can suggest leukemia; overproduction of white

	12–18 g/dL; hematocrit (Hct) 37%–54%; reticulocyte count 0.5%–2.5% of total RBCs; platelets 150,000–400,000/μL	platelets	blood cells halts production of RBCs and platelets
Bone marrow aspiration/bone marrow biopsy	No leukemia cells present	Leukemia cells present; 30% blast cells required for diagnosis of acute leukemia; < 5% blast cells for diagnosis of remission	A thin needle is used to draw up a small amount of liquid bone marrow; a small cylinder of bone and marrow (about ½" long) is removed with a slightly larger needle. The site of both samples is usually at the back of the hipbone.

Other Tests: Other supporting tests include x rays, lymph node biopsy, computed tomography (CT) scan, magnetic resonance imagery (MRI), ultrasound, cytochemistry, flow cytometry, immunocytochemistry, and lumbar puncture.

PRIMARY NURSING DIAGNOSIS

Risk for infection related to decreased primary and secondary responses

OUTCOMES. Immune status; Knowledge: Infection control; Risk control; Risk detection; Nutrition status; Treatment behavior: Illness or injury; Hydration; Knowledge: Infection control

INTERVENTIONS. Infection control; Infection protection; Surveillance; Fluid/electrolyte management; Medication management; Temperature regulation

☐ PLANNING AND IMPLEMENTATION

Collaborative

The treatment for acute leukemia occurs in three phases: induction,consolidation, and maintenance. During the induction phase, the patient receives an intense course of chemotherapy that is meant to cause a complete remission of the disease. Complete remission occurs when the patient has less than 5% of the bone marrow cells as blast cells and the peripheral blood counts are normal. Once remission has been sustained for 1 month, the patient enters the consolidation phase, during which he or she receives a modified course of chemotherapy to eradicate any remaining disease. The maintenance phase may continue for more than a year, during which time the patient receives small doses of chemotherapy every 3 to 4 weeks.

Some patients also need transfusions with blood component therapy to control infection and prevent bleeding and anemia. Bone marrow transplantation (BMT) is an option for some patients. Early BMTs were allogenic transplants using stem cells that had been harvested from bone marrow from siblings or matched from unrelated relatives. In autologous BMTs in the 1980s, physicians began using frozen cells harvested from the donor's own marrow during remission. More recently, a newer form of transplant has occurred with peripheral blood stem cell transplant (SCT) or peripheral blood progenitor cell transplant. Multiple pheresis, or removal of cells from the blood, provides the stem cells from the patient for transplantation. SCT permits the use of doses of chemotherapy and radiation therapy high enough to destroy the patient's bone marrow; after the treatment is completed SCT restores blood-producing bone marrow stem cells. Radiation treatment is sometimes used to treat leukemic cells in the brain, spinal cord, or testicles.

PHARMACOLOGIC HIGHLIGHTS

Medication or Drug Class	Dosage	Description	Rationale
Chemotherapeutic agents	Varies with drug; treatment for AML generally uses higher doses over a shorter period of time, whereas treatment for ALL uses lower doses over a longer period of time	*Adult:* AML remission induction: cytarabine in combination with daunorubicin or idarubicin AML consolidation: cytarabine ALL remission induction: cytoxan, vincristine, prednisone, L-asparaginase, doxoxrubicin ALL consolidation: same as remission induction with addition of 6MP, 6TG, methotraxate, and cytarabine Central nervous system prophylaxis: intrathecal methotrexate *Child:* AML induction: daunomycin, cytosine arabinoside, etoposide AML intensification: cytarabine, daunomycin ALL induction: prednisone, asparaginase, vincristine ALL consolidation/ intensification: methotrexate, 6 mercaptopurine ALL maintenance: add vincristine and predisone	Decrease replication of leukemia cells and kill them

Other Treatment: Supportive care and management of complications from chemotherapy are handled pharmacologically with antibiotics, antifungals, and antiviral drugs. Growth factors may be given to elevate blood counts.

Independent

Focus on providing comfort and support, managing complications, and providing patient education. Determine how the patient is coping with the disease and where you can best provide support. For some patients, improving their comfort is the highest priority, either physically, such as with a bed bath or back rub, or emotionally, such as by listening to fears and concerns and providing interesting distractions. Teach the patient stress- and pain-reduction techniques. Provide mouth care to lessen the discomfort from oral lesions. Support the patient's efforts to maintain grooming and a positive body image. If the patient is a child, provide age-appropriate diversions, and work with the parents or caregivers to keep the significant others present and involved in the child's care.

Protect the patient from injury and infection. To limit the risk of bleeding, hold firm pressure on all puncture wounds for at least 10 minutes or until they stop oozing. Limit the use of intramuscular injections and intravenous catheter placement when the patient is pancytopenic. Avoid taking rectal temperatures, using rectal suppositories, or performing a rectal examination. If the patient does not respond to treatment, be honest about the patient's prognosis. Determine from parents how much information they want to share with the child about a terminal disease. Work with the patient, significant others, and chaplain to help the patient plan for a terminal illness and achieve a compassionate death.

DOCUMENTATION GUIDELINES

- Physical response: Vital signs, physical assessment, signs of infection, signs of bleeding, ability to tolerate activity
- Response to chemotherapy or radiation treatments
- Emotional response to the diagnosis of cancer or the use of reverse isolation
- Comprehension of treatment plan, including care: Purpose and potential side effects of radiation and chemotherapy; bone marrow transplant
- Presence of complications: Infection, bleeding, poor wound healing, ineffective coping by the patient or significant others

DISCHARGE AND HOME HEALTHCARE GUIDELINES

Teach the patient and significant others about the course of the disease, the treatment options, and how to recognize complications. Explain that the patient or parents need to notify the physician if any of the following occur: fever, chills, cough, sore throat, increased bleeding or bruising, new onset of bone or abdominal pain. Discuss the patient's home environment to limit the risk of exposure to infections. Encourage the patient to avoid close contact with family pets because dogs, cats, and birds carry infections. Animal licks, bites, and scratches are sources of infection. The patient should not clean birdcages, litter boxes, or fish tanks. Additional sources of bacteria in the home include water in humidifiers, standing water in flower vases, and water in fish tanks. Encourage the patient to have air filters in furnaces and air conditioners changed weekly. Explain that raw fruits, vegetables, and uncooked meat carry bacteria and should be avoided. If the patient becomes injured, encourage the patient or significant others to apply pressure, use ice, and report excessive bleeding. Teach the patient to avoid blowing or picking the nose or straining at bowel movements to limit the risk of bleeding.

Explain the proper administration and potential side effects of any medications. Teach the patient how to manage pain with the prescribed analgesics and other side effects specific to each chemotherapeutic agent. Explain that the chemotherapy may cause weight loss, even anorexia. Encourage the patient to eat a diet high in calories and protein and to drink at least 2000 mL of fluids per day. If the chemotherapy leads to anorexia, encourage the patient to eat frequent, small meals several times a day. Arrange for a dietary consultation if needed before discharge. If the patient has oral lesions, teach the patient to use a soft toothbrush or cloth and to avoid hot, spicy foods and commercial mouthwashes, which can irritate mouth ulcers. Encourage the patient to take frequent rest periods during the day and to space activities with rest.

Urge the patient to maintain a realistic but positive attitude. The return to an independent lifestyle is possible with the efforts of a competent healthcare team and the patient's cooperation. Provide a list of referral agencies as appropriate, such as the American Cancer Society, hospice, and support groups.

Leukemia, Chronic

DRG Category: 403
Mean LOS: 7.4 days
Description: MEDICAL: Lymphoma and Non-Acute Leukemia with CC

Leukemia is a malignant disease of the blood-forming organs that leads to a transformation of stem cells or early committed precursor cells and thus to an abnormal overproduction of certain leukocytes. Two types of chronic leukemia commonly occur: chronic lymphocytic leukemia (CLL) and chronic myelogenous leukemia (CML).

CLL involves lymphocytes (B cells)—cells that derived from stem cells and which circulate among blood, lymph nodes, and lymphatic organs. In CLL, an uncontrollable spread of abnormal, small lymphocytes occurs in the bone marrow, lymphoid tissues, and blood. In CLL, an underproduction of immunoglobulins (antibodies) leads to increased susceptibility to infections. Some patients also develop antibodies to red blood cells and platelets, which then leads to anemia and thrombocytopenia.

CML is characterized by the abnormal overgrowth of myeloblasts, promyelocytes, metamyelocytes, and myelocytes (all granulocytic precursors) in body tissues, peripheral blood, and bone marrow. In CML the bone marrow becomes 100% cellular (rather than 50% cellular and 50% fat, the normal composition). The spleen enlarges with a greatly expanded red pulp area. CML has two phases: insidious chronic phase and acute phase. In the insidious chronic phase, chronic leukemia originates in the pluripotent stem cell, with an initial finding of hypercellular marrow with a majority of normal cells. After a relatively slow course for a median of 4 years, the patient with chronic leukemia invariably enters a blast crisis, or acute phase.

Both CLL and CML may metastasize to the blood, lymph nodes, spleen, liver, central nervous system, and other organs. The American Cancer Society predicts approximately 30,800 new cases of all types of leukemia will occur in the

United States annually. Approximately 12,500 cases were projected to be chronic leukemia, 8,100 cases of CLL and 4,400 cases of CML.

CAUSES

Several risk factors have been identified, but they do not account for all cases of chronic leukemia. Environmental factors such as exposure to high-dose radiation may increase the risk of CML. In more than 90% of patients with CML, there is the presence of the abnormal Philadelphia (Ph[1]) chromosome, which may be induced by radiation or carcinogenic chemicals. Long-term contact with herbicides and pesticides may increase the risk of CLL. Heredity is a factor: members of the immediate family (parents, siblings, children) who have had CLL create an inherited risk factor. Finally, smoking has been shown to increase the risk of leukemia.

GENDER AND LIFE SPAN CONSIDERATIONS

Chronic leukemia affects mostly older adults, overage 50 years. Only about 2% of chronic leukemia patients are children. CLL affects adults, and CML affects mostly adults and rarely children. Twice as many males as females develop chronic leukemia.

☐ ASSESSMENT

HISTORY. Often symptoms of chronic leukemia are nonspecific and vague. In CML sometimes the first symptom is a dragging sensation caused by extreme splenomegaly, or it may be left upper quadrant pain that is caused by a splenic infarct. In CLL, swollen lymph nodes or enlarged liver and spleen may cause discomfort.

Elicit a history of signs and symptoms such as fatigue and anorexia. Some patients may report any of the following symptoms that are associated with either anemia or increased metabolism because of rapid cell turnover: weakness, weight loss, dyspnea, decreased stamina during exercise, or headache. Ask about bleeding from the gums or nose or easy bruising (signs of thrombocytopenia), abdominal discomfort, or pain in the chest and rib areas. Question the patient about recent weight loss or appetite loss; blood in the urine; or black, tarry stools. Bone and joint tenderness may occur from marrow involvement. Determine if the patient has been running a low-grade fever. Take an occupational history to determine possible exposure to radiation or carcinogenic chemicals.

PHYSICAL EXAMINATION. Observe the patient's general appearance for pallor, and inspect for ecchymoses and bruises. Examine the patient's eyes for retinal hemorrhage. Palpate the lymph nodes to determine the presence of lymphadenopathy and palpate the abdomen for enlargement of the spleen or liver. Palpate the patient's thorax for signs of sternal or rib tenderness, which may be indications of infiltration of the periosteum. Inspect the ankles for edema. Note a low-grade fever. Examine the skin for macular to nodular eruptions, signs of skin infiltrations, bruising, and opportunistic fungal infections. Pulmonary infiltrates may appear when lung parenchyma is involved. Assess the patient's breathing for dyspnea. Auscultate the heart for signs of tachycardia and palpitation.

PSYCHOSOCIAL. Despite advances in treatment and cure, the diagnosis of cancer is an emotionally laden one. Determine the past coping mechanisms used to manage situations of severe stress. Assess the patient's home situation to determine the possibility of home health care. Assess the support systems available, including emotional, religious, financial, and social.

DIAGNOSTIC HIGHLIGHTS

Test	Normal Result	Abnormality with Condition	Explanation
Complete blood count	Red blood cells (RBCs) 4.0–5.5 million/μL; white blood cells 4,500–11,000/μL; hemoglobin (Hg) 12–18 g/dL; hematocrit (Hct) 37–54%; reticulocyte count 0.5–2.5% of total RBCs; platelets 150,000–400,000/μL	Increased white blood cell counts; may be only slightly increased or >200,000/μL; RBCs, decreased; platelets, increased (early in CML) or decreased (CLL and late CML)	Overproduction of white blood cells halts production of RBCs and platelets
Bone marrow aspiration/bone marrow biopsy	No leukemia cells present	Leukemic blast phase cells present; leukemic surface markers on cells	Thin needle used to draw up small amount of liquid bone marrow. In biopsy, small cylinder of bone and marrow (about ½" long) is removed. Site of both samples is usually at back of the hipbone

Other Tests: Coagulation studies (prothrombin time, activated partial thromboplastin time), chromosomal analysis, x rays, computed tomography (CT) scan, magnetic resonance imagery (MRI), ultrasound

PRIMARY NURSING DIAGNOSIS

Risk for infection related to decreased primary and secondary responses

OUTCOMES. Immune status; Knowledge: Infection control; Risk control; Risk detection; Nutrition status; Treatment behavior: Illness or injury; Hydration; Knowledge: Infection control

INTERVENTIONS. Infection control; Infection protection; Surveillance; Fluid/electrolyte management; Medication management; Temperature regulation

☐ PLANNING AND IMPLEMENTATION

Collaborative

The objective of treatment for CLL is palliation. Because treatments destroy normal cells along with malignant ones, therapy focuses on the prevention and resolution of complications from induced pancytopenia (anemia, bleeding, and infection in particular). Chemotherapy is employed to reduce symptoms. Total body irradiation or local radiation to the spleen may also be given as a palliative treatment to reduce complications. Two complications during later stages of CLL are hemolytic anemia (caused by autoimmune disorder) and hypogammaglobulinemia, which further increases the patient's susceptibility to infection. Antibiotics, transfusions of red blood cells, and injections of gamma globulin concentrates may be required for patients with these problems.

Therapy in the chronic phase of CML focuses on controlling leukocytosis and thrombocytosis. Leukapheresis (separation of leukocytes from blood and then returning remaining blood to patient) may be performed to lower an extremely high peripheral leukocyte count quickly and to prevent acute tumor lysis syndrome, but the results are temporary. Plateletpheresis (separation of platelets from blood and then returning remaining blood to patient) may be required for thrombocytosis as high as 2 million. Apheresis (separating blood into components) is usually performed with the use of automated blood cell separators that are designed to remove the selected blood element and return the remaining cells and plasma to the patient.

Bone marrow transplantations before blast crisis offer the best treatment option. Chemotherapy is used in treating CML, but at this time, it has not proven satisfactory in producing long-term remission. Supportive care and management of complications from chemotherapy are handled pharmacologically with antibiotics, antifungals, and antiviral drugs. Some patients also need transfusions with blood component therapy to control infection and prevent bleeding and anemia. To relieve the pain of splenomegaly, irradiation or removal may be used.

PHARMACOLOGIC HIGHLIGHTS

Medication or Drug Class	Dosage	Description	Rationale
Chemotherapy	Varies with drug		Controls symptoms and prevents proliferation of white blood cells
		CLL: chlorambucil (Leukeran) and cyclophosphamide (Cytoxan)	CLL: The patient is generally on chemotherapy for 2 weeks and off for 2 weeks
		CML: busulfan (Myleran) and hydroxyurea; when a blast crisis occurs, other drugs are used: cytosine arabinoside, daunorubicin, methotrexate, prednisone, vincristine, and	CML: Drugs can destroy blast cells, prevent leukemic cells from inhibiting formation of normal granulocytes, or transform the blast cells into normal granulocytes
Prednisone	1 mg/kg po qd	Corticosteroid	Manages immune hemolytic anemia or immune thrombocytopenia

complicating CLL; manages lymphoblastic crisis in CML. Prednisone has a marked lymphocytic effect and may stimulate the production of red blood cells and platelets

Other Drugs: Interferon therapy

Independent

Management focuses on providing comfort, support, and patient education and managing complications. Determine how the patient is coping with the disease and where you can best provide support. For some patients, improving their comfort is the highest priority, either physically, such as with a bed bath or back rub, or emotionally, such as by listening to fears and concerns and providing interesting distractions. Teach stress- and pain-reduction techniques. Provide mouth care to lessen the discomfort from oral lesions. Support the patient's efforts to maintain grooming and a positive body image.

Institute measures to control infection and maintain a safe environment. To limit the risk of bleeding, hold firm pressure on all puncture wounds for at least 10 minutes or until they stop oozing. Limit the use of intramuscular injections and intravenous catheter placement when the patient is pancytopenic. Avoid taking rectal temperatures, using rectal suppositories, or performing a rectal examination.

Assist the patient in minimizing the discomfort of splenomegaly. Provide small, frequent meals. Maintain adequate fluid intake and a high-bulk diet. Prevent constipation. Encourage the patient to cough and perform deep-breathing exercises as a prophylactic for atelectasis.

For patients who are undergoing outpatient chemotherapy, teach about side effects, emphasizing dangerous ones such as bone marrow suppression. Emphasize that the physician should be called in case of a fever over 100°F, chills, redness or swelling, a sore throat, or a cough. Explain the signs of thrombocytopenia. Emphasize that the patient needs to avoid aspirin or aspirin-containing compounds that might exacerbate bleeding. Emphasize the need for adequate rest and the importance of a high-calorie, high-protein diet.

If the patient does not respond to treatment, be honest about prognosis. Implement strategies to manage pain, fever, and infection to ensure the patient's comfort. Work with the patient, significant others, and chaplain to help the patient plan for a terminal illness and achieve a compassionate death.

DOCUMENTATION GUIDELINES

- Physical response: Vital signs, physical assessment, signs of infection, signs of bleeding, ability to tolerate activity
- Response to chemotherapy or radiation treatments
- Comprehension of treatment plan, including care: Purpose and potential side effects of radiation and chemotherapy; bone marrow transplant
- Presence of complications: Infection, bleeding, poor wound healing, ineffective coping by the patient or significant others

DISCHARGE AND HOME HEALTHCARE GUIDELINES

Teach the patient and significant others about the course of the disease, the treatment options, and how to recognize complications. Explain that the patient or family needs to notify the physician if any of the following occur: fever, chills, cough, sore throat, increased bleeding or bruising, new onset of bone or abdominal pain. Urge the patient to maintain a realistic but positive attitude. The return to an independent lifestyle is possible with the efforts of a competent healthcare team and the patient's cooperation. Provide a list of referral agencies as appropriate, such as the American Cancer Society, hospice, and support groups.

Discuss the patient's home environment to limit the risk of exposure to infections. Encourage the patient to avoid close contact with family pets because they carry infections. The patient should not clean birdcages, litter boxes, or fish tanks. Additional sources of bacteria in the home include water in humidifiers, standing water in flower vases, or water in fish tanks. Encourage the patient to have air filters in furnaces and air conditioners changed weekly. Explain that raw fruits, vegetables, and uncooked meat carry bacteria and should be avoided. If the patient is injured, encourage him or her to apply pressure, use ice to the area, and report excessive bleeding. Teach the patient to avoid blowing or picking the nose or straining at bowel movements to limit the risk of bleeding.

Explain the proper administration and potential side effects of any medications. Teach the patient how to manage pain with the prescribed analgesics and other side effects specific to each chemotherapeutic agent. Explain that the chemotherapy may cause weight loss and anorexia. Encourage the patient to eat a diet high in calories and protein and to drink at least 2000 mL of fluids per day. If the chemotherapy leads to anorexia, encourage the patient to eat frequent, small meals several times a day. Arrange for a dietary consultation if needed before discharge. If the patient has oral lesions, teach the patient to use a soft toothbrush or cloth and to avoid hot, spicy foods and commercial mouthwashes, which can irritate mouth ulcers.

Liver Failure

DRG Category: 205
Mean LOS: 6.1 days
Description: MEDICAL: Disorders of Liver Except Malignancy, Cirrhosis, Alcoholic Hepatitis with CC

Liver (hepatic) failure is a loss of liver function because of the death of many hepatocytes. The damage can occur suddenly, as with a viral infection, or slowly over time, as with cirrhosis. Fulminant liver failure occurs with sudden, severe liver decompensation that is caused by massive necrosis of the liver.

Because of the complex functions of the liver, liver failure leads to multiple system complications. When ammonia and other metabolic byproducts are not metabolized, they accumulate in the blood and cause neurologic deterioration. Without normal vitamin K activation and the production of clotting factors, the patient has coagulation problems. Patients are at risk for infections because of general malnutrition, debilitation, impairment of phagocytosis, and decreased liver production of immune-related proteins. Fluid retention occurs because of decreased albumin production, leading to decreased colloidal osmotic pressure with failure to retain fluid in the bloodstream. Renin and aldosterone production cause sodium and water retention. Ascites occurs because of intrahepatic vascular obstruction with fluid movement into the peritoneum.

Complications of liver failure include bleeding esophageal varices, hemorrhagic shock, hepatic encephalopathy, hepatorenal syndrome, coma, and even death. (See Box 8.)

BOX 8   BLEEDING ESOPHAGEAL VARICES

Esophageal varies (fragile, distended, and thin-walled veins in the esophagus) occur in patients with liver failure because of portal hypertension. Obstructed blood circulates to low-resistance alternate vessels around the portal circulation in the liver, which is a high-pressure system. One of these routes is through the esophageal veins, which become distended with blood, irritated from pressure, and susceptible to rupture. Treatment of esophageal varices includes:

Surgery: Procedures include placing a portal caval shunt or distal splenorenal shunt, esophageal repair, or devascularization.

Endoscopic sclerotherapy: To cause fibrosis of the varices, they are injected with solutions during an endoscopy procedure.

Esophageal balloon tamponade: A multilumen gastrointestinal tube with an esophageal and gastric balloon is passed into the upper gastrointestinal tract through the patient's mouth. The gastric balloon, which is filled with 250 to 300 mL of air, acts as an anchor; the esophageal balloon, which is filled with enough air to cause 20 to 75 mm Hg pressure, compresses the esophageal varices to decrease bleeding. Traction may be inserted by taping the outer portions of the multilumen tube to the face mask of a football helmet.

Parenteral therapy: Maintain a large-bore intravenous line and keep several units of packed cells on call from the blood bank at all times.

Vasopressin (Pitressin) therapy: A continuous infusion of this vasoconstrictor causes constriction of the mesenteric circulation and decreased blood flow to the portal circulation.

CAUSES

Although viral hepatitis can lead to liver failure, fewer than 5% of patients with viral hepatitis actually develop it. Other causes include chronic alcohol abuse, hepatotoxic drug reactions, acute infection or hemorrhage that leads to shock, prolonged cholestasis (arrest of bile excretion), and metabolic disorders. Many of these lead to cirrhosis, a chronic liver disease that results in widespread tissue fibrosis, nodule formation, and necrosis of the liver tissue.

GENDER AND LIFE SPAN CONSIDERATIONS

Although acute liver failure can occur at any age, infants and children are more likely to have an inherited disease, whereas adult men are more likely to have alcohol-related disease. Worldwide statistics indicate that postnecrotic cirrhosis is more common in women than in men and is the most common type of liver failure worldwide. Cirrhosis is the tenth leading cause of death in the United States and occurs most commonly between the ages of 35 and 55.

☐ ASSESSMENT

HISTORY. Take a detailed medication history with particular attention to hepatotoxic medications, such as anesthesia agents, analgesics, antiseizure medications, cocaine, alcohol, isoniazid (INH), and oral contraceptives. Ask about any recent travel to China, southeast Asia, sub-Saharan Africa, the Pacific Islands, and areas around the Amazon River, which may have exposed the patient to hepatitis B. Explore the patient's occupational history for hepatitis exposure; patients who are day-care workers, dental workers, physicians, nurses, or hospital laboratory workers are particularly at risk. Ask the patient if he or she has experienced previous liver or biliary disease. Intravenous drug users and male homosexuals are at risk for hepatitis and, therefore, liver failure. Those who eat raw shellfish are at similar risk.

Early symptoms include personality changes (agitation, forgetfulness, disorientation), fatigue, anorexia, drowsiness, and mild tremors. Some patients experience sleep disturbance and low-grade fevers. As larger areas of the liver are destroyed, the patient has increasing fatigue, confusion, and lethargy. If the patient has long-standing liver failure, he or she experiences jaundice, dry skin, early-morning nausea, vomiting, anorexia, weight loss, altered bowel habits, and epigastric discomfort. If sudden fulminant liver failure occurs, the patient may develop encephalopathy (decreased mental status, fixed facial expression), peripheral swelling, ascites, and bleeding tendencies. Urine is often dark from bilirubin, and stools are often light-colored because of the absence of bilirubin.

PHYSICAL EXAMINATION. The patient with acute liver failure usually has jaundiced skin and sclera. Fluid retention results in ascites and peripheral edema. The patient's facial expression appears fixed, his or her movements are hesitant, and speech is slow. Usually the patient's mental status is markedly decreased, and you may smell fetor hepaticus, a sweet fecal odor, on the patient's breath. The patient may have multiple bruises, a bloody nose, or bleeding gums.

The patient's peripheral pulses are bounding and rapid, indicating fluid overload and a hyperdynamic circulation. You may also palpate peripheral edema, an enlarged firm liver in acute failure and a small hard liver in chronic failure, an enlarged spleen, a distended abdomen, and an abdomen with shifting dullness to percussion and a positive fluid wave because of ascites. As ascites worsens, the patient develops hernias, an everted umbilicus, and an elevated and displaced heart because of a raised diaphragm. Usually the patient with late disease has neck vein distension, and men develop gynecomastia (enlarged breasts), testicular atrophy, and scant body hair. When you monitor the patient's vital signs, you may find an elevated temperature and a low-to-normal blood pressure; if the physician initiates hemodynamic monitoring, the cardiac output may be low if ascites is decreasing the right ventricular filling pressure and if the systemic vascular resistance is low.

PSYCHOSOCIAL. The patient may feel upset or guilty if he or she contracted the disease while traveling. Use a nonjudgmental approach to elicit the patient's feelings if the condition is related to alcohol abuse. If the patient is a candidate for a liver transplant, determine the patient's emotional stability, ability to cope with a complex medical regimen, and ability to rely on significant others.

DIAGNOSTIC HIGHLIGHTS

Test	Normal Result	Abnormality with Condition	Explanation
Prothrombin time (PT)	Varies by laboratory; generally 11–13 seconds	Prolonged > 15 seconds	Prothrombin is formed in the liver and is a vitamin K–dependent glycoprotein that is necessary for firm clot formation
Viral hepatitis seriologies: hepatitis A virus (HAV); hepatitis B virus (HBV); hepatitis C virus (HCV); hepatitis D virus (HDV); hepatitis E virus (HEV) (See Hepatitis entry)	Negative results	If patient has hepatitis: acute HAV: positive anti-HAV IgM; acute HBV: anti-HBV IgM; HB surface antigen; acute HCV: anti-HCV antibody, HCV RNA; HDV: Anti HDV IgM, HDV antigen; HEV: not available; Non A Non B: all tests negative	Identify patients with hepatitis; virus leads to markers such as immunoglobulins (IgG and IgM), antigens, antibodies
Liver function tests	Alanine aminotrans-ferase (ALT), 4–46 U/L; aspartate aminotransferase (AST), 8–20 U/L; alkaline phosphatase, 32–92 U/L	ALT elevated as high or higher than 1000 U/L; AST elevated as high or higher than 1000 U/L; alkaline phosphatase mildly elevated	Determine the extent of liver damage

Other Tests: Bilirubin, lactate dehydrogenase, complete blood count, serum glucose, serum sodium and potassium, ammonia, albumin, and liver biopsy

PRIMARY NURSING DIAGNOSIS

Fluid volume excess related to water and sodium retention

OUTCOMES. Fluid balance; Hydration; Nutrition management; Nutrition therapy; Knowledge: Treatment regime

INTERVENTIONS. Fluid/electrolyte management; Fluid monitoring; Medication administration

◻ PLANNING AND IMPLEMENTATION

Collaborative

Patients are managed with supportive therapy, depending on their symptoms. Fluid and electrolyte imbalances, malnutrition, ascites, respiratory failure, and bleeding esophageal varices can all occur with liver failure. Unless the patient has clinically significant hyponatremia, the patient usually receives limited intravenous fluids and food that contains sodium because increased sodium intake makes peripheral edema and ascites worse. Patients with ascites are usually restricted to 500 mg of sodium per day. A paracentesis may be used to remove 4 to 6 L of fluid. If the ascites is refractory, surgical placement of a peritoneal-venous shunt may be needed. Hypokalemia usually needs to be corrected with intravenous (IV) replacements. If the patient has serious fluid imbalances, a pulmonary artery catheter may be inserted for hemodynamic monitoring.

If respiratory failure is present, the patient may need endotracheal intubation and mechanical ventilation with supplemental oxygen. To manage nutrition in patients without evidence of hepatic encephalopathy, a high-calorie, 80- to 100-g protein diet is prescribed to allow for cellular repair. Some patients may need enteral or total parenteral nutrition to maintain calorie and protein levels. Hepatorenal failure is treated by fluid restriction, maintenance of fluid and electrolyte balance, and withdrawal of nephrotoxic drugs. Renal dialysis is generally not used because it does not improve survival and can lead to additional complications.

If the patient develops hepatic encephalopathy, serial neurological assessments are needed. In patients with signs of elevated intracranial pressure or hepatic coma, the physician may place an intracranial monitoring system. Some patients with liver failure are candidates for transplantation. A liver transplant is indicated for patients with irreversible progressive liver disease who have no alternatives to transplantation.

PHARMACOLOGIC HIGHLIGHTS

Medication or Drug Class	Dosage	Description	Rationale
Histamine receptor (H₂) antagonists	Varies with drug	Ranitidine and famotidine	Decrease gastric secretion; used as prophylaxis for ulcers
Thiamine	100 mg qd for several days or longer, depending on nutritional deficiencies	Vitamin supplement	Reduces risk for neuropathies
Vitamin K	Up to 10 mg IV as needed	Vitamin supplement	Supplement vitamin K, which is needed for prothrombin production

Other Drugs: Sedatives and acetaminophen are avoided because poor metabolism can precipitate encephalopathy. Aspirin is usually avoided because of the action on platelets, which can lead to increased bleeding. If ascites is present, diuretics, particularly aldosterone antagonists such as spironolactone (Aldactone), may be prescribed and, if ineffective, more potent loop diuretics may be added.

Independent

The most common problem for patients with liver failure is fluid volume excess. Measure the patient's abdominal girth at the same location daily, and mark the location as a reference point for future measurements. Notify the physician if the girth increases by 2 inches in 24 hours. Provide the required fluid allotment over the three meals and at night. If the patient desires, reserve some fluids to be used as ice chips. Provide mouth care every 2 hours. Because areas of edema are likely to be fragile and prone to skin breakdown, provide skin care.

One of the most life-threatening complications of liver failure is airway compromise because of neurological or respiratory deterioration. Keep endotracheal intubation equipment and an oral airway at the bedside at all times. Elevate the head of the patient's bed to 30 degrees to ease respirations, and support the patient's arms on pillows to decrease the work of breathing. It is essential to be at the bedside and to perform serial assessments of all critical systems. Space all activities and limit visitors as needed so that the patient gets adequate rest. Consider nonpharmacologic methods to encourage rest, such as diversionary activities and relaxation techniques.

The patient may be anxious, depressed, angry, or emotionally labile. Allow the patient to verbalize anxieties and fears. If needed, refer the patient to a counselor. Evaluate thoroughly anyone who is a candidate for a liver transplant to ensure that he or she has the ability to cope with a complex situation. Answer all questions, and explain the risks and benefits. Refer to an alcohol counselor if appropriate.

DOCUMENTATION GUIDELINES

- Physical responses: Vital signs, ease of respirations, breath sounds, heart sounds, level of consciousness, gastrointestinal distress, abdominal girth, daily weights, color of skin and sclera
- Nutrition: Tolerance of diet, appetite, ability to maintain body weight or to decrease fluid retention, presence of muscle wasting or signs of malnutrition, albumin level
- Response to therapy: Clearing of mental status, improvement in infection, decreased or stable blood ammonia level

DISCHARGE AND HOME HEALTHCARE GUIDELINES

Teach the patient to follow prescribed sodium and fluid restrictions. Assist the patient to individualize a diet plan to maximize personal choices, including a dietitian if necessary. Encourage sodium-restricted patients to read labels on all canned soups, sauces, and vegetables and on all over the counter medications. Be sure the patient understands any pain medication prescribed, including dosage, route, action, and side effects. Teach the patient and family the need to limit the rise of infections by good hand washing, avoidance of others with colds, and prompt treatment by a healthcare provider when an infection occurs. Refer the patient to an alcohol support group.

Lung Cancer

DRG Category: 082
Mean LOS: 6.3 days
Description: MEDICAL: Respiratory
Neoplasms
DRG Category: 075
Mean LOS: 9.9 days
Description: SURGICAL: Major Chest
Procedures

Lung cancer is the leading cause of cancer death among both men and women. Anually, over 156,000 deaths from lung cancer occur, which are 28% of all cancer deaths. Lung cancer accounts for more deaths than prostate, breast, and colon cancer combined. The 1-year survival rate remains approximately 41% and the 5-year survival rate is 14%. Only 15% of lung cancers are found at an early, localized stage.

There are two major types of lung cancer: small cell lung cancer (SCLC) and non-small cell lung cancer (NSCLC). Sometimes a lung cancer shows characteristics of both types and is labeled small cell / large cell carcinoma.

SCLC accounts for 20% of all lung cancers and is almost always caused by smoking. In SCLC, small cells start multiplying quickly into large tumors, generally beginning in the bronchi and the center of the lungs. SCLC can spread to the lymph nodes and other organs. SCLC is sometimes called small cell undifferentiated carcinoma and oat cell carcinoma.

NSCLC accounts for almost 80% of all lung cancers and includes three subtypes: squamous cell carcinoma, adenocarcinoma, and large cell undifferentiated carcinoma. Squamous cell carcinoma, also associated with smoking, tends to be located centrally, near a bronchus, and comprises approximately 30% of all lung cancers. Adenocarcinoma, usually found in the outer region of the lung, accounts for close to 40% of all lung cancers. One type of adenocarcinoma, bronchioloalveolar carcinoma, tends to produce a better prognosis than other types of lung cancer. Large cell undifferentiated carcinoma starts in any part of the lung, grows quickly, and results in a poor prognosis; approximately 10% of lung cancers are large cell undifferentiated carcinoma.

The hilus of the lung, close to the larger divisions of the bronchi, is the most frequent site of lung cancer. Abnormal cells divide and accumulate over time. As the cells grow into a carcinoma, they make the bronchial lining irregular and uneven. The tumor may penetrate the lung wall and surrounding tissue or grow into the opening (lumen) of the bronchus. In more than 50% of patients, the tumor spreads into the lymph nodes and then into other organs.

Systemic effects of the lung tumor that are unrelated to metastasis may affect the endocrine, hematologic, neuromuscular, and dermatologic systems. These changes may cause connective tissue and vascular abnormalities, referred to as paraneoplastic syndromes. In lung cancer, the most common endocrine syndromes are inappropriate anti-diuretic hormone secretion, Cushing's syndrome, and gynecomastia. Complications of lung cancer include emphysema, bronchial obstruction, atelectasis, pulmonary abscesses, pleuritis, bronchitis, and compression on the vena cava.

CAUSES

Approximately 80% of lung cancers are related to cigarette smoking. Lung cancer is 10 times more common in smokers than in nonsmokers. In particular, squamous cell and small cell carcinoma are associated with smoking. Other risk factors include exposure to carcinogenic industrial and air pollutants— such as asbestos, coal dust, radon, and arsenic—and family history.

GENDER AND LIFE SPAN CONSIDERATIONS

The average age of people diagnosed with lung cancer is 60, and it is an unusual diagnosis for people under 40. Of the total number of deaths from lung cancer each year, 57% are men and 43% are women. There has been an observable decline in deaths among younger men, and this is probably related to the diminishing number of young men who smoke. Deaths among women have been rising, although the rate of increase has slowed in recent years. Squamous cell carcinoma is most common in male smokers. Adenocarcinoma is equally common in men and women.

⬜ ASSESSMENT

HISTORY. Establish a history of persistent cough, chest pain, dyspnea, weight loss, or hemoptysis. Ask if the patient has experienced a change in normal respiratory patterns or hoarseness. Some patients initially report pneumonia, bronchitis, epigastric pain, symptoms of brain metastasis, arm or shoulder pain, or swelling of the upper body. Ask if the sputum has changed color, especially to a bloody, rusty, or purulent hue. Elicit a history of exposure to risk factors by determining if the patient has been exposed to industrial or air pollutants. Check the patient's family history for incidence of lung cancer.

PHYSICAL EXAMINATION. The clinical manifestations of lung cancer depend on the type and location of the tumor. Because the early stages of this disease usually produce no symptoms, it is most often diagnosed when the disease is at an advanced stage. In 10% to 20% of patients, lung cancer is diagnosed without any symptoms, usually from an abnormal finding on a routine chest x ray.

The clinical findings of lung cancer may be localized to the lung or may result from the regional or distant spread of the disease. Auscultation may reveal a wheeze if partial bronchial obstruction has occurred. Auscultate for decreased breath sounds, rales, or rhonchi. Note rapid, shallow breathing and signs of an airway obstruction, such as extreme shortness of breath, the use of accessory muscles, abnormal retractions, and stridor. Tumor involvement of the pleura and chest wall may cause pleural effusion. Typically, pleural effusion causes dullness on percussion and breath sounds that are decreased below the effusion and increased above it. Monitor the patient for oxygenation problems, such as increased heart rate, decreased blood pressure, or an increased duskiness of the oral mucous membranes. Metastases to the mediastinal lymph nodes may involve the laryngeal nerve and may lead to hoarseness and vocal cord paralysis. The superior vena cava may become occluded with enlarged lymph nodes and cause superior vena cava syndrome; note edema of the face, neck, upper extremities, and thorax.

PSYCHOSOCIAL. The patient undergoes major lifestyle changes as a result of the physical side effects of cancer and its treatment. Interpersonal, social, and work role relationships change. The patient is faced with a psychological adjustment to the diagnosis of a chronic illness that frequently results in death. Evaluate the patient for evidence of altered moods such as depression or anxiety, and assess the patient's coping mechanisms and support system.

DIAGNOSTIC HIGHLIGHTS

Test	Normal Result	Abnormality with Condition	Explanation
Chest x ray	Clear lung fields; patent bronchi	Presence of tumors; compression of vital structures	Air-filled lungs are radiolucent (x rays pass through tissue, which appears as a dark area), but tumors or masses may appear more dense.
Computed tomography (CT) scan	Normal organ and tissues	Presence and size of tumor; enlarged lymph nodes; compression of pulmonary structures	Sequential x rays combined by computer to produce a detailed cross-sectional image of lungs
Cytologic sputum analysis	No cancer cells present in sputum	Presence of cancer cells in sputum	Microscopic examination of sputum sample to determine presence of cancer cells; even with large tumors cells may not be obtained in sputum
Bronchoscopy	No tumors or lung blockages	Visualization of tumors or blockages	Visual examination of the lungs through the use of a flexible fiberoptic lighted tube; microscopic examination of cells taken by biopsy and bronchial brushings

Other Tests: Magnetic resonance imaging (MRI), thoracentesis, closed-check needle biopsy, fluoroscopy, positron emission tomography (PET), bone scan, mediastinoscopy, bone marrow biopsy, complete blood count, arterial blood gas

PRIMARY NURSING DIAGNOSIS

Ineffective airway clearance related to obstruction caused by secretions or tumor

OUTCOMES. Respiratory status: gas exchange; respiratory status: ventilation; symptom control behavior; treatment behavior: illness or injury; comfort level

INTERVENTIONS. Airway management; Anxiety reduction; Oxygen therapy; Airway suctioning; Airway insertion and stabilization; Cough enhancement; Mechanical ventilation; Positioning; Respiratory monitoring

☐ PLANNING AND IMPLEMENTATION

Collaborative

The treatment of lung cancer depends on the type of cancer and the stage of the disease. Surgery, radiation therapy, and chemotherapy are all used. Unless the tumor is small without metastasis or nodes when discovered, it is often not curable.

Surgical treatment ranges from segmentectomy or wedge resection (removal of a part of a lobe) to lobectomy (removal of a section of the lung) to pneumonectomy (removal of an entire lung). These procedures all require general anesthesia and a thoracotomy (surgical incision in the chest). If patients are unable to undergo a thoracotomy because of other serious medical problems or widespread cancer, laser surgery may be performed to relieve blocked airways and diminish the threat of pneumonia or shortness of breath. Chemotherapy is used for cancer that has metastasized beyond the lungs. It is used both as a primary treatment and an adjuvant treatment to surgery. The chemotherapy most often uses a combination of anticancer drugs; different combinations are used to treat NSCLC and SCLC.

Radiation therapy is sometimes the primary treatment for lung cancer, particularly in patients who are unable to undergo surgery. It is also used palliatively to alleviate symptoms of lung cancer. In conjunction with surgery, radiation is sometimes used to kill deposits of cancer that are too small to be seen and thus to be surgically removed. Radiation therapy takes two forms: external beam therapy delivers radiation from outside the body and focuses on the cancer and is most frequently used to treat a primary lung cancer or its metastases to other organs; brachytherapy uses a small pellet of radioactive material that is placed directly into the cancer or into the nearby airway.

PHARMACOLOGIC HIGHLIGHTS

Medication or Drug Class	Dosage	Description	Rationale
Chemotherapy	Varies with drug	Cisplatin or carboplatin in combination with gemcitabine, paclitaxel, docetaxel, etoposide, or vinorelbine	More effective in treating NSCLC
		Etoposide and cisplatin or etoposide and carboplatin, ifosfamide, carboplatin, and etoposide, or cyclophosphamide, doxorubicin, and vincristine	More effective in treating SCLC

Independent

Maintain a patent airway. Position the head of the bed at 30 to 45 degrees. Increase the patient's fluid intake, if possible, to assist in liquefying lung secretions. Provide humidified air. Suction the patient's airway if necessary. Assist the patient in controlling pain and managing dyspnea. Assist the patient with positioning and pursed-lip breathing. Allow extra time to accomplish the activities of daily living. Teach the patient to use guided imagery, diversional activities, and relaxation techniques. Provide periods of rest between activities.

Discuss the expected preoperative and postoperative procedures with patients who are undergoing surgical intervention. Emphasize the importance of coughing and deep breathing after surgery. Splinting the patient's incision may decrease the amount of discomfort the patient feels during these activities. Monitor closely the patency of the chest tubes and the amount of chest tube drainage. Notify the physician if the chest tube drainage is greater than 200 mL per hour for more than 2 to 3 hours, which may indicate a postoperative hemorrhage. Early in the postoperative period, begin increasing the patient's activity. Help the patient sit up in the bedside chair, and assist the patient to ambulate as soon as possible.

Explain the possible side effects of radiation or chemotherapy. Secretions may become thick and difficult to expectorate when the patient is having radiation therapy. Encourage the patient to drink fluids to stay hydrated. Percussion, postural drainage, and vibration can be used to aid in clearing secretions.

The patient may experience less anxiety if allowed as much control as possible over his or her daily schedule. Explaining procedures and keeping the patient informed about the treatment plan and condition may also decrease anxiety. If the patient enters the final phases of lung cancer, provide emotional support. Refer the patient and family to the hospice staff or the hospital chaplain. Encourage them to verbalize their feelings surrounding impending death. Allow for the time needed to adjust while you help the patient and family begin the grieving process. Assist in the identification of tasks to be completed before death, such as making a will; seeing specific relatives and friends; or attending an approaching wedding, birthday, or anniversary celebration. Urge the patient to verbalize specific funeral requests to family members.

DOCUMENTATION GUIDELINES

- Physical findings: Adequacy of airway and breathing; vital signs; heart and lung sounds; pain (nature, location, duration, and intensity); intake and output
- Complications: Pneumonia, hypoxia, infection, dehydration, poor wound healing
- Response to interventions: Response to pain medication
- Response to treatment: Chest tube drainage; wound healing; condition of skin following radiation; side effects from chemotherapy

DISCHARGE AND HOME HEALTHCARE GUIDELINES

Teach the patient to recognize the signs and symptoms of infection at the incision site, including redness, warmth, swelling, and drainage. Explain the need to contact the physician immediately. Be sure the patient understands any medication prescribed, including dosage, route, action, and side effects. Provide the patient with the names, addresses, and phone numbers of support groups, such as the American Cancer Society, the local hospice, and the Visiting Nurses Association. Teach the patient how to maximize his or her respiratory effort.

Lupus Erythematosus

DRG Category: 272
Mean LOS: 6.3 days
Description: MEDICAL: Major Skin Disorders with CC
DRG Category: 240
Mean LOS: 6.4 days
Description: MEDICAL: Connective Tissue Disorder with CC

Lupus erythematosus is an autoimmune disease that affects the connective tissue of the body. The course of disease is variable and unpredictable, with episodes of remission and relapse. Only a small percentage of patients (< 10%) have long-lasting remissions.

Lupus takes two forms. Systemic lupus erythematosus (SLE) is a multisystem inflammatory disease that affects any body system but primarily the musculoskeletal, cutaneous, renal, nervous, and cardiovascular systems. Discoid lupus erythematosus (DLE) is a less serious form of the disease that primarily affects the skin. DLE is characterized by skin lesions of the face, scalp, and ears. Long-standing lesions can cause scarring, hypopigmentation, and redness. Only 5% to 10% of patients with DLE develop SLE. The multisystem nature of SLE places the patient at risk for multiple complications, and the disease is ultimately fatal. The survival of patients with SLE is about 90% in 5 years and 80% in 10 years. The most common causes of death are renal failure and infections, followed by neurological and cardiovascular disorders.

CAUSES

The cause of lupus erythematosus is not known. A familial association has been noted that suggests a genetic predisposition, but a genetic link has not been identified. Environmental factors, susceptibility to certain viruses, and an immune system dysfunction with production of autoantibodies are possible causes. Hormonal abnormality and ultraviolet radiation are considered possible risk factors for the development of SLE. Some drugs have been implicated as initiating the onset of lupus-like symptoms and aggravating existing disease; they include hydralazine hydrochloride, procainamide hydrochloride, penicillin, isonicotinic acid hydrazide, chlorpromazine, phenytoin, and quinidine.

GENDER AND LIFE SPAN CONSIDERATIONS

SLE occurs most frequently in females between the ages of 15 and 45, with the average age of onset at 30 years. SLE affects women at least four times more frequently than men and up to 15 times more often than men during childbearing years. It is also more prominent in Asians and African-Americans. DLE is more common in women than in men, and approximately 60% of cases are female patients in their late 20s or older.

☐ ASSESSMENT

HISTORY. Initial symptoms may involve one organ only or multiple systems. Symptoms vary from mild and infrequent to persistent and life-threatening. Take a careful history with a focus on both systemic and single organ symptoms. Systemic symptoms include fatigue, malaise, weight loss, anorexia, and fever.

Musculoskeletal and cutaneous symptoms include joint and muscle pain, puffiness of hands and feet, joint swelling and tenderness, hand deformities, and skin lesions such as the characteristic "butterfly rash" (fixed reddish and flat rash that extends over both cheeks and the bridge of the nose), maculopapular rash (small colored area with raised red pimples), sensitivity to the sun, photophobia, vascular skin lesions, leg ulcers, oral ulcers, and hair loss.

Other symptoms originate in the genitourinary track (menstrual abnormalities, amenorrhea, spontaneous abortion), central nervous system (visual problems, memory loss, mild confusion, headache, seizures, psychoses, loss of balance, depression), hematologic system (venous or arterial clotting, bleeding tendencies), cardiopulmonary system (chest pain, shortness of breath, lung congestion), and gastrointestinal system (nausea, vomiting, difficulty swallowing, diarrhea, and bloody stools).

Ask if there is a family history of SLE. Establish any immune system dysfunction or recent viral infections. Ask if the patient has a history of hormonal abnormality or ultraviolet radiation. Ask the patient if he or she is taking or has taken any of the medications implicated as initiating lupus-like symptoms.

PHYSICAL EXAMINATION. Inspect the integumentary system thoroughly, including the mucous membranes, to determine the site of skin rashes and lesions. Check for lesions and necrosis on the fingertips, toes, and elbows; these may be caused by inflammation of terminal arterioles. Examine the hairline for any signs of hair loss. Assess the patient's extremities and joints for signs of arthritis, lymphadenopathy, and peripheral neuropathy. Determine the extent of range of motion and movement of extremities and level of joint discomfort. Auscultate the lungs and heart to determine the presence of a pleural or pericardial friction rub. Palpate the spleen and liver to determine the presence of tenderness, splenomegaly, or hepatomegaly. Examine the patient's urine for hematuria, proteinuria, and casts.

Assess for fever, pallor, and signs of bleeding, including petechiae and bruising. Check the patient's blood pressure because increased blood pressure might indicate kidney involvement.

PSYCHOSOCIAL. A patient is facing a chronic—and, many times—debilitating disease that can be fatal. The patient may have problems maintaining professional and family roles and may experience loss over a deteriorating health status. The loss of childbearing potential is another loss experienced for some women. Lupus is associated with an increased incidence of spontaneous abortion, fetal death, and prematurity. Assess the patient's and family's ability to cope with the illness. Determine the level of anxiety, fear, and depression.

DIAGNOSTIC HIGHLIGHTS

Tests: Complete blood count, antinuclear antibody, urinalysis, anti-DNA antibody, blood urea nitrogen, creatinine, creatinine clearance

BOX 9   DIAGNOSIS OF SYSTEMIC LUPUS ERYTHEMATOSUS

In order to make the diagnosis of SLE, the patient needs to have at least 4 of the following criteria.

Criteria	Explanation
Malar rash	Flat or raised rash on the cheeks or cheekbones
Discoid rash	Disk-like circular raised patches or rashes, often on the face or scalp
Photosensitivity	Skin rash as a result of an unusual reaction to sunlight
Oral ulcers	Sores, usually painless, on the lips and in the mouth
Arthritis	Tenderness or swelling of two or more peripheral joints
Serositis	Pleuritis or pericarditis
Renal disorder	Urinalysis shows proteinuria or cellular casts (red blood cell, hemoglobin, granular, tubular, or mixed casts)
Neurologic disorder	Seizures, psychosis
Hematologic disorders	Hemolytic anemia, leukopenia (decreased white blood cell count), lymphopenia (decreased lymphocytes), thrombocytopenia (decreased platelets)
Immunologic disorder	Presence of anti-DNA antibody (antibodies to native DNA that indicate autoimmune activity), Anti-Sm nuclear antigen (antinuclear antibody active against acidic nuclear proteins), antiphospholipid antibodies (family of immunoglobulins active against phospholipids)
Antinuclear antibody	Presence of antinuclear antibody (antibodies the body produces against its own DNA and nuclear material; antibodies cause tissue damage)

PRIMARY NURSING DIAGNOSIS

Alteration in comfort related to joint pain or peripheral nerve inflammation or dysfunction; pain (acute) related to inflammation

OUTCOMES. Comfort level; Pain control behavior; Pain level; Symptom severity

INTERVENTIONS. Analgesic administration; Anxiety reduction; Environmental management: Comfort; Pain management; Medication management; Teaching: Individual; Prescribed activity/exercise

☐ PLANNING AND IMPLEMENTATION

Collaborative

Much of the therapy is pharmacologic. General supportive therapy includes adequate sleep and avoidance of fatigue because mild disease exacerbations may subside after several days of bed rest. A physical therapy program is important to maintain mobility and range of motion without allowing the patient to get overtired. If the kidneys are involved, renal dialysis or transplantation may be required.

PHARMACOLOGIC HIGHLIGHTS

Medication or Drug Class	Dosage	Description	Rationale
Nonsteroidal anti-inflammatory drugs (NSAIDS)	Varies with drug	Salicylates: aspirin, choline, salslate; nonsalicylates: diclofenac, ibuprofen, indomethacin, naproxen, sulindac, sulindac	Treat the joint pain and swelling; should be avoided in patients with active nephritis
Hydroxychloroquine (Plaquenil)	400–600 mg po daily for 5–10 days, gradually increasing dose until effective; maintenance is usually 200–400 mg/day po	Antimalarial	Reduces rash, photosensitivity, arthralgias, arthritis, alopecia, and malaise
Corticosteroids	Varies with drug	Prednisone, 1–2 mg/kg po qd; methylprednisolone 500 mg IV	Control SLE in most severe or life-threatening cases (glomerulonephritis, debilitation from symptoms)

Other Therapy: Topical steroids are often used to treat skin rashes. Anticonvulsants may be necessary if seizures occur. When the disease is not responsive to conventional therapies, trials of immunosuppressive (cytotoxic or alkylating) agents may be considered. These agents, however, have serious side effects, including the risk of malignancy and bone marrow suppression.

Independent

The pain and discomfort of SLE can be physically and mentally debilitating. Encourage the patient to maintain activity when the symptoms are mild or in remission. Encourage patients to pace all activity and to allow for adequate rest. Hot packs may relieve joint pain and stiffness. If the patient has Raynaud's phenomenon (abnormal vasoconstriction of the extremities), use warmth to relieve symptoms and protect the patient's hands from injury.

Support the patient's self-image by encouraging good grooming. Suggest hypoallergenic cosmetics, shaving products, and hair products. Encourage the patient to use a hair stylist or barber who specializes in caring for people with scalp disorders and to protect all body surfaces from direct sunlight. The patient should use sunscreen with a protective factor of at least 20 and wear a hat and long sleeves while in the sun. Note that certain drugs (tetracycline) and food (figs, parsley, celery) augment the effects of ultraviolet light and therefore should be avoided.

Fatigue and stress can lead to exacerbations of the illness. Explore ways for the patient to get adequate rest. Because the patient's immune system may have a diminished capacity, encourage the patient to avoid exposure to illness.

Explore the meaning of the chronic illness and coping strategies with the patient. Allow adequate time to discuss fears and concerns. A referral to a support group or counselor may also be necessary.

DOCUMENTATION GUIDELINES

- Physical changes: Vital signs, particularly blood pressure and temperature; daily weight, intake and output; signs of bleeding or tarry stools, petechiae, bruising, pallor
- Physical changes: Location site and description of any skin lesions or rashes and overall condition of the skin
- Physical changes: Presence of any seizure activity, visual disturbances, headaches, personality changes, or memory deficits
- Tolerance to activity, level of fatigue, patient's ability to perform activities of daily living and range of motion of extremities; note the extent of joint involvement and the presence of tingling, numbness, or weakness

DISCHARGE AND HOME HEALTHCARE GUIDELINES

Teach the patient the purpose, dosage, and possible side effects of all medications. Explain to the patient the disease process, the purpose of treatment regimens, and the importance of compliance. Teach the patient when to seek medical attention. Teach the patient to wear a Medic Alert bracelet noting the disease and medications so appropriate action can be taken in an emergency.

Teach the female patient the importance of planning pregnancies with medical supervision because pregnancy is likely to cause an exacerbation of the disease.

Discuss all precipitating factors that need to be avoided, including fatigue, vaccination, infections, stress, surgery, certain drugs, and exposure to ultraviolet light. Teach the patient how to minimize ultraviolet exposure. Teach the patient to avoid strenuous exercise, instead striving for a balance. Stress the importance of adequate nutrition. Small, frequent meals may be better tolerated. Any cosmetics should be approved by the physician and should be hypoallergenic. Encourage the patient to contact the Arthritis Foundation, the Lupus Foundation, and other appropriate support groups that are available in the area.

Lyme Disease

DRG Category: 423
Mean LOS: 7.1 days
Description: MEDICAL: Other Infectious and Parasitic Diseases Diagnoses

Lyme disease is a tick-borne illness that is an acute recurrent inflammatory disease characterized by periods of exacerbation and remissions. This disease is named for the town in Connecticut where it was first recognized in the 1970s. In the last 10 years, the number of cases has ranged from approximately 5000 to 8000 in the United States, making it the leading tick-borne disease in the U.S.

Lyme disease typically begins in summer or early fall and develops in three stages with varying, progressive symptoms over weeks and months if untreated. The most frequent carrier of the disease is the deer tick, a small insect the size of a poppy seed. The deer tick is predominantly found in the New England and mid-Atlantic states, Wisconsin, Minnesota, and northern California, although cases of Lyme disease have been documented in 48 states. Severe long-term effects occur in fewer than 10% of untreated cases. Complications include pericarditis and myocarditis, cardiac dysrhythmias, encephalitis, peripheral neuropathies, and arthritis. Incubation lasts 7–10 days, but diagnosis generally must wait for 4–6 weeks after being bitten by a tick in order to make laboratory tests reliable.

CAUSES

Lyme disease is caused by a spirochete, *Borrelia burgdorferi*. This organism can be transmitted through the saliva of the tick while it is ingesting blood from a host. Not all ticks carry this spirochete, and all bites from infected ticks do not lead to Lyme disease. Burning a tick off or smothering it with petroleum jelly potentiates the spirochete injection via reflux regurgitation.

GENDER AND LIFE SPAN CONSIDERATIONS

The general population of all ages and both sexes are at risk for Lyme disease, especially those who are exposed to infested geographic locations. Reinfection via new contaminated bites is possible throughout one's lifetime.

☐ ASSESSMENT

HISTORY. Note that this disease progresses in stages, each having its own unique symptoms. The first stage involves skin invasion. A characteristic "bull's eye" rash (erythema migrans) and flu-like symptoms may occur within days to weeks of the tick bite. During the second stage, the nerve tissue is invaded, and the patient experiences neurological symptoms and possibly cardiac problems. The most common neurological complications are Bell's palsy and aseptic Lyme meningitis, which can progress to encephalitis. Without treatment at this stage, 8% of patients develop cardiac complications such as heart block, pericarditis, congestive heart failure, dizziness, shortness of breath, and palpitations. Final progression of the untreated disease results in arthritis, which sometimes becomes chronic. Tendons, bursae, and joints (most commonly the knees) may subsequently become infected and result in the arthritic symptoms characteristic of stage three.

Obtain a thorough history regarding the patient's recall of a tick bite within the past 3 to 30 days and recall of exposure to geographic "hot spots." Note that there is a seasonal component to exposure (May to August). Question the patient carefully about presence of malaise, muscle and joint pain, stiff neck, headache, and fatigue, all of which are early symptoms.

PHYSICAL EXAMINATION. Inspect the skin for the characteristic rash, a reddened expanding ring with a lighter center. The rash may be warm to touch, but it is usually painless and may grow to be inches in diameter. Inspect the face for any signs of paralysis; determine if the patient can open and close the eyes and mouth symmetrically. Determine the patient's temperature. Auscultate the patient's heart rate for irregularity and the presence of tachycardia. Progressive symptoms in untreated patients involve neurologic and musculoskeletal symptoms. Perform a complete neurologic examination. Assess the range of motion of the neck and other joints, and determine the patient's muscle strength.

PSYCHOSOCIAL. Anxiety of the unknown—both the fear of disease progression and the fear of the potential for reinfection—contributes to the psychological effect of this disease. Patients may be frustrated with experiencing memory loss; determine the family's understanding and ability to support the patient with an altered mental status.

DIAGNOSTIC HIGHLIGHTS

Test	Normal Result	Abnormality with Condition	Explanation
Enzyme-linked immunosorbent assay (ELISA)	Nonreactive	Levels of specific IgM antibodies peak during the 3rd to 6th week after onset and then gradually decline	Best diagnostic test; measures levels of specific IgM antibodies
Indirect immunofluorescent lyme antibody titer	Negative	Presence of antibodies	Identifies antibodies to a spirochete, *Borrelia burgdorferi,* the agent of Lyme disease

Other Tests: Culture from skin lesions (impractical and rarely performed)

PRIMARY NURSING DIAGNOSIS

Anxiety related to knowledge deficit of disease progression, treatment, and prevention

OUTCOMES. Anxiety control; Coping; Symptom control behavior; Knowledge: Disease process, Medication, Treatment regime

INTERVENTIONS. Anxiety reduction; Calming technique; Coping enhancement; Teaching: Disease process, Individual, Prescribed medications

◻ PLANNING AND IMPLEMENTATION

Collaborative

Oral antibiotics are usually started as early as possible. Tetracycline is the primary choice, but doxycycline, penicillin, and ceftriaxone are also given. Children are usually treated with oral penicillin. Fever is treated with antipyretics and sometimes cooling blankets.

Research is being done on using the protein "Osp A" from the Lyme spirochete as a potential vaccination for this disease. Surprisingly, Osp A vaccination in mice has kept them free from Lyme disease after infected tick bites, but it also killed the spirochete that was present in the ticks who bit the vaccinated mice. Use of this vaccine might be considered in plant and water supplies to help stop the spread of Lyme disease.

PHARMACOLOGIC HIGHLIGHTS

Medication or Drug Class	Dosage	Description	Rationale
Tetracycline	250 mg po qid	Antibiotic	Combats infection; course of antibiotics is generally for 10–20 days; may need home IV therapy if chronic Lyme disease occurs
Analgesics	Varies with drug	Acetaminophen, aspirin, ibuprofen	Relieve joint discomfort

Independent

Nursing care varies, depending on the disease stage. Manage fever with cool sponge baths and limited bedding. Maintain a cool temperature in the environment if possible. Manage fatigue with promotion of rest and comfort. Ice bags are effective for headache. Arthralgia may require immobilization of the painful joint, warm moist applications, and other nonpharmacologic measures to control pain. Assist the patient with range-of-motion exercises and activities to strengthen muscles and joints, being careful not to overexert the patient.

Provide emotional support to patients who are experiencing memory loss and confusion. Determine the patient's chance for injury and plan accordingly by instituting safety measures. Frequently reorient the patient to his or her surroundings. Encourage the patient to share any concerns about his or her mental status. Explain the reason for the mental status changes to the patient and significant others, and answer any questions about the long-range complications of the disease.

DOCUMENTATION GUIDELINES

- Skin assessment: Presence of rash; description and location of rash
- Musculoskeletal assessment: Warmth, tenderness, stiffness, swelling of involved joints
- Cardiac assessment: Rate and regularity of rhythm; presence of chest pain, shortness of breath, palpitations, dizziness
- Neurological assessment: Headache, stiff neck, confusion, sensory loss, memory loss, facial weakness or paralysis, limb weakness
- Response to therapy: Relief of presenting symptoms (fever control, pain relief, resolved neurological and cardiac complications)

DISCHARGE AND HOME HEALTHCARE GUIDELINES

Teach the patient strategies to prevent tick bites:

Wear protective clothing in at-risk areas, such as long sleeves and long pants (pant legs should also be tucked inside of socks), full-cover shoes (not sandals), and light-colored clothing to help make identification of the tiny dark ticks easier.

Use chemical repellents such as DEET, but note they may cause respiratory distress if too much is used, especially in children.

Stay on cleared paths and avoid wandering through grass and woods.

Inspect the body daily. Prime location for bites include the back, axilla, neck, ankle, groin, scalp, and back of the knees.

Wash and dry exposed clothing for at least 30 minutes to kill concealed ticks. Inspect pets as well, not only for carrying ticks into the house but also because Lyme disease is a prime cause of animal arthritis.

If a tick is attached to the skin, remove it carefully to avoid causing it to regurgitate saliva and spirochetes into the host. Use tweezers close to the skin to pull the head or jaw out of the skin. Cleanse the site with antiseptic agent. Do not try to burn off the tick or to smother it with kerosene or petroleum jelly. Emphasize that the patient should finish the entire course of antibiotics, even if he or she is asymptomatic. Inform the physician of recurrent or progressive symptoms for consideration of reinfection

---

Lymphoma, Non-Hodgkin's

DRG Category: 403
Mean LOS: 7.4 days
Description: MEDICAL: Lymphoma and Non-Acute Leukemia with CC
DRG Category: 401
Mean LOS: 9.2 days
Description: SURGICAL: Lymphoma and Non-Acute Leukemia with Other O. R. Procedures with CC

Malignant lymphoma, also called lymphosarcoma or non-Hodgkin's lymphoma (NHL), is a diffuse group of neoplastic diseases that are characterized by rampant proliferation of lymphocytes. Lymphomas fall into two main categories: Hodgkin's and non-Hodgkin's lymphomas, based primarily on the presence or absence of the Reed-Sternberg cell; when the cells are absent, the disease is classified as NHL. (See Table 33.) Of the more than 60,000 new cases of lymphoma that are diagnosed each year in the U.S., approximately 55,000 of them will be NHL.

TABLE 33 | **Comparison of Hodgkin's Disease and Non-Hodgkin's Lymphoma**

CHARACTERISTIC	HODGKIN'S	LOW-GRADE NON-HODGKIN'S	ALL OTHER NON-HODGKIN'S
Site(s) of origin	Nodal	Extranodal, about 10%	Extranodal, about 35%
Nodal distribution	Axial (centripetal)	Centrifugal	Centrifugal
Nodal spread	Contiguous	Noncontiguous	Noncontiguous
Central nervous system involvement	Rare, < 1%	Rare, < 1%	Uncommon, < 10%
Hepatic involvement	Uncommon	Common, > 50%	Uncommon, <1 0%
Bone marrow involvement	Uncommon, < 10%	Common, > 50%	Uncommon

| Marrow involvement adversely affects prognosis | Yes | No | Yes |
| Curable by chemotherapy | Yes | No | Yes |

Malignant lymphoma, or NHL, is a heterogeneous grouping of several disease types that range from the aggressive, rapidly fatal diffuse histiocytic lymphoma to the indolent nodular varieties. Still, all have a less promising prognosis than Hodgkin's disease. Complications of NHL include hypercalcemia, increased uric acid levels, meningitis, and anemia. As tumors grow, they may compress the vital organs and cause organ dysfunction; problems from organ compression include complications such as increased intracranial pressure.

CAUSES

The cause of NHL is unknown. Exposures to viruses and immunosuppression are thought to be related to NHL. Organ transplantation, a history of cancer treated with radiation, acquired immune deficiencies, and autoimmune disorders are considered risk factors. Some believe that both Hodgkin's disease and NHL result from an immune defect or from the activation of an oncogenic virus. One form of NHL, Burkitt's lymphoma, found primarily in Africa, provides a strong case for viral involvement. A herpes virus (Epstein-Barr virus) is probably the causative agent in Burkitt's lymphoma. Exposure to nuclear explosions or reactor accidents, certain pesticides and herbicides, and chemicals (benzene, lead, paint thinner, and formaldehyde) may place patients at risk.

GENDER AND LIFE SPAN CONSIDERATIONS

The peak incidence of NHL occurs later than with Hodgkin's disease. About 25% of cases develop in patients between ages 50 and 59. Maximal risk is between the ages 60 and 69. Small lymphocytic lymphomas occur in the elderly. Lymphoblastic lymphoma has a predilection for males younger than age 20. Follicular lymphomas are uncommon in the young and occur mainly in mid-adult life. Burkitt's lymphoma occurs in children and young adults.

☐ ASSESSMENT

HISTORY. Note any history of infection with the human immunodeficiency virus (HIV), acquired immunodeficiency syndrome (AIDS), organ transplant, congenital immunodeficiency, autoimmune diseases, or other treatment with immunosuppressive drugs. Patients often have complaints of painless enlarged lymph nodes (commonly in the neck, mediastinum, or chest wall), fevers, night sweats, weight loss, weakness, and malaise. Because nodes and extranodal sites are more likely to be involved in NHL, the patient may also report vague abdominal distress (bleeding, bowel obstruction, cramping, ascites), symptoms of spinal cord compression, or back pain. Cough, dyspnea, and chest pain occur about 20% of the time and are indicative of lung involvement.

PHYSICAL EXAMINATION. Carefully inspect all the locations for lymph nodes and the abdomen for signs of hepatosplenomegaly and ascites. Skin lesions that look like nodules or papules with a tendency to ulcerate appear in about 20% of cases. When palpating lymph node chains, examine the submental, infraclavicular, epitrochlear, iliac, femoral, and popliteal nodes. Involved nodes are characteristically painless, firm, and rubbery in consistency; they are in contrast to the rock-hard nodes of carcinoma because they are freely movable and of varying size. Palpate the liver or spleen, which may be enlarged. The patient may also have weight loss and fever.

PSYCHOSOCIAL. The diagnosis of cancer is devastating at any time of life. Because the disease is most common in the older adult, the patient may be planning retirement. The diagnosis of NHL throws all retirement plans into disarray and may lead to feelings of loss, grief, and anger.

DIAGNOSTIC HIGHLIGHTS

Test	Normal Result	Abnormality with Condition	Explanation
Lymph node biopsy; bone marrow biopsy	Normal cells	Positive for lymphoma cells	Determines extent of disease and allows for staging of disease; bone marrow biopsy is generally done only for patients with anemia or fever and night sweats
Computed tomography (CT) or magnetic resonance imaging (MRI) of chest, abdomen, and pelvis	Normal structures	Spread of NHL into organs and body cavities	Used to assist with staging; common sites of extra-lymphatic involvement include spleen, stomach, small intestine; combined with lymphangiography, can predict nodal involvement in 90% of cases
Lymphangiography: a radiographic test of lymphatic vessels and nodes; radiopaque iodine contrast medium is injected into lymphatics of foot or hand	Normal lymphatic system	Identification of structural abnormalities or tumor involvement	Test has been replaced in many situations by CT scanning but may still be used for staging; not usually performed in children

Other Tests: Complete blood cell count and erythrocyte sedimentation rate (shows anemia, leukocytosis, elevated platelet count and erythrocyte sedimentation rate), chest x ray; tests for liver and renal function, including lactate dehydrogenase, alkaline phosphatase, blood urea nitrogen, and creatinine; gallium scan

PRIMARY NURSING DIAGNOSIS

Risk for infection related to impaired primary and secondary defenses

☐ PLANNING AND IMPLEMENTATION

Collaborative

Treatment is based on classification of the cell and staging of the disease. Some of the indolent types of NHL do well with only supportive therapy. The disease process may be slow enough that treatment is saved until the disease takes a more aggressive path. Most patients with intermediate-grade and high-grade lymphomas receive combination chemotherapy.

Radiation is effective for many patients with stage I or stage II NHL. Radiation is delivered to the chest wall, mediastinum, axilla, and neck (the region known as the mantle field). Most patients, however, are at stage III or IV at diagnosis. Surgery has limited use in the treatment of NHL. It may be part of the diagnostic and staging process, but diagnostic laparotomy is much less common than in Hodgkin's disease. A therapeutic splenectomy may be performed for severe spleen enlargement. Gastric or bowel resection may be done if the patient has a primary gastrointestinal lymphoma or has obstructions from bulky nodes. Stem cell transplantation may be considered for patients who have relapsed, are at high risk for relapse, or have tried conventional therapy without success.

OUTCOMES. Immune status; Knowledge: Infection control; Risk control; Risk detection; Nutritional status; Tissue integrity: Skin and mucous membranes; Treatment behavior: Illness or injury

INTERVENTIONS. Infection control; Infection protection; Surveillance; Nutritional management; Medication management; Teaching: Disease process

PHARMACOLOGIC HIGHLIGHTS

Medication or Drug Class	Dosage	Description	Rationale
Chemotherapy	Varies with drug	Some common regimens are CHOP (cyclophosphamide, doxorubicin, vincristine, prednisone); BACOP (bleomycin, doxorubicin, cyclophosphamide, vincristine, prednisone); and MACOP-B (methotrexate with leucovorin rescue factor, doxorubicin, cyclophosphamide, vincristine, prednisone, bleomycin, plus trimethoprim-sulfamethoxazole and ketoconazole)	Chemotherapy is used for stage IVA and all stage B patients; usually lasts for 6–8 months

Other Therapy: Common side effects are alopecia, nausea, vomiting, fatigue, myelosuppression, and stomatitis. Patients who are receiving chemotherapy are administered antinausea drugs, antiemetics, and pain medicines as needed to help control adverse experiences. Experimental drugs currently in clinical trials include paclitaxel, topoisomerase-3 inhibitors, nucleoside analogues, monoclonal antibodies, and interferon.

Independent

Maintain the patient's comfort, protect the patient from infection, provide teaching and support about the complications of the treatment, and provide emotional support.

Fatigue, one of the most common side effects of cancer treatment, can last for several months to several years. A program entitled "Fatigue Initiative Research and Education" (FIRE) is available through the Oncology Nurses Society (www.ons.org).

During irradiation, the patient may suffer from dry mouth, loss of taste, dysphagia, nausea, and vomiting, which can be managed with frequent mouth care. Explore ways to limit discomfort, such as ice chips. Attempt to provide desired foods to support the patient's nutrition. Keep any foul-smelling odors clear of the patient's environment, particularly during meals. Manage skin irritation and redness by washing the skin gently with mild soap, rinsing with warm water, and patting the skin dry. Encourage the patient to avoid applying lotions, perfumes, deodorants, and powder to the treatment area. Explain that the patient needs to protect the skin from sunlight and extreme cold. Before starting treatments, arrange for the patient to have a wig, scarf, or hat to cover any hair loss, which occurs primarily at the nape of the neck.

If the patient develops bone marrow suppression, institute infection controls. Treat the discomfort that may arise from chemotherapy—joint pain, fever, fluid retention, and a labile emotion state (euphoria or depression)—all of which need specific interventions, depending on their incidence and severity. The complexity of the diagnostic and staging process may make the patient feel lost in a crowd of specialists. It is important for the nurse to provide supportive continuity. Patience and repeated explanations are needed. Provide the patient with information about support groups, and refer the patient to a clinical nurse specialist, support groups associated with the American Cancer Society (www.cancer.org), or counselors.

DOCUMENTATION GUIDELINES

- Emotional and physical response to diagnostic testing; healing of incisions; signs of ineffective coping; response to diagnosis; ability to participate in planning treatment options; response of significant others
- Effects of chemotherapy or radiation therapy; response to treatment of symptoms; presence of complications (weight loss, infection, skin irritation)
- Effectiveness of coping; presence of depression; interest in group support of counseling; referrals made

DISCHARGE AND HOME HEALTHCARE GUIDELINES

Teach the patient the following strategies to limit infections:
Avoid crowds, avoid infected visitors, particularly children with colds, wash the hands frequently.
When an infection occurs, report it to a physician immediately.
Avoid direct contact with pets to limit the risk of infections from licks, scratches, or bites. Do not change the cat litter or clean a birdcage.
Maintain a high-calorie and high-protein diet. Take sips of grapefruit juice, orange juice, or ginger ale if nausea persists. Drink at least 2000 mL of fluid a day unless on fluid restriction.
Perform frequent mouth care with a soft toothbrush and avoid commercial mouthwashes.
Contact support groups, the American or Canadian Cancer Society, or counselors as needed.

Mallory-Weiss Syndrome

DRG Category: 174
Mean LOS: 4.9 days
Description: MEDICAL: Gastrointestinal Hemorrhage with CC
DRG Category: 154
Mean LOS: 13.3 days
Description: SURGICAL: Stomach, Esophageal, and Duodenal Procedures, Age > 17 with CC

Mallory-Weiss syndrome is a tear or laceration, usually singular and longitudinal, in the mucosa at the junction of the distal esophagus and proximal stomach. Esophageal lacerations account for between 5% and 10% of upper gastrointestinal (GI) bleeding episodes. Approximately 60% of the tears involve the cardia, the upper opening of the stomach that connects with the esophagus. Another 15% involve the terminal esophagus, and 25% involve the region across the epigastric junction. In a small percentage of patients, the tear leads to upper GI bleeding. Most episodes of bleeding stop spontaneously, but some patients require medical intervention. If bleeding is excessive, hypovolemia and shock may result. Esophageal rupture (Boerhaave syndrome) is rare but catastrophic when it does occur. If esophageal perforation occurs, the patient may develop abscesses or sepsis.

CAUSES

The most common cause of Mallory-Weiss syndrome is failure of the upper esophageal sphincter to relax during prolonged vomiting. This poor sphincter control is more likely to occur after excessive intake of alcohol. Any event that increases intra-abdominal pressure can also lead to an esophageal tear, such as persistent forceful coughing, trauma, seizure, pushing during childbirth, or a hiatal hernia. Other factors that may predispose a person to Mallory-Weiss syndrome are esophagitis, gastritis, and atrophic gastric mucosa.

GENDER AND LIFE SPAN CONSIDERATIONS

Mallory-Weiss syndrome, first described in alcoholics, is now recognized across the life span but is most common in men over the age of 40.

□ ASSESSMENT

HISTORY. The patient may report a history of retching and vomiting, followed by vomiting bright red blood. Ask the patient about the appearance of the vomitus. Hematemesis has a "coffee-ground" appearance if it is of gastric origin and is often a sign of brisk bleeding, usually from an arterial source or esophageal varices. Ask about passage of blood with bowel movements, either a few hours to several days after vomiting. Although vomiting and retching before the onset of bleeding can be indicative of a Mallory-Weiss tear, some patients with Mallory-Weiss syndrome do not present with such a history. Inquire about weakness, fatigue, and dizziness, any and all of which can result with chronic blood loss. Ask about a history of alcoholism, hiatal hernia, seizures, or a recent severe cough.

PHYSICAL EXAMINATION. Inspect the patient's nasopharynx to rule out the nose and throat as the source of bleeding. Assess the patient for evidence of trauma to the head, chest, and abdomen as well. Note that manifestations of GI bleeding depend on the source of bleeding, the rate of bleeding, and the underlying or co-existing diseases. Patients with massive bleeding have the clinical signs of shock, such as a heart rate greater than 110 beats per minute, an orthostatic blood pressure drop of 16 mm Hg or more, restlessness, decreased urine output, and delayed capillary refill.

PSYCHOSOCIAL. The sudden admission to an acute care facility for GI bleeding is stressful and upsetting. Assess the patient's anxiety level, along with his or her understanding of the treatment and intervention plan. Because Mallory-Weiss syndrome is associated with alcohol use and abuse, determine if the patient is a problem drinker and assess the family's and significant others' responses to the patient's drinking.

DIAGNOSTIC HIGHLIGHTS

Test	Normal Result	Abnormality with Condition	Explanation
Fiberoptic endoscopy	Visualization of normal tissue	Mucosal tear at gastroesophageal junction	Small fiberoptic tube is inserted into the esophagus to permit visual inspection
Complete blood count	Red blood cells (RBCs) 4.0–5.5 million/µL; white blood cells 4,500–11,000/µL; hemoglobin (Hg) 12–18 g/dL; hematocrit (Hct) 37%–54%; reticulocyte count 0.5%–2.5% of total RBCs; platelets 150,000–400,000/µL	Decreased RBCs, Hg, and Hct because of upper GI bleeding	Serial monitoring to monitor the extent of blood loss; assesses the response to therapy

Other Tests: Arteriography, coagulation studies

PRIMARY NURSING DIAGNOSIS

Airway clearance, ineffective, related to aspiration of blood

OUTCOMES. Respiratory status: Gas exchange and ventilation; Safety status: Physical injury

INTERVENTIONS. Airway insertion; Airway management; Airway suctioning; Oral health promotion; Respiratory monitoring; Ventilation assistance; Surveillance; Respiratory monitoring; Anxiety reduction

□ PLANNING AND IMPLEMENTATION

Collaborative

Bleeding often subsides spontaneously, but if it does not, a Sengstaken-Blakemore or Minnesota tube is inserted to provide pressure at the source of bleeding by using a balloon tamponade. For continued bleeding, a nasogastric tube may be placed and connected to continuous low suction with periodic lavages. Intra-arterial infusion of vasopressin or therapeutic embolization into the left gastric artery during arteriography has also been shown to be effective in controlling bleeding in some patients. Other strategies to halt bleeding include endoscopy with electrocoagulation for hemostasis or transcatheter embolization with an autologous blood clot or artificial material, such as a gelatin sponge. On rare occasions, the patient may require surgery to suture the laceration.

If the patient has excessive blood loss, institute strategies to support the circulation. To stabilize the circulation and replace vascular volume, place a large-bore (14- to 18-gauge) intravenous catheter and maintain replacement fluids such as 0.9% sodium chloride and blood component therapy as prescribed. With continued or massive bleeding, the patient may be supported with blood transfusions and admitted to an intensive care unit for close observation.

PHARMACOLOGIC HIGHLIGHTS

No medications are used to manage Mallory-Weiss syndrome directly. Patients may be placed on vasopressin to reduce upper GI bleeding, antacids or histamine$_2$ blockers to decrease gastric acidity, and in unusual cases of severe hemorrhage, fluid resuscitation and vasopressors to support the circulation.

Independent

A major cause of morbidity and mortality in patients with active GI bleeding is aspiration of blood with subsequent respiratory compromise, which is seen in patients with inadequate gag reflexes or those who are unconscious or obtunded. Constant surveillance to ensure a patent airway is essential. Check every 8 hours for the presence of a gag reflex. Maintain the head of the bed in a semi-Fowler position unless contraindicated. If the patient needs to be positioned with the head of the bed flat, place the patient in a side-lying position.

Encourage bed rest and reduced physical activity to limit oxygen consumption. Plan care around frequent rest periods, scheduling procedures so the patient does not overtire. Avoid the presence of noxious stimuli that may be nauseating. Support nutrition by eliminating foods and fluids that cause gastroesophageal discomfort. Encourage the patient to avoid caffeinated beverages, alcohol, carbonated drinks, and extremely hot or cold food or fluids. Help the patient understand the treatments and procedures. Provide information that is consistent with the patient's educational level and which takes into account the patient's state of anxiety.

DOCUMENTATION GUIDELINES

- Physical response: Frequency and amount of hematemesis; laboratory values of interest; presence of blood in the stool; degree of discomfort (location, duration, precipitating factors)
- Response to treatments: Success of interventions to stop bleeding; response

to fluids and blood component therapy; function of tamponade tubes; ability to maintain rest and conserve energy
- Ability to tolerate food and fluids; nausea and vomiting

DISCHARGE AND HOME HEALTHCARE GUIDELINES

Teach the patient to avoid foods and fluids that cause discomfort or irritation. Determine the patient's understanding of any prescribed medications, including dosage, route, action or effect, and side effects. Review signs and symptoms of recurrent bleeding and the need to seek immediate medical care. Provide a phone number for the patient to use if complications develop.

Mastitis

DRG Category: 276
Mean LOS: 4.0 days
Description: MEDICAL: Nonmalignant Breast Disorders

Mastitis refers to infection of the glandular tissue of the breast and is seen primarily in lactating women. Approximately 1% of lactating women develop mastitis, which is more common in primiparas. Typically the lactation process is well established before mastitis develops; the highest incidence is seen in the second and third weeks postpartum. If it is left untreated, mastitis may develop into a breast abscess.

CAUSES

Mastitis is usually caused by the introduction of bacteria from a crack, fissure, or abrasion through the nipple that allows the organism entry into the breast. The source of organisms is almost always the nursing infant's nose and throat; other sources include the hands of the mother or birthing personnel and maternal circulating blood. The most common bacterial organism to cause mastitis is *Staphylococcus aureus;* others include beta-hemolytic streptococcus, *Escherichia coli, Candida albicans,* and, rarely, streptococcus. Common predisposing factors relate to milk stasis and include incomplete or inadequate drainage of a breast duct and alveolus that occurs as a result of missed feedings; prolonged delay in infant feeding; abrupt weaning of the infant; and blocked ducts caused by tight clothing or poor support of pendulous breasts. Other predisposing factors include a history of untreated or undertreated infections and a lowered maternal immune function caused by fatigue, stress, or other health problems.

GENDER AND LIFE SPAN CONSIDERATIONS

Although mastitis can occur in both men and women, it is uncommon in nonlactating women and rare in men.

☐ ASSESSMENT

HISTORY. Usually the infection is unilateral; localized symptoms include intense pain, tenderness, redness, and heat at the infection site. In addition, the woman often feels as if she has the flu, with symptoms of muscular aching, fatigue, headache, and fever.

In reviewing breastfeeding history, note if the frequency or regularity of feedings has changed. Fully investigate (1) the length of time the infant spends feeding; (2) the time between feedings; (3) if the infant is falling asleep at the breast; (4) if the infant is sleeping through the night; (5) if the infant receives supplementary water, juice, or formula; (6) if the infant receives bottled breast milk.

Ask the family if schedule changes have occurred that may cause the woman to nurse her infant less frequently. In addition, ask if family members have cold or flu symptoms.

PHYSICAL EXAMINATION. The breast may have a pink or red area that is swollen and often wedge-shaped, resulting from the septal distribution of the connective breast tissue. Most often, the upper outer quadrant is involved, but any area of the breast may be infected. You may also note cracked or sore nipples. Palpation of the area reveals a firm, tender area that is often warm to the touch. During palpation you may also feel enlarged axillary lymph nodes. Fever and tachycardia are also present.

PSYCHOSOCIAL. The transition to motherhood is a time of many changes in the woman's relationships: with the infant, the father, other children, and grandparents. It is important that the mother realize that mastitis is not a reason to discontinue breastfeeding and that her mothering skills are not inadequate because of it.

DIAGNOSTIC HIGHLIGHTS

General Comments: The diagnosis of mastitis is made based on the presenting symptoms and lactation history. Mammography is generally not used to diagnose mastitis, unless malignancy is suspected.

Test	Normal Result	Abnormality with Condition	Explanation
Culture of the breast milk	No growth	Shows growth of the organism causing the infection; confirms the diagnosis	Determines the appropriate antibiotic to treat the infection
Bacterial colony count	No growth	> 1000/mL	Indicates presence of infection
White blood cells	5,000–10,000/μL	> 10,000/μL	Increase in WBCs indicates the magnitude of the infection

PRIMARY NURSING DIAGNOSIS

Breastfeeding, ineffective related to change in feeding patterns, inadequate sucking, incorrect positioning, or infrequent feedings

OUTCOMES. Maternal and infant breastfeeding establishment; Breastfeeding maintenance

INTERVENTIONS. Breastfeeding assistance; Emotional support; Lactation counseling; Nutrition management

☐ PLANNING AND IMPLEMENTATION

Collaborative

Pharmacologic treatment involves the use of antibiotics that are tolerated by the infant and mother. Acetaminophen can be taken for discomfort; nonsteroidal anti-inflammatory drugs can be taken for fever and inflammation.

PHARMACOLOGIC HIGHLIGHTS

Medication or Drug Class	Dosage	Description	Rationale
Penicillinase-resistant penicillins (cloxacillin, dicloxacillin, oxacillin)	Varies by drug	Broad spectrum antibiotic	Fight off infection by damaging the cell wall of the infective agent
Cephalosporins	Varies by drug	Broad spectrum antibiotic	Damage the cell wall of the infective agent

Independent

Prevention is the most important aspect for nursing care. To prevent the development of mastitis, encourage frequent unrestricted nursing. The infant should be observed while nursing for techniques related to latching on, placement, positions, and suck. At the end of the feeding, evaluate the breast for emptiness. Instruct the woman to rotate feeding position of the infant to promote effective emptying of all lobes and to palpate her breast to evaluate emptiness after each feeding. If clogged ducts are noted, she should massage the area before the feeding and assess the area following subsequent feedings to see that it is completely emptied.

If mastitis has developed, encourage the woman to go to bed and stay there. She should only provide care for her infant, with a focus on frequent feeding and complete rest for her. Encourage the mother to continue breastfeeding frequently. Recommend that the woman massage her breasts before breastfeeding when she feels that her breasts are overly full or were not completely emptied at the previous feeding. In addition, instruct the woman to apply heat to the affected area, followed by gentle massage with the palm of the hand, immediately before feeding the infant to promote drainage. Encourage the woman to remove her brassiere during feedings so that constriction of the ducts does not occur from pressure.

Infant position during feeding is critical for effective drainage of the breast. Teach the woman to turn the infant fully on his or her side with the head placed at the mother's breast. The head should face the areola without turning. One or more inches of the areola should be in infant's mouth, and the baby's chin and nose should rest lightly on the breast. In addition, the infant's lips should be flared during nursing. As the infant nurses, the mother should hear swallowing. Encourage the mother to vary the infant's position (cradle, cross-cradle, football, side-lying) at feedings so that all ducts of the breast are effectively emptied. Feeding should always begin on the affected breast.

Teach the mother that she needs to nurse the infant a minimum of every 2 to 3 hours around the clock. Frequent feedings may mean that the mother needs to wake the infant during the night. Pain is managed through the use of ice packs or warm packs applied to the breast. A supportive, well-fitting brassiere may also reduce pain if it does not apply pressure to the infected area. In addition, over the counter analgesics may be used. Encourage the mother to drink at least 3000 mL of fluid per day; light straw-colored urine is an indication of adequate hydration. The mother's diet should meet the nutritional requirements for lactation.

DOCUMENTATION GUIDELINES

- Physical findings: Redness, pain, swelling, appearance of nipples, vital signs
- Ability to nurse: Position, frequency, latching on, sucking
- Infant's response

DISCHARGE AND HOME HEALTHCARE GUIDELINES

PREVENTION. Teach the patient to prevent mastitis by the following interventions:
Continue breastfeeding frequently.
Wash hands before touching breast or beginning breastfeeding.
Breastfeed every 2 to 3 hours around the clock (wake up the baby at night).
Remove brassiere before beginning feeding.
Always begin breastfeeding on the affected side.
To promote emptying of the breast at a feeding, apply warmth to the breast immediately before feeding (a disposable diaper may be wet with warm water and wrapped around the breast) and massage the breast before placing the infant at the breast.
Change the infant's feeding position; use cradle, side-lying, cross-cradle, and football positions to promote emptying of the breast.
Increase the mother's fluid intake.
Evaluate the breast after the feeding to see if the infant has completely emptied the breast. If the baby does not completely empty the breast, finish emptying the breast with a breast pump or manual expression.
Rest and avoid fatigue.

MEDICATIONS. All medications should be taken until the prescription is finished, even if symptoms disappear.

Melanoma Skin Cancer

DRG Category: 272
Mean LOS: 6.3 days
Description: MEDICAL: Major Skin Disorders with CC
DRG Category: 269
Mean LOS: 7.4 days
Description: SURGICAL: Other Skin, Subcutaneous Tissue, and Breast Procedures with CC

Melanoma skin cancer is a type of skin cancer that originates from the melanocytes, frequently a nevus or mole. Melanocytes are melanin-producing cells that are interspersed in the inner layer of the epidermis. Melanin is a dark brown pigment that protects the epidermis and the superficial vasculature of the dermis. Nevi or moles are small, circumscribed aggregates of melanocytes. These skin lesions tend to be hereditary, begin to grow in childhood, and become more numerous in young adulthood.

Skin cancer is the most common cancer in the United States, and melanoma accounts for 4% of all skin cancer cases. Although the lifetime melanoma risk for the overall population is only 1.4%, melanoma is responsible for 79% of skin cancer deaths. According to the American Cancer Society, approximately 47,700 new diagnoses of melanoma were expected in the year 2000, with 7,700 deaths anticipated. Diagnoses of melanoma continue to increase; the number of new melanomas diagnosed per 100,000 people has jumped from 5.76 to 13.8 since 1973. The mortality rate per 100,000 people has increased from 1.6 to 2.3 since 1973, a 44% rise.

CAUSES

Characteristics that are associated with an increased risk for melanoma include fair skin that does not tan well and burns easily, blond or red hair, the tendency to develop freckles, and the presence of a large number of nevi. A strong association exists between exposure to ultraviolet light and the development of cutaneous melanoma, but the exact nature of this relationship is unclear. Other risk factors include a positive family history and immune suppression.

GENDER AND LIFE SPAN CONSIDERATIONS

The incidence of melanoma increases with age; 50% of cases occur in people who are older than age 50. Mortality rates are increasing most rapidly among European-American men older than age 50. Although melanomas are rare in children, the incidence among today's younger people, however, is proportionally higher than among people of the same age decades ago. Melanoma is one of the most common cancers in people who are younger than age 30. European-Americans have a 20 times higher risk factor for melanoma than do African-Americans. Melanoma most often appears on the trunks of fair-skinned men and the lower legs of fair-skinned women; however, people with more darkly pigmented skin do develop melanoma on their palms, soles, and under the nails.

◻ ASSESSMENT

HISTORY. Reports of a change in a nevus or mole or a new skin lesion require careful follow-up. Ask the patient the following questions: When did the lesion first appear or change? What is the specific nature of the change? What symptoms and characteristics of the lesion has the patient noticed? What is the patient's history of exposure to ultraviolet light or radiation? What is the history of thermal or chemical trauma? What personal or family history of melanoma or precancerous lesions exists?

PHYSICAL EXAMINATION. To identify potentially cancerous lesions, inspect and palpate the scalp, all skin surfaces, and the accessible mucosa. Examine preexisting lesions, scars, freckles, moles, warts, and nevi closely. The "ABCD rule" can be useful in identifying distinguishing characteristics of suspicious lesions. (See Table 34.)

TABLE 34 | **ABCD Rule of Assessment for Melanoma**

A = Asymmetry	Change in shape
	Unbalanced or irregular shape
B = Border Irregularity	Indistinct or splayed margins
	Notching of the borders
C = Color Variation	Spread of color from the edge of the lesion into the surrounding skin
	Multiple shades or colors within a single lesion
	Dark brown or black
	Red, white, or blue
D = Diameter	Sudden or continuous increase in size
	Diameter greater than 6 mm (although there has been an increase in 3–6 mm melanomas)

PSYCHOSOCIAL. For many people, the diagnosis of any type of cancer is associated with death. Because cancerous skin lesions are readily visible, the patient with melanoma may experience an altered body image. Ask open-ended questions as you assess the patient's emotional response to the diagnosis of melanoma.

DIAGNOSTIC HIGHLIGHTS

Test	Normal Result	Abnormality with Condition	Explanation
Shave biopsy	No cancer cells present	Presence of melanoma cells	Scrapes off the top layers of skin; may not be thick enough to determine the degree of cancer invasion
Punch biopsy	No cancer cells present	Presence of melanoma cells	Removes a deep sample of skin after numbing the site; cuts through all layers of skin
Incisional and excisional biopsy	No cancer cells present	Presence of melanoma cells	Uses a surgical knife to cut through the full thickness of skin and removes a wedge of skin: incisional biopsy removes

			only a portion; excisional biopsy removes entire tumor
Fine-needle aspiration biopsy	No cancer cells present	Presence of melanoma cells	Uses a thin needle to remove a very small tissue fragment; may be used to biopsy a lymph node near a melanoma to determine the extent of the disease

Other Tests: To diagnose metastases: computed tomography (CT) scan, magnetic resonance imaging (MRI), x rays

PRIMARY NURSING DIAGNOSIS

Impaired skin integrity related to cutaneous lesions

OUTCOMES. Tissue integrity: Skin and mucous membranes; Wound healing: Primary intention; Knowledge: Treatment regime; Nutritional status; Treatment behavior: Illness or injury

INTERVENTIONS. Incision site care; Wound care; Skin surveillance; Medication administration; Infection control; Nutrition management

▢ PLANNING AND IMPLEMENTATION

Collaborative

After diagnostic testing, the cancer is staged. Because the thinner the melanoma, the better the prognosis, the Clark level of a melanoma may be used. This system uses a scale of 1 to 5 to describe which layers of skin are involved. The higher the number, the deeper the melanoma.

The primary treatment for melanoma is surgical resection. Excision of the cancerous lesion with a 2- to 5-cm margin is recommended when feasible. The width of the surrounding margin should be wider for larger primary lesions. When the melanoma is on a finger or toe, surgical treatment is to amputate as much of the finger or toe as is necessary. Elective regional lymph node removal is controversial. Proponents believe that this procedure decreases the possibility of distal metastases, but scientific evidence to support this belief is lacking.

The prognosis for metastatic melanoma is poor; it is highly resistant to currently available chemotherapeutic agents. Radiation is not often used to treat the original melanoma, but is rather used for symptom management as a palliative measure if the cancer has spread to the brain.

PHARMACOLOGIC HIGHLIGHTS

General Comments: Cytokines may cause side effects such as chills, aches, fever, severe fatigue, and swelling.

Medication or Drug Class	Dosage	Description	Rationale
Chemotherapeutic agents	Varies with drug	"Dartmouth Regimen": dacarbazine (DTIC),	Decrease replication of malignant cells and

		carmustine, cisplatin, and tamoxifen	kill them
		Other: cisplatin, vinblastine, DTIC	
Immunotherapy (adjuvant immunotherapy with cytokines)	Varies with drug	interferon-alpha; interleukin-2	Enhances immune system to recognize and destroy cancer cell; shrinks metastatic melanomas (effective in 10%–20% of patients)

Independent

Patient and family education is the most important nursing responsibility in preventing, recognizing, and treating the disorder. Educational materials and teaching aids are available from various community and national organizations, the local or state branch of the American Cancer Society, and online computer services. Nursing care of patients who have had surgery is focused on patient education because most of these patients are treated in an ambulatory or short-term stay setting. Instruct patients to protect the site and inspect the incision and graft sites for bleeding or signs of infection. Immobilize recipient graft sites to promote engraftment. Evaluate limbs that have surgical incisions or local isolated chemotherapy to prevent edema.

Reactions to skin disfigurement that occur with some treatments may vary widely. Determine what the cancer experience means to the patient and how it affects the patient's perception of his or her body image. Help the patient achieve the best possible grooming as treatment progresses. Suggest a support group, or if the patient is coping ineffectively, refer for counseling.

DOCUMENTATION GUIDELINES

- Description of any suspicious lesions: Specific location, shape, size, color, condition of surrounding skin, sensations reported by the patient
- Description of incision sites: Presence of redness, swelling, drainage, warmth, tenderness
- Pain: Description of the qualities and location of the pain, effectiveness of pain relief measures

DISCHARGE AND HOME HEALTHCARE GUIDELINES

Teach the patient to protect the incision site from thermal, physical, or chemical trauma. Instruct the patient to inspect the incision site for signs of bleeding or infection. Teach the patient to notify the physician for fever or increased redness, swelling, or tenderness around the incision site. Provide instructions as indicated for specific adjuvant therapy: chemotherapy, radiation, immunotherapy.

Teach the patient strategies for prevention and for modifying the risk factors:

SKIN SELF-EXAMINATION AND IDENTIFICATION OF SUSPICIOUS LESIONS: Moles or nevi that change in size, height, color, texture, sensation, or shape; development of a new mole.

LIMITATION OF ULTRAVIOLET LIGHT EXPOSURE: Avoid the sun between the hours of 10 a.m. and 3 p.m. when the ultraviolet radiation is the strongest; Wear waterproof sunscreen with a sun protection factor of greater than 15 before going outdoors; Apply sunscreen on cloudy days because roughly 70%–80% of ultraviolet rays can penetrate the clouds; Reapply sunscreen every 2 to 3 hours during long sun exposure; Be aware that the sun's rays are reflected by such surfaces as concrete, snow, sand, and water, thereby increasing exposure to ultraviolet rays; Wear protective clothing when outdoors, particularly a wide-brimmed hat to protect the face, scalp, and neck area; Wear wrap-around sunglasses with 99%–100% UV absorption to protect the eyes and the skin area around the eyes; Be aware of medications and cosmetics that increase the sensitivity to ultraviolet rays; Minimize ultraviolet exposure as much as possible and use sunscreen that contains benzophenones; Avoid tanning booths or sunlamps.

Meningitis

DRG Category: 020
Mean LOS: 8.2 days
Description: MEDICAL: Nervous System Infection Except Viral Meningitis
DRG Category: 021
Mean LOS: 8.4 days
Description: MEDICAL: Viral Meningitis

Meningitis is an acute or subacute inflammation of the meninges (lining of the brain and spinal cord). The bacterial or viral pathogens responsible for meningitis usually come from another site, such as those that lead to an upper respiratory infection, sinusitis, or mumps. The organisms can also enter the meninges through open wounds. Bacterial meningitis is considered a medical emergency because the outcome depends on the interval between the onset of disease and the initiation of antimicrobial therapy. In contrast, the viral form of meningitis is sometimes called aseptic or serous meningitis. It is usually self-limiting and, in contrast to the bacterial form, is often described as benign.

In the bacterial form, bacteria enter the meningeal space and elicit an inflammatory response. This process includes the release of a purulent exudate that is spread to other areas of the brain by the cerebrospinal fluid (CSF). If it is left untreated, the CFS becomes thick and blocks the normal circulation of the CFS, which may lead to increased intracranial pressure (ICP) and hydrocephalus. Long-term effects of the illness are predominantly caused by a decreased cerebral blood flow because of increased ICP or toxins related to the infectious exudate. If the infection invades the brain tissue itself, the disease is then classified as encephalitis. Other complications include visual impairment, cranial nerve palsies, deafness, chronic headaches, paralysis, and even coma.

CAUSES

Meningitis is most frequently caused by bacterial or viral agents. In newborns, *Streptococcus pneumoniae* is the most frequent bacterial organism; in other age groups, it is *S. pneumo*niae and *Neisseria meningitidis*. Viral meningitis is caused by many viruses. Depending on the cause, isolation precautions may be indicated early in treatment. There has been a decrease in viral meningitis in locations where immunizations have become routine.

GENDER AND LIFE SPAN CONSIDERATIONS

Meningitis occurs most frequently in young children, elderly people, and persons in a debilitated state. Infants and the very old are at the most risk for pneumococcal meningitis, whereas children from 2 months to 3 years most frequently have haemophilus meningitis. Prognosis is poorest for patients at the extremes of age: the very young and the very old of both sexes.

◻ ASSESSMENT

HISTORY. The history varies according to which form of meningitis the patient has: acute or subacute. For the subacute form, the patient or family may describe vague, mild symptoms such as irritability, loss of appetite, and headaches. With an acute infection, there may be reports of a headache that became progressively worse, with accompanying vomiting, disorientation, or delirium. The patient may also note an increased sensitivity to light (photophobia), chills, fever, and even seizure activity.

Frequently the patient or family describe a recent upper respiratory or other type of infection. A patient with pneumococcal meningitis may have had a recent ear, sinus, or lung infection or endocarditis. It is sometimes associated with other conditions, such as sickle cell disease, basilar skull fracture, splenectomy, or alcoholism. *Haemophilus influenzae* meningitis is also associated with lung and ear infections.

PHYSICAL EXAMINATION. Classically the signs of meningitis are progressive headache, high fever, vomiting, nuchal rigidity (stiff neck that creates pain when flexed toward chest), and change in the patient's level of consciousness or disorientation. Other signs include photophobia (sensitivity of eyes to light), a positive Kernig's sign (inability to extend legs fully when lying supine) and Brudzinski's sign (flexion of the hips when neck is flexed from a supine position), and seizures. Some patients develop signs of increased ICP, such as mental status deterioration with restlessness, confusion, delirium, stupor, and even coma. Patients often experience visual changes; during ophthalmoscopic examination, you may note papilledema and unreactive pupils. Examine babies for bulging fontanels; nuchal rigidity may not be present if the fontanels are open.

An ongoing assessment throughout the patient's hospitalization is important to detect changes in the condition. Serial monitoring for symptoms such as head and neck pain, vomiting, fever, and alterations in fluid and electrolytes is essential. Neurological assessments are completed at timely intervals (every 1 to 2 hours or as indicated by the symptoms), and changes are reported to the physician when appropriate.

PSYCHOSOCIAL. Provide ongoing evaluations to determine the anxiety level and need for information and support. Anxiety is generally present any time there is an illness associated with the brain. Note that some patients or parents feel guilty because of some delay in accessing the healthcare system. Family members may be particularly upset if they witness a seizure.

DIAGNOSTIC HIGHLIGHTS

Test	Normal Result	Abnormality with Condition	Explanation
Lumbar puncture for cerebrospinal fluid (CSF) analysis	Red blood cells: 0–10/μL; white blood cells: 0–10/μL; routine culture: no growth; fungal culture: no growth; mycobacteria culture: no growth; color: clear; protein: 15–50 mg/dL; glucose: 40–80 mg/dL; pressure: 5–13 mm Hg; gram stain: no	Positive cultures with invading micro-organism; sensitivities identify antibiotics that will kill bacteria; cells: > 200/μL; protein: elevated > 50 mg/dL (viral) and > 500 mg/dL (bacterial); glucose: < 45 mg/dL; color: may be cloudy or hazy; pressure: elevated; gram stain: bacteria stain either gram positive (blue) or gram negative (red)	Identifies invading microorganisms. Increased protein occurs as the result of the presence of viruses or bacteria; glucose is decreased as microorganisms use glucose for metabolism. Lumbar puncture is not done in the presence of known increased intracranial pressure.

Other Tests: Brain scan, computed tomography (CT) scan, magnetic resonance imaging (MRI), cultures and sensitivities (blood, nasal swab, urine), C-reactive protein, complete blood count, counterimmunoelectrophoresis (to determine presence of viruses or protozoa in CSF)

PRIMARY NURSING DIAGNOSIS

Infection related to pathogens in the CSF

OUTCOMES. Immune status; Knowledge: Infection control; Risk control; Risk detection; Nutrition status; Treatment behavior: Illness or injury; Hydration; Knowledge: Infection control

INTERVENTIONS. Infection control; Infection protection; Surveillance; Fluid/electrolyte management; Medication management; Temperature regulation

☐ PLANNING AND IMPLEMENTATION

Collaborative

The most critical treatment is the rapid initiation of antibiotic therapy. In addition, assessment and maintenance of airway, breathing, and circulation (ABCs) are essential. Treatment with intubation, mechanical ventilation, and hyperventilation may occur if the patient's airway and breathing are threatened. Serial neurological assessments and vital signs not only monitor critical changes in the patient but also monitor the patient's response to therapy. Supportive measures such as bed rest and temperature control with antipyretics or hypothermia limit oxygen consumption. Gradual treatment of hyperthermia is required to prevent shivering.

Other strategies to manage increased ICP include osmotic diuretics, such as mannitol, or intraventricular CSF drainage and ICP pressure monitoring. Fluids are often restricted if signs of cerebral edema or excessive secretion of antidiuretic hormone are present. If the patient experiences seizures, the physician prescribes anticonvulsant medications. Surgical interventions or CSF drainage may be required to prevent permanent neurologic deficits as a result of complications such as hydrocephalus or abscesses. The patient is likely to have a severe headache from increased ICP. Because large doses of narcotic analgesia mask important neurologic changes, most physicians prescribe a mild analgesic to decrease discomfort. In children, pain relief decreases crying and fretting, which, if left untreated, have the potential to aggravate increased ICP.

Rehabilitation begins with the acute phase of the illness but becomes increasingly important as the infection subsides. If residual neurological dysfunction is present as a result of irritation, pressure, or brain and nerve damage, an individualized rehabilitation program with a multidisciplinary team is required. Vision and auditory testing should be done at discharge and at intervals during long-term recovery because early interventions for these deficits are needed to prevent developmental delays.

PHARMACOLOGIC HIGHLIGHTS

Medication or Drug Class	Dosage	Description	Rationale
Antibiotics	High dose parenteral therapy IV for 2 weeks	Choice of antibiotic depends on gram stain and culture and sensitivities; if no organisms are seen on gram stain, a third-generation cephalosporin is often used while culture results are pending. Broad spectrum coverage such as vancomycin and ceftazidime may be chosen	Cause bacterial lysis and prevent continuation of infection; initial dosages are based on weight or body surface area and then are adjusted according to peak and trough results to maintain therapeutic levels.

Other Drugs: Adjunct corticosteroid therapy has been reported to decrease the inflammatory process and decrease incidence of sensorineural hearing loss but is controversial.

Independent

Make sure that the patient has adequate airway, breathing, and circulation. In the acute phase, the primary goals are to preserve neurologic function and to provide comfort. The head of the bed should be elevated 30 degrees to relieve ICP. Keep the patient's neck in good alignment with the rest of the body and avoid hip flexion. Control environmental stimuli such as light and noise, and institute seizure precautions. Soothing conversation and touch and encouraging the family's participation are important; they are particularly calming with children who need the familiar touch and voices of parents. Children are also reassured by the presence of a security object.

Institute safety precautions to prevent injury, which may result from either he seizure activity or the confusion that is associated with increasing ICP. Take into account an increase in ICP if restraints are used and the patient fights them. Implement measures to limit the effects of immobility, such as skin care, range-of-motion exercises, and a turning and positioning schedule. Note the effect of position changes on ICP, and space activities as necessary.

Explain the disease process and treatments. Alterations can occur in thought processes when ICP begins to increase and the level of consciousness begins to decrease. Reorient the patient to time, place, and person as needed. Keep familiar objects or pictures around. Allow visitation of significant others. Establish alternate means of communication if the patient is unable to maintain verbal contact (for example, the patient who needs intubation). As the patient moves into the rehabilitative phase, developmentally appropriate stimuli are needed to support normal growth and development. Determine the child's progress on developmental tasks. Make appropriate referrals if the child is not progressing or if the child or family evidence signs of inability to cope.

DOCUMENTATION GUIDELINES

- Physiologic response: Neurologic examination; vital signs; presence of fever; adequacy of airway, breathing, and circulation
- Fluid and electrolyte balance: Intake and output, body weight, skin turgor, abnormal serum electrolytes
- Complications: Seizure activity, decreased mental status, fever, increased ICP

DISCHARGE AND HOME HEALTHCARE GUIDELINES

Explain all medications and include the mechanism of action, dosage, route, and side effects. Explain any drug interactions or food interactions. Instruct the patient to notify the primary healthcare provider for signs and symptoms of complications, such as fever, seizures, developmental delays, or behavior changes. Provide referrals and teaching specific to the identified neurologic deficits. Encourage the parents to maintain appropriate activities to facilitate the growth and development of the child.

Migraine Headache

DRG Category: 025
Mean LOS: 3.3 days
Description: MEDICAL: Seizure and Headache Age > 17 without CC

Migraine headache is a primary headache syndrome that is an episodic vascular disorder with or without a common aura. A migraine headache is a prototype of a vascular headache, which involves vasodilation and localized inflammation. Ultimately, arteries are sensitized to pain. Cerebral blood flow is diminished before the onset of the headache and is increased during the actual episode. Most migraine sufferers have a trigger, or precipitating factor, that is associated with the onset of symptoms

There are two types of migraine headaches: classic migraine and common migraine. Classic migraine has a prodromal (pre-headache) phase that lasts approximately 15 minutes and is accompanied by disturbances of neurologic functioning such as visual disturbances, speech disturbances, and paresthesias. Neurologic symptoms cease with the beginning of the headache, which is often accompanied by nausea and vomiting. Common migraine does not have a preheadache phase but is characterized by an immediate onset of a throbbing headache.

CAUSES

Although the causes of migraine headache are uncertain, a commonly held theory is that early vasoconstriction and subsequent vasodilation occur because of the release of biologically active amines such as serotonin, norepinephrine, and epinephrine. These amines are powerful vasoconstrictors, and after their release, degradation and depletion may lead to vasodilation and the headache syndrome. Another theory suggests that neurokinin, a biological substance similar to bradykinin, may be responsible for the inflammatory response.

GENDER AND LIFE SPAN CONSIDERATIONS

Migraine headaches generally begin in childhood or near puberty, affect females more than males, and continue episodically and with decreasing severity until middle age. It is uncommon for migraine headaches to occur throughout old age. Migraine headaches often increase in frequency during pregnancy in the first trimester for those who have experienced them before pregnancy. Oral contraceptives and hormone replacement therapy also increase the frequency of headaches.

☐ ASSESSMENT

HISTORY. Elicit a history of contributing, or triggering, factors such as consumption of red wine, chocolate cake, cheese, alcohol, caffeine, and foods high in refined sugar. Other triggers are the smell of perfume, presence of flickering lights, intake of nicotine, hunger, fatigue, sleep deprivation, physical exertion, and emotional stress. Ask the patient to describe the symptoms that are associated with the headache. Generally, migraine headaches are unilateral with pulsating or throbbing pain and are associated with nausea, vomiting, and phonophotophobia (intolerance to light and noise). Duration lasts from 4 to 72 hours, although the pain builds over minutes to hours.

Elicit a description from the patient of all symptoms. Classic migraines are associated with a transient visual, motor, sensory, cognitive, or psychic disturbance that lasts up to 15 minutes and precedes the headache. A second phase occurs with numbness or tingling of the lips, changes in mental status (confusion, drowsiness), aphasia, and dizziness. Common migraines have an immediate onset of throbbing pain. Early warning is often a mood change, and pain is often accompanied by nausea and vomiting. Elicit the timing and pattern of episodes. Two to four attacks a month, often beginning in the mornings and usually lasting a day or two, are a common pattern. If the patient is a female, determine the timing of the menstrual cycle, any birth control pills or hormone replacement therapy, and if the patient is pregnant.

PHYSICAL EXAMINATION. Perform a neurologic assessment to determine focal neurologic dysfunction (such as drowsiness, vertigo, aphasia, unilateral weakness, confusion) and visual disturbances (such as spots, lines, or shimmering light). Test the cranial nerves, particularly cranial nerves V, IX, and X. The patient has no signs and symptoms when the headache is not present, but other disorders need to be ruled out before the initial diagnosis of migraine headache is made.

PSYCHOSOCIAL. Psychosocial assessment should include assessment of the degree of stress the person experiences and the strategies he or she uses to cope with stress. Determine the patient's lifestyle patterns, such as exercise patterns, family relationships, rest and work patterns, and substance abuse patterns.

DIAGNOSTIC HIGHLIGHTS

No test is diagnostic for migraine headaches. The following tests may be necessary for differential diagnosis: computed tomography scan, skull x ray, cranial nerve testing, arteriogram, lumbar puncture, cerebrospinal fluid testing, electroencephalogram, magnetic resonance imaging.

PRIMARY NURSING DIAGNOSIS

Pain related to vasoconstriction or vasodilation

OUTCOMES. Comfort level; Pain control behavior; Pain level; Symptom control behavior; Symptom severity; Pain: Disruptive effects; Well-being

INTERVENTIONS. Medication administration; Medication management; Pain management; Comfort; Nutritional monitoring; Environmental management: Comfort; Biofeedback; Sleep enhancement; Guided imagery

☐ PLANNING AND IMPLEMENTATION

Collaborative

Most patients can have their migraine headaches managed pharmacologically. Dietary modification may decrease symptoms; this includes reducing the intake of caffeinated beverages, monosodium glutamate, cheese, sausage, sauerkraut, citrus fruit, chocolate, and red wine.

PHARMACOLOGIC HIGHLIGHTS

Medication or Drug Class	Dosage	Description	Rationale
Nonnarcotic analgesics	Varies with drug	Either aspirin, acetaminophen, or nonsteroidal anti-inflammatory agents may abort a migraine headache if it is taken early; ketorolac tromethamine, naproxen sodium, flurbiprofen, indomethacin, isometheptene, butalbital with aspirin or acetamin reduce headache pain	Abort or relieve a migraine headache

Prochlorperazine	5–10 mg IV	Anti-emetic, anti-psychotic that terminates migraines and helps alleviate nausea	Relieves a migraine headache
Ergotamine	2–3 mg po; may add additional doses to reach 8–10 mg; dosages exceeding 16 mg per week should	Anti-migraine that may have an agonist/antagonist action with alpha adrenergic, serotonergic, and dopaminergic receptors; directly stimulates vascular smooth muscle, constricting arteries and veins	To prevent or abort migraine headache
Dihydroergotamine (DHE)	1–2 mg IM or SC; during the peak of a headache 5–10 mg or prochlorpera-zine may be given IV followed by 0.75 mg of DHE IV over 3 minutes	Venoconstrictor with minimal peripheral arterial constriction; use with caution with patients with cardiac disease	Relieves the pain of migraine headache
Sumatriptan	25–100 mg po initially and may be repeated in 2 hours; may be given as a 6 mg SC dose	Anti-migraine that acts by binding with vascular receptors producing a vasoconstrictive effect on cranial blood vesssel	Relieves the pain of migraine headache
Beta blockers, tricyclic antidepressants, calcium channel blockers	Varies with drug	Used to prevent headaches, particularly those that do not respond to acute therapy	To prevent migraine headaches

Independent

Teach the patient to avoid triggers that may lead to headaches. Patients may be sensitive to odors from cigarette or cigar smoke, paint, gasoline, perfume, or aftershave lotion. Explain to the patient that at the beginning of an attack, he or she may be able to limit pain by resting in a darkened room. If patients sleep uninterrupted with their eyes covered, symptoms may be alleviated.

A combination of complementary therapies may be successful in managing symptoms. Introduce to the patient the possibility of behavior therapy such as biofeedback, exercise therapy, and relaxation techniques. Explore with the patient some techniques for stress reduction and adequate rest. Discuss family- or work-related stress to determine a regimen that may reduce stress and provide for adequate rest and relaxation. Life style management may be essential to control headaches. Ask a dietician to evaluate the patient's food intake and to work with the patient to develop a diet that will minimize exposure to triggers.

DOCUMENTATION GUIDELINES

- Discomfort: Timing, character, location, duration, precipitating factors
- Nutrition: Food and fluid intake; understanding of dietary restriction
- Medication management: Understanding of drug therapy, response to medications

- Response to alternative treatments: Success of treatment, interest in developing other non-traditional management strategies

DISCHARGE AND HOME HEALTHCARE GUIDELINES

Teach the patient how to maintain lifestyle changes with regard to rest, nutrition, and medication management. Make sure that the patient and family understand all aspects of the treatment regimen. Review dietary limitations and recommendations, and make sure the patient understands the dosage and side effects of all medications. Provide a referral to a headache clinic that teaches alternative therapies.

Mitral Insufficiency (Regurgitation)

DRG Category: 135
Mean LOS: 4.3 days
Description: MEDICAL: Cardiac Congenital and Valvular Disorders, Age > 17 with CC
DRG Category: 105
Mean LOS: 11.0 days
Description: SURGICAL: Cardiac Valve Procedures without CC
DRG Category: 104
Mean LOS: 15.2 days
Description: SURGICAL: Cardiac Valve Procedures with CC

Mitral insufficiency, or mitral regurgitation, is the inadequate closure of the mitral valve, which interferes with expulsion of cardiac output from the left ventricle. The mitral valve is located between the left atrium and left ventricle. When the heart contracts, blood is moved forward from the left ventricle out through the aortic valve and into the aorta. During the high pressures that are generated during contraction, blood flows backward through the regurgant valve into the left atrium. Cardiac output, therefore, is separated into forward systemic flow into the aorta and backward regurgitant flow into the left atrium. The amount of forward versus backward flow depends on the severity of the mitral insufficiency and the afterload (impedance to flow against which the left ventricle pumps).

Mitral insufficiency causes an increase in blood volume in both the left atrium and the ventricle. This situation occurs because of the regurgitant blood that flows from left atrium to left ventricle to left atrium again. The increased volume of blood in chronic mitral insufficiency accumulates slowly, allowing the left atrium and left ventricle to increase in size. The heart, therefore, tolerates the regurgitant blood flow without engorgement of the pulmonary circulation or reduction of cardiac output. In acute mitral insufficiency, the left atrium and ventricle are not able to tolerate the dramatic increase in blood volume, so cardiac output decreases and blood backs up quickly into the pulmonary circulation. Pulmonary congestion and acute illness follows.

CAUSES

Common causes of chronic mitral insufficiency are rheumatic heart disease, endocarditis, congenital anomaly, and idiopathic calcification of the mitral annulus, which inhibits valve closure. Calcification associated with aging has been found on autopsies; however, with most patients there was a minimal functional consequence. Connective tissue diseases (Marfan's syndrome, Ehlers-Danlos syndrome) are also associated with mitral insufficiency. Mitral valve prolapse, a common form of mitral insufficiency, occurs with degeneration of mitral leaflets, which causes a "floppy valve." Acute mitral insufficiency can occur with myocardial infarctions that have been caused by ischemia or necrosis of the papillary muscle or by chordae tendineae that support the mitral leaflets.

GENDER AND LIFE SPAN CONSIDERATIONS

Mitral insufficiency can occur at any age, depending on the cause. Mitral valve prolapse is more common in females and peaks in the 30s. Chronic insufficiency increases with age and is therefore more common in the aging population.

☐ ASSESSMENT

HISTORY. Question the patient about a history of rheumatic fever because 50% of all cases of chronic mitral insufficiency are attributed to rheumatic heart disease. Because mitral valve prolapse, a common form of mitral insufficiency, has a familial association, determine if others in the family have the condition. Coronary heart disease contributes to both chronic and acute disorders; therefore, ask the patient if he or she has chest pain or palpitations. Determine if the patient has the classic symptoms of fatigue and shortness of breath. Other symptoms include orthopnea, palpitations, irregular heartbeat, exertional dyspnea, edema, and weight loss.

PHYSICAL EXAMINATION. Inspection and palpation of the precordium are usually unremarkable except in extreme cases of mitral insufficiency. Auscultation of the chest usually reveals a soft first heart sound and a systolic murmur, which is loudest at the apex. In severe mitral insufficiency, you may hear an S_3 gallop. Auscultation of breathing may reveal fine crackles (rales) if pulmonary congestion is present. When the abdomen is palpated, you may note an enlarged liver if the patient has severe right-sided heart failure. The patient may also have jugular vein distension and a prominent alpha wave.

PSYCHOSOCIAL. In an effort to avoid exertional dyspnea and fatigue, patients usually adjust their lifestyles by restricting their activity and resting frequently. They may not notice the increasing fatigue until it gets debilitating. Assess the patient's level of exercise and how he or she copes with activity intolerance.

DIAGNOSTIC HIGHLIGHTS

Test	Normal Result	Abnormality with Condition	Explanation
Transesophageal echocardiogram	Normal mitral valve	Incompetent mitral valve	Mitral valve is incompetent and during the systolic phase, blood flows

		backward into the left atrium; left-sided heart chambers may be enlarged, with an increased left ventricular end-diastolic volume	
Cardiac catheterization	Normal mitral valve	Systolic regurgitant flow from the left ventricle into left atrium; left sided hypertrophy and/or dilation of heart; may have a decreased left ventricular ejection fraction	Same as above
Doppler echocardiography	Normal mitral valve	Incompetent mitral valve	Same as above

Other Tests: Electrocardiogram (ECG) may show atrial fibrillation, chest radiography, prothrombin time, activated partial thromboplastin time (APPT)

PRIMARY NURSING DIAGNOSIS

Activity intolerance related to diminished cardiac output

OUTCOMES. Energy conservation; Coping; Knowledge: Disease process; Mood equilibrium; Symptom severity; Health beliefs: Perceived control; Knowledge: Medication; Treatment regimen

INTERVENTIONS. Energy management; Counseling; Exercise promotion; Hope instillation; Security management; Security enhancement; Presence; Medication management; Teaching: Prescribed diet and medications

□ PLANNING AND IMPLEMENTATION

Collaborative

Physicians place most patients with advanced mitral insufficiency on activity restrictions to decrease cardiac workload. Research suggests that if the patient is on bed rest, the use of a bedside commode creates less workload for the heart than using a bedpan. Fluid restrictions and diuretics may be ordered to reduce pulmonary congestion. Supplemental oxygen enhances gas exchange and oxygenation to decrease dyspnea and chest pain.

Most patients with mitral insufficiency can compensate or be stabilized with medical treatment for their entire lives. Surgical repair or valve replacement is considered in patients with progressive severe disease. Mitral valve repair (valvuloplasty) is preferred over replacement whenever possible. The choice of valve type is based on the patient's age and the potential for clotting problems. A biologic valve (such as a porcine valve from a pig) usually shows structural deterioration after 6 to 10 years and needs to be replaced. A synthetic valve is more durable but also is more prone to thrombi formation. If the incompetent valve is replaced surgically with a synthetic valve, patients are prescribed long-term anticoagulant therapy, such as warfarin (Coumadin). See "Coronary Artery Disease" for a further discussion of the collaborative and independent management of patients after open heart surgery.

PHARMACOLOGIC HIGHLIGHTS

Medication or Drug Class	Dosage	Description	Rationale
Diuretics	Varies with drug	Thiazides; loop diuretics	Manage fluid overload and congestive symptoms
Coronary vasodilators	Varies with drug	Nitroglycerine, nitroprusside, captopril, enalapril, hydralazine	Decrease preload and afterload; decrease regurgitant blood flow; reduce ventricular size
Warfarin	Initially 10–15 mg, then 2–10 mg per day maintenance	Anticoagulant	Prevents thrombi from forming on the synthetic valve
Heparin	Initially 80 units/kg IV bolus, followed by an infusion of 18 units/kg; serial APPT monitoring to guide future doses	Anticoagulant	Prevents thrombi initially until warfarin therapy is well regulated

Other Drugs: Inotropic agents (dobutamine [Dobutrex], digoxin) are used to enhance the heart's pumping ability. If they are present, dysrhythmias are treated with antidysrhythmics, such as propranolol (Inderal) or quinidine.

Independent

Maintain airway, breathing, and circulation. If the patient is stable, focus on reducing the cardiac workload and psychological stress to reduce the metabolic demands of the myocardium. Provide assistance with activities of daily living, and encourage the patient to abide by activity restrictions to allow for adequate rest. Establish a quiet environment with uninterrupted rest periods, if possible. To ease the patient's breathing, elevate the head of the bed. Encourage the patient to avoid sudden changes in position to minimize increased cardiac demand and dizziness. Instruct the patient to sit on the edge of the bed before standing.

Reduce psychological stress by approaching the patient and family in a calm, relaxed manner. Decrease fear of the unknown by providing explanations and encouraging questions. Help the patient maintain or reestablish a sense of control by participating in decisions about aspects of care. If the patient decides to have valve surgery, offer to let the patient speak with someone who already has had the surgery.

DOCUMENTATION GUIDELINES

- Physical findings: Cardiopulmonary assessment, presence of murmurs and rales, vital signs

- Response to interventions and medications: Diuretics, nitrates, vasodilators, inotropic agents, and antidysrhythmic medications
- Reaction to activity restrictions, fluid restrictions, and cardiac diagnosis
- Presence of complications: Chest pain, bleeding, dyspnea, wound infection

DISCHARGE AND HOME HEALTHCARE GUIDELINES

Be sure the patient understands all medications, including the dosage, route, action, and adverse effects, and the need for routine laboratory monitoring for anticoagulants. Explain the need to avoid activities that may predispose the patient to excessive bleeding; hold pressure on bleeding sites to assist in clotting. Remind the patient to notify healthcare workers of anticoagulant use before procedures. Identify foods high in vitamin K, such as turnips, spinach, liver, and cauliflower, which should be limited so the effect of warfarin is not reversed. Instruct the patient to report the recurrence or escalation of signs and symptoms of mitral insufficiency. The appearance of these symptoms could indicate that the medical therapy needs readjusting or that the replaced valve is malfunctioning. Patients with synthetic valves may hear an audible click from the valve closure. The click sounds like the ticking of a watch.

Patients who have had valvular disorders or valve surgery are susceptible to bacterial endocarditis, which causes scarring or destruction of the heart valves. Bacterial endocarditis may result from dental work, surgeries, and invasive procedures, so people who have repaired or replaced heart valves should be given antibiotics before and after these treatments.

Mitral Stenosis

DRG Category: 135
Mean LOS: 4.3 days
Description: MEDICAL: Cardiac Congenital and Valvular Disorders, Age > 17 with CC
DRG Category: 105
Mean LOS: 11.0 days
Description: SURGICAL: Cardiac Valve Procedures without CC
DRG Category: 104
Mean LOS: 15.2 days
Description: SURGICAL: Cardiac Valve Procedures with CC

Mitral stenosis, a pathologic narrowing of the orifice of the mitral valve, occurs when the mitral valve is unable to open fully. The opening of the mitral valve, normally 4 to 6 cm^2 in area, is decreased to half normal size or even smaller because of a series of changes in valve structure. The mitral valve leaflets fuse together and become stiff and thickened by fibrosis and calcification. The chordae tendineae fuse together and shorten, and the valvular cusps lose their flexibility.

The mitral valve is located between the left atrium and the left ventricle. When mitral stenosis occurs, blood can flow from the left atrium to the ventricle only if it is moved forward by an abnormally elevated left atrial pressure. The elevated left atrial pressure leads to increased pulmonary venous and capillary pressures, decreased pulmonary compliance, and exertional dyspnea. Left atrial dilatation, an increase in pulmonary artery pressure, and right ventricular hypertrophy follow as the heart compensates for the stenotic valve.

Complications of mitral stenosis can be serious. Pulmonary edema develops with sudden changes in flow across the mitral valve, such as the increased flow that occurs in exercise. Atrial dysrhythmias, particularly paroxysmal atrial tachycardia, atrial flutter, and atrial fibrillation, occur with more long-standing disease. Pulmonary hypertension can cause fibrosis of the alveoli and pulmonary capillaries. Recurrent pulmonary emboli, pulmonary infections, infective endocarditis, and systemic embolization are all potential complications.

CAUSES

The predominant cause of mitral stenosis is rheumatic fever. Approximately 40% of individuals with rheumatic heart disease have pure or predominant mitral stenosis. A congenital absence of one of the papillary muscles, resulting in a parachute deformity of the mitral valve, is rare. This deformity is observed almost exclusively in infants and young children. Other uncommon causes of mitral stenosis include malignant carcinoid syndrome, systemic lupus erythematosus, rheumatoid arthritis, thrombus formation, and the mucopolysaccharidoses of the Hunter-Hurley phenotype.

GENDER AND LIFE SPAN CONSIDERATIONS

Approximately two-thirds of the patients with mitral stenosis are female. Two-thirds of all women with rheumatic mitral stenosis are younger than age 45.

☐ ASSESSMENT

HISTORY. Because patients generally have a history of either rheumatic fever or a genetic predisposition to valvular heart disease, ask about specific dates and treatments related to the initial episode of rheumatic fever. Note the use of prophylactic antibiotics against the recurrence of rheumatic fever.

Patients may remain asymptomatic for a period of 10 to 15 years after the diagnosis. Once the valve orifice decreases to less than 2.5 cm^2, however, any physiologic state that causes an increase in cardiac output (exercise, fever, anxiety, pain, pregnancy) or a decrease in diastolic filling time (tachycardias, atrial fibrillation) may cause the patient to complain of excessive fatigue, malaise, decreased tolerance to exercise, dyspnea on exertion, orthopnea, paroxysmal nocturnal dyspnea, and dry cough.

PHYSICAL EXAMINATION. As the valve orifice becomes increasingly narrowed, symptoms of right-sided heart failure may occur. Inspect the patient for neck vein distension and pitting peripheral edema. Pulmonary edema may also occur and lead to orthopnea, tachypnea, diaphoresis, pallor, cyanosis, and pink frothy sputum. Palpate the patient's abdomen for hepatomegaly, and auscultate the patient's lungs for crackles.

You may note a normal apical pulse or an irregular rate associated with atrial fibrillation when the heart is auscultated. There are four principal findings: (1) a loud apical first heart sound (closure of the stenotic mitral valve); (2) an opening snap (the snapping of the stenotic mitral valve); (3) a rumbling, apical diastolic low-frequency murmur (blood flowing with difficulty and under increased pressure through the stenotic mitral valve); (4) an increased pulmonic second sound associated with pulmonary hypertension.

PSYCHOSOCIAL. Often patients have been living with the diagnosis for more than 10 years. The possibility of open-heart surgery presents a crisis for patients who fear for their lives. In addition, their symptoms may interfere with activities of daily living. Assess the patient's degree of anxiety and ability to cope with the disease.

DIAGNOSTIC HIGHLIGHTS

Test	Normal Result	Abnormality with Condition	Explanation
Transesophageal echocardiogram	Normal mitral valve	Stenotic mitral valve, left atrial enlargement	Opening of mitral valve is narrow, which elevates left atrial pressure and leads to left atrial hypertrophy and right ventricular hypertrophy
Cardiac catheterization	Normal mitral valve	Stenotic mitral valve; elevation of left atrial pressure, elevation of pulmonary capillary pressures and venous pressures, left atrial enlargement	Same as above
Doppler echocardiography	Normal mitral valve	Stenotic mitral valve; left atrial enlargement	Same as above

Other Tests: Electrocardiogram (ECG) may show atrial fibrillation, chest radiography, prothrombin time, activated partial thromboplastin time (APPT)

PRIMARY NURSING DIAGNOSIS

Activity intolerance related to pulmonary congestion and decreased blood supply to meet the demands of the body

OUTCOMES. Energy conservation; Coping; Knowledge: Disease process; Mood equilibrium; Symptom severity; Health beliefs: Perceived control; Knowledge: Medication; Treatment regimen

INTERVENTIONS. Energy management; Counseling; Exercise promotion; Hope instillation; Security management; Security enhancement; Presence; Medication management; Teaching: Prescribed diet and medications

☐ PLANNING AND IMPLEMENTATION

Collaborative

Once symptomatic, a patient usually progresses from mild to total disability in 5 to 10 years. This downhill course can be accelerated by conversion from a normal cardiac rhythm to atrial fibrillation or by pregnancy, bacterial endocarditis, or embolization.

Definitive therapy for mitral stenosis is surgical replacement of the stenotic valve, particularly when the valve has marked stenosis with an oriface less than 1 cm². Postoperative anticoagulation is not required. Therefore, even patients with mild symptoms are candidates for surgery. Patients who have more severe, disabling symptoms are more likely to require valve replacement. Either a bioprosthetic or a mechanical valve is used by the surgeon, depending on the patient's condition and the surgeon's preference. Percutaneous valvuloplasty may be used in young patients without calcification, by symptomatic pregnant women, and by elderly individuals who are poor risks for open heart surgery. (See "Coronary Artery Disease," for collaborative and independent interventions for the patient who is undergoing open heart surgery.)

PHARMACOLOGIC HIGHLIGHTS

Medication or Drug Class	Dosage	Description	Rationale
Diuretics	Varies with drug	Thiazides; loop diuretics	Manage fluid overload and congestive symptoms
Warfarin	Initially 10–15 mg, then 2–10 mg per day maintenance	Anticoagulant	Prevents thrombi from forming on the synthetic valve; indicated for patients with atrial fibrillation
Heparin	Initially 80 units/kg IV bolus, followed by an infusion of 18 units/kg; serial APPT monitoring to guide future doses	Anticoagulant	Prevents thrombi initially until warfarin therapy is well regulated

Other Drugs: Inotropic agents (dobutamine [Dobutrex], digoxin) are used to enhance the heart's pumping ability. If they are present, dysrhythmias are treated with antidysrhythmics, such as propranolol (Inderal) or quinidine.

Independent

Focus on early detection and management of symptoms and the prevention of complications. Interventions depend on the stage of the disease process. If the patient is newly diagnosed, patient teaching becomes important because of the patient's knowledge deficit. If the patient has severe symptoms that interfere with the ability to perform daily functions, strategies to maintain rest and conserve energy become important. If the patient is a surgical candidate, preoperative and postoperative management are the priority.

During periods of activity intolerance, encourage the patient to maintain bed rest and to allow full assistance with hygiene activities. Provide a bedside commode rather than a bedpan to decrease energy expenditure during voiding. Encourage the patient to keep the head of the bed elevated to at least 30 degrees. Support both arms with pillows to ease breathing and to augment chest excursion. Explore with the patient preferred diversionary activities, such as reading, watching television, needlework, listening to the radio, or quiet visitation with friends and family. Monitor the number of visitors to ensure that the patient is not overfatigued.

Encourage the patient and family to discuss their fears about the progress of the symptoms or the possibility of surgery. Answer questions honestly, provide accurate information, and allow the patient and significant others time to digest information before adding additional content. If the patient needs surgical intervention, evaluate the patient's home situation to determine if additional home assistance will be needed after discharge.

DOCUMENTATION GUIDELINES

- Physical findings of the cardiopulmonary and renal systems: Heart and breath sounds, vital signs, capillary refill, pulmonary artery pressure readings if applicable, intake and output, daily weights
- Presence of complications that are associated with mitral stenosis: Atrial fibrillation, pulmonary edema, heart failure
- Response to medications used to treat the symptoms and complications that are associated with mitral stenosis
- Tolerance to activity
- Response to surgical intervention: Wound healing, fluid balance, pulmonary artery pressures and cardiac output, urine output, chest tube drainage

DISCHARGE AND HOME HEALTHCARE GUIDELINES

Assess the patient's home environment to determine if additional assistance will be needed after discharge. Be sure the patient understands all medications, including the dosage, route, action, and adverse effects. Instruct the patient to report orthopnea, tachypnea, diaphoresis, frothy sputum, irregular pulse, and chest discomfort.

Mononucleosis, Infectious

DRG Category: 421
Mean LOS: 4.0 days
Description: MEDICAL: Viral Illness, Age > 17

The term *mononucleosis* refers to the presence of an abnormally high number of mononuclear leukocytes (white blood cells) in the body. Infectious mononucleosis (IM) results from a viral syndrome that is caused by the Epstein-Barr virus (EBV). The virus is introduced into the host by close contact with another individual who is shedding EBV in the oropharynx. The virus replicates in epithelial cells of the pharynx and salivary glands. A localized inflammatory response produces the pharyngeal exudate. The virus is then carried via the lymphatics to the lymph nodes. Local and generalized lymphadenopathy (disease of the lymph nodes) develops.

Major complications are rare but may include splenic or liver rupture, aseptic meningitis or encephalitis, pericarditis, or hemolytic anemia. EBV has been linked to Burkitt's lymphoma, in Africa, and to nasopharyngeal carcinoma, particularly in Asians. Mononucleosis can also lead to Guillain-Barré syndrome.

CAUSES

Infection with EBV, a herpes virus, is common throughout the world in humans. EBV is probably spread via the oropharyngeal or respiratory route. EBV is also transmitted by blood transfusion.

GENDER AND LIFE SPAN CONSIDERATIONS

IM rarely occurs in children under 5 years old. Infection occurs early in life, however, among individuals of lower socioeconomic groups and in developing countries. IM is most often diagnosed in adolescents who come from higher socioeconomic groups and in college students. The peak incidence of IM is ages 16 to 18 in boys and 14 to 16 in girls. Approximately 12% to 30% of the total cases of IM occur among university students and military cadets. By adulthood, most individuals have had at least one infection with EBV.

☐ ASSESSMENT

HISTORY. The patient often reveals contact with a person who has had IM. Although children have a short incubation period of about 10 days, symptoms in adults may not appear until 1 to 2 months after exposure to the EBV. The patient with suspected IM typically reports a history of fever and fatigue for 1 week, followed by a sore throat (often described as the most painful the patient has ever experienced). Other symptoms include anorexia, painful swallowing, and swelling of the lymph nodes.

PHYSICAL EXAMINATION. Note the redness of the pharynx and observe for exudate. Observe for petechiae that may appear at the junction of the hard and soft palates (occurs in 25% of patients). Note any facial edema, particularly eyelid edema. Facial edema is rarely encountered in other illnesses of young adults and is suggestive of IM. Some patients have a maculopapular rash (discolored patches of skin mixed with elevated red pimples). Palpate for enlarged lymph nodes in the cervical and epitrochlear (around the elbow) areas. Significant adenopathy is almost always present, and its absence should make one doubt the diagnosis of IM. During an abdominal examination, palpate for an enlarged spleen (occurring in 50% of patients) and liver.

PSYCHOSOCIAL. The patient with IM has a viral illness that may last up to 4 weeks. Since most cases occur in college students, IM may prevent the student from performing academically at pre-illness levels. If the student falls behind in his or her studies, the student or parents may feel anxious or stressed. Assess the patient's ability to cope with the interference with school tasks. Determine if the patient has discussed the illness with his or her professors and if arrangements have been made to make up work or withdraw from school if needed. If the young adult is employed rather than in school, determine if the patient has told the employer of his or her healthcare needs.

DIAGNOSTIC HIGHLIGHTS

Test	Normal Result	Abnormality with Condition	Explanation
Complete blood count with	Red blood cells (RBCs) 4.0–5.5	Lymphocytosis with characteristic	Determines extent of viral infection and

differential	million/μL; white blood cells 4,500–11,000/μL; hemoglobin (Hg) 12–18 g/dL; hematocrit (Hct) 37%–54% reticulocyte count 0.5%–2.5% of total RBCs; platelets 150,000–400,000/μL; segmented neutrophils 54%–62%; band neutrophils 3%–5%; eosinophils 1%–3%; basophils < 1%; monocytes 3%–7%; lymphocytes 25%–33%	atypical lymphocytes in peripheral blood	immune dysfunction
IgM antibodies	Negative	Presence of specific antibodies for EBV antigens (viral capsid antigens, early antigents, or Epstein-Barr nuclear antigen)	Identifies presence of Epstein-Barr virus
Monospot	Negative	Presence of heterophil antibodies	Identifies 90% of adult cases with Epstein-Barr virus

PRIMARY NURSING DIAGNOSIS

Risk for ineffective airway clearance related to oropharyngeal swelling

OUTCOMES. Respiratory status: Gas exchange and ventilation; Safety status: Physical injury; Comfort level

INTERVENTIONS. Airway insertion; Airway management; Airway suctioning; Oral health promotion; Respiratory monitoring; Ventilation assistance; Surveillance; Pain management; Analgesic administration; Anxiety reduction

◻ PLANNING AND IMPLEMENTATION

Collaborative

Most patients require nothing more than supportive therapy, such as acetaminophen for fever and bed rest for fatigue. Pain relief is essential if the patient is to maintain fluid intake to prevent fluid volume deficit and dehydration.

To prevent upper airway obstruction from severe tonsillar enlargement, treatment with corticosteroids (prednisone 40 mg per day for 5 to 7 days) is sometimes indicated. If the patient is at risk for airway obstruction (a rare complication), endotracheal intubation may be necessary. About 20% of patients also need a 10-day course of antibiotic therapy because of streptococcal pharyngotonsillitis. Ruptured spleen is an unusual but serious complication that causes sudden abdominal pain and is managed surgically by removal of the spleen.

PHARMACOLOGIC HIGHLIGHTS

No specific pharmacologic therapy treats mononucleosis; anti-viral medications do not limit the EBV infection. Patients usually require analgesia with acetaminophen, propoxyphene (Darvon), or even oral narcotics. Some patients may also be placed on corticosteroids or antibiotics.

Independent

Most patients do not require hospitalization for IM. Focus on supportive care and teaching. Encourage the patient to use anesthetic lozenges or warm saline gargles for pharyngitis. A soft diet such as milkshakes, sherbets, soups, and puddings provides additional liquid and nutritional supplements. Teach patients to avoid strenuous activities and contact sports until liver and spleen enlargement subsides.

DOCUMENTATION GUIDELINES

- Physical findings of pharyngitis, lymphadenopathy, splenomegaly, fever, fatigue
- Reaction to activity and immobility
- Plan to deal with prolonged confinement and possible suspension of activities

DISCHARGE AND HOME HEALTHCARE GUIDELINES

Teach the patient to prevent splenic rupture by avoiding minor trauma, heavy lifting, overexertion, and contact sports for 1 to 2 months. Teach strategies to avoid constipation and straining because these problems cause increased pressure on the spleen. Suggest over-the-counter medications for comfort. Encourage the patient to rest during the acute illness and convalescence period. Note that prolonged fatigue is not uncommon. Encourage students to notify professors about the illness and to arrange for less-demanding assignments during the recovery period. Recommend that the patient plan for a recovery period of several weeks before resuming regular activities, academics, or employment.

Instruct the patient to promptly report to the physician any abdominal and upper quadrant pain radiating to the shoulder. In addition, if the patient reports shortness of breath or inability to swallow, he or she should call 911 for emergency help because tracheostomy or intubation may become necessary.

Multiple Myeloma

DRG Category: 403
Mean LOS: 7.4 days
Description: MEDICAL: Lymphoma and Non-Acute Leukemia with CC

Multiple myeloma, also known as plasma cell myeloma, malignant plasmacytoma, and myelomatosis, is a type of cancer formed by malignant plasma cells (a mature, active B lymphocyte). When a B lymphocyte is stimulated by a T cell, it develops into a mature, antibody-producing factory called a plasma cell. Multiple myeloma results from a transformed plasma cell that multiplies and produces antibody unceasingly, without stimulation. When plasma cells grow out of control, they generate tumors that infiltrate the bone marrow and other sites. Although multiple myeloma could be considered a lymphoma, it is generally classified differently and discussed separately because it presents a different profile of onset, symptoms, treatment, and prognosis.

The disease infiltrates bone and produces osteolytic lesions throughout the skeleton, destroying bones. In later stages, multiple myeloma infiltrates the body organs and destroys them as well. About 3 to 20 years of plasma cell growth may pass before symptoms become apparent. When patients do report symptoms, the disease is well advanced. Survival rates depend on the stage of initial diagnosis. (See Table 35.) The 5-year survival rate for stage I patients is about 50%, with a median survival rate of 60 months. Stage II patients have a 5-year survival rate of 40%, with a median survival rate of 41 months; stage III patients have a 5-year survival rate of 10% to 25%, with median survival time of 23 months.

TABLE 35 | **Staging System for Multiple Myeloma**

STAGE	EXTENT OF DISEASE
I	Low tumor mass ($<0.6 \times 10^{12}$ plasma cells/m^2)
	Must have all of the following:
	Hemoglobin >10 g/dl
	Normal serum calcium (<12 mg/dL)
	Low M-component (IgM) production rates (<0.6) with
	IgG values <5 g/dL
	IgA values <3 g/dL
	Urine light chain M-component <4 g/dL in 24 hours
	Normal x ray or one solitary plasmacytoma
II	Intermediate tumor mass ($<0.6–1.2 \times 10^{12}$ plasma cells/m^2)
	Patients who do not qualify in I and III
III	High tumor mass ($>1.2 \times 10^{12}$ plasma cells/m^2)
	Any one of the following:
	Hemoglobin <8.5 mg/dL
	Serum calcium level >12 mg/dL
	Normal x ray or one solitary plasmacytoma
	High M-component (IgM) production rates (>1.20) with
	IgG values >7 g/dL
	IgA values < or >5 g/dL (depending on variety of multiple myeloma)
	Urine light chain M-component >12 g/dL in 24 hours
	Excessive lytic bone lesions

Multiple myeloma causes a number of complications, including infections such as pneumonia. Other complications are pyelonephritis, renal calculi and renal failure, hematologic imbalance and gastrointestinal or nasal bleeding, hypercalcemia, hyperuricemia, dehydration, and fractures.

CAUSES

The cause is unknown. A variety of factors may predispose an individual to the development of the disease, including exposure to radiation, genetic factors, occupational exposure to petroleum products, other plasma cell diseases, and chronic antigen stimulation. Some patients with multiple myeloma have a history of chronic infections.

GENDER AND LIFE SPAN CONSIDERATIONS

Multiple myeloma is primarily a disease of late middle-aged to elderly persons. The disease may have been developing slowly for many years before diagnosis, however. The average age at diagnosis is 70 years; more men are affected than women. For unknown reasons, rates for African-Americans are twice that of European-Americans.

◻ ASSESSMENT

HISTORY. Establish a history of bone-related pain. Determine if the patient has experienced constant back pain that intensifies with exercise, other aching bone pain, or arthritic-type joint pain. Ask if the patient has experienced any numbness, prickling, or tingling of the extremities (peripheral paresthesia); confusion; fatigue; or weakness. Determine if the patient has experienced weight loss, nausea, vomiting, polyuria, or polydipsia. Ask if the patient has been exposed to radiation on the job or has undergone radiation therapy. Establish a history of body height reduction; vertebral collapse may cause a reduction in height of up to 5 inches or more. Find out if the patient has relatives who have been diagnosed with multiple myeloma.

PHYSICAL EXAMINATION. Examine for signs of pathologic compression fractures of the vertebral column or long bones. Inspect for joint swelling. Note any joint, long bone, or flat bone tenderness. Note cranial nerve palsies, which may be caused by tumor occlusion of vascular flow. Radiculopathies develop from nerve root compression where there is bone infiltration. Carpal tunnel syndrome is common. In advanced cases, noticeable thoracic deformities may be observable. With patients already on chemotherapy for multiple myeloma, note any signs of infection, such as fever and malaise.

PSYCHOSOCIAL. The psychosocial needs of the patient with multiple myeloma may be complex. The patient faces coping with a chronic, painful, and potentially fatal disease that is treated with potentially painful and uncomfortable regimens. Be sensitive to the enormous psychological strain placed on the patient. Consider the effects of the disease on the patient's job status, personal relationships, financial resources, and body image. Assess the patient's support network.

DIAGNOSTIC HIGHLIGHTS

Test	Normal Result	Abnormality with Condition	Explanation
Serum protein electrophoresis; urine protein electrophoresis	Presence of normal immuno-globulins: IgM, IgG, IgE, IgD, IgA	Presence of abnormally low levels of immuno-globulins; presence of abnormal immuno-globulins: monoclonal immunoglobulin	Identifies abnormal proteins produced by cancerous plasma cells as compared to product of normal plasma cells

		(also known as M protein, M spike, paraprotein); presence of abnormal protein, beta$_2$-microglobin	
Bone marrow aspiration; bone marrow biopsy	Presence of normal bone marrow cells	Over 10%–30% of cells in bone marrow sample are plasma cells; biopsy indicates plasma cell tumor	In aspiration, a thin needle is used to draw up a small amount of liquid bone marrow; in biopsy, a small cylinder of bone and marrow (about 1/2" long) is removed. Site of both samples is usually at back of the hipbone
Bone x rays and computed tomography (CT) scan	Normal bone size and structure	Bone destruction and bone lesions	Identifies areas of bone destruction and effects of bone-absorbing hormones
Serum calcium: total calcium, including free ionized calcium and calcium bound with protein	8.6–10.3 mg/dL	> 10.5 mg/dL	Bone destruction causes accumulation of calcium above normal levels in the extracellular fluid compartment
Serum ionized calcium: unbound calcium; level unaffected by albumin level	4.5–5.1 mg/dL	> 5.5 mg/dL	Ionized calcium is approximately 46%–50% of circulating calcium and is the form of calcium available for enzymatic reactions and neuromuscular function

Other Tests: Complete blood cell count, magnetic resonance imaging (MRI), serum creatinine, creatinine clearance, Bence-Jones protein

PRIMARY NURSING DIAGNOSIS

Pain (acute or chronic) related to bone fragility and injury, vertebral collapse, joint swelling, effects of radiation therapy or chemotherapy

OUTCOMES. Comfort Level; Pain control behavior; Pain: Disruptive effects; Pain level

INTERVENTIONS. Pain management; Analgesic administration; Positioning; Teaching: Prescribed activity/exercise; Teaching: Procedure/treatment; Teaching: Prescribed medication

☐ PLANNING AND IMPLEMENTATION

Collaborative

There is no universally accepted staging system for multiple myeloma. (See Table 35.)

Clinicians are most interested in the amount of tumor mass, hemoglobin level, calcium level, serum protein levels, and number of lytic bone lesions. Treatment depends on disease staging and generally consists of chemotherapy, radiation, prednisone, and as much ambulation as the patient can tolerate.

Severe bone pain may be a problem, and pain management may be difficult; nonsteroidal anti-inflammatory drugs (NSAIDs) are the best agents for bone pain but are contraindicated with renal dysfunction, which often accompanies multiple myeloma. Radiation is useful for palliation of bone pain. Radiation therapy may be used for small, local bone lesions or to relieve the pressure that is caused by compression of nerve roots. Surgical treatments in multiple myeloma are limited to any orthopedic fixation procedures that may need to be done in response to pathologic bone fractures. Laminectomy addresses vertebral compression.

Multiple myeloma often leads to bone demineralization and significant amounts of calcium lost into the blood and urine. The patient with multiple myeloma is thus at risk for developing renal calculi, nephrocalcinosis, and renal failure from hypercalcemia. To decrease serum calcium levels that lead to hypercalcemia, the patient is given adequate fluids, diuretics, corticosteroids, or bisphosphonates to decrease demineralization. Plasmapheresis may be used for patients with extremely high immunoglobulin levels that are causing damage to kidneys or patients who have symptoms of hyperviscosity syndrome. Hyperviscosity syndrome results when the plasma proteins (immunoglobulin) contribute more to plasma viscosity than do blood cells.

PHARMACOLOGIC HIGHLIGHTS

Medication or Drug Class	Dosage	Description	Rationale
Chemotherapy	Pulse therapy (4 days of treatment every 4–6 weeks) seems to be as effective as daily therapy	MP: melphalan and prednisone; VBMCP: vincristine, carmustine (BCNU), melphalan, cyclophosphamide, prednisone; VAD: vincristine, doxorubicin, dexamethasone	Suppresses plasma cell growth and controls pain; several single alkylating chemotherapeutic agents produce positive responses in about 30% of patients with multiple myeloma; adding prednisone increases positive responses to about 40% to 50%
Opioids and NSAIDs	Varies with drug	Morphine sulfate, demerol, ibuprofen, aspirin	Manage severe bone pain

Other Drugs: Biphosphonates such as pamidronate and clodronate to reduce bone loss

Independent

Encourage the patient to drink 3000 to 4000 mL of fluids daily. Provide comfort measures for pain, such as repositioning and relaxation techniques. Always accompany the patients as they ambulate, and make sure they use a walker or other supportive aid to prevent falls. Provide corsets or braces as appropriate to assist in weight bearing and to increase bone strength. Provide encouragement and allow the patient to set the pace. If the patient is bedridden, change his or her position every 2 hours and provide passive range-of-motion exercises. Encourage deep-breathing exercises and promote active exercises when tolerable.

Make sure the patient understands the disease process, diagnostic tests, treatment options, and prognosis as previously explained by the physician. Teach the patient what to expect from the treatment and diagnostic tests, including painful procedures such as bone marrow aspiration and biopsy. Explain to the patient what to expect in the event of surgery, emphasizing the need for deep-breathing and changing position every 2 hours after surgery. Emphasize the need to avoid infection by wearing sufficiently warm clothing and by avoiding crowds and people with infections because chemotherapy causes a sensitivity to cold and diminishes the body's natural resistance to infection. Take precautions to prevent infection. Use sterile technique for all procedures, and limit the patient's exposure to visitors, staff, and other patients with infections. Since patients on chemotherapy may develop cold sensitivity, make sure the patient is warm enough.

The patient may experience less anxiety if he or she is allowed as much control as possible over the daily schedule. Explaining procedures and keeping the patient informed about the treatment plan and condition may also decrease anxiety. If the patient enters the final phases of multiple myeloma, provide emotional support. Refer the patient and family to the hospice staff or the hospital chaplain. Encourage the patient and family to verbalize their feelings about impending death. Allow for the time needed to adjust, while helping the patient and family begin the grieving process. Assist in the identification of tasks to be completed before death, such as making a will, seeing specific relatives and friends, and attending an approaching wedding, birthday, or anniversary celebration. Urge the patient to verbalize specific funeral requests to family members. If appropriate, refer the patient and family to the American Cancer Society or another local support group.

DOCUMENTATION GUIDELINES

- Response to chemotherapy or radiation treatments
- Physical findings: Fractures; joint swelling; body height; intake and output; breathing patterns; gastrointestinal bleeding
- Presence of complications: Pneumonia, renal calculi, renal failure, hyperuricemia, ineffective patient or family coping
- Laboratory results: Presence or absence of hypercalcemia; complete blood count; presence of Bence-Jones protein; bone marrow aspirations; globulin levels

DISCHARGE AND HOME HEALTHCARE GUIDELINES

If the patient receives outpatient chemotherapy or radiation, teach the patient the purpose, duration, and potential complications of those treatments. Be sure the patient understands any prescribed pain medication, including dosage, route, action, and side effects. Urge the patient to maintain a realistic but positive attitude; the return to an independent lifestyle is possible with the efforts of a rehabilitation team and the patient's cooperation.

Multiple Organ Dysfunction Syndrome

DRG Category: 101
Mean LOS: 4.6 days
Description: OTHER: Respiratory System Diagnoses with CC (If the patient develops this syndrome during the hospital stay, the reason for admission will determine the DRG assigned.)

Multiple organ dysfunction syndrome (MODS) occurs when altered organ function in an acutely ill patient is present to the extent that homeostasis can no longer be maintained without intervention. MODS was formerly known as multiple system organ failure. The usual sequence of MODS depends somewhat on its cause but often begins with pulmonary failure 2 to 3 days after surgery, followed, in order, by hepatic failure, stress-induced gastrointestinal (GI) bleeding, and renal failure. Mortality rates are linearly related to the number of failed organ systems. Patients with two or more organ systems involved have a mortality rate of approximately 75%, and patients with four organ systems involved have a 100% mortality rate.

MODS was first associated with traumatic injuries in the late 1960s and has subsequently been associated with infection and decreased perfusion to any part of the body. The term *MODS* was adopted in 1991 at a consensus conference of the Society of Critical Care Medicine and the American College of Chest Physicians. The term *MODS* best describes the organ dysfunction that precedes complete failure. Primary MODS, the result of a direct injury or insult to the organ itself, is initiated by a specific precipitating event, such as a pulmonary contusion. The injury or insult causes an inflammatory response within that organ system, and dysfunction develops.

Secondary MODS develops as the result of a systemic response to infection or inflammation. Systemic inflammatory response syndrome (SIRS) is an overwhelming response of the normal inflammatory system, producing systemic effects instead of the localized response normally seen. The inflammatory response is produced by the activation of a series of mediators and results in alterations in blood (selective vasodilation and vasoconstriction), an increase in vascular permeability, white blood cell (WBC) activation, and activation of the coagulation cascade.

CAUSES

The inflammatory response can be triggered by any event, but it is most often associated with a bacterial infection. The events most often associated with the development of SIRS and MODS are shock, trauma, burns, aspiration, venomous snakebites, cardiac arrest, thromboemboli, myocardial infarction, operative procedures, vascular injury, infection, pancreatitis, and disseminated intravascular coagulation (DIC).

GENDER AND LIFE SPAN CONSIDERATIONS

Young adults, males twice as often as females, are at particular risk for MODS because they are the primary trauma population. Increased risk in the trauma patient is related to more prolonged hypotension, extensive amounts of tissue damage, and higher infection rates. Patients over the age of 65 who experience MODS have higher rates of mortality. The normal aging process causes dysfunction of organ systems and, in some patients, immunosuppression. With a significant injury or insult, therefore, it is much easier for organ systems in the elderly to fail. Patients of all ages who abuse alcohol and who are malnourished are also at risk because of the role of alcohol in immunosuppression.

☐ ASSESSMENT

HISTORY. The patient with MODS has a history of infection, tissue injury, or a perfusion deficit to an organ or body part. Often this injury or insult is not life-threatening but exposes the person to bacterial contamination. Question the patient (or if the patient is too ill, the family) to identify the events in the initial insult and any history of pre-existing organ dysfunction, such as chronic lung disease, congestive heart failure, and diabetes mellitus. Elicit a complete medication history and the patient's compliance with medications, and ask if the patient has experienced recent weight loss. Determine the patient's dietary patterns to assess the patient's nutritional status. Take a history of the patient's use of cigarettes, alcohol, and other drugs of abuse.

PHYSICAL EXAMINATION. The physical examination of the patient with MODS varies, depending on the organ systems involved and the severity of their dysfunction. (See Table 36.) Expect the patient to develop signs of pulmonary failure first and then hepatic failure and GI bleeding. Renal failure follows. Note that failures of the central nervous system (CNS) and the cardiovascular system are late signs of MODS.

TABLE 36 | **Organ System Involvement in MODS**

ORGAN SYSTEM	SYMPTOMS OF DYSFUNCTION
Central nervous system	Decreased level of consciousness, confusion, lethargy
Cardiovascular system	Hyperdynamic: tachycardic; normotensive; skin warm and flushed; full bounding pulses
	Hypodynamic: tachycardic; hypotensive; skin cool and mottled; weak, thready pulses
Pulmonary system	Crackles or rales, tachypnea
	Cyanosis of the nail beds and mucous membranes, dyspnea
Gastrointestinal system	Diminished or absent bowel sounds, abdominal distention, intolerance of tube feedings, upper or lower gastrointestinal bleeding, diarrhea.
Hepatic system	Jaundice, petechiae, increased bruising
Renal system	Polyuria, oliguria, or anuria
Coagulation system	Oozing or bleeding from intravenous sites or invasive line sites; bruising and petechiae; bleeding into body parts or cavities; cool, pale to mottled extremites; necrotic digits
General appearance	Weight loss and muscle wasting; temperature <36°C or >38°C

PSYCHOSOCIAL. The patient with MODS may be fully conscious, partially conscious, or unconscious. If the patient is oriented, he or she is likely to be very anxious and fatigued and also confused, lethargic, or comatose. Assess the patient's ability to cope with a prolonged life-threatening illness and the changes in roles that a severe illness brings. The patient may experience fear because of a real threat to his or her life.

DIAGNOSTIC HIGHLIGHTS

General Comments: Diagnostic data are collected to establish the dysfunction of each of the body's systems. (See Table 37.)

Test	Normal Result	Abnormality with Condition	Explanation
Complete blood count	Red blood cells (RBCs) 4.0–5.5 million/μL; white blood cells 4,500–11,000/μL; hemoglobin (Hg) 12–18 g/dL; hematocrit (Hct) 37%–54%; reticulocyte count 0.5%–2.5% of total RBCs; platelets 150,000–400,000/μL	Varies with condition: > 12,000 mm^3 or < 4,000 mm^3 or > 10% band cells (immature cells); red blood cells, Hg, Hct, platelets may be decreased	Underlying disorder may cause alterations in blood cell counts; SIRS leads to production of inflammatory mediators and alterations in white blood cell counts; hematologic failure may lead to suppression of cell production
Partial thrombo-plastin time (activated; APPT)	Varies by laboratory; generally 21–35 seconds	Prolonged; may be prolonged > 80 seconds	May be prolonged if liver failure and hematologic failure occurs
Prothrombin time (PT)	Varies by laboratory; generally 11–13 seconds	Prolonged > 15 seconds	May be prolonged if liver failure occurs

Other Tests: Electrocardiogram, multiple cultures and sensitivities (blood, wound, urine, sputum, catheters), arterial blood gases, pulmonary artery pressure monitoring, cardiac output and index, derived oxygen variables (oxygen delivery, oxygen consumption), electrolytes, glucose.

TABLE 37 | **Definitions of Organ Failure**

ORGAN	DEFINITION OF FAILURE	DIAGNOSTIC FINDINGS
Lungs	Need for ventilator-assisted breathing to treat hypoxemia for 5 days in the postoperative period or until death	Decreased PaO_2 and SaO_2 Decreased $PaCO_2$ Increased shunt fraction Decreased vital capacity and functional residual capacity Decreased static compliance

Kidneys	Serum creatinine concentration >2 mg/dL; for patients with pre-existing renal disease, doubling of admission serum creatinine level	Increased serum creatinine Urine specific gravity < 1.012 Urine sodium > 40 mEq/L
Liver	Serum bilirubin concentration > 2 mg/dL with elevation of either serum aspartate aminotransferase concentration or lactic dehydrogenase concentration above twice normal	See definition
GI tract	Requirement of 2 units of blood replacement within 24 hours for presumed stress bleeding or endoscopic confirmation of upper GI bleeding from acute GI ulcers	Dropping hemoglobin and hematocrit Visualization of ulcers during surgery or endoscopy.

PRIMARY NURSING DIAGNOSIS

Risk for infection related to microorganism invasion, immunosuppression, malnutrition, and presence of invasive monitoring devices

OUTCOMES. Immune status; Knowledge: Infection control; Risk control; Risk detection; Nutrition status; Treatment behavior: Illness or injury; Hydration

INTERVENTIONS. Infection control; Infection protection; Surveillance; Fluid/electrolyte management; Medication management; Temperature regulation

☐ PLANNING AND IMPLEMENTATION
Collaborative

Management of the patient with MODS begins with the recognition of those patients who are at an increased risk for the syndrome. Care must be taken to prevent infection and maintain adequate tissue oxygenation to all body parts. Despite improvement in medical therapies, the mortality rate of MODS remains high.

Treatment of the patient with MODS can be divided into four main areas: anti-infectives, maintenance of tissue perfusion and oxygenation, nutritional support, and immunomodulation. Anti-infective therapy is guided by culture and sensitivity reports. Any potential source of infection should be investigated and eliminated. Antifungal and antiviral agents are used primarily with immunocompromised patients, who are especially susceptible to fungal and viral infections.

Maintaining and monitoring tissue perfusion and oxygenation are crucial to the survival of the patient with MODS. Measurement of oxygen delivery and consumption is necessary to guide fluid replacement therapy and inotropic support of cardiac function. To maximize all components of oxygen delivery (in particular, cardiac index, hemoglobin, and oxygen saturation), the physician maintains the hematocrit within the normal range or even at a supranormal level with blood transfusions. Mechanical ventilation with positive end-expiratory pressure and modes such as pressure control ventilation and inverse ratio inspiration : expiration are used to maintain adequate oxygenation and oxygen delivery. The success of maintaining oxygen delivery is evaluated by following the trend of oxygen consumption. Metabolic demands dramatically increase in

MODS. When oxygen delivery cannot meet the body's metabolic demands, these demands may be decreased with sedation, pharmacologic paralysis, and temperature control.

The goal in the future is to develop medications that allow for immunomodulation therapy to alter the detrimental effects of the systemic immune-inflammatory response. Tumor necrosis factor and interleukin-1 are two cytokines that exert a broad effect on the endothelium, leukocytes, and fibroblasts. Experts hope that modulation of both of these cytokines can decrease many of the body's responses to inflammation. The presence of endotoxin, a substance that is released with the destruction of gram-negative bacteria, stimulates the inflammatory response. Modulation of endotoxin would also decrease many of the body's responses to inflammation.

PHARMACOLOGIC HIGHLIGHTS

Medication or Drug Class	Dosage	Description	Rationale
Anti-infective therapy; antifungal agents; antiviral agents	Varies with drug	Therapy focuses on dysfunctional system and culture results	Prevent and control infection
H_2 receptor antagonist	Varies with drug	Ranitidine (Zantac); cimetidine (Tagamet); famotidine (Pepcid); nizatidine (Axid)	Blocks gastric secretion and maintains the pH of gastric contents above 4.0

Independent

Any potential source of infection should be eliminated if possible. Change the dressing on all invasive line sites and surgical wounds according to protocol to keep the area free of infection and to monitor for early signs of infection. Maintain aseptic technique with all dressing changes and manipulation of intravenous lines. Institute the measures that are necessary to prevent aspiration when patients are placed on enteral feedings. Keep the head of the bed elevated, and check for residual volume and tube placement every 4 hours.

To limit the patient's oxygen expenditure, provide frequent rest periods and create a quiet environment whenever possible. Schedule procedures and nursing care interventions so that the patient has periods of uninterrupted rest. Manage situations of increased metabolic demand—such as fever, agitation, alcohol withdrawal, and pain—promptly so that the patient conserves energy and limits oxygen consumption.

Monitor the patient's environment for sensory overload. Provide purposeful, planned stimuli and keep extraneous, constant noises to a minimum. Provide for planned, uninterrupted rest periods to avoid sleep deprivation. Monitor bony prominences and areas of high risk for skin breakdown. Note that MODS is one of the most critical illnesses that a patient can develop. Although the patient might be well sedated and unresponsive, the family or significant others are generally very anxious, upset, and frightened that the patient might not survive. These fears are realistic, particularly if multiple organs are involved. Provide the significant others with accurate information about the patient's course and his or her prospects for recovery. Encourage the legal representative to participate in decisions about extraordinary measures to keep the patient alive if the patient cannot speak for himself or herself. Determine if the patient has a living will or has discussed his or her desire to be kept alive by technology during a potentially terminal illness. If the decision is to terminate life support, work with the significant others to provide a dignified death for the patient in an environment that allows the family to participate and grieve appropriately. Provide referrals to the chaplain, clinical nurse specialist, or grief counselor as needed.

DOCUMENTATION GUIDELINES

- Physical assessment findings:
  Neurologic: Mental status response to stimuli; if pharmacologically paralyzed, then peripheral nerve stimulation testing
  Pulmonary: Respiratory rate, auscultation findings, amount of ventilatory support, oxygen saturation by pulse oximetry
  Hemodynamics: Cardiac output/index, right and left ventricular measures of preload and afterload; oxygen delivery; oxygen consumption
  Renal function: Fluid intake and urine output
  Hepatic function: Color of skin and sclera, presence of petechiae, bruising, oozing, or frank bleeding
- Response to acute, life-threatening illness: Anxiety level, coping.

DISCHARGE AND HOME HEALTHCARE GUIDELINES

Although no specific adaptive structural changes need to be made, near the time of discharge assess the patient's individual needs. Because organ dysfunction or failure is individualized, home care preparation should be based on meeting the individual's needs. Be sure the patient understands all medications prescribed, including dosage, route, action, and side effects.

Describe the importance of avoiding fatigue and taking frequent rests. Teach the patient to eat small, frequent meals to maintain adequate nutrition. Teach the patient any needed postoperative care: incision care, signs and symptoms of infection, pain management, activity restrictions. Also teach the patient the signs and symptoms of infection and when to report them to the primary healthcare provider.

Multiple Sclerosis

DRG Category: 013
Mean LOS: 5.7 days
Description: MEDICAL: Multiple Sclerosis and Cerebellar Ataxia

Multiple sclerosis (MS) is a chronic, progressive degenerative disease that affects the myelin sheath of the white matter of the brain and spinal cord. Nerve impulses are conducted between the brain and spinal cord along neurons protected by the myelin sheath, which is a highly conductive fatty material. When plaques form on the myelin sheath, causing inflammation and eventual demyelination, nerve transmission becomes erratic. Areas commonly involved are the optic nerves, cerebrum, and cervical spinal cord. MS is the most common demyelinating disorder in the United States and Europe.

Four forms of MS have been identified. Benign MS, which affects approximately 20% of patients, causes mild disability; infrequent, mild, early attacks are followed by almost complete recovery. Exacerbating-remitting MS, which affects approximately 25% of patients, is marked by frequent attacks that start early in the course of the illness, followed by less than complete clearing of signs and symptoms than in benign MS. Chronic relapsing MS, which affects approximately 40% of patients, has fewer, less complete remissions after an exacerbation than has exacerbating-remitting MS. Chronic relapsing MS has a cumulative progression, with more symptoms occurring during each new attack. The fourth form of MS, chronic progressive, afflicts approximately 15% of patients and is similar to chronic relapsing MS except that the onset is more subtle and the disease progresses slowly without remission.

CAUSES

The cause of MS is unknown. Some evidence suggests that an infective agent causes a predisposition to MS, although that agent has not been identified. Some evidence supports immunologic, environmental, or genetic factors as possible causes of the disease. The risk of developing MS is 15 times higher when the disease is present in the patient's immediate family. Conditions such as pregnancy, infection, and trauma seem to precipitate the onset of MS or cause relapses.

GENDER AND LIFE SPAN CONSIDERATIONS

MS is more prevalent in colder climates, in urban areas, and among Caucasians. More than 500,000 Americans have MS. MS affects women more than men in a 2 to 1 ratio. Roughly 70% of patients experience the onset of MS when they are between the ages of 20 and 40, while 20% of patients experience the onset of the disease when they are between the ages of 40 and 60.

□ ASSESSMENT

HISTORY. Vague and unrelated symptoms often dominate the early period of MS before a definitive diagnosis is made. Brain lesions lead to central nervous system signs. Ask the patient about changes in vision and coordination. Determine whether the patient has experienced slurred speech, impotence, ataxia, or double vision (diplopia). Approximately 70% experience involuntary, rhythmic movements of the eyes (nystagmus).

Spinal cord lesions lead to motor and sensory impairment of the trunk and limbs. Ask if problems have occurred with bowel and bladder dysfunction. Determine if the patient has experienced a feeling of heaviness or weakness, numbness or tingling in the extremities. Determine the patient's ability to perform activities of daily living with attention to the fine movement of fingers, as when dressing or picking up small objects. Ask if the patient has experienced burning sensation or pain, decreased temperature sensation, intention tremor (a tremor during a voluntary activity), foot-dragging, staggering, dizziness, or loss of balance. Ask if the patient has experienced decreased motor function after taking a hot bath or shower (Uhthoff's sign), which is caused by the effects of heat on neuromuscular conduction. Roughly 50% of patients with MS lose the ability to sense position, vibration, shape, and texture.

Determine when the patient first noticed any of these difficulties and whether the symptoms later disappeared. Ask about fatigue and its progression throughout the day and what stressors precipitate symptoms. Determine whether there is a family history of the disease. Elicit a history of mild depression and short attention span.

PHYSICAL EXAMINATION. Determine the patient's muscle strength and symmetry, arm and leg movement, and gait. To assess arm strength, have the patient use both hands to push against you. Observe for unilateral or bilateral weakness. Ask the patient to open and close the fist and to move each arm without raising it from the bed. If no purposeful movement occurs, apply light tactile pressure to each arm, gradually increasing the pressure in an attempt to elicit a purposeful response. Assess leg movement in the same way. Ask the patient to move each leg and, if he or she cannot, press the Achilles' tendon firmly between your thumb and index finger, observing for either a purposeful or non-purposeful response.

Assess gait by asking the patient to walk away from you; observe for ataxia, shuffling, or stumbling. Stay close to the patient to prevent falls. If the patient is able to perform these tasks well, test balance by having the patient walk heel-to-toe in a straight line. Observe any leaning to one side.

PSYCHOSOCIAL. When a chronic illness with potential for serious debilitation and possible early death is first discovered, a patient goes through a period of grieving. This grief process may take years. Determine the patient's place on the continuum of shock, denial, or anger, and accept the patient's current stage of coping.

DIAGNOSTIC HIGHLIGHTS

Test	Normal Result	Abnormality with Condition	Explanation
Cerebrospinal fluid (CSF) analysis	Red blood cells: 0–10/µ; white blood cells: 0–10/µ; routine culture: no growth; fungal culture: no growth; mycobacteria culture: no growth; color: clear; protein: 15–50 mg/dL; glucose: 40–80 mg/dL; pressure: 5–13 mm Hg; gram stain: no cells to stain	Elevated protein level, increased white blood cell count. Electrophoresis of CSF shows increased myelin basic protein and IgG bands.	Reflects immune response

Other Tests: No single test reliably diagnoses MS. Supporting tests include electroencephalography, evoked potential studies, computed tomography (CT) scan, and magnetic resonance imaging (MRI).

PRIMARY NURSING DIAGNOSIS

Impaired physical mobility related to fatigue and weakness

OUTCOMES. Ambulation: Walking; Joint movement: Active; Mobility level; Self-care: Activities of daily living; Transfer performance; Balance; Congitive ability; Mood equilibrium; Neurologic status; Muscle function

INTERVENTIONS. Exercise therapy: Ambulation, Joint mobility, Muscle control; Teaching: Prescribed activity/exercise; Energy management; Environmental management; Exercise promotion; Activity therapy; Distraction

▢ PLANNING AND IMPLEMENTATION

Collaborative

Most medical treatment is designed to slow disease progression and address the symptoms of the disease, such as urinary retention, spasticity, and motor and speech deficits. Currently, however, physicians generally prescribe steroid therapy to reduce tissue edema during an acute exacerbation.

Consult with a physical therapist if the patient needs to learn how to use assistive devices or needs to learn exercises to maintain muscle tone and joint mobility. Muscle stretching for spastic muscles and selective strengthening exercises for weakness are prescribed. A social service agency may be required to help the family deal with the often expensive and long-term financial effect of the disease. Vocational redirection may also be required. For a patient who is experiencing depression, consider a referral to a psychiatric clinical nurse specialist. Family counseling is often very helpful.

PHARMACOLOGIC HIGHLIGHTS

Medication or Drug Class	Dosage	Description	Rationale
Corticosteroids	Varies with drug	Prednisone (Orasone); methylprednisolone (Solu-Medrol)	Help decrease symptoms and induce remissions through anti-inflammatory effects
Immunosuppressive agents	Varies with drug	Cyclophosphamide (Cytoxan); interferon beta-1b (Betaseron)	Help decrease symptoms and induce remissions

Other Drugs: Anti-anxiety agents, such as chlordiazepoxide hydrochloride (Librium), may be prescribed to manage mood swings; baclofen (Lioresal) or dantrolene (Dantrium) may be used to relieve muscle spasticity; and patients with urinary symptoms may require behanechol (Urecholine) or oxybutynin (Ditropan).

Independent

Sensory perceptual deficits in the visual fields cause dizziness, headaches, and the potential for injury. Patching each eye, alternating with the other several times a day, improves balance and visualization. Peripheral vision may be affected; teach the patient to scan the environment and to remove potential sources of injury. Ask the patient particularly to look out for hot surfaces and hot water, to which he or she may not be sensitive.

Be sure the patient understands the need to avoid becoming fatigued or overheated. Instruct the patient to alternate periods of activity with periods of rest, discussing the need for frequent rest periods as a permanent lifestyle change.

Explain that baths and showers may prove relaxing but may also exacerbate MS symptoms. Conduct range-of-motion exercises at least twice daily. If necessary, teach the patient how to use a walker or a cane. Care for a neurogenic bladder includes instructing the patient to consume 1500 mL of fluid daily and void every 3 hours. If urine is retained, teach intermittent self-catheterization with clean technique to the patient who is capable. Some patients, however, are incontinent. Teach the patient how to use special pads to avoid skin breakdown. Teach the patient to develop a regular bowel pattern, with bowel elimination about 30 minutes after the morning meal. Insert a glycerine suppository if necessary to stimulate reflex bowel activity. Provide assistance should the patient be unable to perform this self-care.

Teach the patient about the disease process, and be sure he or she knows how to contact the local MS Society. In addition to information and education, the society holds focus group seminars that study relational issues associated with the disease. The society also provides some ongoing therapy and socialization and support for home maintenance. Helping the patient learn to cope with this chronic illness is a major nursing challenge. Listen to the patient's fears; respect his or her abilities and provide positive encouragement. The disabled patient not only loses body function but often his or her role as an active parent and spouse. With the more rapidly progressive forms of MS, the patient may have impairment of cognitive functioning; touch and voice tone can convey concern and care when the meaning of words gets lost.

DOCUMENTATION GUIDELINES

- Physical findings: Muscle strength, gait, muscle symmetry, visual response
- Response to medications, treatments, and special therapies
- Ability to perform self-care, bowel and bladder care
- Presence of complications, infections, contractures

DISCHARGE AND HOME HEALTHCARE GUIDELINES

Be sure the patient understands any pain medication prescribed, including dosage, route, action, and side effects. Be sure the patient understands the need for adequate bladder and bowel elimination. Instruct the patient to notify the primary caregiver of any exacerbation or sudden worsening of the condition. If the patient has difficulty speaking or communicating, be sure that he or she has access to a telephone support network or some other means of calling for assistance when he or she is at home alone for any length of time. Be sure the patient understands that stress, fatigue, and being overheated stimulate exacerbations. Teach the patient how to avoid situations that produce these reactions. Be sure the patient knows how to contact community agencies such as the MS Society for use of such in-home equipment as beds and wheelchairs and home maintenance support. Determine whether a home care agency is needed to provide home supervision and ongoing physical therapy support.

Muscular Dystrophy

DRG Category: 034
Mean LOS: 5.3 days
Description: MEDICAL: Other Disorders of Nervous System with CC

Muscular dystrophy is not a disease but a term applied to a number of genetic disorders that are characterized by gradual progressive weakness and muscle fiber degeneration without neural involvement. The most significant finding in muscular dystrophy is skeletal muscle deterioration. Cardiac and other smooth muscles may be involved as well, leading to serious complications and premature death. To date, there is no cure for any of the muscular dystrophies, but there have been significant research advances related to gene identification for Duchenne's muscular dystrophy (a pseudohypertrophic, progressive form that begins in childhood and is transmitted as a sex-linked recessive trait). The genetic abnormality causes an absence of dystrophia, a protein of muscle cells. This deficit prevents adequate cell functioning, which leads to necrosis of muscle fibers. As the muscle undergoes necrosis, fat and connective tissue replace the muscle fibers. Complications include disabilities, contractures, skeletal deformities, and thoracic muscle weakness. The patient is prone to pulmonary complications such as pneumonia and cardiac dysrhythmias and hypertrophy.

CAUSES

Muscular dystrophy is a progressive degeneration of skeletal muscles from an as yet unknown biochemical defect within the muscle. Duchenne's muscular dystrophy has an incidence of about 3 per 100,000 and is inherited as a recessive single gene defect on the X chromosome, which means it is transmitted from the mother to her male offspring. Another form of dystrophy, Becker's muscular dystrophy, is similarly X-linked but has its onset later in childhood or adolescence and has a slower course. Other heredity disorders include Landouzy-Dejerine dystrophy (facioscapulohumeral) and Erb's dystrophy (limb-girdle).

GENDER AND LIFE SPAN CONSIDERATIONS

In some forms of muscular dystrophy, weakness can appear from infancy to adulthood. The rate of progression varies from rapid to slow, and in many cases the individual may have a normal life span. Muscular dystrophy can affect childen or adults, and both sexes, depending on the type. (See Table 38.)

TABLE 38 | **Four Types of Muscular Dystrophy**

TYPE	GENDER	AGE AT ONSET	CHARACTERISTICS AND PROGRESSION
Duchenne's	Males	Toddler or preschool	Initial loss of pelvic girdle and shoulder muscle control; Gower's sign; rapid progression with death in late adolescence or 20s from cardiac or respiratory complications

Becker's	Males	Early teens	Similar to Duchenne's, no cardiac involvement; slow, near-normal life span
Facioscapulohumeral	Males and females	Children through young adults	Weakness and atrophy of shoulder, face, and eye muscles; slow progression, normal life span
Myotonic	Males and females	Young adults	Muscles remain contracted, atrophy atrophy occurs; life span into the 30s or 40s

☐ ASSESSMENT

HISTORY. A complete family and developmental history provides important diagnostic data for the patient with muscular dystrophy. Since it is a genetic disease, determine if anyone in the family has been previously diagnosed with a musculoskeletal or neuromuscular disease. Children with Duchenne's muscular dystrophy have a history of delayed motor milestones, such as sitting, walking, and standing. Adults may report progressive muscle weakness of the legs, face, and shoulder. The patient may experience difficulty raising the arms over the head or closing the eyes completely. Other early signs include difficulty in puckering the lips, abnormal facial movements, and the inability of facial muscles to change during laughing and crying.

PHYSICAL EXAMINATION. Most dystrophies involve the hip and shoulder girdle musculature, which leads to functional difficulties. Assess the patient's ability to raise the arms above the head, get up from a chair, or walk. Inspect the patient for scoliosis and contractures. For 2- to 5-year-old boys with Duchenne's muscular dystrophy, observe for pelvic and shoulder girdle muscles with distal involvement. Note a waddling, stumbling gait or difficulty climbing stairs. A characteristic sign is the Gower's maneuver: the patient uses his hands to walk up his legs until he is standing erect. His posture may also be distorted, with a lumbar lordosis and protuberant abdomen. He may toe-walk to compensate for quadriceps weakness. Scoliosis occurs after the child is wheelchair-dependent because of weak trunk muscles. Tachycardia occurs as the heart muscle weakens and enlarges. Generally, any cardiac muscle involvement is asymptomatic until late in the course of the disease. Pneumonia develops easily as the child's cough reflex becomes weak and ineffective.

PSYCHOSOCIAL. Since muscular dystrophy is a progressive disease that limits the normal life span, patients and their families will require ongoing emotional support. The genetic nature of the disease frequently creates guilt that often leads to depression. Boys with Duchenne's muscular dystrophy often have an IQ below 90. Frustration, depression, and other signs of emotional immaturity may be present because of the intellectual limitation. Family functioning is challenged because of the progressive losses and prognosis.

DIAGNOSTIC HIGHLIGHTS

Test	Normal Result	Abnormality with Condition	Explanation
Muscle biopsy	Normal muscle fibers	Muscle cell degeneration with	Increased activity of proteolytic enzymes in

		microscopic areas of necrosis and presence of dystrophin	muscle tissue
Electromyogram (EMG)	No electrical activity at rest; orderly recruitment of voluntary motor unit potentials with gradually increasing voluntary motor muscle effort	Progressive muscle weakness	Destruction and deterioration of muscle function

Other Tests: Creatine phosphokinase

PRIMARY NURSING DIAGNOSIS

Impaired physical mobility related to muscle destruction

OUTCOMES. Ambulation: Walking; Joint movement: Active; Mobility level; Self-care: Activities of daily living; Transfer performance; Balance; Cognitive ability; Mood equilibrium; Neurological status; Muscle function

INTERVENTIONS. Exercise therapy: Ambulation, Joint mobility, Muscle control; Teaching: Prescribed activity/exercise; Energy management; Environmental management; Exercise promotion; Activity therapy; Distraction

☐ PLANNING AND IMPLEMENTATION

Collaborative

Currently there is no cure for muscular dystrophy, and therapeutic management is focused on managing the symptoms and maintaining the highest level of functional independence possible. Patients with multiple dystrophy are managed by a multidisciplinary team because of their complex needs. The goals of treatment are to facilitate ambulation and aggressively manage respiratory and cardiac difficulties. With early diagnosis, interventions such as appropriate diet and exercise and social and psychological counseling can begin to prolong the patient's independence and quality of life.

Physical therapy is directed toward keeping functional muscle strength and preventing contractures by passive stretching. Swimming is frequently recommended as an excellent exercise for keeping limber and for allowing participation in athletic events. Gait training and transfer training are important as the patient loses muscle power. Crutches and the use of a powered wheelchair maintain independent mobility for as long as possible. The occupational therapist may fit the patient with braces or splints to prevent or treat contractures. Long leg braces are needed to provide stability for weakened muscles that can no longer provide support for ambulation.

Once the patient is in a wheelchair, obesity frequently becomes a problem. A low-calorie, high-protein diet is recommended to avoid this complication because the additional weight places a strain on already compromised muscles. Constipation may also be a problem that can be managed with added dietary fiber, extra fluids, and stool softeners.

The physician may consider surgery to assist the patient in maintaining a higher quality of life. A spinal fusion may correct abnormal spinal curvatures that occur as the trunk muscles weaken to improve comfort, balanced sitting, and body image. Muscle- and tendon-lengthening procedures may be needed to improve decreased function if contractures form. Preoperative and postoperative preparation is essential to prevent complications. Before a surgical procedure is attempted, an electrocardiogram is needed to determine if the cardiac muscle has been affected by the muscle disease. Malignant hyperthermia (a potentially lethal increase in body temperature in response to certain muscle relaxants or anesthetic agents) is a complication that occurs in children with Duchenne's muscular dystrophy. Early ambulation is necessary to prevent additional weakness, and aggressive respiratory care prevents pneumonia.

PHARMACOLOGIC HIGHLIGHTS

No drugs have been found to slow the progression of the disease.

Independent

Because of the nature of muscular dystrophy, nursing interventions are primarily preventive and supportive. Prevention of complications requires anticipation of problems and systematic monitoring for progression of the disease process. Proper management can increase the length and quality of life. Differences in care can be divided by decreasing mobility into three phases: ambulatory, wheelchair, and bed rest phases.

In the ambulatory phase, when the family first learns of the diagnosis, information about the disease, prognosis, and treatment plans may be overwhelming. Be available to answer questions, provide clarification, and provide emotional support and encouragement related to the family's needs for control in care decisions. The family needs opportunities to express feelings about the genetic transmission, progressive nature, and effect of the disease on the family. The status of younger male children in the family may not be certain; uncertainty creates additional anxiety.

Evaluate safety issues in the home. The child's bedroom should be moved to the first floor if possible, and rugs need to be removed to facilitate mobility. Rubber-soled shoes help prevent slipping. As the disease progresses, home care equipment may be necessary for assistance with mobility and activities of daily living. Nursing interventions are directed toward preventing contractures and encouraging independence and normal development. The patient needs to be monitored for a tendency toward contracture development and range-of-motion exercises instituted as a preventive measure. Stretching exercises and splinting of the arms and legs at night help to slow the progression of contractures. Assist the child and family in developing a plan for both active and passive range-of-motion exercises to do daily; help make reminder sheets so exercises are consistently done.

As the patient becomes dependent in the wheelchair phase, comfort measures become even more critical. Teach the family to make frequent skin assessments to determine evidence of skin breakdown from prolonged sitting. Support stockings, passive exercises, and elevating the lower extremities may decrease pedal edema for patients in wheelchairs. Provide interventions directed toward attaining the child's maximum growth and development level. In the bed rest phase, eventually the patient will be unable to move without assistance. Frequent position changes and meticulous skin care are essential. Proper body alignment in the bed or chair can be maintained by the use of blanket rolls, sandbags, or pillows. Sheepskin or an alternating pressure mattress may provide comfort. Adequate fluid intake is needed to prevent urinary or bowel complications. Use incentive spirometry and diaphragmatic breathing exercises to maintain gas exchange when respiratory muscles are weak. Percussion and postural drainage are used to facilitate effective airway clearance.

Referral needs to be made to the Muscular Dystrophy Association (MDA) and other community agencies. These organizations can provide information about the disease, management, and emotional and social support during the long period of illness. They can also provide financial assistance for treatment needs.

DOCUMENTATION GUIDELINES

- Chronological progression of muscular weakness and decreasing function; cardiac and respiratory involvement
- Responses to treatment plan (exercises, diet, adaptive devices, breathing exercises, growth and development)
- Patient's and family's reactions to disease process, interventions, and role changes

DISCHARGE AND HOME HEALTHCARE GUIDELINES

The child with muscular dystrophy has multiple admissions and discharges. Because multiple dystrophy is a chronic progressive disease, teaching needs to vary according to the interventions and phase of illness. The muscular dystrophy team and the MDA are the best sources of providing information to the patient and family in a timely manner. Encourage the child and parents to maintain peer relationships and foster intellectual development by keeping the child in school as long as possible. Teach the patient and family ways to avoid respiratory problems. Encourage the parents to report respiratory infections as soon as they occur.

Musculoskeletal Trauma

DRG Category: 253
Mean LOS: 5.0 days
Description: MEDICAL: Fracture, Sprain, Strain, and Dislocation of Upper Arm, Lower Leg, or Exterior Foot, Age > 17 with CC

DRG Category: 223
Mean LOS: 2.5 days
Description: SURGICAL: Major Shoulder/Elbow Procedure or Other Upper Extremity Procedure with CC

DRG Category: 210
Mean LOS: 9.0 days
Description: SURGICAL: Hip and Femur Procedures Except Major Joint, Age > 17 with CC

The bony skeleton provides the supporting framework for the human body. Its 206 bones are subject to many stressors, which may result in fractures. Fractures vary in complexity and potential harm to the body. Simple fractures occur with no break from the bone to the outside of the body, whereas compound fractures have an external wound, thus creating contamination of the fracture. Complete fractures occur when bone continuity is completely interrupted, whereas partial fractures (incomplete) interrupt only a portion of bone continuity. Fractures can be classified by fragment position or fracture line. (See Table 39.)

TABLE 39 | **Types of Fractures**

CLASSIFICATION	TYPE	DEFINITION
Fragment position	Angulated	Bone fragments are at an angle to each other
	Avulsed	Bone fragments are pulled from normal position by muscle spasms, muscle contractions, or ligament resistance
	Comminuted	Bone breaks into many small pieces
	Displaced	Bone fragments separate and are deformed
	Impacted	A bone fragment is forced into another bone or bone fragment
	Nondisplaced	After the fracture, two sections of the bone maintain normal alignment
	Overriding	Bone fragments overlap, thereby shortening the total length of the bone
	Segmental	Bone fractures occur in two areas next to each other with an isolated section in the center
Fracture line	Linear	Fracture line is parallel to the axis of the bone
	Longitudinal	Fracture line extends longitudinally but not parallel to the axis of the bone
	Oblique	Fracture line crosses the bone at a 45-degree angle to the axis of the bone
	Spiral	Fracture line coils around the bone
	Transverse	Fracture line forms a 90-degree angle to the axis of the bone

Alcohol consumption is an important cofactor when it is associated with trauma. Acute alcohol intoxication may compound a head or musculoskeletal injury by masking the effects of pain and immobility. In addition, it may modify the patient's ability to tolerate multiple traumas by having a direct cardiodepressant effect. Profound hypotension and bradycardia may result from acute blood loss in the patient with musculoskeletal injury who has been drinking heavily.

Many complications can occur as a result of musculoskeletal trauma. Arterial damage and bleeding can lead to hypovolemic shock. Nonunion of bones, avascular necrosis, bone necrosis, and peripheral nerve damage can lead to lasting deformities and disabilities. Rhabdomyolysis (destruction of skeletal muscle) can lead to renal failure, and bone injury can lead to fat emboli. Infection is the most common complication of trauma and can lead to sepsis and septic shock.

CAUSES

Traumatic injuries can be intentional (assaults, gunshot wounds, stab wounds) or unintentional (falls, motor vehicle crashes [MVCs]). Multiple traumas that result from an MVC often involve several systems of the body and musculoskeletal injury. Falls and MVCs account for a high percentage of the fractures seen today. Children at play take falls as a matter of course, and only occasionally suffer fractures. Their most common fractures are of the clavicle. Adults who fall more often fracture a hip or wrist. Osteoporosis increases the likelihood of fractures from a fall; it even sometimes causes a fracture from a slight shift in the body's position, which then results in a fall, rather than the reverse.

GENDER AND LIFE SPAN CONSIDERATIONS

Multiple musculoskeletal traumas can occur at any time in life—no one is exempt. However, young adults are most at risk. MVCs are the leading cause of death for those between the ages of 4 and 34. Serious industrial accidents are more common in young men, and multiple injuries from falls are especially a problem in older women.

Fractures occur at all ages, with their incidence increasing with age. Osteoporosis, which occurs in many women past menopause and in men somewhat later in life, accounts for the vulnerability to fractures of those past midlife. Fractures in elderly people are often of the wrist, hip, and vertebrae. Healing occurs much more rapidly in the young, and the elderly are more at risk for complications of immobility from both the fracture and its treatment. The high death rate of the elderly within a year after a broken hip is largely from complications of immobility.

☐ ASSESSMENT

HISTORY. Determine the details of the immediate injury. Question the patient if possible, relatives if present, and any witnesses, including bystanders, the police, and the life squad. Note that the obvious injuries may not be the most serious ones. For example, a leg injury may be evident, whereas the pelvic fracture caused by force to the knee or leg during a car crash may be more serious. Obtain information from family or friends about the usual health status. Determine the past medical history, with particular attention to life span considerations such as pregnancy, chronic diseases such as diabetes and hypertension, and patterns of substance abuse.

PHYSICAL EXAMINATION. In the immediate trauma resuscitation, assessment and treatment are merged. Always of first priority is the assessment and management of airway, breathing, and circulation. Neurologic status becomes part of that initial assessment, as the patient is often in a compromised state of consciousness. Monitor the vital signs every 15 minutes or more often until the patient is stabilized. The patient may demonstrate a wide range of blood pressures and heart rates, depending on age, degree of blood loss, baseline vital signs, and degree of alcohol intoxication.

During the physical examination, handle the patient carefully and be aware that any fractures can be made more serious by the manipulation caused by examination. If the cervical spine is injured, movement can lead to lifelong disability. Broken ribs may not initially pose a serious problem for the patient, but with rough handling they may become displaced and cause damage to the pleura and lungs. Manipulation of broken bones also causes increased pain and blood loss. Inspect the patient thoroughly for evidence of fractures, including angulation or shortening of limbs, open wounds, and changes in color from the rest of the body. Note any swelling or muscle spasms of the limbs, which may indicate injuries not apparent initially. Palpate any areas suspected of injury, noting the contour of surrounding bones. Check the range of motion of all joints, listening for crepitus and noting any signs of pain from the patient during the examination, but do not move an obviously injured extremity to test for range of motion. Complete a neurovascular examination, checking pulses, capillary refill, and response to sharp and dull pain stimuli.

PSYCHOSOCIAL. The patient with serious musculoskeletal injury is usually seen in the emergency department and is often in hypovolemic shock. As the patient becomes conscious, the effect of the trauma may be overwhelming; alternatively, the patient may have no memory of the trauma and be distraught to find himself or herself in the hospital. The older patient who has fallen and suffered a broken hip often becomes confused from the trauma. As the situation becomes clearer, the fear of hospitalization and becoming dependent on others poses a real problem. The patient may deny having a fracture or may not realize that fracture and a broken bone are synonymous.

The sudden nature of multiple trauma presents serious psychological stressors to the patient, family, and significant others. Often the victim is young and healthy; parents become extremely anxious, angry, guilty, and even despairing when their child is injured and they cannot protect him or her from danger. Peers often rally to support a classmate; their numbers may overwhelm the visiting area and the hospital's resources. A careful assessment of the family's and peer's response to trauma is important if interventions are to be constructive.

DIAGNOSTIC HIGHLIGHTS

Test	Normal Result	Abnormality with Condition	Explanation
Urine myoglobin	Negative	Positive; > 20 ng/ml	Myoglobin is a heme-containing, oxygen-binding protein that is present in striated and non-striated skeletal and cardiac muscle; it is released into the interstitium fluid after injury to a muscle

| X rays and computed tomography (CT) scan | Intact bones, soft tissues, and joints | Visualization of number and location of fractures | Identifies extent and degree of injury |

Other Tests: Blood alcohol level, urine toxic screen, complete blood count

PRIMARY NURSING DIAGNOSIS

Pain (acute or chronic) related to inflammation and swelling of the tendon

OUTCOMES. Comfort level; Pain control behavior; Pain: Disruptive effects; Pain level

INTERVENTIONS. Pain management; Analgesic administration; Positioning; Teaching: Prescribed activity/exercise; Teaching: Procedure/treatment; Teaching: Prescribed medication

☐ PLANNING AND IMPLEMENTATION

Collaborative

In the emergency situation, planning and implementation are related to the priorities of airway, breathing, circulation, and neurologic status. Unless the musculoskeletal injury is threatening the patient's circulation because of bleeding, management of musculoskeletal injuries usually occurs after the patient is stabilized. When a musculoskeletal injury interrupts a bone or joint, the trauma causes severe muscle spasms that lead to pain, angulation (abnormal formation of angles by the bones), and overriding of the ends of the bones. These complications need to be managed immediately to prevent increased soft tissue injury, decreased venous and lymphatic return, and edema. If the patient has any exposed soft tissue or bone, cover the area with a wet, sterile saline dressing. Prevent reentry of a contaminated bone into the wound if possible.

Early immobilization of the extremity at the trauma scene—which is actually the first step in trauma rehabilitation—preserves the function and prevents further injury. Immobilization limits muscle spasm, decreases angulation and injury from the overriding bone ends, and prevents closed fractures from becoming open fractures. Traction may also be applied to align bone ends in a close-to-normal position. This procedure restores circulatory, nerve, and lymphatic function and limits tissue injury and swelling. Generally, immobilization devices that are applied before the patient is admitted to the hospital are left in place until x rays are performed.

When the fracture is confirmed by diagnostic testing, the bone is reduced by restoring displaced bone segments to their normal position. When the physician restores the bone to normal alignment, venous and lymphatic return improves, as does soft tissue swelling. The orthopedist may perform a closed reduction in which he or she manually manipulates the bones to restore alignment. When closed reduction is not possible, a surgical (open) reduction is performed. The method of reduction depends on the grade, type, and location of the fracture.

External fixation devices are now being used frequently for many fractures that would until recently have been treated with traction. External fixation, such as the Hoffmann device, is a metal system of rods that is designed to maintain alignment of fracture fragments. The patient requires less immobilization and therefore usually suffers fewer of the hazards of immobility. Use the device itself to position limbs, unless it is being used to stabilize a pelvic fracture. External fixation devices may also cause complications, however. Some patients react to them with local irritation, and a few develop infections. Monitor the area every 8 hours while the patient is hospitalized and clean it according to hospital protocol. The most common method is with half-strength hydrogen peroxide. Use of povidore-iodine (Betadine) or Neosporin ointment around the pins after cleansing may also be indicated to prevent infection.

PHARMACOLOGIC HIGHLIGHTS

Medication or Drug Class	Dosage	Description	Rationale
Narcotic analgesia	Varies with drug	Codeine, morphine sulfate, meperidine hydrochloride	Relieve pain

Other Drugs: Antibiotics, antispasmodics

Independent

Follow the priorities of pain management, emotional support to cope with a sudden threat to health status, and prevention of complications. Pain may be caused by ineffective use of some treatment methods for fractures. Casts, traction, and fixation devices, once applied, should not cause pain. Improperly padded casts or ones that have been damaged may cause irritation and pressure to the casted area. Skin traction that causes friction also leads to impaired skin integrity. If the patient has soft tissue wounds that require treatment, a window in the cast may be needed. Maintain the functional integrity of the cast with attention to both immobilization of the fracture and prevention of further damage to the tissues.

Pain that seems extreme when a patient is casted or in skeletal traction may signal the advent of a compartment syndrome, a condition in which an edematous extremity is constricted by the cast. The patient complains of a burning sensation or other paresthesia. Edema may be present; pulses ordinarily remain intact. Even in the presence of substantial edema, the use of ice is contraindicated because of the danger of increased neurovascular compromise. The surgeon may bivalve the cast, remove the traction, or perform a fasciotomy.

The patient and family need a great deal of support to cope with a serious injury. Allow time each day to listen to concerns, discuss the patient's progress, and explain upcoming procedures. If the patient is a young trauma patient, you may need to work out a schedule with the patient's friends so that they can see the patient but also allow the patient adequate rest. Young adults enjoy diversional activities such as a television, tapes, compact discs, and radios. Older patients may experience depression and loss if the injury has long-term implications about their self-care. Consult with social workers and advanced practice nurses if the patient's anxiety or fear is abnormal. If the patient is a heavy drinker or was intoxicated at the time of injury, encourage the patient to evaluate his or her drinking patterns and the link between drinking and injury. If needed, refer the patient appropriately for a full evaluation for substance abuse.

Immobilization involving the whole person, rather than one extremity, requires aggressive prevention of the hazards of immobility. Motivate and educate the patient in order to help him or her anticipate and prevent complications. Delayed healing of either wound or bone may occur as a complication of the patient's status at the time of the fracture or as a result of immobility. Encourage a balanced diet with foods that promote healing, such as those that contain protein and vitamin C. Stimulation of the affected area by isometric and isotonic exercises also helps promote healing. Instruct the patient in those techniques, which may not initially seem possible to him or her. They provide a partial substitute for the stimulation to bone remodeling that is otherwise provided by weight bearing. Remember the design adage that is also useful in orthopedics: Form follows function.

DOCUMENTATION GUIDELINES

- Physiologic response: Adequacy of airway, breathing, circulation; vital signs; serial monitoring of neurological status; urine output; body weight
- History of injury, description, forces applied to the body during the trauma
- Response to treatment/medications: Pain, mobility, range of motion, muscle spasm, response to surgery, tolerance to nutrition
- Presence and response to traction and immobilization devices
- Complications: Infection, bleeding, anxiety, lack of mobility

DISCHARGE AND HOME HEALTHCARE GUIDELINES

Ascertain that the patient is alert and able to care for himself or herself within the limitations that are imposed by treatment of the fracture (e.g., cast or external fixation device) or has adequate home care available. Make sure that the patient and family understand any care that is needed for casts or fixation devices. Arrange with social service for the purchase or rental of any supplies, such as crutches, wheelchairs, or home health devices. Teach the patient the hazards of immobility, the symptoms of complications, and when to seek assistance from a healthcare provider. Teach the patient about the route, dosage, mechanism of action, and side effects of all medications. Make sure the patient understands the basic components of a healthy diet. Explore with the patient the effects of drinking and drug use on long-term health and well-being. Remind the patient that rates of reinjury are very high in those who continue to drink alcohol excessively. Determine that the patient has adequate transportation home and for follow-up appointments.

Myasthenia Gravis

DRG Category: 012
Mean LOS: 5.3 days
Description: MEDICAL: Degenerative Nervous System Disorders

Myasthenia gravis (MG) is an autoimmune disease that produces fatigue and voluntary muscle weakness, both of which become worse with exercise and improve with rest. The muscles that are frequently involved include those for eye and eyelid movement, chewing and swallowing, breathing, and movement of the distal muscles of the extremities. This weakness progressively worsens during the day or at times of stress, so the greatest fatigue is likely to occur at the end of the day. MG frequently accompanies disorders of the immune system or the thyroid gland.

Rapid acute exacerbations result in a 5% mortality rate and are classified as either myasthenic or cholinergic crises. Both crises lead to extreme respiratory distress, difficulty in swallowing and speaking, great anxiety, and generalized weakness, thus making differentiation challenging but crucial for selection of appropriate intensive therapy. Myasthenic crisis is caused by undermedication, whereas a cholinergic crisis results from excessive anticholinesterase medication and is thus likely to occur within 45 to 60 minutes of the last drug dosage. The major complications of MG are respiratory distress or insufficiency, aspiration pneumonia, and the poor nutrition that is linked to eating difficulties.

CAUSES

MG, thought to be an autoimmune disorder, is caused by a loss of acetylcholine (ACh) receptors in the postsynaptic neurons at the neuromuscular junction. About 80% of all MG patients have elevated titers for acetylcholine receptor antibodies, which can prevent the ACh molecule from binding to these receptor sites or can cause damage to them. MG is often associated with thymic tumors.

GENDER AND LIFE SPAN CONSIDERATIONS

The prevalence of MG is estimated to be 5 in 100,000 and the disorder occurs primarily in a bimodal distribution. In people in the age range of 20 to 30 years, women are more often affected than men; in the later years (over 50 years old), men are more likely to be affected than women.

Infants and children are also at risk for MG. Neonatal MG occurs in 10% to 20% of infants with myasthenic mothers. Symptoms occur within a few days after birth and usually last about 1 to 2 weeks. This short-term form of MG in infants is associated with the circulating maternal antibodies. MG may be congenital; in this case, it occurs in two forms. One form primarily consists of ocular weakness with some extremity weakness. The second form primarily involves bulbar weakness (weakness of the lips, tongue, mouth, larynx, and pharynx) with some ocular impairment; it characteristically is not associated with elevated ACh antibody titers. Juvenile MG begins with symptoms in the preteen years.

☐ ASSESSMENT

HISTORY. Elicit a careful history of the patient's symptoms and pay particular attention to changes that involve the eyes, which are often the earliest signs of MG. These changes include ptosis (eyelid drooping), diplopia (double vision), reduced eye closure, and blurred vision. Ask if the patient has to tilt the head back to see properly. Question the patient about weight loss because of problems with chewing and swallowing. Determine the patient's ability to perform sustained or repetitive movements of the extremities, such as brushing the hair or carrying groceries. Determine if the symptoms are milder in the morning, worsen as the day progresses, and subside after short rest periods. Ask the patient if the head bobs when he or she is tired or if the jaw hangs open.

PHYSICAL EXAMINATION. You may note a "mask-like" or "snarling" appearance because of the involvement of the facial muscles. Note if the patient has weak neck muscles that cause difficulty in maintaining head position. Assess the patient's posture and body alignment because the patient may slouch or walk with a slow gait. The patient's voice may fade during conversation. Determine the symmetry of muscle strength and movement. Perform an eye examination to determine visual acuity and eye movement, which are often abnormal. When you auscultate the patient's lungs, you may hear decreased breath sounds resulting from hypoventilation.

The patient who has confirmed MG may develop acute exacerbations, which can occur in two forms: myasthenic or cholinergic crisis. Myasthenic crisis is caused by undermedication and is also characterized by hypoxia (associated with tachycardia and possible elevated blood pressure), absence of the cough and gag reflexes, ptosis, diplopia and mydriasis (large pupils), and a positive response to the medication edrophonium (Tensilon). In comparison, a cholinergic crisis results from excessive anticholinesterase medication and is likely to occur within 45 to 60 minutes after the last drug dose. Side effects of overmedication include diarrhea and abdominal cramping, bradycardia and possible hypotension, a flushed diaphoretic appearance, miosis (small pupils), and increased secretions (saliva, tears, and bronchial secretions). Response to Tensilon is negative, and twitching and "thick tongue" dysphagia may occur.

PSYCHOSOCIAL. The course of MG is unpredictable because of its exacerbations and remissions. Patients live in fear of not being able to breathe adequately. Depression may occur in patients who experience exacerbations and functional limitations in their lifestyles and role responsibilities. Assess the family's support system and ability to deal with chronic disease and any emergency situations that may occur.

DIAGNOSTIC HIGHLIGHTS

Test	Normal Result	Abnormality with Condition	Explanation
Edrophonium (Tensilon) test	No change in strength	Marked, temporary improvement of strength	Administration of 10 mg of edrophonium IV over 30 seconds to determine if blocking cholinesterase improves symptoms temporarily; test results often show false positive results, which limits the diagnostic ability of test
Acetylcholine receptor antibody test	Negative = 0.03 nmol/L	Positive	Detects presence of antibodies against the acetylcholine receptor in serum; antibody interferes with acetylcholine binding, preventing muscle contraction
Electromyography (EMG)	Normal response to repeated nerve stimulation	Decremental response to repetitive nerve stimulation	Skeletal muscle action potential is tested to determine the response to repeated stimulations

PRIMARY NURSING DIAGNOSIS

Ineffective airway clearance related to difficulty in swallowing and aspiration

OUTCOMES. Respiratory status: Gas exchange; Respiratory status: Ventilation; Symptom control behavior; Treatment behavior: Illness or injury; Comfort level

INTERVENTIONS. Airway management; Anxiety reduction; Oxygen therapy; Airway suctioning; Airway insertion and stabilization; Cough enhancement; Mechanical ventilation; Positioning; Respiratory monitoring

◻ PLANNING AND IMPLEMENTATION

Collaborative

There is no cure for MG; treatment is predominantly pharmacologic. Plasmapheresis is reserved for patients who are refractory to conventional therapy, during myasthenic or cholinergic crisis, for prethymectomy stabilization and possible reduction in post-thymectomy ventilator therapy, or if unacceptable drug side effects develop. Plasmapheresis separates and removes circulating acetylcholine receptor antibodies from the patient's blood. A thymectomy is indicated for patients with a thymoma and for other selected patients with generalized MG. Thymectomy increases the chance of remission, increases long-term survival, decreases the chance of relapse after stopping immunosuppressant therapy, and allows better control of the disease. Thymectomy is most effective if it is performed early in the disease course. Improvement is recognized in 60% to 70% of thymectomy patients and coincides with complete remission in 20% to 40% of cases (although this remission may require several years to occur).

PHARMACOLOGIC HIGHLIGHTS

Medication or Drug Class	Dosage	Description	Rationale
Anti-cholinesterase drugs	Varies with drug	Pyridostigmine bromide (Mestinon), neostigmine bromide (Prostigmine); neostigmine methylsulfate can be given as a continuous infusion if the patient cannot take oral medication	Block the action of the enzyme anticholinesterase, thereby producing symptomatic improvement; atropine must be readily available to treat cholinergic side effects and medications must be administered on time, or the patient may be too weak or unable to swallow the drug
Prednisone	60–80 mg po qd followed by tapering to alternate-day regime of	Prednisone	Suppresses the autoimmune activity of MG

	lowest effective dose		
Nonsteroidal immunosuppressants	Varies with drug	Azathioprine (Imuran), cyclophosphamide (Cytoxin)	Suppress autoimmune activity when patients do not respond to prednisone; can produce extreme immunosuppression and toxic side effects

Independent

The primary nursing concerns focus on the adequacy of the patient's airway and breathing. Keep suction equipment and intubation supplies at the patient's bedside. For meals, place the patient in a completely upright position. Instruct the patient to swallow only when the chin is tipped downward and never to speak with food in his or her mouth. To prevent pulmonary complications, encourage the patient to perform deep breathing and coughing to enhance ventilation. If the patient requires surgery, instruct him or her on chest splinting during deep-breathing and coughing exercises. Keep the patient's pain under control before all breathing exercises.

Ensure adequate nutritional intake and observe for signs and symptoms of dehydration or malnutrition. Work with the patient and family to plan for foods that are easy to chew and swallow but are still appealing to the patient. Plan mealtime to make the most of the patient's energy peaks. Assist the patient in developing a method for reliable communication. Fear of sudden respiratory distress and the inability to call for help or to reach a call light is very real. If the patient requires hospitalization, locate the patient near the nurses' station, keep a call light nearby at all times, and provide a secondary "call" system (such as a different-toned bell) for use during times of distress. Emphasize clear, honest communication about the realistic expectations of therapy because the time between initiation of the intervention and when the patient experiences improvement can be quite prolonged.

Because treatment and improvement revolve around receiving the optimal dosages of medication, teach patients to recognize their disease status and the indications for self-determined dosage alterations to achieve an optimally effective drug benefit. Also teach the patients how to recognize the early signs of an overdose in order to prevent cholinergic crisis and when to self-medicate with atropine for relief of side effects. Involve the patient in decision making and recognize the patient's ability to manage his or her disease. Because these patients are frequently responsible for determining drug alterations at home, denying their judgment in determining drug dosages can cause them to feel very vulnerable and insecure. Delays in receiving their medications can cause distrust and may result in significant physical difficulty in swallowing the delayed medication. Incorporate the patient's input on plans for scheduling physical activities around rest periods.

Assist the patient in working through any feelings of depression that can occur because of MG's profound effect on lifestyle, roles, and responsibilities. Depression can also result from the disbelief by others of the MG diagnosis because the patient may appear to have suspiciously fluctuating symptoms. Provide encouragement to these patients to live full, productive lives. Educate the family and significant others on the fluctuation of MG, and place them in contact with support groups and the Myasthenia Gravis Foundation.

DOCUMENTATION GUIDELINES

- Respiratory status: Rate, quality, depth, ease, breath sounds, arterial hemoglobin saturation with oxygen
- Ability to chew, swallow, and speak (swallowing can be subjectively rated by the patient in anticipating ability to swallow food [0 = unable to swallow liquids to 5 = able to swallow regular diet]), food intake, daily weights
- Muscle weakness and strength, speed and degree of fatigue, ability to perform activities of daily living, response to rest, and plans for modification of activity
- Ptosis (can be rated by the nurse [0 = unable to open lid to 5 = uppermost edge of iris visible])

DISCHARGE AND HOME HEALTHCARE GUIDELINES

Instruct the patient and family on the importance of rest and avoiding fatigue. Be alert to factors that can cause exacerbations, such as infection (an annual flu shot is suggested), surgery, pregnancy, exposure to extreme temperatures, and tonic and alcoholic drinks. Instruct the patient and family about drug actions and side effects, the indications for dosage alteration, and the selective use of atropine for any overdose. Stress the importance of taking the medication in a timely manner. It is advisable to time the dose 1 hour before meals for best chewing and swallowing. Explain the potential drug interactions (especially aminoglycosides and neuromuscular blocking agents, which include many pesticides). Encourage the patient to inform the dentist, ophthalmologist, and pharmacist of the myasthenic condition.

Instruct patients about the symptoms that require emergency treatment, and encourage them to locate a neurologist familiar with MG management for any follow-up needs. Suggest that they collect a packet of literature to take to the emergency department in case the available physician is unfamiliar with this disease. (*The Physician's Handbook* is available on request from the MG Foundation.) Instruct patients to wear MG identification jewelry. Suggest having an "emergency code" to alert family if they are too weak to speak (such as ringing the phone twice and hanging up). Instruct the family about cardiopulmonary resuscitation techniques, how to perform the Heimlich maneuver, how to contact the rescue squad, and how to explain the route to the hospital. Make a referral to a vocational rehabilitation center if guidance for modifying the home or work environment, such as a raised seat and handrail for the toilet, would be beneficial.

Myocardial Infarction

DRG Category: 122
Mean LOS: 4.9 days
Description: MEDICAL: Circulatory Disorders with AMI without C.V. Comp Disch Alive
DRG Category: 121
Mean LOS: 7.0 days
Description: MEDICAL: Circulatory Disorders with AMI and C.V. Comp Disch Alive
DRG Category: 107
Mean LOS: 9.3 days
Description: SURGICAL: Coronary Bypass without CC
DRG Category: 106
Mean LOS: 12.1 days
Description: SURGICAL: Coronary Bypass with CC

Myocardial infarction (MI) results when myocardial tissue becomes necrotic because of absent or diminished blood supply. In North America, MI is one of the most common causes of death, with a mortality rate of approximately 25%. In addition, more than 50% of sudden deaths occur within 1 hour of the onset of symptoms.

When myocardial tissue is deprived of oxygenated blood supply for a period of time, an area of myocardial necrosis develops; this necrosis is surrounded by injured and ischemic tissue. Pain usually develops from irritation of nerve endings in the ischemic and injured areas. The typical chest pain for adult males is a substernal, crushing pain that radiates down the left arm and up into the jaw. Women and elderly patients with MIs often experience an indigestion-type discomfort and shortness of breath instead of the "typical" substernal pressure.

Infarctions may be classified according to myocardial thickness and the location of affected tissue. Although the majority of MIs occur in the left ventricle, more right ventricular involvement is being recognized. Left ventricular infarctions are classified as inferior (diaphragmatic), anterior, and posterior. Right ventricular infarctions are usually not differentiated by a specific location. Transmural, or Q-wave infarctions, involve 50% or more of the total thickness of the ventricular wall and are characterized by abnormal Q waves and ST-T wave changes. Partial thickness infarctions (also called subendocardial, nontransmural, and non-Q-wave infarcts) are characterized by ST-T wave changes but no abnormal Q waves.

Complications of MI include cardiac dysrhythmias, extension of the area of infarction, heart failure, and pericarditis. Rupture of the atrial or ventricular septum, valvular rupture, or rupture of the ventricles can occur as well. Other complications include ventricular aneurysms and cerebral and pulmonary emboli.

CAUSES

Infarctions may occur for a variety of reasons, but coronary thrombosis of a coronary artery narrowed with plaque is the most common cause. Other causes include spasms of the coronary arteries; blockage of the coronary arteries by embolism of thrombi, fatty plaques, air, or calcium; and disparity between myocardial oxygen demand and coronary arterial supply. Multiple risk factors have been identified for coronary artery disease and MI. Some factors—such as age, family history, and gender—cannot be modified. Aging increases the atherosclerotic process, family history may increase the risk by both genetic and environmental influences, and males are more prone to MIs than are premenopausal women. Premenopausal women have the benefit of protective estrogens and a lower hematocrit, although heart disease is on the rise in this population, possibly because of an increased rate of smoking in women. Once women become postmenopausal, their risk for MI increases, as it also does for men over age 50.

Modifiable risk factors include cigarette smoking, which causes arterial vasoconstriction and increases plaque formation. A diet high in saturated fats, cholesterol, sugar, salt, and total calories increases the risk for MIs. Elevated serum cholesterol and low-density lipoprotein levels increase the chance for atherosclerosis. Hypertension and obesity increase the workload of the heart, and diabetes mellitus decreases the circulation to the heart muscle. Hostility and stress may also increase sympathetic nervous system activity and pose risk. A sedentary lifestyle diminishes collateral circulation and decreases the strength of the cardiac muscle. Medications can also prevent risks. Oral contraceptives may enhance thrombus formation, cocaine use can cause coronary artery spasm, and anabolic steroid use can accelerate atherosclerosis.

GENDER AND LIFE SPAN CONSIDERATIONS

MI is the single largest cause of death among American men and women. The risk of MI increases with age, but MIs also occur in young adults. Both men and women are at risk for MI. Women have higher morbidity and mortality rates after MI than men, possibly because they are older and have more pre-existing diseases than men when the MI occurs. Women with chest pain also delay seeking treatment longer than men do.

□ ASSESSMENT

HISTORY. Symptomatology is very important in diagnosing MIs. Ask about chest, jaw, arm, and epigastric pain. Remember that not all people have the "typical" chest pain; evaluate the whole clinical picture because some people may experience no pain at all. Ask about shortness of breath, racing heart rate, diaphoresis, clammy skin, dizziness, nausea, and vomiting. Note that sudden death and full cardiac arrest may be the first indication of MI.

Elicit a thorough description of the symptoms by using the P, Q, R, S, T approach. P stands for palliative or precipitating measures (what was occurring when the symptoms began and what made the symptoms better or worse). Q is the quality of the discomfort (sharp, stabbing, or pressure). R represents radiating; S is the severity of the discomfort on a scale such as one from 1 to 10. T stands for time since symptoms and discomfort began. The time is very important because increased time to treatment may mean increased muscle damage; time to treatment dictates management. The timing of asking these questions is also important. If the patient is in acute distress, ask the minimum number of questions that are necessary to treat the pain effectively and ask the additional questions later.

PHYSICAL EXAMINATION. The patient with an MI usually appears acutely ill with diaphoresis, clammy skin, nausea and vomiting, and shortness of breath, but the patient may have mild symptoms such as epigastric discomfort. When you inspect the patient, note the respiratory status, including rate, depth, rhythm, and effort. Observe the patient's skin for color and diaphoresis, and observe the mental status for confusion, dizziness, and anxiety.

When you auscultate the patient's heart, you may hear heart sounds that are irregular if dysrhythmias are present, an S_3 if irregular ventricular filling occurs, and an S_4 if irregular atrial filling occurs. A murmur may be heard if the valves are not closing tightly because of ischemia or injury of the papillary muscle.

PSYCHOSOCIAL. Inquire about stressors in the patient's life and how the patient deals with them. A diagnosis of heart disease and MI is a life-changing event that carries emotionally laden concerns for most patients. Also assess the patient's ability to cope with a sudden illness and the change in roles that an MI involves.

DIAGNOSTIC HIGHLIGHTS

Test	Normal Result	Abnormality with Condition	Explanation
Electrocardiogram	Normal PQRST pattern	ST segment elevation, T-wave inversion, and an abnormal Q wave (wider than 0.04 seconds or more than ⅓ height of QRS complex)	Electrical conduction system adversely affected by myocardial ischemia and necrosis; Q wave occurs because necrotic cells do not conduct electrical stimuli
Creatine kinase isoenzyme (MB-CK)	0%–6% to total CK	Elevated	Elevations occur resulting from tissue damage
Cardiac troponin I (cTnI); cardiac troponin T (cTnT)	< 3.1 µg/L; < 0.2 µg/L	Elevated	Used to differentiate between angina and MI; earliest increases occur in 3–6 hours; peak increase occurs in 10–24 hours

Other Tests: Cholesterol (total, low-density lipoprotein, high-density lipoprotein), triglycerides, lactate dehydrogenase, complete blood count, cardiac catheterziation, thallium scan, radionuclide ventriculography, two-dimensional echocardiography

PRIMARY NURSING DIAGNOSIS

Altered tissue perfusion (myocardial) related to narrowing of the coronary artery(ies) associated with atherosclerosis, spasm, or thrombosis

OUTCOMES. Cardiac pump effectiveness; Circulation status; Comfort level; Pain control behavior; Pain level; Tissue perfusion: Cardiac

INTERVENTIONS. Cardiac care; Cardiac precautions; Oxygen therapy; Pain management; Medication administration; Circulatory care; Positioning

❑ PLANNING AND IMPLEMENTATION

Collaborative

The physician usually prescribes oxygen therapy, often at 2 to 4 L per minute to provide increased oxygen to the myocardial tissue. If it has been less than 4 to 6 hours since pain began, and if the clinical picture suggests an MI, thrombolytic agents may be given to dissolve the coronary thrombus. A cardiac catheterization may be performed when the patient's condition is stable to identify the areas of blockage in the coronary arteries and to assist in determining treatment. Medical treatment with medications as described here may be the treatment of choice if the blockage is extensive and if the patient has conditions that increase mortality or morbidity with surgery. A percutaneous transluminal coronary angioplasty (PTCA) may be performed if the blockages are limited and are accessible with a balloon catheter. The cardiologist inflates the balloon catheter at the area of blockage and compresses the plaque or pushes the arterial wall out to enlarge the arterial lumen. The cardiologist may also place a stent at the area of dilation to maintain patency. An arthrectomy, which involves shaving off the plaque in the coronary artery and removing the debris to obtain arterial patency, is another nonsurgical option.

Continuous cardiac monitoring, along with intermittent 12-lead ECGs, helps the healthcare team monitor the resolution of ischemic and injured areas. Hemodynamic monitoring may be initiated, and a flow-directed pulmonary artery catheter may be used to measure filling pressures in the ventricles, to determine pulmonary artery pressures, and to calculate the cardiac output. Notify the physician for significant signs of decreased cardiac output, such as hypotension, diminished urine output, crackles in the lungs, cool and clammy skin, and fatigue.

The surgical option for patients with coronary blockages caused by plaque is coronary artery bypass grafting (CABG). To restore blood flow to the heart muscle distal to the blockages, the surgeon uses the left internal mammary artery or the saphenous vein to bypass the areas of blockage within the coronary arteries. Diet restrictions begin in the hospital and should be continued at home. A collaborative effort among the patient, dietician, physician, and nurse plans for a diet low in cholesterol, fat, calories, and sodium (salt). Drinks in the coronary care unit are usually decaffeinated and not too hot or cold in temperature, although some experts question the need to restrict extremes of temperature. Foods with fiber may decrease the incidence of constipation.

PHARMACOLOGIC HIGHLIGHTS

Medication or Drug Class	Dosage	Description	Rationale
Recombinant tissue-plasminogen activator (alteplase, rt-PA)	IV bolus followed by IV infusion 0.75 mg/kg over 30 minutes; then 0.50 mg/kg over 60 minutes	Thrombolytic agent	Less likely to cause hypotension and allergic reaction than other drugs; more expensive than other agents and associated with a higher risk of intracranial hemorrhage but more efficacious
Reteplase (r-PA)	10 units IV bolus, repeated 30 minutes later	Thrombolytic agent	Reduced fibrin specificity but longer half life than rt-PA

| Streptokinase | 1.5 million units over 60 minutes IV | Thrombolytic agent | 1%–2% have allergic reactions; 10% have hypotension |
| Heparin | 1000 units per IV started 4 hours after thrombolytic agents and continued for 48 hours | Anticoagulant | Prevents additional thrombus formation in the coronary arteries |

Other Drugs: Vasodilators such as nitrates, beta-adrenergic blockers, calcium antagonists, or angiotensin-converting enzyme inhibitors are given to increase coronary perfusion and decrease afterload if the patient's blood pressure is adequate. Usually the patient requires pain medication, with parenteral morphine the drug of choice. Aspirin is used because of its antiplatelet activity, and antidysrhythmics, sedatives, and stool softeners may be given.

Independent

The focus is to control pain and related symptoms, to reduce myocardial oxygen consumption during myocardial healing, and to provide patient/family education. Remember that chest pain may indicate continued tissue damage; therefore, manage chest pain immediately. In addition to the pharmacologic methods mentioned here, a variety of measures can be used to reduce the cardiac workload during periods of chest pain. To decrease oxygen demand, encourage the patient to maintain bed rest for the first 24 hours; encourage rest throughout the entire hospitalization. Create a quiet, restful environment and encourage family involvement in the patient's care. Discourage any straining such as Valsalva's maneuver.

Because anxiety and fear are common among both patients and families, encourage everyone to discuss their concerns and express their feelings. Use a calm, reassuring voice; give simple explanations about care and procedures; and stay with the patient during periods of high anxiety if possible. Discuss with the patient and family the diagnosis, the activity and diet restrictions, and medical treatment. Numerous lifestyle changes may be needed. A cardiac rehabilitation program is helpful in limiting risk factors and in providing additional guidance, social support, and encouragement.The goals of a cardiac rehabilitation program are to reduce the risk of another MI through re-education and implementation of a secondary prevention program and to improve the quality of life for the MI victim. The program provides progressive monitored exercise, additional teaching, and psychosocial support. An exercise stress test is used before beginning exercise to evaluate the patient's response to physical activity and to determine an appropriate program. There are usually three phases to cardiac rehabilitation: in hospital, outpatient, and follow-up.

DOCUMENTATION GUIDELINES
- Response to vasodilators and pain medications
- Physical findings of cardiac functions: Vital signs, heart sounds, breath sounds, urine output, peripheral pulses, level of consciousness
- Psychosocial response to treatment and diagnosis
- Presence of complications: Bleeding tendencies, respiratory distress, unrelieved chest pain, constipation

DISCHARGE AND HOME HEALTHCARE GUIDELINES

Be sure the patient understands all the medications, including the dosage, route, action, and adverse effects. Instruct the patient to keep the nitroglycerin bottle sealed and away from heat. The medication may lose its potency after the bottle has been opened for 6 months. If the patient does not feel a sensation when the tablet is put under the tongue or does not get a headache, the pills may have lost their potency.

Explain the need to treat recurrent chest pain or MI discomfort with sublingual nitroglycerin every 5 minutes for three doses. If the pain persists for 20 minutes, teach the patient to seek medical attention. If the patient has severe pain or becomes short of breath with chest pain, teach the patient to take nitroglycerin and seek medical attention right away. Explore mechanisms to implement diet control, an exercise program, and smoking cessation if appropriate.

Myocarditis

DRG Category: 144
Mean LOS: 4.5 days
Description: MEDICAL: Other Circulatory System Diagnoses with CC
DRG Category: 103
Mean LOS: 25.4 days
Description: SURGICAL: Heart Transplant

Myocarditis describes the infiltration of myocardial cells by various forms of bacteria or viruses that damage the myocardium by inciting an inflammatory response. Myocarditis results in white blood cell (WBC) infiltration and necrosis of myocytes (heart muscle cells). Although myocarditis commonly is self-limiting, mild, and asymptomatic, it sometimes induces myofibril degeneration, which leads to right- and left-sided heart failure. When myocarditis recurs, it can produce chronic valvulitis (usually when it results from rheumatic fever), dysrhythmias, thromboembolism, or cardiomyopathy.

CAUSES

Myocarditis generally occurs as a result of an infectious agent, but it also can be caused by radiation or other toxic physical agents, such as lead. A variety of drugs, including phenothiazines, lithium, and chronic use of cocaine, may also lead to myocarditis. In the United States the most common cause of myocarditis is viral infection (e.g., coxsackie, Group B, ECHO), but a variety of bacterial, protozoal, parasitic, helminthic (such as trichinosis), and rickettsial infections can produce inflammation of the heart.

GENDER AND LIFE SPAN CONSIDERATIONS

Myocarditis can occur at any age and in both sexes. Infants and immunosuppressed adults are at risk for Chagas's disease (South American trypanosomiasis), a disease that occurs with insect bites, particularly in Brazil, Argentina, and Chile.

☐ ASSESSMENT

HISTORY. Establish a history of malaise, fatigue, dyspnea, palpitations, myalgias, and fever. Ask the patient to describe any chest pain or soreness, including the onset, location, intensity, and duration of the pain. Determine if the patient has experienced excessive tachycardia, both at rest and with effort. Elicit a history of medication use, particularly the use of phenothiazines, lithium, or cocaine. Ask if the patient has been exposed to radiation or lead or has undergone radiation therapy for lung or breast cancer. Determine if the patient has been previously diagnosed with rheumatic fever, infectious mononucleosis, polio, mumps, trichinosis, sarcoidosis, or typhoid. Develop a history of recent upper respiratory tract infections, including viral pharyngitis and tonsillitis. Ask if the patient has recently traveled to South America.

PHYSICAL EXAMINATION. Although myocarditis is generally uncomplicated and self-limiting, it may induce myofibril degeneration that results in right and left heart failure. When heart failure progresses, a number of changes can occur. Inspect the patient for signs of cardiomegaly, neck vein distension, dyspnea, resting or exertional tachycardia that is disproportionate to the degree of fever, and supraventricular and ventricular dysrhythmias. Palpation may reveal a left ventricular heave. Auscultate for pericardial friction rub and, with heart failure, crackles in the lungs and an S_3 heart sound. Auscultate breath sounds and heart sounds one to two times every 8 hours. Assess for signs and symptoms of decreased cardiac output (decreased urine output, delayed capillary refill, dizziness, syncope).

PSYCHOSOCIAL. The patient is likely to be experiencing severe anxiety, even fear, since the condition involves his or her heart. Determine the patient's knowledge of heart disease and the meaning that the diagnosis represents in his or her life. Assess the patient's emotional, financial, and social resources to manage the disease.

DIAGNOSTIC HIGHLIGHTS

Test	Normal Result	Abnormality with Condition	Explanation
Endomyocardial biopsy	Normal myocytes	Presence of abnormal numbers of lymphocytes; degeneration of muscle fibers	Viral infection causes damage to myocytes
Creatine kinase isoenzyme (MB-CK)	0%–6% to total CK	Elevated	Elevations occur resulting from damage

Other Tests: Electrocardiogram, viral antigen, IgM antibody titers, erythrocyte sedimentation rate, troponin levels

PRIMARY NURSING DIAGNOSIS

Decreased cardiac output related to a reduced mechanical function of the heart muscle or valvular dysfunction

OUTCOMES. Cardiac pump: Effectiveness; Circulation status; Tissue perfusion:

Abdominal organs and peripheral; Vital sign status; Electrolyte and acid base balance; Endurance; Energy conservation; Fluid balance

INTERVENTIONS. Cardiac care; Circulatory care: Mechanical assist device; Fluid/ electrolyte management; Medication administration; Medication management: Oxygen therapy; Vital signs monitoring

☐ PLANNING AND IMPLEMENTATION

Collaborative

The primary goal of treatment of myocarditis is to eliminate the underlying cause. Patients admitted to the hospital are placed in a coronary care unit where their cardiac status can be observed via cardiac monitor. Oxygenation and rest are prescribed in order to prevent dysrhythmias and further damage to the myocardium. Apply intermittent compression boots, as prescribed, to prevent the complications of thrombophlebitis.

Congestive heart failure responds to routine management, including digitalization and diuresis, although patients with myocarditis appear to be particularly sensitive to digitalis. Observe for signs of digitalis toxicity such as anorexia, nausea, vomiting, blurred vision, and cardiac dysrhythmias. Patients with a low-cardiac output state, which is commonly associated with severe congestive heart failure, require serial monitoring of cardiac filling pressures; a flow-directed pulmonary artery catheter has the capability of measuring cardiac output. With severe heart failure, dobutamine appears valuable because of its inotropic effects with limited vasoconstrictor and arrhythmogenic properties. Intractable congestive cardiac failure or shock, or both, in a patient with acute myocarditis may indicate the need for temporary partial or total cardiopulmonary bypass and eventual cardiac transplantation.

PHARMACOLOGIC HIGHLIGHTS

Medication or Drug Class	Dosage	Description	Rationale
Antibiotics	Varies with drug and causative agent	Varies with drug and causative agent	Kill pathogens

Other Drugs: The use of immunosuppression therapy is indicated for viral immune-mediated myocardial damage; however, precise drug protocols with corticosteroids, azathioprine, or cyclosporine are controversial and are generally limited to use with life-threatening complications such as intractable heart failure.

Independent

Focus on maximizing oxygen delivery and minimizing oxygen consumption. Encourage the patient to maintain bed rest with the head of the bed elevated. Stress the importance of bed rest by assisting with bathing, as necessary, and providing a bedside commode to reduce stress on the heart. For patients with enough mobility, encourage active range-of-motion activities to prevent blood stasis. For patients who are acutely ill, extremely weak, or in cardiac failure, perform passive range-of-motion exercises. Provide regular skin care for the patient on bed rest to maintain skin integrity.

In addition to any prescribed analgesics, assist the patient with pain management by teaching relaxation techniques, guided imagery, and distractions. Encourage the patient to sit upright, leaning slightly forward, rather than lying supine. Use pillows to increase the patient's comfort.

Before discharge, be sure to teach the patient about the pathophysiology of myocarditis. Explain the prescribed medications, any potential complications, and lifestyle limitations. Reassure the patient that activity limitations are temporary and that myocarditis is generally a self-limiting condition.

DOCUMENTATION GUIDELINES

- Physical findings: Signs of infection, cardiac monitoring results, breath sounds, heart sounds, intake and output, vital signs
- Laboratory results: Hemodynamic results; changes in chest x ray
- Response to pain: Location, description, duration, response to interventions
- Response to treatment: Change in pain, temperature reduction, increased activity tolerance
- Presence of complications: Myofibril degeneration, right- and left-sided heart failure

DISCHARGE AND HOME HEALTHCARE GUIDELINES

Be sure the patient and family understand any medication prescribed, including dosage, route, action, and side effects. If the patient is on immunosuppression therapy, review the medications and strategies to limit infection. Review with the patient all follow-up appointments that are scheduled. Review the need to check with the physician before resuming physical activities. Caution the patient to avoid active physical exercise during and after viral or bacterial infection. Review the nature of the disease process and signs and symptoms to report to the physician.

Nephrotic Syndrome

DRG Category: 331
Mean LOS: 5.1 days
Description: MEDICAL: Other Kidney and Urinary Tract Diagnoses, Age > 17 with CC

Nephrotic syndrome (NS), a clinical syndrome rather than a disease, is characterized by renal glomerular injury and massive loss of protein in the urine. An accompanying loss of serum albumin, an increased level of serum lipids, and massive peripheral edema occur.

Pathophysiologic changes are caused by a defect in the glomerular basement membrane, which results in increased membrane permeability to protein, particularly albumin. Loss of albumin through the glomerular membrane reduces serum albumin and decreases colloidal oncotic pressure in the capillary vascular beds. Subsequently, fluid leaks into the interstitial spaces, collects in body cavities, and creates massive generalized edema and ascites. Interstitial fluid shifts cause a decrease in the fluid volume within the vascular bed. The vascular fluid volume deficits stimulate the renin/angiotensin system and the release of aldosterone. These compensatory mechanisms cause renal tubular reabsorption of sodium and water, which further contributes to edema formation. Some patients become markedly immunosuppressed because of the loss of the immunoglobulin IgG in the urine. Enhanced urinary excretion of transferrin may lead to anemia, and loss of antithrombin III may lead to enhanced coagulation.

Complications occur because of the increased tendency for blood coagulation owing to increased blood viscosity. These changes may result in thromboembolic vascular occlusion in the kidneys, lungs, and lower extremities in particular. Other complications include accelerated atherosclerosis, acute renal failure, malnutrition, and a lowered resistance to infection.

CAUSES

Numerous factors contribute to the development of NS. These factors may be of idiopathic, secondary, or congenital origin. Idiopathic NS, the most common form, occurs in the absence of any systemic pre-existing disease. One type, minimal change NS, is the most frequent form in children and, although the cause is unknown, is associated with autoimmune changes. Other causes of idiopathic NS are several forms of glomerulonephritis and focal sclerosis of the glomeruli. Secondary NS occurs during or following a known disease process, such as cancer, acquired immunodeficiency syndrome, or lupus erythematosus. It also follows drug toxicity, insect stings, and venomous animal bites. Congenital nephrotic syndrome is transmitted by a recessive gene.

GENDER AND LIFE SPAN CONSIDERATIONS

In the pediatric population, 80% of the cases of NS are idiopathic, minimal change NS. Congenital NS also occurs in the pediatric population, although it is usually fatal within the first 2 years of life unless the child receives a renal transplant. Secondary NS occurs in all age groups but is the major etiological factor in adults of both sexes.

☐ ASSESSMENT

HISTORY. Patients may report no illness before the onset of symptoms; others have a history of systemic multisystem disease, such as lupus erythematosus, diabetes mellitus, amyloidosis, or multiple myeloma or have a history of an insect sting or venomous animal bite. Symptoms usually appear insidiously and may include lethargy, depression, and weight gain. The patient may describe gastrointestinal (GI) symptoms of nausea, anorexia, and diarrhea. Initially patients report periorbital edema in the morning and abdominal or extremity edema in the evening.

PHYSICAL EXAMINATION. In the early stages, inspect the patient's appearance for periorbital edema, ascites, and peripheral edema. In later stages, inspect the patient for massive generalized edema of the scrotum, labia, and abdomen. Pitting edema is usually present in dependent areas. The patient's skin appears extremely pale and fragile. You may note areas of skin erosion and breakdown. Often urine output is decreased from normal and may appear characteristically dark, frothy, or opalescent. Some patients have hematuria as well. Patients with severe ascites may be in acute respiratory distress, with an increase in respiratory rate and effort. When you auscultate the patient's lungs, you may hear adventitious breath sounds, such as crackles, or the breath sounds may be distant because of a pleural effusion. When you auscultate the patient's blood pressure, you may find orthostatic changes.

During the acute phases of the illness, assess the patient's fluid status by ongoing monitoring of the patient's weight, fluid intake and output, and degree of pitting edema. Measure the patient's abdominal girth daily and record changes. Monitor for signs of complications, particularly thromboembolic complications such as renal vein thrombosis (sudden flank pain, a tender costovertebral angle, macroscopic hematuria, and decreased urine output) and extremity arterial occlusion (decreased distal pulses, blanched and cold extremities, delayed capillary refill).

PSYCHOSOCIAL. Patients and family members may express fear or display signs of anxiety related to changes in the patient's appearance. The uncertain prognosis and the possibility of lifestyle changes add to their stress. Because of the insidious onset of symptoms, parents and significant others often verbalize guilt over not seeking medical attention sooner.

DIAGNOSTIC HIGHLIGHTS

Test	Normal Result	Abnormality with Condition	Explanation
Urinalysis	Minimal red blood cells; moderate clear protein casts; negative for protein	Increased proteinurea	Protein is lost in urine caused by loss of albumin through the glomerular membrane
24-hour urine collection	Minimal red blood cells; moderate clear protein casts; negative for protein	> 3.5 g per day of proteinuria	Protein is lost in urine caused by loss of albumin through the glomerular membrane
Serum albumin	3.5–5.0 g/dL	Decreased	Albumin is lost in urine

Other Tests: Creatinine, blood urea nitrogen, renal biopsy, cholesterol, triglycerides, serum potassium (hypokalemia is common)

PRIMARY NURSING DIAGNOSIS

Fluid volume excess (total body) related to excessive serum protein loss and resultant volume shifts out of vascular bed

OUTCOMES. Fluid balance; Hydration; Circulation status; Cardiac pump effectiveness

INTERVENTIONS. Fluid monitoring; Fluid/electrolyte management; Fluid resuscitation; Intravenous therapy; Circulatory care

☐ PLANNING AND IMPLEMENTATION

Collaborative

Edema is controlled by restricting salt to 2 to 3 grams per day. Dietary alterations also include a high-protein diet with restrictions of cholesterol and saturated fat. If the patient has accompanying renal insufficiency, restriction of dietary protein may complicate the dietary plan. The amount of protein lost in the urine needs to be added to the calculated protein restriction to arrive at the total daily protein intake. Most patients need nutritional consultation with a dietician to identify an appropriate diet within the restrictions. Involve the patient, parents, or significant others in the meal selection to ensure that the diet is appealing to the patient. Discuss the optimal fluid intake for the patient with the physician so that the patient is well hydrated and yet does not have continued fluid retention.

Other collaborative interventions are primarily pharmacologic. In spite of the excessive edema, patients need to be monitored for dehydration and hypokalemia, particularly when they are on diuretic therapy. Patients need to maintain an adequate fluid intake and a diet high in potassium (unless they have renal insufficiency).

PHARMACOLOGIC HIGHLIGHTS

Medication or Drug Class	Dosage	Description	Rationale
Prednisone (Orasone)	1 mg/kg per day po until < 3 g protein per day in urine	Glucocorticoid	Decreases permeability of glomerulus to protein; initiated as soon as possible after the diagnosis of NS is confirmed
Cyclophosphamide (Cytoxan)	2 mg/kg per day po for 8 weeks	Antineoplastic	For patients who respond poorly to glucocorticoids

Other Drugs: The physician may prescribe diuretics if respiratory compromise from edema occurs or if edema causes tissue breakdown. Some patients may also receive parenteral albumin to raise the oncotic pressure within the vascular bed. To prevent thromboembolic complications, many patients are given anticoagulant therapy with heparin and warfarin. Acute thrombolytic episodes may require fibrinolytic agents such as streptokinase or surgical thrombectomy.

Independent

Focus on maintaining the patient's fluid balance, promoting skin care, preventing nosocomial infection, and providing supportive measures. To maintain the patient's skin integrity, turn patients every 2 hours. Observe the skin closely for areas of breakdown until the edema resolves. Use an egg-crate mattress or specialty bed to limit irritation to skin pressure points, and encourage the patient or parents to avoid tight-fitting clothing and diapers.

Note that both the medications and the disease process may lead to immunosuppression. Implement scrupulous infection control measures, such as hand washing, sterile technique with invasive procedures, and clean technique for all noninvasive procedures to reduce the chance of infection. Do not assign patients to rooms with other patients who have infectious processes. Encourage visitation, but ask visitors with infections to wait until they are infection-free before visiting. To limit the risk of blood clotting, encourage the patient to be as mobile as possible considering his or her underlying condition. If the patient is bedridden, use active and passive range-of-motion exercises at least every 4 hours and have the patient wear compression boots when immobile in bed.

Note that some patients have a disturbed body image because of the side effects of steroid therapy (moon face, increased facial and body hair, abdominal distension, and mood swings). Encourage the patient to express these feelings and note that they are temporary until the condition resolves and the steroids are discontinued. If the patient desires, limit visitation to immediate family only until the patient resolves the anxiety over the body image disturbance.

DOCUMENTATION GUIDELINES

- Fluid volume parameters: Intake and output, urine character, urine specific gravity, urine protein, edema (location and degree of pitting), abdominal girth
- Condition of skin/mucous membranes: Turgor, membrane color and moisture, location of any skin breakdown (location, size, appearance, presence of drainage and character)
- Presence of GI complaints: Nausea, anorexia, diarrhea (if present, amount, frequency, color)
- Respiratory status: Rate and rhythm, lung expansion, presence of retractions or nasal flaring, adventitious breath sounds, type of expectorated secretions
- Comfort level: Type of discomfort, location, and intensity; if pain is present, describe the location, intensity (using a pain scale), and character

DISCHARGE AND HOME HEALTHCARE GUIDELINES

Teach the patient and family about the disease process, prognosis, and treatment plan. Explain that they need to monitor the urine daily for protein and keep a diary with the results of the tests. Have the patient or family demonstrate the testing techniques before discharge to demonstrate their ability to perform these monitoring tasks. Instruct the patient and family to avoid exposure to communicable diseases and to engage in scrupulous infection control measures such as frequent handwashing. Encourage patients with hypercoagulability to maintain hydration and mobility and to follow the medication regimen.

Teach the patient and family the purpose, dosage, route, desired effects, and side effects for all prescribed medications. Inform patients on anticoagulant therapy of the need for laboratory monitoring of activated partial thromboplastin time or prothrombin time. Caution patients who are receiving steroid therapy to take the dosages exactly as prescribed; explain that skipping doses could be harmful or life-threatening. In cases of long-term steroid therapy, explain the signs of complications, such as GI bleeding, stunted growth (children), bone fractures, and immunosuppression. Encourage patients to resume normal activities as soon as possible.

Neurogenic Bladder

DRG Category: 332
Mean LOS: 3.1 days
Description: MEDICAL: Other Kidney and Urinary Tract Diagnoses, Age > 17 without CC
DRG Category: 312
Mean LOS: 3.5 days
Description: SURGICAL: Urethral Procedures, Age > 17 with CC

Neurogenic bladder is defined as an interruption of normal bladder innervation because of lesions on or insults to the nervous system. Neurogenic bladder dysfunctions have been categorized in two ways: according to the response of the bladder to the insult (Classification I) or according to the lesion's level (Classification II). (See Table 40.)

TABLE 40 | **Classifications of Neurogenic Bladder**

CLASSIFICATION	TYPE	CAUSES	RESPONSE
Classification I	Uninhibited	Cerebrovascular accident (CVA), multiple sclerosis; lesions in cortico-regulatory tracts	Can void spontaneously when bladder is full
	Sensory paralytic	Lesions in lateral spinal tract from diabetic peripheral neuropathy, pernicious anemia	Cannot sense a full bladder and has chronic retention and overflow incontinence
	Motor paralytic	Spinal cord lesions at or above sacral level (S-2-S-4; upper motor neuron lesion)	Unable to initiate voiding even when bladder is full and causing extreme pain
	Autonomous	Retention and incontinence occur when a condition such as cancer, trauma, or infection causes destruction of nerve connections between the bladder and the CNS (lower motor neuron lesion)	Cannot perceive bladder fullness or cannot initiate voiding without assistance such as abdominal pressure
	Reflex	Upper neuron lesions above T-12	Cannot perceive bladder filling; bladder contracts on reflex, but often does not empty completely, leading to an increased potential for bladder infection
Classification II	Upper motor neuron	Damage to corticospinal or pyramidal tract in	Bladder tends to respond in a spastic, hypertonic, or

| damage | brain or spinal cord at or above the level of the sacral vertebrae (S-2 to S-4) | hyperreflexic manner; nerve impulses are not transmitted from spinal area to cerebral cortex; no sensation of urge to void; lower cord is unaffected so bladder reflexively empties, resulting in urinary incontinence |
| Lower motor neuron damage | Damage to anterior horn cells, nerve roots, or peripheral nervous system below the sacral vertebrae | Bladder tends to respond in a flaccid, atonic, or hyporeflexic manner; messages related to bladder filling do not reach cerebral cortex, resulting in residual urinary retention |

Many complications can result in patients with neurogenic bladder, such as bladder infection and skin breakdown related to incontinence. In addition, urolithiasis (stones in the urinary tract) is a common complication. Patients with spinal lesions above T-7 are also at risk for autonomic dysreflexia, a life-threatening complication. Autonomic reflexia results from the body's abnormal response to stimuli such as a full bladder or a distended colon. It results in severely elevated blood pressure, flushing, diaphoresis, decreased pulse, and a pounding headache. Chronic renal failure (CRF) can also result from chronic overfilling of the bladder, causing backup pressures throughout the renal system.

CAUSES

See Table 40.

GENDER AND LIFE SPAN CONSIDERATIONS

The incidence and manifestations of neurogenic bladder dysfunction do not change with age, except that older people of both sexes are more at risk for CVAs. They also may have had neurologic diseases longer, resulting in more sequelae such as neurogenic bladder dysfunction. The treatment plan is unmodified for elderly patients, except that self-catheterization may need to be modified, or not used at all, depending on the ability of the individual.

□ ASSESSMENT

HISTORY. Take a full history of urinary voiding, including night/day patterns, amount of urine voided, and number of urinary emptyings per day. Most patients will describe a history of urinary incontinence and changes in the initiation or interruption of urinary voiding. Elicit an accurate description of the sensations during bladder filling and emptying. In patients with spastic neurogenic bladder, expect the patient to describe a history of involuntary or frequent scanty urination without a sensation of bladder fullness. In patients with flaccid neurogenic bladder, expect overflow urinary incontinence. Also ask patients if they have a history of frequent urinary tract infections, a complication that often accompanies neurogenic bladder.

PHYSICAL EXAMINATION. Evaluate the extent of the patient's CNS involvement by performing a complete neurologic assessment, including strength and motion of extremities and levels of sensation on the trunk and extremities. With a spastic neurogenic bladder, the patient may have increased anal sphincter tone so that when you touch the abdomen, thigh, or genitalia, the patient may void spontaneously. Often the patient will have residual urine in the bladder even after voiding. In patients with a flaccid neurogenic bladder, palpate and percuss the bladder to evaluate for a distended bladder; usually the patient will not sense bladder fullness in spite of large bladder distension because of sensory deficits. In patients with urinary incontinence, evaluate the groin and perineal area for skin irritation and breakdown.

PSYCHOSOCIAL. The patient will likely view neurogenic bladder dysfunction as one more manifestation of an already uncontrollable situation. Anxiety about voiding will be added to the anxiety about the underlying cause of the dysfunction. Urinary incontinence leads to embarrassment over the lack of control and concern over the odor of urine that often can permeate clothing and linens. Patients who perceive that the only alternative is urinary catheterization have concerns about being normally active with a catheter and may also fear sexual dysfunction.

DIAGNOSTIC HIGHLIGHTS

Test	Normal Result	Abnormality with Condition	Explanation
Uroflowmetry	> 200 mL, 10–20 mL/second, depending on age	Decreased	Measures completeness and speed of bladder emptying, which are both reduced
Cystometry	Absence of residual urine; sensation of fullness at 300–500 mL; urge to void at 150–450 mL	Varies with type of dysfunction; may have residual urine and lack of sensation or urge to void	Evaluates detrusor muscle function and tonicity; determines etiology of bladder dysfunction; and differentiates among classifications of bladder dysfunction

Other Tests: Urethral pressure profile, urinalysis, excretory urogram, voiding cystourethrogram, cystourethroscopy, electrocyography of pelvic muscles, ultrasound of bladder

PRIMARY NURSING DIAGNOSIS

Altered urinary elimination related to incontinence or retention secondary to trauma or CNS dysfunction

OUTCOMES. Urinary continence; Urinary elimination; Infection status; Knowledge: Disease process, Medication, Treatment regimen; Symptom control behavior

INTERVENTIONS. Urinary retention care; Fluid management; Fluid monitoring; Urinary catheterization; Urinary elimination management

☐ PLANNING AND IMPLEMENTATION

Collaborative

The goals for the medical management of patients include maintaining the integrity of the urinary tract, controlling or preventing infection, and preventing urinary incontinence. Many of the nonsurgical approaches to managing neurogenic bladder depend on independent nursing interventions such as the Crede method, Valsalva's maneuver, or intermittent catheterization (see below).

If all attempts at bladder retraining or catheterization have failed, a surgeon may perform a reconstructive procedure, such as correction of bladder neck contractures, creation of access for pelvic catheterization, or other urinary diversion procedures. Some surgeons may recommend implantation of an artificial urinary sphincter if urinary incontinence continues after surgery.

PHARMACOLOGIC HIGHLIGHTS

Medication or Drug Class	Dosage	Description	Rationale
Bethanechol (Urecholine)	10–50 mg tid to qid po	Parasympathomimetic; cholinergic	Assists in contraction of detrusor (bladder) muscle, especially in flaccid neurogenic bladder disorders
Antimuscarinic (anticholinergic) drugs	Varies with drug	Atropine; propantheline (Pro-Banthine)	Decrease spasticity and incontinence in spastic neurogenic bladder disorders

Independent

Focus on bladder training. The patient may notice bladder dysfunction initially during the acute phase of the underlying disorder, such as during recovery from a spinal cord injury. During this time, an indwelling urinary catheter is frequently in place. Ensure that the tubing is patent to prevent urine backflow and that it is taped laterally to the thigh (in men) to prevent pressure to the penoscrotal angle. Clean the catheter insertion site with soap and water at least two times a day. Before transferring the patient to a wheelchair or bedside chair, empty the urine bag and clamp the tubing to prevent reflux of urine. Encourage a high fluid intake (2 to 3 L per day) unless contraindicated by the patient's condition.

Bladder retraining should stimulate normal bladder function. For the patient with a spastic bladder, the object of the training is to increase the control over bladder function. Encourage the patient to attempt to void at specific times. Various methods of stimulating urination include applying manual pressure to the bladder (Crede's maneuver), stimulating the skin of the abdomen or thighs to initiate bladder contraction, or stretching the anal sphincter with a gloved, lubricated finger. If the patient is successful, measure the voided urine and determine the residual volume by performing a temporary urinary catheterization.

The goal is to increase the times between voidings and to have a concurrent decrease in residual urine amounts. Teach the patient to assess the need to void and to respond to the body's response to a full bladder, as the usual urge to void may be absent. When the residual urine amounts are routinely less than 50 mL, catheterization is usually discontinued.

If bladder training is not feasible (this is more frequently experienced when the dysfunction is related to a flaccid bladder), intermittent straight catheterization (ISC) is necessary. Begin the catheterizations at specific times and measure the urine obtained. Institutions and agencies have varied policies on the maximum amount of urine that may be removed through catheterization at any one time. Self-catheterization may be taught to the patient when he or she is physically and cognitively able to learn the procedure. If this procedure is not possible, a family member may be taught the procedure for home care. Sterile technique is important in the hospital to prevent infection, although home catheterization may be accomplished with clean technique.

If the patient demonstrates signs and symptoms of autonomic dysreflexia, place the patient in semi-Fowler's position, check for any kinking or other obstruction in the urinary catheter and tubing, and initiate steps to relieve bladder pressure. These interventions may include using the bladder retraining methods to stimulate evacuation or catheterizing the patient. The anus should be checked to ascertain if constipation is causing the problem, but perform fecal assessment or evacuation cautiously to prevent further stimulation that might result in increased autonomic dysreflexia. Monitor the vital signs every 5 minutes, and seek medical assistance if immediate interventions do not relieve the symptoms.

The patient's psychosocial state is essential for health maintenance. Teaching may not be effective if there are other problems that the patient believes have a higher priority. The need for a family member to perform catheterization may be highly embarrassing for both the patient and the family. Because anxiety may cause the patient to have great difficulty in performing catheterization, a relaxed, private environment is necessary. Some institutions have patient support groups for people who have neurogenic bladders; if a support group is available, suggest to the patient and significant other that they might attend. If the patient has more than the normal amount of anxiety or has ineffective coping, refer the patient for counseling.

DOCUMENTATION GUIDELINES

- Physical findings related to intake, output, residual urine measures, presence of edema or dehydration, incontinence, autonomic dysreflexia, infection
- Response to cholinergic or anticholinergic medications
- Response to treatment, including patient perceptions of comfort, control of bodily functions, and ability to perform bladder evacuation procedures

DISCHARGE AND HOME HEALTHCARE GUIDELINES

The patient and significant others need to understand that although they have achieved a bladder program in the hospital, their daily rhythm may be quite different at home. They need to be encouraged to adapt the pattern of bladder evacuation to the family schedule. Teach the patient the medication dosage, action, side effects, and route of all prescribed medications.

Discuss potential complications, particularly urinary tract infection, and encourage the patient to report signs of infection to the physician immediately. Teach the patient and significant others preventive strategies, such as keeping equipment clean, good hand-washing techniques, and adequate fluid intake to limit the risk of infection. Refer the patient to an appropriate source for catheterization supplies if appropriate, or refer the patient to social service for help in obtaining supplies. Discuss the potential for sexual activity with the patient; if possible, have a nurse of the same gender talk with the patient to answer questions and provide support.

Osteomyelitis

DRG Category: 238
Mean LOS: 9.1 days
Description: MEDICAL: Osteomyelitis
DRG Category: 233
Mean LOS: 7.4 days
Description: SURGICAL: Other Musculoskeletal System and Connective Tissue O.R. Procedures with CC

Osteomyelitis is an infection of bone, bone marrow, and the soft tissue that surrounds the bone. It is generally caused by pyogenic (pus-producing) bacteria but may be the result of a viral or fungal infection. Osteomyelitis may be an acute or chronic condition. Acute osteomyelitis refers to an infection that is less than 1 month in duration from the time of the initial infection. Chronic osteomyelitis refers to a bone infection that persists for longer than 4 weeks or represents a persistent problem with periods of remission and exacerbations.

Osteomyelitis most commonly occurs in the long bones. The metaphysis (growing portion of a bone) of the distal portion of the femur and the proximal portion of the tibia are the most frequent sites because of the sluggish blood supply that occurs in that area. After gaining entrance to the bone, the bacteria grow and form an abscess, which spreads along the shaft of the bone under the periosteum. Pressure elevates the periosteum, destroying its blood vessels and causing bone necrosis. The dead bone tissue (sequestra) cannot easily be liquefied and removed. The body's healing response is to lay new bone (involucrum) over the sequestra. However, the sequestra is a perfect environment for bacteria, and chronic osteomyelitis occurs if the bacteria are not eliminated. Complications from osteomyelitis include chronic infection, skeletal and joint deformities, immobility, and altered growth and development.

CAUSES

Osteomyelitis is caused by direct or indirect invasion of an organism into the bone or its surrounding tissue. Any break in the skin, which normally acts as a protective barrier, can lead to direct infection. These breaks may be caused by abrasions, open fractures, or surgical instrumentation, such as the insertion of pins for skeletal traction. Indirect infections are caused by organisms that are transported through the bloodstream (hematogenous) from an infection in a distant site, such as otitis media, tonsillitis, or a furuncle (boil). The most common organisms responsible for osteomyelitis are *Staphylococcus aureus* and hemolytic streptococcus.

Previous trauma to a bone may predispose the area to osteomyelitis. Any delay in treatment of a fracture may also contribute to the development of osteomyelitis. Hematogenous osteomyelitis (originating in the blood) may occur in the adult who has undergone surgery or examination of the genitourinary tract, or whose resistance has been lowered by debilitating illness. With older patients, the infection may become localized in the vertebra.

GENDER AND LIFE SPAN CONSIDERATIONS

The acute form of osteomyelitis is most frequently found in children, while the chronic form is most commonly observed in adults. Hematogenous osteomyelitis generally occurs in boys from the age of 1 to 12. Osteomyelitis in a joint is more common in children than in adults. If the epiphyseal plate is heavily infected in the child, one extremity may develop longer than the other. Adults may experience an infection as a result of malignancy, burns, pressure sores, urinary tract infections, or infections as a result of atherosclerosis and diabetes mellitus.

☐ ASSESSMENT

HISTORY. Question the patient about any previous bone trauma, open injuries, or surgical procedures. Elicit information about the patient's general well-being, level of fatigue, and previous illnesses, specifically any infections. In the acute phase, the patient may report the chracteristic signs of an infection: high temperature, chills, fever, increased pulse, nausea, diaphoresis, general weakness, and malaise. In the chronic phase, the patient may report an exacerbation characterized by low-grade fever, fatigue, pain, and purulent drainage from a sinus tract.

PHYSICAL EXAMINATION. Local and systemic signs and symptoms of osteomyelitis are generally present. Examination of the area reveals local infectious symptoms, such as redness or swelling and increased warmth. A foul-smelling draining wound may be present, with an intense pain or tenderness over the affected bone; you may note muscle spasms as well. The patient often protects the extremity by intentionally limiting movement in the joint closest to the affected area. Observe the patient's gait to identify a limp or abnormal gait.

PSYCHOSOCIAL. If the patient has an acute condition, assess the level of anxiety related to treatment plans, potential for sepsis, or potential of the illness to become chronic. In the chronic condition, the patient may be depressed and discouraged. A mistrust of the healthcare team may develop if interventions do not result in permanent resolution of the infection. Chronic pain and decreased mobility can lead to long-term disability, resulting in financial burdens, changes in body image or self-image, and alteration in family or social roles.

DIAGNOSTIC HIGHLIGHTS

Test	Normal Result	Abnormality with Condition	Explanation
Bone scan	Normal bony structures	Bone changes caused by inflammation and infection	Identifies areas of infection; identifies changes in blood flow

			resulting from inflammation
Bone biopsy	Cultures and sensitivities are negative	Positive for infecting organism	Identifies organisms; identifies bacterial sensitivities to antibiotics
Blood cultures and sensitivities	Negative	Positive for infecting organism	Identify organisms; identify bacterial sensitivities to antibiotics

Other Tests: Magnetic resonance imaging, complete blood count, erythrocyte sedimentation rate, x rays, computed tomography (CT) scan

PRIMARY NURSING DIAGNOSIS

Pain (acute) related to swelling and inflammation

OUTCOMES. Comfort level; Pain control behavior; Pain level; Symptom control behavior; Symptom severity; Well-being

INTERVENTIONS. Pain management; Analgesic administration; Cutaneous stimulation; Heat/cold application; Touch; Exercise therapy; Progressive muscle relaxation

☐ PLANNING AND IMPLEMENTATION

Collaborative

The most critical factor in eliminating osteomyelitis is prevention. To prevent direct infections, early care of injuries that break the skin and aseptic care of surgical wounds are essential. Indirect infections may be prevented by aggressive treatment of infections at any location. Early diagnosis and treatment are extremely important to prevent chronic osteomyelitis. With early treatment, the chances of effectively controlling acute osteomyelitis are quite good. The physician who suspects osteomyelitis prescribes broad-spectrum intravenous antibiotics immediately after blood, wound, or bone cultures are obtained to determine the causative organism.

Early and adequate debridement of open fractures to remove necrotic tissue limits bacterial growth. Administration of prophylactic antibiotics in patients with open fractures and after surgery to reduce fractures decreases the incidence of post-traumatic osteomyelitis; it is important for the antibiotics to reach the bone before bone necrosis occurs. If treatment is delayed and necrotic bone develops, there is a decrease in effectiveness of the antibiotic to combat infection.

The physician usually prescribes analgesics for pain. Heat applications may also decrease discomfort. Usually the patient limits his or her own activity, but the joints above and below the affected part are often immobilized with a splint or a bivalved cast to decrease pain and muscle spasm and to support wound healing. No weight bearing is permitted on the affected part. A diet high in calories, protein, calcium, and vitamin C is started as soon as possible to promote bone healing. If there is pus formation under the periosteum, the physician performs a needle aspiration and possibly insertion of a drainage tube to evacuate the subperiosteum area. If the response to antibiotics is slow and an abscess develops, an incision and drainage (I and D) may be done. The surgeon may place catheters in the wound for irrigation or for direct antibiotic instillation. Treatment for chronic osteomyelitis may include surgical debridement of devitalized and infected tissue so that permanent healing can take place. This operation, called a sequestrectomy, consists of the removal of the sequestrum and the overlying involucrum (sheath or covering).

PHARMACOLOGIC HIGHLIGHTS

Medication or Drug Class	Dosage	Description	Rationale
Antibiotics	Varies with drug	Depends on cultures and sensitivities; parenteral antibiotic therapy may be continued for 4–8 weeks, followed by oral antibiotics for 2–3 weeks	Kill bacteria and decrease spread of infection; after open fractures and surgery, used to reduce fractures

Independent

Osteomyelitis often includes a prolonged hospital stay and in-depth preparation for long-term care in the home. Several strategies exist to manage the discomfort of fever and pain nonpharmacologically. Encourage oral fluids to prevent dehydration because of the elevated temperature and infectious process. Frequent positioning and distractions help with pain control. Use imagery and relaxation techniques to help control discomfort.

To prevent contamination to other areas of the body, use various types of sterile dressings to contain the exudate from draining wounds. The most common are dry, sterile dressings; dressings saturated in saline or antibiotic solution; and wet-to-dry dressings. Use aseptic technique when you change dressings, and dispose of contaminated dressings appropriately. Universal precautions are extremely important to prevent cross-contamination of the wound or spread of the infection to other patients.

Handle the involved extremity carefully to avoid increasing pain and the risk of a pathologic fracture. To provide support, immobilization, and comfort, the extremity may be splinted. Proper application of the splint is extremely important because an improperly applied device can result in pressure ulcers or nerve damage. Regular skin assessments and conscientious skin care are important to prevent pressure sores from bed rest. Good body alignment, appropriate positioning of the affected extremity, and frequent position changes for the rest of the body prevent complications and promote comfort. Flexion deformity or contractures may occur if the patient is permitted to maintain a position of comfort instead of a position of function. Foot-drop can develop quickly in the lower extremity if the foot is not correctly supported. Promote range-of-motion, isotonic, and isometric exercises for the rest of the body to maintain joint flexibility and muscle strength.

DOCUMENTATION GUIDELINES

- Appearance of extremity and wound
- Physical signs of infection: Vital signs, appearance of area, presence of weakness or malaise

- Response to medications: Pain, antipyretic, stool softeners
- Response to interventions such as surgery or debridement

DISCHARGE AND HOME HEALTHCARE GUIDELINES

Patient education varies with the etiology of osteomyelitis; an individualized teaching plan needs to be developed for each patient. Regardless of the etiology, prolonged bed rest and parenteral antibiotic therapy are usually a part of the treatment plan. Discuss the cause and treatment of osteomyelitis with the patient, along with the importance of following the treatment plan. The major issues that need to be addressed are medication administration, activity, and signs and symptoms that may require notification of the physician. Discuss the need to contact the physician if increased pain, temperature, drainage, redness, or swelling develops. Also make certain the patient understands the signs of allergic drug reactions.

Emphasize the importance of long-term antibiotics that the patient requires, including the need to continue the medication even after the symptoms disappear. If intravenous or central line antibiotics are prescribed at home, arrange for assistance from home healthcare nurses. Also include the family in all patient teaching. Note that significant others are often responsible for delivering the care. Have the patient or significant other not only explain all procedures but also demonstrate all techniques.

Osteoporosis

DRG Category: 244
Mean LOS: 4.9 days
Description: MEDICAL: Bone Diseases and Specific Arthropathies with CC

Osteoporosis is an age-related metabolic disease that is defined as low bone mass with a normal ratio of mineral to osteoid, the organic matrix of bone. Bone demineralization results in decreased density and subsequent fractures as bone resorption occurs faster than bone formation. The general reduction in skeletal bone mass occurs as bones lose calcium and phosphate, become brittle and porous, and develop an increased susceptibility to fractures. Common sites for fractures are the wrist, hip, and vertebral column.

Osteoporosis can be classified as primary or secondary. Primary osteoporosis is more common and is not associated with an underlying medical condition. Secondary osteoporosis results from an associated underlying condition, such as hyperparathyroidism, or an iatrogenic cause, such as long-term corticosteroid or heparin administration.

CAUSES

The exact cause of osteoporosis is unknown. A mild but prolonged negative calcium balance, resulting from an inadequate dietary intake of calcium, may be an important contributing factor. Declining gonadal adrenal function, faulty protein metabolism because of estrogen deficiency, and a sedentary lifestyle may also contribute. Risk factors that increase the likelihood of osteoporosis also include smoking, advanced age, heavy caffeine consumption, vitamin D deficiency, excess alcohol consumption, long-term heparin or corticosteroid use, and the use of laxatives or antacids. Additionally, patients who are postmenopausal are more susceptible to osteoporosis. Patients who have Cushing's disease or Parkinson's disease, rheumatoid arthritis, scoliosis, or anorexia, or who have had bilateral oophorectomy, are also at greater risk. Paradoxically, both a sedentary lifestyle and excessive exercise are thought to be risk factors for osteoporosis.

GENDER AND LIFE SPAN CONSIDERATIONS

Osteoporosis is the twelfth leading cause of death in the United States and accounts for more than $6 billion in health-related costs each year. More than 1.5 million fractures per year occur in persons over age 45. More than 20 million Americans have osteoporosis, with Caucasians and females being more susceptible than other groups. The incidence in women is five times greater than in men, and approximately 50% of all women over age 65 have symptomatic osteoporosis.

Two types of primary osteoporosis have been identified. Postmenopausal osteoporosis occurs in women between the ages of 60 and 70, with wrist and vertebral fractures a common injury; senile osteoporosis occurs in people over 70, and women are affected twice as often as men are. Senile osteoporosis often produces hip and vertebral fractures. The mortality rate for elderly patients with hip fractures is more than 50%, and the resulting disability can be devastating.

◻ ASSESSMENT

HISTORY. Take a careful history of all traumatic injuries, with a particular focus on previous bone fractures. Collect data about risk factors: age, sex, race, body frame, age of menopause onset, diet, patterns of alcohol intake, caffeine use, smoking, medications, concurrent medical conditions, and exercise habits. Inquire about complaints of back pain while lifting or bending, particularly when assessing elderly women. If the patient has vertebral collapse, he or she may describe backache or pain that radiates around the lower trunk and is aggravated by movement.

PHYSICAL EXAMINATION. Diagnosis of osteoporosis is typically made after the patient sustains a vertebral, wrist, or hip fracture. Often, the patient is asymptomatic before admission with a bone fracture. A typical first sign of osteoporosis is vertebral collapse on bending over; sudden lower back pain that radiates around the trunk is a common symptom.

Inspection of the vertebral column reveals curvature of the dorsal spine, the classic "dowager's hump." Often the patients report a height reduction of 2 to 3 inches over 20 years. Palpation of the vertebrae that is accompanied by back pain and voluntary restriction of spinal movement is indicative of a compression vertebral fracture, which is the most common type of osteoporotic fracture. The most common area for fracture occurrence is between T-8 and L-3. The radius (Colles's fracture), hip, and femur are also gently palpated and assessed for pain and fracture.

PSYCHOSOCIAL. Assess the patient's concept of body image and self-esteem if there is severe curvature of the spine. Inquire about the patient's ability to find clothing to fit, any decrease in social activity, or alterations in sexuality. Evaluate the patient's home environment; inquire about fall risks in the environment—for example, stairs, waxed floors, and scatter rugs.

DIAGNOSTIC HIGHLIGHTS

Test	Normal Result	Abnormality with Condition	Explanation
Dual energy x-ray absorptiometry (DXA)	No bone loss	Bone loss > 3%	Measures bone mineral content at several sites
Bone x rays	No bone loss	Bone loss; cannot determine bone loss until 25%–40% has occurred	Determines structure of bone

Other Tests: Complete blood count, chemistry screening, thyroid stimulating hormone level, urinalysis, serum protein electrophoresis, serum and urine calcium levels, vitamin D level, serum phosphorus levels, alkaline phosphatase, computed tomography (CT) scan

PRIMARY NURSING DIAGNOSIS

Pain (acute) related to fracture

OUTCOMES. Comfort level; Pain control behavior; Pain level; Symptom control behavior; Symptom severity; Well-being

INTERVENTIONS. Pain management; Analgesic administration; Cutaneous stimulation; Touch; Exercise therapy; Progressive muscle relaxation

◻ PLANNING AND IMPLEMENTATION

Collaborative

Nonsurgical management is directed to measures that retard bone resorption, form new bone tissue, and reduce the chance of fracture. These goals are often met through pharmacologic therapy. For the patient who has had a fracture, pain medication is prescribed to relieve pain, and a diet high in protein, vitamin C, and iron is recommended to promote bone healing. Orthotic devices are ordered to stabilize the spine and reduce pain.

Consult with the physical therapist to develop an exercise plan that includes weight-bearing and strengthening exercises. Consult with the occupational therapist if self-care assistive devices are needed. Generally, bowling and horseback riding are discouraged. If your assessment indicates that the patient's home environment places him or her at risk, consult with social services or a public health nurse.

PHARMACOLOGIC HIGHLIGHTS

Medication or Drug Class	Dosage	Description	Rationale
Conjugated estrogen (Provera)	0.625 mg per day cyclically	Estrogen hormone	Prevents bone loss and reduces number of fractures; needs to be initiated within 3–5 years of menopause

Calcium supplements	1000–1500 mg per day po	Mineral supplement	Prevents bone loss and supplements calcium
Alendronate (Fosamax)	5 mg per day po	Bone resorption inhibitor	Prevents bone loss and inhibits bone resorption

Other Drugs: Androgens, calcitonin, and vitamin D metabolites may be ordered to decrease bone resorption. Analgesics also may be needed to manage the pain.

Independent

Stress the need for routine exercise of the upper and lower body and a diet high in calcium for all middle-aged and older women. If the patient is placed on estrogen, encourage her to complete monthly breast self-examinations and immediately report any lumps to the physician. Teach the patient to report abnormal vaginal bleeding immediately. Emphasize the need for regular gynecologic exams. Careful monitoring of patient medications with side effects of weakness and dizziness is also warranted.

To prevent falls and other activities that could cause a fracture, a hazard-free environment is required. If the patient is hospitalized, assist the patient during ambulation in a well-lighted room and provide non-skid shoes. Maintain the patient's activity at the highest level possible. Encourage the patient to perform as many of the activities of daily living as the pain allows. Check the patient's skin daily for redness, warmth, and new sites of pain, which are all indicators of new fractures. Explain to the patient's family how easily an osteoporotic patient's bones can fracture. Check orthotic devices for proper fit, patient tolerance, and skin irritation. If surgery is needed to repair fractures, encourage verbalization of feelings about surgery, change in body image, or inability to cope with the disease progression. The patient may need reassurance to help cope with limited mobility. If possible, arrange for the patient to interact with others who have osteoporosis. Be sure to include the family or significant other in the interactions.

DOCUMENTATION GUIDELINES

- Physical findings of musculoskeletal assessment: Pain, mobility, numbness, curvature of the spine
- Response to pain medications
- Reaction to exercise plan and orthotic devices

DISCHARGE AND HOME HEALTHCARE GUIDELINES

Reinforce the medication, exercise, and diet plan. Provide a hazard-free environment to prevent falls. Apply orthotic devices correctly. Remove scatter rugs, provide good lighting, and install handrails in the bathroom. Be sure the patient understands all medications, including the dosage, route, action, and side effects. If the patient is placed on estrogen therapy, she needs routine gynecologic checkups to detect early signs of cervical cancer. Consider placement in a nursing home if a patient cannot return home. Communicate the special needs of the patient on the transfer chart. The need for physical or occupational therapy, social work, and homemaking personnel is determined by the home care nurse. Facilitate the procurement of needed orthotic devices or ambulation aids before the patient goes home. The Osteoporosis Foundation provides information to clients regarding the disease and its treatment.

Otitis Media

DRG Category: 69
Mean LOS: 3.3 days
Description: MEDICAL: Otitis Media and Upper Respiratory Infection Age > 17 without CC
DRG Category: 62
Mean LOS: 1.3 days
Description: SURGICAL: Myringotomy with Tube Insertion, Age 0–17

Otitis media, the most common cause of antibiotic prescription in the United States, is an infection of the middle ear that can occur in several forms. Acute otitis media (AOM) is a suppurative (pus forming) effusion of the middle ear. Bullous myringitis is AOM that leads to bullae formation between the middle and inner layers of the tympanic membrane. Persistent otitis media occurs when an acute infection does not resolve after 4 weeks of treatment. Recurrent otitis media occurs in children with three separate bouts of AOM within a 6-month period, six within a 12-month period, or six episodes by 6 years of age.

The eustachian tube protects the middle ear from secretions and allows for drainage of secretions into the nasopharynx. It also permits equalization of air pressure with atmospheric pressure in the middle ear. A mechanical obstruction of the eustachian tube can result in infection and middle ear effusion. A functional obstruction can occur with persistent collapse of the eustachian tubes, particularly in infants and young children, because the amount and stiffness of their cartilage is less than that of older children and adults. Eustachian tube obstruction leads to negative middle ear pressure and a sterile middle-ear effusion. Drainage of the effusion is inhibited by impaired mucociliary action and sustained negative pressure. Contamination of the middle ear may occur from nasopharyngeal secretions and lead to infection. Because infants and young children have a shorter eustachian tube than older children, it makes them more susceptible to reflux of nasopharyngeal secretions into the middle ear and development of infection. Other predisposing factors include upper respiratory infections, allergies, Down syndrome, bottle propping during feedings, day-care attendance, and parental smoking. Complications include persistent AOM, tympanic membrane perforation, mastoiditis, hearing loss for several months, speech delay, and cerebral thrombophlebitis.

CAUSES

Bacteria pulled into the eustachian tube leads to the accumulation of purulent fluid in the middle ear. Common bacteria include *Streptococcus pneumoniae, Haemophilus influenzae,* and *Moraxella catarrhalis. S. pneumoniae* is the most common type of infection (40% to 50% of all cases) and is the least likely to resolve without antibiotic treatment.

GENDER AND LIFE SPAN CONSIDERATIONS

Acute otitis media is most common in infants and children. Approximately 70% of children younger than 3 years develop AOM, and 20% of children have recurrent problems with otitis media. The peak number of infections occurs between 6 to 36 months and 4 to 6 years of age. Children who develop OAM during their first 12 months of life have higher risk of recurrent acute or chronic disease. Boys have more infections than girls, and there is also an increased incidence in children with cleft palates and other craniofacial anomalies.

◻ ASSESSMENT

HISTORY. Determine the presence of risk factors by observing the child and asking the parents questions. If the child is not able to speak, ask the parents if the child has had evidence of ear pain (otalgia). In infants and young children ear pain is often manifested by irritability, inability to sleep, and ear pulling. Ask if the child has demonstrated lethargy, dizziness, tinnitus, and unsteady gait. Other symptoms include diarrhea, vomiting, fever, sudden hearing loss, stuffy nose, rhinorrhea, and sneezing.

PHYSICAL EXAMINATION. During an examination with an otoscope, the clinician can see a reddened, bulging tympanic membrane with poor mobility and obscured or absent landmarks. The tympanic membrane is often hypervascular and red, yellow, or purple in color. Note that redness alone should not be used to diagnose AOM, particularly in a crying child. The tympanic membrane may demonstrate thin-walled, sagging bullae filled with yellow fluid if the child has bullous myringitis. Differential diagnosis includes mastoiditis, dental abscesses, sinusitis, parotitis, peritonsillar abscess, trauma, impact teeth, and immune deficiency.

PSYCHOSOCIAL. Evaluate the parental–child interaction to determine how well the parent follows up on the child's cues. Determine the extent of the parent's knowledge about risk factors. Determine the parent's feeding practices.

DIAGNOSTIC HIGHLIGHTS

Test	Normal Result	Abnormality with Condition	Explanation
Tympanocentesis	Negative for fluid and infection	Positive for bacteria and fluid	Used to identify type of bacteria in children < 2 months old. In older infants and children, the procedure is rarely done unless (1) the child is in a toxic state or is immunocompromised; (2) there is the presence of resistant infection; (3) there is acute pain from bullous myringitis; or (4) there is no response to antibiotic therapy

Other Tests: Complete blood count

PRIMARY NURSING DIAGNOSIS

Risk for infection related to invasion or proliferation of microorganisms

OUTCOMES. Immune status; Knowledge: Infection control; Risk control; Risk detection; Nutritional status

INTERVENTIONS. Medication administration; Medication management; Surveillance; Teaching: Disease process

□ PLANNING AND IMPLEMENTATION

Collaborative

Once AOM is diagnosed, the primary treatment is pharmacologic. However, a current debate exists as to whether antibiotics are appropriate because of growing rates of antibiotic-resistant bacteria. Many physicians support the idea that because 60% to 90% of the infections resolve without antibiotics, treatment for all AOM may not be necessary. Antibiotics are recommended for children with clear local signs (bulging membrane with cloudy or yellow fluid, very red membrane, or otorrhea), if systemic signs (fever in particular) are present, if more than three attacks have occurred in the past 18 months, or if otitis media with effusion is present. Decongestants and antihistamines are not considered helpful unless the child has allergies.

In patients with severe pain, therapeutic drainage (myringotomy) may be necessary to provide immediate relief. An incision is made that is large enough of allow for adequate drainage of the middle ear. Children who undergo this procedure need to be evaluated after approximately 14 days to determine that the infection and otoscopic signs are resolving.

PHARMACOLOGIC HIGHLIGHTS

Medication or Drug Class	Dosage	Description	Rationale
Amoxicillin	40 mg/kg per 24 hours tid for 10 days	Antibacterial	Treats AOM because it is usually effective against the most commonly encountered bacteria
Antibacterials	Varies with drug	Many appropriate drugs, including erythromycin, clarithromycin, azithromycin, sulfonamide, cefaclor, cefuroxime	Eradicate the bacterial infection

Other: Antimicrobial ototopical drops are indicated if the tympanic membrane is ruptured. Analgesic eardrops may help with the pain if there has been no perforation of the membrane. Acetaminophen is usually used to reduce fever.

Independent

Explain to the parents that the symptoms should begin to resolve in 24 to 48 hours as the antibiotics take effect. If the acute signs increase in the first 24 hours despite antibiotics, the parents need to bring the child back for a return examination to rule out severe infections such as meningitis or suppurative complications. Make sure that the parents understand that the child needs to receive the entire course of therapy to prevent recurrent infections. Teach the parents that supportive therapy with relief of pain and fever will increase the child's comfort. Application of heat may provide pain relief.

Instruct the parents about bottle propping, feeding infants while they are recumbent, and passive smoke exposure, all of which are risk factors for developing AOM. Breastfeeding until at least 4 to 6 months has a protective effect against AOM. Encourage patients to attend follow up appointments and to avoid requesting antibiotics unless it is absolutely necessary. If repeated infections occur and the child attends day care, parents may want to consider another situation.

DOCUMENTATION GUIDELINES

- Discomfort: Character, location, duration, severity, nonverbal indicators, strategies that reduce discomfort
- Behavior: Manifestations, signs of irritability, gait, amount of crying
- Patterns of rest and activity: Sleep patterns, presence of lethargy or restlessness
- Medication management: Parents' understanding of drug therapy, response to medications
- Response to teaching: Response to parenting suggestions, understanding of follow-up appointments

DISCHARGE AND HOME HEALTHCARE GUIDELINES

Make sure that the parents understand all aspects of the treatment regimen, with particular attention to taking the full course of medication therapy. Make sure the parents understand the necessity of any follow-up visits.

Ovarian Cancer

DRG Category: 366
Mean LOS: 5.9 days
Description: MEDICAL: Malignancy, Female Reproductive System with CC
DRG Category: 357
Mean LOS: 8.9 days
Description: SURIGCAL: Uterine and Adnexa Procedures for Ovarian or Adnexal Malignancy

Ovarian cancer is the primary cause of death from reproductive system malignancies in women. Three types of ovarian cancers exist: primary epithelial tumors, germ cell tumors, and gonadal stromal (sex cord) tumors. Primary epithelial tumors compose approximately 90% of all ovarian cancers and include serous and mucinous cystadenocarcinomas, endometrioid tumors, and mesonephric tumors. They arise in the ovarian epithelium (known as mullerian epithelium). Germ cell tumors, which arise from an ovum, include endodermal sinus malignant tumors, embryonal carcinoma, immature teratomas, and dysgerminoma. Sex cord tumors, which arise from the ovarian stroma (the foundational support tissues of an organ), include granulosa cell tumors, the comas, and arrhenoblastomas.

Ovarian cancers grow and spread silently until they affect the surrounding organs or cause abdominal distension. At the appearance of these symptoms, metastases to the fallopian tubes, uterus, ligaments, and other intraperitoneal organs occur. Tumors can spread through the lymph system and blood into the chest cavity.

As the disease progresses, the patient experiences multiple system complications. Peripheral edema, ascites, and intestinal obstruction can complicate the course of the disease. Patients develop severe nutritional deficiencies, electrolyte disturbances, and cachexia. If the lungs are involved, the patient develops malignant recurrent pleural effusions.

Because of the lack of early detection and the rapid progression of the disease, the number of deaths caused by ovarian cancer has risen. Approximately 25% of women with ovarian cancer survive for 5 years, but no long-term improvement in the survival rate has occurred in the past 30 years.

CAUSES

Although several theories exist, the exact cause of ovarian cancer is unknown; many factors, however, seem to play a role in its development. A family history of ovarian cancer places the patient at risk, as does a diet high in saturated fats. Women who live in industrialized countries have a higher risk than do those in underdeveloped countries. Exposure to asbestos and talc may place the patient at risk. Other associated factors include nulliparity, infertility, celibacy, and heavy menses with pain. Late menarche, early menopause, pregnancy, and oral contraception may offer a protective benefit by effecting ovulation suppression.

GENDER AND LIFE SPAN CONSIDERATIONS

The incidence of ovarian cancer is highest in women between the ages of 20 and 54. In rare instances, the disease can occur in childhood and during pregnancy. In the general population, ovarian cancer occurs in 1 in 70 women; the risk is increased to 5% if one first-degree relative has the disease.

☐ ASSESSMENT

HISTORY. Elicit a detailed family history of all cancer-related illnesses, paying particular attention to the history of female relatives. The patient's descriptions of the signs and symptoms vary with the tumor's size and location; symptoms usually do not occur until after tumor metastasis. The patient may describe urinary frequency, constipation, abdominal distension, and weight loss. Pelvic discomfort and acute pelvic pain may occur, and if infection, tumor rupture, or torsion has resulted, the pain may resemble that of acute appendicitis.

PHYSICAL EXAMINATION. The patient often appears thin and chronically ill. Her abdomen may be grossly distended, but her extremities are thin and even wasted. When you palpate the abdominal organs, you may be able to feel masses. During the vaginal examination, you may be able to palpate an ovary in postmenopausal women that feels like the size of an ovary in premenopausal women. An ovarian tumor may feel hard like a rock or pebble, may feel rubbery, or may have a cyst-like quality. Palpation of an irregular, nodular ("handful of knuckles"), insensitive bilateral mass in the pelvis strongly suggests the presence of an ovarian tumor.

PSYCHOSOCIAL. If the patient is a young woman who needs to undergo surgery and loses her childbearing ability, determine the meaning of children to her and her partner. Consider the patient's developmental level, financial resources, job responsibilities, home care responsibilities, and the degree of independence of any children. If the patient is a child, determine whether or not her parents have told her she has cancer. If the prognosis of the patient's cancer is poor, determine the patient's degree of understanding of the gravity of the prognosis. Determine the effect of the patient's religion and spirituality on the course of the disease.

DIAGNOSTIC HIGHLIGHTS

General Comments: None of the tumor markers is specific enough to be considered for routine screening, but they are helpful in differential diagnosis of pelvic masses and to follow up treated cases.

Test	Normal Result	Abnormality with Condition	Explanation
Cancer antigen 125 (CA-125)	0–35 U/mL	Elevated in 80% of the patients	Serial measured; elevation indicates tumor progression; decrease indicates effective anti-tumor treatment
Human chorionic gonadotropin (hCG); serum alpha-fetoprotein	Normally are not present in non-pregnant women	Elevated in embryonal cell carcinoma and dysgerminoma	Serially measured; elevation indicates tumor progression; decrease indicates effective anti-tumor treatment
Exploratory laparotomy	Negative study	Tumor is visualized	Accurate diagnosing and staging

Other Tests: Computerized tomography (CT) scan, magnetic resonance imagery (MRI) and sonography are useful for monitoring the course of the disease. Upper and lower bowel series and intravenous pyelography, are done to determine the extent of the disease and whether the cancer is primary or metastatic. Liver function studies, blood chemistries, and chest x rays are also done.

PRIMARY NURSING DIAGNOSIS

Pain (acute) related to tumor invasion, tissue destruction, and organ compression

OUTCOMES. Pain control; Pain: Disruptive effects; Well-being

INTERVENTIONS. Analgesic administration; Pain management; Meditation; Transcutaneous electric nerve stimulation (TENS); Hypnosis; Heat/cold application

□ PLANNING AND IMPLEMENTATION

Collaborative

SURGICAL. Aggressive surgical treatment is usually used. If there is a desire to preserve the fertility of young women or girls, however, a conservative approach may be used if they have a unilateral encapsulated tumor. In this approach, the surgeon may resect the ovary, biopsy structures such as the omentum and uninvolved ovary, and perform peritoneal washings for cytologic examination of pelvic fluid. These patients need careful follow-up with periodic diagnostic tests to determine if the tumor is metastasizing.

More typically, the surgeon performs a total abdominal hysterectomy and bilateral salpingo-oophorectomy with tumor resection. In addition, the surgeon performs an omentectomy, appendectomy, lymph node palpation with possible lymphadenectomy, and other biopsies and washings as necessary. Sometimes the surgeon is unable to remove the tumor completely if it is wrapped around or has invaded vital organs. Monitor the patient carefully after surgery for complications such as wound infection, hemorrhage, fluid and electrolyte imbalance, and poor gas exchange.

If a young girl has had both ovaries removed, she needs hormonal replacement beginning at puberty so that she develops secondary sex characteristics. Chemotherapy after surgery prolongs survival time but is primarily palliative rather than curative, although it does provide remissions in some patients.

Although radiation therapy is uncommon because it causes depression of the bone marrow, sometime patients receive it as an option to other treatments.

PAIN MANAGEMENT. No matter which treatment is chosen to manage the patient's cancer, pain management is an issue. Monitor the patient's pain (location, duration, frequency, precipitating factors) and administer analgesics as needed. Determine the patient's response to analgesia by asking the patient to rate her pain on a scale of 0 to 10, with 0 indicating no pain and 10 indicating the worst pain she has experienced. Collaborate with the physician to develop a pain-management strategy that effectively keeps the patient free of pain and yet awake and alert without respiratory complications. Consider patient-controlled analgesia (PCA) as a possibility if intravenous medications are needed. If the patient's disease is terminal, manage the pain so that the patient has a comfortable and dignified death.

PHARMACOLOGIC HIGHLIGHTS

Medication or Drug Class	Dosage	Description	Rationale
Melphalan, chlorambucil, methotrexate, vincristine, vinblastine, bleomycin, cisplatin, and paclitaxel	Drugs are often given in combination, and dosage depends on the stage of the disease, patient status, etc.	Antineoplastic	Used after surgery to destroy cancer cells that may have spread into the abdominal cavity; palliative
Acetaminophen; NSAIDs; opiods;	Depends on the drug and patient	Analgesics	Analgesics used are determined by the severity of

combination of opiod and NSAIDs	condition and tolerance	pain

Experimental Therapy: Other treatments, such as vaccines, lymphokine-activated killer cells, and immunotherapy therapy, are being investigated.

Independent

Prevention and early detection are difficult in ovarian cancer because of the disease's lack of obvious signs and symptoms. Encourage all adolescent girls and women to have regular pelvic examinations as part of an annual checkup. When the patient is diagnosed with ovarian cancer, she has to manage a host of physical and emotional problems. Help the patient manage any accompanying physical discomfort with nonpharmacologic strategies and pain medications. Teach the patient relaxation techniques or guided imagery. Explain the role of diversions as a mechanism to control pain. If the patient requires hospitalization for surgery or chemotherapy, teach her about the route, dosage, action, and complications of her analgesics so that she can manage her pain at home knowledgeably. If the patient is discharged with a PCA system, arrange for her to rent the equipment and obtain the prescriptions she needs to continue using it. If the patient's family does not have the financial resources to manage the needed equipment, discuss her needs with a social worker or contact the American or Canadian Cancer Society for assistance.

Depression, grief, or anger is common in women who have been diagnosed with ovarian cancer. To determine the patient's ability to cope, encourage her to discuss her feelings and monitor her for the physical signs of inability to cope, such as altered sleep patterns. Encourage her to express her feelings without fear of being judged. Note that surgery and chemotherapy may profoundly affect the patient's and partner's sexuality. Answer any questions honestly, provide information on alternatives to traditional sexual intercourse if appropriate, and encourage the couple to seek counseling if needed. If the woman's support systems and coping mechanisms are insufficient to meet her needs, help her find other support systems and coping mechanisms. Provide a list of support groups.

DOCUMENTATION GUIDELINES

- Physiologic response: Vital signs, intake and output if appropriate, weight loss or gain, sleep patterns, incisional healing
- Comfort: Location, onset, duration, and intensity of pain; effectiveness of analgesics and pain-reducing techniques
- Response to therapy: Drugs, surgery, radiation

DISCHARGE AND HOME HEALTHCARE GUIDELINES

PREVENTION. Teach the patient the need to have regular gynecologic examinations and to report any symptoms to her healthcare provider.

MEDICATIONS. Ensure that the patient understands the dosage, route, action, and side effects of any medication she is to take at home. Note that some of the medications require her to have routine laboratory tests following discharge to monitor her response.

COPING. Discuss with the woman helpful coping mechanisms. Encourage her to be open with her partner, her family, and her friends about her concerns. Help the patient cope with hair loss. Teach her cosmetic techniques to deal with hair and body changes. Explore alternative methods to medication to manage nausea and vomiting.

POSTOPERATIVE. Discuss any incisional care. Encourage the patient to notify the surgeon of any unexpected wound discharge, bleeding, poor healing, or odor. Teach her to avoid heavy lifting, sexual intercourse, and driving until the surgeon recommends resumption.

RADIATION. Teach the patient to maintain a diet high in protein and carbohydrates and low in residue to decrease bulk. If diarrhea remains a problem, instruct the patient to notify the physician or clinic because anti-diarrheal agents can be prescribed. Encourage the patient to limit her exposure to others with colds because radiation tends to decrease the ability to fight infections. To decrease skin irritation, encourage the patient to wear loose-fitting clothing and avoid using heating pads, rubbing alcohol, and irritating skin preparations.

Paget's Disease

DRG Category: 244
Mean LOS: 4.9 days
Description: MEDICAL: Bone Disease and Specific Arthropathies with CC

Paget's disease, or osteitis deformans, is a slowly progressing condition of bone structure that is characterized by increased and disorganized bone turnover. The bones affected vary, but those most commonly involved are the femur, tibia, lower spine, pelvis, and skull. Initially, there is an increase in the number of osteoclasts, which leads to excessive bone resorption and a compensatory increase in osteoblastic activity to repair bone matrix. As a result, the bone is enlarged and distorted, with areas of poor mineralization that resemble a mosaic pattern. Consequently, the bone cannot adequately withstand stresses and strains and is weaker.

Paget's disease causes bones to fracture easily, often after only a minor trauma; these fractures heal slowly and often incompletely. If the spine is involved, the vertebrae may collapse, causing paraplegia. If the skull is involved, bony impingements on the cranial nerves can lead to blindness, hearing loss, tinnitus, or vertigo. Other complications of Paget's disease include osteoarthritis, hypocalcemia, renal calculi, bone sarcoma, hypertension, and gout. The disease is most life-threatening when it is combined with congestive heart failure because of the need for increased cardiac output to supply increased blood flow to the bones.

CAUSES

The cause of Paget's disease is not known. One theory suggests that it is the result of a slow viral infection, possibly mumps, with a long dormant period. A familial tendency has also been noted. It appears more commonly in the United States, Australia, South Africa, and New Zealand than in the Middle East, Asia, and Africa.

GENDER AND LIFE SPAN CONSIDERATIONS

Paget's disease occurs most frequently in people over the age of 40 and is more common in men.

◻ ASSESSMENT

HISTORY. Paget's disease is frequently discovered as a result of x rays taken during a routine physical examination. Ask if the patient has experienced deep bone pain. Establish a history of bone fractures. Ask if the patient's hat size has changed or if he or she has experienced headaches. Elicit any history of decreased hearing or vision or of vertigo. Find out if the patient has noticed any changes in gait while walking or has experienced any difficulty breathing (possibly caused by kyphosis of the spine).

PHYSICAL EXAMINATION. Assess the patient's skeleton for deformities. Inspect the skull for enlargement, particularly in the frontal and occipital areas. Check for cranial nerve compression by testing for decreased hearing and vision, difficulty swallowing, and problems with balance. Examine legs and arms for bowing and subsequent deformities. Ask the patient to walk across the room and back to observe a characteristic waddling gait.

Observe for signs of kyphosis. Note if the patient is bent forward with the chin resting on the chest or has a barrel chest. Kyphosis can compromise chest excursion and cause dyspnea. Palpate the affected areas for increased warmth. Paget's disease causes an increase in vascularity of the affected bones, thus causing the skin temperature to rise. Elderly patients or those with large, highly vascular lesions may develop congestive heart failure because of the heart's attempt to pump more blood through bones with increased vascularity. Assess the patient's apical pulse, respirations, and blood pressure. Note the presence of peripheral edema and neck vein distension from right-sided heart failure and pulmonary congestion.

PSYCHOSOCIAL. Because the diagnosis of Paget's disease is unexpected, the patient and family may experience increased anxiety levels. There may be fear related to possible falls with fractures and the possibility of self-care deficits. Social isolation may also occur as a result of increasing bone pain and deformities.

DIAGNOSTIC HIGHLIGHTS

Test	Normal Result	Abnormality with Condition	Explanation
X rays	Normal structure of the skeletal system	Disordered and architecturally unsound	Disease causes increased osteoclastic bone resorption
Bone scans	Normal structure of the skeletal system	Identifies involved areas of the skeleton	Disease causes increased osteoclastic bone resorption

Other Tests: Bone biopsy, complete blood cell count, serum alkaline phosphatase

PRIMARY NURSING DIAGNOSIS

Pain (acute) related to fractures and nerve compression

OUTCOMES. Comfort level; Pain control behavior; Pain level; Symptom control behavior; Symptom severity; Well-being

INTERVENTIONS. Pain management; Analgesic administration; Cutaneous stimulation; Heat/cold application; Touch; Exercise therapy; Progressive muscle relaxation

□ PLANNING AND IMPLEMENTATION

Collaborative

MEDICAL. Generally, patients with Paget's disease who are asymptomatic require no specific treatment but need careful ongoing monitoring. Calcitonin and bisphosphonates are used to treat Paget's disease. Mild pain is usually controlled successfully with nonsteroidal anti-inflammatory drugs. Nonpharmacologic treatment modalities are also prescribed for patients with Paget's disease. Heat therapy and massage can help decrease pain. A physical therapy consultation can provide a protocol of simple strengthening and weight-bearing exercises. Braces and other ambulation aids may help support deformities and improve function.

SURGICAL. Surgery may be needed to reduce or prevent pathologic fractures, to correct secondary deformities, and to relieve neurologic impairment. Unfortunately, joint replacement is difficult because methyl methacrylate (a glue-like bonding material) does not set properly on bone that is affected by Paget's disease.

PHARMACOLOGIC HIGHLIGHTS

Medication or Drug Class	Dosage	Description	Rationale
Calcitonin	100 IU SC or IM qd initially and then 50 IU SC 3 times a week	Calcium regulator	Decreases the number and availability of osteoclasts, thereby retarding bone resorption relieves bone pain; helps the remodeling of pagetoid bone into lamellar bone
Etidronate	5–10 mg/kg per day, not to exceed 3 months	Bisphosphonates; calcium regulator	Slows rate of bone turnover in pagetic lesions; lowers serum alkaline phosphatase; reduces elevated cardiac output by decreasing vascularity of bone, thereby averting high-output cardiac failure

Independent

Focus on reducing pain and immobility, preventing injury, and educating the patient about the disease and treatment regimen. Correlate the patient's pain with his or her activities, and modify schedules as needed. Instruct the patient in the use of relaxation techniques such as guided imagery and music therapy. Evaluate the patient's level of functioning, and encourage the patient to remain as active as possible. Perform range-of-motion exercises to joints, unless contraindicated, progressing from passive to active exercise as tolerated. Encourage the patient to perform self-care activities independently.

For patients on extended bed rest, reposition the patient frequently and use a flotation mattress. Prevent pressure ulcers by providing meticulous skin care.

Institute measures to prevent injury. Instruct the patient to move slowly and avoid sudden movements. Keep the environment free of clutter. Encourage the use of ambulation aids, such as walkers or canes, as needed. Carefully plan exercise protocols and activity regimens to minimize fatigue.

DOCUMENTATION GUIDELINES

- Physical findings: Kyphosis, mobility, gait, presence of skeletal deformities
- Description of physical pain, comfort measures used, and response to interventions
- Sensory disturbances: Vision loss, hearing loss
- Level of tolerance of activity
- Laboratory results: Serum calcium and alkaline phosphatase levels
- Reaction to changes in body image

DISCHARGE AND HOME HEALTHCARE GUIDELINES

Encourage the patient to follow a recommended moderate exercise program. Suggest the use of a firm mattress or bed board to minimize spinal deformities. Emphasize the importance of attending physical therapy sessions and routine follow-up visits with the physician. Stress the importance of assessing the home environment for safety. Teach the patient to maintain adequate lighting, remove scatter rugs, and keep the home uncluttered. Instruct the patient to avoid abrupt movements and to report any increases in bone pain. Teach the patient to use assistive devices for ambulation.

Be sure the patient understands the dosage, route, action, and side effects of all prescribed medications. Instruct the patient in proper self-injection techniques for calcitonin. Educate the patient about side effects, such as nausea, vomiting, itchy hands, fever, inflammation of the injection site, and facial flushing, as well as the signs and symptoms of hypercalcemia. Teach the patient to take EHDP medication with fruit juice on an empty stomach at least 2 hours before meals. Tell the patient to call the physician if he or she experiences stomach cramps, diarrhea, or new bone pain. Educate the patient who is taking plicamycin about the signs and symptoms of infection. Tell the patient to report any easy bruising, bleeding, nausea, or anorexia. Provide information about the Paget's Disease Foundation (165 Cadman Plaza East, Brooklyn, NY 11201).

Pancreatic Cancer

DRG Category: 203
Mean LOS: 6.3 days
Description: MEDICAL: Malignancy of Hepatobiliary System of Pancreas

Pancreatic cancer is currently the fourth most common cause of cancer-related deaths in the United States. Approximately 30,000 Americans are diagnosed each year with pancreatic cancer, and the same number die each year. About 20% of patients survive 1 year after diagnosis, and fewer than 5% of persons with the disease are alive 5 years after diagnosis.

Tumors can develop in both the exocrine and the endocrine tissue of the pancreas, although 95% arise from the exocrine parenchyma (functional tissue). Islet cell tumors, as functioning or nonfunctioning insulinomas, compose 5% of pancreatic tumors. Adenocarcinoma of the ductal origin is the most common cell type (75% to 92%), and it occurs most frequently in the head of the pancreas. Pancreatic adenocarcinoma grows rapidly, spreading to the stomach, duodenum, gallbladder, liver, and intestine by direct extension and invasion of lymphatic and vascular systems. Further metastatic spread to the lung, peritoneum, and spleen can occur. Metastatic tumors from cancers in the lung, breast, thyroid, or kidney or skin melanoma have been found in the pancreas.

CAUSES

Although the exact cause is unknown, associations with cigarette smoking (incidence is more than twice as high for smokers as nonsmokers), diets high in fat or meat, diabetes mellitus, and chronic pancreatitis have been suggested. Persons who have occupational exposure to gasoline derivatives, naphthylamine, and benzidine are considered to be at higher risk. High coffee consumption and alcohol intake have been implicated; however, many believe a direct effect of these substances on the development of pancreatic cancer is questionable.

GENDER AND LIFE SPAN CONSIDERATIONS

Pancreatic carcinoma can occur in persons of all ages but is rare before the age of 45. Its peak incidence is between the ages of 60 and 70. The incidence in men and women is now equal and is attributed to the increase in smoking among women. Pancreatic cancer occurs 50% more frequently among African-Americans than among European-Americans, with the highest incidence in the United States developing among Korean-Americans living in Los Angeles.

☐ ASSESSMENT

HISTORY. Cancer of the pancreas has been called a "silent" disease; one reason for the poor survival rate is that cancer is often not detected during its early stages. The signs and symptoms are vague and frequently disregarded, or they are attributed to some minor ailment. Abdominal pain is a common sign of advanced pancreatic cancer. Unplanned weight loss and epigastric pain that may radiate to the back are common complaints. Ask the patient to describe the type and intensity of the pain and also aggravating and relieving factors. Patients often report a dull intermittent pain that has become more intense. Eating and activity often precipitate pain, whereas lying supine or sitting up and bending forward may offer relief. Question the patient as to the presence of any nausea, vomiting, anorexia, flatulence, diarrhea, constipation, or unusual fatigue.

PHYSICAL EXAMINATION. Inspect the patient for the presence and extent of jaundice, which is the presenting symptom in 80% to 90% of patients with cancer of the pancreatic head. The jaundice may have preceded or followed the onset of pain, but it usually progresses along a distinctive pattern: beginning on the mucous membranes, then on the palms of the hands, and finally becoming generalized. Assess for the presence of pruritus, dark urine, and clay-colored stools.

Early tumors can usually not be palpated but auscultate, palpate, and percuss the abdomen. If the tumor involves the body and tail of the pancreas, an abdominal bruit may be heard in the left upper quadrant (indicating involvement of the splenic artery) and a large, hard mass may be palpated in the subumbilical or left hypochondrial region. Note the presence of liver or spleen enlargement. Dullness on percussion may indicate the presence of ascites or gall bladder enlargement.

PSYCHOSOCIAL. Assess for the presence of irritability, depression, and personality changes. The sudden onset of characteristic symptoms can precipitate these emotional responses. Families and patients often display profound grief and disbelief on receiving the diagnosis of pancreatic cancer and a poor prognosis. Assess the specific feelings and fears of the patient and family and also support systems available and previous coping strategies.

DIAGNOSTIC HIGHLIGHTS

Test	Normal Result	Abnormality with Condition	Explanation
Computed tomography (CT) scan	Normal structure of the pancreas and surrounding organs and structures	Identifies size and location of tumors	Provides detailed images with multiple cross-sections of the pancreas
Magnetic resonance imaging (MRI)	Normal structure of the pancreas and surrounding organs, structures, and vessels	Identifies size and location of tumors; determines if vessels are compressed by tumor	Uses radio waves and strong magnets; computer translates pattern of radio waves into detailed images
Abdominal sonogram (ultrasound)	Normal structure of the pancreas	Although CT is more accurate in locating tumors, may be used to rule out pancreatic pseudocysts	Creates oscilloscopic picture from echoes of high-frequency sound waves passing over pancreatic area
Tumor marker antigen; CA 19–9	< 37 AU/mL	Elevated > 1000 AU/mL indicates metastasis	Elevated levels occur in 80% of patients with pancreatic cancer

Other Tests: Upper GI series, biopsy of pancreatic tissue, angiography, endoscopic retrograde cholangiopancreatography

PRIMARY NURSING DIAGNOSIS

Pain (chronic and acute) related to the effects of tumor invasion and surgical incision

OUTCOMES. Comfort level; Pain control behavior; Pain: Disruptive effects; Pain level

INTERVENTIONS. Pain management; Analgesic administration; Positioning; Teaching: Prescribed activity/exercise; Teaching: Procedure/treatment; Teaching: Prescribed medication

◻ PLANNING AND IMPLEMENTATION

Collaborative

Surgery, radiotherapy, and chemotherapy are the major treatment modalities for pancreatic cancer. A distal pancreatectomy, used more often with islet cell tumors than with exocrine cancer, removes only the tail of the pancreas or the tail and part of the body. The spleen is also removed. A total pancreatectomy or a pancreatoduodenectomy (Whipple procedure) is used when cure is the objective. In a total pancreatectomy, the entire pancreas and spleen are removed. The Whipple procedure involves removal of the head of the pancreas, distal stomach, gallbladder, pancreas, spleen, duodenum, proximal jejunum, and regional lymph nodes. The procedure induces exocrine insufficiency and insulin-dependent diabetes. A pancreatojejunostomy, hepaticojejunostomy, and gastrojejunostomy are performed with the Whipple procedure to reconstruct the gastrointestinal system. A vagotomy is usually done in both procedures to decrease the risk of peptic ulcer.

Careful postoperative management is essential for providing comfort and reducing surgical mortality. Observe vital signs, prothrombin times, drainage from drains, and wounds for signs of infection, hemorrhage, or fistula formation. Report immediately any evidence of increasing abdominal distension; shock; hematemesis, bloody stools; or bloody, gastric, or bile-colored drainage from incision sites. Vitamin K injections and blood components may be needed.

Monitor GI drainage from the nasogastric (NG) or gastrostomy tubes carefully. These tubes are strategically placed during surgery to decompress the stomach and prevent stress on the anastomosis sites. Maintain the tube's patency by preventing kinks or dislodgment; maintain suction at the prescribed level (usually low continuous suction for an NG tube). Secure gastrostomy tubes in a dependent position. Monitor the color, consistency, and amount of drainage from each tube. The presence of serosanguineous drainage is expected, but clear bile-tinged drainage or frank blood could indicate disruption of an anastomosis site and should be reported immediately. Do not irrigate the NG or gastrostomy tube without specific orders. When irrigation is ordered, gently instill 10 to 20 mL of normal saline solution to remove an obstruction.

Because postoperative nutritional requirements for adequate tissue healing approximate 3000 calories per day, parenteral hyperalimentation is often ordered. Monitor the blood and urine glucose levels every 6 hours, and administer insulin as needed. Once oral food and fluids are allowed, the patient is placed on a bland, low-fat, high-carbohydrate, high-protein diet. Administer pancreatic enzyme supplements (pancrelipase [Viokase, Cotazym] and lipase, for metabolism of long-chain triglycerides) with each meal and snack. Observe and report any evidence of diarrhea or frothy, floating, foul-smelling stools (an indication of steatorrhea) because an adjustment in the enzyme replacement therapy may be needed.

A combination of adjuvant chemotherapy and radiation therapy with surgery may increase survival time 6 to 11 months. Most patients receive chemotherapy and radiation therapy on an outpatient basis. Palliative surgical procedures can be used to relieve the obstructive jaundice, duodenal obstruction, and severe back pain that are characteristic of advanced disease.

PHARMACOLOGIC HIGHLIGHTS

Medication or Drug Class	Dosage	Description	Rationale
Chemotherapy	Varies with drug	Gemcitabine; fluorouracil (5-FU)	Kills cancer cells
Pancreatic enzyme supplements	Varies with drug	Pancrelipase; lipase	Aid in digestion of proteins, carbohydrates, and fats

Postoperative Drugs: Narcotic analgesics delivered via a patient-controlled analgesic device or an epidural catheter are usually ordered. Monitor the patient's response to these devices, and encourage their usage to maintain pain at a tolerable level. Administer prophylactic antibiotics as ordered.

Independent

Provide emotional support and information as treatment goals and options are explored. Patients newly diagnosed with pancreatic cancer are often in shock, especially when the disease is diagnosed in the advanced stages. Encourage the patient and family to verbalize their feelings surrounding the diagnosis and impending death. Allow for the time needed to adjust to the diagnosis, while helping the patient and family begin the grieving process. Assist in the identification of tasks to be completed before death, such as making a will; seeing specific relatives and friends; or attending an approaching wedding, birthday, or anniversary celebration. Urge the patient to verbalize specific funeral requests to family members.

Help family members identify the extent of physical home care that is realistically required by the patient. Arrange for visits by a home health agency. Suggest the family seek supportive counseling (hospice, grief counselor) and, if necessary, make the initial contact for them. Local units of the American Cancer Society offer assistance with home care supplies and support groups for patients and families.

Following any surgical procedure, direct care toward preventing the associated complications. Use the sterile technique when changing dressings and emptying wound drainage tubes. Place the patient in a semi-Fowler position to reduce stress on the incision and to optimize lung expansion. Help the patient turn over in bed, and perform coughing, deep-breathing, and leg exercises every 2 hours to prevent skin breakdown and pulmonary and vascular stasis. Teach the patient to splint the abdominal incision with a pillow to minimize pain when turning or performing coughing and deep-breathing exercises. As soon as it is allowed, help the patient get out of bed and ambulate in hallways three to four times each day. Be alert for the sudden onset of chest pain or dyspnea (or both), which could indicate the presence of a pulmonary embolism.

As the disease progresses and pain increases, large doses of narcotic analgesics may be needed. Instruct the patient on the effective use of the pain scale and to request pain medication before the pain escalates to an intolerable level. Consider switching as-needed pain medication to an around-the-clock dosing schedule to keep pain under control. Encourage the patient and family to verbalize any concerns about the use of narcotics, and stress that drug addiction is not a consideration.

DOCUMENTATION GUIDELINES

- Response to the diagnosis of pancreatic cancer, the diagnostic tests, and recommended treatment regimen
- Description of all dressings, wounds, and drainage collection devices: Location of drain, color and amount of drainage, appearance of incision, color and amount of GI drainage
- Physical findings related to the pulmonary assessment, abdominal assessment, presence of edema, and condition of extremities
- Response to pain medications, oral intake, and activity regimen
- Presence of complications: Hemorrhage, infection, pulmonary congestion, activity intolerance, unrelieved discomfort, absence of return of bowel sounds and function, decrease in urinary output
- Bowel pattern: Presence of constipation, diarrhea, steatorrhea

DISCHARGE AND HOME HEALTHCARE GUIDELINES

Reinforce the need for small, frequent meals. Warn against overeating at any one meal, which places too great a demand on the pancreas, and stress limiting caffeine and alcohol. Instruct the patient to inspect his or her stools daily and report to the physician any signs of steatorrhea. Teach the patient and family the care related to surgically induced diabetes: symptoms and appropriate treatment for hypoglycemia and hyperglycemia, procedure for performing blood glucose monitoring, administration of insulin injections. Teach the patient or significant other to change the dressing over the abdominal incision and empty the drains daily (if present).

Teach the patient care of skin in the external radiation field. Instruct the patient to do the following:

Wash the skin gently daily with mild soap, rinse with warm water, and pat the skin dry

Not wash off the dark ink markings outlining the radiation field

Avoid applying any lotions, perfumes, deodorants, or powder in the treatment area

Wear nonrestrictive, soft, cotton clothing directly over the treatment area

Protect the skin from sunlight and extreme cold

Pancreatitis

DRG Category: 204
Mean LOS: 5.7 days
Description: MEDICAL: Disorders of Pancreas Except Malignancy
DRG Category: 191
Mean LOS: 13.6 days
Description: SURGICAL: Pancreas, Liver, and Shunt Procedures with CC

Pancreatitis, acute or chronic, is an inflammation and potential necrosis of the pancreas. Tissue damage from pancreatitis occurs because of activation of proteolytic and lipolytic pancreatic enzymes that are normally activated in the duodenum. Proteolytic enzymes, such as trypsin, elastase, and phospholipase, break down protein; lipolytic enzymes break down fats. The enzymes cause autodigestion (destruction of the acinar cells and islet cell tissue), with leakage of the enzymes and fluid into surrounding tissues. The pancreas can return to normal after an attack of acute pancreatitis with successful treatment, or it may progress to a state of chronic inflammation and disease.

In chronic pancreatitis, there is permanent destruction. Precipitation of proteins causes pancreatic duct obstruction. Edema and distension cause damage and loss of the acinar cells, which normally produce digestive enzymes. The normal cells are replaced with fibrosis and necrosis. As the autodigestion process of the pancreas progresses, the cells form walls around the fluid that contains enzymes and the necrotic debris. These pseudocysts can rupture into the peritoneum and surrounding tissues, resulting in complications of infection, abscesses, and fistulae. The islet cells within the pancreas may also be damaged and destroyed, leading to diabetes mellitus. Other complications include massive pancreatic hemorrhage and shock, acute respiratory distress syndrome, atelectasis, pleural effusion, pneumonia, paralytic ileus, and, rarely, cancer.

CAUSES

Three factors cause premature enzyme activation. Mechanical causes—such as pancreatic duct damage and obstruction—may result from gallstones migrating into the duct, bile reflux from the duodenum into the duct, tumors, radiation therapy, ulcer disease, or inflammation. Metabolic causes result from changes in the secretory processes of the acinar cells in conditions such as alcoholism (90% of the cases), diabetic ketoacidosis, hyperlipidemia, hypercalcemia, and drugs (acetaminophen, estrogen). Miscellaneous causes include infectious diseases (mumps, hepatitis B, coxsackie viral infections) and ischemic injury as a result of lupus erythematosus, cardiopulmonary bypass surgery, post-transplantation complications, or shock.

GENDER AND LIFE SPAN CONSIDERATIONS

The main cause of pancreatitis in adult males is alcoholism and in adult females is cholelithiasis and biliary tract disturbances. The principal cause in children is cystic fibrosis. Pancreatic secretions decrease with age. Elderly persons have decreased ability to tolerate dietary fat and have an increased risk of gallstones that may lead to pancreatitis.

□ ASSESSMENT

HISTORY. Obtain a detailed history of alcohol use and ingestion patterns. Assess for a family history of pancreatitis or a history of external abdominal trauma, surgery, cancer, recent bacterial infections, and biliary or gastrointestinal disease. Obtain a complete medication profile of prescribed and over the counter drugs.

Determine the onset and severity of symptoms. Patients often seek medical attention for severe upper abdominal pain they describe as knifelike, twisting, and deep in the midepigastrium or umbilical region. The pain may radiate to the dorsal area of the back or around the costal margins. Pain begins 12 to 48 hours after excessive alcohol intake or, with gallstone-related pancreatitis, can occur after a large fatty meal. Nausea and vomiting are present in up to 90% of the cases.

PHYSICAL EXAMINATION. The patient appears acutely ill with restless, apprehensive, and agitated behavior. Some become confused and, if shock or hypoxemia is impending, unresponsive. Respirations are often rapid and shallow. The patient may assume a fetal position with legs drawn upward to relieve abdominal pain. You may note mottled or jaundiced skin. You may see a bluish discoloration in the flanks (Grey-Turner's sign) and around the umbilicus (Cullen's sign), which indicates blood accumulation in these areas. Skin may be cold and diaphoretic. You may also note coarse tremors of the extremities as a sign of low calcium. Other findings include tea-colored or foamy urine (indicating the presence of bile) and gray, foul-spelling, foamy stools that indicate the presence of undigested fat.

Asucultate the abdomen before palpation and percussion to check for decreased bowel sounds, which is a common finding in patients with pancreatitis. On palpation, note extreme abdominal tenderness, distension, guarding, and rigidity. Ascites and rebound tenderness are present in severe disease. When you percuss the abdomen, you may find abdominal tympany. The patient often has labile vital signs. During periods of pain, the patient may be hypertensive, but as hypovolemic shock progresses to late stages, blood pressure may fall. Patients usually have rapid heart rates; rapid, thready pulses; and decreased breath sounds in the lower lobes because of shallow respirations, pain, and increased abdominal size.

PSYCHOSOCIAL. Assess the patient's anxieties and coping abilities related to the demands of an acute care environment and a sudden illness. The patient with chronic pancreatitis needs assistance with feelings of hopelessness and apathy that may result from chronic pain and general debilitation. Assess the family's coping with role changes and responsibilities. Alcohol abuse counseling may be necessary.

DIAGNOSTIC HIGHLIGHTS

Test	Normal Result	Abnormality with Condition	Explanation
Serum amylase	50–180 units/dL	> 180 units/dL	Enzyme produced by pancreas that aids digestion of complex carbohydrates; increases 12–24 hours after acute inflammation
Serum calcium	8.6–10.3 mg/dL	< 8.6 mg/dL	Necrosis of fat from release of

			pancreatic enzymes leads to binding of free calcium
Serum lipase	31–186 units/L	> 186 units/L	Enzyme produced by pancreas that aids digestion of fat; specific marker for inflammation of pancreas; begins to elevate within 2 hours of the inflammation
Serum glucose	75–105 mg/dL	> 105 mg/dL	Interference with insulin release leads to hyperglycemia in some patients

Other Tests: Complete blood count, serum bilirubin, alkaline phosphatase, serum liver enzymes, abdominal ultrasound, computed tomography (CT) scan

PRIMARY NURSING DIAGNOSIS

Pain (acute or chronic) related to inflammation, edema, peritoneal irritation

OUTCOMES. Comfort level; Pain control behavior; Pain level; Symptom severity

INTERVENTIONS. Analgesic administration; Anxiety reduction; Environmental management: Comfort, Pain management; Medication management; Patient-controlled analgesia assistance

☐ PLANNING AND IMPLEMENTATION

Collaborative

The immediate goal of therapy is to control and decrease the inflammation of the pancreas. The fluid lost into the retroperitoneal space can be as much as 4 to 12 L with severe disease. Volume replacement with fluids such as lactated Ringer's injection or normal human serum albumin is used to restore blood volume and prevent hypovolemic shock. Normal human serum albumin is often used if low albumin levels lead to a loss of osmotic pressure in the vascular system. Urinary output is monitored hourly to measure volume status: less than 1 mL/kg per hour is a sign of hypoperfusion. The physician may insert a pulmonary artery catheter for hemodynamic monitoring to assess the adequacy of the volume replacement and cardiac output. Patients who develop sepsis and shock may not respond to fluid volume replacement and remain hypovolemic. This complication requires vasoactive parenteral medications.

Hypocalcemia is a common electrolyte imbalance that accompanies pancreatic necrosis and requires calcium replacement. It may cause tetany, seizures, respiratory complications, and myocardial changes. Magnesium deficits often accompany hypocalcemia and need replacement as well. Loss of potassium through vomiting, fluid loss in the third spaces, acidosis, and renal insufficiency can lead to ventricular dysrhythmia. The blood glucose is monitored as a part of the renal profile and by finger sticks every 6 hours to determine the need for exogenous insulin replacement. Respiratory support involves administering oxygen by a variety of routes, which may include mechanical ventilation. Because of inadequate breathing patterns and the risk of laryngospasm, the patient may require endotracheal intubation; also, position end-expiratory pressure,

pressure control ventilation, and inverse inspiratory-to-expiratory ratio ventilation (increasing inspiratory time) may be used.

The goal of therapy is to reduce the secretion of pancreatic enzymes, which stops the inflammatory process. The inflammation leads to nerve irritation and pain. Obtain a baseline pain assessment, and reassess every 4 hours using a pain-rating scale; provide narcotic analgesia as needed. Bed rest is important to decrease the basal metabolic rate, which, in turn, decreases pancreatic secretions. Insertion of a nasogastric tube for intermittent suction also contributes to this goal by preventing the release of secretion in the duodenum. Nothing-by-mouth (NPO) status is strictly maintained, with no ice chips or sips of water during the acute phase. Nutritional support to restore the damaged pancreatic cells is provided by initiating total parenteral nutrition within 3 days of the onset of the acute phase.

Surgical interventions may be indicated for managing the complications that are associated with pancreatic necrosis. The procedures include pancreatic drainage, pancreatic resection or debridement, and removal of obstructions (biliary stones). The current therapy for removal of stones is early endoscopic retrograde cholangiopancreatography and endoscopic sphincterotomy. Peritoneal lavage is used for patients who do not respond to intensive treatment after 3 days; it has significantly decreased the incidence of complications and the mortality rate.

PHARMACOLOGIC HIGHLIGHTS

Medication or Drug Class	Dosage	Description	Rationale
Insulin	Varies with patient	Hypoglycemic	Supplements endogenous hormone to control glucose levels
Opiates	Varies with drug	Meperidine (Demerol); fentanyl (Sublimaze)	Relieve pain; narcotic analgesics that do not cause spasms of the sphincter of Oddi may falsely elevate amylase level, so amylase levels need to be drawn before the pain therapy begins

Other Drugs: Antacids to neutralize gastric secretions; histamine antagonists to decrease gastric acid production; dopamine to improve myocardial contractility, increase cardiac output, and decrease inflammation by reducing permeability in pancreatic ducts. Chronic therapy may include a low-fat diet and oral pancreatic enzyme supplements.

Independent

During the acute phase of pancreatitis, focus on continued monitoring and teaching. Monitor the patient's pain to determine intensity, location, characteristics, and factors that aggravate or relieve the pain. Frequent doses of analgesics are required. Other measures to provide comfort include positioning the patient in a knee-chest posture, stress reduction, and relaxation exercises. Provide a restful environment, but also initiate diversional activities. Monitor the patient's respiratory status continually. Place the patient in high Fowler position to improve lung expansion, and use other mechanisms to enhance gas exchange. If the patient is not intubated, keep emergency intubation equipment close by in case tetany and laryngospasm occur. The risk of tetany is enhanced if the patient hyperventilates. Maintain a calm environment, a constant presence, and medications to assist the patient with quiet breathing.

After the removal of the nasogastric tube, the diet progresses slowly from liquids to a diet high in calories and low in fat. During the immediate recovery period, arrange for small, frequent meals. Explain the need to avoid food and drinks with caffeine, spicy foods, and heavy meals that stimulate pancreatic secretion. Develop a realistic weight gain goal. Assist with dietary teaching by planning a week's menu, incorporating the patient's specific dietary needs and restrictions.

DOCUMENTATION GUIDELINES

- Patient's description of pain and response to medications and alternative comfort measures
- Physical findings: Respiratory rate and rhythm, use of accessory muscles, character of breath sounds, mentation, pertinent laboratory findings, presence of fever
- Intake and output, fluid balance, weight changes, vital signs, results of renal profile laboratory studies
- Presence of nausea and vomiting, nasogastric tube, weight loss to 20% under ideal
- Presence of complications: Hemorrhage, sepsis, shock, respiratory distress syndrome, tetany, hyperglycemia

DISCHARGE AND HOME HEALTHCARE GUIDELINES

Prevention involves correcting the initiating events. If the disease is related to alcohol use, reinforce the importance of abstaining and provide appropriate referrals. Teach the patient to recognize early symptoms that may indicate recurrence and when to contact the physician. Emphasize the importance of follow-up care. Teach the rationale, action, dosage, and side effects of all prescribed medications. Instruct the patient to take prescribed pancreatic enzyme replacements with or immediately after meals and to swallow them whole and not with hot liquids that would disrupt the protective coating. If the patient is being discharged with the requirement for continued insulin injections, the patient and family should demonstrate the injection technique and the procedure for blood glucose self-monitoring. Provide a log and show them how to keep a record of glucose levels and insulin dosages. The patient with a loss of pancreatic endocrine function requires extensive ongoing diabetic teaching after discharge; refer for additional counseling if necessary. Encourage the patient to seek nutritional follow-up with clinic or physician visits, especially for hyperglycemic management.

Parkinson's Disease

DRG Category: 012
Mean LOS: 6.3 days
Description: MEDICAL: Degenerative Nervous System Disorders

Parkinsonism is a clinical condition that is characterized by the following: gradual slowing of voluntary movement (bradykinesia); muscular rigidity; stooped posture; distinctive gait with short, accelerating steps; diminished facial expression; and resting tremor. Parkinson's disease occurs with progressive parkinsonism in the absence of a toxic or known etiology and is a progressively degenerative disease of the substantia nigra and basal ganglia. Parkinson's disease is also called paralysis agitans.

Degeneration of the substantia nigra in the basal ganglia of the midbrain leads to depletion of the neurotransmitter dopamine, which is normally produced and stored in this location. Dopamine promotes smooth, purposeful movements and modulation of motor function. Depletion of dopamine leads to impairment of the extrapyramidal tracts and consequent loss of movement coordination.

Complications include injuries from falls, skin breakdown from immobility, and urinary tract infections. Death is usually caused by aspiration pneumonia or other infection.

CAUSES

The majority of all cases of classic Parkinson's disease are primary, or idiopathic, Parkinson's disease (IPD). The cause is unknown; a few cases suggest a hereditary pattern. Secondary, or iatrogenic, Parkinson's disease is drug- or chemical-related. Dopamine-depleting drugs such as reserpine, phenothiazine, metoclopramide, tetrabenazine, and the butyrophenones (droperidol and haloperidol) can lead to secondary Parkinson's disease.

GENDER AND LIFE SPAN CONSIDERATIONS

Parkinson's disease occurs in 1% of the population over age 50; however, juvenile parkinsonism is associated in people younger than age 40 who have Wilson's disease, progressive lenticular degeneration, or Huntington's disease. Parkinson's disease affects men slightly more often than it does women. Approximately 15% of people with IPD develop dementia as they age.

□ ASSESSMENT

HISTORY. Obtain a family, medication, and occupational history. Parkinson's disease progresses through the following stages: (1) mild unilateral dysfunction; (2) mild bilateral dysfunction, as evidenced by expressionless face and gait changes; (3) increasing dysfunction, with difficulties in walking, initiating movements, and maintaining equilibrium; (4) severe disability, including difficulties in walking and maintaining balance and steady propulsion, rigidity, and slowed movement; and (5) invalidism, which requires total care. Note the timing of progression of all symptoms.

The three cardinal signs of Parkinson's disease are involuntary tremors, akinesia, and progressive muscle rigidity. The first symptom of Parkinson's disease is a coarse, rest tremor of the fingers and thumb (pill-rolling movement) of one hand. It occurs during rest and intensifies with stress, fatigue, cold, or excitation. This tremor disappears during sleep or purposeful movement. The tremor can occur in the tongue, lip, jaw, chin, and closed eyelids. Eventually the tremor can spread to the foot on the same side and then to the limbs on the other side of the body.

PHYSICAL EXAMINATION. Assess the patient for signs of akinesia (complete or partial loss of muscle movement). Perform a passive range-of-motion examination, assessing for rigidity. Rigidity of the antagonistic muscles, which causes resistance to both extension and flexion, is a cardinal sign of Parkinson's disease. Flexion contractures develop in the neck, trunk, elbows, knees, and hips. Note alterations in the respiratory status because rigidity of the intercostal muscles may decrease breath sounds or cause labored respirations. Observe the patient's posture, noting if he or she is stooped, and assess gait dysfunction. Note involuntary movements, slowed movements, decreased movements, loss of muscle movement, repetitive muscle spasms, an inability to sit down, and difficulty in swallowing.

Observe the patient's face, noting an expressionless, mask-like appearance, drooling, and decreased tearing ability; note eyeballs fixed in an upward direction or eyelids completely closed, which are rare complications of Parkinson's disease. Assess for defective speech, a high-pitched monotone voice, and parroting the speech of others. Autonomic disorders that are manifested in Parkinson's disease include hypothalamic dysfunction, so assess for decreased or Parkinson's perspiration, heat intolerance, seborrhea, and excess oil production. Observe the patient for orthostatic hypotension, which manifests in fainting or dizziness. Note constipation or bladder dysfunction (urgency, frequency, retention).

PSYCHOSOCIAL. Parkinson's disease does not usually affect intellectual ability, but 20% of patients with Parkinson's disease develop dementia similar to Alzheimer's disease. The Parkinson's disease patient commonly develops depression later in the disease process, and this is characterized by withdrawal, sadness, loss of appetite, and sleep disturbance. Patients may also demonstrate problems with social isolation, ineffective coping, potential for injury, and sleep pattern disturbance.

DIAGNOSTIC HIGHLIGHTS

The diagnosis of Parkinson's disease is made through clinical findings rather than diagnostic tests. The key to diagnosis is the patient's response to levodopa.

PRIMARY NURSING DIAGNOSIS

Self-care deficit related to rigidity and tremors

OUTCOMES. Self-care: Activities of daily living—Bathing, Hygiene, Dressing, Grooming, Eating; Anxiety control; Endurance; Comfort level; Mood equilibrium; Energy conservation; Muscle function; Mobility level

INTERVENTIONS. Exercise therapy: Ambulation, Balance, Joint mobility, Muscle control; Environmental management, Self-care assistance; Exercise promotion; Energy management; Body image enhancement

◻ PLANNING AND IMPLEMENTATION

Collaborative

To control tremor and rigidity, pharmacologic management is the treatment of choice. Long-term levodopa therapy can result in drug tolerance or drug toxicity. Symptoms of drug toxicity are confusion, hallucinations, and decreased drug effectiveness. Treatment for drug tolerance and toxicity is either a change in drug dosage or a drug holiday. Autologous transplantation of small portions of the adrenal gland into the brain's caudate nucleus of Parkinson's disease patients is offered on an experimental basis in some medical centers as a palliative treatment. In addition, if medications are ineffective, a thalamotomy or stereotaxic neurosurgery may be done to treat intractable tremor.

Physical and occupational therapy consultation is helpful to plan a program to reduce flexion contractures and to maximize functions for the activities of daily living. To prevent impaired physical mobility, perform passive and active range-of-motion exercises and muscle-stretching exercises. In addition, include exercises for muscles of the face and tongue to facilitate speech and swallowing. Use of a cane or walker promotes ambulation and prevents falls.

PHARMACOLOGIC HIGHLIGHTS

Medication or Drug Class	Dosage	Description	Rationale
Antiparkinson	Varies with drug	Levodopa (L dopa); carbidopa-levodopa (Sinemet)	Controls tremor and rigidity; converted to dopamine in the basal ganglia
Amantadine hydrochloride (Symmetrel)	100 mg bid po	Antiviral	Controls tremor and rigidity by increasing the release of dopamine to the basal ganglia
Synthetic anticholinergics	Varies with drug	Trihexyphenidyl (Artane); benztropine mesylate (Cogentin)	Block acetylcholine-stimulated nerves that lead to tremors

Other Drugs: Antihistamines are sometimes prescribed with the anticholinergics to inhibit dopamine uptake; bromocriptine mesylate, a dopamine antagonist, is ordered to stimulate dopaminergic receptors.

Independent

Promote independence in the patient. Encourage maximum participation in self-care activities. Allow sufficient time to perform activities, and schedule outings in late morning or in the afternoon to avoid rushing the patient. Reinforce occupational and physical therapy recommendations. Use adaptive devices as needed. If painful muscle cramps threaten to limit the patient's mobility, consider warm baths or muscle massage.

To facilitate communication, encourage the Parkinson's disease patient to speak slowly and to pause for a breath at appropriate intervals in each sentence. Teach deep-breathing exercises to promote chest expansion and adequate air exchange. Be alert to nonverbal clues, and supplement interactions with a communication board, mechanical voice synthesizer, computer, or electric typewriter.

To maintain nutritional status, monitor the patient's ability to chew and swallow. Monitor weight, intake, and output. Position the patient in the upright position for eating to facilitate swallowing. Offer small, frequent meals; soft foods; and thick, cold fluids. Supplemental puddings or nutritional shakes may be given throughout the day to maintain weight.

Help the patient maintain a positive self-image by emphasizing his or her abilities and by reinforcing success. Encourage the patient to verbalize feelings and to write in a journal. Help the patient maintain a clean, attractive appearance. Caregivers may need a great deal of emotional support. Explore strategies for long-term care with the patient and significant others.

DOCUMENTATION GUIDELINES

- Ability to ambulate, perform the activities of daily living, progress in an exercise program
- Use of verbal and nonverbal communication
- Statements about body image and self-esteem
- Discomfort during activity

DISCHARGE AND HOME HEALTHCARE GUIDELINES

Be sure the patient or caregiver understands all medications, including the dosage, route, action, and adverse reactions. Avoid the use of alcohol, reserpine, pyridoxine, and phenothiazine while taking levodopa. In general, recommend massage and relaxation techniques, and reinforce exercises recommended by the physical therapist. Several techniques facilitate mobility and enhance safety in Parkinson's disease patients. Instruct the patient to try the following strategies: To assist in maintaining balance, concentrate on taking larger steps with feet apart, keeping back straight and swinging the arms.
To overcome akinesia, tape the "frozen" leg to initiate movement.
To reduce tremors, hold objects (coins, keys, or purse) in the hand.
To obtain partial control of tremors when seated, grasp chair arms.
To reduce rigidity before exercise, take a warm bath.
To initiate movement, rock back and forth.
To prevent spine flexion, periodically lie prone and avoid using a neck pillow.
Teach the patient to eliminate loose carpeting, install grab bars, and elevate the toilet seat. Use of chair lifts can also be beneficial.

Explore coping strategies. Support groups for the Parkinson's disease patient and family are available in most cities. Contact the American Parkinson's Disease Association and Referral Center (APDA), 116 John Street, New York, NY (1-800-223-2732). Encourage the patient to be independent in the activities of daily living. Use devices and assistance as necessary. Provide ample time to complete self-care.

Pelvic Fractures

DRG Category: 236
Mean LOS: 5.5 days
Description: MEDICAL: Fractures of Hip and Pelvis

A pelvic fracture is a break in the integrity of either the innominate bones or the sacrum. The innominate bones are connected posteriorly at the level of the sacrum and anteriorly to the symphysis pubis. These structures form a ring of bones with ligaments that are designed to accommodate weight distributed from the trunk to the pelvis across both the sacrum and the joints at the S-1 vertebra. The S-1 joints are maintained by the anterior and posterior ligaments and pelvic floor ligaments. The iliac vascular structures, lumbosacral plexus, lower genitourinary tract, reproductive organs, portions of the small bowel, distal colon and rectum, iliofemoral vessels, and lumbosacral plexus bilaterally all may be affected by a pelvic fracture.

Pelvic fractures account for approximately 3% of all fractures, with an associated mortality rate that ranges from 10% to 50%. The most immediate, serious complications that are associated with pelvic fractures are hemorrhage and exsanguination, which together cause up to 60% of the deaths from pelvic injuries. Pelvic fractures that are associated with sacral and sacroiliac disruption may cause sciatic and sacral nerve injuries.

CAUSES

Two out of three occurrences of pelvic fractures are associated with motor vehicle crashes (MVCs) and automobile-pedestrian trauma. Industrial accidents, falls, crush injuries, and sports injuries also cause pelvic fractures. Pelvic fractures may also occur from a low-impact fall or direct blows to bony prominences. A variety of classification systems have been developed to describe pelvic fractures. See Table 41 for one such classification.

TABLE 41 | **Functional Classification of Pelvic Fractures**

CLASSIFICATION	DESCRIPTION/STABILITY
Lateral compression	Rotationally unstable but vertically stable
	Posterior elements are stable
	May cause soft tissue and genitourinary tract injury
Anterior-posterior compression	"Open book injury" with symphysis pubis disruption
	Posterior element stability is variable
	May be associated with genitourinary tract injury
Vertical shear	Virtually always instability in the posterior elements
	Commonly associated with soft tissue, skin, vascular, genitourinary, gastrointestinal, and neurologic injury
Acetabular disruption	Includes simple fractures, dislocations, and implosion of the head of the femur into the pelvis
	Generally unstable
	May be associated with genitourinary and neurovascular injuries

GENDER AND LIFE SPAN CONSIDERATIONS

Pelvic fractures may occur at any age, from the pediatric to the elderly populations. Complex pelvic fractures are more common in men and women younger than 35 years of age and are less frequent in patients older than 65 years of age. The overall incidence of pelvic fractures is similar for men and women, with an increase in incidence in women older than 85, perhaps because of their increased incidence of osteoporosis.

◘ ASSESSMENT

HISTORY. Establish a history of the mechanism of injury, along with a detailed report from pre hospital professionals. In cases of MVCs, include the type of vehicle and speed at the time of the crash. Determine whether the patient was a driver or passenger and whether he or she was using a safety restraint. If the patient experienced a fall, determine the point of impact, distance of the fall, and type of landing surface. Ask if the patient experienced suprapubic tenderness, the inability to void, or pain over the iliac spikes. Determine if the patient has any underlying medical disorders, such as polycystic kidney disease or frequent urinary tract infections. Take a medication history, and determine if the patient has a current tetanus immunization.

PHYSICAL EXAMINATION. The initial evaluation or primary survey of the trauma patient is centered on assessing the airway, breathing, circulation, disability (neurological status), and exposure (completely undressing the patient). Inspection may reveal abrasions, ecchymosis, or contusions over bony prominences, the groin, genitalia, and suprapubic area. Ecchymosis or hematoma formation over the pubis or blood at the urinary meatus is significant for associated lower genitourinary tract trauma. Palpation of the iliac crests and anterior pubis may suggest underlying injury; however, "rocking of the pelvis" is discouraged because it may cause an increase in vascular injury and bleeding. Internal rotation of the lower extremity or "frog leg positioning" is suggestive of pelvic ring abnormalities.

Perform complete rectal and pelvic examinations to assess for bleeding, rectal tone, and, in women, the presence of vaginal wall disruptions. Check the position of the prostate gland in men and palpate for a "high-riding" prostate, which may indicate genitourinary tract injury. Assess the lower extremities for paresis, hypoesthesia, alterations in distal pulses, and abnormalities in the plantar flexion and ankle jerk reflexes. Inspect the perineum, groin, and buttocks for lacerations that may have been caused by open pelvic fractures. Note that from one-third to one-half of all trauma patients have an elevated blood alcohol level, which complicates assessments and may mask abdominal pain.

Monitor hourly fluid volume status, including hemodynamic, urinary, and central nervous system parameters. Notify the physician if delayed capillary refill, tachycardia, urinary output less than 0.5 mL/kg per hour, or alterations in mental status (restlessness, agitation, and confusion) occur. Body weights are helpful in indicating fluid volume status over time.

PSYCHOSOCIAL. The patient who has a pelvic fracture faces stressors that range from the unexpected nature of the traumatic event and acute pain to potential life-threatening complications. The traditional means of verbal communication are often limited or absent, thus leading to the patient's fear, loss of control, and isolation. Significant lifestyle and functional changes may occur in patients with pelvic fractures and their associated injuries. Assess patients' coping strategies, level of anxiety, and overall understanding of their injuries. Assess patients' ability to adapt to their current circumstances.

DIAGNOSTIC HIGHLIGHTS

Test	Normal Result	Abnormality with Condition	Explanation
Pelvic x rays	Intact bony structure	Evidence of fractures and dislocations	Demonstrates radiographic evidence of pelvic injury
Retrograde urethrography	Intact urethra	Injured or transected urethra	Shows location and extent of genitourinary injury
Computed tomography (CT) scan	Intact bony structure	Evidence of fractures, dislocations, and sacral injuries	Assesses pelvis and sacroiliac joint and sacral injuries

Other Tests: Pregnancy test, hematocrit, hemoglobin, platelet count, prothrombin time

PRIMARY NURSING DIAGNOSIS

Fluid volume deficit related to active hemorrhage secondary to pelvic fracture and adjacent vascular structures

OUTCOMES. Fluid balance; Circulation status; Cardiac pump effectiveness; Hydration

INTERVENTIONS. Bleeding reduction; Fluid resuscitation; Blood product administration; Intravenous therapy; Circulatory care; Shock management

◻ PLANNING AND IMPLEMENTATION

Collaborative

Maintenance of airway, breathing, and circulation are the highest priority. Many patients are in hypovolemic shock (see "Hypovolemic/Hemorrhagic Shock") and require fluid resuscitation. Patients with stable pelvic fractures can be managed with bed rest alone, and early ambulation is guided by their level of pain or associated injuries. Patients with unstable pelvic fractures can also be managed with bed rest, spica casts, or sling traction, but there is an increasing risk of complications associated with prolonged bed rest. Movement, weight-bearing restrictions, and head of bed elevation are prescribed by the orthopedic surgeon. The physician often prescribes sequential compression devices to prevent venous stasis.

External immobilization helps decrease pain, reduce the amount of blood transfusions, and facilitate early ambulation. Immobilization can be achieved through the use of several devices that can be applied externally or percutaneously to the pelvis through the skin into the bony structure. This type of fixation can be performed at the scene of the injury in an attempt to decrease bleeding and to immediately immobilize bony deformities. A pneumatic anti-shock garment (PASG) immobilizes unstable bony injuries and provides a tamponade effect, but it is a controversial intervention because its use has been associated with an increase in pre-hospital time and hemodynamic abnormalities. External stabilization can also be accomplished through the use of an external skeletal fixation device.

Surgical open reduction and internal fixation of pelvic ring disruptions are accomplished with the use of a variety of plates and screws that are secured internally. The goal of internal fixation is to restore the pelvis to its original anatomic configuration. When to perform the open reduction and internal fixation is controversial. Monitor for erythema, drainage, and edema at all wound sites, incision sites, and external fixator appliance insertion sites every 4 hours. Perform pin care as prescribed every 4 to 6 hours.

PHARMACOLOGIC HIGHLIGHTS

General Comments: Surgeons may choose to follow cultures of wounds, urine, blood, and sputum, rather than use prophylactic antibiotics. A tetanus booster may be administered to patients, depending on their history.

Medication or Drug Class	Dosage	Description	Rationale
Narcotic analgesics	Varies with drug but generally given IV in the early phases	Morphine sulfate, fentanyl, demerol	Provide relief of pain

Independent

Maintain the patient in a supine position if it is not contraindicated because of other injuries. Ensure adequate airway and breathing in this position. Because Trendelenburg's position may have negative hemodynamic consequences, may increase the risk of aspiration, and may interfere with pulmonary excursion, it is not recommended. If the PASG has been applied to stabilize the bony fractures and tamponade bleeding, protect the extremities with towels.

Wound care varies, depending on the severity of wounds, the presence of an open fracture, and the type of fixation device applied. Initial debridement may be done in the operating room at the time of the exploratory laparotomy. Wounds and any exposed soft tissue and bone are covered with wet sterile saline dressings. Avoid povidone-iodine (Betadine)–soaked dressings to limit iodine absorption and skin irritation. Use universal precautions to avoid exposing patients to infection.

Extensive periods of bed rest increase the risk of complications. Remove devices every shift to assess the underlying skin and provide skin care. Sequential compression devices may be applied to the upper extremities if the lower extremities are fractured or in skeletal traction. Provide active or passive range-of-motion exercises to uninjured extremities every shift, as appropriate. Maintain traction by keeping it free-hanging; do not remove weights when moving or repositioning the patient. Some patients may benefit from the use of specialty beds, such as a rotating bed that may improve pulmonary status while maintaining bony stability. Do not use external fixation devices to move or turn patients. Maintain skin integrity by using specialty mattresses with pressure-releasing components. Protect the patient from injury by covering all wire ends with plastic tips, corks, or gauze. When positioning the patient with an external fixation device, protect the skin with padding. Keep the patient's skin clean and dry. Gently massage the patient's bony prominences every 4 hours.

DOCUMENTATION GUIDELINES

- Physical findings: Vital signs, urine output, body weight, capillary refill, mental status, quality of peripheral pulses, urethral bleeding, bowel sounds, wound healing, bruising
- Response to bed rest and immobility, position of external fixation device, degree of range of motion, progress toward rehabilitation
- Presence of complications: Infection; pressure sores; inadvertent injury from external fixation devices, hemorrhages
- Pain: Location, duration, precipitating factors, responses to interventions

DISCHARGE AND HOME HEALTHCARE GUIDELINES

To prevent complications of prolonged immobility, encourage the patient to participate in physical and occupational therapy as prescribed. If compression stockings are prescribed, teach the patient or family the correct application. Verify that the patient has demonstrated safe use of assistive devices such as wheelchairs, crutches, walkers, and transfers. Teach the patient the purpose, dosage, schedule, precautions, and potential side effects, interactions, and adverse reactions of all prescribed medications. Review with the patient all follow-up appointments that are arranged. If home care is necessary, verify that appropriate arrangements have been completed.

Pelvic Inflammatory Disease

DRG Category: 368
Mean LOS: 5.6 days
Description: MEDICAL: Infections, Female Reproductive System
DRG Category: 361
Mean LOS: 13.1 days
Description: SURGICAL: Laparoscopy and Incisional Tubal Interruption

Pelvic inflammatory disease (PID) is an infectious inflammatory disease of the pelvic cavity and the reproductive organs. PID may be localized and confined to one area, or it can be widespread and involve the whole pelvic region including the uterus (endometritis), fallopian tubes (salpingitis), ovaries (oophoritis), pelvic peritoneum, and pelvic vascular system. The infection can be acute and recurrent or chronic.

PID can be a life-threatening and life-altering condition. Complications of PID include pelvic (or generalized) peritonitis and abscess formations, with possible obstruction of the fallopian tubes. Obstructed fallopian tubes can cause infertility or an ectopic pregnancy. Other complications of PID are bacteremia with septic shock and thrombophlebitis with the possibility of an embolus.

CAUSES

Many types of microorganisms, such as a virus, bacteria, fungus, or parasite, can cause PID. Common organisms involved in PID include *Chlamydia trachomatis, Neisseria gonorrheae,* staphylococci, streptococci, coliform bacteria, mycoplasmas, and *Clostridium perfringens.* The means of transmission is usually by sexual intercourse, but PID can also be transmitted by childbirth or by an abortion.

GENDER AND LIFE SPAN CONSIDERATIONS

PID predominantly affects women who are sexually active, particularly those who have multiple partners or who change partners frequently. Women who use an intrauterine device (IUD) as a means of birth control are also at a higher risk for developing PID. Other risk factors include age (teenagers in particular), marital status (women who are single have a higher risk), current or recent pregnancy, and previous history of PID.

□ ASSESSMENT

HISTORY. A thorough history of past infections, a sexual history, and a history of contraceptive use are essential to evaluate a woman with PID. The patient may describe a vaginal discharge, but the characteristics of the discharge depend on the causative organism. For example, a gonorrhea or staphylococcus infection causes a heavy, purulent discharge. With a streptococcus infection, however, the discharge is thinner with a mucoid consistency. The woman may also experience pain or tenderness, described as aching, cramping, and stabbing, particularly in the lower abdomen or pelvic region, or both. Low back pain may also be present. Other symptoms include dyspareunia (painful sexual intercourse); fever greater than 100.4°F; general malaise; anorexia; headache; nausea, possibly with vomiting; urinary problems such as dysuria, frequency, urgency, and burning; menstrual irregularity; and constipation or diarrhea.

PHYSICAL EXAMINATION. Observe closely for vaginal discharge and the characteristics of this discharge. Inspect the vulva for signs of maceration. Note if the woman has experienced pruritus that has led to irritated, red skin from scratching. If vomiting is reported, inspect the skin for signs of fluid deficit, such as dryness or poor skin turgor. Rebound tenderness may be noted. When the cervix is manipulated, the woman may complain of pain in this area. Auscultate the bowel; at first the bowel sounds are normal, but as the disease progresses, if it is not treated, the bowel sounds are diminished or even absent if a paralytic ileus is present.

PSYCHOSOCIAL. Because PID may be a life-threatening and life-altering disease, assess the patient's emotional ability to cope with the disease process. In particular, explore the woman's and her partner's concerns about fertility. Because sexual partners need to be treated to prevent reinfection, the patient may have concerns about discussing her illness with her partner or partners.

DIAGNOSTIC HIGHLIGHTS

General Comments: A variety of tests, along with clinical symptoms and sexual history support the diagnosis of PID.

Test	Normal Result	Abnormality with Condition	Explanation
White blood cell count (WBC)	5000–10,000/mm^2	>10,500/mm^2	Infection and inflammation elicit an increase in WBCs
Erythrocyte sedimentation rate (ESR)	Up to 20 mm per hour	>20 mm per hour	Inflammation increases the protein content of plasma, thus increasing the weight of RBCs and causing them to descend faster
Laparoscopy	Normal-appearing reproductive organs	Pelvic structures are red and inflamed; possible adhesions and scarring	Direct visualization of the pelvic cavity is possible

Other Tests: Cultures of drainage/cervix for various STIs.

PRIMARY NURSING DIAGNOSIS

Pain related to infectious process

OUTCOMES. Pain control; Pain level; Comfort level

INTERVENTIONS. Medication administration; Pain management; Heat/cold application; Analgesic administration

☐ PLANNING AND IMPLEMENTATION

Collaborative

Without treatment, this disease process can be lethal for women. The goal is to rid the patient of infection and preserve fertility if possible. Because no single antibiotic is active against all possible pathogens, the CDC recommends combination regimens. These regimens vary if the patient is hospitalized or treated on an outpatient basis. Usually the treatment is broad spectrum antibiotics. Both the affected woman and her sexual partner(s) should be treated with antibiotics. Women with PID are usually treated as outpatients, but if they become acutely ill, they may require hospitalization. The hospitalized patient with PID usually is placed on bed rest in a semi-Fowler position to promote vaginal drainage. IV fluids may be initiated to prevent or correct dehydration and acidosis. If an ileus or abdominal distension is present, a nasogastric tube is usually inserted to decompress the gastrointestinal tract. Urinary catheterization is contraindicated to avoid the spread of the disease process; tampons are also contraindicated. If the woman has an IUD, it is removed immediately.

If antibiotic therapy is not successful and the patient has an abscess, hydrosalpinx (distension of the fallopian tube by fluid), or some type of obstruction, a hysterectomy with bilateral salpingo-oophorectomy (removal of ovaries and fallopian tubes) may be done. A laparotomy may be done to incise adhesions and to drain an abscess. Signs of peritonitis, such as abdominal rigidity, distension, and guarding, need to be reported immediately so that medical or surgical intervention can be initiated. If the patient is poorly nourished, a dietary consultation is indicated.

Analgesics are prescribed to manage the pain that accompanies PID. Comfort measures can include the use of heat applied to the abdomen or, if they are approved by the physician, warm douches to improve circulation to the area. (See other interventions for pain in the following section.)

PHARMACOLOGIC HIGHLIGHTS

Medication or Drug Class	Dosage	Description	Rationale
Cefoxitin and Doxycycline	2 g IM 100 mg po bid × 14 days	Cephalosporin, 2nd generation Tetracycline antibiotic	Outpatient treatment recommended by the CDC
Ofloxacin and Clindamycin or Metronidazole	400 mg po bid × 14 days 450 mg po qid × 14 days 500 mg po bid × 14 days	Antibacterial, fluoroquinolone Antibiotic Systemic trichomonacide	Outpatient treatment recommended by the CDC
Cefoxitin or Cefotetan and Doxycycline	2 g IV q 6 hours 2 g IV q 12 hours 100 mg q 12 hours po × 10–14 days	Cephalosporin, 2nd generation Cephalosporin, 2nd generation Tetracycline antibiotic	Inpatient treatment recommended by the CDC
Clindamycin and Gentamycin and after discharge Doxycycline	900 mg IV q 8 hours 2 mg/kg IV or IM loading dose, then 1.5 mg/kg q 8 hours 100 mg po q 12 hours × 10–14 days	Antibiotic Antibiotic, aminoglycoside Tetracycline antibiotic	Inpatient treatment recommended by the CDC

Independent

Monitor vital signs and the patient's symptoms to evaluate the course of the infection and its response to treatment. Always follow universal precautions; ensure that any item used by the patient is carefully disinfected. Provide perineal care every 2 to 4 hours with warm, soapy water to keep the area clean. Teach the patient that she needs to do these procedures as well. Allow the patient time to express her concerns. If appropriate, include the woman's partner in a question-and-answer session about the couple's potential to have children. Note that the inability to bear children is a severe loss for most couples, and they may need a referral for counseling.

Interventions that can help relieve pain include having the patient lie on her side with the knees flexed toward the abdomen. Massaging the lower back also increases her comfort. Use diversions such as music, television, and reading to take the patient's mind off the discomfort.

Teach the patient interventions to prevent the recurrence of PID: to use condoms, to have all current sexual partners examined, to wash hands before changing pads or tampons, and to wipe the perineum from front to back. Encourage her to obtain immediate medical attention if fever, increased vaginal discharge, or pain occurs. Discuss with the patient when sexual intercourse or douching may be resumed (usually at least 7 days after hospital discharge).

DOCUMENTATION GUIDELINES

- Physical findings: Vital signs, abdominal assessment, condition of integument
- Occurrence of pain: Location, intensity, duration, triggers, response to pain interventions
- Presence of vaginal discharge: Characteristics, amount of discharge

DISCHARGE AND HOME HEALTHCARE GUIDELINES

PREVENTION. To prevent a recurrence of PID, teach the patient the following:
Take showers instead of baths.
Wear clean, cotton, nonconstrictive underwear.
Avoid using tampons if they were the problem.
Change sanitary pads or tampons at a minimum of every 4 hours.
If using a diaphragm, remove it after 6 hours.
If any unusual vaginal discharge or odor occurs, contact a medical care provider immediately.
Maintain a proper diet, with exercise and weight control.
Maintain proper relaxation and sleep.
Have a gynecologic examination at least annually.
Use a condom if there is any chance of infection in the sexual partner.
Use a condom if the sexual partner is not well known or has had another partner recently.

MEDICATIONS. Ensure that the patient knows the correct dosage and time that the medication is to be taken and that she understands the importance of adhering to this regimen.

COMPLICATIONS. Teach all patients who have had PID the signs and symptoms of an ectopic pregnancy, which are pain, abnormal vaginal bleeding, faintness, dizziness, and shoulder pain. Explain alternate means of contraception to the woman if she previously used an IUD. Ensure that the woman is familiar with the manifestation of PID, so she can report a recurrence of the disease.

Peptic Ulcer Disease

DRG Category: 177
Mean LOS: 4.5 days
Description: MEDICAL: Uncomplicated Peptic Ulcer with CC
DRG Category: 154
Mean LOS: 13.3 days
Description: SURGICAL: Stomach, Esophageal, and Duodenal Procedures, Age > 17 with CC

Peptic ulcer disease refers to ulcerative disorders in the lower esophagus, upper duodenum, and lower portion of the stomach. An ulcer is a sharply circumscribed break of the mucosa that may extend through the tissue layers of the muscle and serosa into the abdominal cavity. The types of peptic ulcers are gastric and duodenal, both of which are chronic diseases. Stress ulcers, which are caused by a physiologic response to major trauma, are clinically distinct from chronic peptic ulcers.

Gastric ulcers are less common than duodenal ulcers and usually occur in the lesser curvature of the stomach within 1 inch of the pylorus. The ulcer formation is caused by an inability of the mucosa to protect itself from damage by acid pepsin in the lumen (which is caused by a breakdown of the defensive factors). Duodenal ulcers occur in the proximal part of the duodenum (95%), are less than 1 cm in diameter, and are round or oval. A higher number of parietal cells in the stomach cause hypersecretion, or rapid emptying of the stomach; this may lead to a larger amount of acid being delivered to the first part of the duodenum and result in the formation of an ulcer. Hemorrhage and peritonitis can occur if the peptic ulcer erodes through the intestinal wall. Other complications include abdominal or intestinal infarction or erosion of the ulcer into the liver, pancreas, or biliary tract.

CAUSES

Factors that contribute to the development of peptic ulcers include a genetic predisposition to ulcer formation; poor cell restitution; excessive acid secretion; stress; excessive alcohol intake; smoking; ingestion of aspirin and nonsteroidal anti-inflammatory drugs (NSAIDs); and chronic use of drugs such as steroidal, potassium, or iodine compounds. The *Helicobacter pylori* bacterium, the principal causative agent of type B chronic gastritis, is also thought to be a major cause of peptic ulcers. Associated diseases include hyperparathyroidism, chronic lung disease, and alcoholic cirrhosis.

GENDER AND LIFE SPAN CONSIDERATIONS

The incidence of duodenal ulcers is highest in people 40 to 50 years old and is equally common in men and women. Gastric ulcers, which occur most often in people 60 to 70 years old, are more common in men. Mortality with gastric ulcer perforation is three times greater than that with duodenal ulcer perforation, partly because of the increased age of the patients. Duodenal ulcers occur in approximately 10% of the population at some time in their lives. More than half of the people who have duodenal ulcers heal spontaneously but have a high incidence of recurrence within 2 years.

□ ASSESSMENT

HISTORY. Epigastric pain is the major symptom. Assess pain by obtaining a history of the onset, duration, and characteristics in relation to food intake and medications. Patients may describe pain as sharp, burning, or gnawing, or it may be achy and perceived as abdominal pressure. Pain with duodenal ulcer occurs from 90 minutes to 3 hours after eating, is relieved with food or antacids, and may awaken a person at night. It is located to the right of the midline epigastrium with duodenal ulcers and to the left of the midline with gastric ulcers. Gastric ulcer pain is precipitated by food and is not relieved by antacid use to the same extent as duodenal ulcer pain is. Some patients have constant pain or no clear pattern of discomfort. As a result of the pain, weight loss and anorexia may occur with gastric ulcers. Weight gain may result with duodenal ulcers because food relieves the pain.

Question the patient about a family history of ulcer disease; smoking and alcohol habits; presence of other symptoms, such as nausea and vomiting; and changes in stool color, level of energy, appetite, and body weight. Review the patient's medication profile, both prescribed and over the counter (OTC). Ask about the amounts of caffeinated beverages taken daily. Determine the foods that aggravate the symptoms. Assess the patient's level of stress and coping skills.

PHYSICAL EXAMINATION. On inspection, you may note pale mucous membranes and skin because of anemia from acute or chronic blood loss. Some patients have black or tarry stools. Currant-colored or bright red stools occur only with massive bleeding. During auscultation, you may note that bowel sounds are hyperactive initially but diminish because of a paralytic ileus with ulcer perforation and peritonitis. Palpation in the midline may reveal epigastric tenderness.

PSYCHOSOCIAL. Researchers have not been able to establish a characteristic duodenal ulcer personality. Chronic stress and anxiety, however, are believed to increase gastric secretions and may be factors in exacerbating ulcer recurrence. Assess the patient's response to the disease, and note any unusual stressors that have an effect on the patient's or significant other's life.

DIAGNOSTIC HIGHLIGHTS

Test	Normal Result	Abnormality with Condition	Explanation
Barium radiographic studies	Normal gastrointestinal track	Presence of ulcers often as a protrusion on radiographic examination	Barium study highlights presence of ulcer in stomach or duodenum
Esophagogastro-duodendoscopy (EGD)	Normal gastrointestinal mucosa	Presence of mucosal ulcerations in the stomach or duodenum	Flexible endoscopy to allow visualization of mucosa

Other Tests: Serum gastrin levels, hemoglobin, hematocrit, complete blood count (CBC)

PRIMARY NURSING DIAGNOSIS

Pain (acute) related to inflammation and irritation

OUTCOMES. Comfort level; Pain control behavior; Pain level; Symptom severity

INTERVENTIONS. Analgesic administration; Anxiety reduction; Environmental management: Comfort; Pain management; Medication management; Patient-controlled analgesia assistance

☐ PLANNING AND IMPLEMENTATION

Collaborative

The treatment of choice for patients with peptic ulcers is generally pharmacologic. Drugs can be used to buffer or inhibit acid secretion that leads to ulceration and causes symptoms. Nutritional therapy is also prescribed. The current treatment is to eliminate foods that cause discomfort and symptoms. There is no evidence that bland or soft diets reduce gastric acid, promote healing, or relieve symptoms. Instruct the patient to avoid alcohol, coffee, and other caffeine-containing beverages. Refer patients with significant weight loss to a dietitian.

Most patients do not require surgery. However, in the event of the primary complications of hemorrhage, perforation, or obstruction, surgery may be necessary. Hemorrhage occurs in 15% of patients with duodenal ulcers and occurs more frequently in patients with NSAID-associated ulcers who have no prior symptoms. Perforation into the peritoneal cavity, which occurs in 6% of patients, happens when the ulcer erodes through the entire thickness of the gastric or duodenal wall. Obstruction occurs in 2% to 4% of patients with duodenal or pyloric ulcers. Treatment begins conservatively with gastric suction and fluid and electrolyte therapy. Pyloroplasty may follow.

The most common surgical interventions that are required for persons who do not respond to medical treatments are vagotomy with antrectomy, vagotomy with pyloroplasty, and parietal cell vagotomy (also called superselective or proximal gastric vagotomy). Several important complications can occur after surgery. Bile reflux gastritis, which occurs because of a reflux of duodenal contents into the stomach, occurs after a pyloroplasty or when the pylorus is bypassed or removed. Marginal ulcers are those that develop where gastric acids contact the operative site, usually at the site of anastomosis. Acute gastric dilation occurs in the postoperative period when dilation of the stomach causes reflex hypotension, pain, and tachycardia. The symptoms are relieved with vomiting or gastric suction.

PHARMACOLOGIC HIGHLIGHTS

General Comments: Most duodenal ulcers heal in 4 to 6 weeks, and treatment seldom extends past 8 weeks. Maintenance drug therapy is indicated for at least 1 year for patients with frequent recurrences. Gastric ulcers should heal in 8 to 12 weeks, more rapidly when acid is completely suppressed with use of a proton pump inhibitor such as omeprazole (Prilosec). If gastric ulcers do not heal with treatment, malignancy is suspected. Misoprostol (Cytotec), a prostaglandin E analog, inhibits gastric acid secretion and protects mucosa.

Medication or Drug Class	Dosage	Description	Rationale
H$_2$ antagonist	Varies with drug	Cimetidine, rantidine, famotidine, nizatidine	Reduces acid secretion
Antibiotics (for patients with *H. pylori* bacteria)	Varies with drug	Amoxicillin (Amoxil), tinidazole, metronidazole (Flagyl), tetracycline	Eradicate *H. pylori*; patients usually take two antibiotics, bismuth subsalicylate (Pepto-Bismol) and an H$_2$ antagonist; prevention of recurrence is 92%
Sucralfate (Carafate)	1 gram po bid	Anti-ulcer	Buffers stomach acids and raises gastric pH by acting as a physical barrier to acid, pepsin, and bile salts

Independent

Provide information about the cause and contributing factors as they pertain to the individual patient. Explain the relationship of gastric acidity, mucosal damage, and the significance of the symptoms of ulcer formation (pain, bleeding, nausea and vomiting, black stools). Discuss possible complications of peptic ulcer disease as it progresses: hemorrhage, perforation, and obstruction because of repeated ulcerations and scarring. Emphasize the need to adhere to the medication schedule, even when symptoms subside, to ensure complete healing and to prevent recurrence. Encourage the patient to avoid aspirin and other NSAIDs for aches and pains and suggest alternatives, such as acetaminophen (Tylenol). Provide a list of OTC drugs that contain aspirin.

Explore ways to reduce stress, and emphasize the importance of emotional and physical rest to reduce gastric secretion. Teach relaxation exercises to use during rest periods that fit into daily routines. Explain why elimination of smoking facilitates healing and reduces recurrence. Provide a list of community agencies that have smoking cessation programs. Discuss the patient's concerns openly. Identify attitudes and situations that could interfere with the needed lifestyle changes. Involve the family or significant others in these discussions and plans to gain their support.

DOCUMENTATION GUIDELINES

- Physical findings of epigastric or abdominal pain, nausea, vomiting, tarry stools, bleeding, infection, presence of complications (hemorrhage, perforation, obstruction)
- Response to medication therapy, nutritional therapy, emotional/physical rest
- Response to surgical interventions

DISCHARGE AND HOME HEALTHCARE GUIDELINES

Advise the patient that recurrence is greater than 50% with noncompliance. Reinforce the need to avoid the following: aspirin products and NSAIDs, alcohol intake, caffeine products, and smoking. Review signs and symptoms that should be reported—those that may indicate recurrence or complications, including pain, nausea, vomiting, black tarry stools, fatigue, and frank bleeding. Stress the importance of eating three meals at approximately the same time each day.

Postoperatively, tell the patient what to expect if infection occurs so he or she can tell the healthcare provider when the first signs occurred. The symptoms include pain, redness, swelling, and drainage at the incisional site. After a Billroth II surgical procedure, the patient may develop symptoms of the dumping syndrome. Explain the reason and timing of the symptoms that may occur, noting that the episodes will subside in 6 to 12 months. Teach the patient how to control the problems:

Take fluids only between meals, none with meals
Eat smaller amounts more frequently in a semirecumbent position
Eat a low-carbohydrate diet, concentrating on high-protein and moderate-fat foods
Avoid refined sugars (sweets)
Lie down after meals for 30 minutes
Take anticholinergic drugs 30 minutes before meals as prescribed.
Reinforce the need to stop smoking to promote healing and prevent recurrence.

Pericarditis

DRG Category: 144
Mean LOS: 4.5 days
Description: MEDICAL: Other Circulatory System Diagnoses with CC

Pericarditis is an inflammation of the pericardium, which is the membranous sac that encloses the heart and great vessels. The inflammatory response causes an accumulation of leukocytes, platelets, fibrin, and fluid between the parietal and visceral layers of the pericardial sac, thus producing a variety of symptoms, depending on the amount of fluid accumulation, how quickly it accumulates, and whether the inflammation resolves after the acute phase or becomes chronic.

An acute pericardial effusion is caused by an accumulation of fluid in the pericardial sac. The fluid accumulation interferes with cardiac function by compressing the cardiac chambers. Chronic constrictive pericarditis usually begins as an acute inflammatory pericarditis and progresses over time to a chronic, constrictive form because of pericardial thickening and stiffening. The thickened, scarred pericardium becomes nondistensible and decreases diastolic filling of the cardiac chambers and cardiac output. Chronic pericardial effusion is a gradual accumulation of fluid in the pericardial sac. The pericardium is slowly stretched and can accommodate more than 1 L of fluid at a time.

CAUSES

Pericarditis may also be classified etiologically into three broad categories: infectious pericarditis, noninfectious pericarditis, and pericarditis presumably related to hypersensitivity or autoimmunity. Infectious pericarditis may be caused by a viral infection such as the coxsackie B virus. Pyrogenic, tuberulous, mycotic, syphilitic, and parasitic infections may also cause pericarditis. Noninfectious pericarditis may be caused by a number of factors, including acute myocardial infarction, trauma, aortic aneurysm (with leakage into the pericardial sac), uremia, sarcoidosis, and myxedema. Both primary tumors, either benign or malignant, and metastatic tumors in the pericardium may cause pericarditis. Other causes include cholesterol and chylopericardium.

Pericarditis is also thought to be related to hypersensitivity or autoimmunity. Rheumatic fever and collagen vascular disease, such as systemic lupus erythematosus, rheumatoid arthritis, and scleroderma, may cause pericarditis. Some drugs, such as procainamide and hydralazine, are thought to cause pericarditis, as can postcardiac injury, such as Dressler's syndrome, and postpericardiotomy.

GENDER AND LIFE SPAN CONSIDERATIONS

Pericardial disease can occur at any age. Idiopathic (viral) inflammatory pericarditis occurs most frequently in adults, and more common in men than women. Tuberculous (bacterial) pericarditis is seen most often in children and in immunosuppressed patients.

◻ ASSESSMENT

HISTORY. Acute inflammatory pericarditis is most frequently idiopathic; however, the patient may have a history of a viral, bacterial, fungal, or parasitic infection. Take a detailed history of the patient's symptoms, especially pain. Ask the patient to describe the pain: Is it dull or sharp, and is it persistent? Is the location of the pain retrosternal or left precordial and radiating to the neck, left arm, and trapezius ridge? Ask if the pain is worsened by trunk movement, position, and deep inspiration. Ask about fever, cough, dyspnea, dysphagia, hiccups, nausea, and abdominal pressure (because of the compression of surrounding tissues by the enlarged pericardial sac).

The patient with a chronic pericardial disease may reveal a history of myocardial infarction (Dressler's syndrome), tuberculosis, chronic renal failure, radiation therapy, malignancies, connective tissue disease, and acquired immuno-deficiency syndrome (AIDS). Note a history of increasing dyspnea, fatigue, loss of appetite, nausea, and cough. Chest pain is not usually associated with chronic pericarditis.

PHYSICAL EXAMINATION. Check the patient's vital signs for tachycardia, tachypnea, and fever. If there is an effusion, the blood pressure may be low and a pulsus paradoxus may be present (an abnormal drop in systolic pressure with inspiration). Inspect the patient's neck for vein distension because of elevated jugular venous pressures that are caused by chronic pericarditis. Auscultate for heart sounds to establish a pericardial friction rub. Although the presence of a pericardial friction rub is a significant finding, the absence of a rub is not because pericardial friction rub is transient.

PSYCHOSOCIAL. Because of severe chest pain, patients with acute pericarditis may be in distress. The patient may be fearful of having a myocardial infarction. Assess the patient's ability to cope with a sudden illness and severe pain.

DIAGNOSTIC HIGHLIGHTS

Test	Normal Result	Abnormality with Condition	Explanation
Electrocardiogram	Normal PQRST pattern	ST-T wave elevation and	Results of pericardial thickening and

		eventually T wave inversion when ST segment returns to baseline	diminished diastolic filling
Computed tomography (CT) scan or magnetic resonance imaging (MRI)	Normal cardiac structures	Pericardial thickening	Radiography and three-dimensional evidence of inflamed pericardium

Other Tests: White blood cell count (elevated), cardiac enzymes, chest x ray, intracardiac pressure measurements, cardiac catheterization

PRIMARY NURSING DIAGNOSIS

Pain (acute) related to swelling and inflammation of the heart or surrounding tissue

OUTCOMES. Comfort level; Pain control behavior; Pain level; Symptom severity

INTERVENTIONS. Analgesic administration; Anxiety reduction; Environmental management: Comfort; Pain management; Medication management

□ PLANNING AND IMPLEMENTATION

Collaborative

Pericarditis is treated by correcting the underlying cause and therefore relieving the signs and symptoms. Acute pericarditis is treated with analgesic and anti-inflammatory agents. Acute pericardial effusions are treated according to the hemodynamic effect on the myocardium. An acute effusion that causes a decreased cardiac output is an indication for pericardiocentesis, which allows for fluid to be removed from the pericardial sac. Cardiac compression is relieved, and cardiac output returns. Other alternatives are a pericardiotomy, which is a surgical incision in the pericardial sac, or pericardial window (fenestration), which is the removal of one or more small portions of the pericardial sac. These surgical procedures are used when pericardiocentesis is unsuccessful or must be repeated because of continued accumulation of fluid.

Chronic pericarditis, with or without an effusion, may require a pericardectomy, which involves a thoracotomy incision and carries a much higher mortality (5% to 14%) than the other procedures. Note that, to halt the hemorrhage, a rapidly accumulating tamponade from hemorrhage into the pericardiac space should be managed surgically rather than by pericardiocentesis.

PHARMACOLOGIC HIGHLIGHTS

Medication or Drug Class	Dosage	Description	Rationale
Nonsteroidal anti-inflammatory agents	Varies with drugs	Aspirin, indomethacin, ibuprofen	Reduce pain and inflammation

Other Drugs: Corticosteroids can create gastrointestinal disturbances, which may increase the likelihood of the patient's failure to adhere to the prescribed medical therapy. Bacterial pericarditis is treated with antibiotics.

Independent

Place the patient in a high Fowler position. Use pillows to increase the patient's comfort, and encourage the patient to sit upright and lean slightly forward rather than lie supine. If the upright position does not alleviate the pain, have the patient try a side-lying position for 10 minutes. If the patient needs to perform coughing and deep-breathing exercises, provide instruction on splinting the chest with pillows to decrease the pain.

Remain with the patient during periods of increased pain and discomfort. Encourage the patient and family to verbalize their fears and concerns and to ask questions about the treatment and course of the disorder. Inform the patient and family about pericarditis and its causes. Explain all procedures. Assist the patient and family in distinguishing acute pericarditis from myocardial infarction. Teach them about continuing medications as prescribed even after the pain is gone but to taper use of steroids.

DOCUMENTATION GUIDELINES

- Physical findings: Vital signs, signs of pulsus paradoxus or pericardial friction rub, breath sounds, quality of heart tones
- Assessment of pain: Precipitating factors, quality, radiation, associated signs and symptoms, relief
- Response to medication: Body temperature, pain control

DISCHARGE AND HOME HEALTHCARE GUIDELINES

Be sure the patient understands any pain medication prescribed, including dosage, route, action, and side effects. The patient and family or significant other needs to understand the importance of decreased activity until the chest pain is completely gone. If the patient has undergone a surgical procedure, follow the activity restrictions for a thoracotomy.

Peritonitis

DRG Category: 188
Mean LOS: 4.9 days
Description: MEDICAL: Other Digestive System Diagnoses, Age > 17 with CC
DRG Category: 170
Mean LOS: 9.8 days
Description: SURGICAL: Other Digestive System Operating Room Procedures with CC

Peritonitis is the inflammation of the peritoneal cavity. The peritoneum is a double-layered, semipermeable sac that lines the abdominal cavity and covers all the organs in the abdominal cavity. Between its visceral and parietal layers is the peritoneal cavity. Although the peritoneum walls off areas of contamination to prevent the spread of infection, if the contamination is massive or continuous, this defense mechanism may fail, resulting in peritonitis. Perhaps the most serious complication caused by peritonitis is intestinal obstruction, which results in death in 10% of patients. Other complications include abscess formation, bacteremia, respiratory failure, and shock.

CAUSES

The most common cause is infection with *Escherichia coli,* but streptococci, staphylococci, and pneumococci may also cause the inflammation. The main sources of inflammation are the gastrointestinal (GI) tract, external environment, and bloodstream. Entry of a foreign body—such as a bullet, knife, or indwelling abdominal catheter—and contaminated peritoneal dialysate may precipitate peritonitis. Acute pancreatitis may also cause peritonitis.

GENDER AND LIFE SPAN CONSIDERATIONS

Peritonitis can occur at any age and across both genders. The elderly patient with peritonitis is at greater risk for developing life-threatening complications. The young adult male population is at risk because one of the primary causes of death in this gender and age group (multiple trauma) can lead to peritonitis.

□ ASSESSMENT

HISTORY. Obtain a thorough history and try to determine the possible sources of peritoneal infection. Ascertain any history of GI disorders, penetrating or blunt trauma to the abdomen, or recent abdominal surgery. Ask if the patient has any inability to pass flatulence or stools. Ask if the patient has experienced any weakness, nausea, or vomiting or a recent history of dehydration and high temperatures.

The parietal peritoneum is well supplied with somatic nerves, whereas the visceral peritoneum is relatively insensitive. With peritonitis, stimulation of the parietal peritoneum causes sharp, localized pain, whereas stimulation of the visceral peritoneum results in a more generalized abdominal pain. The pain is a steady ache that occurs directly over the area of inflammation. The intensity depends on the type and amount of foreign substances that are irritating the peritoneum and the somatic nerves supplying the parietal pentoneum. Peritoneal pain is almost always increased by pressure or tension of the peritoneum, such as coughing, sneezing, and palpation. Ask whether abdominal pain is generalized or localized. Inflamed diaphragmatic peritonitis can cause shoulder pain as well.

PHYSICAL EXAMINATION. Visually inspect the abdomen for size and shape. Peritonitis leads to abdominal distension. When assessing the GI system, auscultate before palpation. Bowel sounds are decreased or absent. Palpation reveals abdominal rigidity and elicits rebound tenderness with guarding. The patient may keep movement to a minimum to reduce the pain. Well-localized pain may cause rigidity of the abdominal muscles. The patient is generally in a knee-flexed position with shallow respirations in an attempt to minimize pain.

Check the patient for signs of dehydration, such as a dry and swollen tongue, dry mucous membranes, and thirst. High fever may result in rapid heart rate. The patient may experience hiccups in cases of diaphragmatic peritonitis. Observe the patient for pallor, excessive sweating, or cold skin, which are signs of electrolyte and fluid loss.

PSYCHOSOCIAL. Patients with peritonitis have often been coping with a serious illness or traumatic injury to the abdomen and may already be weary of discomfort and pain. Besides dealing with intensified pain and new complications, the patient with peritonitis is also at risk for life-threatening complications such as shock, renal problems, and respiratory problems. Assess the patient's and family's anxiety and feelings of powerlessness about the illness and potential complications.

DIAGNOSTIC HIGHLIGHTS

Test	Normal Result	Abnormality with Condition	Explanation
White blood cell (WBC) count	Adult males and females 4,500–11,000 mm^3	Elevated	Detects the presence of an infectious process
Abdominal and chest x rays	Normal structures	Dilation, edema, inflammation, fluid or free air in abdominal cavity	Inflammation leads to accumulation of fluid, perforation, or even rupture
Diagnostic peritoneal lavage	Clear return	White blood cells > 500 mm^3; red blood cells > 50,000/mL; presence of bacteria on gram stain; bile-stained fluid	Identifies presence of infection, bleeding or, in the case of bile, ruptured gall bladder or intestines

Other Tests: Serum electrolytes, blood urea nitrogen, creatinine, hemoglobin, hematocrit, blood cultures and sensitivities

PRIMARY NURSING DIAGNOSIS

Pain (acute) related to inflammation of the peritoneal cavity

OUTCOMES. Comfort level; Pain control behavior; Pain level; Symptom severity

INTERVENTIONS. Analgesic administration; Anxiety reduction; Environmental management: Comfort; Pain management; Medication management; Patient-controlled analgesia assistance

☐ PLANNING AND IMPLEMENTATION

Collaborative

Interventions are supportive and include fluid and electrolyte replacement. To rest the GI tract, a nasogastric (NG) or intestinal tube is inserted to reduce pressure within the bowel. Food and fluids are prohibited. Parenteral nutrition is often indicated for nutritional support. Monitor fluid volume by checking the patient's skin turgor, urine output, weight, vital signs, mucous membrane condition, and intake and output including NG tube drainage.

If the peritonitis has been caused by a perforation of the peritoneum, surgery is necessary as soon as the patient's condition has been stabilized to eliminate the source of the infection by removing the foreign contents from the peritoneal cavity and inserting drains. Paracentesis (abdominocentesis) to remove excess fluids may be necessary as well. After surgery, it is important to assess the patient frequently for peristaltic activity. Auscultate for bowel sounds, and check for flatus, bowel movements, and a soft abdomen. When peristalsis resumes, and the patient's temperature and pulse rate become normal, treatment generally calls for a decrease in parenteral fluids and an increase in oral fluids. If the patient has an NG tube in place, clamp it for short intervals. If the patient does not experience nausea or vomiting, begin oral fluids as ordered and tolerated.

PHARMACOLOGIC HIGHLIGHTS

Medication or Drug Class	Dosage	Description	Rationale
Antibiotics	Varies with drug	Cefoxitin with an aminoglycoside or penicillin G; clindamycin with an aminoglycoside	Halt the growth of bacteria and cause bacterial lysis
Analgesics	Varies with drug	Meperidine (Demerol), morphine, fentanyl	Relieve pain; until a firm diagnosis is made, analgesia may be withheld to prevent its masking significant changes in the patient's condition

Independent

Nursing care focuses on providing a stable, comfortable environment for the patient, who is experiencing both physical and psychological stress. To provide relief from pain, maintain bed rest and place the patient in the semi-Fowler position, which helps the patient breathe more deeply. Offer regular oral hygiene and lubrications to counteract mouth and nose dryness that are caused by fever, dehydration, and NG intubation. Provide psychological support by encouraging questions and verbalization of the patient's anxieties and concerns. Teach the patient about peritonitis and what caused it in his or her case, explaining the necessary treatment.

For patients who are undergoing surgery, provide teaching before surgery. Answer questions about the surgical procedure and the potential complications. Review postoperative care procedures. Teach the patient deep-breathing and coughing exercises. Explain the duration of the patient's hospital stay after surgery, which varies, depending on the underlying cause. Postoperatively, because even slight movements intensify the patient's pain, move the patient carefully. Keep the bed's siderails up and implement other safety measures, particularly if fever and pain disorient the patient. Teach the patient how to care for the incision; describe signs of infection. If convalescent services are required after discharge, refer the patient to the hospital's social service department or to a home healthcare agency.

DOCUMENTATION GUIDELINES

- Physical response: Vital signs; signs of pain, guarding, abdominal rigidity; bowel sounds

- Response to medications, including antibiotics and analgesics, blood values (WBC count, electrolytes)
- Presence of complications: Respiratory distress, shock, inadequate renal output, unrelieved discomfort
- Appearance of dressing or wound: Bleeding, drainage, appearance of incision
- Level of activity: Activity tolerance, ability to ambulate

DISCHARGE AND HOME HEALTHCARE GUIDELINES

Be sure the patient understands all medications, including the dosage, route, action, and adverse effects. If the patient is to be discharged while he or she is still on antibiotics, emphasize the need to complete the medication regimen. Teach the patient the signs of resistance (new onset of fever and abdominal pain) and superinfection (oral candida infection, yeast infection in the moist areas of the skin).

Teach the patient to report any nausea; vomiting; abdominal pain; abdominal distension, bloating, or swelling; or bleeding, odor, redness, drainage, or warmth from a surgical incision. Advise the patient to seek emergency treatment for respiratory problems such as dyspnea. Teach the patient to avoid heavy lifting for 6 weeks. Review dietary and activity limitations.

Pernicious Anemia

DRG Category: 395
Mean LOS: 4.3 days
Description: MEDICAL: Red Blood Cell Disorders, Age > 17

Anemia is a condition of reduced hemoglobin levels; pernicious anemia (also known as Addison's anemia) is caused by a deficiency of or inability to use vitamin B_{12}. Normally, vitamin B_{12} combines with the intrinsic factor, a substance that is secreted by the gastric mucosa, and then follows a path to the distal ileum, where it is absorbed and transported to body tissues. In pernicious anemia, intrinsic factor deficiency impairs vitamin B_{12} absorption. The deficiency of vitamin B_{12} inhibits the growth of red blood cells (RBCs) and leads to the production of insufficient and deformed RBCs with poor oxygen-carrying capacity. Because these deformed RBCs are known as megaloblasts (primitive, large, macrocytic cells), pernicious anemia is characterized as one of the megaloblastic anemias. Pernicious anemia is also caused by a deficiency of gastric hydrochloric acid (hypochlorhydria).

Complications caused by pernicious anemia include macrocytic anemia and gastrointestinal disorders. Pernicious anemia impairs myelin formation and thus alters the structure and disrupts the function of the peripheral nerves, spinal cord, and brain. Patients have a high incidence of benign gastric polyps, peptic ulcers, and gastric carcinoma. Low hemoglobin levels and consequent hypoxemia of long duration can result in congestive heart failure and angina pectoris in the elderly. If it is left untreated, pernicious anemia can cause psychotic behavior or even death.

CAUSES

Two causes lead to deficiency of vitamin B_{12}: inadequate intake or poor absorption. Inadequate intake may result from dietary deficiencies. Failure to absorb occurs from a deficiency in intrinsic factor. Pernicious anemia is significantly more common in patients with autoimmune-related disorders, such as thyroiditis, myxedema, and Graves' disease, which, in theory at least, decrease the hydrochloric acid production that is essential for intrinsic factor formation. Gastric resection can also result in the absence of intrinsic factor.

GENDER AND LIFE SPAN CONSIDERATIONS

Pernicious anemia is the most prevalent form of vitamin B_{12} deficiency in the United States and is most common in the Great Lakes region and New England. Still, pernicious anemia occurs only in 0.1% of the population. This disorder most commonly affects people older than age 50 years, and the incidence rises as the age increases. Juvenile pernicious anemia, however, has been found in children younger than 10 years of age; generally it is caused by a congenital stomach disorder that secretes abnormal intrinsic factor.

◻ ASSESSMENT

HISTORY. Because large stores of vitamin B_{12} are present in the body, signs and symptoms of pernicious anemia may not appear for some time. Ask the patient if he or she has experienced repeated infections. Elicit a history of severe fatigue, weakness, anorexia, nausea, vomiting, flatulence, diarrhea, or constipation. Ask the patient if he or she has experienced a sore tongue or heart palpitations or recent difficulties in breathing after exertion.

Central nervous system findings are a hallmark of this anemia. Establish a history of sensory organ disturbance; ask the patient if he or she has experienced blurred or altered vision, altered taste, or altered hearing. Ask the patient if he or she has experienced numbness, tingling, lack of coordination, or lack of position sense. Ask male patients about recent experiences with impotence. Elicit any history of lightheadedness, memory lapses, faulty judgment, irritability, or paranoia.

Elicit a complete history of medical conditions, especially autoimmune-related disorders, such as thyroiditis, myxedema, and Graves' disease. Ask the patient if he or she has undergone a gastric resection or if any members of his or her family have had pernicious anemia.

PHYSICAL EXAMINATION. The patient may appear listless. Note any premature graying or whitening of the hair. The patient may have waxy, pale to light lemon yellow skin and jaundiced sclera. Inspect the patient's mouth and check for pale lips and gums and a beefy, red, smooth tongue as a result of papillary atrophy. Note any incidence of leg edema. Weight loss may be apparent.

Percussion or palpation of the abdomen may reveal an enlarged spleen and liver. You may note tachycardia and a rapid pulse rate. Auscultation of the heart may reveal a systolic murmur. Spinal degeneration may occur, and positive Romberg's and Babinski's signs may be a clinical finding.

PSYCHOSOCIAL. Pernicious anemia produces a variety of distressing signs and symptoms, such as changes in the function of the sensory organs, dietary habits, excretory function, and sexual performance. Appearance changes may disturb the patient as well. Neurological complications may cause paranoia, disorientation, or delirium.

DIAGNOSTIC HIGHLIGHTS

Test	Normal Result	Abnormality with Condition	Explanation
Red blood cell (RBC) count	Red blood cells (4.0–5.5 million/μL	Macrocytic anemia; decreased RBC < 4.0 million/μL	Development of abnormally large red blood cells because of vitamin deficiency
Vitamin B_{12} level	200–1100 pg/mL	Decreased	Deficit in absorption or intake
Schilling test	> 10% absorption of administered dose of B_{12}	< 10% of absorption of administered dose of B_{12}	Pernicious anemia leads to decreased absorption or intake
Serum antibodies to intrinsic factor	Negative	Positive	Type I antibodies occur in 70% of patients with pernicious anemia; Type II antibodies occur in 40% of patients with pernicious antibodies

Other Tests: Complete blood count, bilirubin, lactic dehydrogenase

PRIMARY NURSING DIAGNOSIS

Altered nutrition: Less than body requirements related to anorexia, diarrhea, or achlorhydria

OUTCOMES. Nutritional status: Food and fluid intake; Nutrient intake; Biochemical measures; Body mass; Energy; Endurance,

INTERVENTIONS. Nutrition management; Nutrition therapy; Nutritional counseling and monitoring; Fluid/electrolyte management; Medication management

□ PLANNING AND IMPLEMENTATION

Collaborative

Primary intervention focuses on locating and correcting the contributing causes. Medical therapy centers around vitamin B_{12} replacement. Oral vitamin B_{12} is indicated for rare dietary deficiencies when intrinsic factor is intact. More often, vitamin B_{12} is given parenterally, but because of the risk of allergic reactions, it should be started slowly. A generally well-balanced diet with emphasis on vitamin B_{12}–rich foods, such as animal protein, eggs, and dairy products, is important. Soybean milk may be offered as a source of vitamin B_{12} for strict vegetarians. A low-sodium diet may be imposed.

Begin bed rest to combat fatigue. To reduce the cardiac workload, elevate the head of the bed and administer oxygen as ordered. Oral care may include antifungal preparations and special mouth rinses with hydrogen peroxide and salt water and topical anesthetics, such as magnesium hydroxide and viscous lidocaine, for mouth pain. Ensure that meals do not irritate the patient's mouth by being too hot or cold or too difficult to chew.

PHARMACOLOGIC HIGHLIGHTS

Medication or Drug Class	Dosage	Description	Rationale
Vitamin B$_{12}$ (cyanocobalamin)	Oral 1–25 μg per day; subcutaneous or intramuscular 100 μg per day for 7 days	Vitamin	Replaces vitamin

Other Drugs: Anti-dysrhythmics, cardiotonics, diuretics, or vasodilators may be prescribed. Stool softeners are sometimes ordered to reduce straining during bowel movements. Antibiotics may be prescribed to combat accompanying infections. For critically ill patients with cardiopulmonary distress, blood transfusions and digitalis may be ordered.

Higher doses are administered until RBC regeneration occurs, after which monthly injections are given for life. Iron replacement may be given initially to combat lowered hemoglobin levels.

Independent

Plan undisturbed rest periods to help the patient conserve energy. Provide a safe environment to prevent injury that is caused by neurologic effects. Provide assistance for walking and activities of daily living if necessary. Provide a safe environment because fine motor skills are diminished and paresthesias and balance difficulties occur. Allow time each day to sit with the patient to talk about the response to the illness and to answer questions.

If the patient's mouth and tongue discomfort make speech difficult, provide an alternate means of communication, such as a pad and pencil. Encourage fluid intake. Monitor dietary patterns carefully to determine if the patient is eating easily and tolerating meals.

Patient teaching and discharge planning are priorities. Teach the patient about the disease process of pernicious anemia and its chronic nature. Explore acceptable alternatives to activities of daily living that make living with pernicious anemia easier. Teach the patient to pace all activities and take rest periods. Encourage the patient to avoid extremes in temperature. Recommend that if the patient has developed problems with fine motor control, he or she may have an easier time dressing if clothing is designed without small buttons or hooks. Teach the patient and family to recognize and report immediately any signs of infection or complications (difficulty breathing, chest pain, dizziness, tingling in the extremities). Social service and home care referrals may be needed for follow-up.

DOCUMENTATION GUIDELINES

- Physical findings: Red, swollen tongue; pale yellow lips and gums; skin tone
- Laboratory results: Decreased RBCs, WBCs, platelets, vitamin B$_{12}$
- Presence of complications: Neurologic deficits, congestive heart failure
- Disturbed sensorium: Delirium, irritation, disorientation, paranoia
- Response to vitamin B$_{12}$ therapy

DISCHARGE AND HOME HEALTHCARE GUIDELINES

Teach the patient the relationship between vitamin B_{12} injections and the resolution of signs and symptoms of pernicious anemia. Instruct the patient how to self-administer a B_{12} injection, and establish a calendar for regular monthly injections. Discuss the need for a well-balanced diet.

Teach the route, dosage, side effects, and indications for use of medications. Instruct the patient to report any recurrent episodes of signs and symptoms of pernicious anemia. Patients with pernicious anemia are at risk for developing gastric carcinoma, so encourage twice-a-year complete physical examinations.

If the patient has experienced permanent neurologic disabilities, refer him or her to a physical therapist for an intensive program of rehabilitation.

Pheochromocytoma

DRG Category: 300
Mean LOS: 6.3 days
Description: MEDICAL: Endocrine Disorders with CC

Pheochromocytoma is a rare tumor, most often located in the adrenal gland, that arises from catecholamine-producing chromaffin cells. Although pheochromocytoma occurs in only 0.1% to 0.3% of all hypertensive patients, hypertension may be fatal if the pheochromocytoma goes unrecognized. These tumors secrete large quantities of epinephrine and norepinephrine, resulting in persistent or paroxysmal hypertension. Pheochromocytomas are vascular tumors that contain hemorrhagic or cystic areas and are most often well encapsulated, with 90% of the tumors being benign. The tumors are generally less than 6 cm in diameter and usually weigh less than 100 g.

Some 80% of these tumors arise from the adrenal medulla and are unilateral. These tumors follow the rule of 10s: 10% occur in children, 10% are bilateral or multiple, 10% are familial, 10% are malignant, 10% recur after surgical removal, and 10% are extra-adrenal. The 10% located in extra-adrenal sites are known as paragangliomas. Complications include cerebrovascular accident, retinopathy, heart disease, metastatic cancer, and renal failure. Patients with pheochromocytoma are also at higher risk for complications during operative procedures, pregnancy, and diagnostic testing.

CAUSES

Most patients develop a pheochromocytoma from unknown causes. Approximately 10% to 20% of pheochromocytomas may be associated with an inherited autosomal dominant trait, which resulted in two familial multiple endocrine neoplasia (MEN) syndromes. Type IIa MEN combines pheochromocytoma with hyperparathyroidism and medullary carcinoma of the thyroid. Type IIb MEN combines pheochromocytoma and medullary carcinoma of the thyroid with multiple neuromas, Marfan's syndrome, hypertrophic corneal nerves, and ganglioneuromas.

GENDER AND LIFE SPAN CONSIDERATIONS

Pheochromocytoma occurs equally in men and women, has no racial predominance, and most commonly occurs between the ages of the early 20s and the late 50s. In children, the tumors are more likely to occur bilaterally and in an extraadrenal location than in adults. Pheochromocytoma can occur during pregnancy, most often during the third trimester, and can cause the death of the mother and the fetus.

☐ ASSESSMENT

HISTORY. Although some patients with pheochromocytoma are asymptomatic, about 50% have a history of experiencing "spells" that are characterized by the 5 Ps: sudden increase in blood pressure, palpitations, pallor, profuse perspiration, and pain (chest pain, headache, and abdominal pain). The spells may last 1 minute to several hours and may occur from several times a day to once every several months. The attacks may also be precipitated by heavy lifting, exercise, or distension of the urinary bladder. Medications, such as opiates, histamine, and corticotropin, can also lead to attacks; therefore, take a complete medication history. Ask if the patient has experienced weight loss or constipation because of excessive catecholamine secretion.

A patient's history may include failure to respond to a multiple antihypertensive drug regimen, unusual fluctuations of blood pressure, cardiac dysrhythmias that are resistant to treatment, signs of cardiomyopathy, and a family history of pheochromocytoma or MEN. Hypertension (diastolic pressure higher than 115 mm Hg), which is the single most characteristic clinical sign, is sustained in 50% of the patients and is paroxysmal in the other 50%.

PHYSICAL EXAMINATION. Perform an ophthalmic examination to assess for retinal changes. Note if the patient has a tremor or if the skin feels unusually warm and appears flushed. Auscultate the patient's blood pressure to determine any orthostatic changes (two-thirds of patients with pheochromocytoma experience significant decreases in blood pressure when they stand up). Inspect the patient's urine for hematuria, which is associated with pheochromocytoma of the urinary bladder.

Throughout the time the patient is under your care, monitor serial blood pressures to determine if high or low levels occur. Monitor the heart rate and rhythm, assessing for sinus tachycardia and other cardiac dysrhythmias. Avoid palpation over the bladder or deep palpation of the kidneys and the adrenal gland, which can lead to a severe hypertensive attack.

PSYCHOSOCIAL. If the tumor is resectable, determine the patient's degree of anxiety about the illness, surgery, and recovery. If the tumor if malignant, assess the patient's ability to cope with lifestyle changes, possibly including early retirement. Assess the patient for extreme anxiety, emotional lability, personality changes, and psychosis.

DIAGNOSTIC HIGHLIGHTS

Test	Normal Result	Abnormality with Condition	Explanation
Free urine catecholamines,	Epinephrine 0–15 μg; norepinephrine	Elevated	Elevated amount of catecholamines are

vanillylmandelic acid (VMA) and metanephrines (24 hour)	0–100 μg; VMA less than 7 μg/mg; metanephrines < 1 mg per day		excreted in the urine
Plasma catecholamine levels	Epinephrine 0–110 pg/mL; norepinephrine 70–750 pg/mL	Slight increase	Tumor releases epinephrine and norepinephrine
Computed tomography (CT) scan	Normal adrenal structure	Location and size of tumor and metastases	Identifies tumor

Other Tests: Serum calcitonin, ultrasound, magnetic resonance imaging

PRIMARY NURSING DIAGNOSIS

Altered tissue perfusion (cerebral) related to impaired cerebral blood flow

OUTCOMES. Circulation status; Cognitive ability; Neurological status; Tissue perfusion: Peripheral

INTERVENTIONS. Cerebral perfusion promotion; Circulatory care; Circulatory precautions; Neurological monitoring; Resuscitation; Vital signs monitoring; Hemodynamic regulation

◻ PLANNING AND IMPLEMENTATION

Collaborative

More than 90% of pheochromocytomas can be cured by surgical removal. Patients who do not have operative tumors are treated pharmacologically. Preoperative treatment goals are to lower blood pressure, increase intravascular volume, and prevent paroxysmal hypertension. Before surgery, the patient's blood pressure needs to be controlled pharmacologically. To prevent intraoperative and postoperative hypotension, the patient may require IV plasma volume expanders or blood transfusions. In addition, a high-salt diet is recommended to help expand blood volume.

Postoperatively the patient is usually admitted to an intensive care unit for continuous cardiac and respiratory monitoring. Because of the rapid decrease in circulating catecholamines, hypovolemic shock and hypotension are critical concerns; however, most patients have persistent hypertension in the immediate postoperative period. Often the patient requires continuous pulmonary and systemic arterial monitoring to determine the hemodynamic response to tumor removal. Hypoglycemia can occur after the tumor is removed because of excessive insulin secretion; close monitoring of blood glucose and sustained infusion of glucose-containing fluids are necessary for several days after surgery. If a bilateral adrenalectomy is performed, iatrogenic adrenocortical insufficiency results, necessitating adrenocortical hormone replacement for life. In this instance, glucocorticoids are administered during and after surgery.

Monitor the blood pressure continuously after surgery, and expect it to be labile. The patient may need IV anti-hypertensives but may also be sensitive to IV analgesics, which may cause hypotension. Observe the patient for complications such as paralytic ileus (absent bowel sounds, abdominal distension), hemorrhage (delayed capillary blanching, piloerection [gooseflesh], diminished urinary output, increased heart rate), infection (wound drainage, poor wound healing, fever), and low glucose (dizziness, irritability, tachycardia, palpitations).

PHARMACOLOGIC HIGHLIGHTS

Medication or Drug Class	Dosage	Description	Rationale
Phentolamine	2.5–5 mg IV 1–2 hours before surgery	Alpha-adrenergic blocking agent	Blocks catecholamine synthesis during a hypertensive crisis
Phenoxybenzamine	10 mg po bid	Alpha-adrenergic blocking agent	Controls blood pressure for a period of 1 day to 2 weeks preoperatively
Beta-adrenergic blockers	Varies with drug	Propranolol or atenolol	Manage hypertension for patients with a heart rate > 110, history of dysrhythmias, or epinephrine-secreting tumor; instituted several days after the alpha-adrenergic blockade

Other Drugs: Patients for whom surgery is not an option can be managed with metyrosine, which controls hypertensive episodes by decreasing catecholamine synthesis. If malignancy occurs, the patient can be treated with radiation therapy followed by chemotherapy, consisting of cyclophosphamide (Cytoxan), vincristine, and decarbazine.

Independent

Before the surgical procedure, document the number and type of attacks the patient experiences. Ask the patient to immediately report signs such as headache, palpitations, and nervousness. Remain with the patient during the acute attack and monitor serial vital signs. Maintain a quiet environment to limit the development of stressful episodes, which could precipitate a spell. If the patient experiences signs and symptoms, document the duration, type of symptoms, and precipitating factors. Promote rest, and encourage the patient to avoid stressors; explore relaxation techniques such as breathing exercises, music therapy, and guided imagery.

If the patient is facing surgery, encourage the patient to verbalize his or her feelings and concerns about the surgery. Explain the procedure, what the patient can expect preoperatively and postoperatively, and how long the patient should anticipate being in an intensive care unit. Explore how the patient may feel postoperatively, and remind the patient that pain medication is available to manage postoperative discomfort.

Expect the postoperative patient to have a labile blood pressure for the first 48 hours. Maintain a quiet environment because increased noise and stress may precipitate a hypertensive episode. Postoperative diaphoresis and intolerance to heat often occur; if possible, lower the room temperature to fit the patient's comfort level, and assist the patient with dry linens at least every 8 hours. Before the patient's discharge, make sure the patient and significant others understand all medications and postoperative home care.

DOCUMENTATION GUIDELINES

- Physical findings related to pheochromocytoma: Blood pressure and heart rate; presence of flushing or pallor; nausea and vomiting; palpitations; pain (headache, chest pain, abdominal pain); profuse perspiration, orthostatic hypotension, and significant changes in blood pressure; hypoglycemic reactions; fever; extreme anxiety; changes in mental capacity
- Response to alpha-adrenergic and beta-adrenergic drug therapy, fluid replacement, and pain medications
- Response to the removal of the tumor: Severe hypotension, signs and symptoms of adrenal insufficiency, hypoglycemia, absence of symptoms
- Presence of complications: Hemorrhage, hypovolemia, shock, profound hypotension, adrenal insufficiency, infection

DISCHARGE AND HOME HEALTHCARE GUIDELINES

Teach the patient the importance of compliance with re-evaluation studies of catecholamine and metanephrine levels. Teach the patient that pheochromocytoma can recur and that pheochromocytoma left undetected can cause encephalopathy, high-grade fever, multisystem failure, and death. Teach patients to monitor their blood pressure at home, to report subnormal measurements or diastolic pressures over 115 mm Hg, and to notify the physician immediately for other symptoms of an attack. Be sure the patient understands all medications, including the dosage, route, action, and adverse effects.

Pituitary Tumor

DRG Category: 300
Mean LOS: 6.3 days
Description: MEDICAL: Endocrine Disorders with CC
DRG Category: 286
Mean LOS: 7.6 days
Description: SURGICAL: Adrenal and Pituitary Procedures

Pituitary tumors, which are generally anterior lobe adenomas, make up from 10% to 15% of all intracranial neoplasms. Approximately 15% of all intracranial tumors are pituitary tumors that cause symptoms. About 2,000 new pituitary tumors are diagnosed each year in the United States, but very few are fatal.

Pituitary adenomas are divided into two categories by their size. Microadenomas are smaller than 1 centimeter, and macroadenomas are larger than 1 centimeter. While microademonas may cause complications because of overproduced pituitary hormones, they generally do not damage surrounding tissue. Because of their size, macroadenomas can be locally invasive, often damaging normal pituitary tissue and nearby nerves and parts of the brain. Most pituitary tumors are nonmalignant, but because of their invasiveness they are considered neoplastic conditions.

Some 75% of pituitary adenomas are functional (hormone-producing) tumors. Pituitary adenomas are currently classified by the type of pituitary hormone they contain rather than the older terminology (basophilic, eosinophilic, and chromophobic), which was not as useful. Because the hormone produced by an adenoma strongly influences its signs and symptoms, and thus the choice of diagnostic tests and treatment, the new classification system has been developed. Detection of hormone production is based on blood tests or tests of the surgically removed tumor. Based on these results, adenomas are classified as prolactinomas, or prolactin-producing adenomas (30% of pituitary tumors); somatotrophin-secreting adenomas (15%–20%); corticoptrophin, or ACTH-secreting adenomas (10%–15%); gonadotrophin-secreting adenomas (very small percentage); thyrotropin-secreting adenomas (very small percentage); null cell adenomas (15%–20%); and plurihormal (mixed-cell) adenomas. The outlook for survival also varies, depending on what kind of adenoma exists.

Craniopharyngiomas, although they are not actually pituitary tumors in the true sense, sometimes develop next to the pituitary or in other areas within the skull. These tumors do not make pituitary hormones but can disrupt normal hormone production by compressing the pituitary gland or the stalk that connects the pituitary gland to the hypothalamus. Like adenomas, craniopharyngiomas are benign. However, they cause visual and other neurological problems because they can invade the hypothalamus and other parts of the brain. Craniopharyngiomas account for less than 3% of all intracranial tumors, but more than 10% of intracranial tumors in children. Teratomas, germinomas, and choriocarcinomas are all uncommon tumors that occur most often in children or young adults. Rathke's cleft cysts and gangliocytomas to the pituitary are uncommon tumors that are usually found in adults.

Pituitary tumors lead to hormone excess, hormone deficiencies, or any combination of imbalances. In addition, as the tumor grows, it replaces normal pituitary gland tissue. The concave bony portion of the skull where the pituitary gland resides (sella turcica) enlarges, and the tumor may displace other brain tissue as well. Complications from pituitary tumors include loss of hormonal function in all systems of the body and compression of central nervous system structures such as the hypothalamus. Complications of surgery include hemorrhage, infection, cerebrospinal fluid (CSF) leak, and diabetes insipidus.

CAUSES

Although the cause of pituitary tumors is unknown, the patient's heredity may predispose him or her to a tumor.

GENDER AND LIFE SPAN CONSIDERATIONS

Approximately 70% of pituitary tumors occur in people between 30 and 50 years of age. Only 3% to 7% occur in people younger than 20 years. The female-to-male ratio is 2:1.

□ ASSESSMENT

HISTORY. Ask the patient to describe any endocrine or neurologic symptoms. Usually patients give a history of slowly developing, progressive symptoms.

They frequently complain of headaches, visual disturbances (blurred vision or double vision progressing to blindness), decreased sexual interest, menstrual irregularities, and impotence. Family members may report central nervous system (CNS) changes, such as anxiety, personality changes, seizure activity, and even dementia. Depending on tumor type, patients may describe weakness, fatigue, sensitivity to cold, and constipation.

PHYSICAL EXAMINATION. You may note that the skin has a waxy appearance; fewer than normal wrinkles for the patient's age; and a decreased amount of body, pubic, and axillary hair. Assess the patient's skin for hyperpigmentation, oiliness, acne, and diaphoresis. Assessment of visual function is important because pituitary tumors may press on the optic chiasm. Assess the patient's visual fields, visual acuity, extraocular movements, and pupillary reactions. A classic finding is bitemporal hemianopsia (blindness in the temporal field of vision). Perform an assessment of the cranial nerves. The tumor may involve cranial nerves III (oculomotor, which regulates pupil reaction), IV (trochlear, which along with the abducens regulates conjugate and lateral eye movements), and VI (abducens). Examine the patient's musculoskeletal structure, determining whether foot and hand size are appropriate for body size; whether facial features are altered, such as thick ears and nose; and whether the skeletal muscles are atrophied.

PSYCHOSOCIAL. The patient may have personality changes such as irritability and even occasional hostility. Assess the patient's interpersonal relationships, the response of significant others, and the patient's and significant others' abilities to cope with a potentially serious illness. Patients may be concerned about body image, fertility, and sexual performance.

DIAGNOSTIC HIGHLIGHTS

Test	Normal Result	Abnormality with Condition	Explanation
Growth hormone	< 10 ng/mL	Elevated	Functional (hormone-producing) tumor elevates levels of various hormones
Gonadotrophins: Follicle stimulating hormone (FSH)	< 20 inter-national units/L	Elevated	Functional (hormone-producing) tumor elevates levels of various hormones
Luteinizing hormone (LH)	<10 inter-national units/L	Elevated	
Prolactin	< 25 ng/mL	Elevated	Functional (hormone-producing) tumor elevates levels of various hormones
Thyrotropin (thyroid stimulating hormone, TSH)	1.0–6.2 μU/mL	Elevated	Functional (hormone-producing) tumor elevates levels of various hormones
Adrenocorticotropin hormone (ACTH)	< 60 pg/mL	Elevated	Functional (hormone-producing) tumor elevates levels of various hormones

Magnetic resonance imaging (MRI)	No visual evidence of tumors; normal brain structure	Provides visual evidence of tumors	Standard imaging test to identify pituitary tumors; can identify macroadenomas and microadenomas larger than 3 mm; can locate small abnormalities in pituitary gland unrelated to symptoms; 5%–25% of patients have unrelated minor abnormalities of pituitary gland

Other Tests: Biopsy of pituitary tissue

PRIMARY NURSING DIAGNOSIS

Pain (acute) related to pressure from a space-occupying lesion

OUTCOMES. Comfort level; Pain control behavior; Pain: Disruptive effects; Pain level

INTERVENTIONS. Pain management; Analgesic administration; Positioning; Teaching: Prescribed activity/exercise; Teaching: Procedure/treatment; Teaching: Prescribed medication

☐ PLANNING AND IMPLEMENTATION

Collaborative

The treatment of a pituitary tumor is guided by whether it is a carcinoma or an adenoma. Treatment of adenomas is guided by whether or not the adenoma is functional, whether it is a microadenoma or a macroadenoma, and which hormone is being secreted. The main treatment for many pituitary tumors is surgery, while medications can relieve symptoms and sometimes shrink the tumor. With larger and more invasive tumors, the likelihood of cure by surgery decreases. The usual operation for pituitary tumors is a transsphenoidal hypophysectomy (removal of the pituitary gland through a surgical incision in the sphenoid bone). The surgery has a low neurologic complication rate and leaves no visible scar. Cure rates for microadenomas are greater than 80% but are lower if the tumor is large or if it has invaded nearby nerves or brain tissue.

In a newer procedure, surgeons use endoscopic surgery, operating through a fiber optic device that has been inserted through an incision in the lining of the nose. This procedure takes less time and causes fewer complications than transsphenoidal hypophysectomy. For larger or more complicated tumors, a craniotomy is required to remove the tumor, but the surgery exposes patients to a higher incidence of permanent neurologic complications than with transsphenoidal hypophysectomy. The overall surgical cure rate for patients with growth hormone–secreting adenomas is about 60%. The cure rate is slightly higher for corticotrophin-secreting adenomas, because these tend to be smaller tumors. Only complicated prolactinomas are treated surgically.

Complications of pituitary surgery can be serious but, fortunately, are extremely rare. If large arteries, nearby nerves, or nearby brain tissue is damaged, a stroke or blindness is possible. Meningitis can result from damage to the membranes that surround the brain. Much more likely is a temporary onset of diabetes insipidus, which usually resolves itself within 1 to 2 weeks after surgery. Damage to the pituitary thus leading to hypopituitarism may be unavoidable when treating some macroadenomas, but such damage can be treated by medication.

Postprocedural or postsurgical monitoring of the patient is crucial. Make sure the patient has an adequate airway and is breathing at all times. If you suspect airway compromise (changes in mental status, restlessness, confusion, shortness of breath, stridor, apnea), notify the physician immediately. Check with the surgeon to determine the preferred protocol for endotracheal suctioning. Perform serial neurological assessments to identify changes in mental status, pupil reaction, and strength and motion of the extremities. After surgery, maintain the subarachnoid drainage systems, and note the amount, color, and consistency of all drainage. Position the patient by elevating the head of the bed to 30 to 45 degrees to decrease edema and to promote CSF flow to the lumbar cistern. If the patient is not responsive, position the patient in a side-lying position to facilitate drainage from the mouth.

Explain that the patient needs to avoid leaning forward, blowing the nose, or sneezing. Do not remove the nasal packing until the surgeon requests it. Withhold oral fluid intake in the immediately postoperative period because it may stimulate the vomiting center and contribute to increased intracranial pressure. Provide analgesics to manage pain relief, and if the patient does not experience relief, notify the surgeon so that the medication type or dosage can be altered. If CSF drains from the nose, notify the surgeon immediately, and monitor the patient for signs of a CNS infection (changes in level of consciousness, irritability, fever, foul drainage) or pulmonary infection (fever, pulmonary congestion, yellow or white pulmonary secretions). Monitor the patient for diabetes insipidus owing to a lack of anti-diuretic hormone; maintain intake and output records, and notify the physician if a fluid deficit occurs.

PHARMACOLOGIC HIGHLIGHTS

Medication or Drug Class	Dosage	Description	Rationale
Prolactin-inhibitor	Varies with drug	Bromocriptine (Alphagen, Parlodel); cabergoline (Dostinex)	Shrinks prolactin-secreting tumors in 1 to 6 months; ineffective for treating acromegaly; side effects such as nausea and orthostatic hypotension may preclude use of bromocriptine in some patients

Other Drugs: Octreotide, lanreotide is used to inhibit growth hormone (somatotrophin) secretion; cyropheptadine is used to inhibit corticotrophin.

Independent

To limit the risk of injury before surgery, discuss with the patient the best mechanisms to provide a safe environment if his or her vision is impaired. Provide an uncluttered room with a clear pathway to the bathroom. Encourage the patient to wear well-fitting shoes or slippers when ambulating. Keep the call light within reach of the patient at all times.

Postoperatively, elevate the patient's head to facilitate breathing and fluid drainage. Do not encourage the patient to cough, as this interferes with the healing of the operative site. Provide frequent mouth care and keep the skin dry. To promote maximum joint mobility, perform or assist with range-of-motion exercises. Encourage the patient to ambulate within 1 to 2 days of the surgery. To assure healing of the incision site, explain the need to avoid activities that increase intracranial pressure, such as tooth brushing, coughing, sneezing, nose blowing, and bending. Provide a well-organized and stress-free environment. Explain the treatment options and answer questions. Provide periods of uninterrupted rest each day, and schedule diagnostic procedures to allow the patient to recover.

Encourage the patient to use nonpharmacologic methods to control any discomfort. Both patients requiring surgery and patients being managed medically have many emotional needs. Provide privacy so that the patient is able to ask questions about his or her sexual function. Expect that patients may experience loss, grief, or anger if they are dealing with sexual dysfunction such as impotence or infertility. The patient may require support and assistance to develop coping strategies.

DOCUMENTATION GUIDELINES

- Physical findings of hormone excesses or deficiencies: Decreased body hair, hirsutism, altered secondary sexual characteristics, acromegaly, galactorrhea; vital signs; neurologic assessment; visual examination
- Response to therapy: Surgery, radiation, medications, counseling
- Postoperative management: CSF drainage, nasal packing, wound drainage, signs of complications (diabetes insipidus, infection, increased intracranial pressure, hemorrhage, CSF leak, airway compromise)

DISCHARGE AND HOME HEALTHCARE GUIDELINES

Be sure the patient understands all medications, including dosage, route, action, and adverse effects. Explain the symptoms of a CSF leak to the patient. Instruct the patient to notify the physician of fluid drainage from the nares or down the back of the throat, increased temperature, unrelieved headaches, photophobia, nausea and vomiting, or a "stiff neck." Explain the risk for massive fluid loss through urination (diabetes insipidus) and the need to replace this fluid volume. Instruct the patient on a diet that replaces fluid and electrolytes. Instruct the patient to notify the physician of any excess urination.

Placenta Previa

DRG Category: 372
Mean LOS: 2.7 days
Description: MEDICAL: Vaginal Delivery with Complicating Diagnoses
DRG Category: 370
Mean LOS: 4.9 days
Description: SURGICAL: Cesarean Section with CC

Normally the placenta implants in the body (upper portion) of the uterus. Implantation allows for delivery of the infant before the delivery of the placenta. With placenta previa, the placenta is implanted in the lower uterine segment over or near the internal os of the cervix. As the uterus contracts and the cervix begins to efface and dilate, the villi of the placenta begin to tear away from the uterine wall and bright red, painless, vaginal bleeding occurs. Bleeding can occur antepartally or intrapartally. Placenta previa is classified in four ways, depending on the degree of placental encroachment on the cervical os. (See Box 10.) Depending on the amount of blood loss and gestational age of the fetus, placenta previa may be life-threatening to both the mother and the fetus.

BOX 10   CLASSIFICATION OF PLACENTA PREVIA

Low-Lying
The placenta implants in the lower uterine segment but does not reach the cervical os; often this type of placenta previa moves upward as the pregnancy progresses, eliminating bleeding complications later.

Marginal
The edge of the placenta is at the edge of the internal os; the mother may be able to deliver vaginally.

Partial
The placenta partially covers the cervical os; as the pregnancy progresses and the cervix begins to efface and dilate, the bleeding occurs.

Total
The placenta covers the entire cervical os; usually requires an emergency cesarean section.

CAUSES

The cause of placenta previa is unknown, but it is more common in women who have a history of uterine surgeries (cesarean sections, dilation and curettage), infections with endometritis, and a previous placenta previa. It is also more common in those women who currently have a multiple gestation with a large placenta. Smoking and cocaine usage may also be contributing factors.

GENDER AND LIFE SPAN CONSIDERATIONS

Placenta previa is more common in women of advanced maternal age (over 35) and in patients with multiparity. Overall incidence is 1 in 200 term deliveries; risk for recurrence may be as high as 10% to 15%.

◻ ASSESSMENT

HISTORY. Although many women who develop placenta previa have an unremarkable obstetric or gynecologic history, some have had previous uterine surgeries or infections. The prenatal course of the current pregnancy is often uneventful until the patient experiences a bout of bright red bleeding. Question the patient as to the onset and amount of bleeding first noticed. The initial bleeding in placenta previa is often scant because few uterine sinuses are exposed.

PHYSICAL EXAMINATION. The classic sign of placenta previa is painless, bright red bleeding; assess the amount and character of blood loss. Most often this bleeding occurs between 28 and 34 weeks when the lower uterine segment thins and the low implantation site is disrupted. With a marginal or low-lying placenta previa, the bleeding may not start until the patient is in labor. Assess the uterus for contractions; unless the patient is in labor, the uterus is relaxed and nontender. A vaginal examination should not be performed because it increases maternal bleeding and can dislodge more of the placenta.

Check the vital signs; note any symptoms of hypovolemic shock (restlessness, agitation, increased pulse, delayed capillary blanching, increased respirations, pallor, cool clammy skin, hypotension, and oliguria). Monitor the baseline fetal heart rate and the presence or absence of accelerations, decelerations, and variability in the electronic fetal monitoring (EFM).

Ask the patient if she feels the fetus move. Assess the fetal position and presentation by using Leopold's maneuvers. Monitor the patient's contraction status, and palpate the fundus to determine the intensity of contractions. View the fetal monitor strip to assess the frequency and duration of the contractions; more often the uterus is soft and nontender, unless the patient is in labor. Throughout the patient's hospitalization, continue to monitor for signs of hypovolemic shock and the amount and character of bleeding. Maintain continuous EFM until bleeding ceases; then, if hospital policy permits, monitor the fetus for 30 minutes every 4 hours.

PSYCHOSOCIAL. The heavy, bright red bleeding that often accompanies placenta previa is anxiety producing for the mother and significant others. The patient is concerned not only for herself but also for the well-being of the infant. Determine the patient's support system because many of these patients have been on complete bed rest for an extended period of time. Assess the effect of prolonged bed rest on the patient's job, child-care, interpersonal, financial, and social responsibilities.

DIAGNOSTIC HIGHLIGHTS

General Comments: Vaginal exams are contraindicated for a pregnant patient who is bleeding until a previa is ruled out by ultrasound visualization.

Test	Normal Result	Abnormality with Condition	Explanation
Ultrasound	Placental	Placental implantation	Visualization of placenta

(transabdominal, translabial)	implantation visualized in fundus of uterus	visualized in lower uterine segment	determines location and can rule out other causes of bleeding (abruption, cervical lesion, excessive show, etc.)
RBC	4–5.4 ml/mm³	These three values will decrease several hours after significant blood loss has occurred	With active bleeding, RBCs are lost
HGB	12–16 g/dL		
HCT	37%–47%		

Other Tests: Blood type and crossmatch

PRIMARY NURSING DIAGNOSIS

Fluid volume deficit related to blood loss

OUTCOMES. Fluid balance; Hydration; Circulation status

INTERVENTIONS. Bleeding reduction; Blood product administration; Intravenous therapy; Shock management

◻ PLANNING AND IMPLEMENTATION

Collaborative

Management of a patient with placenta previa depends on the admission status of the mother and the fetus, the amount of blood loss, the likelihood that the bleeding will subside on its own, and the gestational age of the fetus. If both the mother and the fetus are stable and the fetus is immature (less than 37 weeks), delivery may be put off and an intravenous (IV) infusion started with lactated Ringer's solution. In addition, the patient is maintained on bed rest with continuous EFM. Closely monitor the fetal heart rate. If any signs of fetal distress are noted (flat variability, late decelerations, bradycardia, tachycardia), turn the patient to her left side, increase the rate of IV infusion, administer oxygen via face mask at 10 L per minute, and notify the physician. Once the bleeding has ceased for 24 to 48 hours, the patient may be discharged to her home on bed rest before delivery. This conservative treatment gives the preterm fetus time to mature. If the patient is in labor and a marginal placenta previa is present, the physician allows her to labor and deliver vaginally, with careful surveillance of maternal and fetal status throughout the labor.

If fetal distress is present or if the patient has lost a significant amount of blood, an immediate cesarean section and, possibly, blood transfusions are indicated. If the patient delivers (vaginally or by cesarean), monitor her for postpartum hemorrhage because contraction of the lower uterine segment is sometimes not effective in compressing the uterine vessels that are exposed at the placental site. Although medication is not given to treat a previa, pharmacologic treatment may be indicated to stop preterm labor (if it is occurring and if bleeding is under control), enhance fetal lung maturity if delivery is expected prematurely, or prevent Rh disease, if the patient delivers.

PHARMACOLGIC HIGHLIGHTS

Medication or Drug Class	Dosage	Description	Rationale
Magnesium sulfate	4–6 g IV loading dose, 1–4 g per hour of IV maintenance	Anti-convulsant	Effective tocolytic, has fewer side effects than beta adrenergic drugs; administered only if bleeding is under control and preterm labor is evident
Betamethasone (Celestone)	12 mg IM q 24 hr × 2 doses	Glucocorticoid	Hastens fetal lung maturity; given if delivery is anticipated between 24 and 34 weeks
RhD immunoglobin (RhoGAM)	120 μg (prepared by blood bank)	Immune serum	Prevents Rh isoimmunizations in future pregnancies; given if mother is Rh negative and infant is Rh positive

Independent

If the patient is actively bleeding, and mother and fetus are stable, maintain the patient on bed rest in the lateral position (preferably left lateral) to maximize venous return and placental perfusion. Because the patient may be on bed rest for an extended period of time, comfort can be increased with back rubs and positioning with pillows. Provide diversional activities and emotional support. The nurse should make every attempt to explain the condition, treatment, and potential outcomes to the patient. Often, if a preterm delivery is unavoidable, a special care nursery nurse comes in and discusses what the mother can expect to happen to her infant on admission to the neonatal intensive care unit.

DOCUMENTATION GUIDELINES

- Amount and character of blood loss; vital signs; presence or absence of signs of hypovolemic shock; fetal heart rate baseline, variability, and presence or absence of accelerations or decelerations; intake and output
- Frequency, intensity, and duration of contractions

DISCHARGE AND HOME HEALTHCARE GUIDELINES

If the patient is discharged undelivered, provide the following instructions:
Notify the physician of any vaginal bleeding, spontaneous rupture of membranes, decreased fetal movement, or regular labor contractions.
Maintain continuous bed rest with bathroom privileges.
Avoid the supine position; use the lateral or semi-Fowler position.
Abstain from sexual intercourse.
Be sure to have the means to reach the hospital at all times.

Pneumocystis carinii Pneumonia

DRG Category: 079
Mean LOS: 8.3 days
Description: MEDICAL: Respiratory Infections and Inflammations, Age > 17 with CC
DRG Category: 489
Mean LOS: 8.3 days
Description: MEDICAL: HIV with Major Related Condition

Pneumocystis carinii pneumonia (PCP) is an acute or subacute pulmonary infection that can be fatal. It is the most common infection in people with HIV infections and is the leading cause of death in this population. PCP is viewed as an opportunistic infection because normal cell-mediated immunity protects most humans from infection. Epidemiologic surveys have found that by age 3 to 4, most humans have been exposed to the pathogen *P. carinii* but have not been seriously affected.

Early in the infection, the organisms line up along the alveolar wall near the type I pneumocytes. The alveoli become infiltrated with a fluid that contains proteins, organisms in varying states of development, cellular debris, and surfactant. As the alveoli become clogged with fluid and wastes, gas exchange is impaired. As the disease progresses, alveoli hypertrophy, type I pneumocytes die, and the patient has markedly diminished gas exchange. PCP affects both lungs and can lead to complications such as pulmonary insufficiency, respiratory failure, and even death.

CAUSES

Although the causative agent, *P. carinii*, is often classified as a protozoa, its structure and function are closer to a fungus. Human transmission occurs by the airborne route, where it multiplies aggressively in the alveoli. Incubation is estimated to be between 4 and 8 weeks. Individuals at risk for PCP are immunocompromised and have conditions such as HIV infection or are premature infants. Other vulnerable populations include patients who receive corticosteroid therapy and organ transplantation.

GENDER AND LIFE SPAN CONSIDERATIONS

Premature infants are at risk for PCP, as are children with immunodeficiency diseases. PCP is the leading cause of death in patients with acquired immunodeficiency syndrome (AIDS); AIDS has become the leading cause of death for certain age groups of young men.

☐ ASSESSMENT

HISTORY. Patients with PCP often appear acutely ill and weak. They often have pallor, weight loss, and fatigue on exertion and become short of breath even when speaking. Determine if the patient has a history of leukemia, lymphoma, organ transplantation, or HIV, all of which compromise the immune system and increase the risk of PCP. Because symptoms of PCP develop over a period of weeks (4 to 8 weeks, generally), initial symptoms may be vague.

Determine if the patient has experienced nonproductive cough or increasing shortness of breath, which are frequent initial symptoms of PCP. Ask about a recent history of anorexia, nausea, vomiting, weight loss, or a low-grade intermittent fever. Note that before PCP prophylaxis in HIV-positive patients, this disease was the first indication of HIV infection in 60% of HIV-positive patients.

PHYSICAL EXAMINATION. Assess for signs of respiratory difficulties, such as stridor, nasal flaring, and rapid breathing. If the patient has a cough, note the type. Examine the patient's skin, noting its color, turgor, temperature, and whether or not it is dry and flaky. Check for pallor, flushing, and cyanosis. Note the type, amount, and color of sputum, which is commonly blood-tinged. Observe the patient's level of consciousness and irritability. Note any muscle wasting or guarding of painful areas. Auscultate the lungs for abnormal breath sounds, crackles, or diminished or absent breath sounds, either unilaterally or bilaterally. Late in PCP, when you percuss the chest, you may hear dullness from lung consolidation.

PSYCHOSOCIAL. PCP is a serious and life-threatening infection; in addition, it may be the defining condition for diagnosis of AIDS, according to the Centers for Disease Control and Prevention. The patient may experience anxiety, depression, or difficulty in coping with the change in heath status. Identify the patient's support system, and evaluate its effectiveness. The diagnosis of AIDS presents many complex familial and societal issues.

DIAGNOSTIC HIGHLIGHTS

Test	Normal Result	Abnormality with Condition	Explanation
Bronchoscopy and bronchoalveolar lavage	Normal pulmonary structures and negative cultures	Washings positive for *Pneumocystis carinii* on immuno-fluorescent stain	Used to view the pulmonary structures and obtain bronchoalveolar washings (more sensitive than standard sputum specimens)
Serum immunofluorescent antibodies	< 1:16; no organisms observed	Presence of organisms	Used to identify antibodies that circulate in blood, formed in response to antigens in protozoan bacterial cell wall

Other Tests: Chest x ray, arterial blood gases, gallium scan, complete blood count

PRIMARY NURSING DIAGNOSIS

Risk for infection related to immunosuppression

OUTCOMES. Immune status; Respiratory status: Gas exchange; Respiratory status: Ventilation; Thermoregulation

INTERVENTIONS. Infection control; Infection protection; Respiratory monitoring; Temperature regulation

☐ PLANNING AND IMPLEMENTATION

Collaborative

Patients require pharmacologic treatment to eradicate the organism. PCP infections may be treated with incentive spirometry, percussion and postural drainage, and humidified oxygen. Some patients may require intubation and mechanical ventilation to maintain gas exchange. If the patient is not intubated and is able to take oral nutrition, a high-calorie, protein-rich diet is recommended. If the patient cannot tolerate large amounts of food, smaller, more frequent meals can be offered. IV fluids and total parenteral nutrition may be needed to maintain fluid balance if the patient cannot tolerate oral enteral feedings.

PHARMACOLOGIC HIGHLIGHTS

Medication or Drug Class	Dosage	Description	Rationale
Trimethoprim-sulfamethoxazole (Bactrim, Septra, TMP/SMX)	5 mg/kg IV every 6–8 hours	Anti-infective	Kills the organism; used for early cases and for prophylaxis
Antibiotics, anti-infectives	Varies with drug	Pentamidine isoehtionate (Nebupent) aerosol treatment; clindamycin;	Kill the organism
Prednisone	40 mg po bid for 5 days and then taper	Corticosteroid	Decreases pulmonary inflammation
Antipyretics, antitussives, analgesics	Prescribed as needed	Oral narcotics	Reduce the respiratory rate and control anxiety, thereby improving comfort and gas exchange

Other Drugs: Antipyretics, antitussives, and analgesics are prescribed as needed. Oral narcotics may be given to reduce the respiratory rate and control anxiety, thereby improving comfort and gas exchange.

Independent

Patients with PCP infection are often weak and debilitated. They may become short of breath even when speaking, and their dyspnea is severe. Discuss your concerns with the physician if the patient remains uncomfortable. Alterations in the medication regimen may be necessary. Position the patient so that he or she is comfortable and breathes with as little effort as possible. Usually if you elevate the bed and support the patient's arms on pillows, the respiration eases. A major nursing responsibility is to coordinate periods of activity and rest. Schedule diagnostic tests and patient care activities with ample rest periods between them. As the patient gains strength, encourage coughing and deep-breathing exercises, and teach him or her how to perform incentive spirometry. Evaluate the patient's gait, and, if it is steady, encourage periods of ambulation interspersed with periods of rest.

Reduce the patient's anxiety by providing a restful environment, including diversional activities. Teach the patient guided imaging or relaxation techniques for nonpharmacologic relief of discomfort. Provide time each day to allow the patient to ask questions and explore fears. Include the family and significant others in all teaching activities as appropriate.

DOCUMENTATION GUIDELINES

- Physical changes: Breath sounds, breathing patterns, sputum production
- Nutritional status: Appetite, body weight, food tolerance
- Complications, changes in oxygen exchange or airway clearance
- Response to medications
- Tolerance to activity, level of fatigue, ability to sleep at night

DISCHARGE AND HOME HEALTHCARE GUIDELINES

Advise the patient to quit smoking, rest, avoid excess alcohol intake, maintain adequate nutrition, and avoid exposure to crowds and others with upper respiratory infections. Teach the patient appropriate preventive measures, such as covering the mouth and nose while coughing when in contact with susceptible individuals. Be sure the patient understands all medications, including the dosage, route, action, and adverse effects. Teach the patient to recognize symptoms, such as dyspnea, chest pain, fatigue, weight loss, fever and chills, and productive cough, that should be reported to health-care personnel.

Pneumonia

DRG Category: 089
Mean LOS: 6.5
Description: MEDICAL: Simple Pneumonia and Pleurisy, Age > 17 with CC
DRG Category: 079
Mean LOS: 8.3 days
Description: MEDICAL: Respiratory Infections and Inflammations, Age > 17 with CC
DRG Category: 475
Mean LOS: 9.5 days
Description: MEDICAL: Respiratory System Diagnosis with Ventilator Support
DRG Category: 483
Mean LOS: 41.9 days
Description: SURGICAL: Tracheostomy Except for Face, Mouth, and Neck Diagnoses

Pneumonia is an inflammatory condition of the interstitial lung tissue in which fluid and blood cells escape into the alveoli. The disease process begins with an infection in the alveolar spaces. As the organism multiplies, the alveolar spaces fill with fluid, white blood cells, and cellular debris from phagocytosis of the infectious agent. The infection spreads from the alveolus and can involve the distal airways (bronchopneumonia), part of a lobe (lobular pneumonia), or an entire lung (lobar pneumonia).

The inflammatory process causes the lung tissue to stiffen, thus resulting in a decrease in lung compliance and an increase in the work of breathing. The fluid-filled alveoli cause a physiologic shunt, and venous blood passes unventilated portions of lung tissue and returns to the left atrium unoxygenated. As the arterial oxygen tension falls, the patient begins to exhibit the signs and symptoms of hypoxemia. In addition to hypoxemia, pneumonia can lead to respiratory failure and septic shock. Infection may spread via the bloodstream and cause endocarditis, pericarditis, meningitis, or bacteremia.

CAUSES

Primary pneumonia is caused by the patient's inhaling or aspirating a pathogen such as bacteria or a virus. Bacterial pneumonia, often caused by staphylococcus, streptococcus, or klebsiella, usually occurs when the lungs' defense mechanisms are impaired by such factors as suppressed cough reflex, decreased cilia action, decreased activity of phagocytic cells, and the accumulation of secretions. Viral pneumonia occurs when a virus attacks bronchiolar epithelial cells and causes interstitial inflammation and desquamation, which eventually spread to the alveoli.

Secondary pneumonia ensues from lung damage that was caused by the spread of bacteria from an infection elsewhere in the body or by a noxious chemical. Aspiration pneumonia is caused by the patient's inhaling foreign matter such as food or vomitus into the bronchi. Factors associated with aspiration pneumonia include old age, impaired gag reflex, surgical procedures, debilitating disease, and decreased level of consciousness.

GENDER AND LIFE SPAN CONSIDERATIONS

Children and young adults up to age 30 are at risk for several forms of viral pneumonia, including mycoplasma pneumonia, adenovirus pneumonia, rubeola pneumonia, and respiratory syncytial virus pneumonia. Adults are at risk for varicella viral pneumonia. People over 40 years of age are at greater risk to contract all forms of bacterial pneumonia, with older men more susceptible to streptococcal bacterial pneumonia and klebsiella bacterial pneumonia. Older people are also at greater risk for viral pneumonia caused by influenza. Neonates with multisystem disease are also at risk for viral pneumonia caused by cytomegalovirus. Staphylococcal pneumonia tends to strike those who are debilitated or who have a history of influenza or intravenous (IV) drug abuse.

▢ ASSESSMENT

HISTORY. The patient may have a history of a recent upper respiratory infection, influenza, or a viral syndrome. Elicit a history of a chronic pulmonary disease, such as asthma, bronchitis, or tuberculosis; prolonged immobility; sickle cell anemia; neurologic disorders that cause paralysis of the diaphragm; surgery of the thorax or abdomen; smoking; alcoholism; IV drug therapy or abuse; and malnutrition. Establish any history of exposure to noxious gases, aspiration, or immunosuppressive therapy. Ask about the major symptoms of pneumonia: cough, fever, sputum production, chest pain, and shortness of breath. Ask the patient to describe the type of cough and the nature of the sputum production. Determine the location of any pain, especially chest pain. Ask about sore throat or chills, vomiting, diarrhea, or anorexia.

PHYSICAL EXAMINATION. Observe the patient's general appearance and respiratory pattern to determine level of fatigue, presence of cyanosis, and presence of dyspnea or tachypnea. Examine the patient's extremities, torso, and face for rash. Assess vital signs for rapid, weak, thready pulse; fever; and blood pressure changes such as hypotension and orthostasis (postural hypotension). Palpate the chest to determine any areas of consolidation or tactile fremitus. Percuss the chest to detect dullness over the area of consolidation. When you auscultate the patient's breathing, listen for rales, crackles, ronchi, and wheezes; "E" to "A" changes; and whispered pectoriloquy.

PSYCHOSOCIAL. The patient with pneumonia may be anxious, fatigued, and in pain from the constant coughing. Assess the patient's ability to cope with a sudden, debilitating illness. The patient may be anxious because of difficulty breathing and be distressed over purulent sputum.

DIAGNOSTIC HIGHLIGHTS

Test	Normal Result	Abnormality with Condition	Explanation
Sputum cultures and sensitivities	Negative cultures and sensitivities (other than	Presence of infecting organisms	Cultures identify organism; sensitivity testing identifies how

	normal bacterial flora)		resistant or sensitive the bacteria are to antibiotics
Chest x ray	Clear lung fields	Areas of increased density; can be a long segment, lobe, one lung, or both lungs	Findings reflect areas of infection and consolidation

Other Tests: Arterial blood gases, complete blood count, blood cultures

PRIMARY NURSING DIAGNOSIS

Ineffective airway clearance related to increased production of secretions and increased viscosity

OUTCOMES. Respiratory status: Gas exchange; Respiratory status: Ventilation; Symptom control behavior; Treatment behavior: Illness or injury; Comfort level

INTERVENTIONS. Airway management; Anxiety reduction; Oxygen therapy; Airway suctioning; Airway insertion and stabilization; Cough enhancement; Mechanical ventilation; Positioning; Respiratory monitoring

☐ PLANNING AND IMPLEMENTATION

Collaborative

Bacterial pneumonia is treated with medications. Physicians may request regular measurements of peak and trough levels, especially for patients who are receiving aminoglycosides, which can produce severe side effects such as renal failure and hearing loss. Many patients need oxygen therapy, even intubation and mechanical ventilation. High fever may be treated with antipyretics or IV hydration to replace fluid loss. Percussion and postural drainage may be prescribed to assist the patient in expectorating secretions.

PHARMACOLOGIC HIGHLIGHTS

Medication or Drug Class	Dosage	Description	Rationale
Antibiotics	Varies with drug	Penicillin G or erythromycin (for patients allergic to penicillin) for streptococcal pneumonia; nafcillin or oxacillin for staphylococcal pneumonia; aminoglycoside or a cephalosporin for klebsiella pneumonia; penicillin G or cylindamycin for aspiration pneumonia	Treat bacterial pneumonia

Independent

Make sure the patient coughs and uses deep-breathing exercises at least every 2 hours. Encourage drinking 3 L of fluid daily, unless contraindicated, to help expectorate secretions. If the patient cannot cough up secretions, you may have to perform nasotracheal or orotracheal suction to maintain an open airway. Turn and position patients on bed rest to help keep the airway open and free of secretions. Elevate the head of the bed to at least 45 degrees to help the patient maintain an open airway, and find positions that ease breathing. Place the patient in an upright position with both arms well supported on pillows, or position the patient to lean forward and rest his or her arms on the overbed table.

Involve the patient in as much decision making as possible, and, when possible, include the family in teaching situations. Explain all procedures, particularly intubation and suctioning. Teach the importance of adequate rest and the deep-breathing and coughing exercises that are designed to clear lung secretions.

Teach proper ways to dispose of secretions and proper hand-washing techniques to minimize the risk of spreading infection. Advise annual influenza vaccinations or avoidance of using antibiotics indiscriminately because such use creates a risk for upper airway colonization by antibiotic-resistant bacteria.

DOCUMENTATION GUIDELINES

- Physical findings of chest assessment: Respiratory rate and depth, auscultation findings, chest tightness or pain, vital signs
- Assessment of degree of hypoxemia: Lips and mucous membrane color, oxygen saturation by pulse oximetry
- Response to deep-breathing and coughing exercises, color and amount of sputum
- Response to medications: Body temperature, clearing of secretions

DISCHARGE AND HOME HEALTHCARE GUIDELINES

Be sure the patient understands all medications, including dosage, route, action, and adverse effects. The patient and family or significant other need to understand the importance of avoiding fatigue by limiting activity and taking frequent rests. Advise small, frequent meals to maintain adequate nutrition. Fluid intake should be maintained at approximately 3000 mL per day so that the secretions remain thin. Teach the patient to maintain pulmonary hygiene measures of coughing, deep breathing, and incentive spirometry at home. Provide information about how to stop smoking.

Pneumothorax

DRG Category: 094
Mean LOS: 6.5 days
Description: MEDICAL: Pneumothorax with CC

Pneumothorax occurs when there is an accumulation of air in the pleural space. Pneumothorax increases intrapleural pressure, thus resulting in the collapse of the lung on the affected side. There are three major types of pneumothorax: spontaneous, traumatic, and tension. Spontaneous pneumothorax is not life-threatening. Traumatic pneumothorax can also be classified as either open (when atmospheric air enters the pleural space) or closed (when air enters the pleural space from the lung). Open traumatic pneumothorax constitutes a life-threatening emergency.

The pleural space between the visceral and parietal pleura exerts negative pressure, which creates a vacuum that keeps the lungs from collapsing. If air accumulates, however, the pressure rises, thus leading to atelectasis (collapsed lung) and ineffective gas exchange. When the air in the pleural space cannot escape, tension pneumothorax occurs. If air accumulation is not stopped, the entire mediastinum shifts toward the unaffected side, thus causing bilateral lung collapse, which is a life-threatening condition. Tension pneumothorax can lead to shock, low blood pressure, and cardiopulmonary arrest.

CAUSES

The cause of a closed or primary spontaneous penumothorax is the rupture of a bleb (vesicle) on the surface of the visceral pleura. Secondary spontaneous pneumothorax can result from chronic obstructive pulmonary disease (COPD), which is related to hyperinflation or air trapping, or from the effects of cancer, which can result in the weakening of lung tissue or erosion into the pleural space by the tumor. Blunt chest trauma and penetrating chest trauma are the primary causes of traumatic and tension pneumothorax. Other possible causes include therapeutic procedures such as thoracotomy, thoracentesis, and insertion of a central line.

GENDER AND LIFE SPAN CONSIDERATIONS

Pneumothorax can occur at any age. Elderly people with COPD and younger people with paraseptal emphysema are susceptible to spontaneous pneumothorax. Spontaneous primary pneumothroax occurs most often in thin men between the ages of 30 and 40. Traumatic injuries are more common in adolescent and young-adult men than in other populations.

☐ ASSESSMENT

HISTORY. Ask about chest pain; determine its onset, intensity, and location. Ask if the patient has shortness of breath or difficulty in breathing or fatigue. Elicit a history of COPD or emphysema or if the patient has had a thoracotomy, thoracentesis, or insertion of a central line. Ask if the patient smokes cigarettes.

For patients who have experienced chest trauma, establish a history of the mechanism of injury by including a detailed report from the pre-hospital professionals, witnesses, or significant others. Specify the type of trauma (blunt or penetrating). If the patient has been shot, ask the paramedics for ballistic information, including the caliber of the weapon and the range at which the person was shot. If the patient was in a motor vehicle crash, determine the type of vehicle (truck, motorcycle, car), the speed of the vehicle, the victim's location in the car (driver vs. passenger), and the use, if any, of safety restraints. Determine if the patient has had a recent tetanus immunization.

PHYSICAL EXAMINATION. The severity of the symptoms depends on the extent of any underlying disease and the amount of air in the pleural space. Examine the patient's chest for a visible wound that may have been caused by a penetrating object. Patients with an open pneumothorax also exhibit a sucking sound on inspiration.

Inspect the patient with pneumothorax for cyanosis, nasal flaring, asymmetric chest expansion, dyspnea, tachypnea, and intercostal retractions. Observe whether the patient has a flail chest, a condition in which the patient has paradoxic chest movement with the chest wall moving outward during expiration and inward during inspiration. On palpation, note any tracheal deviation toward the unaffected side, subcutaneous emphysema (also known as crepitus; a dry, crackling sound caused by air trapped in the subcutaneous tissues), or decreased to absent tactile fremitus over the affected area. Percussion may elicit a hyperresonant or tympanitic sound. Auscultation reveals decreased or absent breath sounds over the affected area and no adventitious sounds other than a possible pleural rub.

Examine the thorax area, including the anterior chest, posterior chest, and axillae, for contusions, abrasions, hematomas, and penetrating wounds. Note that even small penetrating wounds can be life-threatening if vital structures are perforated. Observe the patient carefully for pallor. Take the patient's blood pressure and pulse rate, noting the early signs of shock or massive bleeding, such as a falling pulse pressure, a rising pulse rate, and delayed capillary refill. Continue to monitor the vital signs frequently during periods of instability to determine changes in the condition or the development of complications.

PSYCHOSOCIAL. Patients with a pneumothorax may be confused, anxious, or restless. They may be concerned about their pain and dyspnea and could be in a panic state. Determine the patient's past ability to manage stressors, and discuss with the significant others the most adaptive mechanisms to use. Note that approximately one-half of all traumatic injuries are associated with alcohol and other drugs of abuse.

DIAGNOSTIC HIGHLIGHTS

Test	Normal Result	Abnormality with Condition	Explanation
Chest x ray	Clear lung fields	Lung collapse with air between chest wall and visceral pleura	Lungs are not filled with air but rather are collapsed

Other Tests: Complete blood count, plasma alcohol level, arterial blood gases, computed tomography (CT) scan

PRIMARY NURSING DIAGNOSIS

Impaired gas exchange related to decreased oxygen diffusion capacity

OUTCOMES. Respiratory status: Gas exchange; Respiratory status: Ventilation; Comfort level; Anxiety control

INTERVENTIONS. Airway insertion and stabilization; Airway management; Respiratory monitoring; Oxygen therapy; Mechanical ventilation; Anxiety reduction

□ PLANNING AND IMPLEMENTATION

Collaborative

The priority is to maintain airway, breathing, and circulation. The most important interventions focus on reinflating the lung by evacuating the pleural air. Patients with a primary spontaneous pneumothorax that is small with minimal symptoms may have spontaneous sealing and lung re-expansion. For patients with jeopardized gas exchange, chest tube insertion may be necessary to achieve lung re-expansion.

Maintain a closed chest drainage system; be sure to tape all connections, and secure the tube carefully at the insertion site with adhesive bandages. Regulate suction according to the chest tube system directions; generally, suction does not exceed 20 to 25 cm H_2O negative pressure. Monitor a chest tube unit for any kinks or bubbling, which could indicate an air leak, but do not clamp a chest tube without a physician's order because clamping may lead to tension pneumothorax. Stabilize the chest tube so that it does not drag or pull against the patient or against the drainage system. Maintain aseptic technique, changing the chest tube insertion site dressing and monitoring the site for signs and symptoms of infection such as redness, swelling, warmth, and drainage.

Oxygen therapy and mechanical ventilation are prescribed as needed. Surgical interventions include removing the penetrating object, exploratory thoracotomy if necessary, thoracentesis, and thoracotomy for patients with two or more episodes of spontaneous pneumothorax or patients with pneumothorax that does not resolve within 1 week.

PHARMACOLOGIC HIGHLIGHTS

No routine pharmacologic measures will treat pneumothorax, but the patient may need antibiotics and analgesics, depending on the extent and nature of the injury. Analgesia is administered for pain once the patient's pulmonary status has stabilized.

Independent

Place the patient in a semi-Fowler position to improve lung expansion. Change the patient's position every 2 hours to prevent infection and allow for lung drainage. For patients with traumatic closed pneumothorax, turn the patient onto the unaffected side to improve the ventilation : perfusion ratio. Encourage coughing and deep breathing to remove secretions.

For patients with traumatic open pneumothorax, prepare a sterile occlusive dressing and cover the wound. Monitor carefully for a tension pneumothorax (absent breath sounds, tracheal deviation) because the occlusive dressing prevents air from escaping the lungs. Teach alternative pain relief techniques. Explain all procedures in advance to decrease the patient's anxiety.

DOCUMENTATION GUIDELINES

- Physical findings: Breath sounds, vital signs, level of consciousness, urinary output, skin temperature, amount and color of chest tube drainage, dyspnea, cyanosis, nasal flaring, altered chest expansion, tracheal deviation, absence of breath sounds

- Response to pain: Location, description, duration, response to interventions
- Response to treatment: Chest tube insertion—type and amount of drainage, presence of air leak, presence or absence of crepitus, amount of suction, presence of clots, response to fluid resuscitation; response to surgical management
- Complications: Infection (fever, wound drainage); inadequate gas exchange (restlessness, dropping SaO_2); tension pneumothorax

DISCHARGE AND HOME HEALTHCARE GUIDELINES

Review all follow-up appointments, which often involve chest x rays, ABG analysis, and a physical examination. If the injury was alcohol-related, explore the patient's drinking pattern. Refer for counseling, if necessary. Teach the patient when to notify the physician of complications (infection, an unhealed wound, and anxiety) and to report any sudden chest pain or difficulty breathing.

Polycystic Kidney Disease

DRG Category: 331
Mean LOS: 5.1 days
Description: MEDICAL: Other Kidney and Urinary Tract Diagnoses, Age > 17 with CC
DRG Category: 304
Mean LOS: 8.7 days
Description: SURGICAL: Kidney, Ureter, and Major Bladder Procedures for Nonneopolycystic with CC

Although inherited polycystic diseases are not the only types of cystic diseases of the kidney, all types are a major contributor to chronic renal failure. Infantile autosomal recessive polycystic kidney disease (RPK) and adult autosomal dominant polycystic kidney disease (DPK) are two types of inherited polycystic kidney disease. Infantile (RPK) disease affects both kidneys, leads to renal failure, and causes biliary dilation and fibrosis in the liver. The basic pathology of cyst development is a weakening of the basement membrane, which possibly is caused by an abnormality of the extracellular connective tissue cells. Adult-onset disease (DPK) is a bilateral disorder, although it may have asymmetric progression with multiple expanding cysts that destroy renal function. Renal deterioration eventually leads to uremia, chronic renal failure, and the need for chronic renal dialysis.

Complications include liver, pancreatic, spleen, and lung cysts; aneurysms of the cerebral artery or abdominal aorta; colonic diverticula; and mitral valve prolapse. Approximately 40% of adult patients die of coronary or hypertensive heart disease. About 10% to 40% of people with DPK have berry aneurysms, and 9% die as a result of subarachnoid hemorrhages.

CAUSES

RPK and DPK are genetically inherited. In RPK, siblings of either sex have one chance in four of having the disease. DPK has a 100% incidence because it is an autosomal dominant trait. An average of half of the affected individuals have children with DPK.

GENDER AND LIFE SPAN CONSIDERATIONS

RPK always becomes apparent during childhood in boys and girls, usually before the age of 13. An infant born with active RPK usually dies within the first 2 months of life as a result of uremia or respiratory failure. Renal failure and hypertension develop more slowly when the disease occurs later in childhood. Most patients with DPK are identified between the ages of 30 and 50 years, although newborns can be diagnosed with the disease. A neonate with DPK is likely to be stillborn or die from renal failure within 9 months. In most men and women with DPK, the disease progresses to end-stage renal failure by the time the patient reaches the age of 40 to 50 years.

✷ ASSESSMENT

HISTORY. Children with RPK are apt to have a lengthy medical history, including multiple system complications and frequent hospitalizations. Because children with DPK usually experience cardiopulmonary complications, ask the parents about respiratory distress or increased blood pressure during checkups. The child can also have bleeding varices; ask the parents if the child has ever spit up blood.

When you take a history from adults with DPK who are approximately 40 years old, note that they may have one of two forms of presenting symptoms: pain or hypertension. Pain can occur in one or both kidneys and can vary from a vague sense of heaviness or a dull ache to severe knifelike pain. Some patients describe flank pain from renal colic, bloody urine from the passage of renal calculi, signs of a urinary tract infection (burning or pain on urination, urinary frequency and urgency, fever), and gastrointestinal symptoms (nausea, vomiting, diarrhea, constipation) from compression by the enlarged kidneys. Patients with the second type of DPK often develop hypertension as the initial clinical sign. Changes in urinary output and concentration may accompany hypertension because of developing renal insufficiency.

PHYSICAL EXAMINATION. The infant with RPK has pronounced epicanthal folds (vertical skin folds that extend from the root of the nose to the median end of the eyebrow), a pointed nose and small chin, and low-set ears. When you palpate the child's kidneys, you are able to feel huge, tense bilateral masses on both flanks. These children usually have multiple assessment findings from many malfunctioning organ systems, such as bleeding esophageal varices, pulmonary congestion, hypertension, and oliguria or anuria.

Adult patients with DPK may have a healthy appearance but may have urine that is foul-smelling, cloudy, or bloody because of a urinary tract infection. If the blood vessels that surround the kidney cysts rupture into the renal pelvis, the patient may have moderate-to-severe hematuria. The patient probably has had hypertension for years before any renal damage occurs. As the disease progresses, the patient develops a widening abdomen, which is tender when palpated. In advanced stages, palpation reveals grossly enlarged kidneys.

PSYCHOSOCIAL. When a child is diagnosed with RPK, assess the siblings for the disease as well. With both types of polycystic disease, the patient and partner need genetic counseling. Children of parents diagnosed with DPK should have an ultrasound or genetic testing because approximately half also have DPK. There is a great strain on individuals and their families with both types of polycystic kidney disease because of the poor prognosis of children with RPK and the knowledge that DPK worsens throughout life

DIAGNOSTIC HIGHLIGHTS

Test	Normal Result	Abnormality with Condition	Explanation
Genetic testing	No mutations on genes of interest	PKD1, PKD2, PKD3 genes may have mutations that lead to DPK	Genetic alterations lead to DPK
Computed tomography	Normal renal structure	Markedly enlarged kidney with dilated cysts	Cyst development leads to altered tubular epithelium, cell proliferation, and fluid secretion

Other Tests: Renal ultrasound, serum blood urea nitrogen and creatinine, urinalysis, intravenous pyelogram

PRIMARY NURSING DIAGNOSIS

Pain (acute) related to compression of tissues, trauma to structures from calculi, inflammation, and infection

OUTCOMES. Comfort level; Pain control behavior; Pain: Disruptive effects; Pain level

INTERVENTIONS. Pain management; Analgesic administration; Positioning; Teaching: Prescribed activity/exercise; Teaching: Procedure/treatment; Teaching: Prescribed medication

☐ PLANNING AND IMPLEMENTATION

Collaborative

Because there is no cure for polycystic kidney disease, care centers around alleviating symptoms and slowing the onset of renal impairment. Infants with RPK need management of airway, breathing, and circulation because of the extent of the multiple system involvement. Patients who survive past infancy need treatment for hypertension, congestive heart failure, renal failure, and hepatic failure.

As renal impairment progresses, patients require hemodialysis and renal transplantation. Allografts from siblings may be used only after appropriate genetic screenings have ruled out the possibility that the sibling also has the disease. For those with DPK, surgery may decrease the pressure that is caused by enlarging cysts. This procedure sometimes removes functioning nephrons and may contribute to the loss of renal function, but it also controls hypertension and decreases pain. An alternative is percutaneous aspiration of the cysts.

Infections need to be prevented when possible and treated vigorously because they are difficult to cure and the residual scarring can further worsen the disease. Usually the patient needs a diet high in carbohydrate content and with prescribed limits of fluid, sodium, potassium, phosphorus, and protein.

PHARMACOLOGIC HIGHLIGHTS

Medication or Drug Class	Dosage	Description	Rationale
Antibiotics	Varies with drug	Trimethoprim-sulfamethoxazole; chloramphenicol	Prevent or treat infections; lipid soluble antibiotics are usually used

Other Drugs: Analgesic drugs may be needed for control of the flank pain associated with enlarged kidneys, and antihypertensives are used to manage hypertension.

Independent

One of the most important nursing roles is to promote the patient's comfort. Encourage tepid baths, relaxation techniques, and other nonpharmacologic methods to improve comfort. Because many patients retain fluid from impaired renal regulatory mechanisms, fluid restriction may be necessary. Work with the patient to determine a personal schedule for fluid intake. If the patient desires, allot some of the fluid intake for ice chips. If possible, administer medications with meals to allow the patient to consolidate fluid intake.

The disease can be emotionally draining for the patient and family. Try to provide quiet time each day to talk with the patient. Answer questions, provide teaching materials, and listen to concerns. If the patient or family is not able to cope effectively, refer for counseling.

Teach the patient to use measures to prevent urinary tract infections. Explain the need to empty the bladder completely when voiding. Encourage female patients to wipe from front to back after having a bowel movement. Explain the mechanism of action of all antibiotics to the patient, and stress the need to take them on schedule to maintain blood levels and to take all of them. Teach the patient to notify the primary healthcare provider if symptoms of any of the following recur: burning, frequency, urgency, cloudy or red urine, foul-smelling urine.

DOCUMENTATION GUIDELINES

- Physical findings: Pain, fluid intake and output, daily weights, serial vital signs, laboratory findings (renal function tests and electrolytes in particular), appearance of urine
- Response to pain medications and nonpharmacologic methods of pain relief, fluid and dietary restrictions
- Presence of complications: Urinary tract infection, edema, cardiac disease, intracranial hemorrhage

DISCHARGE AND HOME HEALTHCARE GUIDELINES

Teach the patient how to recognize a urinary tract infection and prevent its recurrence: maintain fluid intake as allowed; complete perineal cleansing; avoid long hot baths; empty the bladder completely. Teach the patient to notify the physician about the following because of possible deterioration in renal function: nausea, vomiting, and weight loss; changes in the pattern or urinary elimination; pruritus; headaches; a weight gain of more than 5 pounds in 1 week; edema; difficulty in breathing; and decreasing urine output. Stress the need to keep follow-up appointments. Teach the patient how to maintain any prescribed diet restrictions, and include the family. Explain all medications, including the dosage, action, side effects, and route.

Polycythemia

DRG Category: 403
Mean LOS: 7.4 days
Description: MEDICAL: Lymphoma and Non-Acute Leukemia with CC

Polycythemia as a generic term refers to an increased concentration of red blood cells (RBCs, or erythrocytes). This blood disorder has several causes and can be classified as primary, secondary, and relative polycythemia. (See Table 42.)

TABLE 42 | **Types of Polycythemia**

TYPE	DEFINITION	SIGNS AND SYMPTOMS	PHYSICAL EXAMINATION
Primary polycythemia (Polycythemia vera)	Chronic proliferative bone marrow disorder that leads to overproduction of RBCs, WBCs, and platelets; results in increased blood viscosity and platelet dysfunction	Early: feeling of fullness in the head, tinnitus, headache, dizziness, hypertension, blurred vision, night sweats, epigastric pain, joint pain, pain on walking Late: pruritus (abnormal histamine metabolism), abdominal fullness, pleuritic pain, epistaxis, gingival bleeding	Engorged veins in the fundus and retina of the eye on fundoscopic examination, congestion of conjunctiva, congested oral mucous membranes, tenderness of ribs and sternum on palpation, ruddy cyanosis, enlarged liver and spleen
Secondary polycythemia	Excessive production of RBCs because of hypoxemia, tumors; often triggered by overproduction of erythropoietin (hormone produced primarily in the kidney and necessary for RBC production)	Shortness of breath from underlying pulmonary disease, symptoms from underlying disease processes	Ruddy cyanosis, ecchymosis, spoon-shaped nails, clubbing of fingers
Relative polycythemia (spurious polycythemia)	Caused by reduced plasma volume; actual RBC count is normal or even reduced; increased blood concentration	Symptoms often vague: headache, dizziness, fatigue, dyspnea, diaphoresis, claudication, ruddy appearance, enlarged	Ruddy appearance, enlarged live and spleen, hypoventilation

occurs because	liver and spleen,
of increased	hypoventilation
concentration of	
cells compared to	
plasma	

Most complications of all types of polycythemia occur as a result of increased blood viscosity (hyperviscosity) or sudden blood loss (hemorrhage). Hyperviscosity may lead to thromboembolic events, such as organ thromboses or splenomegaly. Hemorrhage in any system can occur from platelet dysfunction. Hemorrhage and vasculitis may occur together because an excessive number of RBCs exert pressure on capillary walls. Specific complications include gangrene of the fingers and toes, hypertension, peptic ulcer disease, and cerebrovascular accident. Life expectancy for patients with polycythemia if it is left untreated is roughly 2 years.

CAUSES

The cause of primary polycythemia is unknown; the condition is considered idiopathic. A current theory is that the disease is caused by a stem call defect. Secondary polycythemia is caused by excessive production of erythropoietin. Decreased oxygen delivery leads to appropriate overproduction of erythropoietin in the following diseases: chronic obstructive pulmonary disease, cyanotic heart disease, congestive heart failure, drug toxicities inducing hypoventilation, and prolonged exposure to high altitudes. Overproduction of erythropoietin occurs inappropriately in the following conditions: renal carcinoma, renal cysts, hepatoma, uterine fibroids, and endocrine disorders.

Relative polycythemia is caused by dehydration from the following conditions: decreased plasma volume because of diuretic therapy, persistent nausea and vomiting, decreased fluid intake, diabetic ketoacidosis, diabetes insipidus, plasma loss after thermal injury, and excessive drainage from drains or tubes.

GENDER AND LIFE SPAN CONSIDERATIONS

The incidence of primary polycythemia is the highest in middle-aged and older European-American men, with a median onset age of 60. It is rare in children except in those with cyanotic heart disease. Babies who are small for their gestational age and infants of diabetic mothers may also be at risk.

☐ ASSESSMENT

HISTORY AND PHYSICAL EXAMINATION. The history, symptoms, and clinical findings vary slightly with the three types of polycythemia and degree of increased blood viscosity. A thorough family, environmental, and occupational history is necessary. Many patients with polycythemia have a history of cardiac and pulmonary disease, particularly emphysema.

PSYCHOSOCIAL. Assess the effects of a chronic illness on the patient and family; if the patient does not get enough rest or relaxation, suggest lifestyle changes that might decrease stress. Heavy smokers may acquire certain hemoglobin abnormalities that can lead to SP.

DIAGNOSTIC HIGHLIGHTS

Test	Normal Result	Abnormality with Condition	Explanation
Bone marrow biopsy	Normal bone marrow cells	Hypercellular bone marrow with residual fat; increased in erythroid progenitors, increased maturing granulocytic precursors and megakaryocytes	Thin needle is used to draw up small amount of liquid bone marrow; a small cylinder of bone and marrow (about 1/2" long) is removed; site of both samples is usually at the back of the hipbone
Complete blood count (CBC)	Red blood cells (RBCs) 4.0–5.5 million/μL; white blood cells 4,500–11,000/μL; hemoglobin (Hg) 12–18 g/dL; hematocrit (Hct) 37%–54%; reticulocyte count 0.5%–2.5% of total RBCs; platelets 150,000–400,000/μL	Hg 14–28 g/dL; Hct $\geq$ 55%; RBC $\geq$ 6 million/ mm^3; WBC 12,000–50,000 cells/mm^3; platelet count > 500,000 mm^3	Increased proliferation and production of bone marrow elements

Other Tests: Vitamin B_{12} level

PRIMARY NURSING DIAGNOSIS

Altered protection related to abnormal blood profiles (coagulation)

OUTCOMES. Circulation status; Tissue integrity; Tissue perfusion; Fluid balance

INTERVENTIONS. Bleeding precautions; Fluid management; Surveillance; Medication management; Teaching: Disease process, Prescribed medication; Environmental management; Wound care

☐ PLANNING AND IMPLEMENTATION

Collaborative

Table 43 contains the collaborative interventions for primary, secondary, and relative polycythemia.

TABLE 43 | **Interventions for Polycythemia**

TYPE	OBJECTIVE	INTERVENTIONS
Primary polycythemia	Reduce blood viscosity	• Periodic phlebotomies (removing approximately 350–500 mL of blood) to help the patient maintain normal hemoglobin and hematocrit levels, usually repeated every other day

- Bone marrow suppression with radioactive phosphorus (^{32}P) or chemotherapy (melphalan, busulfan, and chlorambucil) can usually control the disease process (medications can cause leukemia and therefore only used in most seriously ill or elderly patients)
- Pheresis techniques are used to remove RBCs, WBCs, and platelets and to return plasma to blood.

Secondary polycythemia	Treat disease that acts as a hypoxic trigger or causes increased production of erythropoietin	• Change of location for those who live at high altitudes if that is the hypoxic trigger • May be treated by phlebotomy or pheresis if the patient has not responded to treatment or if increased blood viscosity is considered dangerous.
Relative polycythemia	Prevent dehydration and thromboembolic conditions; to correct fluid volume deficits	• Rehydration with fluids and replacement of electrolytes to manage dehydration • Treat underlying cause • Low-cholesterol, low-fat, low-sodium diet; low-purine diet modifies high uric acid levels and limits the risk of calculus formation

PHARMACOLOGIC HIGHLIGHTS

Medication or Drug Class	Dosage	Description	Rationale
Warfarin sodium (Coumadin)	Maintenance: 2–10 mg daily po	Anticoagulant	Assists in preventing clot formation

Other Drugs: For symptom management—increased serum uric acid levels can be treated with allopurinol or cyproheptadine, and pruritus can be managed with antihistamines or phenothiazines.

Independent

The patient's activity level is a primary concern. Allow for periods of rest because the patient may have both hypoxemia and a low hemoglobin count. At the same time, the patient needs to maintain mobility to prevent thrombosis because of increased blood viscosity. If rest and activity are balanced, the patient has the energy to be active for part of the day to limit complications. If the patient is bedridden, a program of active and passive range-of-motion exercises is essential. If the patient's appetite is dulled, encourage small, frequent feedings followed by a rest period to decrease nausea and vomiting. Fluid intake should be at least 3000 mL per day to decrease blood viscosity and limit uric acid calculus formation; work with the patient to determine the best method to prevent fluid volume deficit.

Monitor the patient carefully for signs of bleeding tendencies. Common bleeding sites include the nose, gingiva, and skin. Teach the patient to monitor these sites carefully after hospital discharge and to report any increased bleeding immediately. If the patient experiences minor trauma, teach him or her to apply pressure to the puncture site. In addition, encourage the patient to avoid razors or handling sharp objects. Make sure that the patient's environment is safe to limit the risk of falls or injury. If the patient develops pruritus, discourage scratching of the skin, use skin emollients, and work with the patient to determine a medication schedule that limits discomfort.

DOCUMENTATION GUIDELINES

- Physical findings of skin and mucous membranes: Presence of redness, tenderness, swelling, temperature changes, scratch marks, bleeding ecchymosis
- Response to medications, fluids, diet, and treatments such as phlebotomy or pheresis
- Presence of complications: Bleeding tendencies, respiratory distress, mental status changes, gastric distress, infections

DISCHARGE AND HOME HEALTHCARE GUIDELINES

Teach the patient to avoid the following: crossing the legs, prolonged periods of sitting or standing, and leg positions that put pressure on the popliteal space. Be sure the patient understands all medications, including the dosage, route, action, and adverse effects. Be sure the patient understands all diet and fluid therapy.

Instruct the patient to report leg pain or swelling, skin discoloration, bleeding, decreases in peripheral skin temperature, or signs of possible infection to the physician. For patients with primary polycythemia, genetic counseling may be necessary.

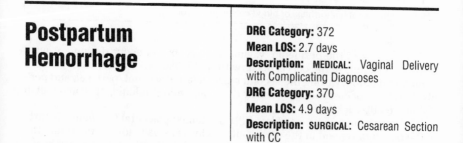

Postpartum Hemorrhage

DRG Category: 372
Mean LOS: 2.7 days
Description: MEDICAL: Vaginal Delivery with Complicating Diagnoses
DRG Category: 370
Mean LOS: 4.9 days
Description: SURGICAL: Cesarean Section with CC

A postpartum hemorrhage (PPH) is frequently defined as a blood loss of greater than 500 mL after giving birth vaginally or a blood loss of greater than 1000 mL after a cesarean section. Because many women lose at least 500 mL of blood during childbirth and do not experience any symptoms, a more accurate way to define PPH is losing 1% or more of the body weight after delivering a baby (1 mL of blood weighs 1 g). For example, a patient weighing 175 lb, or 80 kg, would need to lose 800 mL of blood to be classified as having a postpartum hemorrhage.

PPH is classified as either an early hemorrhage (occurring during the first 24 hours after delivery) or a late hemorrhage (occurring more than 24 hours after delivery). With the current trend in obstetric practice of sending postpartum patients home in 24 hours or less after delivery, the significance of PPH, particularly late hemorrhage, is profound. Often the severity of the hemorrhage depends on the expediency with which it is diagnosed and treated; if the patient hemorrhages at home, her risk increases significantly.

CAUSES

There are several causes of PPH, particularly uterine atony, trauma, and retained placental fragments. Several predisposing factors related to these causes can be found in Box 11. The number one cause of early PPH is uterine atony. After the placenta is delivered, the uterus needs to contract to seal off the blood vessels. If the uterus is contracted, the placental site is smaller, causing less bleeding.

BOX 11 PREDISPOSING FACTORS TO POSTPARTUM HEMORRHAGE

Overdistention of the uterus (multiple gestation, hydamnios)

Grand multiparity

Use of anesthetic agents, especially halothane

Forceps or vacuum delivery

Prolonged or rapid labor

Extended used of oxytocin (Pitocin) during labor

Delivery of large infant

Manual removal of the placenta

Placenta accreta (separation of the placenta is difficult or impossible

Mismanagement of the third stage of labor

Maternal malnutrition or anemia

Pregnancy-induced hypertension

Maternal history of hemorrhage or blood coagulation problems

Lacerations of the perineum, vagina, and cervix can occur during a vaginal birth. Lacerations of the cervix occur with rapid dilation or with pushing before complete dilation. During the second stage of labor, vaginal, perineal, and periurethral tears occur. Failure to repair these lacerations adequately can result in a slow, steady trickle of blood.

The most common cause of late PPH is retained placental fragments. If parts of the placenta remain in the uterus after delivery, small clots form around the retained parts, sealing off the bleeding. After a while the clots slough, and heavy bleeding occurs. Subinvolution (delayed involution) can also be a causative factor in a late PPH.

GENDER AND LIFE SPAN CONSIDERATIONS

PPH is linked not to age but to risk factors. (See Box 11.)

□ ASSESSMENT

HISTORY. Because PPH can be repeated in subsequent pregnancies, always ask a multipara if she had a previous PPH. Ask if the patient has perineal pain. Although some discomfort is expected after a vaginal delivery, severe pain or pressure is uncommon and often indicates a hematoma.

PHYSICAL EXAMINATION. Observe the amount and characteristics of blood loss;

sometimes there is a pooling of blood and the passage of large clots. Usually complete saturation of one perineal pad within 15 minutes or saturation of two or more pads in 1 hour suggests hemorrhage. Palpate the fundus, noting if it is firm or boggy, if it is midline or deviated laterally, and if it is above or below the umbilicus. Normally after delivery, the fundus is firm, midline, and at the level of the umbilicus. A fundus above the umbilicus and deviated laterally may indicate a full bladder. A boggy uterus is indicative of uterine atony and, if it is not corrected, results in a PPH. If the fundus is firm, midline, and at or below the umbilicus and if there is steady, bright red bleeding, further assessment for trauma is necessary. Inspect the perineum carefully to discern any unrepaired lacerations or bleeding from a repaired episiotomy. If a hematoma is suspected, the patient is placed in lithotomy position, and the vagina and perineal area are carefully inspected. A bulging and discoloration of the skin is noted if a hematoma is present. Assess the patient's vital signs. A temperature above 100.4°F may indicate uterine infection, which decreases the myometrium's ability to contract and makes the patient more susceptible to PPH. Note any foul vaginal odor that may accompany the fever with infection. Elevated heart rate, delayed capillary refill, decreased blood pressure, and increased respiratory rate may be noted if PPH is occurring. Assess the patient's color and skin temperature; pallor and cool clammy skin also indicate hypovolemic shock.

PSYCHOSOCIAL. PPH is a traumatic experience because medical complications are unexpected during what is anticipated as a happy time. Assess the anxiety level of the patient; the patient going into hypovolemic shock is highly anxious and then may lose consciousness. The significant others experience a high level of anxiety as well and need a great deal of support.

DIAGNOSTIC HIGHLIGHTS

General Comments: Diagnosis of PPH is usually based on the estimated blood loss, which eventually is reflected in serum laboratory tests.

Test	Normal Result	Abnormality with Condition	Explanation
RBC	4–5.4 million/μL	These three values will decrease several hours after significant blood loss has occurred	With active bleeding RBCs are lost
HGB	12–16 g/dL		
HCT	37%–47%		

PRIMARY NURSING DIAGNOSIS

Fluid volume deficit related to blood loss

OUTCOMES. Fluid balance; Hydration; Circulation status

INTERVENTIONS. Bleeding reduction; Blood product administration; Intravenous therapy; Shock management

□ PLANNING AND IMPLEMENTATION

Collaborative

The goal of treatment is to correct the cause and replace the fluid loss. Expedient diagnosis and treatment of the cause reduce the likelihood of a blood transfusion. Treatment for uterine atony involves performing frequent fundal massage, sometimes bimanual massage (by the medical clinician only), and pharmacologic therapy. Fluid replacement with normal saline solution, lactated Ringer's injection, volume expanders, or whole blood may be necessary.

Monitor the hematocrit and hemoglobin to determine the success of fluid replacement and the patient's intake and output. If an infection is the cause of the atony, the physician prescribes antibiotics. PPH caused by trauma requires surgical repair with aseptic technique. Hematomas may absorb on their own; however, if they are large, an incision, evacuation of clots, and ligation of the bleeding vessel are necessary. Administer analgesics for perineal pain. If retained fragments are suspected at the time of delivery, the uterine cavity should be explored. Cervical dilation and curettage is indicated to remove retained fragments. If the PPH is uncontrollable, a hysterectomy is done as a last resort.

PHARMACOLOGIC HIGHLIGHTS

Medication or Drug Class	Dosage	Description	Rationale
Oxytocin (Pitocin)	Mix 10–40 U in 1000 cc, give 20–40 mU/min	Oxytocic	Controls bleeding by producing uterine contractions
Methylergonovine (Methergine)	0.2 mg IM	Oxytocic	Controls bleeding by producing uterine contractions
Prostaglandins	Suppository, varies by drug		Used when oxytocin and methylergonovine are not effective

Independent

Be alert for PPH in any postpartum patient, especially those who have any of the predisposing factors. It is often the nurse who discovers the hemorrhage. For the first 24 hours postpartum, perform frequent fundal checks. If the fundus is boggy, massage until it feels firm; it should feel like a large, hard grapefruit. When massaging the fundus, keep one hand above the symphysis pubis to support the lower uterine segment, while gently but firmly rubbing the fundus, which may lose its tone when the massage is stopped. Explain that cramping or feeling like "labor is starting again" is expected with liberal administration of the oxytocic drugs used to manage the bleeding. Encourage the patient to void; a full bladder interferes with contractions and normal uterine involution. If the patient is unable to void on her own, a straight catheterization is necessary.

Monitor vaginal bleeding; the lochia is usually dark red and should not saturate more than 1 perineal pad every 2 to 3 hours. Notify the physician if the bleeding is steady and bright red in the presence of a normal firm fundus; this usually indicates a laceration. Ice packs and sitz baths may relieve perineal discomfort. The patient is usually on complete bed rest. Rooming in with the infant may be difficult; provide for safe care for the infant while it is in the mother's room. Assist the patient and significant others as much as possible with newborn care to facilitate quality time between the mother and her newborn. Assist the patient with ambulation the first few times out of bed; syncope is common after a large blood loss. Ensure adequate rest periods.

DOCUMENTATION GUIDELINES

- Bleeding: Amount, characteristics, precipitating factors
- Fundus: Location (above or below umbilicus, midline or lateral) and firmness
- Vital signs and any signs and symptoms of hypovolemic shock
- Appearance of the perineum, episiotomy, laceration repair (use REEDA [redness, edema, ecchymosis, drainage, approximation] to guide the documentation); fluid intake and output
- Absence or presence of vaginal odor

DISCHARGE AND HOME HEALTHCARE GUIDELINES

TEACHING. Teach the patient how to check her own fundus and do a fundal massage; this is especially important for patients at risk who are discharged early from the hospital. Advise the patient to contact the physician for the following: a boggy uterus that does not become firm with massage, excessive bright red or dark red bleeding, many large clots, fever above 100.4°F, persistent or severe perineal pain or pressure.

MEDICATIONS. If iron supplements are provided, teach the patient to take the drug with orange juice and expect some constipation and dark-colored stools. If oxytocics are ordered, emphasize the importance of taking them around the clock as prescribed. If antibiotics are ordered, teach the patient to finish the prescription, even though the symptoms may have ceased.

Pregnancy-Induced Hypertension

DRG Category: 373
Mean LOS: 1.9 days
Description: MEDICAL: Vaginal Delivery without Complicating Diagnoses
DRG Category: 370
Mean LOS: 4.9 days
Description: SURGICAL: Cesarean Section with CC

Pregnancy-induced hypertension (PIH) is a multisystem disorder of pregnancy that affects approximately 7% of all pregnant women. PIH is characterized by a classic triad of symptoms that manifest after 20 weeks gestation: hypertension, proteinuria, and edema. Hypertension is defined as an increase of 30 mm Hg in the systolic pressure, or an increase of 15 mm Hg in the diastolic pressure, or an elevation of the blood pressure to 140/90; this elevated reading must be observed two times at least 6 hours apart. PIH most often occurs in the last 10 weeks of gestation, during labor, or in the first 48 hours after delivery.

PIH is divided into three categories: (1) preeclampsia, which is characterized by elevated blood pressure, edema (especially facial), and proteinuria, all of which occur after 20 weeks; (2) eclampsia, the development of seizures along with preeclampsia; and (3) chronic hypertension, which is elevated blood pressure before the 20th week of pregnancy that can also develop into preeclampsia.

If untreated (or sometimes even with aggressive treatment), the symptoms get progressively worse. The devastating sequence of events after preeclampsia is as follows: eclampsia, HELLP syndrome (hemolysis, elevated liver enzyme levels, low platelet count), followed by disseminated intravascular coagulation (DIC), which is often fatal. Not only is PIH life-threatening for the mother, but it can also cause intrauterine growth retardation, decreased fetal movement, chronic hypoxia, or even death in the fetus caused by decreased placental perfusion.

CAUSES

The cause of PIH is unknown; it is often called the "disease of theories" because many causes have been proposed, yet none has been well established. Experts believe that decreased levels of prostaglandins and a decreased resistance to angiotensin II lead to a generalized arterial vasospasm that then causes endothelial damage. The brain, liver, kidney, and blood are particularly susceptible to multiple dysfunctions. Several risk factors have been identified that may predispose a woman to developing PIH: nulliparity; familial history; multiple gestation; patient history of diabetes mellitus, chronic hypertension, renal disease, trophoblastic disease, and malnutrition.

GENDER AND LIFE SPAN CONSIDERATIONS

PIH tends to occur most frequently in pregnant adolescents and in women over age 35.

☐ ASSESSMENT

HISTORY. Obtain a thorough medical and obstetric history early in the pregnancy to determine if the patient has any of the risk factors. If she had a previous delivery, obtain information on any problems that occurred. Assess the patient's level of consciousness and orientation because her mental status may deteriorate as PIH progresses. Ask the patient if she has noticed an increase in edema, especially in her face; nondependent edema is more significant than dependent edema. The significant other may report that the patient's face is "fuller." Ask the patient if her hands and feet swell overnight and if her rings feel tight; she may even report that she is unable to take off her rings. Question her about any nausea, headaches, visual disturbances (blurred, double, spots), or right upper quadrant pain. Ask the patient and significant others if she has had seizures.

PHYSICAL EXAMINATION. Inspect the patient for pitting edema. Although most pregnant women experience some edema, it has a more abrupt onset in PIH. Weigh the patient daily, in the same clothes, at the same time, to help estimate fluid retention; often the patient gains several pounds in 1 week. Blood pressure should be taken on the right arm while the patient is supine and also in the left lateral position. Compare blood pressure readings to determine increasing trends.

A funduscopic inspection of the retina may reveal vascular constriction and narrowing of the small arteries. Auscultate the patient's lungs bilaterally to assess for pulmonary edema. Assess the deep tendon reflexes and assign a rating from 1 to 4; with PIH, reflexes are brisker than normal. Check for clonus bilaterally by dorsiflexing the foot briskly and checking if the foot comes back and "taps" your hand. Count the beats of clonus present; presence of clonus is indicative of central nervous system (CNS) involvement. Perform a sterile vaginal examination to determine if the patient is in labor or to determine the "ripeness" of her cervix for labor. Also note if the amniotic sac is intact or ruptured and if there is any bloody "show," which signals the onset of labor. If the amniotic sac is ruptured, note the color, amount, and presence of odor of the fluid. Assess the uterus for the presence of contractions, noting the frequency, duration, and intensity. Place the patient on the fetal monitor immediately to determine the status of the fetus. Provide ongoing assessments of the baseline fetal heart rate and of the presence or absence of variability, accelerations, and decelerations in the heart rate. Often a nonstress test (NST) is done on admission to assess the fetus' well-being.

Remember that the patient's condition can deteriorate rapidly. Vigilantly monitor for signs and symptoms of progressive disease and impending eclampsia and HELLP. Assess the blood pressure, pulse, respirations, and urine output hourly. Check deep tendon reflexes and for clonus hourly or as ordered. Report upward trends. Be alert for such signs and symptoms of impending eclampsia as accelerating hypertension, headache, epigastric pain, nausea, visual disturbances, and altered sensorium, and also increased bleeding tendencies.

PSYCHOSOCIAL. Many women expect pregnancy to be a happy and normal process; the hospitalization is unexpected. Assess the patient's ability to cope with the disorder and her social supports. In addition to concern about the pregnancy, she may have other children that need care while she is hospitalized. Assess the resources of the patient and significant others to manage job, child-care, financial, and social responsibilities.

DIAGNOSTIC HIGHLIGHTS

General Comments: Although this condition is primarily diagnosed by symptoms, several lab profiles indicate the severity of the disease. Serial laboratory tests are done to assist with diagnosis and monitoring of the disease. Increasing and decreasing trends indicate improvement or worsening of the disease state and help diagnose multiorgan involvement.

Test	Normal Result	Abnormality with Condition	Explanation
Dip/24 hour urine for protein and creatinine	Dip–negative 80–125 mL/min	2+ or higher >3g/L for 24 hours elevated	Increase in protein and creatinine in the urine indicates renal disease
Uric acid	2.0–6.6 mg/dL	Elevated	Indicates renal disease
Blood urea nitrogen (BUN)	10–20 mg/dL	Elevated	Indicates renal disease
Liver enzymes		Elevated	Increases indicate liver involvement
• AST	5–40 IU/L		
• ALT	5–35 IU/L		
• LDH	115–225 IU/L		
• Bilirubin	0.1–1.0 mg/dL		

Platelets	150,000–400,000/ mm³	Decreased	Decrease caused by endothelial damage and activation of thrombin
Coagulation studies	WNL values	Prolonged bleeding times; decrease in clotting factors	Abnormalities occur with HELLP and DIC
RBC HGB HCT	4.2–5.4 mil/mm³ 11–16 g/dL 33%–36%	Decreased	Hemolysis occurs if the condition worsens

Other Tests: Fetal testing to assess well-being includes a nonstress test, stress test biophysical profile, ultrasound, and, if the woman is in labor, continuous fetal monitoring and possible scalp pH. If the fetus is premature, an amniocentesis may be done to obtain amniotic fluid for fetal lung maturity tests.

PRIMARY NURSING DIAGNOSIS

Altered tissue perfusion (cardiopulmonary, cerebral, peripheral, renal) related to arterial vasospasm and obstruction to flow

OUTCOMES. Vital signs status; Urinary elimination; Fluid balance; Neurological status; Coagulation status; Tissue perfusion: Abdominal organs; Fetal status: Intrapartum

INTERVENTIONS. Fluid monitoring; Fluid/electrolyte management; Seizure precautions; Medication administration; Vital signs monitoring; Fluid management; Bedside laboratory testing; Electronic fetal monitoring

☐ PLANNING AND IMPLEMENTATION

Collaborative

Often, PIH occurs before the fetus is term. The goals of treatment are to treat the mother safely and keep the infant in utero as long as possible, so long as the fetus is not showing any signs of distress and maternal condition is stable. If the symptoms in PIH are mild, often the patient is treated at home on bed rest, with careful instructions and education on the danger signs and frequent prenatal visits to monitor progression of the disorder.

Maintain the patient on complete bed rest. If the urine output is below 30 mL/hr, suspect renal failure and notify the physician. Readings of 2+ to 4+ protein in the urine and urine-specific gravities of greater than 1.040 are associated with proteinuria and oliguria. Hemodynamic monitoring with a central venous pressure catheter or a pulmonary artery catheter may be initiated to regulate fluid balance.

If the patient is receiving a magnesium sulfate drip, serum magnesium levels are done to determine if the level has reached the therapeutic level; serum levels also alert the caregiver of a move toward toxicity. If the magnesium sulfate infusion does not prevent seizure, the physician may order the administration of phenobarbital or benzodiazepines. Using either low doses of aspirin or dietary calcium supplementation is being explored as means to prevent PIH.

If the patient is alert and is not nauseated, a high-protein, moderate-sodium diet is appropriate. Low-salt diets are not indicated. Glucocorticoids may be given to the mother intramuscularly at least 48 hours before delivery to assist in maturing fetal lungs to decrease the severity of respiratory difficulties in the neonate. A cesarean section is indicated if the fetus is showing signs of distress or if PIH is severe and the patient is not responding to aggressive treatment. All efforts are made to stabilize the patient's condition before surgery.

PHARMACOLOGIC HIGHLIGHTS

Medication or Drug Class	Dosage	Description	Rationale
Magnesium sulfate	6 g IV PB loading dose; 2 g per hour IV maintenance dose	Anticonvulsant	PIH can progress to eclampsia; drug of choice to prevent seizures
Calcium gluconate	1 g IVP slowly over 3 minutes	Antidote for magnesium sulfate	Respiratory depression occurs with magnesium toxicity
Methyldopa (Aldomet) normodyne (Labetalol) nifedipine (Procardia) hydralazine (Apresoline)	Varies with drug (po) (po) (po) (po or IV)	Antihypertensive	Given if diastolic is > 110 mm Hg; IV medication is used if oral is ineffective

Independent

Maintain the patient on bed rest in the left lateral position as much as possible. This position assists with venous return and organ perfusion. Maintain a quiet, dim environment for rest, close to the nurse's station. Eliminate extraneous noises, lights, visitors, and interruptions that might precipitate a seizure. Plan assessments and care to ensure optimal rest. Pad the side rails, and keep the bed in the low position with the call light in reach at all times. To be prepared for emergencies, keep a "toxemia kit" at the bedside, which includes an artificial airway, calcium gluconate, syringes, alcohol pads, and other medications.

If the patient is in labor, closely monitor fetal heart rate patterns and contractions. If the fetal heart rate shows signs of stress, turn the patient to her left side, increase the rate of the IV fluids, administer a humidified oxygen per mask at 10 L/min, and notify the physician. Because abruptio placentae is a potential complication of PIH, be alert for any of the following signs of placental detachment: profuse vaginal bleeding, increased abdominal pain, and a rigid abdomen. The fetus also shows signs of distress (late decelerations, bradycardia).

Provide emotional support to the patient and family. The onset and severity of PIH, along with its potential outcomes for the infant, are worrisome. If delivery of a preterm infant is imminent, educate the family on the environment and care given in the neonatal intensive care unit (NICU). Tour the NICU with the father, and explain what can be expected after the birth. This preparation helps alleviate some of the new parents' fears after the delivery.

After delivery, complications of PIH can still manifest over the next 48 hours.

Continue ongoing monitoring; be alert for seizures and indications that the patient is going into HELLP syndrome.

DOCUMENTATION GUIDELINES

- Vital signs: Blood pressure (value and patient's position); heart rate; daily weights; intake and output
- Edema: Location, presence or absence of pitting, numerical rating (1 to 4)
- Reflexes rated on a 1 to 4 scale and presence or absence of clonus
- Presence or absence of headache, visual disturbances, altered sensorium, epigastric discomfort, nausea
- Response to treatment: Anticonvulsants, antihypertensives, sedatives, bed rest
- Fetal assessment: Baseline heart rate; presence or absence of accelerations, decelerations, variability, fetal movement; response to movement
- Patient's response to pain during labor and to pain relief measures (analgesics, epidural)

DISCHARGE AND HOME HEALTHCARE GUIDELINES

HOME CARE IF UNDELIVERED. If the patient is discharged undelivered, emphasize that follow-up appointments are important for timely diagnosis of progressive PIH. Educate the patient on the importance of the left lateral position for bed rest. Tell the patient to notify the physician immediately for any of the following symptoms: headache; visual disturbance; right upper quadrant pain; change in level of consciousness or "feeling funny"; decreased urine output; increase in edema, especially facial; or any decrease in fetal movement. Tell the patient to weigh herself daily and notify the physician of a sudden weight gain. Be sure the patient understands the seriousness of the disorder and the potential complications to her and her infant.

HOME CARE IF DELIVERED. If the patient is discharged delivered, she needs to receive similar teaching because PIH does not resolve immediately after delivery.

Premature Rupture of Membranes

DRG Category: 373
Mean LOS: 1.9 days
Description: MEDICAL: Vaginal Delivery without Complicating Diagnoses
DRG Category: 370
Mean LOS: 4.9 days
Description: SURGICAL: Cesarean Section with CC

Premature rupture of membranes (PROM) refers to the spontaneous rupturing of the amniotic membranes ("bag of water") before the onset of true labor. It can occur at any gestational age; however, between the end of the 20th week and the end of the 36th week, it is referred to as preterm premature rupture of membranes (PPROM). PPROM occurs in 33% of all preterm births and is a major contributor to perinatal morbidity and mortality. PROM can result in two major complications. First is the delivery of a preterm infant, which can have many problems, the most frequent being respiratory distress because of lung immaturity. Second is that the mother and fetus can develop an infection. The amniotic sac serves as a barrier to prevent bacteria from entering the uterus from the vagina; once the sac is broken, bacteria can move freely upward and cause infection in the mother and the fetus. Furthermore, if the labor must be augmented because of PROM, and the cervix is not ripe, the patient is at a higher risk for a cesarean delivery.

CAUSES

Although the specific cause of PROM is unknown, there are many predisposing factors. An incompetent cervix leads to PROM in the second trimester. Infections such as cervicitis and amnionitis—and also placenta previa, abruptio placentae, and a history of induced abortions—may be involved with PROM. Additionally, any condition that places undue stress on the uterus, such as multiple gestation, polyhydramnios, or trauma, can contribute to PROM. Fetal factors involved are genetic abnormalities and fetal malpresentation. A defect in the membrane itself is also a suspected cause.

GENDER AND LIFE SPAN CONSIDERATIONS

PROM occurs in 3% to 17% of all deliveries, but it is not associated with maternal age.

☐ ASSESSMENT

HISTORY. Ask the patient the date of her last menstrual period to determine the fetus's gestational age. Ask her if she has been feeling the baby move. Review the prenatal record if it is available, or question the patient about problems with the pregnancy, such as high blood pressure, gestational diabetes, bleeding, premature labor, illnesses, and trauma. Have the patient describe the circumstances leading to PROM. Determine the time the rupture occurred, the color of the fluid and the amount, and if there was an odor to the fluid. Patients can report a sudden gush of fluid or a feeling of "always being wet." Inquire about any urinary, vaginal, or pelvic infections. Ask about cigarette, alcohol, and drug use and exposure to teratogens.

PHYSICAL EXAMINATION. The priority assessment is auscultation of the fetal heart rate (FHR). Fetal tachycardia indicates infection. FHR may be decreased or absent during early pregnancy or if the umbilical cord prolapsed. If bradycardia is noted, perform a sterile vaginal examination to check for an umbilical cord. If a cord is felt, place the patient in Trendelenburg's position, maintain manual removal of the presenting part off of the umbilical cord, and notify the physician immediately.

Note the frequency, duration, and intensity of any contractions. With PROM, contractions are absent. Perform a sterile vaginal examination if the patient is term (> 37 weeks), and note the dilation and effacement of the cervix and the station and presentation of the fetus. If the patient is preterm, notify the physician before doing a vaginal examination, which is often deferred in preterm patients to decrease the likelihood of introducing infection.

It is important in the initial examination to determine if PROM actually occurred. Often, urinary incontinence, loss of the mucous plug, and increased leukorrhea, which are common occurrences during the third trimester, are mistaken for PROM. Inspect the perineum and vaginal vault for presence of fluid, noting the color, consistency, and any foul odor. Normally, amniotic fluid is clear or sometimes blood-tinged with small white particles of vernix. Meconium-stained fluid, which results from the fetus passing stool in utero, can be stained from a light tan to thick green, resembling split pea soup. Take the patient's vital signs. An elevated temperature and tachycardia are signs that infection is present as a result of PROM. Auscultate the lungs bilaterally. Palpate the uterus for tenderness, which is often present if infection is present. Check the patient's reflexes, and inspect all extremities for edema.

PSYCHOSOCIAL. If the pregnancy is term, most patients are elated with the occurrence of rupture of membranes, even though they are not having contractions. If the patient is preterm, PROM is extremely upsetting. Assess the patient's relationship with her significant other and available support.

DIAGNOSTIC HIGHLIGHTS

Test	Normal Result	Abnormality with Condition	Explanation
Nitrazine test tape	Yellow to olive green indicates acidic, and intact membranes	Blue-green to deep blue indicates alkaline, membranes probably ruptured	Amniotic fluid is alkaline and thus turns the yellow paper blue
Speculum exam and fern test	No fluid is seen in vaginal vault, fern pattern is not noted on slide	Fluid is visualized at cervical os; microscope slide reveals fern pattern	Amniotic fluid possesses ferning capacity evident by microscopic examination of a prepped slide

Other Tests: Complete blood count (CBC), cervical cultures for infections, amniocentesis (to check lung maturity if PPROM has occurred), ultrasound

PRIMARY NURSING DIAGNOSIS

Risk for infection related to loss of protective barrier

OUTCOMES. Risk control; Risk detection; Knowledge: Infection control

INTERVENTIONS. High-risk pregnancy care; Infection control; Labor induction: surveillance; Electronic fetal monitoring: Intrapartum

☐ PLANNING AND IMPLEMENTATION

Collaborative

Treatment varies, depending on the gestational age of the fetus and the presence of infection. If infection is present, the fetus is delivered promptly, regardless of gestational age. Delivery can be vaginal (induced) or by cesarean section. Intravenous antibiotics are begun immediately. The antibiotics cross the placenta and are thought to provide some protection to the fetus.

If the patient is preterm (< 37 weeks) and has no signs of infection, the patient is maintained on complete bed rest. A weekly nonstress test, contraction stress test, and biophysical profile are done to continually assess fetal well-being. If the gestational age is between 28 and 32 weeks, glucocorticoids are administered to accelerate fetal lung maturity. Use of tocolysis to stop contractions if they begin is controversial when rupture of membranes has occurred. Some patients are discharged on bed rest with bathroom privileges if the leakage of fluid ceases, no contractions are noted, and there are no signs and symptoms of infection; however, most physicians prefer to keep the patient hospitalized because of the high risk of infection.

If the patient is term and PROM has occurred, the labor can be augmented with oxytocin. It is always desirable to deliver a term infant within 24 hours of rupture of membranes because the likelihood of infection is decreased. Some patients and physicians prefer to wait 24 to 48 hours and let labor start on its own without the use of oxytocin. If this is the case, monitoring for signs and symptoms of infection and fetal well-being is critical. If the patient has an epidural, turn her from side to side hourly to ensure adequate distribution of anesthesia. Use pillows to support the back and abdomen and between the knees to maintain proper body alignment. Most patients are unable to void and require a straight catheter every 2 to 3 hours to keep the bladder empty; if a long labor is anticipated, sometimes a urinary catheter is inserted. Maintain the infusion of intravenous (IV) fluids to prevent hypotension, which can result from regional anesthesia.

Determine the patient's preference for pain relief during labor. If IV narcotics are used, assess the effects of these drugs on the respiratory status of the neonate upon birth. The neonatal nurse or nurse practitioner should be on hand to reverse respiratory depression at delivery. Many patients who receive oxytocin request an epidural because IV narcotics do not provide effective pain relief.

PHARMACOLOGIC HIGHLIGHTS

Medication or Drug Class	Dosage	Description	Rationale
Ampicillin, or Other antibiotics	1–2 g q 6 hours IVPB Dosage varies with drug	Antibiotic	Prophylaxis; treatment for infection
Oxytocin (Pitocin)	Mix 10 U in 500 mL of IV solution, begin infusion at 1 mU per minute and increase 1–2 mU per minute q 30 minutes	Oxytocic	Brings on labor contractions
Meperidine (Demerol);	25 mg IVP q 3–4 hours	Opiod analgesic	Pain relief of labor contractions
Butorphanol tartrate (Stadol)	1–2 mg q 3–4 hours IVP		

Independent

Teach every prenatal patient from the beginning to call the physician if she suspects rupture of membranes. If rupture of membranes occurs, monitor for signs and symptoms of infection and the onset of labor. Maintain the patient in the left lateral recumbent position as much as possible to provide optimal uteroplacental perfusion.

Assist the patient who is having natural childbirth in breathing and relaxation techniques. Often the coach plays a significant role in helping the patient deal with the contractions. The nurse should become involved only when necessary. If a preterm delivery is expected, educate the patient and family on the expected care of the newborn in the neonatal intensive care unit (NICU). If possible, allow the patient to visit the NICU and talk to a neonatologist.

Hospital stay for a vaginal delivery is 24 hours and for a cesarean section 72 hours. Teach the patient as much as possible about self-care and newborn care while in the hospital. Arrange for a follow-up home visit by a perinatal nurse. If the baby is retained in the NICU after the patient is discharged, support and educate the family as they return to the hospital to visit their newborn.

DOCUMENTATION GUIDELINES

- Time of rupture of membranes, color of fluid, amount of fluid, presence of any odor
- Contractions: Frequency, duration, intensity, pattern, patient's response
- FHR assessment: Baseline, accelerations, decelerations, variability
- Patient's comfort level in labor, response to medications, vital signs

DISCHARGE AND HOME HEALTHCARE GUIDELINES

HOME CARE IF UNDELIVERED. The patient should maintain bed rest, check her temperature four times per day, abstain from intercourse, not douche or use tampons, and have a WBC count drawn every other day. Tell her to notify the physician immediately of any fever, uterine tenderness or contractions, leakage of fluid, or foul vaginal odor.

HOME CARE IF DELIVERED. Teach the patient to be aware of signs and symptoms that indicate postpartum complications. Teach her not to lift anything heavier than the baby and not to drive until after the postpartum checkup with the

Pressure Ulcer

DRG Category: 271
Mean LOS: 7.5 days
Description: MEDICAL: Skin Ulcers
DRG Category: 263
Mean LOS: 12.5 days
Description: SURGICAL: Skin Graft and/or Debride for Skin Ulcer or Cellulitis with CC

A pressure ulcer is an irregularly shaped, depressed area that resulted from necrosis of the epidermis and/or dermis layers of the skin. Prolonged pressure causes inadequate circulation, ischemic ulceration, and tissue breakdown. Muscle tissue seems particularly susceptible to ischemia. Pressure ulcers may occur in any area of the body but occur mostly over bony prominences that can include the occiput, thoracic and lumbar vertebrae, scapula, coccyx, sacrum, greater trochanter, ischial tuberosity, lateral knee, medial and lateral malleolus, metatarsals, and calcaneus. Some 96% of pressure ulcers develop in the lower part of the body. Pressure ulcers have been staged by the National Ulcer Advisory Panel, but the stages serve as a description only and do not necessarily provide an order for progression. (See Table 44.)

TABLE 44 | **Staging of Pressure Ulcers**

STAGE	DESCRIPTION
I	Nonblancable erythema; involves changes in the underling vessels of the skin; bright red color that does not resolve after 30 minutes of pressure relief; can be painful and tender
II	Partial thickness skin loss of epidermis and dermis; cracks or blisters on skin with erythema and/or indurations.
III	Full-thickness skin loss of epidermis and dermis; extends down to subcutaneous tissue; appears as a crater or covered by black eschar, wound base usually not painful; indistinct borders; may have sinus tracts or undermining present.
IV	Full-thickness skin loss with extensive destruction of tissue, muscle, bone, and/or supporting structures; appears as a deep crater or is covered by thick eschar; wound base not painful; may have sinus tracts and undermining present

CAUSES

When external pressure exceeds normal capillary pressure of 25 mm Hg, blood flow in the capillary beds is decreased. When the external pressure surpasses arteriole pressure, blood flow to the area is impaired. Ischemia occurs when the pressure exceeds 50 mm Hg and blood flow is completely blocked. Pressure from the bony prominence is transmitted from the surface of the body to the underlying bone, and all underlying tissues are compressed.

Pressure ulcers caused by shearing or friction result when one tissue layer slides over another. Shearing results in stretching and angulating of blood vessels, causing injury and thrombosis to the area. These injuries commonly occur when the head of the bed is elevated, causing the torso to slide downward.

GENDER AND LIFE SPAN CONSIDERATIONS

Pressure ulcers can occur at any age and across both genders but are more prevalent in the elderly population over 70 years of age. About 25% of the elderly have some type of pressure ulcer.

□ ASSESSMENT

HISTORY. Generally, patients have a history of a condition that causes decreased circulation and sensation leading to inadequate tissue perfusion. Associated diseases and conditions include diabetes mellitus, arterial insufficiency, peripheral vascular disease, and decreased activity and mobility or spinal cord injury. Patients with casts, braces, and splints are also predisposed to developing pressure ulcers.

PHYSICAL EXAMINATION. The clinical manifestations of pressure ulcers are generally described in four stages that reflect the amount of tissue injury and the degree of underlying structural damage. Assess the wound to determine the precise location, along with size and depth. The color of the wound (whether pink, red, yellow, or black) indicates the stage of healing and the presence of epithelial tissue. A beefy red color signifies the presence of granulation tissue and denotes adequate healing. Black tissue indicates necrotic and devitalized tissue and signifies delayed healing. Observe for areas of sinus tracts and undermining, which indicate deeper involvement under intact wound margins. Determine the amount of drainage and the type, color, odor, consistency, and quantity. Assess the area around the wound for redness, edema, indurations, tenderness, and breakdown of healed tissues to identify signs and symptoms of infection.

PSYCHOSOCIAL ASSESSMENT. The patient may exhibit signs of anxiety and depression because of the potential setback in an already long list of medical problems. The condition may slow the patient's progress toward independence or necessitate a move from home to a nursing home for an elderly patient.

DIAGNOSTIC HIGHLIGHTS

Test	Normal Result	Abnormality with Condition	Explanation
Skin or wound culture and sensitivity	Negative for microorganisms	Positive for microorganisms	Some pressure ulcers become infected, which slows healing

Other Tests: Supporting tests include hemoglobin and hematocrit levels (weekly), white blood cell differentials, and albumin and total protein levels.

PRIMARY NURSING DIAGNOSIS

Impaired skin integrity related to pressure over bony prominences or shearing forces

OUTCOMES. Tissue integrity: Skin and mucous membranes; Wound healing: Primary intention; Immobility consequences: Physiological; Knowledge: Treatment regime; Nutritional status; Tissue perfusion: Peripheral; Treatment behavior: Illness or injury

INTERVENTIONS. Wound care; Skin surveillance; Positioning; Pressure management; Pressure ulcer prevention; Medication administration: Topical; Circulatory precautions; Infection control; Nutrition management

◘ PLANNING AND IMPLEMENTATION

Collaborative

In the early stages pressure ulcers are best handled by nursing rather than medical interventions. Surgical intervention may be necessary to excise necrotic tissue in late stages of ulcer development. Skin grafts or musculocutaneous flaps may be indicated in very deep wounds in which healing is difficult or has been unsuccessful in completely covering the area. Drains may be inserted to prevent fluid buildup in the wound. The drains facilitate the removal of blood and bacteria from the wound that can increase the risk of infection.

Mechanical debridement by an enzymatic agent (collagenase [Santyl]) may be ordered. Other types of wound care dressings include hydrocolloid, hydrogels, calcium alginates, film dressings, and topical agents and solutions. The type of dressing depends on the depth of the wound and the amount of debridement of necrotic tissue or support of granulation tissue required. In general, the following guidelines might be helpful in ulcer management, although management may depend on the particular ulcer and patient:

Stage I ulcers require no type of dressings.

Stage II pressure ulcers are treated with moist or occlusive dressings to maintain a moist, healing environment.

Stage III ulcers require debridement, usually with an enzymatic agent or wet-to-moist normal saline soak.

Stage IV ulcers are treated like stage III ulcers or by surgical excision and grafting. All wounds, however, are assessed before treatment because all wounds are different, and similar treatments may not be successful for dissimilar wounds.

A dietitian may assess the nutritional state of the patient to determine adequate vitamin and nutrient intake, with a particular focus on vitamins A, C, and B complex.

Hyperbaric oxygen therapy may be indicated for wounds that are deep and difficult to treat. This method delivers 100% oxygen to wounds at greater than atmospheric pressure several times a week or every day until healing or other treatments are indicated. Do not use lotions, cosmetics, perfume, hair spray or petroleum-based products on the patient's skin before the treatment. Monitor the patient for anxiety and claustrophobia when he or she is placed in an enclosed chamber. Electrotherapy is a method of delivering low-intensity direct current to wounds in attempts to assist the healing process. The amount of electricity is determined by the depth of the injury. Treatments vary from 15 minutes each day to 2 hours of stimulation twice a day.

PHARMACOLOGIC HIGHLIGHTS

Medication or Drug Class	Dosage	Description	Rationale
Hydrocolloids	No dosage; prepackaged wafers	Occlusive, adhesive wafers such as	Provides a moist and protective

		DouDerm or ConvaTac	environment for shallow wounds with light exudates; may remain in place for 3–5 days
Hydrogels	No dosage; topical gel	Glycerin-based gel such as IntraSite	Gel promotes healing by rehydrating necrotic tissue, facilitating debridement, and absorbing exudates to maintain moist environment
Alginates	No dosage; prepackaged pads	Pads formed from brown seaweed; Kaltostat	Absorbent; used to treat deep wounds with heavy drainage
Adhesive films	No dosage; prepackaged pads	Plastic, self-adhering membrane; Tegaderm	Self-adhering but waterproof wafers that are permeable to oxygen and water vapor; appropriate for partial-thickness wounds; useful as secondary dressings for wounds treated with hydrocolloids or alginates

Independent

The most important nursing intervention is prevention. Identify patients who are at risk by using assessment tools such as the Braden scale or the Norton scale, which determine the sensory and physiologic factors that increase the incidence of pressure ulcers. The high-risk patient needs turning and proper positioning at least every 2 hours. Pressure-relieving devices, such as silicone-filled pads and foam mattresses, may be helpful. Dynamic devices include specialty beds (low-air-loss, air-fluidized, and air cushions). Airflow pressure mattresses are also useful preventive strategies.

Keep the patient's skin dry. Patients who are incontinent of feces and urine should be cleaned as soon as possible to prevent skin irritation. When soiling of the skin cannot be controlled, use absorbent underpads and topical agents that act as moisture barriers. Avoid the use of hot water, and use a mild cleansing agent to minimize dryness and irritation in high-risk patients. Treat dry skin with moisturizers, but use care in massaging bony prominences as this may impede capillary blood flow and increase the risk of deep tissue injury. Lift high-risk patients up in bed instead of pulling them, which increases the risk of shearing and friction forces on the skin's surfaces. To prevent the patient from sliding down in bed, do not elevate the patient's head more than 20 degrees unless this angle is contraindicated because of other medical problems or treatment modalities. Keep linens dry and wrinkle-free. When skin breakdown occurs, apply appropriate dressings using clean technique or, in cases which infection is present, sterile technique.

Teach the caregiver preventive strategies, and determine if the patient's situation is in jeopardy because of inadequate care. Note that the caregiver may have feelings of guilt because of the failure to prevent complications of immobility; the caregiver may need support rather than teaching, depending on the situation.

DOCUMENTATION GUIDELINES

- Physical findings of assessment for potential skin breakdown: Redness and dryness
- Physical findings of direct wound assessment: Size, depth, type of tissue present (granulation, necrotic), drainage; signs of infection
- Type and frequency of dressing changes with sequencing of how the wound was cleaned and the dressing applied
- Response to treatments: Surgery, wound debridement, dressing, medication application

DISCHARGE AND HOME HEALTHCARE GUIDELINES

Refer patients at increased risk for skin breakdown to a home healthcare agency to assist with monitoring skin and providing pressure-relieving devices in the home environment. Teach the patient or caregiver about frequent turning and positioning, how to keep the skin clean and dry, signs and symptoms of early breakdown and complications of existing ulcers, strategies to manage redness or skin breakdown, appropriate wound care and dressing techniques. Use a return demonstration before discharge to assess the understanding and ability to perform wound care.

Preterm Labor

DRG Category: 379
Mean LOS: 2.1 days
Description: MEDICAL: Threatened Abortions
DRG Category: 373
Mean LOS: 1.9 days
Description: MEDICAL: Vaginal Delivery without Complicating Diagnoses

Preterm labor (PTL) refers to labor that occurs after the completion of the 20th week and before the beginning of the 37th week of gestation. In order to be considered preterm labor, the uterine contractions must occur at a frequency of 4 in 20 minutes or 8 in 60 minutes. Spontaneous rupture of the membranes often occurs in PTL. If the membranes are intact, documented cervical change (80% effacement or 2-cm dilation) must be noted during a vaginal examination for the situation to be classified as PTL.

PTL is the number one cause of the high infant morbidity and mortality rate in the United States. From 8% to 10% of all births in the United States are preterm. The major fetal risk of preterm delivery is related to immaturity of the lungs and respiratory system. Preterm infants can have many other problems as well, such as neurologic complications, thermoregulation problems, and immaturity of major organ systems. Maternal risks of preterm labor are related to the pharmacologic treatment involved in stopping the labor.

CAUSES

In many cases, the cause cannot be identified. Preterm premature rupture of membranes occurs in about one-third of the cases, but its causes are also unknown. Intrauterine infection can precede or follow premature rupture of membranes. Several risk factors have been identified. (See Box 12.)

BOX 12   RISK FACTORS FOR PRETERM LABOR
Historical
Preterm labor
Preterm delivery
Cone biopsy
Induced or habitual abortions
Diethystilbesterol exposure
Uterine leiomyomas or cervical anomalies
Renal disease
Hypertension
Prepregnancy weight < 100 lb
Obstetric-Related
Cervical incompetence
Placenta previa or abruption
Hydramnios
Maternal infection
Abdominal surgery during pregnancy
Fetal-Related
Multiple gestation
Fetal anomalies

GENDER AND LIFE SPAN CONSIDERATIONS

Women who are younger than 19 or older than 35 years of age are more likely to have PTL. PTL is more prevalent in African-Americans than in European-Americans; it is also associated with low socioeconomic status, low educational level, and single parenthood.

☐ ASSESSMENT

HISTORY. Ask the date of the patient's last menstrual period to estimate delivery date. If the patient reports using cigarettes, alcohol, or other harmful substances, determine the amount and frequency. Ask about the onset of contractions and their frequency, duration, and intensity. (See Box 13.)

BOX 13	SIGNS AND SYMPTOMS OF PRETERM LABOR

Uterine contractions, cramping, lower back pain
Feeling of pelvic pressure or fullness
Change in the amount or character of amniotic fluid
Blood show
Gastrointestinal upset: Nausea, vomiting, diarrhea
General sense of discomfort or "just feeling bad"
Sensation that baby is frequently "balling up"

Have the patient describe the contractions; sometimes false labor is felt in the lower abdomen and is irregular. Ask if the patient feels the baby move. Ask about any medical problems because some pharmacologic treatment may be contraindicated in certain instances (cardiac disease, hypertension, renal disease, uncontrolled diabetes, and asthma).

PHYSICAL EXAMINATION. A thorough initial examination is needed to help determine if the patient is in PTL or in false labor. Apply a fetal monitor to determine the frequency and duration of contractions. Palpate the fundus of the uterus; if the patient is having PTL, note uterine firmness. Obtain the fetal heart rate with an electronic fetal monitor, noting baseline, presence or absence of accelerations or decelerations, and variability. After checking with the physician, perform a sterile vaginal examination to determine dilation, station, and effacement. Note any vaginal bleeding, bloody show, or leakage of amniotic fluid. Nitrazine (pH) paper can be used during the examination to detect if the membranes have ruptured (paper turns blue because pH is alkaline). Note that an elevated temperature indicates infection or dehydration.

PSYCHOSOCIAL. The reality of a premature delivery and a sick newborn in a neonatal intensive care unit (NICU) creates a tremendous amount of stress and emotion for the parents and significant others. Assess the patient's and the significant others' abilities to cope. The patient may experience guilt, suspecting that she did something wrong during the pregnancy to precipitate the labor.

DIAGNOSTIC HIGHLIGHTS

General Comments: Preterm labor is generally diagnosed by the presence of contractions accompanied by cervical change. Testing is done to examine the possibility of delivery and cervical ripeness.

Test	Normal Result	Abnormality with Condition	Explanation
Fetal fibronectin (fFN)	Absent in cervico-vaginal secretions between 20 and 37 weeks	Positive	If positive, 60%, will deliver within 1 week; if negative, 99.3% do not deliver within 1 week
Cervical length (via transvaginal	> 30 mm; no evidence of a	< 25 mm (10th percentile) or	Cervical effacement indicates that the

ultrasound)	bulging bag of water or leakage of fluid	evidence of funneling or leaking of the amniotic fluid at the internal os	cervix is ripening for labor

Other Tests: An abdominal ultrasound to assess the size and well-being of the infant, amniocentesis to obtain amniotic fluid to perform tests to determine fetal lung maturity; complete blood count (CBC); vaginal/cervical/urine cultures (infections often precede preterm labor)

PRIMARY NURSING DIAGNOSIS

Fear related to uncertainty of outcome and complexity/effects of treatments

OUTCOMES. Fear control; Anxiety control; Comfort level; Coping

INTERVENTIONS. Labor suppression; High-risk pregnancy care; Security enhancement; Resuscitation: Fetus

☐ PLANNING AND IMPLEMENTATION

Collaborative

The goals of treatment are to stop the contractions and to prevent the cervix from dilating, thereby keeping the fetus in utero as long as possible until term. Once the cervix reaches 4 cm in dilation, treatment is stopped and the delivery is allowed to occur. Ideally, delivery is in a hospital with the expertise necessary to treat a preterm neonate.

About 50% of all PTL can be halted with the conservative treatment of bed rest and hydration. Administer intravenous (IV) fluids, usually a crystalloid such as lactated Ringer's solution. If the patient is anxious, sedatives are used cautiously. Terbutaline sulfate subcutaneously is often given, along with hydration. If the contractions stop and the labor is not progressing, patients are discharged home on complete bed rest. Home monitoring of uterine contractions with transmission of data to the physician is possible. Also, patients may be discharged with a terbutaline pump, which infuses 3 to 4 mg of terbutaline subcutaneously each day.

If labor continues, IV medications are indicated. Tocolysis (inhibition of uterine contractions) is contraindicated in cases of maternal infection, pregnancy-induced hypertension, hypovolemia, and fetal distress. During the initial period of infusion of beta-adrenergic drugs, auscultate the patient's lungs for rales and rhonchi; observe for dyspnea and chest discomfort; determine the fetal heart rate, maternal pulse, blood pressure, and respiratory rate; and monitor the status of contractions every 10 minutes. Monitor serum glucose and potassium levels, as ritodrine often increases glucose levels and decreases potassium. If glucocorticoids are administered concurrently, monitor the patient for signs and symptoms of pulmonary edema. If magnesium sulfate is used for tocolysis, closely monitor deep tendon reflexes; hyporeflexia occurs if the patient is becoming toxic and precedes respiratory depression. If tocolysis is successful, and contractions are under control, the infusion is discontinued by gradually decreasing the rate, and converting to oral administration.

Monitor the fetal heart rate variability and for the absence or presence of accelerations and decelerations. If signs of fetal stress occur, turn the patient on her left side, increase the rate of the IV hydration, administer oxygen at 10 L per minute per mask, and notify the physician.

Delivery of the preterm infant can be done vaginally or by cesarean. The decision for the method of delivery is often made jointly by the physician, neonatologist, and parents. If the fetus is very premature, often the neonatologist suggests a cesarean to prevent trauma to the fetal head and an increased risk of intraventricular hemorrhage.

PHARMACOLOGIC HIGHLIGHTS

Medication of Drug Class	Dosage	Description	Rationale
Ritodrine (Yutopar)	Initially, .05–.10 mg per minute; then increase .05 mg per minute q 10 minutes, for a maximum dose .35 mg per minute; after IV is discontinued, 10 mg po q 2 hours for 24 hours, then, 10–20 mg q 4–6 hours	Beta-adrenergic, uterine relaxant (only FDA approved drug for PTL)	Relaxes the uterus
Terbutaline (Brethine)	Initially, 2.5 µg per minute; increase to a max of 20 µg per minute OR 0.25 mg SQ q 20 minutes × 3 doses, then q 3 hours; after IV is dc/d, follow with 5 mg po q 4–6 hours	Beta-adrenergic	Less expensive than ritodrine, effective tocolytic
Magnesium sulfate	4–6 g IV loading dose, 1–4 g per hour of IV maintenance	Anticonvulsant	Effective tocolytic, has fewer side effects than beta-adrenergic drugs
Nifedipine	10–20 mg q 6 hours	Calcium channel blocker	Considered second line therapy; only recently used for PTL
Betamethasone (Celestone)	12 mg IM q 24 hours × 2	Glucocorticoid	Hastens fetal lung maturity; indicated if delivery is anticipated between 24 and 34 weeks

dc/d: discontinued

Independent

Prevention of PTL is an important function of the nurse. During the initial prenatal visit, educate the patient on the signs and symptoms of PTL and ask the patient on subsequent visits if she is experiencing any of these indicators. If a patient reports alcohol, cigarette, or drug use any time during the pregnancy, work with her to modify her behavior. A referral to a drug treatment, smoking cessation, or alcohol counseling program may be indicated. Encourage patients to stay well hydrated, especially during the warm weather, because dehydration can cause contractions. Additionally, nurses can become involved in community education of adolescents and women about the symptoms, risk factors, and consequences of PTL.

Admission to the hospital for PTL is often a first hospitalization for many young patients. Provide emotional support and educate the patient on simple procedures that may seem routine (drawing laboratory work, frequent assessments done by nurses and physicians, mealtimes and menus). Discuss the implications and expectations of preterm delivery. Be realistic in the discussions and, if possible, arrange for a visit to the NICU and a talk with the neonatologist. Include the family in conversations with the patient, and encourage them to assist with caring for the patient while she is on bed rest. Often the patient is on bed rest for several days in the hospital and at home. While she is in the hospital, suggest diversional activities, such as videos, special visitors, games, etc.

DOCUMENTATION GUIDELINES

- Contraction status: Frequency, intensity, duration
- Fetal heart rate: Baseline, variability, accelerations, decelerations
- Patient's response to bed rest and hydration
- Patient's response to tocolysis: vital signs, anxiety, ability to sleep, deep tendon reflexes, lung sounds, intake and output

DISCHARGE AND HOME HEALTHCARE GUIDELINES

HOME CARE IF UNDELIVERED. Discuss the importance of maintaining bed rest in the lateral position. Teach the patient to remain well hydrated, take all medications exactly as prescribed, and report any uncomfortable side effects to the physician. Teach the patient to avoid any activity that could possibly initiate labor (sexual intercourse, nipple stimulation). Explain that the patient should check daily to determine whether the fetus is moving or the uterus is contracting. Teach the patient how to palpate the fundus and judge the intensity of a contraction. Teach the patient how to use the home monitor for uterine contractions and the terbutaline pump if ordered. Review the warning signs of PTL and when she should call the physician.

HOME CARE IF DELIVERED. Teach the patient to be aware of signs and symptoms that indicate postpartum complications: a hard, reddened area on the breast; pain in the calf of the leg; increase in bleeding; foul odor to vaginal discharge; fever; burning with urination; or persistent mood change. Teach her not to lift anything heavier than the baby and not to drive until after the postpartum checkup with the physician. Encourage her to maintain a healthy diet and adequate nutrition and to schedule rest time around the baby's sleeping times. Elicit the help of family members if needed.

Prostate Cancer

DRG Category: 346
Mean LOS: 5.3 days
Description: MEDICAL: Malignancy, Male Reproductive System with CC
DRG Category: 336
Mean LOS: 4.0 days
Description: SURGICAL: Transurethral Prostatectomy with CC

Prostate cancer is the most common type of cancer in men and the third leading cause of death among men in the United States. Adenocarcinomas compose 95% of the prostate cancers. They most frequently begin in the outer portion of the posterior lobe of the prostate gland. Local spread occurs to the seminal vesicles, bladder, and peritoneum. Prostate cancer metastasizes to other sites via the hematologic and lymphatic systems, following a fairly predictable pattern. The pelvic and perivesicular lymph nodes and bones of the pelvis, sacrum, and lumbar spine are usually the first areas to be affected. Metastasis to other organs usually occurs late in the course of the disease, with the lungs, liver, and kidneys being most frequently involved.

Although the recommendation is controversial, the American Cancer Society now advises screening for prostate cancer in asymptomatic men beginning at age 40. American Cancer Society guidelines include an annual digital rectal examination beginning at age 40 and annual serum prostate-specific antigen (PSA) testing beginning at age 50.

CAUSES

The cause of prostate cancer remains unclear, but age, viruses, and androgens are thought to have contributing roles. A family history of prostate cancer, a high-fat diet, and environmental exposure to cadmium (an element found in cigarettes and alkaline batteries) are also considered risk factors.

GENDER AND LIFE SPAN CONSIDERATIONS

The peak incidence of prostate cancer is in men between the ages of 60 and 70; 80% of the cases are diagnosed in men over the age of 65. The highest incidence of prostate cancer occurs in African-American men. Prostate cancer is rare in men under the age of 40, but when the disease occurs in younger men, it is generally more aggressive.

□ ASSESSMENT

HISTORY. Ask about family history of prostate cancer, an occupational exposure to cadmium, and the usual urinary pattern. A patient may report symptoms such as urinary frequency, nocturia, dysuria, slow urinary stream, or hematuria if the disease has spread beyond the periphery of the prostate gland or if benign prostatic hypertrophy is also present. Presenting symptoms that include weight loss and back pain are often indicative of advanced disease.

PHYSICAL EXAMINATION. The physician palpates the prostate gland via a digital rectal examination. A normal prostate gland feels soft, smooth, and rubbery. Early-stage prostate cancer may present as a non-raised, firm lesion with a sharp edge. An advanced lesion is often hard and stone-like with irregular borders. A suspicious prostatic mass is further evaluated by extending the examination to the groin to look for the presence of enlarged or tender lymph nodes.

PSYCHOSOCIAL. Men have reported not having a rectal examination because of embarrassment. Additionally, treatment for prostate cancer can be accompanied by distressful side effects, such as sexual dysfunction and urinary incontinence. Assess the patient's knowledge and feelings related to these issues and the presence of support systems. Note the coping strategies the patient has used in the past to manage stressors. Include the patient's spouse or significant other in conversations.

DIAGNOSTIC HIGHLIGHTS

General Comments: Positive findings during the digital rectal exam and an elevated PSA suggest the diagnosis. Other tests may be needed to confirm and determine metastasis.

Test	Normal Result	Abnormality with Condition	Explanation
Prostate specific antigen (PSA)	< 4 ng/mL	Increased levels, > 10 ng/mL	The higher the level, the greater the tumor burden; can be used to monitor response to treatment or recurrent CA
Transrectal ultrasound (TRUS)	Prostate gland is of normal size, contour, and consistency	Enlarged, solid prostate mass is noted	Can identify prostatic CA early; very small tumors can be detected
Biopsy	Benign	Malignant	Confirms the diagnosis

Other Tests: Computed tomograpy (CT) scan of the abdomen and pelvis, magnetic resonance imaging (MRI), lymphangiogram, intravenous pyelogram, chest x ray, bone scan, laparoscopic pelvic lymphadenectomy, serum reverse transcriptase-polymerase chain reaction (RT-PCR), and acid phosphatase level.

PRIMARY NURSING DIAGNOSIS

Pain (chronic bone) related to metastatic spread of disease

OUTCOMES. Pain control; Pain: Disruptive effects; Well-being

INTERVENTIONS. Analgesic administration; Pain management; Meditation; Transcutaneous electric nerve stimulation (TENS); Hypnosis; Heat/cold application

☐ PLANNING AND IMPLEMENTATION

Collaborative

CONSERVATIVE. Periodic observation, or "watchful waiting," may be proposed to a patient with early-stage, less aggressive prostate cancer. With this option, no specific treatment is given, but the progression of the disease is monitored via periodic diagnostic tests.

SURGICAL. Radical prostatectomy has been the recommended treatment option for men with middle-stage disease because of high cure rates. This procedure removes the entire prostate gland, including the prostatic capsule, the seminal vesicles, and a portion of the bladder neck. Two common side effects of prostatectomy are urinary incontinence and impotence. The urinary incontinence usually resolves with time and after performing Kegel exercises, although 10% to 15% of men continue to experience incontinence 6 months after surgery. Impotence occurs in 85% to 90% of patients. All men who undergo radical prostatectomy lack emission and ejaculation because of the removal of the seminal vesicles and transection of the vas deferens.

Transurethral resection of the prostate (TURP) may be recommended for men with more advanced disease, especially if it is accompanied by symptoms of bladder outlet obstruction. This procedure is not a curative surgical technique for prostate cancer but does remove excess prostatic tissue that is obstructing the flow of urine through the urethra. The incidence of impotence following TURP is rare, although retrograde ejaculation (passage of seminal fluid back into the bladder) almost always occurs because of the destruction of the internal bladder sphincter during the procedure. Many men equate ejaculation with normal sexual functioning, and to some the loss of the ejaculatory sensation may be confused with the loss of sexual interest or potency. Also, a bilateral orchiectomy may be done to eliminate the source of the androgens since 85% of prostatic cancer is related to androgens.

All patients return from surgery with a large-lumen three-way Foley catheter. The large lumen of the catheter and the large volume in the balloon (30 mL) help splint the urethral anastomosis and maintain hemostasis. Blood-tinged urine is common for several days after surgery, but dark red urine may indicate hemorrhage. If continuous urinary drainage is used, maintain the flow rate to keep the urine light pink to yellow in color and free from clots, but avoid overdistension of the bladder.

Antispasmodics may be ordered for bladder spasms. Anticholinergic and antispasmodic drugs may also be prescribed to help relieve urinary incontinence after the Foley catheter is removed. Because of the close proximity of the rectum and the operative site, trauma to the rectum should be avoided as a means of preventing hemorrhage. Stool softeners and a low-residue diet are usually ordered to limit straining with a bowel movement. Rectal tubes, enemas, and rectal thermometers should not be used.

RADIATION. Both external beam radiotherapy and internal implant (brachytherapy) are used in the treatment of prostate cancer. Radiation therapy is also used in areas of bone metastasis. The goal in extensive disease is palliation: Reduce the size of the prostate gland and relieve bone pain. Brachytherapy involving the permanent (iodine-125 or gold-198) or temporary (iridium-192) placement of radioactive isotopes can be used alone or in combination with external radiation therapy.

Patients who receive permanently placed radioisotopes are hospitalized for as long as the radiation source is considered a danger to persons around them. The principles of time, distance, and shielding need to be implemented. Care needs to be exerted so that the radioisotope does not become dislodged. Dressings and bed linens need to be checked by the radiation therapy department before these items are removed from the patient's room.

PHARMACOLOGIC HIGHLIGHTS

Medication or Drug Class	Dosage	Description	Rationale
Acetaminophen/ NSAIDs; opiods; combination opiod/ NSAIDs	Depends on drug	Analgesic	Analgesic is determined by severity of pain; pain may be postoperative or caused by metastasis
Cyclophosphamide (Cytoxan); fluo-rouracil; doxorubi-cin hydrochloride (Adriamycin); paclitaxel (Taxol)	Depends on drug; may be given singly or in combination	Antineoplastic	Used to treat or stabilize the disease
Leuprolide (Lupron)	1 mg per day SQ	Antineoplatic, hormonal agent	Blocks the action/ secretion of androgens, that stimulate tumor growth
Goserelin acetate (Zoladex)	Depends on stage of CA and treatment combination		
Flutamide (Eulexin)	250 mg tid, q 8 hours	Antineoplastic, hormonal agent	Blocks androgens; often given with other similar agents

Experimental Therapy: Finasteride (Proscar), an androgen hormone inhibitor is being investigated as an adjuvant monotherapy following a radical prostatectomy and to prevent progression of first stage prostate cancer.

Independent

Dispel misconceptions, and explain all diagnostic procedures. Patients with early-stage disease need support while they make decisions about treatment options. Encourage the patient and his partner to verbalize their feelings and fears. Clarify the differences between the various treatment options and reinforce the treatment goals. Provide written materials, such as *Facts on Prostate Cancer* published by the American Cancer Society or *What You Need to Know about Prostate Cancer* published by the National Cancer Institute. Suggest that the patient write down questions that arise so they are not forgotten during visits with the physician.

Ask about pain regularly, and assess pain systematically. Believe the patient and family in their reports of pain. Inform the patient and family of options for pain relief as proposed by the National Cancer Institute (pharmacologic, physical, psychosocial, and cognitive-behavioral interventions), and involve the patient and family in determining pain relief measures.

Implement postoperative strategies to decrease complications. Patients are usually able to ambulate on the first day after surgery. Help the patient to get out of bed and walk in the halls to his tolerance level, usually three or four times a day. Once nausea has passed, bowel sounds are present, and fluids are allowed, encourage a fluid intake of 2500 to 3000 mL per day to maintain good urine output. Adequate fluid intake, and thus output, minimizes the formation of blood clots in the urinary bladder that can obstruct the Foley catheter.

Be alert for behavior indicating denial, grief, hostility, or depression. Inform the physician of any ineffective coping behaviors and the patient's need for more information or a referral for counseling. Suggest alternative sexual behaviors, such as touching and caressing. Patients who are undergoing orchiectomy need extensive emotional support. Establish a therapeutic relationship to promote the expression of feelings. Be sensitive to the patient's fear of his loss of masculinity. Reinforce that having the testes removed in adulthood does not affect the ability to have an erection and orgasm.

Stress to patients who are hospitalized for insertion of a radioactive implant that, while the temporary implant is in place, interactions with nurses and other individuals occur only during brief time periods. Attempt to relieve feelings of abandonment and isolation by communicating with the patient via the hospital intercom system. Once the temporary implant has been removed or the permanent radioactive substance has decayed, remind the patient that he is no longer a danger to others.

DOCUMENTATION GUIDELINES

- Description of all dressings, wounds, drainage collection devices, and urinary output; location, color, and amount of drainage; appearance of incision; color and amount of urine; presence of clots in the urine; urinary pattern after catheter removal
- Physical findings related to the pulmonary assessment, abdominal assessment, presence of edema, condition of extremities, bowel patterns, presence of complications (hemorrhage, infection, pulmonary congestion, activity intolerance, unrelieved discomfort, blockage of Foley catheter)
- Urinary pattern following removal of Foley catheter
- Response to potential for alteration in sexual function
- Description of the skin in the radiation field or site of insertion of radiation implant

DISCHARGE AND HOME HEALTHCARE GUIDELINES

TEACHING. Provide the following instructions to patients who have undergone a radical prostatectomy:

Perform Kegel exercises to enhance sphincter control after the Foley catheter is removed. Establish a voiding pattern of every 2 hours during the day and every 4 hours during the night. With each voiding, contract the pelvic muscles to start and stop urinary flow several times. Contract the pelvic floor muscles and the muscle around the anus as though to stop a bowel movement 10 to 20 times, four times each day.

Maintain an oral fluid intake of 2000 to 3000 mL per day. Avoid alcoholic and caffeinated beverages.

Eat high-fiber foods and take stool softeners to prevent constipation. Avoid straining with bowel movements and do not use suppositories and enemas.

Avoid strenuous exercise, heavy lifting, and driving an automobile until the physician allows.

Avoid sitting with the legs in a dependent position for 3 to 4 weeks, and avoid sexual intercourse for 6 weeks.

CARE OF SKIN IN EXTERNAL RADIATION FIELDS. Instruct the patient to do the following: Wash the skin gently with mild soap, rinse with warm water, and pat dry daily.

Leave (not wash off) the dark ink markings that outline the radiation field.

Avoid applying any lotions, perfumes, deodorants, or powder to the treatment area.

Wear soft, nonrestrictive cotton clothing directly over the treatment area.

Protect the skin from sunlight and extreme cold.

CARE AFTER THE INSERTION OF A PERMANENT RADIOISOTOPE. Instruct the patient to observe for lost seeds in bed linens. Teach the patient to use tweezers to place lost seeds in aluminum foil, wrap them tightly, and take them to the radiation oncology department at the hospital. Teach the patient to call the physician if he experiences a temperature over 100°F, burning or difficulty with urination, excessive bleeding or clots in urine, or rectal bleeding.

FOLLOW-UP CARE. Teach the patient when to see the physician for follow-up care and to watch for any sign of recurrent disease.

Prostatitis

DRG Category: 350
Mean LOS: 4.5 days
Description: MEDICAL: Inflammation of the Male Reproductive System
DRG Category: 336
Mean LOS: 4.0 days
Description: SURGICAL: Transurethral Prostatectomy with CC

Prostatitis, an inflammation of the prostate gland is classified in four categories. Acute bacterial prostatitis is an acute, usually gram-negative, bacterial infection of the prostate gland, generally in conjunction with acute bacterial cystitis. Chronic bacterial prostatitis is a subclinical chronic infection of the prostate by bacteria that can be localized in prostatic secretions. Nonbacterial prostatitis is a chronic prostatitis for which there is no identifiable organism. Prostatodynia is a condition in which the patient experiences irritation and pelvic pain on voiding; the symptoms suggest an acute inflammatory process, but there is no evidence of inflammatory cells in the prostatic secretions.

The most common complication of prostatitis is a urinary tract infection. If it is left untreated, a urinary tract infection can progress to prostatic edema, urinary retention, pyelonephritis, epididymitis, and prostatic abscess.

CAUSES

Both acute and chronic prostatitis can result from either the ascent of bacteria in the urethra, the reflux of infected urine, or the spread of bacteria from the rectum via the lymph nodes. Instrumentation (the process of spreading infection during procedures such as cystoscopy or urinary catheterization) is a less common cause. Prostatitis can also occur from sexual intercourse. *Escherichia coli* causes approximately 80% of bacterial prostatitis. Other common bacteria that are involved include pseudomonas, klebsiella, proteus, *Serratia,* and *Enterobacter.* The cause of prostatodynia is uncertain.

GENDER AND LIFE SPAN CONSIDERATIONS

Acute bacterial prostatitis occurs more frequently in older men, probably because of the enlargement of the prostate gland with age. Acute bacterial prostatitis should also be considered as a source of infection in all men with fever of unknown origin. Bacterial prostatitis or abscesses have been found to be more prevalent in patients with acquired immunodeficiency syndrome (AIDS) than in other individuals. Chronic prostatitis affects up to 35% of all men over the age of 50 but is not necessarily associated with infection.

◻ ASSESSMENT

HISTORY. Take a careful history to elicit genitourinary symptoms. Generally, patients with suspected acute bacterial prostatitis have symptoms that are similar to those of a urinary tract infection: dysuria, frequency, urgency, and nocturia. Additionally, patients report perineal pain radiating down to the sacral region of the back, down the penis and suprapubic area, and possibly into the rectal area. Hematuria or a purulent urethral discharge may be present. The patient may also complain of fever, chills, myalgia (muscle aches), arthralgia (painful joints), and malaise. Patients with chronic bacterial prostatitis are usually asymptomatic but complain of chronic cystitis.

PHYSICAL EXAMINATION. Although some patients are asymptomatic, the patient may appear acutely ill with fever, muscle ache, weakness, and malaise. Inspect the urethra for redness, swelling, or discharge. Inspect the urine for cloudiness, purulence, or hematuria. The nurse practitioner or physician palpates the prostate rectally to determine the degree of tenderness and consistency of the gland and to rule out the presence of a perirectal abscess, tumor, or foreign body. In acute bacterial prostatitis, the prostate may feel warm, firm, indurated, swollen, and tender to palpation. In chronic prostatitis, the prostate may be normal or feel boggy or indurated. Prostatic massage should not be performed because of the risk of bacteremia. Patients with chronic bacterial prostatitis have varying symptoms, often symptoms similar to those of acute bacterial prostatitis but milder.

PSYCHOSOCIAL. Discuss the patient's fear of sexually transmitted disease and impotence related to this illness. Assess the patient's ability to cope with a painful, prolonged illness with a high probability of recurrence or chronicity. If the patient has chronic bacterial prostatitis, assess the patient's and partner's coping strategies and support systems.

DIAGNOSTIC HIGHLIGHTS

General Comments: Prostatitis is primarily diagnosed by symptoms; however, a urine culture will confirm the diagnosis and identify the causative organism. Although prostatic massage is not recommended to obtain prostatic fluid, if this is done and leukocytes are present with a negative culture, a diagnosis of non-bacterial prostatitis can be made.

Test	Normal Result	Abnormality with Condition	Explanation
Urine culture	Negative findings	Positive for bacteria growth, > 10,000 bacteria/ mL of urine	The causative pathogen is identified

PRIMARY NURSING DIAGNOSIS

Pain (acute/chronic) related to prostate inflammation and infection

OUTCOMES. Pain control; Pain level; Pain: Disruptive effects

INTERVENTIONS. Analgesic administration; Medication administration; Pain management; Positioning

☐ PLANNING AND IMPLEMENTATION

Collaborative

Most physicians prescribe antibiotic therapy based on the results of the bacterial cultures; sometimes parenteral antibiotics are required if the infection is systemic. Bed rest and local measures such as 20-minute sitz baths two or three times a day can assist in reducing pain. Regular sexual intercourse or ejaculation helps drainage of prostatic secretions and lessens infection and pain after the acute inflammation subsides. For acute episodes, and once antibiotics have been started, some physicians recommend regular prostatic massage for several weeks.

If drug therapy for chronic bacterial prostatitis is unsuccessful, on rare occasions the patient may undergo a transurethral resection of the prostate (TURP) to remove all infected tissue. Because this procedure may lead to retrograde ejaculation and sterility, it is usually done on older men. A total prostatectomy also has the risk of causing impotence and incontinence and is performed only when necessary.

PHARMACOLOGIC HIGHLIGHTS

Medication or Drug Class	Dosage	Description	Rationale
Trimethoprim-sulfamethoxazole (Bactrim, Septra)	1 DS tablet bid for 30 days	Antibacterial	Eliminates causative organism
Ciprofloxacin hydrochloride (Cipro)	500 mg bid for 28 days	Fluoroquinolone anti-infective	Eliminates causative organism

Nitrofurantoin (Macrodantin)	100 mg qd for 4–16 weeks	Urinary antiseptic	Given for chronic prostatitis along with Bactrim
Stool softeners	Varies with drug	NA	Constipation is very painful for patients with prostatitis
Analgesics	Varies with drug	NA	Relieve pain

Independent

The most important nursing interventions for patients with acute or chronic bacterial prostatitis focus on preventing complications. Monitor for urinary retention; for persistence of fever, perineal pain, or difficulty voiding; and for recurring urinary tract infection. If the patient is not on fluid restriction, encourage the patient to drink at least 3 L of fluid a day to facilitate elimination.

Suggest strategies to increase comfort. If the patient exhibits a decreased ability to void, encourage him to void while in a warm water bath with the pelvic muscles relaxed. To assist with pain control, use relaxation techniques and diversionary activities.

Patient teaching is essential. Some patients prefer to have someone of the same gender talk about sexual functioning. In periods of acute infection and inflammation, the patient is usually encouraged to abstain from sexual intercourse. If the patient has chronic bacterial prostatitis, encourage him to be sexually active to promote drainage of the prostate gland. During periods of known infection, the patient should use a condom. Answer the patient's and partner's questions thoroughly. If possible, encourage the patient to speak with other men with prostatitis to learn how others have coped with the illness.

DOCUMENTATION GUIDELINES

- Physical findings: Pain, bladder distension, hematuria, enlarged and tender prostate
- Response to therapy: Pain medication, sitz baths, fluids, antibiotics
- Urinary output: Characteristics, color, amount
- Presence of complications: Urinary retention, persistence of fever, perineal pain, dysuria
- Response to treatment: TURP or surgery

DISCHARGE AND HOME HEALTHCARE GUIDELINES

PREVENTION. Explain the need to drink fluids to facilitate kidney function and to avoid food and drinks that have diuretic action or are prostatitic. If the physician has prescribed sitz baths, the patient or family needs to know that sitz baths should be taken for 10 to 20 minutes several times daily.

MEDICATIONS. Be sure the patient understands the need to take all prescribed antibiotics. The patient should understand all medications, including the dosage, route, action, and any adverse effects. Remind the patient that the entire course of antibiotics should be completed before stopping the drug.

COMPLICATIONS. Instruct the patient to report fever, hematuria, urinary retention, or difficulty voiding. The patient needs to understand the need for prolonged follow-up to avoid recurrence.

POSTPROCEDURE. If the patient has had surgery or a TURP, teach that urinary dribbling, frequency, and occasional hematuria are not unusual. Explain that the patient will gradually regain urinary control. Remind the patient to avoid heavy lifting, strenuous exercise, or long automobile or plane trips. These situations may place the urinary system under high pressures from bladder distension or abdominal pressure that may lead to bleeding. Usually the physician requests that the patient abstain from sexual activity for several weeks after the procedures.

Psychoactive Substance Abuse

DRG Category: 434
Mean LOS: 4.9 days
Description: MEDICAL: Alcohol/Drug Abuse or Dependence, Detoxification, or Other Symptom Treatment with CC

Psychoactive substances are drugs or chemicals that have an effect on the central nervous system (CNS). The National Institute of Drug Abuse defines drug abuse or drug dependence as a condition in which the use of a legal or illegal drug causes physical, mental, emotional, or social harm. Drug usage impairs one's ability to function in daily activities of living and in work environments. Relationships with family and friends become impaired and dysfunctional.

Most of the abused drugs fall into two main categories, CNS depressants and CNS stimulants. CNS depressants include narcotics, sedatives, barbiturates, tranquilizers, and inhalants. The desired effect by the user is a sense of increased self-esteem, euphoria, relaxation, and relief from pain and anxiety. CNS stimulants include amphetamines, hallucinogens, and cocaine. The desired effect by the user is a sense of well-being, alertness, excitation, overconfidence, and increased initiative.

Tolerance to the drug results in the need for increasing amounts, and the physiological and psychological dependence on the drug leads to maladaptive behaviors. Attempts to discontinue or control use of the drug lead to withdrawal symptoms, which if left untreated can range from feeling flu-like symptoms to coma and possible death. The withdrawal from a drug produces feelings and sensations opposite of the effects produced by using the drug. Withdrawal can be treated to avoid withdrawal symptoms. Chronic abuse of psychoactive substances may lead to complications, including pulmonary emboli, respiratory infections, trauma, musculoskeletal dysfunctions, psychosis, malnutrition disturbances, gastrointestinal disturbances, hepatitis, thrombophlebitis, bacterial endocarditis, gangrene, and coma.

CAUSES

The cause of substance abuse is complex and involves many factors, including the type and availability of the drug, personality type, environmental factors, peer pressure, coping abilities of the individual, genetic factors, and sociocultural influences. Cocaine dependence is thought to be associated with a deficiency in dopamine and norepinephrine neurotransmitters. Use of narcotics and opiates may interfere with the biochemical factors that are related to the body's own production of opiate-like substances.

A psychological factor that seems common to all forms of substance abuse is low self-esteem. Also found are feelings of inadequacy, loneliness, shame, and guilt that lead to depression and a sense of hopelessness and despair. Sociocultural factors have significant influence. Increasing numbers of individuals experience family breakup and separation, school failure, poverty, unemployment, "living in the fast lane," and stressors related to highly competitive work environments. Teenagers and young adults often begin experimenting as a result of peer pressure and the easy availability of drugs.

GENDER AND LIFE SPAN CONSIDERATIONS

Drug use and abuse are prevalent across the life span from young adolescents to the elderly. Increasing numbers of the elderly are abusing drugs as a way of coping with the stressors of aging. Young teens are vulnerable to experimentation as they attempt to conform to group norms and peer pressure. The typical users of barbiturates, sedatives, and tranquilizers are middle-class, middle-aged women. Cocaine use is often seen in younger adult professionals, entertainers, and business executives. Marijuana usage is seen most frequently in teens and young adults.

◻ ASSESSMENT

HISTORY. The physiological signs and symptoms of use or intoxication vary, depending on the substance. Consequently, when a person is admitted in an intoxicated state or in withdrawal, it is important to know what drug or drugs have been used, the route used, and, if possible, the amount of drug used. Determine if alcohol is also being used because there is a synergistic effect that increases the effect of both drugs.

Some patients may be misusing and abusing psychoactive drugs through ignorance. Others may have begun using them as part of a physician-prescribed treatment regimen and then became addicted. If the individual is unable to give a history because of overdose, friends or family members may provide needed information and clothing can be checked for drug paraphernalia. Elicit a history of previous detoxification treatments, effectiveness, length of recovery, and what influenced a return to drug usage.

PHYSICAL EXAMINATION. If the patient is admitted with intoxication and a drug history cannot be obtained, signs and symptoms can be indicators of the type of drug used. (See Table 45.) Inspect the patient for evidence of how the drug is used, such as needle marks from mainlining, nasal irritation caused by snorting, ulcerations on lips and tongue from chewing, cellulitis from injecting drugs and missing the vein, and infections from sites used for mainlining.

TABLE 45 | **Signs and Symptoms of Drug Use and Withdrawal**

DRUG	OVERDOSE	WITHDRAWAL
Narcotics	Constricted pupils, slow shallow breathing, coma, seizures, possible death	Watery eyes, runny nose, nausea, cramping, loss of appetite, yawning, irritability, tremors, panic, chills, sweating

Depressants/barbituates	Dilated pupils, shallow breathing, clammy skin, weak and rapid pulse, coma, possible death	Anxiety, insomnia, delirium, tremors, seizures, possible death (see "Alcohol Withdrawal")
Stimulants/amphetamines, cocaine	Elevated temperature, agitation, hallucinations, seizures, possible death	Apathy, depression with sleep for long periods of time, irritability, disorientation.
Hallucinogens	"Bad trip," longer with episodes of psychosis, possible death	No apparent withdrawal symptoms
Marijuana	Fatigue, paranoia, psychosis	Hyperactivity, insomnia, loss of appetite

Adapted from Kneisl, CR: Nursing care of clients with substance abuse. In Black, JM, and Matassarin-Jacobs, E: Medical-Surgical Nursing, A Psychophysiologic Approach. Philadelphia, WB Saunders, 1993.

PSYCHOSOCIAL. Obtain information on how the patient perceives the effect drugs have on his or her life, work, and the relationship with family and friends. Identify strengths and limitations. Assess the patient's emotional state before admission, especially noting depression and thoughts about suicide. If the patient is involved in a relationship, determine the degree of stability. Ask whether the partner uses drugs and what his or her attitude is toward the patient's drug use. If the patient is a parent, find out the children's ages and investigate how the children are affected by the patient's drug use.

Elicit an employment history, including the type and length of employment. Determine how the use of drugs has affected the patient's work. Determine how much time off from work has been caused by the drug use. Establish a history of the financial effects of the drug use; ask how much the patient spends on drugs and if he or she has developed other sources of income besides his or her job. Determine how the use of drugs has affected the patient's financial resources.

DIAGNOSTIC HIGHLIGHTS

Test	Normal Result	Abnormality with Condition	Explanation
Serum and urine drug screens	Negative for screened substance	Positive for screened substance	Identify drugs that have been ingested

Other: For unresponsive patients with suspected drug overdose—serum glucose, complete blood count, blood urea nitrogen, serum electrolytes, arterial blood gases, electrocardiogram, chest x ray

PRIMARY NURSING DIAGNOSIS

Self-esteem disturbance related to immaturity, personal vulnerability

OUTCOMES. Self esteem; Body image; Hope; Mood equilibrium; Role performance; Social interaction skills

INTERVENTIONS. Counseling; Substance use treatment: Withdrawal and/or overdose; Therapy group; Support group; Emotional support; Mood management; Substance use treatment and prevention

□ PLANNING AND IMPLEMENTATION

Collaborative

The immediate goal after depressant ingestion is to keep the individual safe during a drug overdose or withdrawal. The long-term goal is for the patient to remain drug-free. In the acute phase, the immediate effects of narcotics can be reversed with naloxone (Narcan). In the case of barbiturate overdose when the patient is conscious, mild intoxication can be treated by letting the individual "sleep it off." More severe cases of overdoses need to be handled in an acute or critical care environment where continuous monitoring can occur. Of paramount importance is to make sure the patient has adequate airway, breathing, and circulation during the time period that depressants may lead to severe respiratory depression.

Generally if the patient is unconscious and the substance is unknown, the following steps are taken in management: (1) begin supplemental oxygen; (2) insert intravenous line with saline infusion or dextrose in water; (3) administer dextrose, thiamine, and naloxone; (4) protect airway with endotracheal intubation; (5) pass orogastric tube, lavage and administer activated charcoal; (6) admit the patient for ongoing observation and management. Activated charcoal is produced from the destructive distillation of organic materials. The substance absorbs toxic substances because of large external pores and a large internal surface area that binds with toxic ions. A cathartic such as magnesium citrate is given to help GI excretion of the toxic substance bound with activated charcoal. Activated charcoal is also given for overdoses when the substance is known, such as phenobarbital, carbamazepine, cyclic antidepressants, amphetamines, and cocaine.

Management of stimulants can be similar to that of depressants, with the administration of activated charcoal. Seizures are a possibility in the case of an overdose with stimulants, but note that amphetamines and cocaine have a short duration time of 2 to 4 hours. Phenytoin (Dilantin) can be ordered to prevent seizure activity, and benzodiazepines are also used to treat agitation or seizures. External cooling may be used to reduce hyperthermia, and intravenous fluids may be used to replace fluid loss and to prevent myoglobin damage in the kidneys. All patients with substance abuse and overdoses need counseling and therapy to manage their substance use patterns.

PHARMACOLOGIC HIGHLIGHTS

Medication or Drug Class	Dosage	Description	Rationale
Naloxone	2 mg IV; use smaller doses for patients who are not apneic to avoid withdrawal	Opioid antagonist	Blocks the action of opioids that can lead to respiratory depression and apnea
Dextrose	100 mL IV 50% solution	Sugar	Rules out hypoglycemia as a cause for coma; given to patients who are known not to be hyperglycemic

Thiamine	100 mg IV	Vitamin	Prevents Wernicke-Korsakoff syndrome (encephalopathy associated with thiamine deficiency that is often seen with chronic alcohol use)
Haloperidol	2–5 mg IV or IM	Antipsychotic	Controls combative or agitated behavior during withdrawal or treatment
Pentobarbital	100–200 initially po and then in decreasing doses over 10 days	Barbiturate	Protects the patient from seizure activity
Phenytoin	300–400 mg daily in divided doses po or IV	Anticonvulsant	Prevents and limits seizures related to drug withdrawal

Other Drugs: Desipramine hydrochloride (Norpramin), bromocriptine mesylate (Parlodel), amantadine hydrochloride (Symmetrel), and melphalan (phenylalanine mustard) have been prescribed to decrease the craving for cocaine during withdrawal. Antidepressants may also be prescribed for the depression that accompanies the withdrawal from stimulants. Diazepam (Valium) or diphenhydramine hydrochloride (Benadryl) is administered to calm the individual who is experiencing a bad trip from hallucinogens. Phenothiazines in low doses may be ordered to control the flashbacks that can occur after the last dose of a hallucinogen. Because the patient has built up a tolerance for drugs, the amount of medication needed to keep the patient safe may be more than what is considered a safe dosage. Methadone is used to stabilize individuals during withdrawal from narcotics, which is then followed by withdrawal of the methadone over a period of a week. Other methods, such as the "cold turkey" approach, require abstinence from the drug, with phenothiazines administered to reduce anxiety and nausea and to keep the patient sedated. Clonidone (Catapres) has also been used to decrease discomfort during the withdrawal process.

Independent

During the acute phase, keep the patient safe. Use strategies for continuous monitoring of airway, breathing, and circulation, and implement emergency measures as needed to support life. Monitor for seizure activity and place the patient on the seizure precautions regimen. Examine the environment for safety risks such as falls from the bed or self-discontinuation of tubes. Assess the potential for a suicide attempt and, if necessary, initiate suicide precautions and never leave the patient unattended.

Meet the self-care deficits related to hygiene, nutrition, and elimination. Promote a sense of security: approach the patient in a calm, nonthreatening, and nonjudgmental way. Building a trusting relationship with the patient provides a foundation for addressing the more long-term goals that are associated with becoming drug-free.

Following the acute phase, initiate the process of rehabilitation, and implement a treatment plan to maintain abstinence. The first goal is to work toward getting the individual to break through the denial of drug abuse and take responsibility to begin the recovery process. Provide educational materials and arrange a consultation with a chemical abuse counselor to begin the process before discharge from an acute care setting. Often, individuals are admitted from an acute care setting to an inpatient or outpatient treatment facility where nursing staff and other healthcare providers can begin specialized treatment programs. These programs include peer group programs in which confrontation, support, and hope are part of the treatment process. Treatment goals for the individual include development of a healthy self-concept, self-discipline, adaptive coping strategies, strategies to improve interpersonal relationships, and ways of filling leisure time without the use of drugs.

DOCUMENTATION GUIDELINES

- Physical findings: Vital signs; adequacy of airway, breathing, and circulation; response to medication protocols for overdose or withdrawal, nutrition, intake and output, elimination patterns
- Mental/neurological findings: Anxiety levels, depression, delusions, hallucinations, presence or absence of seizures
- Understanding of the need for consultation with drug abuse counselor
- Understanding of the need for continued treatment for self and family

DISCHARGE AND HOME HEALTHCARE GUIDELINES

The patient should be discharged to an inpatient or outpatient treatment program to address the long-term effects of substance abuse. After discharge from a treatment program, the individual may continue with groups such as Narcotics Anonymous (NA), Cocaine Anonymous (CA), or Alcoholics Anonymous (AA). Family dynamics often play a role in the use of drugs. It is important for the family to be involved in the treatment plan through individual and family therapy and support groups that address issues dealing with family members who abuse drugs.

Pulmonary Embolism

DRG Category: 078
Mean LOS: 7.8 days
Description: MEDICAL: Pulmonary Embolism

Pulmonary embolism (PE) is a potentially life-threatening condition in which a free-flowing blood clot (embolism) becomes lodged within the pulmonary vasculature. Approximately 500,000 cases of PE are reported yearly.

When an embolism becomes lodged within a pulmonary vessel, platelets accumulate around the thrombus and trigger the release of potent vasoactive substances. The pulmonary vasculature constricts, which leads to an increased pulmonary vascular resistance, increased pulmonary arterial pressure, and increased right ventricular workload. Blood flow abnormalities result in a ventilation/perfusion mismatch that is initially dead-space ventilation (ventilation with no perfusion). As atelectasis occurs, shunting (perfusion without ventilation of the alveolus) results. If the right side of the heart (accustomed to pumping out against a relatively low-resistance pulmonary circuit) cannot empty its volume against the increased pulmonary vascular resistance, right-sided heart failure occurs. Ultimately, cardiac function may deteriorate with decreased cardiac output, decreased systemic blood flow, and shock.

CAUSES

A PE usually occurs when a thrombus in the deep veins of the lower extremities loosens or dislodges and begins to move in the bloodstream. The thrombus (now an embolus because it is moving in the bloodstream) floats to the heart, moves through the right side of the heart, and enters the pulmonary circulation through the pulmonary artery. Major risk factors for the development of PE include any condition that produces venous stasis, increased blood coagulability, or venous endothelial (vessel wall) changes. Situations resulting in these pathologic changes include immobility, dehydration, injury, or decreased venous return. Conditions associated with these risk factors include varicosities, pregnancy, obesity, tumors, thrombocytopenia, atrial fibrillation, multiple trauma, presence of artificial heart valves or vessels, sepsis, and congestive heart failure.

GENDER AND LIFE SPAN CONSIDERATIONS

PE may occur in any age group. PE is a frequent cause of sudden death for approximately 50,000 people each year in the United States. PE in children is associated with cardiac conditions and coagulopathic diseases such as sickle cell anemia or cancer. Young women are at risk for PE during pregnancy or while they take high-estrogen-content birth control pills. Adults, particularly the elderly, are at risk for PE because of deep vein thrombosis, cardiac conditions, and increased blood coagulability.

◻ ASSESSMENT

HISTORY. Many patients with PE report a history of deep vein thrombosis, surgery, or some other condition that results in vascular injury or increased blood coagulability. Patients may describe a sudden onset of dyspnea and chest pain for no apparent reason. Some patients report severe symptoms, such as severe pain, wheezing, diaphoresis, and a sense of impending doom. The severity of the symptoms partly depends on the size, number, and location of the emboli.

PHYSICAL EXAMINATION. Patients often appear short of breath, diaphoretic, weak, fearful, and anxious. They may be febrile, or their skin may be cold and clammy. Those in critical condition may develop severe chest pain, syncope, and chest splinting and may cough up bloody sputum. Not all patients become hypoxemic because the increased respiratory rate increases their minute volume and thereby maintains gas exchange. However, some patients have signs of hypoxemia, such as confusion, agitation, and central cyanosis.

When you auscultate the patient's chest, you may note decreased breath sounds, wheezing, crackles, or a transient pleural friction rub. You may also note tachycardia, a third heart sound, or a loud pulmonic component of the second heart sound. You may note a warm, tender area in the leg. Ongoing monitoring during an acute episode of PE is essential for patient recovery. Monitor the patient's vital signs, including temperature, pulse, blood pressure, and respiratory rate, every hour or as needed. Observe the patient continuously for signs of right ventricular failure as evidenced by neck vein distension, rales, peripheral edema, enlarged liver, dyspnea, increased weight, and increased heart rate. Monitor the patient for signs of shock, such as severe hypotension, mottling, cyanosis, cold extremities, and weak or absent peripheral pulses.

PSYCHOSOCIAL. Depending on the severity of symptoms, patients and their families usually display some degree of anxiety. Because PE is life-threatening, their fears are justified and appropriate. Assess the patient's and family's ability to cope.

DIAGNOSTIC HIGHLIGHTS

Test	Normal Result	Abnormality with Condition	Explanation
Arterial blood gases	PaO_2 80–100 mm Hg; $PaCO_2$ 35–45 mm Hg; $SaO_2 > 95\%$	$PaO_2 < 80$ mm Hg in a majority of patients; $PaCO_2$ varies but often < 35 mm Hg; $SaO_2 < 95\%$	Poor gas exchange and shunting leads to hypoxemia; hypocapnea occurs from increased respiratory rate
Ventilation/ perfusion scan	Negative for emboli/ thrombi; uniform uptake of particles and equal gas distribution	Wash out of radioactivity in embolized areas; ventilation defects in embolized areas	Emboli/thrombi lead to lack of perfusion and shunting

Other Tests: Complete blood count, prothrombin time, partial thromboplastin time, echocardiogram, pulmonary angiogram, arterial blood gases, chest x ray, impedence plethysmography and compression ultrasonography for diagnosis of deep vein thrombosis (DVT)

PRIMARY NURSING DIAGNOSIS

Impaired gas exchange related to impaired pulmonary blood flow and alveolar collapse

OUTCOMES. Respiratory status: Gas exchange; Respiratory status: Ventilation; Symptom control behavior; Treatment behavior: Illness or injury; Comfort level

INTERVENTIONS. Airway management; Anxiety reduction; Oxygen therapy; Airway suctioning; Airway insertion and stabilization; Cough enhancement; Mechanical ventilation; Positioning; Respiratory monitoring

◻ PLANNING AND IMPLEMENTATION

Collaborative

Massive PE is a medical emergency. Make sure that the patient's airway, breathing, and circulation are maintained. Administer oxygen immediately to support gas exchange and prepare for the possibility of intubation and mechanical ventilation. Obtain intravenous (IV) access for administration of fluids and pharmacologic agents. Before administration of thrombolytic agents, draw a coagluation profile and complete blood count to obtain a baseline.

Although it is rare, severe cases of PE that are unresponsive to anticoagulant or thrombolytic therapy may require surgery. The least invasive technique is the insertion of a transvenous catheter into the pulmonary vasculature. If the procedure is unsuccessful, however, a thoracotomy may be required to remove the obstructing embolism. Patients prone to PE seeded from deep vein thrombi may have a prosthetic umbrella inserted into the inferior vena cava to trap the emboli.

PHARMACOLOGIC HIGHLIGHTS

Medication or Drug Class	Dosage	Description	Rationale
Anticoagulants	Varies with drug and patient weight; standard heparin dosage is 80 units/kg bolus IV followed by an infusion of 18 units/kg per hour titrated according to coagulation studies; starting dosage of warfarin is 5 mg per day for 2 days po with changes depending on prothrombin time	Sodium heparin; sodium warfarin (Coumadin)	Standard treatment is to initiate intravenous heparin with clinical suspicion of PE to reduce further formation of clots
Thrombolytic agents	Varies with drug	Streptokinase; urokinase; recombinant tissue plasminogen activator	Break down clots previously formed and hasten resolution of clots, but have not been shown to reduce mortality

Other Drugs: Morphine sulfate to manage pain and anxiety, diuretics to reduce edema, inotropic agents for heart failure

Independent

The primary concern for the nurse who is caring for a patient with PE includes the maintenance of airway, breathing, and circulation by support of the cardiopulmonary system. The most important independent measure before PE formation is prevention of thrombus formation. To prevent PE in high-risk patients, encourage early chair rest and ambulation as the patient's condition allows. Even patients who are intubated and mechanically ventilated with multiple catheters can be gotten out of bed without physiologic risk for periods of chair rest. Provide active and passive range-of-motion at least every 8 hours for all patients on bed rest. Teach the family and significant others of an immobile patient how to perform passive range-of-motion exercises. If the patient is not on fluid restriction, encourage drinking at least 2 L of fluids a day to decrease blood viscosity. Use compression boots for patients who are on bed rest to increase venous return.

During anticoagulant therapy, protect patients from injury. Report any signs of increased bleeding, such as ecchymosis, epistaxis, hematuria, mucous membrane bleeding, decreasing hemoglobin or hematocrit, and bleeding from puncture sites. Restrict parenteral injections and venipunctures to essential procedures only. If the patient is ambulatory, provide a safe environment.

Provide information about the diagnosis and prognosis of PE, and explain all procedures and diagnostic tests. Set aside time each day to talk with the patient and family to allow for expression of their feelings. If the patient is a child, monitor the patterns of growth and development using age-appropriate milestones and developmental tasks. Provide age-appropriate play activities for children.

DOCUMENTATION GUIDELINES

- Respiratory response: Rate and rhythm, presence of adventitious breath sounds; retractions or nasal flaring (pediatric); oxygen saturation; character and amount of expectoration; type, location, and patency of the artificial airway
- Cardiovascular response: Skin and oral mucosa color; heart rate and rhythm; peripheral pulses; location and degree of edema
- Presence of pain (chest or extremity), location, character, and intensity; swelling or warmth of the patient's extremities
- Complications: Hematuria, epistaxis, hemoptysis, bloody vomitus, bleeding
- Response to treatment: Anticoagulation, oxygen, sedation, surgery

DISCHARGE AND HOME HEALTHCARE GUIDELINES

Teach the patient and family methods of prevention. Because of the association of deep vein thrombosis and PE, instruct patients to avoid factors that cause venous stasis. Explain that patients should avoid prolonged sitting, crossing of their legs, placing pillows beneath the popliteal fossae, and wearing tight-fitting clothing such as girdles. Encourage hospitalized patients to ambulate as soon as possible after surgery and to wear anti-embolic hose or pneumatic compression boots while they are bedridden. Encourage patients to drink at least 2 L of fluid a day unless they are on fluid restriction. Suggest that obese patients limit calorie intake to reduce their weight.

Discuss all medications with the patient and family. Patients are usually discharged on warfarin. Remind the patient to keep appointments with the healthcare professional. Note that the patient needs periodic blood specimens to monitor drug levels. Explain that warfarin is continued unless the patient consults with the healthcare professional. Explain that the patient cannot take any over the counter drug preparations that contain salicylates without consulting the healthcare provider. Encourage the patient to avoid foods that are rich in vitamin K, such as dark green vegetables, which counteract the effects of warfarin. Encourage the patient to wear a medical identification bracelet that shows he or she is on anticoagulant therapy. Describe the complications of anticoagulant therapy. Instruct the patient to avoid activities that might predispose to injury or bleeding. Children may require helmets and other protective equipment. Encourage the patient to use a soft toothbrush and an electric razor for shaving. Instruct the patient to report any orange or pink-red urine discoloration, blood in the stool, excessive bruising, heavy menses, excessive gum bleeding, hemoptysis, bloody vomitus, and abdominal or flank pain. Encourage the patient to inspect his or her back in the mirror each day to check for bruising. Instruct the patient to inform dentists and other healthcare providers about the anticoagulant therapy before any procedure.

Instruct the patient and family about possible complications. If leg pain or swelling, decreased pulses in the lower extremities, shortness of breath, chest pain, or anxiety occurs, the patient or family should report to an emergency department as soon as possible.

Pulmonary Fibrosis

DRG Category: 483
Mean LOS: 41.9 days
Description: MEDICAL: Interstitial Lung Disease with CC

Pulmonary fibrosis is a restrictive lung disease in which alveolar inflation is reduced, thus impairing lung function. The alveoli are affected by fibrotic tissue, which may develop after inflammation, infection, or tissue damage. The resulting scarring and distortion of pulmonary tissue lead to serious compromise in gas exchange. Fibrosis leads to decreased lung compliance and increased elastic recoil, which increases the overall work of breathing and inefficient exchange of gases.

CAUSES

Pulmonary fibrosis is believed to result from exposure to radiation or inhalation of noxious materials such as silica, asbestos, and coal dust. Pulmonary conditions that can result in pulmonary fibrosis include pneumonia, atelectasis, alveolar cell cancer, pulmonary edema, and lung surgery or trauma. Nonpulmonary causes include neuromuscular disease such as Guillain-Barré syndrome, amyotrophic lateral sclerosis, myasthenia gravis, or muscular dystrophy. Approximately one-third of patients can trace their initial episodes of dyspnea to a viral respiratory illness. Deformities of the bones, such as ankylosing spondylitis and scoliosis, can result in pulmonary fibrosis.

GENDER AND LIFE SPAN CONSIDERATIONS

Although it is possible for pulmonary fibrosis to occur at any age, the average age of patients who are diagnosed with pulmonary fibrosis is 50. Elderly patients or those exposed to risk factors for a prolonged period of time are at the greatest risk. Pulmonary fibrosis occurs in both men and women.

□ ASSESSMENT

HISTORY. Establish a history of work or lifestyle that may have caused the disease. Ask if the patient has worked as a coal miner or with materials such as asbestos or silica or whether he or she has lived near industrial plants that use such materials. Determine if the patient has had respiratory complications or conditions such as pneumonia, atelectasis, alveolar cell cancer, pulmonary edema, and lung surgery or trauma. Ask if the patient has experienced pain while breathing or shortness of breath. Ask if the patient smokes cigarettes. There is some suspicion that genetic factors may determine susceptibility to the disease, so take a family history of pulmonary conditions, including pulmonary fibrosis.

PHYSICAL EXAMINATION. Observe the patient's respiratory status, noting rate, depth, rhythm, and ease of breathing. In the initial phases of the disease, the physical examination may be normal and the lungs may be clear on auscultation. As the disease progresses, individuals with pulmonary fibrosis frequently develop shallow, rapid breathing patterns in an attempt to conserve energy. Note any cough. Auscultate the patient's lungs; listen for diminished or absent breath sounds or coarse crackles, particularly at the lung bases on inspiration. Note chest excursion and symmetry. Check for digital clubbing. Because pulmonary fibrosis in its late stages can cause cor pulmonale, check for signs of cardiac failure, such as elevated neck veins, liver distension, and swelling of the lower extremities.

PSYCHOSOCIAL. Patients may experience a lowering of self-esteem with increased dependence on others and changing roles. In addition, shortness of breath and difficulty in breathing usually cause increased anxiety. If the disease has an occupational source, financial concerns may play an important role if the patient is unable to return to work.

DIAGNOSTIC HIGHLIGHTS

Test	Normal Result	Abnormality with Condition	Explanation
Chest x ray	Clear lung fields	Identification of interstitial infiltrates or ground glass pattern	Fibrotic areas have a changed appearance
Forced expiratory flow (FEF): Maximal flow rate attained during the middle (25% to 75%) of FVC maneuver	Varies by body size	25% of the predicted value	Predicts obstruction of smaller airways
Residual volume (RV): Volume of air remaining in lungs at end of a maximal expiration	1.2 L	Increased up to 400% normal	Increased RV indicates obstruction

Other Tests: Gallium scan, serologic tests, histologic analysis

PRIMARY NURSING DIAGNOSIS

Ineffective breathing pattern related to shortness of breath and difficulty breathing

OUTCOMES. Respiratory status: Gas exchange; Respiratory status: Ventilation; Symptom control behavior; Treatment behavior: Illness or injury; Comfort level

INTERVENTIONS. Airway management; Anxiety reduction; Oxygen therapy; Airway suctioning; Airway insertion and stabilization; Cough enhancement; Mechanical ventilation; Positioning; Respiratory monitoring

□ PLANNING AND IMPLEMENTATION

Collaborative

To relieve breathing difficulties and correct hypoxia, most physicians prescribe low-flow oxygen therapy (2 to 4 L per minute). Corticosteroid therapy is the treatment of choice. If the patient does not respond to the corticosteroid therapy, immunosuppression with cyclophosphamide (Cytoxan) is considered. Cyclophosphamide reduces the white blood cell count, causing a distinct drop in the total blood lymphocyte count. Patients who do not respond to conventional therapy and whose life expectancy is less than 18 months may be candidates for lung transplantation. If cor pulmonale develops, the patient may be placed on diuretics and digitalis. Bronchodilators may improve wheezing and airway obstruction. Infections need to be identified and treated promptly. Pneumococcal and influenza vaccines are important.

PHARMACOLOGIC HIGHLIGHTS

Medication or Drug Class	Dosage	Description	Rationale
Prednisone	5–60 mg per day po; dose is individualized	Corticosteroid	Decreases the inflammatory process
Cyclophosphamide (Cytoxan)	1–5 mg/kg per day; dose is individualized	Antineoplastic	Reduces the white blood cell count, causing a distinct drop in the total blood lymphocyte count

Independent

Focus on relieving respiratory difficulties and caring for the patient's emotional condition. To assist with breathing, assist the patient to attain an upright, supported position to enhance respiratory excursion. Assist the patient into a Fowler or semi-Fowler position. Provide assistance with the activities of daily living as appropriate, and help the patient conserve energy by alternating rest periods with periods of activity. Plan rest time of at least 1 hour after meals before engaging in activities. Teach the patient deep-breathing and coughing exercises. Use humidified air. Provide regular oral hygiene to combat dry mouth.

Because there is no cure for pulmonary fibrosis, dealing with a chronic debilitating disease requires many psychosocial adjustments for the patient and family members. Encourage the patient to verbalize concerns and fears. Encourage the patient to identify actions and care measures that help make him or her comfortable and relaxed. As much as possible, try to include the patient and family in decision making about care measures. Lifestyle changes for the patient may be necessary. A well-balanced diet with adequate fluid intake is important. If the patient smokes cigarettes or pipes, smoking cessation is an essential intervention for the patient's survival. A job counseling session may be helpful if the patient needs to change occupations. If the patient is having trouble coping with role changes, counseling may be helpful.

DOCUMENTATION GUIDELINES

- Physical changes: Skin color, respiratory patterns, breath sounds, breathing difficulties, chest symmetry and excursion, pulse oximetry
- Reaction to diagnosis and coping strategies
- Frequency of oxygen use, noting liter flow and type of delivery device, activity tolerance

DISCHARGE AND HOME HEALTHCARE GUIDELINES

Teach energy conservation methods and relaxation, breathing, and coughing techniques. Explain the importance of pacing activities, avoiding strenuous activity, and providing rest periods. Teach the patient positions that can provide relief during acute episodes of dyspnea. To prevent infection, encourage the patient to receive flu and pneumococcal vaccines and to avoid crowds and people with known respiratory infections. Be sure the patient understands all medications, including the dosage, route, action, and adverse effects. If the patient is using oxygen therapy at home, teach the patient and family appropriate safety precautions. Help the patient understand the equipment and liter flow, and provide information on how to obtain all the necessary equipment. Work with social services to provide for equipment in the home.

Pulmonary Hypertension

DRG Category: 144
Mean LOS: 4.5 days
Description: MEDICAL: Other Circulatory System

Pulmonary hypertension is diagnosed when the systolic pressure in the pulmonary artery exceeds 30 mm Hg. It is most commonly seen in pre-existing pulmonary or cardiac disease but may occur (although rarely) as a primary condition when it is produced by fibrosis and thickening of the vessel intima. An increase in resistance of the vessels in the pulmonary vasculature bed occurs secondary to hypoxemia (oxygen deficiency). Chronic hypoxemia produces hypertrophy of the medial muscle layer in the smaller branches of the pulmonary artery, which decreases the size of the vessel lumen. Vasoconstriction, the pulmonary system's response to hypoxemia, results in a pressure buildup in the right side of the heart because flow through the pulmonary system is impaired. When hypertension in the pulmonary system (measured as pulmonary vascular resistance) is greater than the ability of the right side of the heart to pump, the cardiac output falls and may cause shock.

CAUSES

The cause of primary pulmonary hypertension is unknown, but the disease tends to occur in families. Secondary pulmonary hypertension is caused by conditions that produce hypoxemia, such as chronic obstructive pulmonary disease, obesity, alveolar hypoventilation, smoke inhalation, and high altitude.

GENDER AND LIFE SPAN CONSIDERATIONS

Pulmonary hypertension is most commonly seen in the elderly person with cardiac or pulmonary disease. It may occur at any age, however. Idiopathic primary pulmonary hypertension tends to occur more often in women between 20 and 40 years of age. Congenital causes may lead to occurrence in the pediatric population.

☐ ASSESSMENT

HISTORY. Patients are usually without symptoms until late in the disease. Up to 50% of the pulmonary circulation may be impaired before significant hypertension is produced. Determine the presence of risk factors. Ask if the patient has experienced chest pain, labored and painful breathing (dyspnea), or syncope. Occasionally the enlarged pulmonary artery compresses the left recurrent laryngeal nerve, producing hoarseness. Some patients may describe periods of heart palpitations.

PHYSICAL EXAMINATION. Signs of right ventricular failure are common, such as jugular venous distension, increased central venous pressure, and peripheral edema. Low cardiac output may produce central cyanosis, syncope, or chest pain. Auscultation of the heart may therefore reveal atrial gallop at the lower left sternal border, narrow splitting of S_2 or increased S_2 intensity, or ejection click at the second intercostal space, left sternal border. When palpating the precordium, you may detect a heave over the right ventricle or an impulse from the pulmonary artery itself. Signs of left ventricular failure, such as systemic hypotension (low blood pressure) and low urinary output, may coexist. Presentation may include hyperventilation, coughing, and eventually rapid breathing (tachypnea) or dyspnea. Initially, breath sounds may be clear or decreased, but you may hear crackles or wheezing.

PSYCHOSOCIAL. The patient is experiencing a potentially life-threatening condition that requires the use of complex medical technology. Assess the anxiety level of the patient, and plan interventions to place a minimum demand on the patient's energy. Support of the patient is essential throughout hospitalization, from routine care such as placement and maintenance of the pulmonary artery catheter to attempts at averting a cardiac arrest.

DIAGNOSTIC HIGHLIGHTS

Test	Normal Result	Abnormality with Condition	Explanation
Pulmonary artery pressure and pulmonary vascular resistance (PVR) (measurements made with a pulmonary artery pressure)	Systolic 15–20 mm Hg; diastolic 8–15 mm Hg; PVR- 180–285 dynes/second per cm^{-5} per m^2	Pressures elevated, with systolic pressure < 25 mm Hg; pulmonary artery systolic pressure may approach systemic arterial pressure	Sustained elevation of pulmonary vascular pressures

Other Tests: Pulmonary function tests, exercise testing, electrocardiogram, ventilation perfusion scan, pulmonary angiogram, chest x rays

PRIMARY NURSING DIAGNOSIS

Impaired gas exchange related to changes in the alveolar membrane structure and increased pulmonary vascular resistance

OUTCOMES. Respiratory status: Gas exchange; Respiratory status: Ventilation; Comfort level; Anxiety control

INTERVENTIONS. Airway insertion and stabilization; Airway management; Respiratory monitoring; Oxygen therapy; Mechanical ventilation; Anxiety reduction

☐ PLANNING AND IMPLEMENTATION

Collaborative

Primary pulmonary hypertension has limited therapy, and patients tend to have hemodynamic deterioration in spite of therapy. The median survival rate after diagnosis is 2.5 years. Supportive measures include supplemental oxygen for people who are hypoxemic and the use of diuretics in people who are fluid-overloaded. Relief of hypoxemia helps reduce pulmonary vasoconstriction. If the origin of the problem is structural, surgery may be attempted. Heart-lung transplantation is a consideration for severe conditions.

PHARMACOLOGIC HIGHLIGHTS

Medication or Drug Class	Dosage	Description	Rationale
Diuretics	Varies by drug	Loop diuretics, thiazide diuretics	Reduce both right and left ventricular failure
Sodium warfarin (Coumadin)	5 mg po initially, guided by coagulation studies	Anticoagulant	Prevents microvascular thrombosis, venous stasis, and limitation of physical activity
Vasodilators	Varies by drug	Nitrates; calcium-channel blockers	Improve muscle tone in pulmonary vascular bed and reduce right ventricular workload

Other Drugs: Bronchodilators are used to improve hypoxemia and reduce pulmonary vascular resistance. Note that use of vasodilators is limited because it may produce systemic hypotension. Studies have indicated that infusion of adenosine into the pulmonary artery has a vasodilating effect more specific to the pulmonary circulation. Inhalation of nitric oxide has also been shown to vasodilate the pulmonary vasculature with no effect on systemic vascular resistance.

Independent

To minimize the risk of infection, use the sterile technique during setup and maintenance of the pulmonary artery catheter. Dressings should be changed according to policy, usually every 72 hours. Ask the patient to evaluate chest pain using a scale from 1 to 10, and provide comfort measures in addition to any ordered medication. Reduce energy demands by assisting the patient to a position of comfort, such as the semi-Fowler or Fowler position. Document pulmonary artery catheter readings and report significant changes to the medical team. Monitor the patient for the development of cardiac dysrhythmias.

Allow the patient to verbalize fears, and assist in the development of a realistic perception as the patient appears ready. Incorporate family members and other support system members as appropriate. Help the patient adjust to the limitations imposed by this disorder. Advise against overexertion, and suggest frequent rest periods between activities. The patient may need diversional activities during periods of restricted activity. Be sure the patient understands dietary limitations and medication regimens.

DOCUMENTATION GUIDELINES

- Vital signs, including pulmonary artery catheter readings
- Cardiovascular and pulmonary physical assessment data, including breath and heart sounds as noted in previous sections
- Responses to therapies, including medication, diet, fluids, and oxygen administration

DISCHARGE AND HOME HEALTHCARE GUIDELINES

Risk for recurrent pulmonary embolism can be reduced by teaching the patient to minimize hypercoagulability, to reduce venous stasis, and to control risk factors such as obesity. Teach the patient to drink 2000 mL of fluid a day unless restricted, to rest between activities, and to avoid overexertion. Teach the patient about the prescribed dosage, route, action, and follow-up laboratory work needed for all medications. If the patient is discharged on potassium-wasting diuretics, encourage a diet that is rich in high-potassium foods, such as apricots, bananas, oranges, and raw vegetables. The patient may also need instruction on a low-sodium diet. If the patient needs home oxygen, instruct the patient and significant others in oxygen use and oxygen safety. Arrange with social services for the delivery of oxygen equipment. If the patient smokes, teach strategies for smoking cessation or provide a referral for smoking cessation programs.

Pyelonephritis

DRG Category: 320
Mean LOS: 5.9 days
Description: MEDICAL: Kidney and Urinary Tract Infections, Age > 17 with CC

Pyelonephritis is an inflammation of the renal pelvis and of the renal tissue; it is caused by an invasion of microorganisms. It can be either acute (also known as acute infective tubulointerstitial nephritis) or chronic in nature, as differentiated by the clinical picture and long-term effects. The infection, which primarily affects the renal pelvis, calyces, and medulla, progresses through the urinary tract as organisms ascend the ureters from the bladder because of vesicoureteral reflux (reflux of urine up the ureter during micturition) or contamination.

Acute pyelonephritis occurs 24 to 48 hours after contamination of the urethra or after instrumentation such as a catheterization. Complications include calculus formation, renal abscesses, septic shock, and chronic pyelonephritis. Chronic pyelonephritis is a persistent infection that causes progressive inflammation and scarring. It usually occurs after chronic obstruction or because of vesicoureteral reflux. This destruction of renal cells may alter the urine-concentrating capability of the kidney and can lead to chronic renal failure.

CAUSES

The causative organisms are usually bacteria but can be fungi or viruses. Patients with diabetes, hypertension, chronic renal calculi, chronic cystitis, and congenital or abnormal urinary tract and pregnant women are more likely to acquire pyelonephritis than are other groups. *Escherichia coli* is responsible for 90% of the episodes in a normal anatomic urinary tract system. Proteus, klebsiella, and occasionally gram-positive cocci account for the rest.

GENDER AND LIFE SPAN CONSIDERATIONS

Pyelonephritis occurs more often in women than in men because the female urethra is much shorter than the male urethra. Men, however, are more susceptible if they have an obstruction from prostatic hypertrophy, cancer, urinary stones, or urethral stenosis. Pyelonephritis is also seen in elderly men with indwelling catheters.

◻ ASSESSMENT

HISTORY. Question the patient carefully to determine if he or she has experienced dysuria, frequency, and urgency (signs of an irritative urinary tract) before seeking care. Ask if the patient is voiding in small amounts or experiencing nocturia. It is important to determine if these symptoms are a change from the patient's usual voiding patterns. Ask for a description of the urine, which may be foul-smelling, cloudy, or bloody, and of any pain; discomfort resulting from pyelonephritis usually occurs in the flank, groin, or suprapubic areas. Also question the patient about any flu-like symptoms, such as malaise, nausea, vomiting, chills, headache, and fatigue. The pain may radiate down the ureter toward the epigastrium and may be colicky if it is associated with a renal calculus.

PHYSICAL EXAMINATION. If you suspect acute pyelonephritis, determine if the patient is febrile. Inspect the urine for color, cloudiness, blood, or presence of a foul odor. Percussion or deep palpation over the costovertebral angle elicits marked tenderness. Not all of these signs may be present. Lower urinary tract symptoms are absent in approximately 15% of women. Flank pain, tenderness, and fever may also be absent. In chronic pyelonephritis, the early symptoms are minimal. Assess the blood pressure because often these patients present with hypertension. There may be irritating urinary tract symptoms, but they are milder in nature than in acute pyelonephritis.

PSYCHOSOCIAL. To prevent permanent kidney damage, acute and chronic pyelonephritis needs to be diagnosed promptly and treated appropriately. Assess the patient's ability to care for himself or herself, as well as his or her learning capabilities, support systems, financial resources, and access to health care.

Identify and alleviate barriers to ensure a prompt, efficient plan of care to help the patient regain a sense of wellness.

DIAGNOSTIC HIGHLIGHTS

Test	Normal Result	Abnormality with Condition	Explanation
Urine culture and sensitivity	Negative cultures	Presence of bacteria	Identifies bacterial contaminants; most common is *E. coli*
Urinalysis	Minimal red and white blood cells; moderate clear protein casts; negative for protein	Pyuria, leukocyte castes	Shows the presence of white blood cells and pus

Other Tests: Blood cultures; complete blood count; x ray of kidney, ureter, bladder; blood urea nitrogen; creatinine; renal ultrasound; intravenous pyelogram; cystourethrogram

PRIMARY NURSING DIAGNOSIS

Infection (urinary tract) related to instrumentation, contamination, or obstruction

OUTCOMES. Immune status; Knowledge: Infection control; Risk control; Risk detection; Nutritional status; Treatment behavior: Illness or injury

INTERVENTIONS. Infection control; Infection protection; Medication prescribing; Nutritional management; Surveillance; Nutritional management; Infection control

☐ PLANNING AND IMPLEMENTATION

Collaborative

The goal of therapy is to rid the urinary tract of the pathogenic organisms and to relieve an obstruction if present. The antibiotics chosen depend on the urine culture and sensitivity. Urinary catheterization is used only when absolutely necessary. Surgery is performed only if an underlying defect is causing obstruction, reflux, or calculi. Hypertension is common in patients with chronic pyelonephritis and needs to be controlled with medication. In addition, supportive care is important. If the cause of pyelonephritis is renal calculi, dietary management, such as limiting calcium, oxalate, or purines, may be necessary.

PHARMACOLOGIC HIGHLIGHTS

Medication or Drug Class	Dosage	Description	Rationale
Antibiotics	Varies by drug; generally parenteral antibiotics for 3–5 days until the patient is afebrile	Depends on urine culture and sensitivity	Eradicate bacteria and maintain adequate blood levels; provide accurate results in

| for 24–48 hours, followed by oral administration for 2–4 weeks | serum peak and trough levels |

Other Drugs: Most patients are admitted with nausea and vomiting, and the physician may prescribe IV fluids to balance hydration. Patients are given analgesics, antipyretics, and anti-emetics to control pain, fever, and nausea.

Independent

Provide comfort measures for the patient with flank pain, headache, and irritating urinary tract symptoms. Back rubs may provide some relief of flank pain. Sitz baths may provide some relief if perineal discomfort is present. It is helpful to use a pain management flowsheet and alternative distractions and comfort measures (massage, music, positioning, verbal support, imagery). Because the patient is usually febrile, employ measures that promote heat reduction (cool packs, limited bedding, cool room temperature). To promote nutrition and adequate fluid balance, ask the patient his or her fluid preferences. Encourage the patient to drink at least 2000 mL per day to help empty the bladder and to prevent calculus formation but not more than 4000 mL per day, which would dilute the antibiotic concentration and lessen its effectiveness. Initiate measures to ensure complete emptying of the bladder, such as running water or spraying the perineum with warm water. Ensure the patient's privacy during voiding.

Teach women in the high-risk groups strategies to limit reinfection. Encourage the woman to clean the perineum by wiping from the front to the back after bowel movements. Stress the need for frequent hand washing. Explain the need for routine checkups if the patient experiences frequent urinary tract infections. Encourage the patient to notify the physician if she notes cloudy urine, burning on urination, and urinary frequency or urgency.

DOCUMENTATION GUIDELINES

- Physical appearance of urine: Cloudy, bloody, or malodorous
- Presence of flank or perineal pain, duration of pain, frequency of pain, response of pain to interventions
- Presence of dysuria; frequency and urgency of urination
- Presence of complications: Increasing BUN and creatinine, unresolved infection, urinary tract obstruction, uncontrolled pain or fever

DISCHARGE AND HOME HEALTHCARE GUIDELINES

Instruct the patient on ways to reduce the risk of subsequent infections: increase fluid intake to 2000 to 3000 mL per day to wash the bacteria out of the bladder; avoid caffeine and alcohol; drink juices that acidify the urine (cranberry, plum, and prune); void at the first urge and at least every 2 to 3 hours during the day to prevent bladder distension; void immediately after sexual intercourse and drink two glasses of water as soon as possible; practice good perineal hygiene (wipe labia from front to back).

Explain to the patient that the entire prescription of antibiotics should be taken even if the patient feels better. Emphasize the importance of following the special instructions that accompany the antibiotic. Emphasize the importance of follow-up urine cultures and examinations. Note that recurrent infection may require prolonged antibiotic therapy.

Renal Failure, Acute

DRG Category: 316
Mean LOS: 5.9 days
Description: MEDICAL: Renal Failure
DRG Category: 315
Mean LOS: 6.0 days
Description: SURGICAL: Other Kidney and Urinary Tract Operating Room Procedures

Acute renal failure (ARF) is the abrupt deterioration of renal function that results in the accumulation of fluids, electrolytes, and metabolic waste products. It is usually accompanied by a marked decrease in urinary output. Although ARF is often reversible, if it is ignored or inappropriately treated it can lead to irreversible kidney damage and chronic renal failure. Although the incidence depends on the underlying cause, estimates of prevalence range from 5% to 50% of all hospitalized patients.

Approximately 70% of patients develop oliguric ARF with a urine output < 500 mL per day. The other 30% of patients never develop oliguria and have what is considered non-oliguric renal failure. Oliguric ARF generally has three stages. During the initial phase (often called the oliguric phase), when trauma or insult affects the kidney tissue, the patient becomes oliguric. This stage may last a week or more. The second stage of ARF is the diuretic phase, which is heralded by a doubling of the urinary output from the previous 24 hours. During the diuretic phase, patients may produce as much as 5 L of urine in 24 hours but lack the ability for urinary concentration and regulation of waste products. This phase can last from 1 to several weeks. The final stage, the recovery phase, is characterized by a return to a normal urinary output (about 1500 to 1800 mL per 24 hours), with a gradual improvement in metabolic waste removal. Some patients take up to a year to recover full renal function after the initial insult.

Complications of ARF include severe electrolyte imbalances such as hyperkalemia and hypocalcemia. The patient is also at risk for secondary infections, congestive heart failure, and pericarditis. ARF that does not respond to treatment of the underlying cause can progress to chronic renal failure (CRF; see the next chapter).

CAUSES

The causes of ARF can be classified as prerenal, intrarenal (intrinsic), and postrenal. Prerenal ARF results from conditions that cause diminished blood flow to the kidneys. Disorders that can lead to prerenal failure include cardiovascular disorders (dysrhythmias, cardiogenic shock, congestive heart failure, myocardial infarction), disorders that cause hypovolemia (burns, trauma, dehydration, hemorrhage), maldistribution of blood (septic shock, anaphylactic shock), renal artery obstruction, and severe vasoconstriction.

Intrarenal, or intrinsic, ARF involves the actual destruction of the renal parenchyma (functional cells). The most common cause of intrarenal failure is acute tubular necrosis, or damage to the renal tubules because of either a nephrotoxic or an ischemic injury. Nephrotoxic injuries occur when the renal tubules are exposed to a high concentration of a toxic chemical. Common sources of nephrotoxic injuries include antibiotics (aminoglycosides, sulfon-amides), diuretics, nonsteroidal anti-inflammatory drugs (ibuprofen), and contrast media from diagnostic tests. Ischemic injuries occur when the mean arterial blood pressure is less than 60 mm Hg for 40 to 60 minutes. Situations that can lead to ischemic injuries include cardiopulmonary arrest, hypovolemic or hemorrhagic shock, cardiogenic shock, or severe hypotension.

Postrenal (postobstructive) ARF is caused by a blockage to urine outflow. One of the most common causes of postrenal ARF in hospitalized patients is an obstructed Foley catheter. Other conditions that can lead to postrenal ARF include ureteral inflammation or obstruction, accidental ligation of the ureters, bladder obstruction (infection, anticholinergic drug use, tumors, trauma leading to bladder rupture), or urethral obstruction (prostate enlargement, urethral trauma, urethral strictures).

GENDER AND LIFE SPAN CONSIDERATIONS

Some experts report that the concentrating ability of the kidneys decreases with advancing age. Oliguria in the geriatric patient, therefore, may be diagnosed with urine production of as much as 600 mL per day. Elderly patients may have a decreased blood flow, decreased kidney mass, decreased filtering surface, and decreased glomerular filtration rate. The elderly, therefore, are more susceptible to insults that result in ARF, and their mortality rates tend to be higher. Older men have the added risk of pre-existing renal damage because of the presence of benign prostatic hypertrophy.

◻ ASSESSMENT

HISTORY. When you elicit the patient's history, look for a disorder that can lead to prerenal, intrarenal, or postrenal ARF. Question the patient about recent illnesses, infections, or injuries, and take a careful medication history with attention to maximum daily doses and self-medication patterns. Determine the patient's urinary patterns and document information such as frequency of voiding, approximate voiding volume, and pattern of daily fluid intake. Evaluate the patient for a recent history of gastrointestinal (GI) problems, such as anorexia, nausea, and changes in bowel patterns. Some patients have a recent history of weight gain, edema, headache, confusion, and sleepiness.

PHYSICAL EXAMINATION. The patient appears seriously ill and often drowsy, irritable, confused, and combative because of the accumulation of metabolic wastes. In the oliguric phase, the patient may show signs of fluid overload such as hypertension, rapid heart rate, peripheral edema, and crackles when you listen to the lungs. Patients in the diuretic phase appear dehydrated, with dry mucous membranes, poor skin turgor, flat neck veins, and orthostatic hypotension. The patient may have increased bleeding tendencies, such as petechiae, ecchymosis of the skin, and bloody vomitus (hematemesis).

PSYCHOSOCIAL. The patient with ARF may be highly anxious because of the unknown outcome of the problem. Anxiety may increase as such symptoms as hemorrhage or pain from an obstructing calculus appear. Because ARF may occur as an iatrogenic problem (a problem caused by the treatment of a disease), you may need to explain to the patient or significant others that the problem was not avoidable and is a potential complication of the underlying disorder.

DIAGNOSTIC HIGHLIGHTS

Test	Normal Result	Abnormality with Condition	Explanation
Blood urea nitrogen (BUN)	5–20 mg/dL	Elevated	Kidneys cannot excrete wastes
Serum creatinine	0.5–1.1 mg/dL	Elevated	Kidneys cannot excrete wastes
24 hour urine creatinine	Females 85–125 mL per minute; males 95–135 mL per minute	50% decrease	Acute damage to the kidney limits ability to clear creatinine
Urine sodium	20–40 mEq/L	Prerenal < 20 mEq/L Intrarenal < 20 mEq/L Postrenal > 40 mEq/L	Prerenal and sometime intrarenal leads to sodium retention whereas postrenal leads to sodium loss in urine

Other Tests: Urinalysis; complete blood count; erythrocyte sedimentation rate; hemodynamic monitoring; renal ultrasound; radionuclide scanning; magnetic resonance angiography; renal biopsy; serum levels of sodium, potassium, magnesium, and phosphorus; arterial blood gases

PRIMARY NURSING DIAGNOSIS

Fluid volume deficit related to excessive urinary output, vomiting, hemorrhage

OUTCOMES. Fluid balance; Circulation status; Cardiac pump effectiveness; Hydration

INTERVENTIONS. Bleeding reduction; Fluid resuscitation; Blood product administration; Intravenous therapy; Circulatory care; Shock management

◻ PLANNING AND IMPLEMENTATION

Collaborative

During the oliguric-anuric stage, diuretic therapy with furosemide (Lasix) or ethacrynic acid (Edecrin) may be attempted to convert oliguric ARF to nonoliguric ARF, which has a better renal recovery rate. During the diuretic phase, fluid volume replacement may be ordered to compensate for the fluid loss and to maintain adequate arterial blood flow to the kidneys. A daily record of intake, output, and weights assists the physician in making treatment decisions. During fluid replacement, monitoring with central venous pressures or pulmonary artery catheters helps track the patient's response to interventions. The physician should be notified if the patient's urine output drops below 0.5 mL/kg per hour or if the daily weight changes by more than 2 kg (4.4 lb).

Electrolyte replacement is based on the patient's serum electrolyte values. The physician attempts to limit hyperkalemia because of its potentially lethal effects on cardiac function. Note the excretory route for medications so that the already damaged kidneys are not further damaged by nephrotoxins. The patient's response to medications is important; drug dosages may need to be decreased because of decreased renal excretion. In addition, timing of medications may need to be changed because of increased excretion during dialysis.

Hemodialysis, peritoneal dialysis, or alternative dialysis methods may be used to manage ARF. Indications for dialysis include fluid overload, hyperkalemia, metabolic acidosis, uremic intoxication, and the need to remove nephrotoxic substances such as metabolites or drugs. The diet for the patient with ARF is usually high in carbohydrates to prevent protein breakdown and low in protein to provide essential amino acids but to limit increases in azotemia (increased urea in the body). For patients who lose sodium in the urine, the diet is high in sodium; for patients with sodium and water retention, the diet is low in sodium and may also contain a fluid restriction. Potassium restrictions are frequently ordered, based on laboratory values.

PHARMACOLOGIC HIGHLIGHTS

Medication or Drug Class	Dosage	Description	Rationale
Diuretics	Varies by drug	Furosemide (Lasix); ethacrynic acid (Edecrin); mannitol	Convert oliguria ARF to non-oliguric
Phosphate binders	15–30 mL with meals tid	Aluminum hydroxide (Basaljel, Amphojel)	Enhance GI excretion of phosphorus

Other Therapy: Some physicians prescribe renal dose dopamine (Intropin) to increase urine output. Sodium polystyrene sulfonate (Kayexelate) can be administered orally or rectally to reduce potassium. Sodium bicarbonate may be ordered to correct metabolic acidosis. If the patient is receiving hemodialysis, supplements of water-soluble vitamins are needed because they are removed during dialysis. Other medications include anti-hypertensives to control blood pressure, antibiotics to manage secondary infections, diphenhydramine (Benadryl) to manage itching, and recombinant human erythropoietin to increase red blood cell production.

Independent

Rest and recovery are important nursing goals. By limiting an increased metabolic rate, the nurse limits tissue breakdown and decreases nitrogenous waste production. A quiet, well-organized environment at a temperature comfortable for the patient ensures rest and recovery.

To help the patient deal with fluid restrictions, use creative strategies to increase the patient's comfort and compliance. Give medications with meals or in minimal IV volumes to maximize the amount of fluid available for patient use.

Several factors place the patient with ARF at risk for impaired skin integrity. Uremia results in itching and dryness of the skin. If the patient experiences pruritus, help the patient clip the fingernails short and keep the nail tips smooth. Use skin emollients liberally, avoid harsh soaps, and bathe the patient only when necessary. Frequent turning and range-of-motion exercises assist in preventing skin breakdown. If the patient is taking medications that cause frequent stools, clean the perineum and buttocks frequently to maintain skin integrity.

Note that one of the most common sources of postrenal ARF is an obstructed urinary catheter drainage system. Before contacting the physician about a decreasing urinary output in an acutely or critically ill patient, make sure that the catheter is patent. If institutional policy permits, irrigate the Foley catheter using sterile technique with 30 mL of normal saline to check for obstruction. Note any kinks in the collecting system. If institutional policy permits, replace the indwelling Foley catheter with a new catheter and urinary drainage system to ensure it is functioning adequately. Signs that postrenal ARF is caused by obstruction in the urinary catheter include a sudden cessation of urinary output in a patient whose urinary output has previously been high or average and a urinary output with normal specific gravity and normal urinary sodium.

The patient with ARF is often irritable and confused. Recognize that the irritability is part of the disease process. Keep the environment free of unnecessary clutter to reduce the chance of falls. If the patient is on bed rest, maintain the bed in the low position and keep the side rails up. Keep the patient's call light within easy reach and the patient's belongings on a bedside table close to the bed. The patient with ARF is anxious, not only because of the ambiguity of the prognosis, but also because he or she may be in an acute care environment for treatment. Provide the patient with ongoing, repeated information about what is happening and why. Ongoing reassurance for both the patient and the significant others is essential.

DOCUMENTATION GUIDELINES

- Physical findings: Urinary output and description of urine, fluid balance, vital signs, findings related to original disease process or insult, presence of pain or pruritus, mental status, GI status, and skin integrity
- Condition of peritoneal or vascular access sites
- Nutrition: Response to dietary or fluid restrictions, tolerance to food, maintenance of body weight
- Complications: Cardiovascular, integumentary infection

DISCHARGE AND HOME HEALTHCARE GUIDELINES

All patients with ARF need an understanding of renal function, signs and symptoms of renal failure, and how to monitor their own renal function. Patients who have recovered viable renal function still need to be monitored by a nephrologist for at least a year. Teach the patient that he or she may be more susceptible to infection than previously. Advise daily weight checks. Emphasize rest to prevent overexertion. Teach the patient or significant others about all medications, including dosage, potential side effects, and drug interactions. Explain that the patient should tell the healthcare professional about the medications if the patient needs treatment such as dental work or if a new medication is added. Explain that ongoing medical assessment is required to check renal function.

Explain all dietary and fluid restrictions. Note if the restrictions are life-long or temporary. Patients who have not recovered viable renal function need to understand that their condition may persist and even become chronic. If chronic renal failure is suspected, further outpatient treatment and monitoring are needed. Discuss with significant others the lifestyle changes that may be required with chronic renal failure.

Renal Failure, Chronic

DRG Category: 316
Mean LOS: 5.9 days
Description: MEDICAL: Renal Failure
DRG Category: 315
Mean LOS: 6.0 days
Description: SURGICAL: Other Kidney and Urinary Tract Operating Room Procedures

Chronic renal failure (CRF) refers to irreversible renal dysfunction as manifested by the inability of the kidneys to excrete sufficient fluid and waste products from the body to maintain health. CRF is fatal if it is not treated.

CRF is a progressive process; stages are defined by categorizing how much renal function remains. The first stage of renal deterioration is reduced renal reserve, which occurs when the patient has a glomerular filtration rate (GFR; the amount of filtrate formed by the kidneys each minute; normally 125 mL per minute) of 35% to 50% of normal. The second stage, renal insufficiency, occurs when the patient has a GFR that is 25% to 35% of normal. The patient with renal failure has a GFR of 20% to 25% of normal. The patient with the final stage of renal dysfunction, end-stage renal disease (ESRD) has a GFR of 15% to 20% of normal or less. When patients reach ESRD, treatment with dialysis is commonly initiated. Patients with CRF are generally treated on an outpatient basis unless the patient develops complications or an urgent problem that requires hospitalization.

All individuals with CRF experience similar physiologic changes, regardless of the initial cause of the disease. The kidneys are unable to perform their normal functions of excretion of wastes, concentration of urine, regulation of blood pressure, regulation of acid-base balance, and production of erythropoietin (the hormone needed for red blood cell production and survival). Complications of CRF include uremia (accumulation of metabolic waste products in the blood and body tissues), anemia, peripheral neuropathy, sexual dysfunction, osteopenia (reduction of bone tissue), pathologic fractures, fluid overload, congestive heart failure, hypertension, pericarditis, electrolyte imbalances (hypocalcemia, hyperkalemia, hyperphosphatemia), metabolic acidosis, esophagitis, and gastritis.

CAUSES

CRF may be caused by either kidney disease or diseases of other systems. (See Table 46.)

TABLE 46 | **Causes of Chronic Renal Failure**

CATEGORY	DISEASES
Congenital/hereditary disorders	Polycystic kidney disease, renal tubular acidosis
Connective tissue disorders	Progressive systemic sclerosis, systemic lupus erythematosus
Infections/inflammatory conditions	Chronic pyelonephritis, glomerulonephritis, tuberculosis

Vascular disease	Hyptertension, renal nephrosclerosis, renal artery stenosis
Metabolic/endocrine diseases	Diabetes mellitus, gout, amyloidosis, hyperparathyroidism
Obstructive diseases	Renal calculi
Nephrotoxic conditions	Medication therapy, drug overdose

GENDER AND LIFE SPAN CONSIDERATIONS

Both men and women are at risk for chronic renal failure. Geriatric patients are more susceptible to some of the causes of acute renal failure (ARF) and may therefore experience CRF more frequently. CRF as a result of other diseases (diabetes mellitus or uncontrolled hypertension) is more common in the elderly simply because they have had the disease longer.

◻ ASSESSMENT

HISTORY. The patient may report a history of ARF (see "Renal Failure, Acute"), although usually the patient does not become symptomatic until he or she has a GFR less than 35% of normal. The patient likely complains of oliguria and weight gain. Ask the patient about the color of the urine, whether it is clear or cloudy, and whether it is frothy. The patient may also complain of a metallic taste in the mouth, anorexia, and stomatitis. Elicit a gastrointestinal (GI) history with particular attention to nausea, vomiting, hematemesis, diarrhea, and constipation.

Elicit the patient's description of any central nervous system (CNS) symptoms. Blurred vision is common. Patients may have impaired decision making and judgment, irritability, decreased alertness, insomnia, increased extremity weakness, and signs of increasing peripheral neuropathy (decreased sensation in the extremities, hands, and feet; pain; and burning sensations).

Patients often report changes in other body systems as well. Some have idiopathic bone and joint pain in the absence of a diagnosis of arthritis. Others suffer from loss of muscle mass and nocturnal leg cramping. Men may be impotent or notice gynecomastia, and women may mention amenorrhea (absence of menses). Both may have decreased libido.

PHYSICAL EXAMINATION. CRF affects all body systems. Patients with CRF have significant cardiovascular involvement. Hypertension is usually noted in the patient with CRF and may indeed be its cause. Patients often have rapid, irregular heart rates; distended jugular veins; and, if pericarditis is present, a pericardial friction rub and distant heart sounds. Respiratory symptoms include hyperventilation, Kussmaul breathing, dyspnea, orthopnea, and pulmonary congestion. Rales may signify fluid overload. Frothy sputum combined with shortness of breath may indicate some degree of pulmonary edema.

The renal effects of CRF are pronounced. You may smell a urine-like odor on the breath and notice a yellow-gray cast to the skin. If the patient is producing any urine at all, it may be dilute, with casts or crystals present. The skin is fragile and dry, and there may be uremic frost on the skin or open areas owing to severe scratching (pruritus) by the patient. The patient may have bruising; petechiae; brittle nails; dry, brittle hair; gum ulcerations; or bleeding. If the patient has been followed for CRF, there may already be access sites created in preparation for dialysis. Assess the sites for patency (an arteriovenous fistula should have a palpable thrill and audible bruit) and signs of infection.

When you assess the CNS, you may find that the patient has difficulty with ambulation because of altered motor function, gait abnormalities, bone and joint pain, and peripheral neuropathy. The patient's mental status may range from mild behavioral changes to profound loss of consciousness and seizures. Electrolyte imbalances may result in signs of hypocalcemia (see "Hypocalcemia"), muscle cramps, and twitching.

PSYCHOSOCIAL. Patients with CRF present complex and difficult challenges to caregivers. Many have personality and cognitive changes. Apathy, irritability, and fatigue are common and interfere with interpersonal relationships. Sexual dysfunction is common. A careful assessment of the patient's capabilities, home situation, available support systems, financial resources, and coping abilities is important before any nursing interventions can be planned.

DIAGNOSTIC HIGHLIGHTS

Test	Normal Result	Abnormality with Condition	Explanation
Blood urea nitrogen (BUN)	5–20 mg/dL	Elevated	Kidneys cannot excrete wastes
Serum creatinine	0.5–1.1 mg/dL	> 3.0 mg/dL	Kidneys cannot excrete wastes
24 hour urine creatinine	Females 85–125 mL/min; males 95–135 mL/min	< 95% decrease	Acute damage to the kidney limits ability to clear creatinine

Other Tests: Urinalysis; complete blood count; erythrocyte sedimentation rate; hemodynamic monitoring; renal ultrasound; radionuclide scanning; magnetic resonance angiography; renal biopsy; serum levels of sodium, potassium, magnesium, and phosphorus; arterial blood gases

PRIMARY NURSING DIAGNOSIS

Fluid volume excess related to compromised regulatory mechanisms

OUTCOMES. Fluid balance; Hydration; Circulation status; Cardiac pump effectiveness

INTERVENTIONS. Fluid monitoring; Fluid/electrolyte management; Intravenous therapy; Circulatory care; Medication management; Hemodialysis therapy; Vital signs monitoring

☐ PLANNING AND IMPLEMENTATION

Collaborative

Patients who have progressed to ESRD require either dialysis or renal transplantation. The three basic types of dialysis are peritoneal dialysis, hemodialysis, and continuous hemofiltration. Peritoneal dialysis uses the peritoneum as the semipermeable membrane. Access is achieved with the surgical placement of a catheter into the peritoneal cavity. Approximately 2 L of sterile dialysate is infused into the cavity and left for a variable period of time (usually from 4 to 8 hours). At the end of the cycle, the dialysate is removed and discarded. A fresh amount of sterile dialysate is infused, and the cycle is continued.

Hemodialysis uses a surgically inserted vascular access, such as a shunt, or vascular access into an arterialized vein that was created by an arteriovenous fistula. In emergencies, vascular access through a large artery may be used. The blood is removed through one end of the vascular access and is passed through a machine (dialyzer). The dialyzer contains areas for the dialysate and the blood, separated by a semipermeable membrane. The fluid and waste products move quickly through the membrane because the pressure on the blood side is higher than on the dialysate side. The blood is returned to a venous access site.

Continuous hemofiltration uses vascular access in the same manner as hemodialysis. The patient's heparinized blood goes from an arterial access, through the hemofilter (the semipermeable membrane), and back to the patient through venous access. No dialysate is used. The hemofilter uses the patient's own blood pressure as the source of pressure. One disadvantage is that frequently too much fluid is filtered, thus resulting in the need for intravenous fluid replacement. Other procedures, such as veno-veno dialysis, are also used in some institutions.

Surgical interventions for the patient with CRF consist of creating peritoneal or vascular access for dialysis or renal transplantation. The transplanted kidney may come from a living donor or a cadaver. One-year survival rates are currently 70% to 90%. The new organ is placed in the iliac fossa. The original kidneys are not generally removed unless there is an indication, such as infection, for removing them. The greatest postoperative problem is transplant rejection. The diet for the CRF patient is generally restricted in fluids, protein, sodium, and potassium. It is usually high in calories, particularly carbohydrates. The fluid restriction is generally the amount of the previous day's urine plus 500 to 600 mL. The patient with CRF is frequently taking many medications. A significant concern is that the patient's altered renal function also alters the action and the excretion of medications; toxicity, therefore, is always considered a possibility, and dosages are altered accordingly.

PHARMACOLOGIC HIGHLIGHTS

Medication or Drug Class	Dosage	Description	Rationale
Antihypertensives	Varies by drug	ACE inhibitors; beta-adrenergic antagonists	Treat the underlying hypertension
Diuretics	Varies by drug	Loop and thiazide diuretics	Control fluid overload early in the disease if the patient is not anuric (total absence of urinary output)
Sodium bicarbonate	352–650 mEq/L po tid	Alkalinizing agent	Supplements sodium bicarbonate when serum level falls below 18–20 mEq/L

Sodium polystyrene sulfonate (Kayexalate)	Orally or by enema: 15 g/60 mL in 20–100 mL sorbitol to facilitate passage of resin through the intestinal tract	Cation exchange resin; 0.5–1.0 mEq/L of potassium is removed with each enema, but an equivalent amount of sodium is retained	Exchanges sodium for potassium in the GI tract, leading to the elimination of potassium

Other Drugs: Hypocalcemia and hyperphosphatemia may be treated with aluminum antacids that bind dietary phosphorus. If long-term effects of aluminum hydroxide are a concern, an oral calcium (with vitamin D) preparation may be given. Recombinant erythropoietin (Epogen) may be given for the treatment of anemia. If the patient undergoes renal transplantations, immunosuppressives such as azathioprine (Imuran) or cyclosporine (Sandimmune) are prescribed. Corticosteroids may also be given at this time to decrease antibody formation.

Independent

To help the patient deal with fluid restrictions, use creative strategies to increase the patient's comfort and compliance. Use ice chips, frozen lemon swabs, hard candy, and diversionary activities. Give medications with meals or with minimal fluids to maximize the amount of fluid that is available for patient use. Skin care is important because of the effects of uremia. Uremia results in itching and dryness of the skin. If the patient experiences pruritus, help the patient clip the fingernails short and keep the nail tips smooth. Teach the patient to use skin emollients liberally, to avoid harsh soaps, and to bathe only when necessary. You may need to speak to the physician to request an as-needed dose of an oral antihistamine such as diphenhydramine (Benadryl). If the patient is hospitalized, frequent turning and range-of-motion exercises assist in preventing skin breakdown. If the patient is taking medications that cause frequent stools, teach the patient to clean the perineum and buttocks frequently to maintain skin integrity.

The patient needs to plan the week's activities to incorporate the level of fatigue, the dialysis routine, and any desired activities. The patient may also find that cognitive activities are more easily accomplished on certain days in relationship to dialysis treatments. Reassure the patient that this is not unusual but is caused by the shift of fluid and waste products. Counseling relative to role function, family processes, and changes in body image is important. Sexuality counseling may be required. Reassure the patient that adaptation to a chronic illness with an uncertain future is not easy for either the patient or the significant others. Participate when asked in discussions related to feasibility of home dialysis, placement on the transplant list, and decisions related to acceptance or refusal of dialysis treatment. Encourage decisions that increase feelings of control for the patient.

If the patient undergoes a renal transplantation, provide preoperative and postoperative care as for any patient with abdominal surgery. Monitoring of fluids is more important for these patients than other surgical patients because a decrease in output may be an early sign of rejection. Other signs include weight gain, edema, fever, pain over the site, hypertension, and increased white blood cell count. Emotional support is important for the patient and family, both preoperatively and postoperatively, because both positive and negative outcomes produce emotional turmoil. Teaching about immunosuppressive drugs is essential before discharge.

DOCUMENTATION GUIDELINES

- Physical findings: Urinary output (if any) and description of urine, fluid balance, vital signs, findings related to complications of CRF, presence of pain or pruritus, mental status, GI status, skin integrity
- Condition of peritoneal or vascular access sites
- Nutrition: Response to dietary or fluid restrictions, tolerance to food, maintenance of body weight
- Complications: Cardiovascular, integumentary, infection
- Activity tolerance: Level of fatigue, ability to perform activities of daily living, mobility

DISCHARGE AND HOME HEALTHCARE GUIDELINES

CRF and ESRD are disorders that affect the patient's total lifestyle and the whole family. Patient teaching is essential and should be understood by the patient and significant others. Note that you may need to work collaboratively with social services to arrange for the patient's dialysis treatments. Issues such as the location for outpatient dialysis and follow-up, home health referrals, and the purchasing of home equipment are important. All teaching should be reinforced at intervals during the patient's lifetime.

CARE OF PERITONEAL CATHETER FOR DIALYSIS. The access site is a sterile area that requires a sterile dressing except when the site is being accessed. Teach the patient or significant others the dressing technique recommended by your institution. In addition, the patient needs to learn the signs of an infected access site, such as swelling, redness, drainage, and odor. In addition, teach the patient to avoid restrictive clothing around the waist and to avoid external abdominal pressure.

CARE OF EXTERNAL ARTERIOVENOUS DIALYSIS ACCESS (SHUNT). A shunt can be surgically inserted on any limb, but the dominant arm is usually avoided. The access site is considered sterile and is covered with a sterile dressing at all times. Teach the patient to cover the access site between dialysis treatments with a dressing and further support, such as a non-elastic tensor bandage. Because one end of the shunt is directly inserted into an artery, care must be taken to ensure that the shunt does not accidentally come apart, which would lead to immediate hemorrhage. Teach the patient to carry a clamp to use if the shunt becomes disconnected. Teach the patient to feel for the "thrill" of blood moving through the shunt when it is touched (except during dialysis). The presence of darker blood within the shunt may indicate clotting; if this condition occurs, the patient needs to notify the dialysis staff or physician immediately. Any pressure on that limb—such as blood pressure readings, sleeping with the affected limb under the body, carrying boxes or groceries with that arm, or tight clothing—is contraindicated. Tell the patient not to use creams or lotions on the access site and to protect the site during bathing.

CARE OF THE ARTERIOVENOUS FISTULA. The increased pressure in the arterialized vein creates a large and sometimes unsightly vessel but also creates an access site with enough pressure to complete hemodialysis. Teach the patient to palpate a thrill over the anastomosis or graft site every day. Postoperatively, the patient may be asked to do strengthening exercises (grasping ball) to increase the size of the arterialized vein. After hemodialysis, the nursing staff applies pressure for a lengthy period of time to ensure clotting of the patient's blood. If the patient notices excessive bleeding after a dialysis treatment, he or she must notify the dialysis unit. Teach the patient that the site does not need to be protected during bathing. Tell the patient to remind all healthcare personnel that the involved arm should not be used for blood pressure measurements and phlebotomy.

POST-TRANSPLANTATION TEACHING. Discharge teaching for the patient with a renal transplant includes information about medications and the signs of rejection. The immunosuppressive drugs place the patient at greater risk for infection and skin cancer. Teach the patient to avoid large groups of people in the first 3 to 4 months and strong sunlight for the duration of the transplant. Although most forms of daily activity are restricted only by how the patient is feeling, contact sports and heavy lifting are contraindicated because of the placement of the transplant. Teach the patient to report signs of infection, rejection, and skin changes immediately to the physician. Teach the patient or significant others about all medications, including dosage, potential side effects, and drug interactions.

Retinal Detachment

DRG Category: 046
Mean LOS: 4.4 days
Description: MEDICAL: Other Disorders of the Eye, Age > 17 with CC
DRG Category: 036
Mean LOS: 1.5 days
Description: SURGICAL: Retinal Procedures

A retinal detachment occurs when the retina is pulled away from or out of its normal position. The retina is the innermost lining of the eye and contains millions of photoreceptors, light-sensitive nerve fibers, and cells that are responsible for converting light energy into nerve impulses. The retina functions as film does in a camera: the light enters through the lens to the retina, and an image is transmitted to the brain via the optic nerve. The retina is attached to the choroid (vascular coat of the eye between the sclera and retina) at two locations: at the optic nerve and at the ciliary body. The remaining retina relies on the vitreous (jelly-like mass that fills the cavity of the eyeball) to apply pressure against the lining to maintain its position. The detachment can occur spontaneously as a result of a change in the retina or vitreous; this detachment is referred to as a primary detachment. Secondary detachment occurs as a result of another problem, such as trauma, diabetes, or pregnancy-induced hypertension. Complications from retinal detachment include visual impairment and blindness.

CAUSES

The most common cause of retinal detachment is the formation of a hole or tear, which can occur as part of the normal aging process or during cataract surgery or trauma. The hole allows the vitreous fluid to leak out between the layers, thus separating the sensory retinal layer from its blood supply in the choroid. Patients who have had previous cataract surgery, severe injury, or a family history of detachment, glaucoma, and nearsightedness are more likely to experience a retinal detachment.

GENDER AND LIFE SPAN CONSIDERATIONS

A retinal detachment most often occurs in women and men between the ages of 50 and 70. It can also occur infrequently in children who were born prematurely and are experiencing retinopathies as a result of prolonged oxygenation.

☐ ASSESSMENT

HISTORY. Patients with suspected retinal detachment complain of a painless change in vision. Ask the patient if he or she has experienced "floaters" or black spots, flashing lights, or the sensation of a curtain being pulled over the field of vision. Some patients report feeling as if they are looking through a veil or through cobwebs. Ask the patient if he or she recently experienced any eye trauma.

PHYSICAL EXAMINATION. A thorough visual examination is done to detect changes in vision. Inspect the retina with an ophthalmoscope to determine the extent of the tear. Assess the patient's ability to ambulate safely and to perform the normal activities of daily living.

PSYCHOSOCIAL. If the patient is still employed rather than retired, determine the effect of visual impairment on the patient's ability to perform the job. Determine the effects of visual changes on leisure activities. Assess the patient's support system, access to health care, and financial resources.

DIAGNOSTIC HIGHLIGHTS

Test	Normal Result	Abnormality with Condition	Explanation
Opthalmoscopic examination	Normal retina	Gray bulge or fold in retina; may be able to see jagged or irregularly-shaped tear	Allows examiner to view the internal and external structures of the eye

PRIMARY NURSING DIAGNOSIS

Sensory-perceptual alterations (visual) related to decreased sensory reception

OUTCOMES. Safety behavior: Fall prevention; Body image; Endurance; Rest; Neurological status; Well-being

INTERVENTIONS. Eye care; Fall prevention; Emotional support; Medication management; Self-esteem enhancement

☐ PLANNING AND IMPLEMENTATION

Collaborative

The main objective in treating a tear or hole is to prevent a retinal detachment. Photocoagulation, cryotherapy, and diathermy are used to produce an inflammatory response that creates an adhesion or scar, which seals the edges of the tear. These therapies differ in the mechanism used to cause the scarring effect. Photocoagulation uses light beams; cryotherapy uses cold to freeze the tissues; diathermy uses energy from a high-frequency current. All three result in sealing of the hole to prevent the vitreous from spilling between the layers.

If the retina is detached, surgical repair is required. The objective of the surgical procedure is to force the retina into contact with the choroid. The scleral buckling procedure places the retina back into position.

Preoperatively the patient is on bed rest and has activity restrictions, depending on the size and location of detachment. Total eye rest may be needed. The patient may not read, watch television, or participate in any activity that causes rapid eye movements. An eye patch may be prescribed. It is important to position the patient either to keep the retinal tear lowermost within the eye or in the dependent position to allow the retina to fall back against the epithelium, which prevents further detachment.

When gas or oil is used, the physician asks the patient to remain in a position that keeps the gas or bubble against the repaired area of the retina. The head is usually kept parallel to the floor and turned to the side with the unaffected eye down. It may take 4 to 8 days for the bubble to absorb. The patient cannot fly or travel up to high altitudes until the gas bubble is gone because a rapid increase in altitude can increase the intraocular pressure and result in a re-detachment of the retina. Reading, writing, close work, watching television, shampooing, shaving, and combing the hair may be restricted.

PHARMACOLOGIC HIGHLIGHTS

Medication or Drug Class	Dosage	Description	Rationale
Cyclopentolate hydrochloride (Cyclogyl)	Drops as prescribed	Cycloplegic agent	Causes dilation of the pupil and rest of the muscles of accommodation
Antibiotics	Drops as prescribed	Gentamicin; prednisolone acetate	Prevent eye infections

Other Drugs: Anti-emetics and analgesics are ordered to manage nausea, vomiting, and pain.

Independent

Assure the patient that it is normal for vision to continue to be distorted after surgery because of postoperative inflammation and cycloplegic eye drops. Inform the patient that vision will return to normal over several weeks. During hospitalization, keep the side rails raised, the bed in a low position, and the call light within the patient's reach. Provide a safe environment and identify potential safety hazards.

The patient needs to assume the position that was ordered by the physician for postoperative management. Assist the patient to use an over-the-bed table if necessary, or place pillows to support the arms and lower back. Place a sign at the head of the bed, giving each practitioner instructions on the position to be maintained. Observe the eye patch for drainage and notify the physician for drainage other then serous. Once the initial eye patch has been removed, place cool compresses over the closed eyelid for relief of discomfort. The eye may be swollen, reddened, and ecchymotic for several days, and the conjunctiva may persist for weeks. If the patient experiences postoperative nausea and vomiting, maintain an odor-free environment and apply cool compresses to the forehead.

DOCUMENTATION GUIDELINES

- Visual acuity
- Reaction to activity restrictions; ability of patient to participate in activities of daily living independently
- Complications such as bleeding, infection, decreased visual acuity, falls
- Response to medications and ability of the patient to instill eye drops
- Understanding of eye care at home

DISCHARGE AND HOME HEALTHCARE GUIDELINES

Have the patient or significant others demonstrate the correct technique for instilling eye drops. Instruct the patient to wash his or her hands before and after removing the dressing; using a clean washcloth, cleanse the lid and lashes with warm tap water; tilt the head backward and inclined slightly to the side, so the solution runs away from the tear duct and other eye to prevent contamination; depress the lower lid with the finger of one hand. Tell the patient to look up when the solution is dropped on the averted lower lid; do not the place drop directly on the cornea.

Do not touch any part of the eye with the dropper; close the eye after instillation, and wipe off the excess fluid from the lids and cheeks. Close the eye gently so the solution stays in the eye longer.

Teach the patient to use warm or cold compresses for comfort several times a day. Note that the patient should wear either an eye shield or glasses during the day, during naps, and at night. Teach the patient to avoid vigorous activities and heavy lifting for the immediate postoperative period. Teach the patient the symptoms of retinal detachment and the action to take if it occurs again. Instruct the patient about the importance of follow-up appointments, which may be every few days for the first several weeks after surgery.

Rheumatic Fever, Acute

DRG Category: 240
Mean LOS: 6.4 days
Description: MEDICAL: Connective Tissue Disorders with CC Heart Involvement
DRG Category: 144
Mean LOS: 4.5 days
Description: MEDICAL: Other Circulatory System Diagnosis with CC

Acute rheumatic fever is an autoimmune disorder that follows an upper respiratory infection with group A beta-hemolytic streptococci. Rheumatic fever affects the heart, central nervous system, skin, and musculoskeletal system. In addition to an initial insult, recurrences are common.

Acute rheumatic fever is most destructive to the heart. Rheumatic heart disease occurs in up to 50% of patients with acute rheumatic fever and may affect any of the layers of the heart during the acute phase. Endocarditis leads to leaflet swelling of the valves, leaflet erosion, and deposits of blood and fibrin on the valves; these deposits are called "vegetation." Myocarditis causes cellular swelling, damage to collagen, and formation of fibrosis and scarring. Pericarditis can occur as well, which can lead to pericardial effusion. In addition to valvular disease, acute rheumatic fever can lead to severe carditis and life-threatening heart failure. Complications lead to a 20% death rate within the first 10 years after the initial illness.

CAUSES

Acute rheumatic fever is caused by a prior streptococcal infection and is often associated with nasopharyngitis, or upper respiratory infections. The group A beta-hemolytic streptococcus infection, which may have been mild and even unnoticed and untreated, usually occurred 2 to 6 weeks before the development of symptoms of acute rheumatic fever. Experts suspect that rheumatic fever is an autoimmune response triggered by antibodies that are produced in response to the streptococcal infection. The antibodies react with the body's cells and produce characteristic lesions in the target organs.

GENDER AND LIFE SPAN CONSIDERATIONS

Although acute rheumatic fever primarily targets the school-age population, it also occurs in adults. It is particularly common in children aged 5 to 15 from disadvantaged backgrounds. Valvular heart disease is most likely to damage the mitral valve in females and the aortic valve in males. In both genders, tricuspid and pulmonic valve damage occurs rarely.

◻ ASSESSMENT

HISTORY. Usually the patient has a sore throat and a fever of at least 100.4°F a few days to several weeks before the onset. The patient either may have been treated with antibiotics or may not have completed a full course of treatment. Determine if the patient has experienced migratory joint tenderness (polyarthritis), chest pain, fever, and fatigue. Some patients describe unexplained nosebleeds as well. Patients with pericarditis may describe sharp pain over the shoulder that radiates to the neck, back, and arms. The pain may increase with inspiration and decrease when the patient leans forward from a sitting position. Patients with heart failure may describe shortness of breath, cough, and right upper quadrant abdominal pain. In addition, the patient may describe fatigue or activity intolerance, along with periorbital, abdominal, or pedal edema.

PHYSICAL EXAMINATION. The patient may have a distinctive red rash, referred to as erythema marginatum. This nonpruritic rash appears primarily on the trunk of the body, the buttocks, and the extremities; it appears on the face in only rare instances. In addition, subcutaneous nodules of less than 1 cm in diameter form on the skin. Painless and movable, they usually appear over bony prominences: the hands, wrists, elbows, knuckles, feet, and vertebrae. If the patient has heart failure, there may be peripheral edema.

The patient may also demonstrate chorea (previously referred to as St. Vitus' dance). Mild chorea produces hyperirritability, problems concentrating, and illegible handwriting. Severe chorea causes purposeless, uncontrollable jerky movement and muscle spasms, speech disturbances, muscle fatigue, and inco-ordination. Transient chorea may not appear until several months after the initial streptococcal infection.

When the joints are palpated, the patient may have migratory polyarticular arthritis (more than four joints are progressively involved). The most frequently involved joints include the knees, elbows, hips, shoulders, and wrists. These joints are extremely warm and tender to the touch, and even a light palpation can cause pain. The pain usually subsides after the patient becomes afebrile.

Heart murmurs serve as an indicator that carditis has occurred. The aortic and mitral valves are particularly involved as a result of the Aschoff bodies (small nodules of cells and leukocytes) that form on the tissues of the heart. You are more likely to hear the murmurs at the third intercostal space right of the sternum for the aortic valve and at the apex of the heart if the mitral valve is involved. When you palpate peripheral pulses, you may note a rapid heart rate.

PSYCHOSOCIAL. The disease is likely to occur at an age when children are active and industrious. Those that require extended bed rest may have trouble coping with the limitations placed on them.

DIAGNOSTIC HIGHLIGHTS

Test	Normal Result	Abnormality with Condition	Explanation
Throat cultures	Negative culture	Positive for Group A beta-hemolytic streptococci	Identifies causative organism in the acute phase of pharyngeal infection
ASO titer (antistreptolysin O titer)	< 166 Todd Units	< 250 Todd Units for an inactive infection; 500–5000 Todd Units for an active infection	Antibody to the streptolysin-O enzyme produced by group A beta-hemolytic streptococci; titers raise about 7 days after infection and gradually return to baseline after 12 months

Other Tests: Complete blood count, C-reactive protein, erythrocyte sedimentation rate (ESR) chest x ray, echocardiogram, chest computed tomography (CT) scan, chest magnetic resonance imaging (MRI)

PRIMARY NURSING DIAGNOSIS

Pain (acute) related to tissue swelling

OUTCOMES. Comfort level; Pain control behavior; Pain: Disruptive effects; Pain level

INTERVENTIONS. Pain management; Analgesic administration; Positioning; Teaching: Prescribed activity/exercise; Teaching: Procedure/treatment; Teaching: Prescribed medication

☐ PLANNING AND IMPLEMENTATION

Collaborative

The goal of management is to end the infection, relieve the symptoms, and prevent recurrence. Complete eradication of the streptococcal infection is necessary so that the heart and kidneys are not damaged. The physician may prescribe antibiotic therapy, intramuscular benzathine penicillin G, if the patient has no known history of allergy to penicillin. Reinforce the need for the patient to complete all medications and to watch for potential side effects, such as rash, hives, wheezing, or anaphylaxis. Activity restrictions are required to ensure full recovery. In patients with active carditis, strict bed rest may be needed for approximately 5 weeks. The physician then prescribes a progressive increase in activity. If valvular dysfunction leads to persistent heart failure, the patient may need surgery to correct the deficit in heart function.

PHARMACOLOGIC HIGHLIGHTS

Medication or Drug Class	Dosage	Description	Rationale
Benzathine penicillin G	1.2 million units IM	Antibiotic	Eradicates the infection; injections may be given in the hospital or by a home health nurse; oral penicillin may be given, with erythromycin as an alternative in those allergic to penicillin
Aspirin	650 mg po as needed	Nonsteroidal anti-inflammatory	Treats the arthralgia (muscle achiness); monitor for side effects such as tinnitus, gastric upset, and petechiae

Other Drugs: Prednisone (to treat the carditis); furosemide (for patients with congestive heart failure). After the acute phase of the disease, the physician usually prescribes monthly injections of benzathine penicillin G or daily oral antibiotics. Preventive treatment with antibiotics may last at least for 5 years.

Independent

Explain to the child and the family the need to take all antibiotics until they are completed. This information needs to be conveyed in such a manner so as to promote compliance, not communicate guilt. Remind the parents that failure to seek treatment for a streptococcal infection is common because the symptoms are so mild. The patient is likely to remain on oral antibiotics indefinitely through his or her life.

Managing activity restrictions is a challenging goal in working with a young person of school age who is on bed rest. As the chorea decreases, the child needs to participate in therapeutic play activities that promote a sense of industry and minimize any feelings of inferiority—activities such as reading, board games, and video game play. Encourage the parents to obtain a tutor so the patient can keep up with schoolwork during his or her convalescence. To protect the patient who develops chorea and has an unsteady gait, make sure that all obstructions are cleared out of the way during ambulation to reduce the risk of injury.

DOCUMENTATION GUIDELINES

- The extent of the skin lesions for the erythema marginatum rash and subcutaneous nodules
- The extent of chest pain and cardiac involvement
- The extent of the chorea and joint involvement
- Reaction to bed rest and activity restriction

DISCHARGE AND HOME HEALTHCARE GUIDELINES

Teach the patient or parents to prevent any further streptococcal infections by good hand washing and avoiding people with sore throats. Encourage the patient or parents to contact the primary healthcare provider if a sore throat occurs. Explain all medications, including dosage, action, route, and side effects. Encourage the patient to resume activity gradually and to use an elevator, if one is available, at school. Teach the patient to return to physical education classes or extracurricular sports gradually, with the guidance of the physician. Encourage the patient to take frequent naps and rest periods.

Rheumatoid Arthritis

DRG Category: 240
Mean LOS: 6.4 days
Description: MEDICAL: Connective Tissue Disorders with CC

Rheumatoid arthritis is a chronic, progressive, systemic disease that is characterized by recurrent inflammation of connective tissue, primarily diarthrodial joints (hinged joints that contain a cavity within the capsule that separates the bony elements to allow freedom of movement) and their related structures. The disease generally begins with inflammation of the synovial membrane, which becomes thickened and edematous. The thickened synovium, or pannus, erodes the articular cartilage and underlying bone, thus causing joint destruction. The small peripheral joints of the hand and wrist and the joints of the knees, ankles, elbows, and shoulders are usually affected symmetrically. The cervical spine may also be affected. Extra-articular involvement of the disease includes inflammation of the tendon sheaths; the bursae; and the connective tissue of the heart, lungs, pleurae, and arteries.

If the disease is left untreated, the inflammatory process of rheumatoid arthritis moves through four stages. In the first stage, synovitis is caused by congestion and edema of the synovial membrane and joint capsule. In the second stage, the formation of pannus, thickened layers of granulation tissue that cover and invade cartilage begins, and this leads to eventual destruction of the joint capsule and bone. In the third stage, fibrous ankylosisis noted in the inflammatory process; this is the fibrous invasion of the pannus and scar formation that occludes joint space. In the fourth and final stage, the fibrous tissue calcifies, causing ankylosis and total immobility.

Complications caused by rheumatoid arthritis include temporomandibular joint disease, which impairs the patient's chewing and causes headaches. Infection, osteoporosis, myositis, cardiopulmonary lesions, lymphadenopathy, and peripheral neuritis may also occur.

CAUSES

Although the specific cause of rheumatoid arthritis is unknown, there is speculation about multiple causation, which includes infection, autoimmunity, and genetic factors and also environmental and hormonal factors. The strongest evidence of an autoimmune cause is supported by the findings of rheumatoid factor (RF) in the serum of more than 80% of affected individuals. Studies in immunology have identified the appearance of a relationship between rheumatoid arthritis and the human leukocyte antigen (HLA) system, which is made up of a series of linked genes on the sixth chromosome, indicating a genetic causative factor.

GENDER AND LIFE SPAN CONSIDERATIONS

Rheumatoid arthritis is two to three times more common in women than in men. The disease can occur at any age, although the onset peaks between 30 and 60 years of age.

◻ ASSESSMENT

HISTORY. Determine if the patient has experienced fatigue, malaise, low-grade fever, weight loss, anemia, or anorexia, which are all common early symptoms of rheumatoid arthritis. Ask about stiffness: Does it occur before or after physical activity, and does the patient need to "limber up" after inactivity, such as sleeping? Ask if the patient has experienced paresthesia (tingling) of the hands and feet or joint pain with swelling and warmth in the joint. Determine whether the patient is taking medication for pain, and, if so, ask about the dosage and frequency.

PHYSICAL EXAMINATION. Observe the patient initially for pallor and signs of fatigue and immobility. Assess all joints carefully, looking for deformities, contractures, immobility, and inability to perform the activities of daily living. Inspect the patient's fingers for edema or congestion in the joints. Inspect the elbows for rheumatoid nodules, which are subcutaneous, rounded, non-tender masses. Note skin lesions or leg ulcers caused by vasculitis. Check for a positive Babinski's sign, which is caused by spinal cord compression if the vertebrae are involved. If the patient is able to participate, assess the metacarpophalangeal joints by having the patient dorsiflex, extend, and flex the fingers. Assess the patient's ability to perform radial and ulnar deviation. Also ask the patient to straighten the fingers, then abduct and adduct them. Test the muscle strength of the patient's hand by having the patient squeeze your hands simultaneously. Ask the patient to make a fist and resist your attempt to pry it open.

To assess the patient's elbow and shoulder range of motion, ask the patient to flex and extend the arms and to abduct and adduct each extended arm. Test the trapezius muscles by placing your hands on the patient's shoulders and asking the patient to shrug the shoulders as you press down on them. Look for subcutaneous nodules around the elbows.

Observe the range of motion of the hips, knees, and ankles by asking the patient to walk about and to sit down in a chair. If the patient is in pain, you can defer the examination, relying instead on observations of the patient as you observe him or her in the setting.

PSYCHOSOCIAL. Initially, assess the patient's understanding of what the disease means and what he or she believes life holds in the future. Identify the patient's support system and how available support persons are. If the patient has had rheumatoid arthritis for some time, assess the patient's current level of functioning. Determine if the disease affected relationships, work, or leisure activities.

DIAGNOSTIC HIGHLIGHTS

Test	Normal Result	Abnormality with Condition	Explanation
Rheumatoid factor (Rose Waaler)	Negative < 1:20	1:40–1:60	Identifies unusual IgG and IgM antibodies that develop against connective tissue disease
Antinuclear antibody	Negative	> 1:8	Identifies antibodies to the body's own DNA and nuclear material

Other Tests: Complete blood count, erythrocyte sedimentation rate, serum protein electrophoresis, serum complement, serum protein electrophoresis, synovial fluid analysis, immunoglobulin analysis, bone x rays, computed tomography (CT) scan, magnetic resonance imaging (MRI)

PRIMARY NURSING DIAGNOSIS

Pain (chronic) related to joint swelling and deformity

OUTCOMES. Comfort level; Pain control behavior; Pain: Disruptive effects; Pain level

INTERVENTIONS. Pain management; Analgesic administration; Positioning; Teaching: Prescribed activity/exercise; Teaching: Procedure/treatment; Teaching: Prescribed medication

☐ PLANNING AND IMPLEMENTATION

Collaborative

The goals of treatment are to relieve pain, inhibit the inflammatory response, preserve joint function, and prevent deformity. Initial medical treatment consists of pharmacologic measures. An appropriate ongoing exercise program is prescribed by the physical therapist; this includes teaching proper body mechanics. Therapy may also include the use of moist heat, but ice may be prescribed in some cases. Splints are provided for painful joints. The physical therapist teaches the patient to use a walker and cane if indicated.

Some patients may undergo surgery to restore joint function. One type of procedure, a synovectomy, involves removal of the inflamed synovium early in the disease process. Patients who are in relatively good physical and mental condition may be candidates for joint reconstructive surgery (arthroplasty). The effectiveness of hip and joint replacement is considered quite good, although replacement surgery associated with other joints is less efficacious. Osteotomy involves cutting the bone to realign the joint and to shift the pressure points to a less denuded area of the joint; this shift relieves pain. Tendon transfers may prevent deformities or relieve contractures.

PHARMACOLOGIC HIGHLIGHTS

Medication or Drug Class	Dosage	Description	Rationale
Nonsteroidal anti-inflammatory drugs	Varies with drug	Aspirin, ibuprofen, piroxicam, fenoprofen, phenylbutazone, indomethacin, propoxyphene, or naproxen, if the patient is intolerant to high doses of aspirin	Relieve pain; may be given with misoprostol (Cytotec) to minimize GI symptoms
Prednisone	5–60 mg po daily	Corticosteroid	Reduces inflammation in people who do not respond to nonsteroidal anti-inflammatory drugs

Other Drugs: Remission-producing agents, such as gold salts, d-penicillamine, and anti-malarials, may be prescribed in cases of persistent arthritis that do not respond to conservative therapy. In intractable cases, physicians may prescribe immonosuppressives such as methotrexate.

Independent

Teach the patient assistive techniques to manage joint pain, such as meditation, biofeedback, and distraction. Advise the patient to take warm to hot showers or baths in the morning or evening to help relieve the pain. During acute stages of the disease, encourage the patient to avoid exercising the inflamed joints; help the patient understand the need to rest; however, patients do need to maintain mobility and movement of joints that are not involved. Provide necessary assistance with the activities of daily living, and prevent flexion contractures by having the patient lie prone with the feet hanging between the mattress and footboard several times a day. Keep the patient warm, and provide meticulous skin care.

During subacute and chronic stages of rheumatoid arthritis, the patient needs to return to as much independence as possible. When mobility improves, encourage the patient to assume more responsibility for self-care. Promote adequate rest, especially after activity, and plan rest periods during the day. Assist the patient with nutrition to prevent anorexia, which contributes to anemia, thus causing further weakness and activity intolerance. Determine whether the patient has a firm mattress and straight-back chairs with arm rests at home to support proper positioning. Show the patient how to avoid flexion contractures of the large muscle groups while sleeping and sitting.

Teach the patient to avoid putting pillows under the legs while sitting and sleeping and to avoid sitting in soft, low chairs. When the acute inflammatory stage subsides and the patient is ready for discharge from the hospital, teach him or her to take medications as prescribed, stressing the need to maintain therapeutic blood levels of the drug. Suggest that the patient use dressing aids such as a long-handled shoehorn, elastic shoelaces, a zipper pull, and a buttonhook. Recommend the use of hand-held shower nozzles, grab bars, and hand rails. As rheumatoid arthritis progresses and deformity becomes pronounced, patients may suffer with body image disturbances and inability to engage in sexual activity. Assist the patient and partner to cope with these problems.

DOCUMENTATION GUIDELINES

- Physical findings: Deformed joints, swollen nodes, range of motion, strength and dexterity of extremities
- Response to medication and treatments, level of pain, degree of pain relief
- Ability to perform self-care and tolerance to activity

DISCHARGE AND HOME HEALTHCARE GUIDELINES

Ensure that the patient understands the appropriate methods for pain relief and the need to notify a home care agency or physician if the regimen is ineffective. Be sure the patient understands any pain medication prescribed, including dosage, route, action, and side effects. Ensure that the patient understands the rest-activity cycle, use of assistive devices, exercise routine, and proper body mechanics. Determine whether or not a home care agency needs to evaluate the home for safety equipment such as rails and grab bars and whether ongoing supervision is required. The Arthritis Foundation, which publishes information about arthritis, is engaged in a national education program about living with the condition. Help the patient get in touch with this organization.

Rocky Mountain Spotted Fever

DRG Category: 423
Mean LOS: 7.1 days
Description: MEDICAL: Other Infectious and Parasitic Diseases Diagnoses

Rocky Mountain spotted fever is a tick-borne disease that is found in all 48 contiguous states. A small intracellular parasite, *Rickettsia rickettsii*, is released from the salivary glands of some adult ticks. A concentration of cases occurs in the Southwestern, Southern, and Southeastern United States. The highest incidence of the disease occurs during the months of May, June, and July, the months when North Americans are most likely to be outdoors.

The patient outcome is directly related to accurate, early diagnosis and appropriate treatment. Without treatment, the disease has a mortality rate of up to 40%. With treatment, the mortality rate declines to less than 10%. After exposure, the incubation period is usually about a week, but in cases of severe infection, it can be as short as 2 days. Complications, although uncommon, include pneumonia, pneumonitis, middle-ear infections, and parotitis. If the infection is left untreated, the associated rash may lead to peeling skin and even gangrene of the elbows, fingers, and toes. Life-threatening complications—such as disseminated intravascular coagulation, shock, and acute renal failure—occur rarely.

CAUSES

Rickettsia rickettsii is implicated as the cause of Rocky Mountain spotted fever and is spread by exposure from two types of ticks. The mountain wood tick is found mainly in the West and is called *Dermacentor andersoni.* The dog tick, *Dermacentor variabilis,* is more commonly found in the East. The ticks attach themselves to exposed body areas such as the neck, hair, and ankles. The tick then not only engorges itself on the blood of the host, but also infects the host during a prolonged bite of 4 to 6 hours.

GENDER AND LIFE SPAN CONSIDERATIONS

The clinical symptoms of Rocky Mountain spotted fever vary with age. Most reports indicate that those infected are mostly male (60%) and under the age of 20 years (50%). Patients older than 15 years fit the most common clinical description of the disease (fever up to 104°F, headache, joint and muscle pain, rash), with the mortality rate the highest in patients over the age of 30 years. Patients younger than 15 years of age (and their parents) often wait longer to seek medical treatment, have a later onset of rash, and manifest more severe disease. These younger patients experience cardiac dysrhythmias and pneumonia more often than do mature patients.

◻ ASSESSMENT

HISTORY. At least 50% of patients presenting with Rocky Mountain spotted fever display the classic triad of symptoms: fever, rash, and a history of exposure to ticks. Ask about the dates of recent outdoor activities and known tick exposure. Note that only about 50% of patients actually recall tick exposure when they are diagnosed with Rocky Mountain spotted fever. Determine if the patient has pets because dogs are another source of the infection. Ask about common symptoms such as fever; severe headache; pain of the joints, muscles, and bones; malaise; and lethargy. Gastrointestinal symptoms are also common, including nausea, vomiting, diarrhea, constipation, anorexia, and abdominal pain.

PHYSICAL EXAMINATION. The patient appears acutely ill, with skin that is warm to the touch. Fevers from 102°F to 104°F are almost a universal symptom. The hallmark hemorrhagic rash that is associated with this disease appears 1 to 15 days after the onset of illness, most commonly around day 3, and therefore may not be present on the initial examination. The hands, wrists, feet, and ankles may have pink 2- to 5-mm macules that blanch with pressure. The rash spreads to the trunk, face, palms of the hands, and soles of the feet. Three days after the rash appears, it becomes fixed, a darker red with a petechial appearance. In approximately 10% of confirmed cases, there is no rash.

The patient may develop a rapid respiratory rate, shallow breathing, and a bronchial cough. Changes in mental status, such as confusion, agitation, and restlessness, may indicate a worsening condition. Fever and dehydration can lead to a rapid and thready peripheral pulse, hypotension, delayed capillary blanching, and shock. Late signs of complications include hepatomegaly and splenomegaly on palpation and pitting peripheral edema.

PSYCHOSOCIAL. Assess the patient's social support network and consider the effect the illness has on the patient's family. Expect them to be anxious and fearful about a sudden, unexpected serious illness. The patient may have to take time off from high school, college, or work and may worry about unmet financial, family, or educational obligations. Note the patient's developmental stage, and recognize the age-related concerns that a sudden illness creates.

DIAGNOSTIC HIGHLIGHTS

Most often the diagnosis of Rocky Mountain spotted fever is made as a result of clinical findings because diagnostic titers of antibodies are only detectable 10 days after the onset of illness. Other tests such as complement fixation titer, indirect hemagglutination titer, indirect immunofluorescence titer, and latex agglutination titer may confirm the diagnosis.

PRIMARY NURSING DIAGNOSIS

Impaired gas exchange related to increased alveolar capillary permeability

OUTCOMES. Respiratory status: Gas exchange and ventilation; Symptom control behavior; Comfort level; Treatment behavior: Illness or injury

INTERVENTIONS. Respiratory monitoring; Energy management; Airway management; Anxiety reduction; Oxygen therapy; Airway suctioning; Airway insertion and stabilization; Cough enhancement; Mechanical ventilation

☐ PLANNING AND IMPLEMENTATION

Collaborative

If the patient needs to have a tick removed, wear gloves and place gentle traction on the tick with either tweezers or the fingers. Do not crush the tick because inhaling the bacteria may lead to disease exposure. Do not apply noxious chemicals onto the tick. Because the patient may be further injured if a match is used on the tick, do not apply a match to the skin to remove the tick. Patients who have severe cases of Rocky Mountain spotted fever are admitted to the hospital, possibly to the intensive care unit. Central parenteral administration of fluids and antibiotics is often necessary, and the patient may also be monitored with a pulmonary artery catheter if he or she is hemodynamically unstable.

PHARMACOLOGIC HIGHLIGHTS

Medication or Drug Class	Dosage	Description	Rationale
Antibiotics	Varies with drug; administered for 7–14 days, depending on patient and drug	Tetracycline hydrochloride for patients over the age of 8 orally or parenterally in 4 divided doses; chloramphenicol for patients less than 8 years of age or in adults with severe disease who have central nervous system involvement	Kill the microorganism and fight infection

Other Drugs: Symptom management—Antipyretics are usually necessary for temperature control, and analgesia is used to control discomfort. Usually the physician avoids prescribing aspirin because of the added risk of platelet dysfunction.

Independent

Nursing care focuses on increasing comfort, monitoring for complications, and educating the patient. Implement nonpharmacologic strategies to manage discomfort, such as tepid sponge baths for fever, frequent linen changes for excessive diaphoresis, and age-appropriate diversions for discomfort. Teach the patient guided imagery, deep-breathing techniques, and music therapy to manage pain and boredom. Provide age-appropriate activities for young adults, such as television, radio, compact disks, and videos, to help them pass the time and to take their minds off discomfort. To conserve the patient's energy during a time of increased metabolic demand, assist with activities of daily living and space all care-giving activities with periods of rest to decrease the patient's oxygen expenditure.

Monitor the patient's skin rash for signs of infection, such as sloughing, redness, warmth, and purulent drainage. Help the patient move in bed to positions of comfort every hour or two, and pad the elbows and heels to prevent skin breakdown. Provide mouth care every 4 hours, and offer the patient mentholated lotions to decrease the itching that is associated with the rash. If possible, maintain a cool room temperature to help the patient control the itching. When the patient's condition has stabilized, discuss methods to avoid tick bites in the future. Encourage the patient to avoid tick-infested areas. If the patient chooses to be out of doors in such an area, teach him or her to wear protective clothing (long pants, tucked-in shirt, laced boots) and to inspect the entire body every 4 hours for ticks. If a tick bite occurs, explain that the tick should be removed with a tweezers by steady traction and then discarded immediately without crushing.

DOCUMENTATION GUIDELINES

- Patient history: Recent trips and outdoor activities specific to possible tick exposure, exposure to pets, and early physical signs
- Physical findings: Pink macular rash, trend of vital signs, fluid intake and output, respiratory assessment, and level of oxygenation (measured by pulse oximetry)

- Patient's response to antibiotic treatment, antipyretics, and other measures to control temperature, and analgesics

DISCHARGE AND HOME HEALTHCARE GUIDELINES

To prevent Rocky Mountain spotted fever, teach patients to avoid tick exposure if possible. Encourage them to wear dark, hooded clothing that is tight around the ankles and wrists when walking in wooded areas and tall grasses. Boots that lace provide additional protection. Explain that after spending time in the country, patients should examine their skin and especially hair for the presence of ticks. Remind patients to use a tick repellant spray containing diethyltoluamide on their clothing. Teach patients to avoid spraying tick repellant directly on the skin.

Be sure the patient understands the importance of continuing to take antibiotics for the entire course. The most commonly prescribed antibiotic for adults is tetracycline. Teach the patient to avoid combining tetracycline with milk, antacids, and iron pills because these inactivate the drug. Antibiotics are prescribed for up to 1 week after the fever is gone. Teach the patient to report increasing shortness of breath, inability to take oral food and fluids, or a rash that appears infected. Encourage patients to report a fever that does not respond to every-4-hour doses of acetaminophen.

Salmonella Infection (Salmonellosis)

DRG Category: 423
Mean LOS: 7.1 days
Description: MEDICAL: Other Infectious and Parasitic Diseases Diagnoses

Salmonellosis is a bacterial infection caused by gram-negative bacilli of the genus *Salmonella*. Sometimes classified as food poisoning because it is frequently acquired by ingesting food that has been contaminated with the *Salmonella* bacterium, salmonellosis occurs as either enterocolitis, bacteremia, localized infection, typhoid, or parathyroid fever. The most severe form of salmonellosis is typhoid, which can cause perforation or hemorrhage of the intestines, pneumonia, toxemia, acute circulatory failure, and cerebral thrombosis.

Once the *Salmonella* bacterium is ingested, it multiplies rapidly in the mucosal layers of the stomach and small intestine. The greater the number of organisms ingested, the shorter the incubation period; typically, incubation is 8 to 48 hours after ingestion of contaminated food or liquid, and symptoms usually last for 3 to 5 days. An inflammatory response in the tissues produces gastroenteritis. The infection may stop there, or the salmonella organisms may travel via the lymph and vascular system throughout the body. The dissemination of organisms produces lesions in other organs or, possibly, sepsis. Systemic lesions may result in appendicitis, peritonitis, otitis media, pneumonia, osteomyelitis, or endocarditis. Symptoms of intermittent fever, chills, anorexia, and weight loss indicate sepsis.

CAUSES

Salmonellosis is caused by any of more than 2000 serotypes of *Salmonella* bacteria. Typhoid is transmitted through ingestion of water that has been contaminated with the feces of infected persons. Salmonellosis may also be contracted by eating infected raw eggs or egg products or uncooked meat or poultry, ingesting raw milk, or handling infected animals. *Salmonella* can survive for an extended period of time in water, sewage, ice, and food. Although cooking food thoroughly can reduce the risk of salmonellosis, it cannot eliminate it.

GENDER AND LIFE SPAN CONSIDERATIONS

All people are susceptible. Although the disease is rarely fatal, severity may be pronounced in infants and persons with neoplastic, immunosuppressive, or other debilitating conditions. Enterocolitis and bacteremia are more common among infants. Women over 50 years of age are the most common carriers of typhoid. AIDS patients are susceptible to recurrent bacteremia caused by *Salmonella* bacteria.

☐ ASSESSMENT

HISTORY. Establish a history of fever (often 102°F and higher), nausea, abdominal pain, vomiting, anorexia, and diarrhea that have persisted for at least 4 days. Ask about headache or constipation, which are symptoms of typhoid. The first symptoms generally appear between 8 and 48 hours after ingesting the bacteria; ask the patient about possible sources of the infection. Ask if the patient has had recent contact with an infected person or animal. Determine if the patient has ingested uncooked egg or meat products. If so, ask the patient whether the potentially contaminated food was prepared at home or at another location, such as a restaurant or public gathering. Elicit a history of recent travel to other countries that have endemic typhoid.

PHYSICAL EXAMINATION. The patient appears to be weak and pale because of vomiting and diarrhea. Young children and debilitated patients may show signs of dehydration. Fevers range from 101°F to 105°F. Rose spots may appear on the trunk, and joints may be painful. Palpation of the abdomen may be difficult because of tenderness. Stools are usually greenish-brown, watery, and foul smelling. They contain mucus, pus, or blood.

PSYCHOSOCIAL. The patient with salmonellosis feels ill and may be apprehensive about the diagnosis. The patient feels guilty if he or she has inadvertently exposed others to the disease through food preparation or angry if he or she has been exposed to the illness at a restaurant or other public gathering. Parents of young children are apt to be anxious and afraid for their child's life.

DIAGNOSTIC HIGHLIGHTS

Test	Normal Result	Abnormality with Condition	Explanation
Cultures of feces, urine, vomitus, pus, or blood	Negative for pathogens	Presence of *Salmonella*	Determines presence of *Salmonella* in various samples; stool culture is the definitive diagnostic tool for salmonellosis

Other Tests: Complete blood count to determine the response to infection

PRIMARY NURSING DIAGNOSIS

Infection related to the presence of the infective organism

OUTCOMES. Immune status; Knowledge: Infection control; Risk control; Risk detection; Treatment behavior: Illness or injury

INTERVENTIONS. Infection control; Medication management; Environmental management; Surveillance; Nutrition management; Teaching: Disease process

☐ PLANNING AND IMPLEMENTATION

Collaborative

Patients with systemic infections are placed on the antibiotic that is most appropriate for their condition. Symptom management is accomplished by fluid and electrolyte replacement and control of fever. Because antidiarrheal and antispasmodic agents slow intestinal mobility, some experts do not recommend their use because they retard the intestinal transit of the infecting organisms.

The patient with salmonellosis is placed on bed rest during the acute phase and should be on enteric precautions until the diarrhea stops. Observe the patient's stools for consistency and blood. Bleeding or abdominal pain may indicate the complication of bowel perforation; check for a sudden fall in temperature or blood pressure and a rising pulse rate. Many patients with *Salmonella* infection are not hospitalized but recover at home. Report *Salmonella* infection to the local health authority, particularly if the patient is employed in a food-handling occupation.

PHARMACOLOGIC HIGHLIGHTS

Medication or Drug Class	Dosage	Description	Rationale
Antibiotics	Varies with drug	Ampicillin, third-generation cephalosporins, or chloramphenicol; treatment with antibiotics for gastroenteritis is controversial; experts suggest that antibiotics do not shorten the disease and prolong the time that the patient is a carrier	Kill bacteria and halt infection
Nonsystemic antidiarrheals	60–120 mL after each loose bowel movement po	Kaolin/pectin (Kaopectate)	Coat the intestinal mucosa, decrease intestinal secretions, and reduce discomfort

Independent

Relieve pain and discomfort from diarrhea by using a heating pad on the abdomen and washing and lubricating the anus. Use universal precautions. Employ scrupulous hand-washing techniques before and after working with the patient who has salmonellosis. Wear gloves when you dispose of feces or any objects that have been contaminated by the patient's feces. Provide regular skin and mouth care, and turn the patient often. While the patient is infected, allow him or her as much rest as possible between activities. Provide a restful atmosphere. To help reduce the patient's temperature, apply tepid wet towels to the patient's groin and axillae.

After joint abscesses have been drained, provide heat, elevation, and passive range-of-motion exercises to decrease swelling and maintain mobility. Explain to the patient the need to report salmonella infections to the local health authority. To prevent future infections, instruct the patient and family to wash their hands thoroughly after defecation and before handling food. Also, instruct the patient to avoid raw eggs or foods prepared with raw eggs, to cook meat and poultry thoroughly, to refrigerate food below 46°F, and to wash the hands after handling animals.

DOCUMENTATION GUIDELINES

- Physical findings: Vital signs; dehydration; intake of food and fluids; tolerance of food, including instances of vomiting; output; and diarrhea or constipation with description of stool
- Notification of the local health authority
- Response to treatment: Changes in symptoms, increased comfort, and decrease in body temperature

DISCHARGE AND HOME HEALTHCARE GUIDELINES

Instruct the patient and family about the cause, transmission, and symptoms of the disease and preventive measures. Teach the family how to care for the patient at home. Treat mild fever with antipyretics, and maintain a good fluid intake. Ice pops and soda may increase fluid intake for young children. Avoid the use of laxatives. Gradually increase the patient's activity level as tolerated. Explain the need to report complications of bleeding, dehydration, or the return of symptoms to the physician at once. Be sure the patient understands any medications prescribed, including dosage, route, action, and side effects. Stress the importance of completing the antibiotic regimen even after symptoms diminish.

Sarcoidosis

DRG Category: 092
Mean LOS: 6.4 days
Description: MEDICAL: Interstitial Lung Disease with CC

Sarcoidosis, formerly called Boeck's sarcoid, is a noncontagious multisystem disorder characterized by epithelioid granular tumors (granulomas) that most frequently affect the lung; more than 90% of cases involve lung or intrathoracic lymph node involvement. Pulmonary sarcoidosis is usually a chronic disorder associated with an intense cellular immune response in the alveolar structures of the lungs. A series of interactions between lymphocytes (primarily responsible for the granuloma formation), macrophage/monocytes (primarily responsible for interstitial fibrosis), epithelioid cells, and giant cells lead to the formation of noncaseating granulomas. The granulomas can lead to fibrosis, which affects the lung's ability to exchange gases. Other recurrent sites include the liver, lymph nodes, bone marrow, skin, and eyes. Sarcoidosis is detected occasionally in the spleen, joints, heart, skeletal muscle, phalangeal bones, parotid glands, and central nervous system (CNS).

About 65% to 70% of the cases of sarcoidosis usually resolve spontaneously within 2 years. Without treatment, however, sarcoidosis can lead to chronic progressive sarcoidosis, which is associated with pulmonary fibrosis, scarring, and progressive pulmonary disease. In such cases, when the heart can no longer pump against the noncompliant fibrotic lungs, cor pulmonale can develop. Other potentially lethal complications are superinfections by organisms such as *Aspergillus*.

CAUSES

Sarcoidosis is a complex and mysterious disease of unknown origin, although 80% of patients with sarcoidosis have presented with high titers of the Epstein-Barr virus. There is increasing evidence that a triggering agent strikes and stimulates an enhanced cell-mediated immune process at the site of involvement. The triggering agent may be a fungus, an atypical mycobacterium, pine pollen, or a toxic chemical such as zirconium or beryllium, which can lead to illnesses resembling sarcoidosis. Because there is a slightly higher incidence of sarcoidosis in the same family, the triggering agent may be genetic.

GENDER AND LIFE SPAN CONSIDERATIONS

The disease onset is usually between 20 and 30 years of age or between 45 and 65 years of age and is more frequent among women than men. Frequency is ten times higher in African-Americans than in European-Americans; African-American women of childbearing age develop sarcoidosis twice as frequently as do African-American men.

◻ ASSESSMENT

HISTORY. Sarcoidosis is known as the great masquerader because it presents in a variety of guises from lymphadenopathy to erythema nodosum (red and painful nodules on the legs, associated with rheumatism). Establish a history of arthralgia in the wrists, ankles, and elbows, which is an initial symptom of sarcoidosis. Ask if the patient has experienced fatigue, malaise, weakness, anorexia, or weight loss. Elicit a history of respiratory difficulties, such as breathlessness, cough (generally nonproductive but may be blood-tinged [hemoptysis]), or substernal chest pain. Ask if the patient has had any visual deficits or any eye pain, night sweats, seizures, or cranial or peripheral nerve palsies, which are signs of CNS involvement. Determine if a family history of sarcoidosis exists. Ask if the patient has been exposed to a viral or bacterial infection or to chemicals such as beryllium or zirconium.

PHYSICAL EXAMINATION. Examine the patient's skin for lesions, plaques, papules, and subcutaneous nodules on the face, neck, and extremities. A common skin lesion, erythema nodosum, is seen in 10% of cases; other lesions, such as lupus pernio (hard, blue-purple, swollen, shiny lesions of the nose, cheeks, lips, ears, fingers, and knees), are seen in 15% of patients. When granulomas affect the face, they tend to occur around the nose and may cause nasal destruction and disfigurement. Note the patient's skin tone for signs of jaundice.

Examine the patient's eyes for signs of enlarged tear glands, conjunctival infections, and granulomatous uveitis; if the patient has noted visual difficulties, perform a vision examination. Bilateral granulomatous uveitis occurs in 15% of cases and can lead to loss of vision because of secondary glaucoma. Other ocular symptoms may include retinal periphlebitis, lacrimal gland enlargement, and conjunctival infiltration, which can result in blurred vision, ocular pain, conjunctival infections, and iritis.

Inspect the patient's legs and arms for muscle wasting and enlarged or reddened joints. Ask the patient to move the joints in full range of motion to determine if pain or tenderness occurs. Palpate the salivary and parotid glands to determine if nontender enlargement is present. Palpate the lymph nodes to assess for lymphadenopathy and the abdomen for an enlarged liver and spleen. Auscultate the patient's chest to determine if diminished breath sounds indicate pulmonary fibrosis, infiltration, or restrictive disease. If breath sounds are not audible in one lung, suspect a pneumothorax. If you hear adventitious breath sounds or lung consolidation, suspect pulmonary infection. Auscultate the patient's heart, and note any irregularities that might indicate bundle-branch block or ventricular ectopy.

PSYCHOSOCIAL. As with any chronic disease, the patient and family need continual support and caring from healthcare professionals. Assess the patient's and family's ability to cope with a chronic disease and the change in roles that a chronic disease demands. The patient may also be distressed over changes in his or her appearance that have been caused by lesions on the face in particular.

DIAGNOSTIC HIGHLIGHTS

General Comment: Sarcoidosis is primarily diagnosed by exclusion.

Test	Normal Result	Abnormality with Condition	Explanation
Tuberculin skin test, fungal serologies, and sputum cultures for mycobacteria and fungi	Negative	Used to make a differential diagnosis; positive results indicate diagnosis other than sarcoidosis	Rule out tuberculosis
Tissue biopsy	Negative	Used to make a differential diagnosis; positive results indicate diagnosis other than sarcoidosis	Rules out mediastinal lymphoma and other granuloma lung diseases
Chest x ray	Clear lung fields with no lymphadenopathy	Bilateral hilar lymphadenopathy or lung involvement is visible in 90% of cases	Sarcoidosis is staged by x ray, ranging from Stage 0 (normal chest x ray) through Stage 4 (lung fibrosis)

PRIMARY NURSING DIAGNOSIS

Impaired gas exchange related to altered alveolar-capillary membrane changes and decreased oxygen-carrying ability

OUTCOMES. Respiratory status: Gas exchange and ventilation

INTERVENTIONS. Airway management; Oxygen therapy; Respiratory management; Energy management; Surveillance; Respiratory monitoring; Ventilation assistance; Respiratory monitoring; Anxiety reduction

☐ PLANNING AND IMPLEMENTATION

Collaborative

Asymptomatic sarcoidosis requires no treatment, although ongoing assessment is called for. Sarcoidosis with ocular, respiratory, CNS, cardiac, or systemic symptoms requires treatment with systemic or topical corticosteroids. Other treatment includes a low-calcium, high-calorie nutritional diet with an increase in fluids to prevent malnutrition, hypercalcemia, and dehydration. A low-sodium diet may be indicated if sodium retention occurs because of prednisone. Ongoing monitoring of the patient's physical condition by physical examination and diagnostic tests indicates the patient's response to treatment and the appearance of complications.

PHARMACOLOGIC HIGHLIGHTS

Medication or Drug Class	Dosage	Description	Rationale
Prednisone	May range from 30 to 60 mg per day po, tapering over 4–8 weeks to a maintenance dose of 10–15 mg for 6 months	Corticosteroids remain the mainstay of therapy for the first 1–2 years, but some patients may require lifelong steroid therapy.	Relieves symptoms and reverse fibrosis of pulmonary tissue

Other Drugs: Optic agents such as methylcellulose eye drops and other ophthalmic ointments are used to treat ocular manifestations. Antidysrhythmic agents are used to treat ventricular ectopy. Salicylates and other nonsteroidal anti-inflammatory drugs are used for the treatment of arthritis manifestations.

Independent

Because many patients have pulmonary granulomas that have the potential to affect airway, breathing, and gas exchange, the primary nursing focus is to ensure that these essential functions are preserved. Maintain an oral airway and endotracheal intubation equipment near the patient at all times in case they are needed to clear airway obstruction. Support the patient's breathing by positioning the patient for comfort (often with the head of the bed elevated and the arms raised slightly on pillows). Adjust the patient's activity to reduce oxygen demands. Space all activities with adequate periods of rest. Provide uninterrupted periods of sleep at night and at least one 2-hour rest period during the day. Schedule diagnostic tests to provide adequate rest, and work with the family and other visitors to conserve the patient's energy.

The patient's change in vision places him or her at risk for injury. Teach the patient to scan the area for obstructions before he or she begins to walk. Remove any obstructions or rugs in the path between the patient's bed and the bathroom. Encourage the patient to wear well-fitting shoes or slippers when ambulating. The patient's impaired vision, intolerance to activity, and any lesions on the face may lead to a disturbance in self-concept or body image. Elicit from the patient his or her priorities for a "good" appearance and support those activities that the patient finds beneficial. Those activities may include extra hair care, using makeup, wearing clothing from home, maintaining a beard or moustache, or other similar grooming strategies. Help the patient maintain the highest level of activity that his or her disease allows. As with any chronic, debilitating disease with no cure, the patient is expected to have times of depression and anxiety. Use a supportive, nonjudgmental approach and active listening. Answer the patient's questions honestly, and provide information about the long-range prognosis of the condition. If the patient or family demonstrates ineffective coping, refer the patient or significant others for counseling or to a support group.

DOCUMENTATION GUIDELINES

- Physical findings: Breath sounds, respiratory rate and depth, heart sounds, cardiac rhythm, visual changes, ability to ambulate safely, appearance of skin lesions
- Pain: Degree of joint and muscle pain; location, duration, and type of pain; response to analgesics; degree of mobility or immobility
- Response to corticosteroid therapy, changes in activity tolerance, ability to perform self-care

DISCHARGE AND HOME HEALTHCARE GUIDELINES

Teach the patient the purpose, dosage, schedule, precautions and potential side effects, interactions, and adverse reactions of all prescribed medications. Stress the need for compliance with prescribed steroid therapy. Stress the importance of regular follow-up and treatment. If appropriate, refer the patient with failing vision to community support and resources such as the American Foundation for the Blind, 15 W. 16th Street, New York, NY 10011 (212-620-2000).

Teach the patient the signs and symptoms of possible complications that need to be reported to the primary healthcare provider, such as dizziness, anorexia, and peripheral edema (cor pulmonale); diminished vision and massive urine output (diabetes insipidus); flank pain (kidney stones); headache and fever (meningitis); and fever and productive cough (infection).

Septic Shock

DRG Category: 127
Mean LOS: 5.5 days
Description: MEDICAL: Heart Failure and Shock

Septic shock is a clinical syndrome associated with severe systemic infection. It is a sepsis-induced shock with hypotension despite adequate fluid replacement. Patients have perfusion abnormalities, including lactic acidosis, oliguria (urine output < 400 mL per day), or an acute alteration in mental status. Often septic shock is characterized by decreased organ perfusion, hypotension, and organ dysfunction. Septic shock is the major cause of death in intensive care units; the mortality rate is as high as 50% to 80% depending on the patient population. The incidence has increased during the last 50 years in North America.

The syndrome usually begins with the development of a local infectious process. Bacteria from the local infection enter the systemic circulation and release toxins into the bloodstream. Gram-negative bacteria release endotoxins from their cell membrane as they lyse and die, whereas gram-positive bacteria release exotoxins throughout their life span. These toxins trigger the release of cytokines (proteins released by cells to signal other cells) such as tumor necrosis factor and the interleukins. They also activate phagocytic cells such as the macrophages. The complex chemical reactions lead to multiple system effects. As the syndrome progresses, blood flow becomes more sluggish, tissues become hypoxic, and acidosis develops. Ultimately, major organ systems (such as the lungs, kidneys, liver, and blood coagulation) fail, which leads to multiple organ dysfunction syndrome.

CAUSES

Although any microorganism may cause septic shock, it is most often associated with gram-negative bacteria such as *Escherichia coli, Klebsiella pneumoniae, Pseudomonas,* and *Serratia.* Gram-positive bacteria such as *Staphylococcus aureus* can also cause septic shock and in past years have led to outbreaks of toxic shock syndrome. A fungal infection causes septic shock in less than 3% of the cases. Common factors or conditions that are associated with septic shock include diabetes mellitus, malnutrition, alcohol abuse, cirrhosis, respiratory infections, hemorrhage, cancer, and surgery. People with traumatic injuries with either peritoneal contamination, burns, prolonged intravenous (IV) cannulation, abscesses, or multiple blood transfusions are at particular risk as well.

GENDER AND LIFE SPAN CONSIDERATIONS

Elderly patients, both men and women, are at high risk because of the immunocompromise that is associated with the aging process. In neonates, the most common cause of septic shock is an immature immune system. Clinical manifestations may differ in the adult and pediatric populations. For instance, poor feeding and decreased activity levels may be early indicators of septic shock in infants. Pediatric patients may also maintain vital signs within normal limits for longer periods of time before circulatory failure occurs. Older individuals may never have an increased temperature and may remain hypothermic throughout the course of the disease.

☐ ASSESSMENT

HISTORY. Patients appear critically ill and may have already been intubated and on mechanical ventilation for adult respiratory distress syndrome (ARDS). Because of the severity of the patient's condition, you may not be able to interview him or her for a complete history. You may obtain a great deal of information from the family and from other healthcare providers when the patient is transferred to your care. Because patients with septic shock are among the most critical of all patients treated in a hospital, they are admitted to a critical care unit for management.

Patients often have a history of either an infection or a critical event, such as a traumatic injury, perforated bowel, or acute hemorrhage. Some patients may also have a long-standing IV catheter or a Foley catheter. Determine the cause for the patient's admission to the hospital and any history of a chronic disease such as cancer, diabetes mellitus, or pneumonia. Note any brief periods of decreased tissue perfusion such as hemorrhage, severe hypotension, or cardiac arrest that may demand emergency management before the development of septic shock. Take a thorough medication history, with particular attention to recent antibiotic administration or total parenteral nutrition. Ask if the patient has been exposed to any treatment—such as organ transplantation, radiation therapy, or chemotherapy—that would lead to immunosuppression.

PHYSICAL EXAMINATION. Three stages have been identified, but all patients do not progress with the same pattern of symptoms. In early septic shock (early hyperdynamic, compensated stage), some patients are tachycardic, with warm and flushed extremities and a normal blood pressure. As shock progresses, the diastolic blood pressure drops, the pulse pressure widens, and the peripheral pulses are bounding. The patient's temperature may be within normal limits, elevated, or below normal, and the patient may be confused or agitated. Often the patient has a rapid respiratory rate, and peripheral edema may develop. In the second stage (late hyperdynamic, uncompensated stage), widespread organ dysfunction begins to occur. Blood pressure falls, and the patient becomes hypotensive. Increased peripheral edema becomes apparent. Respirations become more rapid and labored; you can hear rales when you auscultate the lungs; and the patient's sputum may become copious, pink, and frothy. In late septic shock, the blood pressure falls below 90 mm Hg for adults, the patient's extremities become cold, and signs of multiple organ failure (decreased urinary output, abdominal distension, absence of bowel sounds, bleeding from invasive lines, petechiae, cardiac dysrhythmias, hypoxemia, and hypercapnia) develop.

PSYCHOSOCIAL. As the syndrome progresses, patients may develop symptoms that change their behavior and appearance and situations that increase their anxiety and that of their family members. Ultimately the family may be faced with the death of a loved one. Continuously assess the coping mechanisms and anxiety levels in both patients and families.

DIAGNOSTIC HIGHLIGHTS

Test	Normal Result	Abnormality with Condition	Explanation
Cultures and sensitivities	Negative for pathologic bacterial	Positive for pathologic bacterial flora or fungi	Identifies infecting organism in blood,

flora or fungi	urine, sputum, or wounds; note that in 40% of patients who develop septic shock, no bacterium is ever identified in cultures

Other Tests: In the later stages of septic shock, as complications develop, serial chest x rays are essential to follow the progression of conditions such as pulmonary congestion and ARDS.

PRIMARY NURSING DIAGNOSIS

Infection related to exposure to bacteria from trauma, invasive instrumentation, or contamination

OUTCOMES. Immune status; Knowledge: Infection control; Risk control; Risk detection; Treatment behavior: Illness or injury

INTERVENTIONS. Infection control; Medication management; Environmental management; Surveillance; Nutrition management; Teaching: Disease process

□ PLANNING AND IMPLEMENTATION

Collaborative

The primary goals of treatment in septic shock are to maintain oxygen delivery to the tissues and to restore the vascular volume, blood pressure, and cardiac output. IV fluids are administered to increase the volume within the vascular bed; crystalloids (normal saline solution or lactated Ringer's injection) are usually the fluids of choice. Vasopressors, such as dopamine or norepinephrine (Levophed), may also be required to maintain an adequate blood pressure. The patient is also placed on broad spectrum IV antibiotics. If the patient's hemoglobin and hematocrit are insufficient to manage oxygen delivery, the patient may need blood transfusions. A pulmonary artery catheter is inserted to monitor fluid, circulatory, and gas exchange status.

An aggressive search for the source of sepsis is an essential part of the treatment. Any indwelling catheters, whether they are urinary, intravascular, intracerebral, or intra-arterial, are discontinued if possible or moved to another location. A surgical consultation may be performed to search for undrained abscesses or to debride wounds. If complications such as ARDS develop, more aggressive treatment is instituted. Intubation, mechanical ventilation, and oxygenation are required for severe respiratory distress or failure. Patients often need ventilator adjuncts, such as positive end-expiratory pressure, pressure-control ventilation, or inverse inspiration-to-expiration ratio ventilation.

Total parenteral feeding or enteral feedings may be instituted for patients who are unable to consume adequate calories. Monitor the success of nutritional therapy with daily weights. During supportive care, the entire healthcare team needs to monitor the patient's condition carefully with serial cardiopulmonary assessments, including vital signs, physical assessment, and continuous hemodynamic monitoring. Patients should be attached to a pulse oximeter for continuous assessment of the arterial oxygen saturation. The patient's level of consciousness is important. In children, monitor the child's activity level and the response to parents or significant others.

PHARMACOLOGIC HIGHLIGHTS

Medication or Drug Class	Dosage	Description	Rationale
Vasopressors	Varies by drug	Dopamine, dobutamine, phenylnephrine, or norepinephrine	Maintain an adequate blood pressure
Broad spectrum antibiotics	Varies by drug	Examples: vancomycin, gentamicin, penicillin, cephalosporin	Eradicate bacteria

Independent

Priorities of nursing care for the patient with septic shock include maintaining airway, breathing, and circulation; preventing the spread of infection; increasing the patient's comfort; preventing injury; and supporting the patient and family. Monitor the patient continuously for airway compromise and prepare for intubation when necessary. Maintain strict aseptic technique when you manipulate invasive lines and tubes. Use universal precautions at all times. Unless the patient is endotracheally intubated, place patients with a decreased level of consciousness in a side-lying position, and turn them every 2 hours to protect them from aspiration. To increase the intubated patient's comfort, provide oral care at least every 2 hours.

Maintain skin integrity by placing the patient on an every-2-hour turning schedule. Post the schedule at the head of the bed to increase the visibility of the routine. Implement active and passive range of motion as appropriate to the patient's condition. Provide the family with information about diagnosis, prognosis, and treatment. Expect the patient and family to have high levels of anxiety and fear, given the grave nature of septic shock. Support effective coping strategies, and provide adequate time for the expression of feelings.

DOCUMENTATION GUIDELINES

- Cardiovascular response: Heart rate and rhythm; presence and character of peripheral pulses; capillary refill time; pulmonary artery pressure, central venous pressure, left atrial pressure, and right atrial pressure; cardiac output and index; oxygen delivery and oxygen consumption
- Respiratory response: Rate and rhythm; lung expansion; breath sounds; oxygen saturation; color of oral mucosa and skin; type, location, and patency of an artificial airway
- Neurological response: Level of consciousness, orientation, strength and movement of extremities, activity level, response to the parents or significant others
- Signs of infection: Response to antibiotics

DISCHARGE AND HOME HEALTHCARE GUIDELINES

Instruct patients who have been identified as high risk to call the healthcare provider at the first signs of infection. Teach high-risk individuals to avoid exposure to communicable diseases and to use good hand-washing technique. Reinforce the need for immunizations against infectious diseases such as influenza. Encourage patients to consume a healthy diet, get adequate rest, and limit their alcohol intake. Instruct patients and families about the purpose, dosage, route, desired effects, and side effects of all medications. Explain that it is particularly important that the patient take the entire antibiotic prescription until it is finished.

Sickle Cell Disease

DRG Category: 395
Mean LOS: 4.3 days
Description: MEDICAL: Red Blood Cell Disorders, Age > 17

Sickle cell disease is a genetic, autosomal recessive disorder that results in abnormalities of the globin genes of the hemoglobin molecule of the red blood cells (RBCs). It is more common in African-Americans than in other groups in the United States. It can be in the form of sickle cell anemia or either sickle cell thalassemia or sickle cell hemoglobin C. Sickle cell anemia, the severest of the sickle cell disorders, is homozygous and has no known cure. Sickle cell trait occurs when a child inherits normal hemoglobin from one parent and hemoglobin S (Hb S; the abnormal Hb) from the other; people with the sickle cell trait are carriers only and rarely manifest the clinical signs of the disorder.

The RBCs that contain more Hb S than hemoglobin A (Hb A) are prone to sickling when they are exposed to decreased oxygen tension in the blood. The cells become more elongated, thus the term "sickle." Once sickled, RBCs are more rigid, fragile, and rapidly destroyed. The RBCs therefore have a short survival time (30 to 40 days, as compared with a normal 120-day survival rate), a decreased oxygen-carrying capacity, and low hemoglobin content. They cannot flow easily through tiny capillary beds and may become clumped and cause obstructions. The obstructions can lead to ischemia and necrosis, which produce the major clinical manifestations of pain. Complications include chronic obstructive pulmonary disease, congestive heart failure, and infarction of organs such as the spleen, retina, kidneys, and even the brain.

CAUSES

Two factors have been identified as producing sickling, although the exact cause is unknown. The first is hypoxemia, which is caused by low oxygen tension in the blood from high altitudes, strenuous exercise, or low oxygen concentration during anesthesia. The second is a change in the condition of the blood, such as decreased plasma volume, decreased blood pH, or increased plasma osmolality as a result of dehydration.

GENDER AND LIFE SPAN CONSIDERATIONS

Clinical symptoms rarely appear before the child is 6 months old and occur in both boys and girls. Sickle cell occurs most frequently in African-Americans but also occurs in African, Mediterranean, Caribbean, Middle Eastern, and Central American populations. Approximately 1 of 12 African-Americans has sickle cell trait. Many patients die in their teens, although with improved management, up to half can live as long as 40 or 50 years.

☐ ASSESSMENT

HISTORY. Most infants do not develop symptoms during the first 6 months because fetal hemoglobin has a protective effect. The parents or the child may describe a history of lung infections or cardiomegaly (hypertrophy of the heart). Children with the disease may have a history of chronic fatigue, dyspnea, joint pain and swelling, and chest pain.

PHYSICAL EXAMINATION. The extent of the symptoms depends on the amount of Hb S that is present. The general signs are similar to the other types of hemolytic anemia (anemia as a result of destruction of RBCs): malaise, fatigue, pallor, jaundice, and irritability. Children begin to fall below the growth curve in height and weight at around 7 years, and puberty is usually delayed. They are often small for their age and may have narrow shoulders and hips, long extremities, and a curved spine. You may note jaundice and pale skin. Often the children have heart rates that are faster than normal and heart murmurs; you may find a large liver and spleen. Eventually, all body systems, including the heart, lungs, central nervous system, kidneys, liver, bones and joints, skin, and eyes, are affected. The most severe problem is sickle cell crisis. (See Table 47.)

TABLE 47 | **Sickle Cell Crisis**

TYPE/DESCRIPTION	SYMPTOMS
Vaso-occlusive crisis: Most common type; usually appears after age 5; the result of sickling in the microcirculation that leads to vasospasm, thrombosis, and local infection	Severe pain: Joint, abdominal, muscle, and thoracic Jaundice, dark urine Fever, elevated white blood cell count, lethargy, fatigue, sleepiness
Sequestration crisis: Occurs in infants between 8 and 24 months; massive pooling of RBCs in the liver and spleen	Lethargy, pale skin Hypovolemia: Tachycardia, cool extremities, dropping urinary output, delayed capillary refill
Aplastic crisis: Results from bone marrow depression and is associated with viral infections; leads to compensatory increase in RBCs and RBC lysis	Lethargy, pale skin Shortness of breath Altered mental status, sleepiness
Hyperhemolytic crisis: Rare; result of certain medications or infections	Abdominal distension Jaundice, dark urine

Note: Sickle cell crisis may be preceded by a recent infection or a stressor such as dehydration, strenuous activity, or high altitude. Other assessment findings include changes in mental status, such as sleepiness, listlessness, and irritability. Fever, severe pain, bloody urine, and pallor of the lips, tongue, palms, and nails may also occur.

PSYCHOSOCIAL. Children with sickle cell disease have a chronic, potentially fatal genetic disorder. Frequent hospitalizations and delayed growth and development put them at risk for low self-esteem and body image problems. In addition, because of the genetic nature of the disease, parents may experience guilt feelings. Families need extensive genetic and psychological counseling to avoid problems. Assess the child and the family for coping skills and knowledge deficits about the cause and prevention of sickle cell crisis.

DIAGNOSTIC HIGHLIGHTS

Test	Normal Result	Abnormality with Condition	Explanation
Genetic testing	Negative	Mutant gene	Identifies expressed mutations in single genes
Peripheral blood smear	Normal RBCs	Classic distorted sickle-shaped RBCs	RBCs have a characteristic sickle shape caused by structurally abnormally Hb molecules.
Hemoglobin electrophoresis	No Hb S	Presence of Hb S	Identifies sickle cell disease by identifying Hb S; a stained blood smear can show sickling cells
Complete blood count	RBCs: 4.0–5.5 million/µL	Decreased	Chronic hemolytic anemia leads to decreased red blood cells
	Hemoglobin 12–18 g/dL	Decreased, generally 5–10 g/dL	
	White blood cells 4,500–11,000 /µL	Chronic neutrophilia is often present	
	Platelets 150,000–400,000/µL	Often increased	

PRIMARY NURSING DIAGNOSIS

Altered growth and development related to physical disabilities secondary to poor tissue perfusion

OUTCOMES. Child development; Physical maturation; Care-giver patient relationship; Parenting; Psychosocial adjustment

INTERVENTIONS. Nutritional monitoring; Nutrition therapy; Self-responsibility facilitation; Developmental enhancement; Counseling; Caregiver support

☐ PLANNING AND IMPLEMENTATION

Collaborative

Although sickle cell disease cannot be cured, there are many treatment alternatives to prevent exacerbations, limit complications, and manage sickle cell crises. Medical management centers on the treatment of anemia and the prevention of crisis. Families are counseled to avoid the causes of crisis (i.e., dehydration, infection, hypoxia, high altitudes, vigorous exercise, and stress). To prevent aplastic crisis, prophylactic daily doses of penicillin are given to infants beginning when they are about 4 months old.

Sequestration and aplastic crises are treated with transfusions of packed RBCs. A vaso-occlusive crisis is treated with analgesia and increased hydration. Pain levels should be assessed frequently and corrected quickly. Avoid using aspirin, which may increase acidosis. Children may not express the need for pain medication because of fear of the route of administration. Patient-controlled analgesia, therefore, may be used, with morphine sulfate as the drug of choice. Iron supplements may be used if folic acid levels are lower than normal.

PHARMACOLOGIC HIGHLIGHTS

Medication or Drug Class	Dosage	Description	Rationale
Analgesia	Varies by drug	Morphine sulfate, meperidine (Demerol)	Relieves pain

Independent

Counsel children and families on the importance of maintaining hydration even when the child is ill or during hot weather. Encourage oral fluid intake in addition to intravenous fluids when children are in the hospital. Increase fluid intake to 1.5 times the normal maintenance volume if the child's cardiac function is adequate.

In cases of acute crisis, pain is the overriding problem. In addition to prescription medicines, employ other pain-reducing interventions, such as diversion, imagery, and general comfort measures. Keep the pain level within tolerable limits for the individual. Encourage families to maintain a normal life for the child with sickle cell disease. Arrange for genetic counseling so that families can make informed decisions. When appropriate, and depending on the age, include siblings in the care.

DOCUMENTATION GUIDELINES

- Response to pain medication and other pain-reduction methods
- Physical findings of pain: Location and duration
- Response to hydration methods
- Presence of complications: Unresolved pain, cerebrovascular accident, kidney impairment

DISCHARGE AND HOME HEALTHCARE GUIDELINES

Teach the patient and family the causes, signs, and symptoms of crisis and ways to avoid future crisis. Emphasize good nutrition and the avoidance of caffeine and smoking. Patients and families need to be taught the signs and symptoms of complications, such as cardiopulmonary dysfunction, increased intracranial pressure, and renal impairment. The patient and family need to be taught the importance of taking daily antibiotics and the side effects, dosage, and route of medication. If the patient is on pain medications, care should be taken to ensure that the medication is not abused but is taken when the patient is in need. Patients and families need to understand the need for genetic counseling, the potential long-term effects of sickle cell disease, and the possible complications. Older children and parents need to deal with the delayed sexual maturity that occurs. Long-term follow-up care is essential for patients with sickle cell disease.

Sjögren's Syndrome

DRG Category: 240
Mean LOS: 6.4 days
Description: MEDICAL: Connective Tissue Disorders with CC

Sjögren's syndrome (SS) is the most common autoimmune rheumatic disorder after rheumatoid arthritis (RA). It is a chronic, progressive disease that is associated with other diseases such as RA in approximately 50% of the cases.

SS is characterized by failure of exocrine glands and by diminished tearing and salivary secretion (sicca complex). It results from chronic exocrine gland dysfunction, although the disorder may also involve other organs such as the lung and kidney. SS may be a primary disorder or it may be associated with connective tissue disorders, such as rheumatoid arthritis, scleroderma, systemic lupus erythematosus, and primary biliary cirrhosis. Tissue damage results either from infiltration by lymphocytes or from the deposition of immune complexes. The overall prognosis for patients with SS is good, and the disease seldom leads to significant complications.

CAUSES

The direct cause of SS is unknown. It seems likely that both environmental and genetic factors contribute to its development. In a genetically susceptible individual, either bacterial or viral infection or exposure to pollen may be the catalyst for SS.

GENDER AND LIFE SPAN CONSIDERATIONS

SS occurs mainly in women: 9 out of 10 patients are female. The mean age of occurrence is 50. A small percentage of these women may have accompanying non-lymphoma and lymphoid malignancies.

☐ ASSESSMENT

HISTORY. Establish a history of either autoimmune or lymphoproliferative disorders. Rule out other causes of oral and ocular dryness; ask about any history of sarcoidosis, endocrine disorders, anxiety or depression, and radiation therapy to the head and neck. Many commonly used medications produce dry mouth as a side effect, so take a thorough history of medications. In patients with salivary gland enlargement and severe lymphoid infiltration, rule out malignancy. Approximately 50% of patients with SS have confirmed rheumatoid arthritis. When you ask about symptoms, the patient may report gritty or sandy sensations in the eye or a film across the visual field. Patients may also report dryness of the mouth, burning oral discomfort, difficulty in chewing and swallowing dry foods, increased thirst, and reduced taste. The patient may also report the incidence of many dental caries and chronic middle ear infections. Dryness of the vagina and vulva leads to reports of painful urination, itching, and painful or difficult sexual intercourse.

The patient's tongue is often red and dry with atrophic taste buds. Unilateral or bilateral parotid and salivary glands may be hardened and nontender. Dental caries are a common finding. The dryness may make talking difficult. Patients may have a dry chronic cough and an increased incidence of upper and lower respiratory tract infections, which has resulted in a chronic vocal hoarseness. Nasal mucosa may be dry and reddened. Gastrointestinal tract involvement may lead to gastritis, esophageal mucosal atrophy, and difficulty in swallowing. Genitalia may appear dry and possibly ulcerated. Involvement of the exocrine glands leads to dry, tough, scaly skin; decreased sweat; and chronic itching.

The patient with SS has complaints that may have been attributed to multiple causes, possibly over years. Because SS is closely related to systemic lupus erythematosus and rheumatoid arthritis, the patient may have been misdiagnosed, causing considerable emotional distress. Because SS affects senses, such as sight and taste, and also sexuality, assess the patient's ability to cope with the presenting symptoms and other common complaints.

DIAGNOSTIC HIGHLIGHTS

Test	Normal Result	Abnormality with Condition	Explanation
Salivary gland biopsy	Normal salivary gland cells	Presence of inflammatory cells and immune complexes	Identifies abnormal cells in secretory glands and ducts
Slit-lamp examination	Normal examination	Detection of dryness of conjunctiva and reduced tearing	Identifies reduced tear film and dryness of eyes

PRIMARY NURSING DIAGNOSIS

Impaired skin integrity related to diminished or absent glandular secretions

OUTCOMES. Tissue integrity: Skin and mucous membranes; Wound healing: Primary intention; Knowledge: Treatment regime; Self-care: Hygiene; Treatment behavior: Illness

INTERVENTIONS. Skin and membrane surveillance; Skin care; Medication administration; Fluid balance; Surveillance

☐ PLANNING AND IMPLEMENTATION

Collaborative

Care of the patient with SS is designed to treat symptoms. Instill artificial tears as often as every 30 minutes to prevent corneal ulcerations or opacifications that may be caused by insufficient lacrimal secretions.

Patients who also have rheumatoid arthritis may benefit from a combined program of medical, rehabilitative, and surgical treatments. The primary goals are suppression of further joint and tissue inflammation, maintenance of joint and tissue function, repair of joint damage, and relief of pain.

PHARMACOLOGIC HIGHLIGHTS

Medication or Drug Class	Dosage	Description	Rationale
Corticosteroids	Varies with drug	Antiinflammatory agents that are not curative but help the patient manage symptoms	Provide relief of symptoms; reduce constitutional symptoms

Other Therapy: Twice-a-day, sustained-release cellulose capsules (hydroxypropyl cellulose) may be used. If eye infection develops, the patient receives antibiotics; topical steroids are avoided.

Independent

Suggest the use of sunglasses to protect the patient's eyes from strong light, wind, and dust. To reduce the risk of infection caused by dry eyes, advise the patient to keep his or her face clean and to avoid rubbing the eyes. Mouth dryness can be relieved by using a swab or spray and by drinking plenty of fluids, especially at mealtime. Sugarless throat lozenges can also relieve mouth dryness without promoting tooth decay. Meticulous oral hygiene should include regular brushing, flossing, and fluoride treatment at home, along with frequent dental checkups. Teach the patient to avoid medications that decrease saliva production, such as atropine derivatives, antihistamines, anticholinergics, and antidepressants. Suggest high-protein, high-calorie liquid supplements to patients with painful mouth lesions. Soft foods may be easier for patients to swallow. Parotid gland enlargement can be treated with local heat and analgesia.

Respiratory dryness can be reduced by using a humidifier at home and at work. Nasal dryness can be relieved by the use of normal saline solution drops. Moisturizing lotions can ease skin dryness, as can avoiding lengthy hot showers or baths. Patients should avoid sunburn and any lengthy exposure to the sun; recommend using a sunscreen when outdoors. Water-soluble lubricating jelly is an effective lubricant during sexual intercourse.

DOCUMENTATION GUIDELINES

- Physical findings of dysphagia (difficulty swallowing)
- Physical findings of presence of red, irritated, or ulcerated mucosal membranes
- Reaction to remoisturizing the affected areas

DISCHARGE AND HOME HEALTHCARE GUIDELINES

Instruct the patient to avoid sugar, tobacco, alcohol, and spicy, salty, and highly acidic foods. Recommend high-calorie, protein-rich liquid supplements to patients with painful mouth lesions. Teach the patient how to instill eye drops, ointments, or sustained-release capsules. Advise the patient to avoid over-the-counter medications that include saliva-decreasing compounds, such as antihistamines, antidepressants, anticholinergics, and atropine derivatives.

Skin Cancer

DRG Category: 283
Mean LOS: 4.8 days
Description: MEDICAL: Minor Skin Disorders with CC
DRG Category: 272
Mean LOS: 6.3 days
Description: MEDICAL: Melanoma—Major Skin Disorders with CC
DRG Category: 265
Mean LOS: 5.4 days
Description: SURGICAL: Skin Graft and/or Debridement Except for Skin Ulcer or Cellulitis with CC

Skin cancer is the most common malignancy in the United States, accounting for over 40% of all diagnosed cancers. The majority of skin cancers (more than 90%) are classified as nonmelanoma skin cancers (NMSCs) of which there are two types: basal cell carcinoma (BCC) and squamous cell carcinoma (SCC). Approximately 75% of skin cancers are BCC; SCC is the next most common skin cancer, followed in frequency by melanoma. More than 1.3 million cases of NMSC are diagnosed annually. Other less frequently occurring skin cancers include skin adnexal tumors, Kaposi's sarcoma, various types of sarcomas, Merkel cell carcinoma, and cutaneous lymphoma, all of which together account for fewer than 1% of NMSCs.

BCC is a slow-growing tumor that is characterized by the inability of basal cells to mature. Even though 70% of BCC metastases are to regional lymph nodes that can be excised easily, distant metastases to the bone, brain, lung, and liver can also occur; these distant metastases are accompanied by a grave prognosis. Although BCC can be treated effectively, it is not uncommon for it to return after treatment. From 35% to 50% of people diagnosed with one basal cell cancer will develop a new skin cancer within 5 years of the first diagnosis.

SCC leads to an invasive tumor that can metastasize to the lymph nodes and visceral organs. SCC, which constitutes 20% of all skin cancers, is characterized by lesions on the squamous epithelium of the skin and mucous membranes. The risk of metastasis is associated with the size and penetration of the tumor, the tumor morphology, and the causative factors. Complications of NMSCs include disfigurement of facial structures and metastasis to other tissues and organs.

In the year 2000, about 1900 deaths from NMSC were expected by the American Cancer Society. The 5-year survival rate for patients with BCC is greater than 99%; although BCCs rarely spread to lymph nodes or other organs, those patients who do have metastasized BCC have a 5-year survival rate of only 10%. The overall 5-year survival rate for patients with SCC is more than 95%; for patients with spread of SCC to lymph nodes or other organs, the 5-year survival rate is 25%.

CAUSES

The cause of NMSCs may be environmental (ultraviolet radiation or ultraviolet B exposure), occupational (arsenic, mineral oils, or ionizing radiation exposure), viral (human immunodeficiency virus or human papilloma virus), related to medical conditions (immunosuppression or scars from removed SCC or BCC), or related to heredity (xeroderma pigmentosum, or albinism). More than 90% of NMSCs are attributed to exposure to ultraviolet radiation from the sun.

GENDER AND LIFE SPAN CONSIDERATIONS

The incidence of skin cancer is more common between the ages of 30 and 60, with the majority of lesions occurring in patients over 50 years of age. However, younger people are now more likely to develop skin cancer, perhaps because of greater exposure to the sun. Children rarely have the disease, although the incidence increases with each decade of life. The ratio of European-Americans to African-Americans among people who develop skin cancer is 20:1. Males are more likely to develop BCC (2:1 ratio) and SCC (3:1 ratio) than women.

☐ ASSESSMENT

HISTORY. Assess the patient for a personal or family history of skin cancer. Ask if the patient has an exposure to risk factors, including environmental or occupational exposure, at-risk medical conditions, or exposure to viruses. Note that outdoor employment and living in a sunny, warm climate such as the southeastern (Florida) or southwestern (New Mexico, Arizona, California) United States, Australia, or New Zealand place the patient at risk. Question the patient about any bleeding lesions or changes in skin color. Explore the history of non-healing wounds or lesions that have been present for several years without any change. Question the patient about the presence of atypical moles, an unusual number of moles, or any noticeable change in a mole.

PHYSICAL EXAMINATION. Inspect the patient for additional risk factors, such as light skin and hair (red, blond, light brown), freckling, and light eye color (blue or green). Examine the patient's skin for the presence of lesions. Use a bright white light and magnification during the skin examination. Stretch the skin throughout the examination to note any nodules or translucent lesions. Examine folds or wrinkles in the skin. Assess the skin for ulcerations, sites of poor healing, old scars, drainage, pain, and bleeding. Because more than 70% of NMSCs occur on the face, head, and neck, closely examine these areas. Complete the skin assessment, considering that, in order of frequency, the remainder of NMSCs occurs on the trunk, upper extremities, lower extremities, and, lastly, the genitals. Determine if the patient has precursor lesions of SCC, such as actinic keratoses (a hornlike projection on the skin from excessive sun exposure) and/or Bowen's disease (intra-epidermal carcinoma). No assessment of precursor lesions for BCC is necessary because no equivalent lesions exist.

Assess for the characteristic lesions of BCC, which tend to be asymptomatic, grow slowly, be 0.5 to 1.0 cm in size, and have overlying telangiectasis (vascular lesions formed by dilated blood vessels). BCCs are classified as nodular (the most common type), superficial, pigmented, morpheaform, and keratotic. Nodular BCC appears as a translucent, nodular growth. Superficial BCC, frequently appearing on the trunk, presents as a scaly lesion with a distinct, raised, pearly margin. Pigmented BCC has a characteristic dark or bluish color with a raised and pearly border. The morpheaform BCC lesion is poorly demarcated, is light in color, and has a plaque-like appearance. Keratotic BCC lesions appear similar to ulcerating nodular BCC.

Assess for the characteristic lesions of SCC, which are usually found on sun-damaged skin. The lesions tend to be scaly, 0.5 to 1.5 cm in size, and likely to metastasize; they also grow rapidly. SCC lesions are usually covered by a warty scale surrounded by erythema that bleeds easily with minimal trauma. The tumor appears nodular, plaque-like, and without a distinct margin. When SCC is invasive, the lesion appears firm, dome-shaped, erythematous, and with an ulcerating core.

PSYCHOSOCIAL. Determine the patient's willingness to follow primary prevention strategies and to institute changes that decrease the risk of skin cancer or its recurrence. Of particular concern are patients who are adolescents and young adults who place a high premium on physical appearance. If the patient has metastatic disease, assess the ability to cope with highly stressful situations. Determine if the patient has support systems and the ability to cope with major lifestyle changes.

DIAGNOSTIC HIGHLIGHTS

General Comments: The initial diagnosis of skin cancer is made by clinical observation and is confirmed by histologic studies through biopsy.

Test	Normal Result	Abnormality with Condition	Explanation
Shave biopsy	No cancer cells present	Presence of cancer cells	Scraping off the top layers of skin; may not be thick enough to determine the degree of cancer invasion
Punch biopsy	No cancer cells present	Presence of cancer cells	Deep sample of skin is removed after numbing the site; cuts through all layers of skin
Incisional and excisional biopsy	No cancer cells present	Presence of cancer cells	Surgical knife is used to cut through full thickness of skin, and a wedge of skin is removed; incisional biopsy removes only a portion; excisional biopsy removes entire tumor
Fine-needle aspiration biopsy	No cancer cells present	Presence of cancer cells	Thin needle is used to remove very small tissue fragment; may be used to biopsy a lymph node near a melanoma to determine extent of disease

PRIMARY NURSING DIAGNOSIS

Impaired skin integrity related to cutaneous lesions

OUTCOMES. Tissue integrity: Skin and mucous membranes; Wound healing: Primary intention; Knowledge: Treatment regimen; Nutritional status; Treatment behavior: Illness or injury

INTERVENTIONS. Incision site care; Wound care; Skin surveillance; Medication administration; Infection control; Nutrition management

◻ PLANNING AND IMPLEMENTATION

Collaborative

Treatment depends on the patient's characteristics; whether the lesion is a primary or recurrent tumor; and its size, location, and histology. For some primary SCCs and BCCs, therapies may include electrosurgery, surgical excision, cryosurgery, and radiation therapy, which all have comparable cure rates of greater than 90%. Tumors best suited to such methods are generally small, superficial, well defined, and slow growing. Treatment is done on an outpatient basis, unless the tumor involves deep anatomic sites and surgery cannot be performed under local anesthesia. Mohs' micrographic surgery is the preferred procedure for invasive SCCs, incomplete excisions, and recurrences. The procedure is also preferred for BCCs that are greater than 2 cm, are located in high-risk areas, have aggressive morphology, or have ill-defined borders. Reconstructive surgery may be necessary after Mohs' surgery or extensive excision.

Topical fluorouracil may be used to manage some SCC skin lesions. During treatment, the patient's skin is more sensitive than usual to the sun. Healing generally occurs in 1 to 2 months. With metastatic SCC, radiation, chemotherapy, and surgery may be combined. The chemotherapeutic agent commonly used is cisplatin or doxorubicin, or both. External beam radiation therapy may be used in cases where a tumor is difficult to remove surgically because of its size or location and in situations where the patient's health precludes surgery. As an adjuvant therapy after surgery, radiation can be used to kill small deposits of cancer cells that were not visible during surgery. Radiation may also be used when NMSC has spread to other organs or to lymph nodes. If the patient undergoes radiation therapy, prepare the patient for common side effects such as nausea, vomiting, diarrhea, hair loss, and malaise

PHARMACOLOGIC HIGHLIGHTS

Medication or Drug Class	Dosage	Description	Rationale
Chemotherapeutic agents	Topical application	Fluorouracil (5-FU)	Manage premalignant conditions such as actinic keratosis

Independent

Nursing care focuses on wound management, threats to body image and self-esteem, and prevention. Teach the patient how to care for the wound aseptically.

Coordinate a consistent, standard plan so that the patient can begin to assume care for the wound. If the wound is large and infected, keep it dry and clean. If it has an odor, control the odor with odor-masking substances such as oil of cloves or balsam of Peru in the room.

Patients are often upset about the changes in their appearance. Listen to the patient's fears and anxieties and accept the patient's perception of his or her appearance. Assist the patient and significant others to have realistic expectations. Help the patient present a pleasant appearance by assisting with hair care and clothing. Some patients experience increased self-esteem when they wear their own clothing rather than hospital-issued clothing, if hospitalization is needed. If hair loss occurs during radiation, encourage the patient to wear any type of head covering that improves body image, such as baseball caps, wigs, scarves, or bandanas. If it is appropriate, arrange for the patient to interact with others who have a similar problem. If the patient has end-stage disease, listen to the patient's and significant others' fears and concerns. Identify the needs of the family, and investigate mechanisms for support from the chaplain, the American Cancer Society, or a local hospice.

If the patient cannot continue with his or her present occupation, arrange for job counseling to evaluate possible occupational alternatives. Encourage the patient to avoid excessive sun exposure by using sunscreen and wearing protective clothing. Explain the necessity of examining the skin weekly or monthly for precancerous lesions and to obtain health care when any unusual skin changes occur.

DOCUMENTATION GUIDELINES

- Physical findings related to skin cancer: Location and description of lesions, degree of healing, appearance and healing of surgical wound
- Patient's history related to skin cancer and associated risk factors
- Psychological response: Psychosocial state related to diagnosis of skin cancer, self-esteem, body image, level of anxiety and fear about prognosis, coping ability
- Response to diagnostic and treatment interventions: Surgery, chemotherapy, radiation

DISCHARGE AND HOME HEALTHCARE GUIDELINES

Teach the patient primary prevention strategies:

To perform self-skin assessments, including the use of a buddy or a mirror during the self-assessment

To use sunscreens and lip balms with a sun protection factor of 15; to apply sunscreens 15 to 30 minutes before every exposure to the sun, and to follow the reapplication guidelines

To use wrap-around sunglasses with 99%–100% UV absorption to protect the eyes and the skin area around the eyes

To avoid sun exposure, particularly between 10:00 a.m. and 3:00 p.m.

To use available shade, avoid artificial tanning, and wear protective clothing

To be aware of photosensitivity because certain medications and cosmetics can enhance ultraviolet ray exposure

To encourage members of the family to follow all prevention strategies

Spinal Cord Injury

DRG Category: 009
Mean LOS: 6 days
Description: MEDICAL: Spinal Disorders and Injuries

Spinal cord injury (SCI), trauma to the spinal cord, affects approximately 12,000 Americans every year. A physiologic cascade of events occurs at the time of an SCI and leads to neuronal damage and neurologic deficit. The initial injury causes a release of glutamate, which causes cellular damage and petechial hemorrhages at the injury site. Calcium influx into the neuron is caused by thrombus formation. This alteration in calcium triggers the arachidonic acid cascade to be initiated, thus leading to free radical formation, lactic acidosis, and lipid peroxidation. This final series of events hastens ischemia of the white matter and microvasculature destruction, with resultant neuronal damage and permanent neurologic deficit. This series of physiologic and chemical events associated with acute SCI lead to the permanent neurologic deficit. With aggressive medical interventions and nursing management, approximately 90% of patients with acute SCI survive.

SCI can be classified by a variety of methods: complete and incomplete cord injury, mechanism of injury, and the level of injury. In a complete SCI, the patient loses all function below the neurological injury level (the lowest neurological segment with intact motor and sensory function). In an incomplete SCI, some motor or sensory function below the neurological injury level remains intact. (See Table 48.)

TABLE 48 | **Types of Incomplete Spinal Cord Injury**

INJURY	MECHANISM	DESCRIPTION	FUNCTIONS PRESERVED	FUNCTIONS IMPAIRED
Brown-Séquard syndrome	Penetrating trauma	One side of the cord is affected	Opposite side pain and temperature sensation	Opposite side movement, proprioception, light touch
			Same side movement, proprioception, light touch	Same side pain and temperature sensation
Posterior cord syndrome	Extension	Loss of posterior column sensory function; motor paralysis	Pain sensation	Vibratory sensation
			Motor function Temperature sensation	Proprioception
Anterior cord syndrome	Flexion	Hyalgesia; hypesthesia, motor paralysis, posterior column sensory function preserved	Light touch Proprioception Vibratory sensation	Pain sensation Motor function Temperature sensation

Central cord syndrome	Flexion or extension	Injury to central gray matter	Motor functions of lower extremities	Motor functions of upper extremities

CAUSES

Leading causes of SCI include motor vehicle crashes (MVCs), falls, acts of violence, and sporting injuries. SCIs caused by violence have increased dramatically in the last decade. The mechanism of injury influences the type of SCI and the degree of neurologic deficit.

GENDER AND LIFE SPAN CONSIDERATIONS

Acute SCIs occur in both children and adults, although the majority occur between the ages of 16 and 18. The vast majority, approximately 80%, involve men. The financial impact of acute SCIs is tremendous, but it is related to the age of most patients and the degree of disability.

☐ ASSESSMENT

HISTORY. Determine the mechanism of injury in addition to taking a detailed report from pre-hospital professionals about the patient with an acute SCI. Question the pre-hospital care provider, significant others, or witnesses about the situation surrounding the injury. If the patient was in an MVC, determine the speed and type of the vehicle, whether the patient was restrained, the patient's position in the vehicle, and if the patient was thrown from the vehicle on impact. If the patient fell, the distance of the fall is important to know during the initial assessment and evaluation phase. A key component of the history in the patient with a suspected acute SCI is information about the patient's motor and sensory function at the scene of the injury.

PHYSICAL EXAMINATION. Assess the patient as soon as possible after the primary injury and again each hour during the acute period. Neurological assessments usually include the Glasgow Coma Scale and pupil reflexes.

The initial assessment is conducted at the injury site. This primary survey generally takes about 30 seconds and focuses on assessing airway, breathing, and circulation and implementing life-saving intervention. Stabilizing the cervical spine prevents an incomplete SCI from progressing to a complete one. The secondary survey is a complete head-to-toe assessment. Sometime during the first 48 hours, a tertiary survey is performed to discover any subtle injuries that may have been missed during the initial assessment.

Assess the patient's injury level. Test the patient's ability to distinguish a pinprick from dull pain at each level of the dermatomes. Rectal examination helps determine if the sphincter tone is normal and if the SCI is complete or incomplete. Normal sphincter tone and anal winking indicate an incomplete SCI. Evaluate the patient's motor strength to help determine the injury level. Test the patient's motor movement.

Examine the patient for signs of neurogenic shock, which usually occurs within 30 to 60 minutes after the SCI when sympathetic nerves have lost their normal connections to the central nervous system (CNS). Signs to look for include decreased heart rate and pronounced hypotension (systolic pressure below 90 mm Hg).

PSYCHOSOCIAL. Acute SCI is catastrophic and alters not only the lives of patients but also the lives of their families, friends, and the community they live in. Physiologic alterations are significant in patients with acute SCIs, as are the psychosocial adjustments. Ongoing assessment of the patient's and family's coping skills is critical in planning meaningful support and interventions to assist the patient in reaching his or her functional potential.

DIAGNOSTIC HIGHLIGHTS

Test	Normal Result	Abnormality with Condition	Explanation
Spine x rays	Normal body structures	May show spine fractures or injury such as dislocation or subluxation	Determines the integrity of bony structures of spine
Computed tomography (CT) scan	Normal body structures	Determines degree and extent of injury; may show spine fractures or injury such as dislocation or subluxation	Determines the integrity of bony structures of spine
Magnetic resonance imaging (MRI)	Normal body structures	Determines degree and extent of injury; may show spine fractures or injury such as dislocation or subluxation	Determines the integrity of bony structures of spine

Other Tests: Electromyography, somatosensory-evoked potentials, motor-evoked potentials, complete blood count, urinalysis, arterial blood gases

PRIMARY NURSING DIAGNOSIS

Ineffective airway clearance related to hypoventilation or airway obstruction

OUTCOMES. Respiratory status: Gas exchange and ventilation; Safety status: Physical injury

INTERVENTIONS. Airway insertion; Airway management; Airway suctioning; Oral health promotion; Respiratory monitoring; Ventilation assistance

☐ PLANNING AND IMPLEMENTATION

Collaborative

Maintenance of airway, breathing, and circulation are the highest priority in patients with spinal cord injury. The patient with a cervical or high thoracic injury is at risk for developing pulmonary insufficiency, problems with airway clearance, and ineffective breathing patterns. The patient may require endotracheal intubation or tracheostomy with mechanical ventilation. Assess tidal volume and vital capacity every 2 hours in the patient who is not endotracheally intubated. Hydration may be provided by IV crystalloid fluids or by dextran, a plasma expander that may be used to increase capillary blood flow.

The benefits of early spinal stabilization are decreased morbidity and decreased length of hospital stay, but the neurologic benefits are controversial. Although this is a temporary intervention, external stabilization may be accomplished by Gardner-Wells tongs, which can be applied until surgical stabilization can be performed. A halo apparatus can be applied either as a primary intervention or to protect a surgical repair. This device immobilizes the cervical spine but allows the patient increased mobility. Patients with stable thoracolumbar spine fractures only require support with a rigid external brace for several months. Timing for surgical (internal) stabilization of cervical spine injuries is controversial. Some suggest that early surgical stabilization enhances neurologic recovery and decreases morbidity, but others believe that early stabilization may increase biochemical alterations and vascular instability.

Patients with unstable thoracolumbar spine fractures are managed with metal rods and surgical decompression. Neurologic outcome may be improved by postponing surgery until spinal cord edema is decreased.

Postoperative patients may require a rigid cervical collar or rigid external brace to protect the surgical repair. Patients with acute SCI from penetrating trauma may require surgical intervention for debridement and closure of the dura, if cerebrospinal fluid leakage persists. If x-ray films demonstrate that a bullet or other foreign body is within the spinal cord, surgical removal may be recommended to decrease the likelihood of chronic radicular pain.

PHARMACOLOGIC HIGHLIGHTS

Medication or Drug Class	Dosage	Description	Rationale
Methylprednisolone	30 mg/kg IV as a loading dose, followed by a 48-hour intravenous infusion of 5.4 mg/kg per hour	Corticosteroid	Reduces inflammation and improves motor and sensory function
Inotropic agents	Varies by drug	Dopamine, dobutamine	Improve systemic vascular resistance and blood pressure
Atropine	1 mg IV as needed	Anticholinergic	Manage symptomatic bradycardia

Other Drugs: Prophylactic anticoagulants may prevent the formation of deep vein thrombosis when the patient is no longer at risk for hemorrhage. Histamine-receptor antagonists decrease gastric acid secretion by inhibiting the receptor sites in the parietal cells and reducing the risk of stress ulcers. Antacids may be administered to neutralize gastric acid.

Independent

The most critical nursing intervention for the patient with an acute SCI it is critical to maintain airway, breathing, and circulation. Maintain cervical alignment and immobilization. An abdominal binder may be beneficial in patients with SCIs to provide additional support of the abdominal musculature, a major contributor to respiratory excursion. A potentially life-threatening complication associated with acute SCI is autonomic dysreflexia. This dysfunction may occur after the acute phase and is characterized by a hypersympathetic response to some noxious stimuli; this response is commonly found in patients with SCIs above the T-8 level. (See Box 14.) Deep vein thrombosis may also occur. Apply sequential compression devices or foot pumps as prescribed.

BOX 14 AUTONOMIC DYSREFLEXIA	
Precipitating Factors	*Clinical Manifestations*
Bladder distension or urinary tract infection	Paroxysmal hypertension
Bowel distension	Pounding headache
Pressure ulcers	Blurred vision
Thrombophlebitis	Bradycardia
Gastric ulcers, gastritis	Diaphoresis above the level of injury
Pulmonary emboli	Piloerection
Menstruation	Nasal congestion
Constrictive clothing	Nausea
Pain	Pupillary dilation
Sexual activity; ejaculation	
Manipulation of bowel or bladder	
Spasticity	
Exposure to hot or cold stimuli	

Check bony prominences and areas under the brace or jacket for skin breakdown. Aggressive physical and occupational therapy early in the acute phase may be beneficial to the patient's overall rehabilitation. Joint range-of-motion exercises prevent contractures and severe muscle wasting. Some patients may require splints for the upper and lower extremities to prevent flexion contractures and footdrop.

Prevent urinary tract infections by instituting an intermittent catheterization protocol early. Protocols vary, but most begin with catheterizing every 4 hours. Monitor the residual urine volume; when it is less than 400 mL, catheterization can be done every 6 hours. Record the amount of urine voided and the post-void residuals. As the amount of residual volume decreases, increase the time intervals between catheterizations. Before catheterization, assist the patient in emptying the bladder by Crede's method or by gently tapping or percussing the bladder. Establish bowel continence early in the acute phase.

When the patient is eating by mouth or is being tube fed, administer stool softeners as ordered. If the patient has not had a bowel movement, administer bisocodyl (Dulcolax) suppository. If the patient is NPO (nothing by mouth), administer bisocodyl every other night. Digital stimulation is used in conjunction with the bowel program. Adequate fluid volume status is important for a successful bowel and bladder program.

Provide diversionary activities to help pass the time. Arrange for the patient or family to consult with a clinical nurse specialist, chaplain, or social worker to assist in coping with anxiety and stress, if it is deemed necessary. If the patient has little hope for recovery, consider speaking with the family about donating the patient's organs, if appropriate.

If the patient is scheduled for discharge, teach the patient and family about the recommended activity level and rehabilitative exercises. Explain how to recognize the signs and symptoms of infection or a deteriorating level of consciousness. Instruct the patient and family in the name, dosage, action, and potential adverse effects of all prescribed medications. Show them the proper care for wounds and lacerations. Make sure the patient and family are aware of the schedule for follow-up medical care.

DOCUMENTATION GUIDELINES

- Physical findings: Vital signs, hemodynamic parameters, urinary output, tidal volumes, vital capacity, level of consciousness
- Presence of complications: Pulmonary infections, urinary tract infection, deep vein thrombosis, alterations in skin integrity, autonomic dysreflexia
- Presence of bowel and bladder continence

DISCHARGE AND HOME HEALTHCARE GUIDELINES

Encourage the patient to participate in therapies. Instruct the patient to communicate any abnormalities that are recognized. Explain the use of compression stockings as prescribed, with correct application. Teach the patient to maintain the bowel and bladder program. Verify that the patient and family understand the causes and symptoms of autonomic dysreflexia. Be sure the patient understands any medication prescribed. Verify that the patient and family have demonstrated safe use of all assistive devices: wheelchair, transfers, adaptive feeding equipment, and toileting practices. Review with the patient and family all follow-up appointments that are arranged. Verify that all at-home arrangements have been completed.

Subarachnoid Hemorrhage

DRG Category: 014
Mean LOS: 6.4 days
Description: MEDICAL: Specific Cerebrovascular Disorders Except Transient Ischemic Attack
DRG Category: 001
Mean LOS: 9.6 days
Description: SURGICAL: Craniotomy Except for Trauma, Age > 17

Subarachnoid hemorrhage (SAH) is the direct hemorrhage of arterial blood into the subarachnoid space. Immediately after rupture, intracranial pressure (ICP) rises, resulting in a fall in cerebral perfusion pressure (CPP = mean arterial pressure − ICP). Furthermore, the expanding hematoma acts as a space-occupying lesion, as it compresses or displaces brain tissue. Blood in the subarachnoid space may impede the flow and reabsorption of cerebrospinal fluid (CSF), thus resulting in hydrocephalus. The bleeding ceases with the formation of a fibrin-platelet plug at the point of the rupture and by tissue compression. As the clot, which forms initially to seal the rupture site, undergoes normal lysis or dissolution, the risk of rebleeding increases.

Cerebral vasospasm, or narrowing of the vessel lumen, is another common complication of SAH; it occurs in 35% to 49% of individuals. The pathophysiology of vasospasms is not clearly understood, but it is believed that they are precipitated by certain vasoactive substances (e.g., prostaglandins, serotonin, and catecholamines), which are released by the blood into the subarachnoid space. When vasospasm develops, it may last for several days or even several weeks. By decreasing cerebral blood flow, a vasospasm produces further neurological deterioration, cerebral ischemia, and cerebral infarction.

CAUSES

SAH typically results from cerebral aneurysm rupture (70%), which occurs when the blood vessel wall becomes so thin that it can no longer withstand the surrounding arterial pressure. Because aneurysm-forming vessels usually lie in the space between the arachnoid and the brain, hemorrhage from an aneurysm usually occurs in the subarachnoid space. Another less common cause of SAH is arteriovenous malformation.

GENDER AND LIFE SPAN CONSIDERATIONS

The peak incidence of aneurysm rupture is between 40 and 65 years of age. Under the age of 40, SAH occurs more commonly in men, but after the age of 50, it is more common in women. Few aneurysms rupture in persons younger than the age of 20. The peak incidence of SAH from arteriovenous malformation is between 30 and 40 years of age.

◻ ASSESSMENT

HISTORY. Ask if the patient has had a sudden brief loss of consciousness followed by a severe headache; this sign has been reported by 45% of patients who survive SAH. Many also report a severe headache associated with exertion but no loss of consciousness. Establish any recent history of vomiting, stiff neck, photophobia, seizure, or partial paralysis. Establish any history of cerebral aneurysms.

PHYSICAL EXAMINATION. Observe the patient for signs and symptoms of cranial nerve deficits, especially cranial nerves III, IV, and VI. Meningeal irritation may lead to nausea, vomiting, stiff neck, pain in the neck and back, and possible blurred vision or photophobia. Examine for symptoms of stroke syndrome, such as hemiparesis, hemiplegia, aphasia, and cognitive deficits. Cerebral edema, increased ICPs, and seizures may also occur. Assess the vital signs for bradycardia, hypertension, and a widened pulse pressure. Other symptoms may result from pituitary dysfunction, caused by irritation or edema, leading to diabetes insipidus (excessive urinary output, hypernatremia) or hyponatremia.

PSYCHOSOCIAL. Provide emotional support for the patient and family. Encourage the patient to verbalize his or her fears of death, disability, dependency, and becoming a burden. Answer the patient's and family's questions, and involve both the patient and family or significant others in all aspects of planning care. If necessary, make home health referrals before the patient's discharge.

DIAGNOSTIC HIGHLIGHTS

Test	Normal Result	Abnormality with Condition	Explanation
Computed tomography (CT) scan	Normal brain and supporting structures	Blood collection in subarachnoid space often in the cisterns or sylvian fissure	Identifies areas of bleeding

Other Tests: Lumbar puncture; complete blood count; arterial blood gases; serum electrolytes

PRIMARY NURSING DIAGNOSIS

Alteration in tissue perfusion (cerebral) related to interruption in cerebral blood flow or increased ICP

OUTCOMES. Circulation status; Cognitive ability; Neurological status; Tissue perfusion: Peripheral; Communication: Expressive ability; Communication: Receptive ability

INTERVENTIONS. Cerebral perfusion promotion; Circulatory care; Intracranial pressure monitoring; Neurological monitoring; Peripheral sensation management; Circulatory precautions; Hypovolemia management; Vital signs monitoring; Emergency care; Medication management

□ PLANNING AND IMPLEMENTATION

Collaborative

Surgery is the treatment of choice for a cerebral aneurysm that has ruptured into the subarachnoid space. Until a decision about surgery is made, however, the management of the patient is focused on preventing secondary injury and relieving symptoms.

Monitor ICP to detect brain swelling and hydrocephalus. Maintain fluid volume within a normal range because dehydration increases hemoconcentration, which may increase the incidence of vasospasm. If cerebral edema is present, maintain moderate fluid restriction and administer prescribed steroids; dexamethasone (Decadron) and methylprednisolone (Solu-Medrol) are the drugs of choice. Steroid therapy is continued for at least 1 week postoperatively. Pharmacologic management is also used to control hypertension to prevent rebleeding. The goal of therapy is to maintain the systolic blood pressure at 150 mm Hg. Hypotension must be avoided at all costs because it worsens ischemic deficits. Assess the intravascular volume status with either a central venous access monitor or pulmonary artery catheter, depending on the patient's condition.

Complications during the immediate postoperative period include brain swelling, bleeding at the operative site, fluid and electrolyte disturbances, hydrocephalus, and the onset of cerebral vasospasm. If an intracranial monitoring system is in place, report ICP rises over 15 mm Hg. Calculate the CPP, and maintain the CPP greater than 50 mm Hg.

PHARMACOLOGIC HIGHLIGHTS

Medication or Drug Class	Dosage	Description	Rationale
Nimodipine	60 mg po every 4 hours	Calcium channel blocker	Reduces venospasm and cerebral ischemia
Antihypertensives	Varies by drug	Nitroprusside; propranolol; hydralazine	Lower blood pressure, but only used with extreme hypertension (when diastolic BP > 130 mm Hg)

Other Drugs: Mannitol (osmotic diuretic) may be ordered to decrease cerebral edema; stool softeners; sedatives may be used to induce rest; anticonvulsants; analgesics (acetaminophen or codeine) to control headache

Independent

Accurate, detailed, and serial assessments are essential. Frequently the first signs of rebleeding and vasospasm are evidenced through subtle changes in the neurologic examination. At any time during the course of SAH, maintenance of airway, breathing, and circulation is the top priority. In the postoperative period, unless otherwise indicated, maintain the bed at an elevation of 30 to 40 degrees. Prevent flexion of the head, and maintain proper alignment of the head and neck with towel rolls or sandbags. Avoid hip flexion greater than 90 degrees. Suction the patient as needed to keep the airway open. If deep endotracheal suctioning is indicated, hyperventilate and hyperoxygenate the patient before suctioning and limit suctioning to less than 30 seconds.

To prevent complications from postoperative immobility, turn the patient often and provide skin care. Perform active or passive range-of-motion exercises, and encourage deep-breathing exercises when the patient is able. Space all nursing care activities to maintain ICP less than 15 mm Hg. Allow ICP to drop between all activities. Encourage other departments to space x rays, therapies, and interviews to allow adequate rest and to avoid ICP elevations. Avoid conversations at the bedside that might be disturbing to the patient. Explain all procedures even if the patient does not appear to respond. Use soft restraints only when absolutely necessary; fighting restraints raises ICPs and thereby impedes venous outflow from the brain.

After surgery, monitor the dressing for bleeding or cerebrospinal fluid leakage. If either occurs, notify the physician and reinforce the dressing. Inspect the surgical site with all dressing changes for redness, drainage, poor wound healing, and swelling.

DOCUMENTATION GUIDELINES

- Neurological findings: Level of consciousness; pupillary size, shape, and reaction to light; motor function of extremities; other cranial nerve deficits (blurred vision, extraocular movement deficits, drooping eyelids, facial weakness); speech loss; headache and facial pain; photophobia; and stiff or painful neck; deterioration of neurological status

DISCHARGE AND HOME HEALTHCARE GUIDELINES

Prepare the patient and family for the possible need for rehabilitation after the acute care phase of hospitalization. Instruct the patient to report any deterioration in neurologic status to the physician. Teach the patient signs and symptoms of deterioration in neurologic status. Stress the importance of follow-up visits with the physician. If the patient has had surgery, teach the patient or caregiver to notify the physician for any signs of wound infection or poor incisional healing. Be sure the patient understands all medications, including dosage, route, action, adverse effects, and the need for routine laboratory monitoring for anticonvulsants.

Subdural Hematoma

DRG Category: 014
Mean LOS: 6.4 days
Description: MEDICAL: Specific Cerebrovascular Disorders, Except TIA
DRG Category: 002
Mean LOS: 9.8 days
Description: SURGICAL: Craniotomy for Trauma, Age > 17

Subdural hematoma (SDH) is an accumulating mass of blood, usually clotted, or a swelling that is confined to the space between the dura mater and the subarachnoid membrane. SDHs are space-occupying lesions and thus categorized as focal brain injuries, which account for approximately 50% of all head injuries and 60% of the mortality in head-injured patients. Sometimes an SDH is referred to as a mass lesion because it occupies critical space in the cranial vault. Deaths from SDH usually occur because of the expanding mass lesion that leads to excessive brain swelling and herniation, thus causing brain stem ischemia and hemorrhage.

SDHs are classified as either acute or chronic based on when symptoms appear. Acute SDHs have clinical findings that are evident within 24 to 72 hours after the traumatic event. A subacute SDH produces symptoms within 2 to 10 days; symptoms appear in chronic SDH within weeks or months. (See Table 49.) Generally, head trauma involves both a primary injury and a secondary injury. The primary injury results from the initial impact, which causes immediate neurologic damage and dysfunction. The secondary injury follows the initial trauma and probably stems from cerebral hypoxia and ischemia that then lead to cerebral edema, increased intracranial pressure (ICP), and brain herniation. A consequence of increased ICP, brain herniation is a life-threatening condition in which brain structures protrude through an opening in the brain cavity.

TABLE 49 | **Types of Subdural Hematomas**

TYPE	DESCRIPTION	ONSET OF SYMPTOMS	SYMPTOMS
Acute	Usually results from brain laceration with injury to the small pial veins	24–72 hours	Decreased level of consciousness, hemiparesis, unilateral pupil dilation, extraocular eye movement, paralysis, cranial

	bridging the subdural space		nerve dysfunction
Subacute	Similar to acute	2–10 days	Similar to acute
Chronic	Usually occurs in the elderly or in problem drinkers who experience atrophy of the brain; often associated with falls	2 weeks or more	Interval when patient appears to recover and then progressive deterioration occurs. Drowsiness, inattention, personality changes, headache; progresses to hemiparesis, pupil changes, decreased mental status

CAUSES

The mechanisms of injury that are associated with the development of SDH are a strong direct force to the head or an acceleration-deceleration force. These can occur in motor vehicle crashes (MVCs), auto-pedestrian crashes, falls, and assaults. Chronic SDH is most commonly associated with falls in the elderly and in problem drinkers.

GENDER AND LIFE SPAN CONSIDERATIONS

Traumatic injuries, which are usually preventable, are the leading cause of death in Americans aged 1 through 44 years and the fourth leading cause of death for all age groups. Most head injuries are associated with MVCs, which in the 15- to 24-year-old age group are three times more common in males than in females. In the 15- to 34-year-old age group, European-Americans have a death rate from MVCs that is 40% higher than the rate of African-Americans. The elderly population and chronic abusers of alcohol have cortical atrophy, which places them at risk for SDH.

☐ ASSESSMENT

HISTORY. Question the pre-hospital care provider, significant others, or witnesses about the situation when the injury occurred. If the patient was in an MVC, determine the speed and type of vehicle, whether the patient was restrained, the patient's position in the vehicle, and if the patient was thrown from the vehicle on impact. If the injury occurred in a motorcycle crash, ask if the patient was wearing a helmet. If the patient fell, determine the point of impact, distance of the fall, and type of landing surface. Ask if the patient experienced momentary loss of reflexes or momentary arrest of respiration, followed by loss of consciousness. If the patient was unconscious at any time, find out for how long. Determine if the patient experienced a headache, nausea, vomiting, dizziness, convulsions, decreased respiratory rate, or progressive insensitivity to pain (obtundity).

PHYSICAL EXAMINATION. The initial evaluation or primary survey of the patient with a head injury is centered on assessing the airway, breathing, circulation, and disability (neurologic status). Exposure (undressing the patient completely) is incorporated as part of the primary survey. The secondary survey, a head-to-toe assessment including vital signs, is then completed.

The initial neurologic assessment of the patient with SDH includes monitoring the vital signs, assessing the level of consciousness, examining pupil size and level of reactivity, and assessing on the Glasgow Coma Scale, which evaluates eye opening, best verbal response, and best motor response. Clinical findings may include a rapidly changing level of consciousness from confusion to coma, ipsilateral pupil dilation, hemiparesis, and abnormal posturing, including flexion and extension. A neurologic assessment is repeated at least hourly during the first 24 hours after the injury.

Examine the entire scalp and head for lacerations, abrasions, contusions, and bony abnormalities. Take care to maintain cervical spine immobilization during the examination. Patients with SDH may have associated cervical spine injuries or thoracic, abdominal, or extremity trauma. Examine the patient for signs of basilar skull fractures, such as periorbital ecchymosis (raccoon's eyes), subscleral hemorrhage, retroauricular ecchymosis (Battle's sign), hemotympanum (blood behind the eardrum), and leakage of cerebrospinal fluid (CSF) from the ears (otorrhea) or nose (rhinorrhea). Gently palpate the facial bones, including the mandible and maxilla, for bony deformities and step-offs. Examine the oral pharynx for lacerations, and check for any loose or fractured teeth.

PSYCHOSOCIAL. The patient may be anxious about his or her condition during intervals of lucidity. Assess the patient's ability to cope with a sudden illness and the change in roles that a sudden illness demands. Determine the significant others' responses to the injury. Expect parents of children who are injured to feel anxious, fearful, and sometimes guilty. Note if the injury was related to alcohol consumption (approximately 40% to 60% of head injuries occur when the patient has been drinking), and elicit a drinking history from the patient or significant others. Assess the patient for signs of alcohol withdrawal 2 to 14 days after admission.

DIAGNOSTIC HIGHLIGHTS

Test	Normal Result	Abnormality with Condition	Explanation
Computed tomography (CT) scan	Normal brain and supporting structures	Blood collection on brain surface	Identified mass lesion

Other Tests: Cervical spine x rays to rule out cervical spine injury; transcranial Doppler ultrasound; skull x rays; complete blood count; arterial blood gases; plasma electrolytes

PRIMARY NURSING DIAGNOSIS

Ineffective airway clearance related to hypoventilation or airway obstruction

OUTCOMES. Respiratory status: Gas exchange; Respiratory status: Ventilation; Symptom control behavior; Treatment behavior: Illness or injury; Comfort level

INTERVENTIONS. Airway management; Anxiety reduction; Oxygen therapy; Airway suctioning; Airway insertion and stabilization; Cough enhancement; Mechanical ventilation; Positioning; Respiratory monitoring

☐ PLANNING AND IMPLEMENTATION

Collaborative

MEDICAL. Endotracheal intubation and mechanical ventilation are critical to ensure oxygenation and ventilation and to decrease the risk of pulmonary aspiration. A PaO_2 greater than 100 mm Hg and $PaCO_2$ between 28 and 33 mm Hg may decrease cerebral blood flow and intracranial swelling. The routine use of hyperventilation is controversial, and some physicians are using $SjvO_2$ (saturation of jugular venous bulb) monitoring to assess the response to changes in PaO_2 and $PaCO_2$. Generally the $PaCO_2$ is maintained at 35 to 40 mm Hg.

SURGICAL. Surgical management is the evacuation of the clot, control of the hemorrhage, and resection of nonviable brain tissue. Rapid surgical intervention is essential. If surgical evacuation is delayed for more than 4 hours, these lesions produce a higher mortality rate. The surgeon exposes the area involved, the clot is evacuated, bleeding from surface vascular structures is controlled with bipolar coagulation, and bridging veins are controlled with Gelfoam or muscle tissue. The surgical site may be drained postoperatively by using a Jackson-Pratt drain for 24 to 48 hours. Possible postoperative complications include intracranial hypertension, reaccumulation of the clot, intracerebral hemorrhage, and development of seizures.

Patients with critical head injuries who have a high probability of developing intracranial hypertension may require invasive ICP monitoring with an intraventricular catheter. Some physicians use a Glasgow Coma Scale score of less than 7 as an indicator for monitoring ICP. The goal is to maintain the ICP at less than 10 mm Hg and the CPP greater than 80 mm Hg. Management of intracranial hypertension may also be done by draining CSF through a ventriculostomy, either intermittently or continuously according to a predetermined ICP measurement.

PHARMACOLOGIC HIGHLIGHTS

Medication or Drug Class	Dosage	Description	Rationale
Diuretics	Varies by drug	Furosemide, mannitol	Assist in managing intracranial hypertension (although their use remains controversial)
Sedatives	Varies by drug	Short-acting sedatives: midazolam, propofol (Diprivan), fentanyl	Control intermittent increases in ICP with a resultant decrease in CPP; short action of drugs allows for temporarily stopping infusion so that neurological assessment can be performed
Chemical paralysis	Varies by drug	Mivacurium, atracurium (short-acting agents that have few hypotensive effects)	Improves oxygenation and ventilation for some patients with severe head injuries
Anticonvulsants	Prophylactically	Phenytoin (Dilantin)	Controversial in the routine management of SDH; overall

> effectiveness has yet
> to be determined

Other Drugs: Antibiotics, barbiturates (persistently elevated ICP despite routine interventions may be managed with the induction of a barbiturate coma, which reduces the metabolic rate of brain tissue)

Independent

The highest priority in managing patients with SDH is to maintain a patent airway, appropriate ventilation and oxygenation, and adequate circulation. Make sure the patient's endotracheal tube is anchored well. If the patient is at risk for self-extubation, maintain him or her in soft restraints. Note the lip level of the endotracheal tube to determine if tube movement occurs. Notify the physician if the patient's PaO_2 drops below 80 mm Hg, $PaCO_2$ exceeds 40 mm Hg, or severe hypocapnia ($PaCO_2 < 25$ mm Hg) occurs.

Help control the patient's ICP. Maintain normothermia by avoiding body temperature elevations. Avoid flexing, extending, or rotating the patient's neck because these maneuvers limit venous drainage of the brain and thus raise ICP. Avoid hip flexion by maintaining the patient in a normal body alignment, thus limiting venous drainage. Maintain a quiet, restful environment with minimal stimulation; limit visitors as appropriate. Time nursing care activities carefully to limit prolonged ICP elevations. Use caution when suctioning the patient: hyperventilate the patient beforehand, and suction only as long as necessary. When turning the patient, prevent Valsalva's maneuver by using a draw sheet to pull the patient up in bed. Instruct the patient not to hold on to the side rails.

Strategies to maximize the coping mechanisms of the patient and family are directed toward providing support and encouragement. Provide simple educational tools about head injuries. Teach the patient and family appropriate rehabilitative exercises, as necessary. Help the patient cope with long stretches of immobility by providing diversionary activities appropriate to the patient's mental and physical abilities. Head injury support groups may be helpful. Referrals to clinical nurse specialists, pastoral care staff, and social workers are helpful in developing strategies for support and education.

DOCUMENTATION GUIDELINES

- Trauma history, description of the event, time elapsed since the event, whether or not the patient had a loss of consciousness, and, if so, for how long
- Adequacy of airway, breathing, and circulation; serial vital signs
- Appearance, bruising or lacerations, drainage from the nose or ears
- Physical findings related to the site of head injury: Neurological assessment, presence of accompanying symptoms, presence of complications (decreased level of consciousness, unequal pupils, loss of strength and movement, confusion or agitation, nausea and vomiting), CPP, ICP
- Signs of complications: Seizure activity, infection (fever, purulent discharge from any wounds), aspiration pneumonia (shortness of breath, pulmonary congestion, fever, productive cough), increased ICP
- Response to surgery and clot evacuation: Mental status changes, incisional healing, presence of complications (infection, hemorrhage)

DISCHARGE AND HOME HEALTHCARE GUIDELINES

Review proper care techniques for wounds and lacerations. Discuss the recommended activity level, and explain rehabilitative exercises as appropriate. Teach the patient and family to recognize symptoms of infection or a deteriorating level of consciousness. Stress the need to contact the physician on the appearance of such signs or symptoms. Teach the patient the purpose, dosage, schedule, precautions and potential side effects, interactions, and adverse reactions of all prescribed medications. Review with the patient and family all follow-up appointments that have been arranged. If the patient is a problem drinker, refer the patient to a counselor.

Sudden Infant Death Syndrome

DRG Category: 34
Mean LOS: 5.5 days
Description: MEDICAL: Other Disorders of the Nervous System with CC

Sudden infant death syndrome (SIDS) is the sudden, unexplained death of an infant under 1 year of age, for reasons that remain unexplained even after autopsy. A typical scenario is when a seemingly healthy infant of 2 to 3 months of age is put to bed without concern over illness but is later found dead. SIDS occurs worldwide with an incidence of 0.2 to 3.0 per 1,000 live births. SIDS is the most common cause of death in infants under 6 months of age.

Although there is great uncertainty in the scientific community about risk factors for SIDS, several genetic, environmental, and social factors have been linked with SIDS. Risk factors include premature births (particularly associated with apnea or bronchopulmonary dysplasia); low birth weight; young, unmarried mother; lack of prenatal care; maternal smoking or anemia; maternal substance use; cold weather; and low-income housing.

CAUSES

A wide variety of findings have been reported in infants who have died of SIDS. Some of these findings include retarded postnatal growth, low APGAR scores at birth, increased pulmonary arterial smooth muscle, increased right ventricular muscle mass, and a variety of cardiopulmonary and neurological cellular abnormalities. The cellular findings suggest that SIDS may be caused by exposure to chronic hypoxia and respiratory failure. However, the direct evidence is controversial and has led to multiple theories. Several theories suggest that SIDS may be caused by sleep apnea, congenital central nervous system anomaly, neuromuscular infantile botulism, accidental suffocation, abnormal upper airway dysfunction, cardiac abnormalities, or inborn errors of metabolism.

GENDER AND LIFE SPAN CONSIDERATIONS

Boys are more affected than girls. The incidence is highest during the second and third months of life; few cases occur in the first 2 weeks of life or after 6 months of age. More SIDS deaths occur between the hours of midnight and 9 A.M., and more occur in the colder than warmer months.

☐ ASSESSMENT

HISTORY. If you suspect that an infant is at risk for SIDS, elicit a history of risk factors. Determine if the infant has a history of apparent life-threatening events (ALTE). In this situation, the infant may cease to breathe, develop pallor or cyanosis, have a marked change in muscle tone, choke or gag, or become unresponsive, and yet the child is successfully resuscitated. This "near miss" is thought to be a warning sign for future SIDS. If parents have lost a child to SIDS, the history of the event needs to be elicited carefully and with compassion because of the loss and grief patients are experiencing.

PHYSICAL EXAMINATION. Infants with ALTE have a number of physical findings. Neurologic examination has identified abnormalities of muscle tone, particularly with shoulder hypotonia. Other published reports describe increased incidence of periodic breathing during sleep with pauses of up to 10 seconds and possibly increased respiratory rates. Some infants have faster heart rates than normal, less heart rate variability, and shorter Q-T intervals. Some children, before the incident, have cold symptoms a week to a few days before SIDS.

PSYCHOSOCIAL. If an infant has had an ALTE, parents are likely to be anxious and afraid. Provide a referral to a support group and consider providing them with counseling to deal with their anxiety. For a family who has lost a child to SIDS, management is directed to assisting the family to cope with loss of an infant. Sadness and feelings of despair or hopelessness may evolve; patients and families should be encouraged to discuss these openly. Parents and siblings will likely experience feelings of guilt or anger and will need opportunities to express these feelings.

DIAGNOSTIC HIGHLIGHTS

No test is diagnostic for ALTE or SIDS. In suspected cases of ALTE, a full diagnostic investigation should include complete blood count, blood chemistries, blood urea nitrogen, blood gas analysis, chest x ray with magnification of the upper airways, upper GI barium study, electrocardiogram, 24-hour monitoring electrocardiogram, a variety of respiratory studies, electroencephalogram, esophageal pH, and sleep studies.

PRIMARY NURSING DIAGNOSIS

Grief related to the loss of an infant through SIDS

OUTCOMES. Coping; Grief resolution; Psychosocial adjustment: Life change; Self-esteem; Mood equilibrium

INTERVENTIONS. Counseling; Family support; Active listening; Coping enhancement; Crisis intervention; Emotional support; Family support; Grief work facilitation: Perinatal death

☐ PLANNING AND IMPLEMENTATION

Collaborative

Following an ALTE or with infants at risk for SIDS, a number of preventive measures can occur. Positioning is one measure that appears to aid in the prevention of SIDS. Encourage all parents to place infants on their backs to sleep until at least 6 months of age. Because of publicity on the link between sleep position and SIDS, the use of a prone sleeping position for infants has decreased in the United States from 70% to 24%. At the same time, the Centers for Disease Control and Prevention have reported that the SIDS rate has fallen by 38% in the United States.

Encourage parents to use a firm mattress for their infants. Explain that they should not use soft bedding or have stuffed animals in the bed with the infant, and infants should not sleep on a waterbed or with parents. Parents should avoid overheating the infant's room (temperature should be in the range of 68°F to 72°F). Recommend that mothers avoid alcohol and drug use during pregnancy and breastfeeding; explain that parents should not allow passive inhalation of cigarette smoke by the infant.

Home monitoring may be recommended for infants with ALTE or for siblings of infants who have died from SIDS. However, the rate of SIDS in succeeding children is very low (<2%). Because monitoring cannot prevent the occurrence of SIDS, some controversy exists about home monitoring for succeeding infants. Monitors exist to measure heart rate, heart rate variability, and respiratory rate. Apnea monitors, however, may not detect complete airway obstruction as infants continue to make respiratory efforts even when the airway is obstructed. There is little information available to determine whether home monitoring is necessary, and the decision is generally made by the physician or nurse practitioner and the parents. If monitoring is initiated, the abilities of members of the household to handle and interpret monitors becomes important so that true and false alarms may be handled appropriately. In addition, parents should receive appropriate training in cardiopulmonary resuscitation and proper use of monitoring equipment.

PHARMACOLOGIC HIGHLIGHTS

No pharmacologic management is known to prevent SIDS and ALTE.

Independent

Management after the death of an infant from SIDS is focused on helping the family cope with the infant's loss. Parents often react with disbelief, anger, or shock. Confusing the situation with child abuse, which will compound the family's emotional trauma, should be avoided.

A thorough investigation of the incident is important, but questions need to be asked carefully and with compassion. Obtain a thorough history from the caretaker about the situation, but be careful not to accuse the family of mistakes in care giving. Obtain the information within a few hours of the event so as to obtain a thorough history. Reassure the family or caretaker that SIDS was not their fault and was unpreventable. Offer support and counseling, and provide a referral as appropriate. Support groups and resources include the following:
Compassionate Friends, www.compassionatefriends.org
National SIDS Resource Center, 800-821-8955
Sudden Infant Death Syndrome Alliance, 800-221-7437, www.sidsalliance.org
Remember to assist the surviving siblings, who may need referrals for counseling to understand their feelings of guilt, loss, or vulnerability. Help parents deal with their other children and with their own need for extra attention and concern.

DOCUMENTATION GUIDELINES

- Description of the SIDS event: Precipitating factors, risk factors, situation, timing, sleep and wake patterns of infant, position during sleep, type of mattress
- Health history of infant: Previous illnesses, birth weight and length of gestation, history of ALTE
- Maternal health history: Tobacco and substance use, parity, nutrition, socioeconomic status

DISCHARGE AND HOME HEALTHCARE GUIDELINES

Make sure that the caregiver and family have contact information for support services. Encourage the family to receive grief counseling and let them know that grieving takes many months or even more time. Arrange for a visit with the primary care provider at the end of a year to evaluate family functioning. If home monitoring is instituted for succeeding children, make sure the caregiver understands the monitors and can make decisions about true and false alarms. Teach the caregiver cardiopulmonary resuscitation if it is deemed appropriate.

Syndrome of Inappropriate Antidiuretic Hormone (SIADH)

DRG Category: 300
Mean LOS: 6.3 days
Description: MEDICAL: Endocrine Disorders with CC

Syndrome of inappropriate antidiuretic hormone (SIADH), a disorder of the posterior pituitary gland, is a condition of excessive release of antidiuretic hormone (ADH) that results in excessive water retention and hyponatremia. SIADH occurs when ADH secretion is activated by factors other than hyperosmolarity or hypovolemia. Excess ADH secretion increases renal tubular permeability and reabsorption of water into the circulation, resulting in excess extracellular fluid volume, reduced plasma osmolality, increased glomerular filtration rates, and decreased sodium levels. Without treatment, SIADH can lead to life-threatening complications. Water intoxication accompanied by sodium deficit may lead to free water movement into cerebral cells, which can cause cerebral edema and result in coma and even death.

CAUSES

Several conditions contribute to SIADH. Central nervous system (CNS) responses to fear, pain, psychoses, and acute distress are known to increase the rate of ADH secretion by the posterior pituitary gland. Physiological conditions that increase intracranial pressure, such as acute CNS infections, brain trauma, anoxic brain death, cerebrovascular accident, and brain surgery, may lead to SIADH. Other conditions associated with SIADH include peripheral neuropathy, delirium tremens, and Addison's disease and also certain medications such as analgesics, anesthetics, thiazide diuretics, and nicotine. Some tumors have been associated with ADH production, such as small cell carcinoma of the lungs, pancreatic cancer, prostate cancer, and Hodgkin's disease. Positive pressure ventilation can also lead to SIADH in normovolemic individuals.

GENDER AND LIFE SPAN CONSIDERATIONS

Both children and adults are at risk. Typical childhood conditions that can lead to SIADH include pneumonia, meningitis, head trauma, and subarachnoid bleeding. In adults, the condition is most commonly associated with CNS disorders.

☐ ASSESSMENT

HISTORY. Ask if the patient has experienced alterations in urinary patterns. Question the patient about recent weight gain.

PHYSICAL EXAMINATION. Signs of sodium deficit generally occur slowly. Ask if the patient has experienced recent fatigue, weakness, or headaches. Late signs include nausea, vomiting, muscle weakness, decreased level of consciousness, seizures, and even coma. Note that the most severe, life-threatening signs of SIADH are not fluid overload and pulmonary congestion but, rather, the CNS effects from acute sodium deficiency. The severity of hyponatremia determines the severity of findings on physical assessment. Perform a neurologic assessment to determine if the patient has experienced changes in the level of consciousness, which can range from confusion to seizure activity. Life-threatening symptoms such as seizures may indicate acute water excess, whereas nausea, muscle twitching, headache, and weight gain are more indicative of chronic water accumulation.

PSYCHOSOCIAL. The family and significant others may be fearful if the patient has experienced CNS changes that alter behavior and alertness. If the patient has had seizures, note that family members may have many questions. The patient's and family's responses to SIADH are often a reflection of their responses to these other conditions, which are important to consider in any evaluation of patient and family coping.

DIAGNOSTIC HIGHLIGHTS

Test	Normal Result	Abnormality with Condition	Explanation
Urine osmolality (osmolality refers to a solution's concentration of solute particles per kilogram of solvent)	200–1200 mOsm/L	> 100 mOsm/L	Excretion of inappropriately concentrated urine and hyponatremia caused by overproduction of ADH
Blood osmolality	275–285 mOsm/L	< 275 mOsm/L	Water loss in urine and hypernatremia lead to hemo-concentration; levels above 320 mOsm/L are considered "panic levels" and require

			immediate intervention
Serum sodium	136–145 mEq/L	< 120 mEq/L	Sodium loss in the urine leads to hyponatremia and hemodilution

Other Tests: Blood urea nitrogen, urine specific gravity, urine sodium, radio-immunoassay of ADH

□ PLANNING AND IMPLEMENTATION

Collaborative

Restoration of normal electrolyte and fluid balance and normal body fluid concentration are the treatment goals. Treatment involves correction of the underlying cause and correction of hyponatremia. If the patient's life is not in danger from airway compromise or severe hyponatremia, the physician often restricts fluids initially to 600 to 800 mL per 24 hours or less. With fluid restriction, the hormone aldosterone is released by the adrenal gland and the patient begins to conserve sodium in the kidneys. As serum sodium increases, SIADH gradually corrects itself. The patient needs assistance to plan fluid intake, and a dietary consultation is also required for consistency in fluid management.

If fluid restriction is unsuccessful, the physician may prescribe an intravenous (IV) infusion of a 3% to 4.5% saline solution. Use caution in administering these hypertonic solutions, and always place them on an infusion control device to regulate the infusion rate precisely. Monitor the patient carefully because sodium and water retention may result, thus leading to pulmonary congestion and shortness of breath.

Diuretics to remove excess fluid volume may be used in patients with cardiac symptoms.

PHARMACOLOGIC HIGHLIGHTS

Medication or Drug Class	Dosage	Description	Rationale
Diuretics	Varies with drug	Thiazide diuretics	Remove excess fluid volume (may be used in patients with cardiac symptoms)
Demeclocycline (Declomycin)	600 mg–1200 mg per day in 2–3 divided doses po	Antibiotic: tetracycline derivative	Blocks action of ADH at distal and collecting tubules of the kidney

Other Drugs: If excessive diuresis is caused by diuretics, potassium supplements are given. Phenytoin (Dilantin) may be prescribed to limit or prevent seizures and to prevent further release of ADH in patients with low sodium levels.

PRIMARY NURSING DIAGNOSIS

Fluid volume excess related to retention of free water

OUTCOMES. Fluid balance; Hydration; Circulation status; Cardiac pump effectiveness

INTERVENTIONS. Fluid monitoring; Fluid/electrolyte management; Circulatory care; Vital signs monitoring; Medication management

Independent

If the patient is at risk for airway compromise because of low serum sodium levels or seizure activity, maintaining a patent airway is the primary nursing concern. Insert an oral or nasal airway if the patient is able to maintain his or her own breathing, or prepare the patient for endotracheal intubation if it is needed. If the patient is able to maintain airway and breathing, consider positioning the patient so that the head of the bed is either flat or elevated no more than 10 degrees. This position enhances venous return and increases left atrial filling pressure, which, in turn, reduce the release of ADH.

Explore with the patient methods to maintain the fluid restriction. If thirst and a dry mouth cause discomfort, try alternatives such as hard candy (if the patient is awake and alert) or chewing gum. Allocate some of the restricted fluids for ice chips to be used throughout the day at the patient's discretion. Work with the patient to determine the amount of fluid to be sent on each tray so that fluid intake is spread equitably throughout the day. If the patient is receiving fluids in IV piggyback medications, consider those volumes as part of the 24-hour intake. Work with the pharmacy to concentrate all medications in the lowest volume that is safe for the patient.

Promote range-of-motion exercises for patients who are bedridden, and turn and reposition them every 2 hours to limit the complications of immobility. Maintain side rails in the up position to prevent injury if the patient has a decreased mental status. Initiate seizure precautions to ensure the patient's safety.

DOCUMENTATION GUIDELINES

- Physical findings: Status of airway, assessment of CNS, fluid volume status (presence of edema, skin turgor, intake and output), serum sodium level
- Response to fluid restriction, diuretics, and other medications
- Presence of complications: Changes in lung or cardiac sounds; changes in level of consciousness; seizures

DISCHARGE AND HOME HEALTHCARE GUIDELINES

Be sure the patient or significant others understand the medication regimen, including the dosage, route, action, adverse effects, and need for follow-up laboratory tests (ADH level, serum sodium and potassium, blood urea nitrogen and creatinine, urine and serum osmolality). Instruct the patient to report changes in voiding patterns, level of consciousness, presence of edema, symptoms of hyponatremia, reduced neurologic functioning, nausea and vomiting, and muscle cramping. If the patient is going home on fluid restriction, be sure to discuss methods of limiting fluid intake and encourage the patient to weigh himself or herself daily to monitor for fluid retention.

Syphilis

DRG Category: 423
Mean LOS: 7.1 days
Description: MEDICAL: Other Infectious and Parasitic Diseases Diagnoses

Syphilis is a chronic, infectious, systemic, sexually transmitted vascular infection that is characterized by five stages: incubation, primary, secondary, latency, and late. The incubation stage begins with the penetration of the infecting organism, the spirochete *Treponema pallidum,* into the skin or mucosa of the body. Within 10 to 90 days after the initial infection, the primary stage begins with the appearance of a firm, painless lesion called a chancre at the site of entry. If it is left untreated, the chancre heals spontaneously in 1 to 5 weeks. As this primary stage resolves, systemic symptoms appear, thus signaling the start of the secondary stage. Secondary stage symptoms include malaise, headache, nausea, fever, local or generalized rash, and silver-gray eroded patches on the mucous membranes. These symptoms subside in 2 to 6 weeks, and the infected person enters a latent stage, which may last from 1 to 40 years. During latency, periodic symptoms of secondary syphilis may recur.

Approximately one-third of untreated syphilis patients eventually progress to the late stage of syphilis; the complications are often disabling and life-threatening. In this stage, destructive lesions called gummas develop in either the skin, bone, viscera, central nervous system, or cardiovascular system. Three subtypes of late syphilis are late benign syphilis, cardiovascular syphilis, and neurosyphilis. Late benign syphilis can result in destruction of the bones and body organs, which leads to death. Cardiovascular syphilis develops in approximately 10% of untreated patients and can cause aortitis, aortic regurgitation, aortic valve insufficiency, and aneurysm. Neurosyphilis develops in approximately 8% of untreated patients and can cause meningitis and paresis.

CAUSES

Syphilis is a communicable disease caused by the organism *T. pallidum.* Transmission usually occurs through direct contact with open lesions, body fluids, or the secretions of infected persons during sexual contact. Blood transfusions, placental transfer, and, in rare cases, contact with contaminated articles are also modes of transmission. Susceptibility to syphilis is universal, but only 10% of exposures lead to active infection.

GENDER AND LIFE SPAN CONSIDERATIONS

Syphilis is most commonly reported in the 15- to 30-year-old age group. It occurs more frequently in men, but the incidence in women is steadily rising. Incidence is highest among urban populations. Prenatal transmission from an infected mother to her fetus is possible. In the past, one-third of fetal demises were caused by maternal syphilis, but this number has decreased significantly with less incidence in pregnant women today.

□ ASSESSMENT

HISTORY. Establish a sexual history, including the number of sexual partners and whether the patient was protected by a condom. Determine if any of the patient's partners were infected with a sexually transmitted infection (STI). Question the patient about intravenous (IV) drug use and previous STIs. With an infant, establish the sexual history of the mother.

Elicit a history of chancres. Ask the patient to describe the appearance, location, and duration of any chancres, particularly if they are no longer present. Establish a history of fever, headaches, nausea, anorexia, weight loss, sore throat, mild fever, hair loss, or rashes, symptoms of the primary and secondary stages. Determine if the patient has experienced paresis, seizures, arm and leg weakness, alterations in judgment, or personality changes, all of which are symptoms of late-stage syphilis.

PHYSICAL EXAMINATION. Carefully inspect the patient's genitalia, anus, mouth, breasts, eyelids, tonsils, or hands for a primary lesion. With female patients, be sure to determine if chancres have developed on internal structures such as the cervix or the vaginal wall. Chancres vary in appearance and location, depending on which stage the disease has entered, so record a detailed description of any lesions (Table 50).

TABLE 50 | **Syphilitic Lesions**

STAGE OF DISEASE	DESCRIPTION OF LESION
Primary	Chancres that start as painless papules and then erode; have indurated, raised edges and clear bases. Found on genitals, lips, tongue, nipples, tonsils, anus, fingers, and eyelids
Secondary	Macular, papular, pustular, or nodular rash. Lesions are uniform in size, well defined, generalized. Lesions may enlarge and erode, producing highly contagious pink or grayish-white lesions (condylomata lata). Found on palms, arms, soles, face, scalp, perineum, scrotum, vulva, and between rolls of body fat.
Latent	Absence of lesions.
Late	Gummas: Chronic, superficial nodules or deep, granulomatous lesions. Solitary, asymmetric, painless, indurated. Found on bones and in organs.

If a chancre exists, palpate the surrounding lymph nodes for hard, painless nodules. Also inspect the scalp, skin, and mucous membranes for hair loss, rashes, or mucoid lesions, which are characteristic of the secondary stage. Inspect the fingernails for signs of pitting.

If late syphilis is suspected, assess the patient for the characteristic complications. Observe for joint deformities or disfiguring lesions on the palate. Note areas of numbness or paralysis and hyperactive reflexes. Assess the pupils for size and reaction to light. Assess the patient for pulmonary congestion. Auscultate for heart sounds to determine irregularities, which may indicate valvular degeneration.

PSYCHOSOCIAL. The patient with syphilis is usually embarrassed by the infection and may be reluctant to seek out and continue treatment. Be nonjudgmental. Assure the patient that his or her privacy and confidentiality will be maintained during examination, diagnosis, and treatment, although all sexual partners need to be notified so that they can be examined and treated as needed.

DIAGNOSTIC HIGHLIGHTS

General Comments: Diagnostic tests for syphilis include nontreponemal serology tests.

Test	Normal Result	Abnormality with Condition	Explanation
Venereal disease research laboratory (VDRL)	Negative or nonreactive	Positive	Detects *Treponema* antibodies; becomes positive 2 weeks after inoculation
Rapid plasma reagin (RPR)	Negative or nonreactive	Positive	A sensitive test that detects a non-treponemal antibody called reagin
Fluorescent treponemal antibody absorption test (FTA-ABS)	Negative	Positive	Done if VDRL or RPR is positive; sensitive test that confirms the diagnosis of syphilis 4–6 weeks after inoculation

PRIMARY NURSING DIAGNOSIS

Infection

OUTCOMES. Risk control: Sexually transmitted diseases

INTERVENTIONS. Medication management; Teaching: Safe sex

☐ PLANNING AND IMPLEMENTATION

Collaborative

Medical treatment for syphilis infection at any stage consists of antibiotic therapy to destroy the infecting bacteria. After treatment, patients are instructed to refrain from sexual contact for at least 2 weeks or until lesions heal and to return for serology testing in 1 month and then every 3 months for 1 year.

Carefully question patients about penicillin sensitivity before treatment. They should also be warned about the Jarisch-Herxheimer reaction, which is believed to be caused by toxins that are released from dying spirochetes. The reaction develops 6 to 12 hours after the initial penicillin dose and causes fever, headache, nausea, tachycardia, and hypotension. Instruct the patient to rest, drink fluids, and take antipyretics.

Tell the patient that the disease must be reported to the local health authority but that confidentiality will be maintained. Identifying and treating sexual partners of the infected patient is an important intervention. If the patient is treated in the primary or secondary stage, attempt to contact all sexual partners from the past 3 months. If the patient is in the later stages of the disease, contacts from the previous year are screened. Handle the "contact discovery" interview carefully, and, if possible, have a public health professional conduct the interview.

PHARMACOLOGIC HIGHLIGHTS

Medication or Drug Class	Dosage	Description	Rationale
Benzathine penicillin G	2.4 million units IM, single dose (some recommend a second dose 1 week later)	Antibiotic, penicillin	Effective for primary, secondary, and latent syphilis of less than 1 year duration
Benzathine penicillin G	2.4 million units, IM, weekly, × 3 doses	Antibiotic, penicillin	Effective treatment for latent syphilis of more than 1 year duration, or cardiovascular or late benign syphilis
Aqueous crystalline penicillin G	2–4 million units IV q 4 h for 10–14 days	Antibiotic, penicillin	Recommended to treat neurosyphilis

Independent

Provide care for the patient's lesions. Keep them clean and dry. Properly dispose of contaminated materials from draining lesions. Use universal precautions when you come in direct contact with the patient, when collecting specimens, and when caring for the lesions.

Focus on prevention. Educate patients about the course of the disease and the need to return for follow-up treatment or blood tests. Patients need to understand that although their lesions may heal, the infection may not be gone. Approximately 10% of patients do not respond to the first round of antibiotics, so additional treatment may be necessary.

Teach patients how to reduce risk factors to prevent future infections by limiting the number of sexual partners and practicing safer sex. Using condoms with spermicide and inspecting partners for any rashes or lesions may reduce exposure to the disease. Patients need ongoing emotional support to make lifestyle changes. Explain the need for regular laboratory testing (VDRL) every 3 months for 2 years to detect a relapse. Urge patients in the latent or late stages to have blood tests every 6 months for 2 years. Explain the relationship between HIV and syphilis and perform HIV testing if the patient wishes.

DOCUMENTATION GUIDELINES

- Description of lesions; rashes; and any neurologic, visual, or cardiac abnormalities
- Reaction to medications, including the site and dosage of IM injections
- Information for follow-up, including report of disease incidence to the local health authority and names of patient contacts (to maintain confidentiality, this information may not be kept in the patient's treatment record)

DISCHARGE AND HOME HEALTHCARE GUIDELINES

PREVENTION. Instruct the patient to avoid sexual contact for at least 2 weeks or as prescribed by the physician. Tell the patient to contact the physician if any new lesions or rashes are noted. Teach the patient how to prevent infection from STIs through safer sex practices.

MEDICATIONS. Teach the patient the purpose, dosage, schedule, precautions, and potential side effects, interactions, and adverse reactions of all prescribed medications. Recommend that patients treated as outpatients wait in the clinic or office for at least 30 minutes after administration of penicillin IM or IV to make sure there is no allergic reaction. Instruct patients given oral tetracycline to take the medication 1 hour before or 2 hours after meals and to avoid dairy products, antacids, iron, and sunlight while taking the drug.

PATIENT TEACHING. Teach the patient the importance of follow-up care, and make sure the patient knows the dates and times for follow-up appointments. Teach the patient the cause, symptoms, and mode of transmission for syphilis. Emphasize the importance of testing and treating all of the patient's sexual partners; urge the patient to provide the names of sexual partners.

Tendinitis

DRG Category: 248
Mean LOS: 4.4 days
Description: MEDICAL: Tendinitis, Myositis, and Bursitis
DRG Category: 232
Mean LOS: 3.2 days
Description: SURGICAL: Arthroscopy

Tendinitis is a painful inflammation or tearing of tendons, tendon-muscle attachments, or tendon sheaths. Commonly affected joints include the shoulder (rotator cuff), hip, heel (Achilles' tendinitis), and hamstring. The disorder is characterized by restricted joint movement and pain in the joint area. Fluid accumulation causes swelling early in the course of the disorder, but calcium deposits can increase swelling and cause further joint immobility or acute calcific bursitis.

It can be difficult to differentiate tendinitis from bursitis in the initial stages of both conditions. Bursitis is an inflammation of one or more bursae, the pad-like sacs that contain synovial fluid; these sacs reduce the friction between tendons, ligaments, and bones. Untreated tendinitis can result in bursitis, which can cause joint immobilization.

CAUSES

Tendinitis may result from a traumatic injury, strenuous exercise, or repetitive movement at a rapid pace. It can also be caused by postural misalignment, defective body development, or complications from another disease process such as any of the rheumatic diseases.

GENDER AND LIFE SPAN CONSIDERATIONS

Tendinitis can occur in any age group in anyone who performs an activity that stresses or overloads a joint on a repetitive basis. Women are more prone to tendinitis in their middle and older years. Elderly men also develop the disorder as their joints and soft tissues undergo the changes that occur with aging.

☐ ASSESSMENT

HISTORY. Ask the patient to describe normal and unusual exercise and activity patterns. Determine if the patient has had localized joint swelling, pain, and restricted movement and which joints have been affected. Ask if the pain has affected sleeping patterns. Establish a history of repetitive joint stress or trauma. Determine if the patient has either a congenital musculoskeletal condition that might have caused the tendinitis or a history of rheumatic disease. Determine if the patient has allergies to specific corticosteroids or local anesthetics, which are sometimes prescribed for tendinitis.

PHYSICAL EXAMINATION. The affected joint may be red, warm, and tender to touch. Note to what degree mobility is restricted and the number and location of joints that are involved.

PSYCHOSOCIAL. Patients may be concerned about permanent long-term immobility or restricted movement and how it will affect their lives. Assess their coping abilities.

DIAGNOSTIC HIGHLIGHTS

Test	Normal Result	Abnormality with Condition	Explanation
X rays	Normal bone and soft tissue structure and alignment	Detects bony abnormalities and arthritic changes	Excludes bony abnormalities and arthritis. Tendons are generally not visible on x rays.
Arthrogram	Intact soft tissue structures of the joint; absence of lesions or tears	Detects damage to tendons	Fluoroscopic and radiographic examination of a joint after injection of air and/or radiographic dye

Other Tests: Arthrocentesis, ultrasound.

PRIMARY NURSING DIAGNOSIS

Pain (acute or chronic) related to inflammation and swelling of the tendon

OUTCOMES. Comfort level; Pain control behavior; Pain: Disruptive effects; Pain level

INTERVENTIONS. Pain management; Analgesic administration; Positioning; Teaching: Prescribed activity/exercise; Teaching: Procedure/treatment; Teaching: Prescribed medication

☐ PLANNING AND IMPLEMENTATION

Collaborative

First-line therapy is often pharmacologic. Applications of heat, cold, ice, or ultrasound may be indicated to promote relief of pain and inflammation. The physician may also prescribe immobilization using a sling, splint, or cast. Fluid removal by aspiration and physical therapy to prevent "frozen" joints and preserve motion constitute supplementary treatment. In extremely rare situations, surgery may be necessary to loosen calcification.

PHARMACOLOGIC HIGHLIGHTS

Medication or Drug Class	Dosage	Description	Rationale
Analgesics	Varies with drug	Aspirin, 650 mg po q 4 hours as needed; propoxyphene hydrochloride (Darvon), 500 mg capsule every 6 hours; acetaminophen with 15 or 30 mg of codeine po every 4–6 hours; oxycodone, 5 mg every 6 hours po	Relieve pain and reduce inflammation
Nonsteroidal anti-inflammatories drugs (NSAIDs)	Varies with drug	Sulindac, 150 mg po bid; indomethacin, 25 mg po qid	Relieve pain and reduce inflammation

Other Drugs: Corticosteroids, local injection with corticosteroids or lidocaine for immediate pain relief

Independent

Focus on symptom relief. Encourage the patient to elevate the affected joint as often as possible to promote venous drainage and decrease the swelling. After the patient has received an intra-articular injection, apply ice for about 4 hours to help control the pain. Teach the patient how to apply ice and heat properly to prevent burning or chilling.

Explain to the patient the need to rest and reduce stress on the affected joints by modifying his or her lifestyle or activities until the condition has improved. If a sling is prescribed, teach the patient how to wear it properly. Instruct the patient to wear a splint during sleep to protect an affected shoulder. When the patient's joint pain has diminished, assist with range-of-motion and strengthening exercises. To limit the risk of re-injury, encourage the patient to use proper shoes for exercise and to lose weight if needed.

Explain the importance of anti-inflammatory medications, and teach the patient to take them with milk to minimize gastrointestinal (GI) distress. Also caution the patient to report distress, GI upset, nausea, and vomiting. Explain the seriousness of vomiting coffee-ground-like material and the need to seek medical help immediately. Encourage the patient to take medications with food to minimize gastric distress.

DOCUMENTATION GUIDELINES

- Physical findings: Joint mobility, tenderness, color, warmth
- Response to analgesic and anti-inflammatory medications, change in symptoms, and presence of side effects
- Tolerance of immobility and exercise regimen

DISCHARGE AND HOME HEALTHCARE GUIDELINES

Help the patient find alternatives to repetitive or stressful joint movement. Be sure the patient understands any medications prescribed, including dosage, route, action, and side effects. Caution the patient not to take aspirin with other NSAIDs. Encourage the patient to use heat or cold therapy as prescribed. Teach the patient to use a barrier between the skin and heat or to use cold therapy to prevent burning or frostbite. Remind the patient to keep follow-up appointments with the physician.

Testicular Cancer

DRG Category: 346
Mean LOS: 5.3 days
Description: MEDICAL: Malignancy, Male Reproductive System, with CC
DRG Category: 338
Mean LOS: 3.7 days
Description: SURGICAL: Testes Procedures, for Malignancy

Testicular cancer is a rare tumor that arises from the germinal cells of the embryonal tissues and causes less than 1% of all cancer deaths in men. Testicular tumors are classified as seminomas or nonseminomas. Seminomas are composed of uniform, undifferentiated cells that resemble primitive gonadal cells. This type of tumor represents 40% of all testicular cancer and is usually confined to the testes and retroperitoneal nodes. Nonseminomas show varying degrees of cell differentiation. Sometimes, testicular tumors are "mixed," containing elements distinctive to both groups.

CAUSES

Although specific causative factors for testicular cancer are unknown, research findings suggest a connection between the incidence of cryptorchidism (failure of testicles to descend) and testicular cancer. If an undescended testis is noted in a child, orchiopexy (surgical descent of the testes into its normal position within the scrotum) is recommended as soon as possible after birth. Although orchiopexy does not completely eliminate the risk of testicular cancer, it is believed that the sooner after birth orchiopexy is performed, the less the chance of developing testicular cancer later in life.

Exogenous estrogen has also been linked to testicular cancer. Male offspring of mothers who took diethystilbestrol (DES) during their pregnancy have an increased risk of developing testicular cancer. Additionally, patients who have had mumps, orchitis, or a childhood inguinal hernia are also considered to be at higher risk for developing testicular cancer.

GENDER AND LIFE SPAN CONSIDERATIONS

Testicular cancer is the most common solid tumor malignancy in men aged 15 to 40 years. It is less common in African-American and Asian men.

☐ ASSESSMENT

HISTORY. Obtain a thorough health history, particularly about the occurrence of risk factors. Any male born between 1940 and 1971 should be asked if his mother took any drugs to maintain her pregnancy. The earliest sign of testicular cancer is a small, hard, painless lump that cannot be separated from the testicle; it is occasionally accompanied by low back pain. Men often describe a feeling of "heaviness" or "dragging" in the testicles. These symptoms are often mistaken for epididymitis or muscle strain. Tenderness in the breast may also be present. Inquire about back pain, vague abdominal pain, nausea and vomiting, anorexia, and weight loss, all findings that suggest metastasis.

PHYSICAL EXAMINATION. The testes may be enlarged and swollen. A hydrocele or hematocele may be present. A testicular tumor can be distinguished from a hydrocele by transillumination (inspection of the testes by passing a light through its walls): a tumor does not transilluminate, whereas a hydrocele appears red and a normal testicle illuminates clearly. Because the tumor produces estrogen, inspect the patient for gynecomastia.

A testicular examination is accomplished by placing the index and middle finger on one side of the testicle with the thumb on the other side. Digital separation of the anterior testes from the posterior elements, including the epididymis and cord, is performed with care so that the intrascrotal contents can be palpated. A gentle rolling motion enables the examiner to palpate each testicle completely. A normal testicle is egg-shaped and feels smooth and firm but not hard. One testicle may naturally be larger than the other. A change in size or the presence of a lump is considered to be an abnormal finding. With testicular cancer, the lump is generally painless. Also, palpate the surrounding area for the presence of enlarged lymph nodes. Lymphadenopathy, especially in the abdominal and supraclavicular regions, is also found in more advanced disease.

PSYCHOSOCIAL. The diagnosis of cancer at any time is a lifestyle-altering event, but it is particularly disrupting to this young population. Interruption of schooling or work schedules, financial coverage for medical expenses, transportation to and from scheduled therapies, and child-care issues are a few of the concerns expressed by patients.

DIAGNOSTIC HIGHLIGHTS

General Comments: Most testicular tumors are found in routine checkups or by self examination; they often cause no symptoms.

Test	Normal Result	Abnormality with Condition	Explanation
Scrotal ultrasound	Normal size, shape, and configuration of the testicles	Solid, malignant mass is identified	Noninvasive visualization of the testicles
Radical orchiectomy, followed by a biopsy	NA	Solid mass is removed, 100% prove to be malignant	Needle biopsy would lead to open spread of the cancer cells, thus the biopsy is done after the testicle is removed

Other Tests: Serum laboratory analysis of beta-subunit human chorionic go-nadotropin (hCG) and alpha-fetoprotein (AFP); chest x ray or computed tomography (CT) for lung metastasis; abdominal and pelvic CT or magnetic resonance imaging (MRI) to check for retroperitoneal lymph node metastasis; intravenous pyelography to check for urinary tract involvement

PRIMARY NURSING DIAGNOSIS

Pain (acute) related to inflammation, tissue damage, tissue compression, or nerve irritation from tumor metastasis in the perineum, groin, or abdomen

OUTCOMES. Pain control; Pain: Disruptive effects; Well-being

INTERVENTIONS. Analgesic administration; Pain management; Meditation; Transcutaneous electric nerve stimulation (TENS); Hypnosis, Heat/cold application

☐ PLANNING AND IMPLEMENTATION

Collaborative

SURGICAL. The initial treatment for testicular cancer is surgical resection of the involved testicle (orchiectomy). A testicular prosthesis can be placed if the patient so desires. If a bilateral orchiectomy is performed, the patient may need hormonal replacement. It is controversial whether or not the retroperitoneal nodes should be resected or treated with chemotherapy. Surgical resection carries with it the likelihood of impotence and a significant mortality rate.

Postoperatively, edema and intrascrotal hemorrhage are the two most common problems. Monitor the patient closely for swelling and bleeding. Elevate the scrotum on a rolled towel, and apply ice to assist with discomfort and decrease swelling. Observe for signs of infection. Encourage the patient to wear an athletic supporter during ambulation to minimize discomfort. Usually the patient is encouraged to do so within 12 hours of surgery.

RADIATION AND CHEMOTHERAPY. Depending on staging of the disease, radiation or chemotherapy may also be used. Tumors classified as seminomas are especially radiosensitive. External beam radiation is usually given after surgery if the peritoneal lymph system is disease-positive or if the pelvis and mediastinal and supraclavicular lymph nodes are involved. Inform the patient that although the unaffected testicle is shielded during radiation, it does receive some radiation that is scattered, which may decrease spermatogenesis. Nonseminomatous tumors are not radiosensitive, and chemotherapy is the preferred treatment.

PHARMACOLOGIC HIGHLIGHTS

Medication or Drug Class	Dosage	Description	Rationale
Cisplatin	20 mg/m^2 per day IV for 5 days/cycle	Antineoplastic, alkylating agent	Increases the long-term survival rate when any type of metastasis is found
Vinblastine	Individualized using WBC count as guide	Antineoplastic, plant alkaloid	Most effective at treating metastasis when given in combination
Etoposide	50–100 mg/m^2 per day on days 1–5	Antineoplastic, miscellaneous	Used in combination
Acetaminophen/ NSAIDS; opiods; combination opiods/ NSAIDs	Depends on the drug	Analgesic	Analgesics used are determined by the severity of pain; pain may be postoperative or caused by metastasis

Independent

Nurses can play a role in the early detection of testicular cancer. Patients should be taught how to do a testicular self-examination and should be encouraged to perform the examination monthly. Provide private time for the patient and his partner to ask questions, express concerns, and clarify information. Offer the patient an opportunity for sexuality and fertility counseling after discussing the impact of the surgery on his anatomy and function. Make sure the patient understands the need to perform coughing and deep-breathing exercises to limit pulmonary complications. Before surgery, instruct the patient on the use of an incentive spirometer.

Because stomatitis is a common occurrence, check the mouth regularly for open irritated areas and encourage the patient to use warm mouthwashes. If the patient becomes nauseated, offer small, frequent feedings and eliminate any noxious stimuli such as bad odors. In addition, have the patient drink at least 3 L of fluid per day to ensure adequate hydration. If the patient is receiving radiation, monitor for side effects. Avoid rubbing the skin near the site of radiation to prevent discomfort and skin breakdown.

Ask about pain regularly and assess pain systematically. Believe the patient and family in their reports of pain. Inform the patient and family of options for pain relief as proposed by the National Cancer Institute (pharmacologic, physical, psychosocial, and cognitive-behavior interventions) and involve the patient and family in determining pain relief measures. To manage the discomfort of chemotherapy in addition to medications, consider the use of biofeedback or other alternative relaxation techniques.

The diagnosis of testicular cancer is a devastating one to most men. Discuss the patient's concerns with him. Explain the role of hormonal replacement in maintaining the secondary sex characteristics. If the patient is at risk for sterility, explain sperm banking procedures before treatment if infertility and impotence may result from surgery. Refer the patient to a support group or ask that another man who has experienced a similar diagnosis and treatment share his experiences to provide support. If the patient or partner is struggling to cope with the diagnosis, arrange for a counselor.

DOCUMENTATION GUIDELINES

- Physical findings: Operative incisions, patency of intravenous lines, healing of incisions, vital signs, testicular assessment findings
- Response to treatments: Side effects from medications or radiation therapy; management and control of symptoms
- Presence of complications: Infection, bleeding, respiratory distress, unrelieved pain or nausea

DISCHARGE AND HOME HEALTHCARE GUIDELINES

MEDICATIONS. If hormonal replacement is ordered, be sure the patient understands the dosage, schedule, actions, and side effects of the medication.

PREVENTION. Have the patient demonstrate a testicular self-examination before leaving the hospital. The patient should understand that testicular cancer can recur in the remaining testes and that early detection is a critical factor in the outcome.

SEXUALITY. Inform the patient that if a unilateral orchiectomy was performed, he is still fertile and should not experience impotence. Make sure the patient understands that he has the option of undergoing reconstructive surgery and placement of a testicular prosthesis. Refer the patient to the American Cancer Society to assist with obtaining information and support.

HOME CARE. Teach the patient to do the following:
Avoid prolonged standing because this can increase scrotal edema.
Wear an athletic supporter or snug-fitting undershorts until the area is completely healed.
Avoid heavy lifting for 4 to 6 weeks.
Take a 20-minute tub bath three times a day for 1 week after discharge.

Tetanus

DRG Category: 423
Mean LOS: 7.1 days
Description: MEDICAL: Other Infectious and Parasitic Diseases Diagnoses

Tetanus, or lockjaw, is a preventable but often fatal disorder that is caused by the bacterium *Clostridium tetani,* a spore-forming anaerobe. The bacterium exists in spore form in an aerobic environment until it is exposed to an anaerobic environment. The organism then changes to the vegetative form, multiplies, and produces neurotoxins.

When the tetanus bacteria enter an open wound, they multiply and produce a potent neurotoxin called tetanospasmin, which enters the bloodstream and acts on the spinal ganglia and central nervous system by interfering with the function of the postsynaptic inhibitory potentials. The anterior horn cells become overstimulated, thus resulting in excessive muscle contraction. Toxins may also act directly on skeletal muscle and cause muscle contraction. Complications include lung disorders such as pneumonia, pulmonary emboli, atelectasis, cardiac dysrhythmias, gastric ulcers, and flexion contractures.

CAUSES

Because *C. tetani* is commonly found in soil, tetanus is more common in agricultural regions. Any break in the skin or mucous membrane can result in a tetanus infection, but wounds that are contaminated with soil or those that produce a relatively anaerobic environment are at greater risk. Wounds that produce an anaerobic environment include those with purulent or necrotic tissue, puncture wounds, burns, gunshot wounds, animal bites, and complex fractures. Drug abusers who engage in "skin popping," or subcutaneous injections, are also at risk for a tetanus infection.

GENDER AND LIFE SPAN CONSIDERATIONS

People of all ages and sexes are at risk for tetanus if they have not been vaccinated. In developing countries, tetanus is a common cause of neonatal death when infants are delivered in unsterile conditions. The elderly in developed countries are also at risk even when they are immunized because of the waning effects of past immunizations.

◻ ASSESSMENT

HISTORY. Classically, patients have a dirty (often soil-contaminated) puncture wound or laceration and describe pain or paresthesia at the puncture site. A history of intravenous drug abuse, dental infection, umbilical stump infection (infants), or penetrating eye infection and inadequate tetanus immunization may also be reported. If the wound has been left untreated, early symptoms include difficulty chewing or swallowing. The patient may have a mild fever or painful muscle contractions or spasms in the affected region. Infants may be unable to suck.

PHYSICAL EXAMINATION. Because most cases of tetanus result in a systemic reaction, inspect the patient for neuromuscular changes. Spasms begin in the facial and jaw muscles and progress to muscles of the neck, extremities, and respiratory/pharyngeal regions. Muscles ultimately become rigid, with painful spasms in response to any external stimuli. You may note seizures, posturing, and muscle rigidity; during seizure activity, the patient is awake and in severe pain. Autonomic disturbances include diaphoresis, increased heart rate, cardiac dysrhythmias, and blood pressure fluctuations. Spasms of respiratory and pharyngeal muscles may make it difficult to maintain a patent airway. Patients may exhibit increased respiratory rate, increased inspiratory effort, poor lung expansion, and decreased airflow. Late findings include risus sardonicus (a grotesque, grinning expression), trismus (lockjaw), and opisthotonos (rigid somatic muscles that lead to an arched-back posture). With supportive care, signs and symptoms reverse after the toxin has been metabolized in about 6 weeks.

PSYCHOSOCIAL. The family may feel guilty if the patient has not been vaccinated. Assess the patient's and family's levels of anxiety and their ability to cope. The length of hospitalization and the seriousness of the diagnosis place the patient and family at risk for alterations in growth and development. Assess levels of growth and development using age-appropriate milestones and developmental tasks as guidelines.

DIAGNOSTIC HIGHLIGHTS

General Comments: There are no definitive tests for tetanus.

Test	Normal Result	Abnormality with Condition	Explanation
Lumbar puncture	Normal opening pressures and clear and sterile cerebrospinal fluid (CSF)	Normal opening pressures and clear and sterile CSF	Procedure is used to differentiate between meningitis (positive CSF cultures) and tetanus (negative CSF cultures)

PRIMARY NURSING DIAGNOSIS

Ineffective airway clearance related to muscle spasms and trismus

OUTCOMES. Respiratory status: Gas exchange and ventilation; Symptom control behavior; Treatment behavior: Illness; Comfort level

INTERVENTIONS. Airway management; Airway suctioning; Artificial airway management; Environmental management: Safety; Teaching: Disease process, Prescribed medication; Emotional support

☐ PLANNING AND IMPLEMENTATION

Collaborative

To prevent tetanus, within 3 days of a puncture wound, patients with no previous tetanus immunization require tetanus immune globulin or tetanus antitoxin for temporary protection. Active immunization with tetanus toxoid is also provided. If the patient had a previous immunization more than 5 years before the injury, a booster injection of tetanus toxoid is warranted at the time of injury. Goals of treatment include neutralizing the toxin, preventing complications, and eliminating the source of the toxin. Human tetanus immune globulin is administered immediately. One-half of the dose is administered by infiltrating the wound, and the remaining half is administered intramuscularly into three limbs. Active immunity is given by administering tetanus toxoid at a site remote from the globulin injections. The affected wound is thoroughly debrided after the antitoxin has been administered. Cultures of the wound may be obtained at that time. Parenteral antibiotics (penicillin in particular if the patient has no allergies to the drug) are administered for 10 days.

Respiratory distress may necessitate intubation or tracheostomy and mechanical ventilation with supplemental oxygen. Nasogastric tubes are inserted to prevent gastric distension. Patients with difficulty swallowing may require nutritional support with total parenteral nutrition or enteral feeding by a nasogastric or nasointestinal tube.

PHARMACOLOGIC HIGHLIGHTS

Medication or Drug Class	Dosage	Description	Rationale
Human tetanus immune globulin	One-half dose is administered by infiltrating the wound; remaining half is administered intramuscularly into three limbs; total dose is 3000–10,000 U	Immuno-globulin	Provides passive immunization; administered immediately
Tetanus toxoid absorbed (absorbed onto aluminum hydroxide, phosphate, or potassium sulfate)	Series of three 0.5 mL doses provide protection in 90% of patients; administered at a site remote from globulin injections	Toxoid	Provides active immunization against tetanus; affected wound is debrided after antitoxin has been administered
Penicillin G (or tetracycline; erythromycin)	2 million units IV q 6 hours for 10 days	Antibiotic	Prevent or combat infection (if the patient has no allergies to the drug)

Other Drugs: Neuromuscular blocking agents; antipyretics; analgesics; anticoagulants; sedatives, anti-anxiety agents, and muscle relaxants such as diazepam are administered to decrease muscle spasms. Neuromuscular blocking agents may be required to paralyze the patient if other agents cannot control the spasms or seizures. Antidysrhythmic drugs are given if cardiac rhythm disturbances arise, antipyretics are administered for fever, and analgesics are provided for relief of pain. Prophylactic anticoagulation therapy may be instituted to prevent thrombus formation.

Independent

Nursing care focuses on maintaining a patent airway, regular breathing, and adequate circulation and on providing comfort management, protection from injury, and psychosocial support of the patient and family. If muscle spasms or seizure activity places the patient at risk for airway compromise, use the chin lift or jaw thrust to maintain an open airway if possible. Insert an oral or nasal airway before seizures, but if the patient has lockjaw do not attempt to force an airway in place because you may injure the patient and worsen the airway patency. Have intubation and suction equipment immediately available at the bedside should the patient require it. Anchor the endotracheal tube firmly, and document the lip level of the endotracheal tube in the progress notes for continuity.

Institute seizure precautions as soon as the patient is admitted to the unit.

Pad the side rails of the bed, and provide immediate access to oxygen, suction, intubation equipment, artificial airways, and a resuscitation bag. Place the patient in a quiet, dark room to reduce environmental stimuli. Position the patient who is unconscious or paralyzed from pharmacologic agents in a side-lying position and turn the patient every 2 hours.

Provide clarification of information about the patient's diagnosis, prognosis, and treatment to the patient and family. Make sure that the family has adequate time for expression of their feelings each day. Support effective coping mechanisms and provide appropriate referrals to the chaplain, clinical nurse specialist, or counselor if the patient or family demonstrates ineffective coping behaviors.

DOCUMENTATION GUIDELINES

- Respiratory response: Rate and rhythm; lung expansion, respiratory effort, presence of retractions or nasal flaring (infants); presence of adventitious breath sounds; oxygen saturation; placement and patency of an artificial airway; character and amount of respiratory secretions; color of mucous membranes
- Presence, location, duration, and description of muscle spasms or seizures
- Physical responses: Condition of skin; bowel and urinary elimination patterns; description of stool and urine; pain and comfort level; condition of wound and dressings; weight; response to feedings; response to intravenous infusions, analgesics, muscle relaxants, and antipyretics
- Growth and development level, growth and development activities, response

DISCHARGE AND HOME HEALTHCARE GUIDELINES

Teach the patient and family that tetanus is a preventable disease. Inform them of the appropriate immunization and booster schedule, and encourage them to follow it. Note that the patient may experience pain, tenderness, redness, and muscle stiffness in the limb in which the tetanus injection(s) is (are) given. Explain that the convalescent period following tetanus may be prolonged. The patient may need multidisciplinary rehabilitation and home nursing.

Thoracic Aortic Aneurysm

DRG Category: 130
Mean LOS: 5.8 days
Description: MEDICAL: Peripheral Vascular Disorders with CC
DRG Category: 110
Mean LOS: 9.1 days
Description: SURGICAL: Major Cardiovascular Procedures with CC

A thoracic aortic aneurysm is an abnormal widening of the aorta between the aortic valve and the diaphragm. Thoracic aneurysms account for approximately 25% of all aneurysms. Although aneurysms may be located on the ascending, transverse, or descending part of the aorta or may involve the entire thoracic aorta, they commonly develop between the origin of the left subclavian artery and the diaphragm.

Aneurysm formation is caused by a weakening of the medial layer of the aorta, which stretches outward, causing an outpouching of the aortic wall. Thoracic aortic aneurysms take four forms: fusiform, saccular, dissecting, and false aneurysms. (See Table 51.) Dissection of the aorta can occur with or without an aneurysm but is most often associated with the presence of a pre-existing aneurysm. Thoracic aortic aneurysms may lead to serious or fatal complications if they are left untreated. For example, a thoracic dissecting aneurysm may rupture into the pericardium, thus resulting in cardiac tamponade, hemorrhagic shock, and cardiac arrest.

TABLE 51 | **Forms of Thoracic Aortic Aneurysm**

TYPE	DESCRIPTION
Fusiform	Spindle-shaped bulge that encompasses the entire circumference of the aorta
Saccular	Unilateral pouchlike bulge with a narrow neck, most frequently at a bifurcation that involves only a portion of the vessel circumference
Dissecting	Hemorrhagic separation of the medial and intimal layers, creating a false lumen
False	Pulsating hematoma that results from a rupture of the aorta, secondary to trauma

CAUSES

The single most important cause is atherosclerosis. The atherosclerotic process damages the arterial wall by weakening the medial muscle layer and distending the lumen. Destruction of the medial layer allows the artery to increase in size circumferentially (a fusiform shape), or the artery develops a saccular outpouching at the weakened area. Other factors that contribute include Marfan's syndrome (hereditary musculoskeletal disorder), Ehlers-Danlos syndrome (an inherited disorder of elastic connective tissue), coarctation of the aorta, fungal infections (mycotic aneurysms) of the aortic arch, a bicuspid aortic valve, aortitis, and trauma (external, blunt trauma or iatrogenic trauma that occurs during invasive diagnostic procedures).

GENDER AND LIFE SPAN CONSIDERATIONS

The most common thoracic aortic aneuyrsm is an ascending aortic aneurysm, which is usually seen in hypertensive men under 60 years of age. A descending aortic aneurysm is most common in elderly hypertensive men or younger patients with a history of traumatic chest injury. The incidence of thoracic aortic aneurysm is higher in men than women by a ratio of 3 to 1.

☐ ASSESSMENT

HISTORY. Establish a history of atherosclerosis, hypertension, hypercholesteremia, smoking, obesity, diabetes, and familial tendencies. Elicit a history of pain, including a description and location. (See Table 52.) Establish a history of pulmonary symptoms, such as wheezing, coughing, hemoptysis, dyspnea, or stridor, which may be caused by a descending thoracic aortic aneurysm that compresses the tracheobronchial tree. Ask if the patient has had difficulties swallowing, hoarseness, dyspnea, or dry cough, all of which may be caused by a transverse arch thoracic aortic aneurysm.

TABLE 52 | **Characteristic Signs and Symptoms of Thoracic Aortic Aneurysms**

LOCATION OF ANEURYSM	LOCATION OF PAIN	TYPE OF PAIN
Ascending aorta	Substernal chest pain (reminiscent of angina), extending to the neck, shoulders, lower back, or abdomen but not generally to the jaw or arms; more severe on right side	Severe, boring, ripping
Transverse arch of aorta	Neck pain radiating to the shoulders	Sudden, sharp tearing
Descending aorta	Back and shoulder pain radiating to the chest	Sharp, tearing

PHYSICAL EXAMINATION. The physical examination of a patient with a thoracic aortic aneurysm does not reveal the presence of the aneurysm itself. Certain physical findings, however, should raise your level of suspicion. Complete a neurological examination to determine the adequacy of tissue perfusion. Take the patient's blood pressure in both arms because an ascending thoracic aortic aneurysm may cause a contralateral (opposite side) difference. Take both the patient's right carotid and left radial pulses and note any differences. Auscultate for pericardial friction rub and aortic valve insufficiency murmur, indicating the extension of an ascending aortic aneurysm proximally into the aortic valve. Note any signs of bradycardia.

PSYCHOSOCIAL. Assess the patient's and significant others' understanding of the implications of the condition. Assess the ability of the patient and significant others to cope with a sudden life-threatening illness, a prolonged hospitalization, and the role changes that a sudden illness requires. Assess the patient's level of anxiety about the illness, potential surgery, and complications.

DIAGNOSTIC HIGHLIGHTS

General Comments: Because this condition causes no symptoms, it is often diagnosed through routine physical exams or chest x rays.

Test	Normal Result	Abnormality with Condition	Explanation
Computed tomography (CT) scan	Negative study	Locates outpouching within the aortic wall	Assesses size and location of aneurysm
Chest x ray	Negative study	May show widened mediastinum or enlarged calcified aortic shadow.	Assesses size and location of aneurysm

Traumatic aneurysm may be associated with skeletal fractures

Other Tests: Electrocardiogram, chest x ray, magnetic resonance imaging (MRI), transthoracic echocardiography with Doppler color flow mapping, transesophageal echocardiography, aortic angiography

PRIMARY NURSING DIAGNOSIS

Potential for altered tissue perfusion (cerebral, peripheral, cardiopulmonary, gastrointestinal, renal) related to fluid volume deficit and hemorrhage

OUTCOMES. Cardiac pump effectiveness; Circulation status; Tissue perfusion: Cerebral, Peripheral, Cardiopulmonary, Gastrointestinal, Renal; Vital sign status; Fluid balance; Cognitive status

INTERVENTIONS. Circulatory care; Cardiac care; Airway management; Fluid monitoring; Medication management and administration; Intravenous insertion and therapy; Neurologic monitoring; Oxygen therapy; Emergency care; Laboratory data interpretation; Surveillance

☐ PLANNING AND IMPLEMENTATION

Collaborative

A thoracic aortic aneurysm that is 4 cm in size or less may be treated with oral antihypertensives or a beta-blocking agent to control hypertension. Frequent diagnostic testing (every 6 months) is necessary to determine the size of the aneurysm. A thoracic aortic aneurysm that is 5 cm or greater in diameter is usually treated surgically. Other indications for surgical intervention include dissection, intractable pain, and an unstable aneurysm (one that is changing size). The primary complication for thoracic aortic aneurysms is dissection. Monitor the patient for any changes in the quality of peripheral pulses; changes in vital signs; changes in the level of consciousness; and onset of sudden, severe, ripping, or tearing pain in the chest, neck, back, or shoulders. A ruptured thoracic aortic aneurysm requires immediate surgical intervention.

Preoperatively, assess the patient's peripheral pulses, taking care to compare one side to the other. Take the patient's blood pressure measurement in both arms, and auscultate for an aortic insufficiency murmur to establish a baseline for postoperative comparison. Also, administer large volumes of intravenous fluids and blood products to maintain circulation until surgery is performed. Surgical procedures vary, depending on the location of the aneurysm. An ascending arch aneurysm may be replaced with an interposition graft, a composite valved conduit, or a supracoronary graft with separate aortic valve replacement. A transverse arch aneurysm is usually repaired with anastomoses and reconstructions. A graft is used to repair descending thoracic and thoracoabdominal aneurysms. Postoperatively, monitor cardiopulmonary states, especially for patients with congestive heart failure (CHF), because beta-blocking agents may worsen CHF. If the patient has hypercholesteremia that cannot be controlled with diet, a cholesterol-lowering agent may be prescribed by the physician.

PHARMACOLOGIC HIGHLIGHTS

Medication or Drug Class	Dosage	Description	Rationale
Nitroprusside	0.5–10 μg/kg per minute, titrated to reduce blood pressure IV	Antihypertensive	Reduces blood pressure in acute or critical situations
Morphine	1–10 mg IV	Opioid analgesic	Relieves surgical pain
Fentanyl	50–100 μg IV	Opioid analgesic	
Antihypertensives; diuretics	Varies by drug	Beta blockers	Reduce blood pressure so that hypertension does not stress graft suture lines

Independent

Focus on maintaining adequate circulation, preventing complications, and implementing patient education. For the nonsurgical patient, patient teaching includes information about low-fat, low-cholesterol diets to prevent progression of the atherosclerotic process and to treat hypercholesteremia. Urge the patient to stop smoking cigarettes and provide information about smoking cessation.

For the surgical patient, focus on maintaining adequate circulation preoperatively and postoperatively, preventing complications, and patient teaching. Preoperative care of the elective surgical patient is the same as for any patient who undergoes general anesthesia. Postoperatively, care is similar to that of a patient who undergoes any chest surgery. Provide aggressive pulmonary hygiene every 1 to 2 hours to prevent pulmonary complications. Assist with range-of-motion exercises to limit the effects of immobility. Provide emotional support for the patient and significant others.

DOCUMENTATION GUIDELINES

- Physical findings: Vital signs, pain (location, onset, severity), heart sounds, urine output, healing of incision
- Assessment of circulation: Blood pressure in both arms, quality of peripheral pulses in all extremities, capillary blanch test
- Response to acute, life-threatening illness: Anxiety, fear, coping
- Response to surgery: Incision, wound healing, wound drainage, signs of complications

DISCHARGE AND HOME HEALTHCARE GUIDELINES

The nonsurgical patient is discharged to the home setting. The surgical patient is usually discharged to the home setting if a support system can be identified. An extended-care facility may be required for a short time if a support system is not in place for the patient at the time of discharge. Be sure the patient understands all medications prescribed, including dosage, route, action, and side effects. Provide patients and their families with information about a low-fat, low-cholesterol diet (reduced-calorie if obese). Be sure the patient understands the importance of controlling blood pressure and blood cholesterol levels in the prevention of progression of the atherosclerotic process.

Provide patients who smoke and their families with information about how to stop smoking. Be sure the patient understands that smoking is a risk factor for hypertension and atherosclerosis. Make sure the nonsurgical patient with a thoracic aortic aneurysm understands the necessity for follow-up examinations at regular intervals to determine the size of the aneurysm and the rate of enlargement. The surgical patient is restricted from activity for 6 to 12 weeks postoperatively. Teach the patient to restrict activities by avoiding heavy lifting, pushing or pulling strenuously, and straining. Give the surgical patient specific instructions for wound care. Teach the patient to examine the incision site for signs of infection and to report any to the physician.

Thrombophlebitis

DRG Category: 130
Mean LOS: 5.8 days
Description: MEDICAL: Peripheral Vascular Disorders with CC
DRG Category: 478
Mean LOS: 6.3 days
Description: SURGICAL: Other Vascular Procedures with CC

Thrombophlebitis, inflammation of a vein with an associated blood clot (thrombus), typically occurs in the veins of the lower extremities when fibrin and platelets accumulate at areas of stasis or turbulence near venous valves. Deep vein thrombophlebitis (deep vein thrombosis [DVT]) occurs more than 90% of the time in small veins, such as the lesser saphenous, or in large veins, such as the femoral and popliteal.

DVT is potentially more serious than that of the superficial veins because the deep veins carry approximately 90% of the blood flow as it leaves the lower extremities. Once a thrombus begins to move, it becomes an embolus (a detached intravascular mass carried by the blood). If it reaches the lungs, a pulmonary embolus, it is potentially fatal.

CAUSES

Venous stasis, hypercoagulability, and vascular injury are major causes of thrombophlebitis. Venous stasis results from prolonged immobility, pregnancy, obesity, chronic heart disease such as congestive heart failure or myocardial infarction, recovery from major surgery (surgical procedures lasting more than 30 minutes), cerebrovascular accidents, and advanced age. Hypercoagulability is associated with pregnancy, cigarette smoking, dehydration, deficiencies of substances involved in clot breakdown, disseminated intravascular coagulation, estrogen supplements and oral contraceptives, and sepsis. Vascular injury can occur with lower extremity fractures, surgery, burns, multiple trauma, childbirth, infections, irritating intravenous solutions, venipuncture, and venulitis. Other diseases that may lead to thrombus formation are cancer of the lung, gastrointestinal tract, and genitourinary tract and also atrial fibrillation; individuals older than 55 years are also particularly susceptible to thrombophlebitis.

GENDER AND LIFE SPAN CONSIDERATIONS

Young women and the elderly are more likely to develop thrombophlebitis than adult men because young adult women may have many risk factors (pregnancy, oral contraceptives, smoking, obesity). Women over 30 who smoke and use oral contraceptives are at particular risk. The elderly person's increased tendency for platelet aggregation and elevated fibrinogen levels increases their risk.

☐ ASSESSMENT

HISTORY. Although almost half of the patients with deep and superficial thrombophlebitis are asymptomatic, patients with DVT may have complaints of calf muscle or groin tenderness, pain, fever (rarely above 101°F), chills, general weakness, and lethargy.

PHYSICAL EXAMINATION. Observe both legs, noting alterations in symmetry, color, and temperature of one leg as compared to the other. In DVT, the affected limb may reveal redness, warmth, swelling, and discoloration when compared with the contralateral limb. In addition, superficial veins over the area may be distended. Note the presence of calf pain with dorsiflexion of the foot of the affected extremity, which is a positive Homans' sign. This positive finding occurs in 33% of patients with DVT and is considered an inconsistent and unreliable physical sign.

Superficial vein thrombosis may be asymptomatic or may lead to pain, redness, induration, and swelling in the local area of the thrombus. Note the presence of local redness and nodules on the skin or extremity edema, which is rare. Palpate over the suspected vein involved. It may feel like a cord or thickness that extends upward along the entire length of the vein.

PSYCHOSOCIAL. The patient has not only an unexpected, sudden illness, but also an increased risk for life-threatening complications such as pulmonary embolism. Assess the patient's ability to cope. In addition, assess the patient's degree of anxiety about the illness and potential complications.

DIAGNOSTIC HIGHLIGHTS

Test	Normal Result	Abnormality with Condition	Explanation
Doppler ultrasound; duplex Doppler venous scanning	Normal blood flow velocity	Diminished flow caused by phlebitis	Records sound waves reflected from moving red blood cells in arteries and veins
Radio-opaque venography	Negative	Detection of presence and site of venous thrombosis of lower extremities	Invasive, radiographic procedure with injection of contrast media; lower extremities are radiographed for detection of venous thrombosis

I-125-labeled fibrinogen leg scan	Negative; no evidence of thrombi	Identification of deep vein thrombosis or thrombophlebitis	Nuclear medicine test that involves intravenous injection of redionuclide-labeled fibrinogen and scanning with a counter to measure uptake of radio-active material by the clot

Other Tests: Impedence plethysmography, compression ultrasonography

PRIMARY NURSING DIAGNOSIS

Altered peripheral tissue perfusion related to obstructed venous blood flow

OUTCOMES. Tissue integrity: Peripheral; Tissue integrity: Skin and mucous membranes; Circulation status

INTERVENTIONS. Circulatory care; Laboratory monitoring; Peripheral sensation management; Positioning; Skin surveillance; Embolus precautions; Embolus care: Peripheral

☐ PLANNING AND IMPLEMENTATION

Collaborative

To prevent thrombus formation, most physicians prescribe compression of the legs by graduated compression stockings to reduce venous stasis in low-risk general surgical patients. In higher-risk patients, intermittent pneumatic compression boots prevent venous stasis and increase the normal breakdown of fibrin in the body with increased fibrinolytic activity.

Most patients who develop thrombophlebitis are placed on bed rest with extremity elevation to avoid dislodging the thrombus. Local heat with warm soaks may also be used to reduce venospasm and decrease inflammation. Generally the patient is given analgesics for pain control and anticoagulant therapy, initially with heparin, to prevent further clot formation. From 1 to 3 days later, warfarin (Coumadin) therapy is started. Heparin is usually discontinued 48 hours after the patient's prothrombin time (PT) reaches a therapeutic value. (See Box 15.)

BOX 15   CARING FOR THE PATIENT ON ANTICOAGULANTS

Assessment

Monitor coagulation profile (prothrombin time, partial thromboplastin time, INR) daily and report values below and above the therapeutic range to the physician.

Monitor for overt bleeding such as bruising, tarry stools, coffee-ground or bloody vomitus, oozing gums, hematuria, vaginal bleeding, and heavy menstruation.

Monitor for occult bleeding demonstrated by flank pain or abdominal pain and for changes in mental status.

Management Considerations

Have the antidote for heparin (protamine sulfate) and warfarin (vitamin K) available for emergency use in case of hemorrhage.

Avoid administering aspirin to patients on anticoagulants because the synergistic effect may induce bleeding.

Avoid the following procedures if possible because of the risk of increased bleeding: Intramuscular injections, central line insertions, arterial cannulation, lumbar puncture, and surgical procedures.

Note that the following conditions are relative contraindications to anticoagulant therapy: Active bleeding, cerebrovascular accident, severe hypertension, pericarditis and endocarditis, pregnancy (particularly warfarin therapy), and chronic alcoholism.

Note that the following medications may interact with warfarin:

Increased activity: Allopurinal, cimetidine, indomethacin, metronidazole, oral hypoglycemic agents, phenothiazines, quinidine, tricyclic antidepressants

Decreased activity: Barbiturates, oral contraceptives, rifampin. Apply pressure on all punctures for 5 minutes or as long as needed to stop bleeding.

Some patients may continue heparin subcutaneously for several weeks before changing to warfarin. Because prothrombin assays are performed in various ways, PT results are now also reported as an International Normalized Ratio (INR). The target INR for oral anticoagulation is at least 2.0; current recommendations are to stop heparin therapy after 5 to 7 days of joint therapy when the INR is 2.0 to 3.0 with the patient off heparin.

For patients with massive DVT in proximal veins, thrombolytic therapy may be considered. Before initiating therapy, the risk that the clot presents to the patient is compared to the risk of bleeding from thrombolytic agents.

SURGICAL. Other treatments that may be used for severe, obstructive DVT are thrombectomy (surgical clot removal) and surgical prophylaxis against pulmonary embolism (implantation of a Greenfield filter or an umbrella filter in the inferior vena cava). If a filter device cannot be placed, the inferior vena cava may be tied off (ligated) or stitched (plicated) to limit movement of emboli.

PHARMACOLOGIC HIGHLIGHTS

Medication or Drug Class	Dosage	Description	Rationale
Anticoagulants	Varies with drug and patient weight; standard heparin dose is 80 units/kg bolus IV followed by an infusion of 18 units/kg per hour titrated according to coagulation studies; starting dosage of warfarin is 5 mg per day for 2 days po with changes depending on prothrombin time	Sodium heparin; sodium warfarin (Coumadin)	Standard treatment is to initiate intravenous heparin to reduce further formation of clots

Other Drugs: Analgesics, low molecular weight heparin (enoxaparin or dalteparin, 100 units/kg) is a safe and effective alternative and leads to early discharge for some patients.

Independent

The most important nursing interventions focus on prevention. Decrease the risk of venous stasis in a bedridden patient by performing early ambulation and active or passive range-of-motion exercises several times a day. Avoid using the knee gatch because of the risk of popliteal pressure and venous stasis; encourage patients not to cross their legs, especially when sitting. If pillows are needed to elevate extremities, position them along the entire length of the extremity to prevent additional pressure on veins and to allow for adequate venous drainage. If the patient is immobile and not on fluid restriction, encourage the patient to drink at least 3 L of fluid a day to prevent dehydration and venous stasis.

To prevent injury to vessel walls, monitor intravenous (IV) cannulas to prevent infiltration. If IV medications are irritating to the vein, IV cannulas should be changed and rotated to new sites more often than the standard procedure.

Discuss activity restrictions with the patient and family. The patient usually feels confined and may become resentful because of the need for absolute bed rest. To increase mobility in bed, install an orthoframe and trapeze system to the bed. A sheepskin, air mattress, foam pad, foot cradle, or heel pads can reduce the risk of skin breakdown while the person is on bed rest. Provide diversional activities to reduce anxiety.

DOCUMENTATION GUIDELINES

- Physical findings of affected extremity: Presence of redness, tenderness, swelling
- Response to pain medications, heat application, elevation, rest
- Reaction to immobility and bed rest
- Presence of complications: Bleeding tendencies, respiratory distress, unrelieved discomfort

DISCHARGE AND HOME HEALTHCARE GUIDELINES

Teach the patient preventive strategies. Demonstrate how to apply compression stockings correctly, if they have been prescribed. Be sure the patient understands all medications, including the dosage, route, action, adverse effects, and need for routine laboratory monitoring for anticoagulants. If the patient is being discharged on subcutaneous heparin, the patient or family needs to demonstrate the injection technique. The patient also needs to know to avoid over-the-counter medications, particularly those that contain aspirin. Explain the need to avoid activities that could cause bumping or injury and predispose the patient to excessive bleeding. Instruct the patient to notify the physician if abdominal or flank pain, heavy bleeding during menstruation, and bloody urine or stool occurs.

Recommend using a soft toothbrush and an electric razor to limit injury. Remind the patient to notify the physician or dentist of anticoagulant use before any invasive procedure. Instruct the patient to report leg pain or swelling, skin discoloration, or decreases in peripheral skin temperature to the physician. In addition, if the patient experiences signs of possible pulmonary embolism (anxiety, shortness of breath, pleuritic pain, hemoptysis), he or she should go to the emergency department immediately.

Thyroid Cancer

DRG Category: 300
Mean LOS: 6.3 days
Description: MEDICAL: Endocrine Disorders with CC
DRG Category: 290
Mean LOS: 2.4 days
Description: SURGICAL: Thyroid Procedures

Although thyroid cancer is the most common endocrine cancer, its incidence among all cancers is low: it affects approximately 10,000 people each year in the United States. Most thyroid nodules or tumors develop from thyroid follicular cells; 95% of these nodules and tumors are benign. The remaining 5% of thyroid nodules or tumors are cancerous, and there are several forms of thyroid cancer. Papillary carcinoma is the most common form of primary thyroid cancer. It is also the slowest-growing thyroid cancer and is usually multifocal and bilateral in distribution. Papillary carcinoma metastasizes slowly into the cervical lymph nodes and the nodes of the mediastinum and lungs. Follicular cancer is the next most common form. It is more likely to recur than other forms; it generally metastasizes to the regional lymph nodes and is spread by the blood to distant areas such as the bones, liver, and lungs. More than 90% of patients treated for either papillary or follicular carcinoma will live for 15 years or longer after their diagnosis.

Anaplastic carcinoma of the thyroid is a less common form of thyroid cancer and is resistant to both surgical resection and radiation; the 5-year survival rate is between 3% and 17%. Anaplastic cells metastasize quickly, invade the trachea and surrounding tissues, and compress vital structures. Medullary cancer is even less common; it originates in the parafollicular cells of the thyroid. Metastasis occurs to the bones, liver, and kidneys if the disease is not treated. In addition to metastases, other life-threatening complications include compression of surrounding structures (particularly in the neck), thus leading to difficulty swallowing and breathing. Surgery can cure medullary thyroid cancer, and more than 80% of patients will live at least 10 years after surgery.

The American Cancer Society expected that in the year 2000 roughly 18,400 new cases of thyroid cancer would be diagnosed in the United States. An estimated 700 women and 500 men were expected to die of thyroid cancer during the year 2000.

CAUSES

People who have been exposed to radiation therapy to the neck are particularly susceptible to thyroid cancer, including those exposed to low-dose radiation as children and others exposed to high-dose radiation for malignancies. About 25% of individuals who had radiation in the 1950s to shrink an enlarged thymus gland, tonsils, or adenoids develop thyroid nodules; approximately 25% of those with nodules actually develop thyroid cancer (6% of those exposed to neck radiation in the first place). Other causes of thyroid cancer include prolonged secretion of thyroid-stimulating hormone (TSH) because of radiation, heredity, or chronic goiter.

GENDER AND LIFE SPAN CONSIDERATIONS

Although benign thyroid nodules and thyroid cancers can occur in people of all ages, those between 30 and 50 years old are most likely to develop papillary and follicular thyroid cancer. Women are three times as likely as men to have thyroid cancer.

◻ ASSESSMENT

HISTORY. Most patients present with an asymptomatic neck mass. They may also have complaints of neck discomfort, hoarseness, dysphagia (difficulty swallowing), and rapid nodule growth. Elicit a family history because some forms of thyroid cancer are inherited. If the thyroid has been completely destroyed by cancer cells, the patient may report a history of sensitivity to cold, weight gain, and apathy from hypothyroidism. If the thyroid has become overstimulated, the patient may describe signs of hyperthyroidism: sensitivity to heat, nervousness, weight loss, and hyperactivity. Changes in thyroid function may also lead to gastrointestinal changes such as diarrhea and anorexia.

PHYSICAL EXAMINATION. Observe the patient's neck, noting any mass or enlargement. Patients with anaplastic thyroid cancer may have a rapidly growing tumor that distorts the neck and surrounding structures. Palpate the thyroid gland for size, shape, configuration, consistency, tenderness, and presence of any nodules. Describe the number of nodules present and whether the nodule is smooth or irregular, soft or hard, or fixed to underlying tissue. Note the presence of enlarged cervical lymph nodes, which occur in 25% of patients with the disease. Auscultation may reveal bruits if the thyroid enlargement results from an increase in TSH, which increases thyroid circulation and vascularity.

PSYCHOSOCIAL. Assess the patient's ability to cope with the sudden illness and the diagnosis of cancer. Determine what a diagnosis of cancer means to the patient. Consider the type of cancer (and the speed of cancer growth) when assessing the patient's and family's response to the disease.

DIAGNOSTIC HIGHLIGHTS

Test	Normal Result	Abnormality with Condition	Explanation
Fine-needle aspiration (FNA) biopsy	Microscopic viewing reveals no cancerous cells	Microscopic viewing reveals cancer cells	A thin needle is placed directly into the nodule several times to sample different areas; 5% of FNA biopsies reveal cancer, while 60%–80% clearly show that the nodule is benign
Thyroid scan	Homogenous uptake of radioactive tracer; normal size and shape of thyroid	Abnormal areas of the thyroid may contain less radioactivity (cold nodules with	A small quantity of radioactive iodine is taken orally or by injection; after the chemicals

		decreased uptake) or more radioactivity (hot nodules with increased uptake)	concentrate in the thyroid, a special camera measures the amount of radiation in the thyroid gland
Thyroid stimulating hormone (TSH; thyro-tropin)	< 10 μU/mL	Normal or elevated	Used to determine if radioactive iodine will work as therapy
Serum calcitonin	< 40 pg/mL	Increased in medullary cancer of thyroid; levels 500–2000 pg/mL are often associated with cancer	Thyroid gland polypeptide hormone that is produced by thyroid even when no mass is palpable

Other Tests: Sonogram, computed tomography (CT) scan, magnetic resonance imaging (MRI) used for determining cancer staging, serum calcium

PRIMARY NURSING DIAGNOSIS

Ineffective airway clearance related to swelling and obstruction

OUTCOMES. Respiratory status: Gas exchange; Respiratory status: Ventilation; Symptom control behavior; Treatment behavior: Illness or injury; Comfort level

INTERVENTIONS. Airway management; Anxiety reduction; Oxygen therapy; Airway suctioning; Airway insertion and stabilization; Cough enhancement; Mechanical ventilation; Positioning; Respiratory monitoring

☐ PLANNING AND IMPLEMENTATION

Collaborative

Most physicians prescribe surgical treatment of thyroid cancer, with the definitive treatment depending on the size of the nodule. Surgical interventions range from a thyroid lobectomy to a total thyroidectomy, depending on tissue type. To prevent complications after the thyroidectomy, careful monitoring for airway obstruction and stridor is essential. A tracheostomy tray should be kept near the patient at all times during the immediate recovery period. In addition, monitor for signs of thyrotoxicosis (tachycardia, diaphoresis, increased blood pressure, anxiety) and hypocalcemia (tingling of the fingers and toes, carpopedal spasms, and convulsions). The surgical dressing and incision also need to be assessed for excessive drainage or bleeding during the postoperative period. If the patient complains that the dressing feels tight, the surgeon needs to be alerted immediately.

Generally, after surgery is completed, the patient is started on synthetic levothyroxine therapy to suppress TSH levels and establish a euthyroid (normal) state. Most patients do not have chemotherapy or radiotherapy because these modalities are usually ineffective with rapidly growing thyroid cancers. Chemotherapy is usually reserved as an adjuvant measure to halt the spread of metastasis.

Radioactive iodine (^{131}I) may be used to destroy any remaining thyroid tissue. For radioiodine therapy to be most effective, patients have to have high serum TSH levels. TSH in an injectable form is given to increase its level before radioiodine therapy; withholding thyroid hormone replacement is usually not necessary.

PHARMACOLOGIC HIGHLIGHTS

Medication or Drug Class	Dosage	Description	Rationale
Levothyroxine (Synthroid)	2.6 μg/kg per day for 7–10 days	Synthetic T_4 hormone	Suppresses TSH levels and establishes a euthyroid state postoperatively

Independent

The most important nursing interventions focus on teaching and prevention of complications. When you prepare patients before surgery, discuss not only the procedure and aftercare but also the methods for postoperative communication such as a magic slate or a point board. Explain that the patient will be able to speak only rarely, will need to rest the voice for several days, and should expect to be hoarse. Answer all questions before surgery. After the procedure, monitor the patient's ability to speak with each measurement of vital signs. Assess the patient's voice tone and quality, and compare it with the preoperative voice.

Maintain the bed in a high Fowler position to decrease edema and swelling of the neck. To avoid pressure on the suture line, encourage the patient to avoid neck flexion and extension. Support the head and neck with pillows or sandbags; if the patient needs to be transferred from stretcher to bed, support the head and neck in good body alignment.

Before discharge, make sure that the patient has a follow-up appointment for a postdischarge assessment. Make sure that the patient has the financial resources to obtain all needed medications; some patients require thyroid supplements for the rest of their lives. Refer the patient or family to the American Cancer Society for additional information.

DOCUMENTATION GUIDELINES

- Physical findings: Patency of airway, breathing patterns, voice
- Physical findings of incision: Wound edges, hematoma formation, bleeding, infection
- Presence of complications: Thyrotoxicosis, hypocalcemia, hypothyroidism
- Reaction to diagnosis of thyroid cancer
- Understanding of, and interest in, cancer support groups

DISCHARGE AND HOME HEALTHCARE GUIDELINES

To maintain a euthyroid state, teach the patient and family the symptoms of hypothyroidism for early detection of problems: weakness, fatigue, cold intolerance, weight gain, facial puffiness, periorbital edema, bradycardia, and hypothermia. Be sure the patient understands all medications, including the dosage, route, action, and adverse effects. Explain that the patient needs routine follow-up laboratory tests to check TSH and T_4 levels. Be sure the patient knows when the first postoperative physician's visit is scheduled. Explain any wound care and that the patient should expect to be hoarse for a week or so after the surgical procedure.

Tonsillitis

DRG Category: 60
Mean LOS: 1.5 days
Description: SURGICAL: Tonsillectomy and/or Adenoidectomy Only Age 0–17

Tonsils are defined as the masses of lymphatic tissue that are located in the depressions of the mucous membranes of the fauces (constricted opening, leading from the mouth to the oral pharynx) and pharynx. The tonsils act as a filter to protect the body from bacterial invasion via the oral cavity and also to produce white blood cells. Tonsillitis is generally referred to as an inflammation of a tonsil, particularly a faucial tonsil. Acute tonsillitis is considered acute pharyngitis. When tonsillar involvement is severe, the term tonsillopharyngitis or tonsillitis is used; when the involvement is minor, the term nasopharyngitis is used.

CAUSES

Viral infection is the leading cause of nasopharyngitis. Adenovirus is the most common infecting agent, but other viruses include enteroviruses, herpesvirus, and Epstein-Barr virus. A nonviral cause is *Mycoplasma pneumoniae*. Bacterial causes include group A beta-hemolytic streptococci (GABHS), *Neisseria gonorrheae,* and *Corynebacterium diptheriae.*

GENDER AND LIFE SPAN CONSIDERATIONS

Viral tonsillitis is unusual in infants and is most common in children of both genders who are 4 to 5 years of age. Bacterial infections are uncommon in children under 2 years of age, and are most common in children 5 to 11 years of age.

☐ ASSESSMENT

HISTORY. Usually the symptoms of viral tonsillitis have a gradual onset. Elicit a description of the history and progression of the signs and symptoms. Expect that the predominant symptom is rhinorrhea, (a runny nose), which is the key symptom. Ask parents if the child also demonstrates other common symptoms: sore throat, dysphagia, mild cough, hoarseness, and a low- grade fever. Ask if any members of the household have had a cold or upper respiratory infection. Bacterial infections have an abrupt onset without rhinorrhea. Generally parents will describe fever, weakness, sore throat, dysphagia, nausea, abdominal discomfort, and vomiting.

PHYSICAL EXAMINATION. Children with viral and bacterial infections will have symptoms that reflect the infecting organism. (See Table 53.)

TABLE 53 | **Symptoms of Tonsillitis Based on Causative Agent**

MICROORGANISM	TONSIL APPEARANCE	OTHER FINDINGS
Epstein-Barr virus	Exudate on tonsils, petechiae on soft palate	Diffuse adenopathy

Adenovirus	Exudate on tonsils	Cervical adenopathy
Enterovirus	Vesicles and sores on tonsils	Vomiting, diarrhea, rhinorrhea
Herpesvirus	Tonsil ulcers	Diffuse adenopathy
Bacteria	Red tonsils and uvula, exudates on tonsils	Anterior cervical adenopathy, rash

PSYCHOSOCIAL. The parents and child will be apprehensive. Assess the parents' ability to cope with the acute situation and intervene as appropriate. Note that many children are treated at home rather than in the hospital; your teaching plan may need to consider home rather than hospital management.

DIAGNOSTIC HIGHLIGHTS

General Comments: Diagnostic testing involves identifying the causative organism, determining oxygenation status, and ruling out masses as a cause of obstruction.

Test	Normal Result	Abnormality with Condition	Explanation
Throat culture	Negative for bacteria	Positive for bacteria	To differentiate between viral and bacterial infections (particularly viral from GABHS)

Other Tests: Complete blood count, heterophil antibody test to rule out mononucleosis

PRIMARY NURSING DIAGNOSIS

Pain related to inflammation and infection of the throat and tonsils

OUTCOMES. Comfort level; Pain control behavior; Pain level; Symptom control behavior; Symptom severity; Well-being

INTERVENTIONS. Analgesic administration; Coping enhancement; Oral health restoration; Presence; Positioning, Touch

☐ PLANNING AND IMPLEMENTATION

Collaborative

The aim of treatment for a viral infection is to provide supportive care. Usually fever and sore throat pain can be managed with over the counter analgesia.

Antibiotic therapy is appropriate for bacterial infections. Allow the child to get rest and provide adequate fluid intake. If the child continues to have symptoms in spite of appropriate antibiotic therapy after cultures and sensitivities, the child may represent a "treatment failure" and may need a different antibiotic. If a relapse occurs, a second course of antibiotics may be needed and a family member may be a carrier.

Chronic tonsillitis occurs in children with recurrent throat infections (seven in the past year or five in each of the past 2 years). Tonsillectomy and adenoidectomy decrease the incidence of these problems during childhood, although those who do not have surgery also have a decreased incidence of infection as well. Current recommendations generally encourage physicians to avoid surgery in most cases. The decision to remove the tonsils relates directly to hypertrophy, obstruction, and chronic infection.

PHARMACOLOGIC HIGHLIGHTS

Medication or Drug Class	Dosage	Description	Rationale
Nonnarcotic analgesia and antipyretics	Varies with drug	Acetaminophen, ibuprofen	Relieve aches and pains and reduce fever
Antibiotics	Varies with drug	Benzathine pencillin G, potassium penicillin V, erythromycin, first-generation cephalosporin, amoxicillin-clavulanate, dicloxacillin	Halt replication of the bacteria in bacterial infections

Independent

Children should be allowed to rest as much as possible to conserve their energy; organize your interventions to limit disturbances. Provide age-appropriate activities. Crying increases the child's difficulty in breathing and should be limited if possible by comfort measures and the presence of the parents; parents should be allowed to hold and comfort the child as much as possible. Provide adequate hydration to liquefy secretions and to replace fluid loss from increased sensible loss (increased respirations and fever). The child might also have a decreased fluid intake during the illness. Apply lubricant or ointment around the child's mouth and lips to decrease the irritation from secretions and mouth breathing.

DOCUMENTATION GUIDELINES

- Pain and sore throat: Type, location, severity, response to medications
- Respiratory status: Rate, quality, depth, ease, breath sounds
- Child's response to illness, feeding, rest, and activity
- Parent's emotional response

DISCHARGE AND HOME HEALTHCARE GUIDELINES

Most children will be managed at home. Caregivers need to understand the rationale for all medications. If the child has a viral infection, explain to the parents why an antibiotic is not indicated. If the child has a bacterial infection, make sure the parents understand the importance of taking the entire prescription and to report new onset of symptoms if they occur. Reassure parents that frequent infections are not unusual, but if the infections persist they need to report them to a health care provider.

Toxoplasmosis

DRG Category: 423
Mean LOS: 7.1 days
Description: MEDICAL: Other Infectious Diseases Diagnosis

Toxoplasmosis, a parasitic infection that is widespread throughout the world, is caused by *Toxoplasma gondii,* an intracellular protozoan parasite. Toxoplasmosis refers to clinical or pathologic manifestations of a *T. gondii* infection, which occurs when the protozoa invade the cells but does not usually cause symptoms in patients with normal immune systems. Conversion of chronic *T. gondii* infection into active toxoplasmosis occurs primarily in severely immunocompromised hosts.

There are three forms of *T. gondii:* oocysts, tissue cysts, and tachyzoites. Oocysts are oval-shaped and have been found only in cats; this form of *T. gondii* can live outside of the host in a warm, moist environment for over a year and therefore may play a major role in transmission of *T. gondii* infection. Tissue cysts can contain up to 3000 organisms. Tachyzoites are the crescent-shaped invasive form of *T. gondii:* this form is seen in acute *T. gondii* infection and invades all mammalian cells except nonnucleated red blood cells.

CAUSES

The prevalence of a *T. gondii* infection seems to be highest in warm, humid climates at lower altitudes. The two major routes of *T. gondii* transmission to humans are oral and congenital. Tissue cysts are found in a large percentage of meat used for human consumption, especially in lamb and pork. Vegetables and other food products contain a large number of oocysts. Exposure to cat feces also plays a major role in transmission of infection.

GENDER AND LIFE SPAN CONSIDERATIONS

Toxoplasmosis can occur in at-risk patients of any age and both genders. Neonatal toxoplasmosis may occur as a result of acute maternal infection during pregnancy. Congenitally infected infants who are symptomatic at birth have an 80% chance of developing severe disabilities, such as mental retardation, epilepsy, spasticity, palsies, and impaired vision. Adults with multiple organ involvement are at high risk for mortality or permanent organ failure. Death is almost a certainty in patients with AIDS with toxoplasmic encephalitis; mean survival for treated patients is 7 to 16 months.

☐ ASSESSMENT

HISTORY. Signs of low-grade *T. gondii* infection include fever of unknown origin, asymptomatic lymph node enlargement, malaise, headache, sore throat, rash, and muscle soreness. Question mothers of infants about potential exposure or manifestations of *T. gondii* infection that may have occurred during pregnancy. Explore the presence of conditions that cause an immunocompromised state, such as AIDS, organ transplantation accompanied by immunosuppressive therapy, cancer chemotherapy, and hematologic malignancies.

If you suspect congenital toxoplasmosis, which is transmitted in utero from mother to fetus, ask the parent(s) to describe any central nervous system (CNS) or ocular dysfunction. Clinical manifestations may include microcephalus, hydrocephalus, strabismus, cataracts, glaucoma, deafness, or psychomotor retardation. The term acquired toxoplasmosis is reserved for immunocompetent individuals who have developed clinical manifestations in response to acute infection. Ask about enlarged lymph nodes; a rash; or problems with the heart, liver, lungs, brain, or muscles. Because ocular toxoplasmosis occurs in both acquired and congenital toxoplasmosis, ask the patient if he or she has experienced blurred vision, pain, photophobia, and visual impairment.

PHYSICAL EXAMINATION. In infants with congenital toxoplasmosis, you may note changes in the shape of the head denoting microcephalus or hydrocephalus, or you may find jaundice and a rash. When you palpate the infant's abdomen, you may feel an enlarged liver or spleen. There may also be signs of myocarditis, pneumonitis, and lymphadenopathy (enlarged lymph nodes).

In patients with acquired toxoplasmosis, the most common finding is asymptomatic lymphadenopathy, either confined to a single area or region or generalized. Usually the lymph nodes normalize within a few weeks, but the problem may recur over several months. You may be able to see a rash and palpate an enlarged liver and spleen. Some patients also have signs of dysfunction of the organ or tissue involved (heart, liver, lungs, brain, or muscle).

Ocular toxoplasmosis, which occurs in both acquired and congenital toxoplasmosis, typically causes a lesion on the retina that leads to inflammation of the retina and choroid (retinochoroiditis). An ophthalmoscopic examination reveals patches of yellow-white cotton-like lesions on the retina. The area around the lesions is usually engorged with blood. Acute toxoplasmosis in the immunocompromised patient is associated with a unique set of clinical manifestations. The patient may have any of the signs and symptoms seen in patients with normal immunity but is more likely to have serious organ involvement as well. More than 50% of these patients have manifestations of CNS involvement, such as altered consciousness, motor impairment, neurological deficits, and seizures. These findings indicate a large *T. gondii* brain abscess, or meningoencephalitis. Severe myocarditis and pneumonitis also are common findings in immunocompromised patients with toxoplasmosis. During the management of patients with acute neurologic changes, assess the neurologic status at least hourly. Include assessments of orientation, memory, and thought processes; the strength and motion of the extremities; sensory alterations; pupil response; and the patient's speech, emotional response, and behaviors.

PSYCHOSOCIAL. Death is a real possibility in toxoplasmosis patients with immune dysfunction. Fear of death and feelings of despair or hopelessness may evolve; patients and families should be encouraged to discuss these openly. Mothers of infants with congenital toxoplasmosis may experience feelings of guilt because of their transmission of the infection.

DIAGNOSTIC HIGHLIGHTS

Test	Normal Result	Abnormality with Condition	Explanation
Enzyme-linked immunosorbent assay (ELISA)	Negative	Pinpoints specific toxoplasmosis antibody (IgG and IgM)	Identify presence of antibodies to parasitic infection

Serum toxo plasmosis antibody assay	IgM titer < 1:64	IgM titer increased	Identify presence of antibodies to parasitic infection
Immuno-fluorescence	IgG titer < 1:1024	IgG titer increased	
Tests for hemagglutination (Sabin-Feldman dye test)	Indirect hemagglutination < 1:4	Indirect hemagglutination: past infection > 1:4 and < 1:256; recent infection > 1:256	
Tissue and fluid cultures; fluids are cerebrospinal fluid, lymph node aspirate	Negative for *T. gondii*	Positive for *T. gondii*	Identify presence of parasitic infection

Other Tests: Serum globulin (increased), complete blood count, lymph node biopsy, brain biopsy, computed tomography (CT) scan of the brain, magnetic resonance imaging (MRI) of the brain

PRIMARY NURSING DIAGNOSIS

Sensory-perceptual alterations (visual and auditory) related to inflammation and damage of ocular nerves and tissues and the CNS

OUTCOMES. Cognitive ability; Distorted thought process; Cognitive orientation; Neurological status; Rest; Anxiety control

INTERVENTIONS. Cognitive stimulation; Surveillance: Safety; Sleep enhancement; Reality orientation; Fall prevention; Neurologic monitoring; Medication management; Communication enhancement: Hearing deficit; Emotional support

☐ PLANNING AND IMPLEMENTATION

Collaborative

The challenge in treating toxoplasmosis is that *T. gondii* protozoa are resistant to many antimicrobial agents, and they typically invade tissue that is difficult for many drugs to reach. The ideal duration for pharmacotherapy has not been established. Acute acquired toxoplasmosis should be treated only if the patient is extremely symptomatic or severely immunodeficient. The duration of treatment for immunosuppressed patients depends largely on the duration of the immuno-compromised state. Patients with permanent immunocompromised states, such as AIDS patients, usually need prophylactic antitoxoplasmosis therapy for the rest of their lives. Because the immune-inflammatory response is thought to be responsible for the pathologic processes in ocular toxoplasmosis, glucocorticoid steroids may be ordered in some situations. Steroids have been shown to decrease retinochoroiditis and improve vision but cause further decreased immune function in the immunocompromised patient.

PHARMACOLOGIC HIGHLIGHTS

General Comments: The combination of pyrimethamine and sulfadiazine is the treatment of choice for AIDS patients with toxoplasmic encephalitis. Trimethoprim-sulfamethoxazole is effective in preventing toxoplasmosis encephalitis in AIDS patients who are at risk.

Medication or Drug Class	Dosage	Description	Rationale
Pyrimethamine	75 mg po loading dose; then 25 mg po qd	Antiprotozoal	Eradicates the protozoa; given together with sulfonamides; folinic acid may be given to reduce bone marrow toxicity
Sulfonamides	Varies with drug	Sulfadiazine, sulfamethoxazole	Eradicates the protozoa; given together with sulfonamides; folinic acid may be given to reduce bone marrow toxicity
Azithromycin	500 mg loading po; then 250 mg po qd	Antibiotic	Eradicates the tissue cyst form of *T. gondii;* used with atovaquone
Atovaquone	750 mg with food bid po	Antiprotozoal	Eradicates the tissue cyst form of *T. gondii;* used with azithromycin

Independent

Patients with toxoplasmosis do not require any special precautions to prevent the spread of infection; universal precautions are sufficient. There is no evidence that toxoplasmosis can be spread from person to person. The sensory and neurologic deficits that are associated with acute disseminated toxoplasmosis present the greatest nursing challenges. Provide adequate safety measures as indicated: side rails up, bed location where the patient can be closely monitored, padding of side rails, and assistance with ambulation or activities of daily living. Reorient the patient as often as necessary, provide opportunities for undisturbed sleep, and ensure appropriate amounts of sensory stimulation. Have the patient talk about topics of interest and importance to him or her, such as hobbies, family, occupation, or current sports and news. Encourage family members to bring pictures and other items from home that help the patient focus on pleasant memories. Institute active or passive range-of-motion exercises to maintain neuromuscular function and prevent contractures. Initiate seizure precautions for patients with suspected brain involvement.

Because toxoplasmosis can affect virtually every tissue in the body, the patient often experiences pain and nausea. Choice of analgesic and antinausea agents requires close consultation with the physician, taking into consideration actual or potential neurologic alterations. Nonpharmacologic pain relief methods can be instituted to augment the effect of analgesics, such as relaxation techniques, frequent repositioning to level of comfort, soothing music, and massage therapy. If vision is impaired, the patient needs assistance with activities of daily living. Everyone entering the room should identify themselves by name. Referral to social work services or community organizations for the blind may be indicated if ocular involvement is severe.

DOCUMENTATION GUIDELINES

- Neurologic status: Memory, orientation, thought processes, behaviors, emotions, motor function, sensory function, speech, pupil response
- Patient's or family members' mood and emotional response to the diagnosis of toxoplasmosis and the associated poor prognosis
- Physical responses: Status of lymph nodes (enlargement, any changes from baseline), presence of fever, response to interventions
- Abnormal assessment findings from organs commonly affected by acute toxoplasmosis: Heart, liver, lungs, eyes (visual disturbances)

DISCHARGE AND HOME HEALTHCARE GUIDELINES

Teach the patient and family about the medications. Pyrimethamine can cause folic acid deficiency. The patient should report bleeding, bruising, visual changes, and feelings of fatigue. Folic acid supplements may be recommended by the physician. Pyrimethamine should be taken just before or after meals to minimize gastric distress. Sulfadiazine can cause decreased white blood cell count, cause fever and rash, and lead to crystals in the urine; it should be taken with a full glass of water, and daily fluid intake should be at least 2000 mL. Sulfadiazine causes increased sensitivity to the sun; the patient should avoid prolonged sun exposure and wear sunscreen when going outdoors.

If the patient has AIDS or some other condition that causes a permanent immunocompromised state, emphasize that these drugs probably are needed throughout the patient's lifetime.

If the patient has neuromuscular defects, teach family members the exercises needed to maintain muscle strength and joint range of motion. If the patient has neurological involvement and is not on antiseizure medications, teach the patient and significant others how to recognize a seizure and what to do if it occurs. Discuss the long-term prognosis for acquired toxoplasmosis; assist the patient and family in drawing up an appropriate plan of action.

Tuberculosis

DRG Category: 079
Mean LOS: 8.3 days
Description: MEDICAL: Respiratory Infections and Inflammations, Age > 17 with CC

Tuberculosis (TB) is an infectious disease caused by *Mycobacterium tuberculosis,* an aerobic acid-fast bacillus. Although it is most frequently a pulmonary disease, more than 15% of patients experience extrapulmonary TB that can infect the meninges, kidneys, bones, or other tissues. Pulmonary TB can range from a small infection of bronchopneumonia to diffuse intense inflammation, necrosis, pleural effusion, and extensive fibrosis.

Although TB was thought to be preventable and treatable, the number of cases since 1986 has increased. In 1990 more than 25,000 cases were reported, which is a 10% increase from the previous year. A high infection rate in patients with the human immunodeficiency virus (HIV) and in patients exposed to others hospitalized with TB and a new strain of the disease that is resistant to traditional drugs such as isoniazid (INH) and rifampin, has made TB more prevalent today.

CAUSES

TB is transmitted by respiratory droplets through sneezing or coughing by an infected person. Most infected persons have had a sustained exposure to the active agent, rather than a single one. The *M. tuberculosis* bacilli are inspired into the respiratory tract and usually lodge in the lower part of the upper lobe or the upper part of the lower lobe. The TB bacilli need high levels of oxygen to survive. When they reach the lungs, they multiply rapidly.

Mycobacteria that are not destroyed lie dormant until there is a decrease in the host's resistance. Of individuals who inhale mycobacteria 5% develop clinical TB at that time, 95% have been infected and have no clinical symptoms but enter a latent phase and are at risk to develop TB later.

GENDER AND LIFE SPAN CONSIDERATIONS

TB can affect both genders at any age but is most common in the elderly population and in those who are immunosuppressed.

☐ ASSESSMENT

HISTORY. Ask patients about a previous history of TB or Hodgkin's disease, diabetes mellitus, leukemia, gastrectomy, silicosis (a disease resulting from inhalation of quartz dust), and immunosuppressive disorders. A history of corticosteroid or immunosuppressive drug therapy can also increase the likelihood of TB infection. Other risk factors include a history of multiple sexual partners and abuse of drugs or alcohol. Determine if the patient has had recent contact with a newly diagnosed TB patient or has resided in any type of long-term facility. Take an occupational history as well to determine if the patient is a healthcare worker and therefore at risk.

Ask the patient to describe any symptoms. The patient often reports generalized weakness and fatigue, activity intolerance, and shortness of breath on exertion. Anorexia and weight loss occur because of altered taste and indigestion. The patient may also describe difficulty sleeping, chills or night sweats (or both), and either a productive or nonproductive cough.

PHYSICAL EXAMINATION. The patient looks acutely ill on inspection, with muscle wasting, poor muscle tone, loss of subcutaneous fat, poor skin turgor, and dry flaky skin. When you auscultate the chest, you may hear a rapid heart rate, rapid and difficult breathing, and stridor. Diminished or absent breath sounds may be present bilaterally or unilaterally from pleural effusion or pneumothorax. Tubular breath sounds or whispered pectoriloquies may be heard over large lesions, as may crackles over the apex of the lungs during quick inspiration after a short cough.

The sputum appears green, purulent, yellowish mucoid, or blood tinged. The patient may have pain, stiffness, and guarding of the affected painful area. Accumulation of secretions can decrease oxygenation of vital organs and tissues. You may note cyanosis or a change in skin color, mucous membranes, or nail beds and changes in mental status, such as distraction, restlessness, inattention, or marked irritability.

PSYCHOSOCIAL. Patients dependent on alcohol or drugs, those who are economically disadvantaged, and those who live in crowded conditions are at risk. The living environment needs careful assessment. Ask about living conditions, including the number of people in the household. Patients may have recent or longstanding stress factors, financial concerns, and feelings of helplessness or hopelessness. They may experience feelings of alienation or rejection because they have a communicable disease and are in isolation. They may have changes in patterns of responsibility, physical strength, and capacity to resume roles because of TB. Assess the patient's ability to cope. Assess the degree of anxiety or depression about the illness, the change in health status, and the change in roles.

DIAGNOSTIC HIGHLIGHTS

Test	Normal Result	Abnormality with Condition	Explanation
Fluorochrome or acid fast sputum	Negative	Positive; 3 samples are often obtained	Mycobacterium tuberculosis is a bacterium that resists decolarizing chemicals after staining
Chest x ray	Normal lung structures	Identification of active TB or old lesions	Radiographic assessment of the lungs

Other Tests: Mantoux test, histology or tissue analysis, needle biopsy

PRIMARY NURSING DIAGNOSIS

Risk of infection related to tissue inflammation and infiltration caused by the TB bacilli

OUTCOMES. Immune status; Knowledge: Infection control; Risk control; Risk detection; Treatment behavior: Illness or injury

INTERVENTIONS. Infection control; Medication management; Environmental management; Surveillance; Nutrition management; Teaching: Disease process

☐ PLANNING AND IMPLEMENTATION

Collaborative

Because TB typically becomes resistant to any single-drug therapy, patients generally receive a combination of drugs. The most common combination of drugs prescribed in the United States is isoniazid (INH), rifampin, pyrazinamide, and either ethambutol or streptomycin. Some experts recommend up to 9 months of drug therapy, whereas patients with drug-resistant strains of TB may require as much as 18 months of treatment. Intravenous fluids, total parenteral nutrition, and food supplements may be needed for those with nutritional compromise. Humidity and oxygen are administered to correct hypoxia and to decrease the thickness of secretions. Emergency intubation and mechanical ventilation may be needed in extreme cases.

Teach the patient how and when to take medication and to complete the course of drug therapy because one of the primary reasons for the development of drug-resistant TB strains is the failure of patients to complete medication regimens. If you suspect that the patient may not adhere to the medication regimen, a home health referral is important after the patient is discharged.

PHARMACOLOGIC HIGHLIGHTS

Medication or Drug Class	Dosage	Description	Rationale
Isoniazid (INH)	5 mg/kg per day po once a day	Antitubercular	Inhibits synthesis of bacterial cell wall and hinders cell division
Rifapin	10 mg/kg per day po once a day	Antitubercular	Interferes with RNA synthesis; able to kill slower growing organisms that reside in granuloma in lungs or other organs
Pyrazinamide	15–30 mg/kg po once a day	Antitubercular	Bacteriostatic or bacteriocidal
Ethambutol	15 mg/kg po once a day	Antitubercular	Interferes with cell metabolism and multiplication by inhibiting bacterial metabolites
Streptomycin	1000 mg IM or IV daily	Aminoglycoside antibiotic	Transported across cell membrane, binds to receptor proteins, and prevents cell reproduction

Other Drugs: Second-line medications include cycloserine, ethionamide, and capreomycin sulfate. Mucolytics are used to thin secretions and facilitate expectoration. Increased fluid intake decreases secretions. Bronchodilators increase the lumen size of the bronchial tree and decrease resistance to airflow. Corticosteroids are used in extreme cases when inflammation causes life-threatening hypoxia.

Independent

Nursing priorities are to maintain and achieve adequate ventilation and oxygenation; prevent the spread of infection; support behaviors to maintain health; promote effective coping strategies; and provide information about the disease process, prognosis, and treatment needs.

Use respiratory isolation precautions (masks only) for all patients with pulmonary TB who require hospitalization. Whenever they leave their rooms or receive treatment from the hospital staff, patients should wear masks to help prevent transmission of TB. The masks need to fit tightly and not gap. Teach the patient to cover the mouth when coughing and to dispose of all tissues. For patients with excessive secretions or those who are unable to cooperate with respiratory isolation, gowns and gloves may be necessary for hospital staff. The nurse should always remember to wash the hands before and after patient contact.

Position the patient in a Fowler or semi-Fowler position, and assist with coughing and deep-breathing exercises. Demonstrate and encourage pursed-lip breathing on expiration, especially for patients with fibrosis or parenchymal destruction. Promote bed rest and activity restrictions, and assist with self-care activities as needed.

Teach the patient and family how to use proper protection methods to prevent infection or reinfection. In the case of treatment at home, the family has probably already been exposed to the patient before diagnosis, so wearing masks is not necessary. Advise the family members that they need regular TB testing to ensure that they have not contracted TB. Teach the patient about complications of TB, such as recurrence and hemorrhage, and the need for proper nutrition.

DOCUMENTATION GUIDELINES

- Physical changes: Breath sounds, quality and quantity of sputum, vital signs, mental status
- Tolerance to activity and level of fatigue
- Complications and changes in oxygen exchange or airway clearance

DISCHARGE AND HOME HEALTHCARE GUIDELINES

Advise the patient to quit smoking, avoid excess alcohol intake, maintain adequate nutrition, and avoid exposure to crowds and others with upper respiratory infections. Teach appropriate preventive measures. Be sure the patient understands all medications, including the dosage, route, action, and adverse effects. Instruct the patient to abstain from alcohol while on INH, and refer for eye examination after starting, then every month while taking, ethambutol. Teach the patient to recognize symptoms such as fever, difficulty breathing, hearing loss, and chest pain that should be reported to healthcare personnel. Discuss the patient's living condition and the number of people in the household. Give the patient a list of referrals if he or she is homeless or economically at risk.

Ulcerative Colitis

DRG Category: 188
Mean LOS: 4.9 days
Description: MEDICAL: Other Digestive System Diagnoses, Age > 17 with CC
DRG Category: 148
Mean LOS: 12.2 days
Description: SURGICAL: Major Small and Large Bowel Procedures with CC

Ulcerative colitis is a chronic, inflammatory disease of the colon. Usually the disease begins in the rectum and sigmoid colon and gradually spreads up the colon in a continuous distribution pattern. The inflammatory process involves the mucosa and submucosa of the colon. Gradually, multiple ulcerations and abscesses form at the inflamed areas. As the disease progresses, the colon mucosa becomes edematous and thickened with scar tissue formation, which results in altered absorptive capabilities of the colon. The severity of the disease ranges from a mild form that is localized in specific areas of the bowel to a critical syndrome with life-threatening complications. The most common complications are nutritional deficiencies; others include sepsis, fistulae, abscesses, and hemorrhage. For unknown reasons, patients with ulcerative colitis also have a high risk for arthritis and cancer.

CAUSES

Research has not established a specific cause for ulcerative colitis. Several theories are being pursued, including infectious agents such as a virus or bacteria, an autoimmune reaction, environmental factors such as geographic location, and genetic factors. Current thinking holds that psychosomatic factors such as emotional stress are a result of the chronic and severe symptoms of ulcerative colitis rather than a cause, as was once thought.

GENDER AND LIFE SPAN CONSIDERATIONS

The peak incidence occurs during the early adolescent and young adult years, often between the ages of 10 and 15 years, thus hampering normal growth and development. Girls are infected more often than boys. There is also evidence of a second peak incidence among those 55 to 60 years of age. Two factors that may predispose the elderly population to ulcerative colitis are their increased vulnerability to infection and their susceptibility to inadequate blood supply to the bowel.

☐ ASSESSMENT

HISTORY. A patient with acute ulcerative colitis typically reports numerous episodes of bloody diarrhea. The number of stools may range from 4 to 5 to 10 to 25 per day during severe episodes, often causing sleepless nights. In addition, the patient may report abdominal pain and cramping that is relieved with defecation. Other symptoms may include fatigue, diminished appetite with weight loss, low-grade fever, and nausea with vomiting.

PHYSICAL EXAMINATION. Because ulcerative colitis is a chronic disease, which may cause periods of anorexia, diarrhea, and intestinal malabsorption, inspect for the signs of malnutrition and dehydration: dry mucous membranes, poor skin turgor, muscle weakness, and lethargy.

Palpate the patient's abdomen for tenderness and pain. Typically, pain is noted in the left lower quadrant of the abdomen. Auscultate the patient's abdomen; bowel sounds are often hyperactive during the inflammatory process.

Assess the patient for infection. During the acute inflammatory process, monitor the patient's vital signs every 4 hours or more frequently if the patient's condition is unstable. Watch for temperature elevations and rapid heart rate, which often indicate an infectious process.

PSYCHOSOCIAL. The effects of chronic illness and debilitating symptoms often result in psychological problems for the patient with this disease. Note the patient's current psychological status because depression is common for those with ulcerative colitis. Because emotional stress increases bowel activity and plays a critical role in the exacerbation of the disease, it is also important to assess the patient's current life stressors. In addition, determine the need for instruction on stress reduction techniques.

DIAGNOSTIC HIGHLIGHTS

Test	Normal Result	Abnormality with Condition	Explanation
Colonoscopy; sigmoidoscopy	Normal bowel mucosa	Edematous, friable bowel mucosa with loss of vascular pattern and frequent ulcerations	Direct visualization of mucosa by endoscopic exam
Barium enema with air contrast	Normal bowel	Identifies distribution and depth of disease involvement	Fluoroscopic and radiographic exam of large intestine after rectal instillation of barium sulfate to identify structural abnormalities

Other Tests: Complete blood count, plasma electrolytes, stool culture and sensitivity, biopsy

PRIMARY NURSING DIAGNOSIS

Alteration in nutrition: Less than body requirements related to anorexia, diarrhea, and decreased absorption of the intestines

OUTCOMES. Nutritional status: Food and fluid intake; Nutrient intake; Biochemical measures; Body mass; Energy; Bowel elimination; Endurance

INTERVENTIONS. Nutrition management; Nutrition therapy; Nutritional counseling and monitoring; Fluid/electrolyte management; Medication management; Enteral tube feeding; Intravenous therapy; Total parenteral nutrition administration

☐ PLANNING AND IMPLEMENTATION

Collaborative

MEDICAL. Drug therapy is the typical method used to control the inflammatory process. Sulfasalazine is the primary drug used to achieve remission. After remission is established, dosages are generally reduced, and patients continue on this agent for at least 1 year after an acute attack.

To maintain fluid and electrolyte balance during acute attacks, IV fluids are generally prescribed, and electrolytes may be added to the solutions as needed. Blood transfusions may also be prescribed if the patient is anemic because of numerous bloody diarrheal stools. To achieve bowel "rest," the patient is usually given nothing by mouth. During this time, nutritional deficits may be managed through the use of total parenteral nutrition with vitamin supplements. Helping patients maintain an adequate nutritional status, fluid balance, and electrolyte balance is a priority nursing measure. Record intake and output accurately every shift. Note the number of stools and stool characteristics.

Gradually, as the acute attack subsides and inflammation clears, the patient is placed on a low-residue, low-fat, high-calorie, high-protein, lactose-free diet.

SURGICAL. Surgery may be performed when patients fail to respond to conservative treatment, if acute episodes are frequent, or when a complication such as bleeding or perforation occurs. The standard surgical procedure, when performed, is a total proctocolectomy with ileostomy. This procedure is considered a permanent cure for ulcerative colitis. To prepare the patient for surgery, administer bowel preparations such as laxatives and enemas.

PHARMACOLOGIC HIGHLIGHTS

Medication or Drug Class	Dosage	Description	Rationale
Mesalamine (5-aminosalicylic acid; 5-ASA)) (Asacol, Pentasa)	800–1600 mg po tid	Anti-inflammatory agent, 5-ASA	5-ASA preparations like mesalamine have become treatment of choice and can be used in people who cannot tolerate sulfasalazine
Other anti-inflammatories	Varies with drug: sulfasalazine, 0.5–1.0 g po qid; prednisone, 10–40 mg po tid; methyl-prednisolone, 20–40 mg IV q 12 hours; hydrocortisone, 100 mg IV q 6 hours	Sulfasalazine (Azulfidine); corticosteroids	Slow the inflammatory process; sulfasalazine is not used in treatment of disease confined to small intestine; glucocorticoids such as prednisone are used in acute exacerbations—agents are administered until clinical symptoms subside, at which time steroidal

			agents are tapered off
Immunosuppressive agents	Varies with drug	Azathioprine (Imuran) 6-mercaptopurine	Decrease inflammation and symptoms if steroids fail; decrease steroid requirements

Other Drugs: Anti-diarrheal agents to alleviate symptoms of abdominal cramping and diarrhea in patients with mild symptoms or post-resection diarrhea. Metronidazole (Flagyl) is effective in colon disease; it treats infections with fistulae and perianal skin breakdown and is beneficial in patients who have not responded to other agents. Some patients suffering with severe abdominal pain may require narcotic analgesics such as meperidine (Demerol). Also, patients who develop deficiencies because of problems of malabsorption may require vitamin B_{12} injections monthly or iron replacement therapy. Other nutritional supplements include calcium, magnesium, folate, and other micronutrients.

Independent

Promote patient physical and emotional comfort. Encourage the patient to assume the position of comfort. Instruct in distraction techniques as needed. Promote mental comfort by encouraging the patient to share thoughts and feelings and provide supportive, empathetic care. Discuss measures to decrease life stressors. Teach the patient about the disease process and the typical treatment regimen. Areas to include in the teaching plan include the signs of disease complications, the importance of rest and stress reduction, and any dietary adjustments.

If the patient requires surgery, several nursing interventions are important in the preoperative phase. First, conduct preoperative teaching sessions on deep-breathing techniques and leg exercises. Also, discuss the operative procedure and the typical postoperative course. When appropriate, discuss with the patient information on stoma placement and stoma care. After surgery, ensure a healthy respiratory status for the patient by encouraging the patient to cough and deep-breathe every 1 to 2 hours. Manage patient pain and discomfort with prescribed analgesics and proper positioning techniques. Monitor for adequate wound healing by checking the color and approximation of the wound and noting any wound drainage or odor. Note the stoma size and color during every shift and immediately report any duskiness noted at the stoma site. Note the condition of the skin around the stoma; protect the skin with appropriate barrier products because ileostomy drainage is extremely caustic to skin tissues. Finally, encourage the patient's participation in ostomy care. Assess whether a community resource person from the United Ostomy Association is needed to offer the patient additional support.

DOCUMENTATION GUIDELINES

- Evidence of stability of vital signs, hydration status, bowel sounds, and electrolytes
- Response to medications, tolerance of foods, and ability to eat and select a well-balanced diet
- Location, intensity, frequency of pain, and factors that relieve pain

- Number of diarrheal episodes and stool characteristics
- Description of discharge and follow-up instructions given to the patient
- Presence of complications: Hemorrhage, bowel strictures, bowel perforation, infection
- Patient participation in care of stoma and periostomal skin

DISCHARGE AND HOME HEALTHCARE GUIDELINES

The patient must understand all prescribed medications, including actions, side effects, dosages, and routes. Emphasize ways to prevent future episodes of inflammation (rest, relaxation, stress reduction, well-balanced diet). Review the symptoms of inflammation. Teach the patient to seek medical attention if such symptoms occur. Be certain the patient understands symptoms of complications, such as hemorrhage, bowel strictures and perforation, and infection. The patient must know to seek medical attention if these complications should occur. Ensure that the patient understands the importance of close follow-up because of the high incidence of colon and rectal cancer in patients with ulcerative colitis.

Urinary Tract Infection

DRG Category: 320
Mean LOS: 5.9 days
Description: MEDICAL: Kidney and Urinary Tract Infections, Age >17 with CC

Urinary tract infections (UTIs) are common and usually occur because of the entry of bacteria into the urinary tract at the urethra. Approximately 25% of women have a UTI sometime during their lifetime, and acute UTIs account for approximately 7 million healthcare visits per year for young women. About 20% of women who develop a UTI experience recurrences. Women are more prone to UTIs than men because of natural anatomic variations. The female urethra is only about 1 to 2 inches in length, whereas the male urethra is 7 to 8 inches long. The female urethra is also closer to the anus than is the male urethra, increasing women's risk for fecal contamination. The motion during sexual intercourse also increases the female's risk for infection.

Urinary reflux is one reason that bacteria spread in the urinary tract. Vesicourethral reflux occurs when pressure increases in the bladder from coughing or sneezing and pushes urine into the urethra. When pressure returns to normal, the urine moves back into the bladder, taking with it bacteria from the urethra. In vesicoureteral reflux, urine flows backward from the bladder into one or both of the ureters, carrying bacteria from the bladder to the ureters and widening the infection. If they are left untreated, UTIs can lead to chronic infections, pyelonephritis, and even systemic sepsis and septic shock. If infection reaches the kidneys, permanent renal damage can occur, which leads to acute and chronic renal failure.

CAUSES

The pathogen that accounts for about 90% of UTIs is *Escherichia coli*. Other organisms that are commonly found in the gastrointestinal tract and may contaminate the genitourinary tract include *Enterobacter, Pseudomonas,* group B beta-hemolytic streptococci, *Proteus mirabilis, Klebsiella* species, and *Serratia*. Two growing causes of UTI in the United States are *Staphylococcus saprophyticus* and *Candida albicans.*

Predisposing factors are urethral damage from childbirth, catheterization, or surgery; decreased frequency of urination; other medical conditions such as diabetes mellitus; and, in women, frequent sexual activity and some forms of contraceptives (poorly fitting diaphragms, use of spermicides).

GENDER AND LIFE SPAN CONSIDERATIONS

UTIs are uncommon in children. Once women become sexually active, the incidence of UTI increases dramatically. UTIs are common during pregnancy and are caused by the hormonal changes and urinary stasis that results from ureteral dilation. Men secrete prostatic fluid that serves as an antibacterial defense. As men age past 50, however, the prostate gland enlarges, which increases the risk for urinary retention and infection. As women age, vaginal flora and lubrication change; decreased lubrication increases the risk of urethral irritation in women during intercourse. By age 70, prevalence is similar for men and women.

☐ ASSESSMENT

HISTORY. The patient with a UTI has a variety of symptoms that range from mild to severe. The typical complaint is of one or more of the following: frequency, burning, urgency, nocturia, blood or pus in the urine, and suprapubic fullness. If the infection has progressed to the kidney, there may be flank pain (referred to as costovertebral tenderness) and low-grade fever.

Question the patient about risk factors, including recent catheterization of the urinary tract, pregnancy or recent childbirth, neurologic problems, volume depletion, frequent sexual activity, and presence of a sexually transmitted infection (STI). Ask the patient to describe current sexual and birth control practices because poorly fitting diaphragms, the use of spermicides, and certain sexual practices such as anal intercourse place the patient at risk for UTI.

PHYSICAL EXAMINATION. Physical examination is often unremarkable in the patient with a UTI, although some patients have costovertebral angle tenderness in cases of pyelonephritis. On occasion, the patient has fever, chills, and signs of a systemic infection. Inspect the urine to determine its color, clarity, odor, and character. Surveillance for STIs is recommended as part of the examination.

PSYCHOSOCIAL. UTIs rarely result in disruption of the patient's normal activities. The infection generally is acute and responds rapidly to antibiotic therapy. The general guidelines to increase fluid intake and concomitant frequent urination may be problematic for some patients in restrictive work environments. The accompanying discomfort may result in temporary restriction of sexual activity, especially if an STD is diagnosed.

DIAGNOSTIC HIGHLIGHTS

General Comments: UTIs are very easy to diagnose; follow-up testing demonstrates the effectiveness of treatment.

Test	Normal Result	Abnormality with Condition	Explanation
Urine dip	Negative	Positive (purple shade)	Presence of leukocyte esterase

			indicates UTI; 90% accurate in detecting WBCs in the urine
Urine culture and sensitivity	< 10,000 bacteria/ mL	> 10,000 bacteria/ mL or > 100 in acutely symptomatic patients	Identifies causative organism; determines appropriate antibiotic
Urinalysis	WBC 0–4; RBC ≤ 2; nitrites-none; pH 4.6–8.0; no crystals; clear, aromatic	Increased WBC, RBC, pH, nitrites, crystals; cloudy, odor present	Presence of bacteria in the urine is indicated by several changes noted in a urinalysis

Other Tests: Voiding cystoureterography may detect congenital anomalies that predispose patients to recurrent UTI.

PRIMARY NURSING DIAGNOSIS

Altered urinary elimination related to infection

OUTCOMES. Urinary elimination; Knowledge: Medication, Symptom control

INTERVENTIONS. Medication prescribing; Urinary elimination management

☐ PLANNING AND IMPLEMENTATION

Collaborative

An acid-ash diet may be encouraged. A diet of meats, eggs, cheese, prunes, cranberries, plums, and whole grains can increase the acidity of the urine. Foods not allowed on this diet include carbonated beverages, anything containing baking soda or powder, fruits other than those previously stated, all vegetables except corn and lentil, and milk and milk products. Because the action of some UTI medications is diminished by acidic urine (nitrofurantoin), review all prescriptions before instructing patients to follow this diet.

UTIs are treated with antibiotics specific to the invading organism. Usually a 7- to 10-day course of antibiotics is prescribed, but shortened and large single-dose regimens are currently under investigation. Most elderly patients need a full 7- to 10-day treatment, although caution is used in their management because of the possibility of diminished renal capacity. Women being treated with antibiotics may contract a vaginal yeast infection during therapy; review the signs and symptoms (cheesy discharge and perineal itching and swelling), and encourage the woman to purchase an over-the-counter antifungal or to contact her primary healthcare provider if treatment is indicated.

PHARMACOLOGIC HIGHLIGHTS

Medication or Drug Class	Dosage	Description	Rationale
Cephalexin monohydrate (Keflex)	250 mg–1 g po q 6 h	Antibiotic, first-generation cephalosporin	Bacteriocidal

Sulfisoxazole (Gantrisin)	Initially 2–4 g po, then 1–2 g qid for 10–14 days	Anti-infective, Sulfonamide	Bacteriocidal
Co-trimoxazole (Bactrim, Septra)	160 mg q 12 h for 7–14 days	Anti-infective, Sulfonamide	Bacteriocidal
Nitrofurantoin (Macrodantin)	50–100mg po qid for 10–14 days	Urinary antiseptic	Bacteriocidal; concentrates in the urine and kidneys to kill bacteria
Phenazopyridine (Pyridium)	100–200 mg po tid until pain subsides	Urinary analgesic	Relieves pain

Independent

Encourage patients with infections to increase fluid intake to promote frequent urination, which minimizes stasis and mechanically flushes the lower urinary tract. Strategies to limit recurrence include increasing vitamin C intake, drinking cranberry juice, wiping from front to back after a bowel movement (women), regular emptying of the bladder, avoiding tub and bubble baths, wearing cotton underwear, and avoiding tight clothing such as jeans. These strategies have been beneficial for some patients, although there is no research that supports the efficacy of such practices.

Encourage the patient to take over the counter analgesics unless contraindicated for mild discomfort but to continue to take all antibiotics until the full course of treatment has been completed. If the patient experiences perineal discomfort, sitz baths or warm compresses to the perineum may increase comfort.

DOCUMENTATION GUIDELINES

- Physical response: Pain, burning on urination, urinary frequency; vital signs; nocturia; color and odor of urine; patient history that may place the patient at risk
- Location, duration, frequency, and severity of pain; response to medications
- Absence of complications such as pyelonephritis

DISCHARGE AND HOME HEALTHCARE GUIDELINES

Treatment of a UTI occurs in the outpatient setting. Teach the patient an understanding of the proposed therapy, including the medication name, dosage, route, and side effects. Explain the signs and symptoms of complications such as pyelonephritis and the need for follow-up before leaving the setting.

Explain the importance of completing the entire course of antibiotics even if symptoms decrease or disappear. If the patient experiences gastrointestinal discomfort, encourage the patient to continue taking the medications but to take them with a meal or milk unless contraindicated. Warn the patient that drugs with phenazopyridine turn the urine orange.

Urinary Tract Trauma

Renal and Ureter Trauma
DRG Category: 331
Mean LOS: 5.1 days
Description: MEDICAL: Other Kidney and Urinary Tract Diagnoses, Age > 17 with CC
DRG Category: 304
Mean LOS: 8.7 days
Description: SURGICAL: Kidney, Ureter, and Major Bladder Procedures for Non-Neoplasms with CC

Bladder Trauma
DRG Category: 331
Mean LOS: 5.1 days
Description: MEDICAL: Other Kidney and Urinary Tract Diagnoses, Age > 17 with CC
DRG Category: 308
Mean LOS: 5.4 days
Description: SURGICAL: Minor Bladder Procedures with CC

Urinary tract trauma includes injury to the kidneys, ureters, urinary bladder, and urethra. Although these injuries occur in fewer than 3% of patients admitted to the hospital for trauma, the damage can threaten life and lead to life-long impaired genitourinary (GU) dysfunction. Most urinary tract trauma affects the kidneys (80%). Blunt renal injury is classified as minor, major, and critical trauma. Minor renal trauma occurs when organ tissue is bruised or when superficial lacerations of the renal cortex occur without disruption of the renal capsule. Major renal trauma occurs with major lacerations that extend through the renal cortex, medulla, and renal capsule. Critical renal trauma occurs when the kidney is shattered or when the renal pedicle (stem that contains the renal artery and vein) is injured.

Bladder injury occurs in 8% of GU trauma, usually involves bladder rupture, and can be either intraperitoneal or extraperitoneal. Intraperitoneal bladder rupture occurs with blunt trauma to the lower portion of the abdomen, usually when the bladder is full. The bladder ruptures at the dome (the point of least resistance), and blood and urine collect in the peritoneal cavity. Extraperitoneal bladder rupture usually occurs in conjunction with a pelvic fracture when a sharp bone fragment perforates the bladder at its base. Blood and urine then collect in the space surrounding the bladder base. Urethral injury occurs in 8% of cases of GU tract trauma, whereas ureteral trauma is rare.

Although renal trauma is unusual, it is associated with a 6% to 12% mortality rate, possibly because of the kidneys' high vascularity. Complications of urinary tract trauma include hemorrhage and exsanguination, hypovolemic shock, peritonitis, septic shock, acute renal failure, urinary incontinence, pyelonephritis, and impotence.

CAUSES

Urinary tract trauma is caused by either blunt or penetrating trauma. Motor vehicle crashes are the most common cause of blunt trauma. Other causes include falls, assaults, occupational (crush) injuries, and sports injuries. The energy of the trauma is dissipated throughout the cavity, which frequently causes rupturing of the bladder or kidney or tearing of the urethra. Penetrating trauma to the urinary tract is frequently the result of a gunshot wound or a stabbing injury. The degree and severity of the damage from a gunshot wound depend on the velocity and trajectory of the bullet. The result is usually localized tissue damage and potential hemorrhage in the highly vascular kidney or the distended bladder.

GENDER AND LIFE SPAN CONSIDERATIONS

Trauma is the leading cause of death and disability in individuals from the ages of 1 to 44 years. Although trauma to the urinary tract is relatively rare, young men remain the largest group of individuals admitted to the hospital for the management of multiple trauma. Because urinary tract trauma is not usually an isolated injury, young men are the population at highest risk for this type of trauma.

❏ ASSESSMENT

HISTORY. Obtain a relevant history from the patient or significant others. If the patient is critically injured, note that the history, assessment, and early management merge in the primary survey. Determine as much as you can from witnesses to the trauma or the life squad.

If the patient's condition is stable enough to warrant a separate history, ask questions about allergies, current medications, pre-existing medical conditions, and factors surrounding the injury. Note that patients with pre-existing renal diseases such as polycystic kidney disease and pyelonephritis are at higher risk for renal injury than are those with normal kidneys. If you suspect a lower urinary tract injury, ask if the patient has experienced suprapubic tenderness, the inability to void spontaneously, or bloody urine. If you suspect kidney injury, ask the patient if he or she is experiencing flank pain, pain at the costovertebral angle, back tenderness, colicky pain with the passage of blood clots, or bloody urine. Note that if the patient has a positive blood alcohol level, the patient may not be sensitive to painful stimuli even if he or she has experienced a severe injury.

PHYSICAL EXAMINATION. If the patient is stable enough for you to perform a complete head-to-toe assessment, determine if there are any physical signs indicating kidney injury. Note, however, that physical signs may be masked because of the protection of the kidneys by the abdominal organs, muscles of the back, and bony structures. Inspect the area over the 11th and 12th ribs and flank area for obvious hematomas, wounds, contusions, or abrasions. Inspect the lower back and flank for Grey-Turner's sign, or bruising because of a retroperitoneal hemorrhage. Note any abdominal distension. To identify lower urinary tract trauma, inspect the urinary meatus to determine the presence of blood. Note any bruising, edema, or discoloration of the genitalia or tracking of urine into the tissues of the thigh or abdominal wall.

Auscultate for the presence of bowel sounds in all quadrants. Although the absence of bowel sounds does not indicate urinary tract injury for certain, increase your index of suspicion when bowel sounds are absent because abdominal injury often accompanies urinary tract injury. If you note a bruit near the renal artery, notify the physician at once because an intimal tear may have occurred in the renal artery. Percussion may reveal excessive dullness in the lower abdomen or flank. When you palpate the flank, upper abdomen, lumbar vertebrae, and lower rib cage, the patient may experience pain. Other signs of urinary tract trauma include crepitus and a flank mass. Bladder rupture leads to severe pain in the hypogastrium on palpation or swelling from extravasation of blood and urine in the suprapubic area. Signs of peritoneal irritation (abdominal rigidity, rebound tenderness, and voluntary guarding) may also be present because of extravasation of blood or urine into the peritoneal cavity.

PSYCHOSOCIAL. The patient with urinary tract trauma requires immediate emotional support because of the nature of any sudden traumatic injury. The sudden alteration in comfort, potential body image changes, and possible impaired functioning of vital organ systems often can be overwhelming and can lead to maladaptive coping. Determine the patient's and family's level of anxiety and their ability to cope with stressors.

DIAGNOSTIC HIGHLIGHTS

Test	Normal Result	Abnormality with Condition	Explanation
Retrograde urethrogram	Normal structure of urethra	Transected or torn urethra	Urethra irrigated with contrast media to determine location and extent of injury
Kidney-ureter-bladder x ray and radionuclide imaging	Normal structures of urinary tract	Location and extent of injury	Contrast media and radiography used to identify areas of injury
Renal and lower urinary tract computed tomography	Normal structures of urinary tract	Location and extent of injury	Identifies radio graphic slices with or without contrast

Other Tests: Complete blood count, urinalysis, renal ultrasound, excretory urogram (intravenous pyelogram)

PRIMARY NURSING DIAGNOSIS

Pain (acute) related to tissue damage and swelling

OUTCOMES. Comfort level; Pain control behavior; Pain: Disruptive effects; Pain level

INTERVENTIONS. Pain management; Analgesic administration; Positioning; Teaching: Prescribed activity/exercise; Teaching: Procedure/treatment; Teaching: Prescribed medication

☐ PLANNING AND IMPLEMENTATION

Collaborative

MEDICAL. The initial care of the patient with urinary tract trauma involves airway, breathing, and circulation. Measures to ensure adequate oxygenation and tissue perfusion include establishing an effective airway and supplemental oxygen source, supporting breathing, controlling the source of blood loss, and replacing intravascular volume. As with any traumatic injury, treatment and stabilization of any life-threatening injuries are completed immediately.

SURGICAL. Patients with renal trauma may need urinary diversion with a nephrostomy tube, depending on the location of injury or in situations when pancreatic and duodenal injury coexist with renal trauma. If the patient is unable to void, the trauma team considers urinary catheterization. If the patient has blood at the urinary meatus or if there is any resistance to catheter insertion, a retrograde urethrogram is performed to evaluate the integrity of the urethra. In the presence of urethral injury, an improperly placed catheter can cause long-term complications, such as incontinence, impotence, and urethral strictures. A suprapubic catheter may be used to manage severe urethral lacerations and urethral disruption. Extraperitoneal bladder rupture is usually managed without surgery but, rather, with urethral or suprapubic catheter drainage. Ongoing monitoring of the amount, character, and color of the patient's urine is important during treatment and recovery. In a patient without renal impairment, the physician usually maintains the urine output at 1 mL/kg per hour. Note any blood clots in the urine, and report an obstructed urinary drainage system immediately.

The indications for surgery depend on the severity of injury. Patients with major renal trauma who are hemodynamically unstable and patients with critical trauma need surgical exploration. Patients with urethral disruption and severe lacerations may have surgery delayed for several weeks or even months, or the surgeon may choose to perform surgical reconstruction immediately. Patients with an intraperitoneal bladder rupture have the bladder surgically repaired, with the extravasated blood and urine evacuated during the procedure. Usually suprapubic drainage is used during recovery. Laceration of the ureter is immediately repaired surgically or the patient risks loss of a kidney.

Minor renal trauma is usually managed with bed rest and observation. Minor extraperitoneal bladder tears can be managed with insertion of a Foley catheter for drainage, along with antibiotic therapy. Many urethral tears can be managed with insertion of a suprapubic catheter and delayed surgical repair or plasty, provided that bleeding can be controlled. The patient needs to be monitored for complications throughout the hospital stay, such as infection (dysuria, low back pain, suprapubic pain, and foul or cloudy urine), impaired wound healing (seepage of urine from repair sites, flank or abdominal mass from pockets of urine, and crepitus from urine seepage into tissues), and impaired renal function (nausea, irritability, edema, hypertension, oliguria, and anuria).

PHARMACOLOGIC HIGHLIGHTS

Medication or Drug Class	Dosage	Description	Rationale
Phenazopyridine hydrochloride (Pyridium)	200 mg tid po	Urinary analgesic	Decreases burning, urgency, and frequency

Other Drugs: Antibiotics for patients with penetrating injuries or suspected contamination of wounds, analgesia, antispasmodics may be needed for bladder spasm.

Independent

The most important priority is to ensure the maintenance of an adequate airway, oxygen supply, breathing patterns, and circulatory status. If the patient is stable, apply ice to the perineal area, the scrotum, or the penis to help relieve pain and swelling. Use care to avoid cold burns from ice packs that are in contact with the skin for a prolonged period of time. For severe scrotal swelling, some experts recommend a scrotal support to reduce pain. Use either a commercially available support or a handmade support using an elastic wrap as a sling.

Patients may or may not have residual problems with urinary incontinence or sexual functioning. Loss of urinary continence leads to self-esteem and body image disturbances. Provide the patient with information on reconstructive techniques and methods to manage incontinence. Listen to the patient, and offer support and understanding. Patients often view injury to the urinary tract system as a threat to their sexuality. Reassure patients who are not at risk for sexual dysfunction that their sexuality is not impaired. Sexual concerns should not be ignored during the acute phase of recovery. Be alert to questions about sexuality, which may be phrased in terms that are familiar in the patient's culture. Answer questions honestly, and listen to the patient's questions and responses carefully to understand the full meaning.

Note that the inability to function sexually is an enormous loss to patients of both sexes. It may occur with posterior urethral injury in men when nerve damage occurs in the area. Urinary tract injury in men is often associated with injury to the penis and testes as well. Sexual dysfunction may also occur in women if the ovaries, uterus, vagina, or external genitalia are damaged along with urinary tract structures or the pelvis. Provide specific answers to the patient's questions, such as alternative techniques to intercourse (oral sex, use of a vibrator, massage, or masturbation). Give the patient information about the feasibility and safety of resuming sexual activity, and include the partner in all discussions.

Emotional support of the patient and family is also a key intervention. Patients and their families are often frightened and anxious. If the patient is awake as you implement strategies to manage the airway, breathing, and circulation, provide a running explanation of the procedures to reassure the patient. Explain to the family the treatment alternatives, and keep them updated as to the patient's response to therapy.

DOCUMENTATION GUIDELINES

- Urinary tract assessment: Urinary drainage system (patency, color of urine, presence of bloody urine or clots, amount of urine, appearance of catheter insertion site); fluid balance (intake and output, patency of intravenous catheters, speed of fluid resuscitation); wound healing (wound drainage, extravasation of urine from wound, tracts of urine extending beneath the skin)
- Assessment of level of anxiety, degree of understanding, adjustment, family or partner's response, and coping skills
- Concern over sexual dysfunction, content of conversations, and content taught

DISCHARGE AND HOME HEALTHCARE GUIDELINES

Provide a complete explanation of all emergency treatments, and answer the patient's and family's questions. Explain the possibility of complications to recovery, such as poor wound healing, infection, and anemia. As needed, provide information about any follow-up laboratory procedures that might be required after discharge from the hospital. Provide the dates and times that the patient is to receive follow-up care with the primary healthcare provider or the trauma clinic. Give the patient a phone number to call with questions or concerns. Provide information on how to manage urinary drainage systems if the patient is discharged with them in place. Demonstrate catheter care, emptying the bag, and the need for frequent hand washing. Explain when the patient can resume sexual activity. If the patient has sexual dysfunction, provide the patient with information about alternatives to intercourse; refer the patient to a support group if he or she is interested.

Uterine Cancer

DRG Category: 366
Mean LOS: 5.9
Description: MEDICAL: Malignancy, Female Reproductive System with CC
DRG Category: 354
Mean LOS: 5.9
Description: SURGICAL: Uterine, Adnexa Procedure for Nonovarian, Adnexal Malignancy with CC

Uterine cancer most commonly occurs in the endometrium, the mucous membrane that lines the inner surface of the uterus. Endometrial cancer, specifically adenocarcinoma (involving the glands) accounts for more than 90% of the diagnosed cases of uterine cancer. There has been an increase noted in the number of women with endometrial cancer, partly owing to women living longer and more accurate reporting. Endometrial cancer is the fourth most common cause of cancer in women, ranking behind breast, colorectal, and lung cancer. It is the most common neoplasm of the pelvic region and reproductive system of the female, and it occurs in 1 in 100 women in the United States. Other uterine tumors include adenocarcinoma with squamous metaplasia (previously referred to as adenoacanthoma), endometrial stromal sarcomas, and leiomyosarcomas.

Endometrial cancer can infiltrate the myometrium, thus resulting in an increased thickness of the uterine wall, and it can eventually infiltrate the serosa and move into the pelvic cavity and lymph nodes. It also can spread by direct extension along the endometrium into the cervical canal; pass through the fallopian tubes to the ovaries, broad ligaments, and peritoneal cavity; or move via the bloodstream and lymphatics to other areas of the body. It is a slow-growing cancer, taking 5 or more years to develop from hyperplasia to adenocarcinoma. Endometrial cancer is very responsive to treatment, provided it is detected early. Prognosis depends on the stage, uterine signs, and lymph node involvement.

The overall mortality rate of uterine cancer is 3000 women per year. There are 1.9 deaths per 100,000 noted.

CAUSES

The exact cause of uterine cancer is not known, although it is considered to be dependent on endogenous hormonal levels for growth. Risk factors associated with the development of uterine adenocarcinoma include age, genetic and familial factors, early menarche, late menopause (after 52 years), hypertension, nulliparity, unopposed estrogen hormonal replacement therapy, pelvic irradiation, polycystic ovarian disease, obesity, and diabetes mellitus.

GENDER AND LIFE SPAN CONSIDERATIONS

Uterine cancer occurs primarily in women who are postmenopausal, with a peak incidence occurring between 58 and 60 years of age. Only 10% of the cases occur in women under 50 years of age, and it is rare in women under 30.

◻ ASSESSMENT

HISTORY. Establish a history of risk factors. The major initial symptom of endometrial cancer is abnormal, painless vaginal bleeding, either menometrorrhagia or postmenopausal. A mucoid and watery discharge may be noted several weeks to months before this bleeding. Postmenopausal women may report bleeding that began a year or more after menses stopped. A mucosanguineous, odorous vaginal discharge is noted if metastases to the vagina has occurred. Younger women may have spotting and prolonged, heavy menses.

Inquire about pain, fever, and bowel/bladder dysfunction, which are late symptoms of uterine cancer. Assess the use and effectiveness of any analgesics for pain relief and also the location, onset, duration, and intensity of the pain.

PHYSICAL EXAMINATION. Conduct a general physical and gynecologic examination. The woman should be directed to not douche or bathe for 24 hours before the examination so that tissue is not washed away. Inspection of any bleeding or vaginal discharge is imperative. The characteristics and amount of bleeding should be noted. Upon palpation, the uterus will feel enlarged and may reveal masses.

PSYCHOSOCIAL. Women with the disease often exhibit depression and anger. Therefore a thorough assessment of the woman's perception of the disease process and her coping mechanisms is required. The family should also be included in the assessment to examine the extent of support they can provide for the patient. Family anger, ineffective coping, and role disturbances may interfere with family functioning and need careful monitoring.

DIAGNOSTIC HIGHLIGHTS

General Comments: Several diagnostic tests may be done to confirm the diagnosis and to check for metastases.

Test	Normal Result	Abnormality with Condition	Explanation
Fractional dilatation and curettage of the uterus	No malignant cells found	Malignant cells found	Obtain specimen of endometrium and endocervix for pathological examination
Papanicolaou examination (Pap	No abnormality or atypical cells noted	High-class/grade cytologic results	Initial screening; can detect 50% of

| smear) | cases of uterine cancer |

Other Tests: Sonography, sonohysterography, hysteroscopy, chest x ray, intravenous pyelography

PRIMARY NURSING DIAGNOSIS

Knowledge deficit related to treatment procedures, treatment regimens, medications, and disease process

OUTCOMES. Knowledge: Treatment procedures; Knowledge: Treatment regimens; Knowledge: Medications; Knowledge: Disease process

INTERVENTIONS. Teaching: Disease process; Teaching: Prescribed medication; Teaching: Procedure/treatment; Teaching: Preoperative

☐ PLANNING AND IMPLEMENTATION

Collaborative

SURGICAL. If uterine cancer is detected early, the treatment of choice is surgery. A total abdominal hysterectomy (TAH) with removal of the fallopian tubes and ovaries, bilateral salping-oophrectomy (BSO) is generally performed. Common complications after a hysterectomy are hemorrhage, infection, and thromboembolitic disease. Premenopausal women who have a BSO become sterile and experience menopause. Hormone replacement therapy may be warranted and is appropriate. In a total pelvic exenteration (evisceration or removal of the contents of a cavity), the surgeon removes all pelvic organs, including the bladder, rectum, and vagina. This procedure is performed if the disease is contained in the areas without metastasis. If the lymph nodes are involved, this procedure is usually not curative.

RADIATION. Radiation therapy may also be given in combination with the surgery (before or after) or it may be used alone, depending on the staging of the disease, whether the tumor is not well differentiated, or whether the carcinoma is extensive. Radiation may be the treatment of choice for the very elderly woman with an advanced stage of endometrial cancer for whom surgery would not improve quality of life. With radiation, the possible complications are hemorrhage, cystitis, urethral stricture, rectal ulceration, or proctitis.

Intracavity radiation or external radiation therapy may be given 6 weeks before surgery to limit recurrence or to improve the chance of survival. An internal radiation device may be implanted during surgery (preloaded) or at the patient's bedside (afterloaded). If the device is inserted during the surgical procedure, the postoperative management needs to include radiation precautions. Provide a private room for the patient and follow the key principle to protect against radiation exposure: distance, time, and shielding. The greater the distance from the radiation source, the less exposure to ionizing rays. The less time spent providing care, the less radiation exposure. The source of radiation determines if lead shields are necessary to provide care. All healthcare workers coming in contact with a "hot" patient (a patient with an internal radiation implant) need to monitor their exposure with a monitoring device such as a film badge. Nursing care of patients with radiation implants is detailed in Table 54.

TABLE 54 | **Nursing Care of Patients with Radiation Implants**

STRATEGY	RATIONALE
Place patient in a private room	A private room limits radiation exposure for guests, other patients, and staff
Identify the difference between a sealed and unsealed source	
Sealed sources of internal radiation are completely enclosed by nonradioactive material. The radioactive isotope cannot circulate through the patient's body and cannot contaminate urine, blood, feces, or other secretions. *Unsealed sources,* colloid suspensions that come in direct contact with body tissues, are administered intravenously or orally or instilled into a body cavity. The isotope may be excreted into any body fluid	
Dispose of all wastes according to hospital protocol if the patient has an unsealed source	Decrease the risk of radiation exposure to those other than the patient
Teach the patient to flush the toilet several times after voiding if appropriate	
If the patient has a discharge, discard the linen according to hospital standards	
Plan care so as to spend a minimal amount of time in the room	Limits radiation exposure
Do not spend more than 30 min in the room per shift. Strategies to maximize time:	
Fix food trays outside the room	
Work as quickly as possible	
Take a prepared bed roll into the room for linen changes	
Do not care for more than one patient per shift with radiation implants	
Reassign pregnant staff to other assignments	
Notify the patient that young children and pregnant family or friends should not visit until after the implant is removed	
Use distance between the nurse and patient during caregiving activities (*note:* social isolation may result):	Limits radiation exposure
If patient can be out of bed, have her sit as far as possible from the bed during linen changes	
Provide care standing at the patient's shoulder, where exposure is low; this technique also uses the patient's body as a shield	
Encourage the woman to limit body movements while the source is in place. Keep all personal items within easy reach to limit stretching or straining. Limit lower extremity exercises. Provide diversionary activity such as reading, television, radio, tapes	Decreases the risk of dislodging the implant
Wear a radiation monitoring device at all times when in the room	Records exposure
Mark the room with radiation safety signs	Limits the risk of accidental exposure
Keep long-handled forceps and a lead-lined container on the unit at all times	If the implant is accidentally dislodged, use the forceps to place it in the container and notify radiation safety and the physician immediately

Request that radiation safety monitor all unit procedures for compliance	Limits the risk of accidental exposure

PHARMACOLOGIC HIGHLIGHTS

Medication or Drug Class	Dosage	Description	Rationale
Doxorubicin; cisplantin; carboplatin	Given in combination	Antineoplastic	Response rate of 15%
Paclitaxel (Taxol)	Depends on patient tolerance and condition	Antineoplastic	Response rate of 35%; premedicate with corticosteroids, diphenhydramine, and H2 antagonists
Acetaminophen; NSAIDs; opiods; combination	Depends on the drug and patient condition and tolerance	Analgesics	Analgesics used are determined by the severity of pain

Experimental Therapy: The use of tamoxifen (Nolvadex) to treat advanced or recurrent endometrial cancer is being investigated.

Independent

The major emphasis is prevention, either primary by reduction of risk factors or secondary by early detection. Encourage women to seek regular medical check-ups, which should include gynecologic examination. Discuss risk factors associated with the development of endometrial cancer, particularly as they apply or do not apply to the particular woman. Encourage the older menopausal woman to continue with regular examinations. If the woman is bleeding heavily, monitor her closely for signs of dehydration and shock (dry mucous membranes, rapid and thready pulses, delayed capillary refill, restlessness, and mental status changes). Encourage her to drink liberal amounts of fluids, and have the equipment available for intravenous hydration if necessary. A balanced diet promotes wound healing and maintains good skin integrity.

Patients require careful instruction before radiation therapy or surgery. Explain the procedures carefully, and notify the patient what to expect after the procedure. For surgical candidates, teach coughing and deep-breathing exercises. Fit the patient with antiembolism stockings. If the patient is premenopausal, explain that removal of her ovaries induces menopause. Unless she undergoes a total pelvic exenteration, her vagina is intact and sexual intercourse remains possible. During external radiation therapy, the patient needs to know the expected side effects (diarrhea, skin irritation) and the importance of adequate rest and nutrition. Explain that she should not remove ink markings on the skin because they direct the location for radiation. If a preloaded radiation implant is used, the patient has a preoperative hospital stay that includes bowel preparation, douches, an indwelling urinary catheter, and diet restrictions the day before surgery.

If the woman has pain from either the surgical procedure or the disease process, teach her pain-relief techniques such as imagery and deep breathing.

Encourage her to express her anger and feelings without fear of being judged. Note that surgery and radiation may profoundly affect the patient's and partner's sexuality. Answer any questions honestly, provide information on alternatives to traditional sexual intercourse if appropriate, and encourage the couple to seek counseling if needed. If the woman's support systems and coping mechanisms are insufficient to meet her needs, help her find others. Provide a list of support groups that may be helpful.

DOCUMENTATION GUIDELINES

- Physiologic response: Amount and characteristics of any vaginal bleeding or discharge, vital signs, intake and output if appropriate, weight loss or gain, sleep patterns
- Emotional response: Signs of stress, ability to cope, degree of depression, relationship with partner and significant others
- Comfort: Location, onset, duration, and intensity of pain; effectiveness of analgesics and pain-reducing techniques

DISCHARGE AND HOME HEALTHCARE GUIDELINES

PREVENTION. Teach the need for regular gynecologic examinations, even though she had a hysterectomy. Teach the patient to report any abnormal vaginal bleeding to the healthcare provider. The woman who has had a TAH with BSO is at risk for developing osteoporosis. Recommend a daily intake of up to 1500 mg of calcium through diet and supplements. Recommend vitamin D supplements to enable the body to use the calcium. Stress the need for regular exercise, particularly weight-bearing exercise. Discuss the exercise schedule and type with the patient in light of her treatment and expected recovery time.

MEDICATIONS. Ensure that the patient understands the dosage, route, action, and side effects of any medication she is to take at home. Note that, to monitor her response, some of the medications require her to have routine laboratory tests following discharge from the hospital.

POSTOPERATIVE. Discuss any incisional care. Encourage the patient to notify the surgeon for any unexpected wound discharge, bleeding, poor healing, or odor. Teach the patient to avoid heavy lifting, sexual intercourse, and driving until the surgeon recommends resumption.

RADIATION. To decrease bulk, teach the patient to maintain a diet high in protein and carbohydrates and low in residue. If diarrhea remains a problem, instruct the patient to notify the physician or clinic because anti-diarrheal agents can be prescribed. Encourage the patient to limit her exposure to others with colds because radiation tends to decrease the ability to fight infections. To decrease skin irritation, encourage the patient to wear loose-fitting clothing and avoid using heating pads, rubbing alcohol, and irritating skin preparations.

FOLLOW-UP CARE. Teach the patient appropriate self-care for her specific treatment. Teach the patient to be able to identify where she can obtain assistance should postoperative or posttreatment complications occur. Make sure that the significant others are aware of the expectations of a normal convalescence and whom to call should concerns arise.

Vaginal Cancer

DRG Category: 366
Mean LOS: 5.9 days
Description: MEDICAL: Malignancy, Female Reproductive System with CC
DRG Category: 353
Mean LOS: 8.0 days
Description: SURGICAL: Pelvic Evisceration, Radical Hysterectomy, and Radical Vulvectomy

Vaginal cancer (VC) is a neoplastic disease of cells within the vaginal canal. Because primary cancer of the vagina is rare, VC is usually secondary as a result of metastasis from choriocarcinoma (cancer of the cervix or adjacent organs). VC often extends to the bladder and rectum, which makes treatment difficult.

VC is rare and accounts for only 1% of all gynecologic malignancies. It is most commonly located in the upper one-third of the posterior vagina. The vagina has a thin wall and extensive lymphatic drainage; the severity of the cancer, therefore, varies, depending on its location in relation to the lymphatic system and the thickness of the neoplastic involvement. Stage 0 VC is limited to epithelial tissue. Stage 1 VC is limited to the vaginal wall. Stage 2 VC involves the subvaginal tissue but not the pelvic wall. Stage 3 VC extends to the vaginal wall. Stage 4 VC extends beyond the pelvis or involves the bladder or rectum.

The overall survival rate for VC is 35%. Low survival rates are caused by the advanced stage of the disease at the time of diagnosis, difficulty in treatment resulting from the proximity of important structures, and the rarity of the disease that makes it difficult to determine the best treatment.

CAUSES

The cause of VC is not known, although ingestion of diethylstilbestrol (DES), a drug at one time given to women to limit spontaneous abortion, has been identified as one possible cause. Risk factors include a previous malignancy of the vagina, vulva, or cervix and advancing age. Women who have had cervical cancer previously should be examined on a regular basis to assess for vaginal lesions. Other risk factors include exposure to DES in utero, the improper use of pessaries (infrequent cleaning, infrequent examination to ensure proper fit), exposure to radiation therapy, trauma, exposure to chemical carcinogens found in some sprays and douches, and a history of human papillomavirus.

GENDER AND LIFE SPAN CONSIDERATIONS

VC occurs in menopausal and postmenopausal women, typically over 50 years of age. VC is rare in African-American and Jewish women.

☐ ASSESSMENT

HISTORY. A complete reproductive history of the patient and the patient's mother is important. Evaluate the patient for any risk factors. Ask if the patient's mother was taking DES when pregnant with the patient. Determine a thorough history of the patient's physical symptoms. One of the symptoms of VC is spontaneous vaginal bleeding after either intercourse or a pelvic examination. Vaginal discharge of a watery nature may also be present. Other symptoms include pain, urinary or rectal symptoms, pruritis, dyspareunia (pain during sexual intercourse), and groin masses.

Question the patient about any pain. Assess the use and effectiveness of any analgesics for pain. Document the location, onset, duration, and intensity of the pain. The patient may also describe urinary retention or urinary frequency if the lesion is near the bladder neck.

PHYSICAL EXAMINATION. Inspection of any bleeding or vaginal discharge, with particular attention to the characteristics and amount of bleeding, is imperative. Palpate the groin area to detect any masses. An internal pelvic examination may reveal an ulcerated vaginal lesion.

PSYCHOSOCIAL. A thorough assessment of each woman's perception of the disease process and her coping mechanisms is required. Changes in sexual patterns and body image present stressors to patients. The family of the patient should also be included in the assessment to examine the extent of support they can provide. Her partner may experience anxiety over the potential loss of his mate or fear about altered patterns of sexuality.

DIAGNOSTIC HIGHLIGHTS

General Comments: VC is often well advanced before diagnosis is made.

Test	Normal Results	Abnormality with Condition	Explanation
Lugol's solution applied to vaginal areas	Normal tissue stains	Areas that do not stain indicate suspect areas	Identifies areas to be biopsied
Colposcopy	Normal structures visualized	Lesions noted	Identifies areas that should be biopsied
Biopsy	Benign	Malignant	Confirms the diagnosis

Other Tests: Papanicolaou (Pap) test, barium enema

PRIMARY NURSING DIAGNOSIS

Altered sexuality patterns related to tissue damage, pain, and change in body structures

OUTCOMES. Sexual functioning; Anxiety control

INTERVENTIONS. Sexual counseling; Coping enhancement

☐ PLANNING AND IMPLEMENTATION

Collaborative

Treatment decisions are made based on the extent of the lesion and the age and condition of the patient. Patients with early-stage disease are treated so that the malignant area is removed but the vagina is preserved. Laser surgery is often used during stages 0 and 1. Patients in the later stages of disease are treated with surgery or radiation. The type of surgery or radiation depends on the extent of the disease, the patient's desire to preserve a functional vagina, and the location of the lesion. A radical hysterectomy may be done with removal of the upper vagina and dissection of the pelvic nodes. Most patients receive total external pelvic radiation therapy to shrink the tumor before surgery or before internal intracavity radiation. Internal radiation can be provided for 2 to 3 days with radium or cesium into the vagina. Current survival rates are similar for patients with VC whether they are treated with radiation or surgery.

Collaborative postoperative management includes analgesics for pain relief and careful assessment for signs of postoperative infection or poor wound healing. Before discharge, discuss with the physician the patient's timetable for resumption of physical and sexual activity, and be certain that the patient understands any limitations. For the management of patients with internal radiation, see **Uterine Cancer,** p. 973.

PHARMACOLOGIC HIGHLIGHTS

Medication or Drug Class	Dosage	Description	Rationale
Fluorouracil	Topical	Antineoplastic	Used topically in stages 0 and 1
Acetaminophen; NSAIDs; opiods; combinations of opiods and NSAIDs	Depends on the drug and patient condition and tolerance	Analgesics	Choice of drug depends on the severity of pain

Independent

The nursing management of patients with VC is challenging because of the interaction between the patient's physical and emotional needs. If the woman has pain from either the surgical procedure or the disease process, explore pain-control methods such as imagery and breathing techniques to manage discomfort. The woman may be depressed and angry. Allow the patient to express her anger and concerns without fear of being judged or discouraged. Provide a private place for her to discuss her concerns with the nurse or significant others. Provide a list of support groups for the patient and her partner.

Teach all female patients to be alert for signs of VC, particularly any unusual discharge or bleeding. Encourage all women over the age of 18 to seek annual check-ups, including gynecologic examination. Women should also be taught to perform a genital self-examination at the same time they perform breast self-examination. Teach them to use a mirror to inspect for any changes in the female anatomy and to report any lesions, sores, lumps, or the presence of a persistent itch.

DOCUMENTATION GUIDELINES

- Physical response: Amount and characteristics of any vaginal bleeding or discharge, vital signs, pain (location, onset, duration, intensity, response to interventions)

- Emotional response: Support system, ability to deal with terminal diagnosis, emotional well-being
- Patient's appetite, general appearance, and sleep patterns

DISCHARGE AND HOME HEALTHCARE GUIDELINES

TEACHING. Explain any procedures such as wound care or skin care that need to be continued at home. If the patient has had internal radiation therapy, teach her to use a stent or dilator to prevent vaginal stenosis; sexual intercourse also prevents vaginal stenosis. Teach the patient any limitations on the resumption of sexual activity or activity such as lifting or driving.

COMPLICATIONS. Teach the woman with VC to report any further vaginal bleeding or signs of infection (fever, poor wound healing, fatigue, drainage with an odor).

COPING. Discuss helpful coping patterns with the patient if this was not done previously. Encourage her to be open about her concerns and needs with her family and friends. Provide her with a referral to the American Cancer Society if appropriate.

PREVENTION. Teach teenage and preteenage girls who have been exposed to DES to have examinations at least once annually beginning at menarche regardless of the absence of symptoms of VC.

Vaginitis

DRG Category: 369
Mean LOS: 2.4 days
Description: MEDICAL: Menstrual and Other Female Reproductive System Disorders

Vaginitis is an inflammation of the vagina. Generally it occurs with a hormonal imbalance and an infection with a microorganism. Vaginitis is associated with changes in normal flora, alkaline pH, insertion of foreign bodies such as tampons and condoms, chemical irritations from douches and sprays, and medications such as antibiotics.

CAUSES

Trichomoniasis is a parasitic infection caused by *Trichomonas vaginalis*. Vulvovaginal candidiasis is caused by *Candida* species and commonly occurs when women are taking contraceptives or antibiotics. Repeated candida infections may be an indicator of unrecognized human immunodeficiency viral (HIV) infections. Bacterial vaginosis is characterized by an imbalance in the vaginal flora and occurs with an overgrowth of *Gardnerella* or *Mycoplasma* species. Cervicitis and urethritis are frequent manifestations of gonococcal or chlamydial infections and result from infection by *Neisseria gonorrhoeae* or *Chlamydia trachomatis*, but other agents may also cause vaginitis.

GENDER AND LIFE SPAN CONSIDERATIONS

Vaginitis usually occurs in women after puberty, particularly during pregnancy and when women are taking oral contraceptives. It is also more common in female diabetics than in the general population.

☐ ASSESSMENT

HISTORY. Elicit a history of the onset and description of symptoms, with particular attention to the nature and amount of vaginal discharge, which may be frothy, thick, or malodorous. Question the patient to determine if she is experiencing discomfort such as external inflammation and pain, and pruritus. Patients may describe exertional dysuria, dyspareunia, and vulvular inflammation. Determine the medications that the patient is taking, with particular attention to antibiotics, hormone replacement therapy, and contraceptives. Take a menstrual history. Ask about the patient's rest, sleep, nutrition, exercise, and hygiene practices. Ask the patient if she is pregnant or a diabetic, both of which place the patient at risk for vaginitis.

PHYSICAL EXAMINATION. Physical examination generally reveals some type of discharge, such as frothy, malodorous, purulent vaginal discharge (trichomoniasis); thick, cottage cheese–like discharge (candidiasis); or malodorous, thin, milk-white discharge (bacterial). The external and internal genitalia are often reddened, inflamed, and painful on examination. Women with candidiasis often have patches on vaginal walls and cervix and signs of inflammation. Women with trichomoniasis have a strawberry spot on the vaginal surface and cervix. Bacterial vaginitis often is asymptomatic with a normal vaginal mucosa. Palpate the patient's abdomen for tenderness or pain, which may indicate pelvic inflammatory disease.

PSYCHOSOCIAL. Psychosocial assessment should include evaluation of the patient's home situation and a sexual history. Ask the patient about the type of contraception she and her partner use. Provide a private environment to allow the patient to answer questions without being embarrassed.

DIAGNOSTIC HIGHLIGHTS

Test	Normal Result	Abnormality with Condition	Explanation
Saline wet mount (wet prep)	Negative for *Trichomonas* or *Candida*	Positive for *Trichomonas* or *Candida*	Identifies a sexually transmitted protozoan infection, *Trichomonas* or *Candida*
Potassium hydroxide preparation (KOH)	Negative for fungus	Positive for fungus	Identifies candidiasis (*Candida* species)
Vaginal pH	4.5–5.5	< 4–5 *Candida*; 6–7 *Trichomonas*; 5–6 bacterial vaginosis	Identified microorganization

PRIMARY NURSING DIAGNOSIS

Risk for infection related to invasion or proliferation of microorganisms

OUTCOMES. Immune status; Knowledge: Infection control; Risk control; Risk detection; Nutritional status; Risk control: Sexually transmitted disease; Tissue integrity: Skin and mucous membranes

INTERVENTIONS. Medication administration; Medication management; Perineal care; Surveillance; Bathing; Teaching: Sexuality; Teaching: Disease process

◻ PLANNING AND IMPLEMENTATION

Collaborative

Once vaginitis is diagnosed, the primary treatment is pharmacologic. Patients are told to stop using any douches and feminine hygiene sprays, to observe good nutrition, and to maintain healthy exercise patterns.

PHARMACOLOGIC HIGHLIGHTS

Medication or Drug Class	Dosage	Description	Rationale
Antifungals	Varies with drug; given as a vaginal cream or suppository	Miconazole nitrate, clotrimazone, nystatin, terconazol, tioconazole	Treat vaginal candidiasis
Metronidazole	Single 2 gram dose po for patient and sexual partner; 500 mg qid for 7 days for bacterial vaginosis	Antibacterial	Disrupts susceptible microorganisms and acts as a bactericidal drug; used to treat trichomoniasis or bacterial vaginosis

Other Drugs: Bacterial vaginosis may also be treated with ampicillin or tetracycline.

Independent

Encourage the patient to get adequate rest and nutrition. Encourage the patient to use appropriate hygiene techniques by wiping from front to back after urinating or defecating. Teach the patient to avoid wearing tight-fitting clothing (pantyhose, tight pants or jeans) and to wear cotton underwear rather than synthetics. Explain to patients that the risk of getting vaginal infections increases if one has sex with more than one person. Teach the patient to abstain from sexual intercourse until the infection is resolved. If the patient has *Trichomonas,* her partner needs treatment as well.

The pain and itching from vaginitis may be quite intense until the medication is effective. Some women find that by applying wet compresses and then using a hair dryer on a cool setting several times a day provides some relief of itching. Other women find that a cool sitz bath provides comfort. Be informed about which sexually transmitted diseases need to be reported to the local health department.

DOCUMENTATION GUIDELINES

- Discomfort: Character, location, duration, precipitating factors
- Discharge: Odor, amount, color
- Medication management: Understanding of drug therapy, response to medications
- Response to teaching: Safe sex behaviors, response to life style recommendations

DISCHARGE AND HOME HEALTHCARE GUIDELINES

Teach the patient how to maintain lifestyle changes with regard to rest, nutrition, and medication management. Make sure that the patient understands all aspects of the treatment regime with particular attention to taking the full course of medication therapy. Make sure the patient understands the necessity of any follow-up visits.

Varicose Veins

DRG Category: 130
Mean LOS: 5.8 days
Description: MEDICAL: Peripheral Vascular Disorders with CC
DRG Category: 119
Mean LOS: 3.3 days
Description: SURGICAL: Vein Ligation and Stripping

Varicose veins (varicosities) are abnormally dilated tortuous veins. They occur most often in the lower extremities but can appear anywhere in the body. Primary varicosities are caused by incompetent valves in the superficial saphenous veins, whereas secondary varicosities are the result of impaired blood flow in the deep veins. Primary varicosities tend to occur in both legs, whereas secondary varicosities usually occur in only one leg.

In a ladderlike fashion, perforator veins connect the deep vein and the superficial vein systems, promoting drainage of the lower extremities. Blood can be shunted from one system to the other in the event of either system's being compressed. Incompetence in one system can lead to varicosities. Varicose veins are considered a chronic disease.

CAUSES

Several factors cause increased venous pressure and venous stasis that result in dilation and stretching of the vessel wall. Increased venous pressure results from being erect, which shifts the full weight of the venous column of blood to the legs. Prolonged standing increases venous pressure because leg muscle use is less; therefore, blood return to the heart is decreased.

Heavy lifting, genetic factors, obesity, thrombophlebitis, pregnancy, trauma, abdominal tumors, congenital or acquired arteriovenous fistulae, and congenital venous malformations are among the causes of varicose veins. Chronic liver diseases such as cirrhosis can cause varicosities in the rectum, abdomen, and esophagus.

GENDER AND LIFE SPAN CONSIDERATIONS

Varicose veins affect an estimated one in five persons in the world. About 15% to 20% of all adults in the United States have varicose veins. Prevalence increases with age, peaking in the 50s and 60s and decreasing dramatically after age 70. Varicose veins are more common in women; in the population over age 30, four times as many women as men are affected.

☐ ASSESSMENT

HISTORY. Elicit a history of symptoms, with particular attention to pain and discomfort, changes in appearance of vessels and skin, and complaints of a sensation of fullness of the lower extremities. Ask the patient to describe the amount of time each day spent standing. Take an occupational history with particular attention to those jobs that require long hours of walking or standing. Question the patient about lifetime weight changes, such as changes during pregnancy and sustained periods of being overweight. Ask the patient if there is a personal or family history of heart disease, obesity, or varicose veins.

PHYSICAL EXAMINATION. The number, severity, and type of varicosities determine the symptoms experienced by the individual. With the patient standing, examine the legs from the groin to the foot in good lighting. Inspect the ankles, measure the calves for differences, and assess for edema. Time of examination is a factor because secondary varicosities are more symptomatic earlier in the day. Palpate both legs for dilated, bulbous, or corkscrew vessels. Patients may complain of heaviness, aching, edema, muscle cramps, increased fatigue of lower leg muscles, and itching. Severity of discomfort may be difficult to assess and is unrelated to the size of the varicosity.

PSYCHOSOCIAL. The patient with varicose veins usually has been dealing with a progressively worsening condition. Assess the patient for any problems with body image because of the changed appearance of skin surface that is caused by varicose veins. Question the patient to determine possible lifestyle adjustments to decrease symptoms. The patient may need job counseling or occupational retraining.

DIAGNOSTIC HIGHLIGHTS

General Comments: Incompetency of the deep and superficial veins can be diagnosed by several tests.

Test	Normal Result	Abnormality with Condition	Explanation
Tendelenburg's test	Veins fill from below in about 30 seconds after the tourniquet is in place and the client stands; no further blood fills the veins from above	Additional blood flows into the vein from above, indicating a valve is incompetent and has allowed a backflow of blood	Detects abnormal filling time and incompetent valves; veins normally fill from below; if the vein fills from above, the incompetent

	after the tourniquet is released		valve is allowing blood to flow backward
Doppler ultrasound flow studies	Normal doppler venous signal with spontaneous respirations; no evidence of occlusion	Reversal of blood flow is noted as a result of incompetent valves in varicose veins	Detects moving RBCs, thus demonstrating venous patency
Venous plethysmography (cuff pressure test)	Patent venous system without evidence of thrombosis or occlusion	Venous obstruction	Measures the volume of an extremity; rules out a deep vein thrombosis
Magnetic resonance imaging (MRI)	Normal blood flow without evidence of occlusion	Reversal of blood flow noted	Examines blood flow in extremities
Venography	No evidence of obstruction	Abnormal venous flow seen	X ray study designed to locate thrombi in lower extremities

PRIMARY NURSING DIAGNOSIS

Altered tissue perfusion (peripheral) related to increased venous pressure and obstruction

OUTCOMES. Tissue perfusion: Peripheral

INTERVENTIONS. Circulatory care; Positioning; Pain management

□ PLANNING AND IMPLEMENTATION

Collaborative

MEDICAL. Treatment for varicose veins is aimed at improving blood flow, reducing injury, and reducing venous pressure. Pharmacologic treatment is not indicated for varicose veins. To give support and promote venous return, physicians recommend wearing elastic stockings. If the varicosities are moderately severe, the physician may recommend anti-embolism stockings or elastic bandages or, in severe cases, custom-fitted heavyweight stockings with graduated pressure. When obesity is a factor, the patient is placed on a weight loss regimen. Experts also recommend that the patient stop smoking to prevent vasoconstriction of the vessels.

A nonsurgical treatment is the use of sclerotherapy for varicose and spider veins. Sclerotherapy is palliative, not curative, and is often done for cosmetic reasons after surgical intervention. A sclerosing agent, such as sodium tetradecyl sulfate (Sotradecol), hypertonic saline, aethoxysclerol, or hyperosmolar salt-sugar solution, is injected into the vein, followed by a compression bandage for a period of time.

SURGICAL. A surgical approach to varicose veins is vein ligation (tying off) or stripping (removal) of the incompetent veins. Removal of the vein is performed through multiple short incisions from the ankle to the groin. A compression dressing is applied after surgery and is maintained for 3 to 5 days. Patients are encouraged to walk immediately postoperatively. Elevate the foot of the bed 6 to 9 inches to keep the leg above the heart when the postoperative client is in bed.

Independent

Nursing interventions are aimed at educating the patient to decrease venous stasis, promote venous return, and prevent tissue injury. To prevent vein distension by compression of superficial veins, teach the patient to apply elastic support stockings before standing and to avoid long periods of standing. The patient should be encouraged to engage in an exercise program of walking to strengthen leg muscles. Teach the patient to avoid crossing the legs when sitting and to elevate the legs when sitting or lying down. The patient should be taught to observe the skin when removing stockings to check for signs of irritation, edema, decreased nerve sensation, and discoloration. Preventive measures are similar to those for a patient with thrombophlebitis.

For patients who have had sclerotherapy, teaching should focus on activity restrictions. The patient should learn to avoid heavy lifting. Teach the patient to wait 24 to 48 hours after the procedure before showering and to avoid tub baths. Teach the patient to wear supportive stockings as ordered. Prepare the patient by advising him or her to expect ecchymosis and some scarring, which will fade in several weeks. Caution the patient that some residual brown staining may remain at the injection sites. Inform the patient that the sclerotherapy may need to be repeated in other areas.

DOCUMENTATION GUIDELINES

- Physical assessment of both extremities: Presence of edema, pain, discoloration
- Reaction to the medications used for sclerotherapy and pain management
- Tolerance to activity and exercise

DISCHARGE AND HOME HEALTHCARE GUIDELINES

PREVENTION. To prevent worsening of varicosities, teach the patient to avoid prolonged standing in one place, to avoid sitting with the legs crossed, to elevate the legs frequently during the day, to wear support stockings as ordered, and to drink 2 to 3 L of fluid daily. The patient should wear shoes that fit comfortably and are not too tight.

MEDICATIONS. Teach the patient the purpose, dosage, route, and side effects of any medications ordered.

COMPLICATIONS. Teach the patient to recognize, and observe daily for, signs of thrombophlebitis, which include redness, local swelling, warmth, discoloration (not related to surgery area), and back pain on bending. Teach the patient which signs to report to the physician.

POSTOPERATIVE COMPLICATIONS. Teach the patient to report any signs of infection, such as redness at incision sites or injection sites, severe pain, purulent drainage, fever, or swelling.

Ventricular Dysrhythmias

DRG Category: 138
Mean LOS: 3.9 days
Description: MEDICAL: Cardiac Arrhythmia and Conduction Disorders with CC

A ventricular dysrhythmia is a disturbance in the normal rhythm of the electrical activity of the heart that arises in the ventricles. (See Figure 2.) Types of ventricular dysrhythmias include premature ventricular contractions (PVCs), which can have one focus or can arise from multiple foci; ventricular tachycardia (VT), which can lead to ventricular fibrillation or sudden cardiac death; ventricular fibrillation (VF), which results in death if not treated immediately; and ventricular asystole (cardiac standstill), in which no cardiac output occurs and full cardiopulmonary arrest results. (See Table 55.)

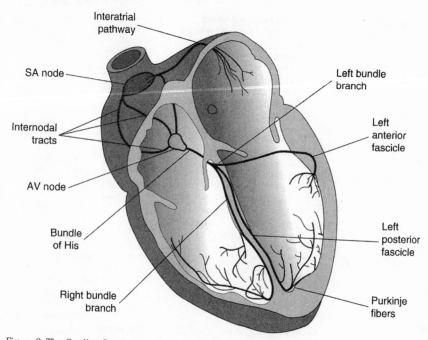

Figure 2 The Cardiac Conduction System
The heart's electrical impulses normally originate spontaneously in the sinoatrial node, located high in the right atrium. The impulse travels along special conduction pathways in the right and left atria and stimulates the atria to contract. The impulse then travels through the atrioventricular node, through the bundle of His, and then down the right bundle branch into the right ventricle and down the anterior fascicle and the left posterior fascicle. The impulse terminates in the Purkinje fibers in the ventricle, stimulating ventricular contraction.

TABLE 55 | **Types of Ventricular Dysrhythmias**

TYPE	DESCRIPTION	CAUSE
Premature ventricular contractions	Early ectopic beats that arise from the ventricles Atrial rate: Regular Ventricular rate: Irregular QRS complex; wide and distorted, usually longer than 0.14 seconds Occurrence: Singly, in pairs, or alternating with regular sinus beats	Heart failure Myocardial infarction Cardiac trauma Myocardial irritation from pacemaker or pulmonary artery catheter insertion Hypercapnia, hypokalemia, or hypocalcemia Medication toxicity (digitalis, aminophylline, tricyclic antidepressants, beta-adrenergic stimulants) Caffeine, tobacco, or alcohol use Physiologic and psychological stress
Ventricular tachycardia	Three or more premature ventricular contractions in a row dissociated from the atrial contraction P waves: In sustained ventricular tachycardia, none are identifiable; usually buried within aberrant, bizarre ventricular contractions Ventricular rate: usually 100–220 beats per minute Ventricular rhythm: May start and stop suddenly	Myocardial ischemia Myocardial infarction Rheumatic heart disease Mitral valve prolapse Heart failure Cardiomyopathy Electrolyte imbalances such as hypokalemia, hypomagnesemia, and hypercalcemia Medication toxicities: Digitalis, procainamide, epinephrine, or quinidine
Ventricular fibrillation	Disorganized, ineffective contraction of the ventricle P waves: None QRS complex: None Ventricular rhythm: Chaotic rhythm with a wavy baseline	Medication toxicities: Digitalis, procainamide, epinephrine, or quinidine
Ventricular asystole (cardiac standstill)	Atrial rhythm: None P, QRS, T waves: None Ventricular rhythm: None	Myocardial ischemia Myocardial infarction Valvular disease Severe heart failure pH and electrolyte imbalances (severe acidosis, hypokalemia, or hyperkalemia in particular) Electric shock Pulmonary embolism Cardiac rupture Cardiac tamponade Cocaine overdose

CAUSES

Conditions that are associated with cardiac dysrhythmias include myocardial ischemia, myocardial infarction, electrolyte imbalance, drug toxicity, and degeneration of the conduction system by necrosis. A dysrhythmia can be the result of a disturbance in the ability of the myocardial cell to conduct an impulse (conductivity), a disturbance in the ability to initiate and maintain an inherent rhythm spontaneously (automaticity), or a combination of both.

GENDER AND LIFE SPAN CONSIDERATIONS

Although these rhythms can occur at any point in the life span and in both sexes, they are more common in the elderly population because of the increased incidence of cardiac diseases, atherosclerosis, and degenerative hypertrophy of the left ventricle. Intrinsic degeneration of the conduction system and a higher propensity toward drug toxicity because of altered metabolism and excretion are contributing factors as patients age. In addition, many of the medications that aging people take to manage heart failure (digitalis and diuretics in particular) place them at risk for drug toxicities and electrolyte imbalances.

☐ ASSESSMENT

HISTORY. If the patient is unable to provide a history of the life-threatening event, obtain it from a witness. Many patients with suspected cardiac dysrhythmias describe a history of symptoms indicating periods of decreased cardiac output. Although occasional PVCs do not usually produce symptoms, some patients report a history of dizziness, fatigue, activity intolerance, a "fluttering" in their chest, shortness of breath, and chest pain. In particular, question the patient about the onset, duration, and characteristics of the symptoms and the events that precipitated them. Obtain a complete history of all illnesses, dietary and fluid restrictions, activity restrictions, and a current medication history.

PHYSICAL EXAMINATION. If the patient does not have adequate airway, breathing, or circulation, initiate cardiopulmonary resuscitation (CPR) as needed. If the patient is stable, complete a general head-to-toe physical examination. Pay particular attention to the cardiovascular system by inspecting the skin for changes in color or the presence of edema. Auscultate the heart rate and rhythm, and note the first and second heart sounds and also any adventitious sounds. Auscultate the blood pressure. Perform a full respiratory assessment, and note any adventitious breath sounds or labored breathing.

PSYCHOSOCIAL. Ventricular dysrhythmias may cause a life-threatening event and a great deal of anxiety and fear because of the potential alterations to current lifestyle and functioning. Assess the ability of the patient and significant others to cope. If the dysrhythmia requires a pacemaker insertion or an automatic implantable cardioverter defibrillator (ICD), determine the patient's response.

DIAGNOSTIC HIGHLIGHTS

Test	Normal Result	Abnormality with Condition	Explanation
12-Lead electrocardiogram (ECG)	Regular sinus rhythm	Varies with dysrhythmias (Table 55)	Detects specific conduction defects; monitors the

> patient's cardiac response to electrolyte imbalances, drug effects, and toxicities

Other Tests: Resting and exercise ECG, Holter monitoring, electrophysiologic studies

PRIMARY NURSING DIAGNOSIS

Altered tissue perfusion (cardiopulmonary, cerebral, renal, peripheral) related to rapid heart rates or the loss of the atrial kick

OUTCOMES. Circulation status; Cardiac pump effectiveness; Tissue perfusion: Cardiopulmonary, Cerebral, Renal, Peripheral; Vital sign status

INTERVENTIONS. Circulatory care; Dysrhythmia management; Emergency care; Vital signs monitoring; Cardiac care; Cardiac precautions; Oxygen therapy; Fluid/electrolyte management; Fluid monitoring; Shock management: Volume; Medication administration; Resuscitation; Surveillance

☐ PLANNING AND IMPLEMENTATION

Collaborative

The first step of treatment is to maintain airway, breathing, and circulation. Low-flow oxygen by nasal cannula or mask may decrease the rate of PVCs. Higher flow rates are usually needed for the patient with VT, and if pulseless VT or VF occurs, the patient needs immediate endotracheal intubation, support of breathing with a manual resuscitator bag, and closed chest compressions (CPR). The most important intervention for a patient with pulseless VT or VF is rapid defibrillation (electrical countershock). If a defibrillator is not available, give a sharp blow to the precordium (precordial thump or thumpversion) to try to convert VT or VF into a regular sinus rhythm. Maintain CPR between all other interventions for patients without adequate breathing and circulation.

The drug of choice to manage PVCs or VT with a pulse is lidocaine at 1.0 to 1.5 mg/kg of body weight given intravenously (IV). If the patient has pulseless VT or VF, the treatment of choice is to defibrillate the patient as discussed previously, intubate the patient, administer epinephrine, and then administer lidocaine. If the patient has electrolyte imbalances, or they are suspected, supplemental potassium and magnesium are administered IV.

In stable patients, trials of various medications or combinations of medications may be used to control the dysrhythmia. Antidysrhythmics, such as bretylium and procainamide, may be used if lidocaine is not successful. Other drugs such as quinidine, propranolol, metoprolol, and verapamil may be used, depending on the cause and nature of the dysrhythmia. Other alternatives include surgical implantation of either a pacemaker or an ICD and surgical ablation of aberrant electrical conduction sites.

The patient with ventricular asystole is managed with CPR. Initiate CPR, intubate the patient immediately, provide oxygenated breathing with a manual resuscitator bag, and obtain IV access. Confirm the ventricular asystole in a second lead to make sure the patient is not experiencing VF, which would indicate the need to defibrillate. If the rhythm still appears as ventricular asystole, administer epinephrine and then atropine in an attempt to have the patient regain an effective cardiac rhythm. The physician may consider a transcutaneous or transvenous pacemaker, but if efforts do not convert the cardiac rhythm, the physician may terminate resuscitation efforts.

PHARMACOLOGIC HIGHLIGHTS

Medication or Drug Class	Dosage	Description	Rationale
Lidocaine	1.0–1.5 mg/kg of body weight given intravenously (IV)	Antidysrhythmic agent	Manages PVCs or VT; inhibits conduction of nerve impulses
Bretylium	5 mg/kg undiluted by rapid IV injection	Antidysrhythmic agent	Manages PVCs or VT; directly affects myocardial cell membrane; initially releases norepine-phrine, then inhibits release
Procainamide	17 mg/kg up to 50 mg per minute in divided doses IV injection	Antidysrhythmic agent	Manages PVCs or VT; prolongs refractory period by direct effect, decreasing myocardial excitability and conduction velocity

Other Drugs: Quinidine, propranolol, metoprolol, flecainide, propafenone, amiodarone, sotalol, ibutilide, verapamil

Independent

As with all potentially serious conditions, the first priority is to maintain the patient's airway, breathing, and circulation. If the patient is not having a cardiopulmonary arrest, maximize the amount of oxygen available to the heart muscle. During periods of abnormal ventricular conduction, encourage the patient to rest in bed until the symptoms are treated and subside. Remain with the patient to ensure rest and to allay anxiety.

For some patients with PVCs, strategies to reduce stress help limit the incidence of the dysrhythmia. A referral to a support group or counselor skilled at stress reduction techniques is sometimes helpful. Teach the patient to reduce the amount of caffeine intake in the diet. Explain the need to read the ingredients of over the counter medications to limit caffeine intake. If appropriate, encourage the patient to become involved in an exercise program or a smoking cessation group.

Patients who experience dysrhythmias are often facing alterations in their lifestyle and job functions. Provide information about the dysrhythmia, the precipitating factors, and mechanisms to limit the dysrhythmia. If the patient is placed on medications, teach the patient and significant others the dosage, route, action, and side effects. If the patient is at risk for electrolyte imbalance, teach the patient any dietary considerations to prevent electrolyte depletion of vital substances.

The most devastating outcome of a ventricular dysrhythmia is sudden cardiac death. If the patient survives the episode, provide an honest accounting of the incident and support the patient's emotional response to the event. If the patient does not survive, remain with the family and significant others, support their expression of grief without being judgmental if it varies from your own ways to express grief, and notify a chaplain or clinical nurse specialist if appropriate to provide additional support.

DOCUMENTATION GUIDELINES

- Cardiopulmonary assessment: Heart and lung sounds, cardiac rate and rhythm on the cardiac monitor, blood pressure, quality of the peripheral pulses, capillary refill, respiratory rate and rhythm
- Activity tolerance and ability to perform self-care
- Complications: Dizziness, syncope, hypotension, electrolyte imbalance, loss of consciousness, uncorrected cardiac dysrhythmias, ineffective patient or family coping

DISCHARGE AND HOME HEALTHCARE GUIDELINES

Explain to the patient the importance of taking all medications. If the patient needs periodic laboratory work to monitor the effects of the medications (such as serum electrolytes or drug levels), discuss with the patient the frequency of these laboratory visits and where to have the tests drawn. Explain the actions, the route, the side effects, the dosage, and the frequency of the medication. Discuss methods for the patient to remember to take the medications, such as numbered medication boxes or linking the medications with other activities such as meals or sleep. Teach the patient how to take the pulse and recognize an irregular rhythm. Explain that the patient needs to notify the healthcare provider when symptoms such as irregular pulse, chest pain, shortness of breath, and dizziness occur.

Stress the importance of stress reduction and smoking cessation. If the patient has the placement of a pacemaker or an ICD, provide teaching about the settings, signs of pacemaker failure (dizziness, syncope, palpitations, fast or slow pulse rate), and when to notify the physician. Explain any environmental hazards based on the manufacturer's recommendations, such as heavy machinery and airport security checkpoints. Make sure the patient understands the schedule for the next physician's checkup. If the patient has an ICD, encourage the patient to keep a diary of the number of times the device discharges. Most physicians want to be notified the first time the ICD discharges after implantation.

Volvulus

DRG Category: 180
Mean LOS: 5.2 days
Description: MEDICAL: Gastrointestinal Obstruction with CC
DRG Category: 148 Mean LOS: 12.2 days
Description: SURGICAL: Major Small and Large Bowel Procedures with CC

A volvulus is a mechanical obstruction of the bowel that occurs when the intestine twists at least 180 degrees on itself. Although it can occur in either the large or small bowel, the most common areas in adults are the sigmoid and ileocecal areas. Compression of the blood vessels occurs, and an obstruction both proximal and distal to the volvulus also occurs. The direction of the chyme flow is obstructed, but the secretions of bile, pancreatic juices, and gastric juices continue. The internal pressure of the bowel rises when fluids and gases accumulate, thus causing a temporary stimulation of peristalsis that increases the distension of the bowel and causes colicky pain. The bowel wall becomes edematous and capillary permeability increases, causing fluid and electrolytes to enter the peritoneal cavity.

These changes place the patient at risk for severe electrolyte imbalance, decreased circulating blood volume, and development of peritonitis. When the volvulus is near or within the ileum, regurgitation and vomiting increase fluid, electrolyte, and acid-base imbalances. Blockage within the cecum or large intestine leads to bowel distension and eventual perforation. Reflux can occur if the ileocecal valve is incompetent. Perforation of the bowel releases bacteria and endotoxins into the peritoneal cavity, causing endotoxic shock and even death.

CAUSES

In some patients, the cause of a volvulus is never discovered. In most cases, however, the condition occurs at the site of an anomaly, tumor, diverticulum, foreign body (dietary fiber, fruit pits), or surgical adhesion.

GENDER AND LIFE SPAN CONSIDERATIONS

Intestinal obstructions can occur at any age and in both sexes. A volvulus can occur in infants with cystic fibrosis because of a meconium ileus. Elderly people are at risk because of the increased incidence of constipation and diverticula in that age group. In children, the most common site is the small bowel. Cecal volvulus is most common in adults in their 50s, whereas sigmoid volvulus is more common in the elderly.

☐ ASSESSMENT

HISTORY. Take a complete history of the patient's eating patterns, bowel patterns, onset of symptoms, and distension. Elicit a gastrointestinal history from the patient, with particular attention to those with a history of constipation and Meckel's diverticulum (a blind pouch found in the lower portion of the ileum). Ask if the patient has had abdominal surgery because adhesions make the patient at risk for a volvulus. Ask the patient to describe any symptoms, which may include abdominal distension, thirst, and abdominal pain. Patients may also report anorexia and food intolerance, with vomiting after eating. Late signs include colicky abdominal pain of sudden onset and vomiting with sediment and a fecal odor. The patient may also describe chronic constipation with no passage of gas or feces, or when a stool is passed, there may be blood in it.

PHYSICAL EXAMINATION. The patient usually appears in acute distress from abdominal pain and pressure. The patient's abdomen appears distended, and the patient may show signs of dehydration such as poor skin turgor and dry mucous membranes. Measure the abdominal girth to identify the amount of distension. When you auscultate the abdomen, you may hear no bowel sounds at all, indicating a paralytic ileus, or you may hear high-pitched peristaltic rushes with high metallic tinkling sounds, indicating intestinal obstruction. You may be able to palpate an abdominal mass, although the patient experiences pain and guarding on palpation.

PSYCHOSOCIAL. The patient may have lived with constipation for a long time and may be embarrassed to discuss the issue of bowel movements or may hold certain beliefs about the frequency and consistency of bowel movements. Assess the patient's self-image and the patient's ability to cope with possible body disfigurement from surgical correction. If the patient is an adult, determine the patient's ability to provide self-care.

DIAGNOSTIC HIGHLIGHTS

Test	Normal Result	Abnormality with Condition	Explanation
Abdominal x rays	Normal abdominal structures	Distended loops of bowel; may be normal x ray	Identifies blockage of lumen of bowel with distal passage of fluid and air (partial) or complete obstruction
Barium enema	Normal abdominal structures	Partial or complete blockage of lumen of bowel	Identifies site of volvulus

Other Tests: Complete blood count, colonoscopy, sigmoidoscopy, abdominal computed tomography (CT) scan

PRIMARY NURSING DIAGNOSIS

Pain (acute) related to inflammation

OUTCOMES. Comfort level; Pain control behavior; Pain level; Symptom severity

INTERVENTIONS. Analgesic administration; Anxiety reduction; Environmental management: Comfort; Pain management; Medication management; Patient-controlled analgesia assistance

□ PLANNING AND IMPLEMENTATION

Collaborative

A tube that is inserted into the small intestine (such as a Miller-Abbott) may be used to decompress the bowel and relieve the volvulus. If a lower bowel volvulus is suspected, a proctoscopy is performed to check for an infarcted bowel, followed by a sigmoidoscopy with a flexible scope to deflate the bowel. If these procedures are successful, the patient immediately expels gas and receives relief from abdominal pain.

Children with small bowel volvulus generally require immediate surgery. In adults, when nonsurgical treatments fail to resolve the volvulus, surgery is performed. The objective of treatment is to relieve the obstruction, although the cause is not always apparent and sometimes is discovered only during surgery. Vascular and mechanical obstructions are relieved by the surgeon, who excises the affected bowel. Depending on the location and extent of the bowel resection, a colostomy or bypass procedure may be performed.

The collaborative postoperative management often includes intravenous analgesia with narcotic agents or patient-controlled analgesia, antibiotic therapy, nasogastric drainage to low continuous or intermittent suction, and intravenous fluids. Monitor the patient for complications such as wound infection (fever, wound drainage, poor wound healing), pneumonia (lung congestion, shallow breathing, fever, productive cough), and bleeding at the surgical site.

PHARMACOLOGIC HIGHLIGHTS

Medication or Drug Class	Dosage	Description	Rationale
Antibiotics	Varies with drug	Broad spectrum	Prevent peritonitis or postoperative infection

Other Therapy: Patient-controlled anesthesia in adults

Independent

When the patient is first admitted to the hospital, he or she is in acute discomfort. Usually, strategies are initiated immediately to correct the underlying condition rather than provide analgesia to minimize the discomfort. Explain to the patient that large doses of analgesics mask the symptoms of volvulus and may place the patient at risk for perforation. Remain with the patient as much as possible until the decision is made to use surgical or nonsurgical treatment to correct the volvulus. If the patient receives successful nonsurgical treatment, the symptoms subside immediately. At that time, provide teaching about strategies to limit constipation, such as diet, adequate fluid intake, and appropriate exercise.

If the patient requires surgery, provide a brief explanation of the procedures and what the patient can expect postoperatively. Have the patient practice coughing and deep breathing, and reassure the patient that postoperative analgesia will be available to manage pain. When the patient returns from surgery, use pillows to splint the abdomen during coughing and deep-breathing exercises. Get the patient out of bed for chair rest and ambulation as soon as the patient can tolerate activity. Notify the physician when bowel sounds resume, and gradually advance the patient from a clear liquid diet to solid food. If the patient experiences any food intolerance at all (nausea, vomiting, pain), notify the surgeon immediately.

If a colostomy or other surgical diversion is needed, work with the patient to accept the change in body image and body function. Allow the patient to verbalize his or her feelings about the ostomy and begin a gradual program to assist the patient to assume self-care. Be honest and explain whether the ostomy is temporary or permanent. If the patient or significant other is going to care for the ostomy at home and is having problems coping, contact the enterostomal therapist or clinical nurse specialist to consult with the patient.

DOCUMENTATION GUIDELINES

- Physical response: Abdominal assessment (return of bowel sounds, relief of distension, and elimination patterns), vital signs, intake and output, pertinent laboratory findings
- Comfort: Location, type, and degree of pain; response to analgesia and other interventions
- Nutrition: Presence of nausea and vomiting, food tolerance, daily weights
- Postoperative recovery: Status of incisions and dressings, presence of complications (infection, lung collapse, hemorrhage), intractable pain

DISCHARGE AND HOME HEALTHCARE GUIDELINES

Teach the patient about strategies to maintain healthy bowel function, such as diet, exercise, drinking fluids, and avoiding laxatives. Provide phone numbers and agencies that can be supportive, such as colostomy and ileostomy groups. Encourage the patient to report any recurrence of symptoms immediately, particularly if the patient has been treated nonsurgically. Encourage patients who have had surgery to avoid strenuous activity for up to 6 weeks.

BIBLIOGRAPHY

Alspach, J. G. (2001). *Instructor's resource manual for the AACN Core Curriculum for Critical Care Nursing* (5th ed.). Philadelphia: W.B. Saunders.

American Cancer Society. (2001). www.cancer.org.

American Heart Association. (2001). www.americanheart.org.

Behrman, R. E., Kliegman, R. M., & Jenson, H. B. (2000). *Nelson textbook of pediatrics* (16th ed.). Philadelphia: W.B. Saunders.

Burns, C. E., Brady, M. A., Dunn, A. M., & Starr, N. B. (2000). *Pediatric primary care.* Philadelphia: W.B. Saunders.

Carey, C. F., Lee, H. H., & Woeltje, K. F. (1998). *The Washington manual of medical herapeutics* (29th ed.). Philadelphia: Lippincott Williams & Wilkins.

Chernecky, C. C., & Berger, B. J. (1997). *Laboratory and diagnostic procedures* (2nd ed.). Philadelphia: W.B. Saunders.

Clark, M. J. (1999). *Nursing in the community* (3rd ed.). Stamford, CT: Appleton & Lange.

Cotran, R. S., Kumar, V., & Collins, T. (1999). *Robbins pathologic basis of disease* (6th ed.). Philadelphia: W.B. Saunders.

Deglin, J. H., & Vallerand, A. H. (2000). *Davis's drug guide for nurses* (7th ed.). Philadelphia: F.A. Davis.

Dipiro, J. T., Talbert, R. L., Yee, G. C., Matzke, G. R., Wells, B., & Posey, L. M. (1999). *Pharmacotherapy: A pathophysiologic approach* (4th ed.). Stamford, CT: Appleton & Lange.

Doherty, G. M., Meko, J. B., Olson, J. A., Peplinski, G. R., & Worrall, N. K. (1999). *The Washington manual of surgery* (2nd ed.). Philadelphia: Lippincott Williams & Wilkins.

Hodgson, B. B., & Kisior, R. J. (2000). *Saunders nursing drug handbook, 2000.* Philadelphia: W.B. Saunders.

Ignatavicius, D. D., Workman, M. L., & Mishler, M. A. (1999). *Medical surgical nursing across the health care continuum* (3rd ed.). Philadelphia: W.B. Saunders.

Johnson, M., Maas, M., & Moorhead, S. (1999). *Nursing outcomes classification* (2nd ed.). St. Louis: Harcourt.

McCloskey, J. C., & Bulechek, G. M. (1999). *Nursing interventions classification* (3rd ed.). St. Louis: Harcourt.

Price, S. A., & Wilson, L. M. (1997). *Pathophysiology* (5th ed.). St. Louis: Mosby.

Smeltzer, S. C., & Bare, B. G. (2000). *Brunner and Suddarth's medical-surgical nursing* (9th ed.). Philadelphia: Lippincott Williams & Wilkins.

Sommers, M. S. (1998). Multisystem. In J. G. Alspach (Ed.). *Core curriculum for critical care nurses.* Philadelphia: W.B. Saunders.

Swearingen, P. L., & Keen, J. H. (2000). *Manual of critical care nursing* (4th ed.). St. Louis: Mosby.

Swearingen, P. L., & Ross, D. (1999). *Manual of medical surgical nursing care* (4th ed.). St. Louis: Mosby.

Venes, D., & Thomas, C. L. (2001). *Taber's cyclopedic medical dictionary* (19th ed.). Philadelphia: F.A. Davis.

Wallach, J. (2000). *Interpretation of diagnostic tests* (7th ed.). Philadelphia: Lippincott Williams & Wilkins.

INDEX

An "f" following a page number indicates a figure; a "t" following a page number indicates a table; and a "b" indicates a box